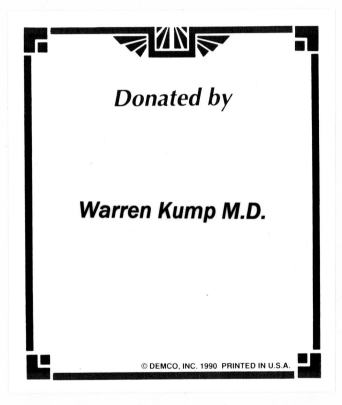

Donated by

Warren Kump M.D.

AN INTRODUCTION

TO THE

HISTORY OF MEDICINE

*WITH MEDICAL CHRONOLOGY, SUGGESTIONS
FOR STUDY AND BIBLIOGRAPHIC DATA*

BY

FIELDING H. GARRISON, A.B., M.D.

LIEUTENANT-COLONEL, MEDICAL CORPS, U. S. ARMY, SURGEON GENERAL'S OFFICE,
WASHINGTON, D. C.

FOURTH EDITION, Reprinted

PHILADELPHIA AND LONDON
W. B. SAUNDERS COMPANY

To

GENERAL WALTER D. McCAW, U. S. ARMY
LIBRARIAN OF THE SURGEON GENERAL'S OFFICE (1903–13)
CHIEF SURGEON, AMERICAN EXPEDITIONARY FORCES (1918–19)

IN ACKNOWLEDGMENT

OF HIS KIND ENCOURAGEMENT

AND

HIS MANY COURTESIES

IN AID OF THE COMPLETION OF THIS BOOK

PREFACE TO THE FOURTH EDITION

THE present revision of this book has been made as exhaustive and searching as has been possible in the extra-official time at the author's disposal. Since the last edition (1922) much water has flown under the bridges and some striking realignments (changes of viewpoint) have been effected in the fundamental disciplines of medicine. To render a clear account of these is no easy matter; to deal adequately and exhaustively with *nuances* of such complexity would require whole-time labor over a number of years, in a work of several volumes. For such a task the present writer has neither the time nor the inclination. It is an open question whether civilization itself has advanced or retrogressed in the decade following the World War and it is dubious whether the gigantic literature of general biology and medicine (a chaotic welter) will ultimately overreach itself, like an inundation, or tends already to the self-sterilization and terminal petrifaction predicted by Spengler for the total West. In this volume the author has endeavored to feature the various new departures in recent medicine by salient examples, realizing that to attempt exhaustive handling would be premature and only confusing to the reader. All attempts at ultimate appraisals of recent happenings as finalities have been futile and valueless, while some of the great expectations entertained of our vaunted post-bellum period are already "sad with sick leavings of the sterile sea." The concluding chapter is therefore submitted, with all due modesty, in the spirit of the Latin device once inscribed on the graduating dissertations of Russian medical students. *Feci quod potui: faciant meliora potentes.*

In addition to the new material in the terminal chapters, a section on medicine in prehistoric times has been added; effort has been made to do justice to the recent medicine of Russia, Italy, Spain, and the Latin-American countries, and the chronology and bibliographies in the appendices have been increased nearly twofold. To include all this material in one volume it has been necessary to throw some of it into smaller type; indeed, with proper consideration for the reader's eyesight, chronologies and bibliographies of such length are more suitable for occasional consultation than for continuous reading. The student who wishes to know the important happenings in a given year, quinquennium, decade, or other period will now find them available, particularly in the decade 1918–28, in which it is attempted to give a picture of the proliferations of socialized and Soviet medicine not possible in the narrative. The "Test Questions," printed in the first edition, have

5

been revamped, with some new features.   Here the design is obviously
not pedagogic, but, in conformity with the original intention of the book,
to help the student to devise ways and means of testing and expanding
his own knowledge and of blocking out lines of independent investigation for himself.   Such questions as Nos. 26 and 44 (pp. 925–928) are
not to be taken seriously, as dry husks to chew, but are merely suggestive
of a phase of mental exercise which is more an ambition of continental
Europeans than of Americans, viz., capacity to deal with ideas.   In
like manner, a close examination of the mottoes immediately facing
the narrative will demonstrate a remarkable consistency and continuity of reasoned doctrine, showing that through the centuries the
greater thinkers on medicine really confirm and sustain one another's
views, albeit in utterances seemingly disparate.   In 1849 Virchow wrote:

> "Should medicine ever fulfil its great ends, it must enter into the larger political
> and social life of our time; it must indicate the barriers which obstruct the normal
> completion of the life-cycle and remove them.   Should this ever come to pass, medi-
> cine, whatever it may then be, will become the common good of all.   It will cease
> to be medicine and will be absorbed into that general simplified body of knowledge
> which is identifiable with power. . . .   When we have exact knowledge of the
> conditions of existence of individuals and of peoples, then only will it be possible
> for the laws of medicine and philosophy to gain the credence of general laws of
> humanity.   Then only will the Baconian 'Knowledge is Power' become accom-
> plished fact."

This first brief for the socialization of medicine, faintly adumbrated
by Descartes, voices an unattainable ideal, just in its beginnings and
far from realization.   But our *kyrielle* of consistent mottoes, the basic
postulates of what is now called "medical philosophy," will leave no
doubt, for our own profession, at least, that

> "Through the ages an increasing purpose runs."

It is hardly necessary to enlarge upon the heuristic value of all this
for the few medical students who will acquire permanent interest in
our subject, but such students are apt to develop literary, editorial,
and philosophic tastes later on.   Recent investigations of the mechanisms of thought tell us very plainly that the mind is seldom, if ever,
self-starting, but is apt to become idle, inert, or incompetent unless
activated by stimuli from within or without.   Stimuli from within, the
voice of the hidden *alter ego*, are too often springs of worry, more
inimical to clear thinking than the street noises and other major and
minor nuisances cursed by Schopenhauer.   Many people in modern
life have become virtual neurotics through this conflict, which is the
special bane and gadfly of the intellectual.   Worry is now known to be
the basic coefficient in mental fatigue and Gillespie affirms that "For
practical purposes the mind is almost tireless."[1]   A study of the history
of science and general culture indicates, moreover, that the human mind
is apparently capable of only a limited number of ideas in any space-
time relation, so that what seems new is really old in a deceptive, novel

[1] R. D. Gillespie: Brit. Med. Jour., Lond., 1928, ii, 366.

guise. Any one who studies secular literature, with reference to medicine, will find that the wisest heads and shrewdest wits of important periods were perfectly aware of the salient lines of medical doctrine current in their time. In poetry, drama, and novels, or what Swinburne called "creative and imaginative literature," we often get, in fact, the very best sidelights on the medicine of the period. Certain devitalized texts and text-books (Spengler's petrifacts) convey the dry husks of medical doctrine, the medicine of the time as it ought to have been or might have been; whence they are seldom studied, except by professional historians. But the secular writers tell us what actually is or was. This fact has been brilliantly illustrated in the series of lectures delivered by Dr. John R. Oliver to his Baltimore classes in 1927–28. Ideas become dynamic in applied science only, or as Virchow expressed it: "The touchstone of true science is power of performance, for it is a truism that what can, also will, and thus attains to real existence." The doctrine of Conservation of Energy is already in the poetic fragments of Empedocles, as well as in the adage *Ex nihilo nihil fit* or even in a queer mechanical contrivance made by Melanesian savages; but it was in the universal application of this idea, as a going, working principle in applied science, that Helmholtz towered above all his contemporaries. Again, the greater physicians of the past, reasoning from what seem to us very faulty premises, somehow got their patients well, otherwise they would have had no clientèle or following. The thing is to ascertain, if possible, just how they did it. Medical history, then, is coming to be taught as a discipline for the mind; for if the student grasps the basic idea latent in anything, he will be in position to apply it or expand it, as occasion arises, without reference to books; and the hope of the future will turn largely upon the intelligent application of worthwhile ideas by intelligent people. As a consequence of our changeable climate and political system, some Americans tend to become infatuated temporarily with particular ideas or cults,[1] which they drop just as speedily when buncoed by them, like Lowell's archetypal journalist, who is "very much of his present way of thinking, whatever that happens to be." This is what Renan implied by *"la dure inintelligence des Américains du Nord."* One remedy for shallow, superficial reactions, essentially different from Scotch or French tenacity of purpose and opinion, English conservatism in action, or even the flightiness of the quick-witted, imaginative Celt, is to be found in the memorable sentence of Joubert: "Experience in dealing with many opinions makes the mind more flexible and confirms it in its final choice of the best course to take," which is only another way of saying: "Prove all things: hold fast to that which is good." Errors in medical reasoning are obviously due to the same cause which the great intellect of Spinoza assigned for all human mishaps: "inadequate ideas." Cardinal Newman affirmed that human beings, at large, are influenced by types rather

[1] See Gilbert Seldes: The Stammering Century, New York, 1928, and Morris Fishbein: The Medical Follies, New York, 1925–27.

than by arguments, and not so much by ideas and pure reason as by prevailing fashions. For the medical student and practitioner the study of the history of his profession, dealing, as it does, with all aspects of human culture, affords one of the best outlets for ideation, and is also one of the best offsets to the mental staleness and ennui which result from narrow specialism and infatuation with a single idea.

During the seven years elapsing since the last edition of this book many remarkable advances have been made in the study of medical history. Most important of these, for our own country at least, is the recent establishment of an Institute and Library of the History of Medicine by the Johns Hopkins University, under direction of Professor William H. Welch, a departure which guarantees, for the first time, the possibility of whole-time study for graduate students, under the guidance of a great master, organizer and teacher, whose wide knowledge of the history of science, medicine, and general culture is probably unsurpassed among American physicians. The *Festschrift* recently presented to the veteran teacher, Professor William S. Miller, of Madison, Wisconsin, is a deserving tribute to a Western pioneer in *Seminar* training of graduate students. The Mayo Foundation (Rochester, Minnesota) has organized annual courses of lectures on medical history, to be delivered by approved authorities at stated intervals. This is the most important and significant advance in the "Old Northwest," which has already distinguished itself through the excellent work of such men as W. S. Miller, Ludwig Hektoen, H. M. Brown, Edward Kremers, T. H. Shastid, LeRoy Crummer, Charles R. Bardeen (Madison), and others. The Medical History Societies in Boston, New York, Philadelphia, Baltimore, Chicago, St. Louis, and other American cities are still flourishing and there are already encouraging developments on the Pacific Coast.

Professor Henry E. Sigerist (Leipzig), who succeeded to Sudhoff's chair and Institute in 1925, has made a statistical study of the status of university teaching of medical history in European and American cities. He finds that the subject is now taught in no less than 63 academic institutions, of which Germany leads with fifteen chairs, Italy has eight, Poland five, and Switzerland three. It is gratifying to learn that our own country stands second on the list (nine chairs).

Among the outstanding teachers are Tricot-Royer (Liège), Maar (Copenhagen), Sigerist (Leipzig), Sticker (Würzburg), Diepgen (Freiburg i. Br.), Hubötter (Berlin), Schmiz (Bonn), Haberling (Düsseldorf), Koch (Frankfurt a. M.), Honigmann (Giessen), Meyer-Steineg (Jena), von Brunn (Rostock), Ménétrier (Paris), Singer (London), Comrie (Edinburgh), Capparoni (Pisa), Corsini (Florence), Castiglioni (Padua), Giuffrè (Palermo), Cardini (Rome), de Lint (Leyden), Fonahn (Oslo), Neuburger (Vienna), Garcia del Real (Madrid), von Györy (Budapest), and Wehrle. (Zürich).

This is a noble and impressive record if we remember that, since the World War, many continental Europeans have maintained their culture at a terrible price, often in the face of extreme privation and even want. It is pleasing to think that even as the names of great

French physicians are commemorated in the streets of Paris, so, too, there is a Beethoven House at Bonn, a Goethe National Museum at Weimar, a Musée Flaubert at Rouen, that there are archæological stations at all the old Ægean and Ionian shrines, with ephors in charge, and even postage stamps commemorating Pasteur, the centenary of the Lisbon School of Surgery (1926) and the great composers and men of letters of Germany, real benefactors of our race, whom the children of the future are called upon to revere and admire. We should have John Morgan, Ephraim McDowell, Daniel Drake, O. W. Holmes, and Marion Sims stamps also, to commemorate the pioneers of American medicine, among other national celebrities.

Of newer text-books on the history of medicine, the recent crop seems as plentiful as the shower of curates over North England at the beginning of Charlotte Bronte's *Shirley*. Not all of these are of equal merit, nay, one we have seen is made up of irresponsible newspaper paragraphing; but special commendation is due to the admirable and informing book of Professor Arturo Castiglioni (Padua), the remarkable contributions of Professors Georg Honigmann and August Bier on the cultural and philosophic aspects of medicine, the effective primer of Professor Charles Singer and the compact History of Surgery by Professor Walter von Brunn. An interesting and valuable History of Scottish Medicine by Dr. John C. Comrie (1927) has been withdrawn from publication pending revision and enlargement. A History of Medicine in the United States up to 1876 by Dr. Francis R. Packard (an enlargement of his book of 1901) is in preparation. A History of Pathology by Dr. Esmond R. Long (Chicago) is just out and a History of Psychiatry by Drs. Gregory Zilboorg and George W. Henry is in preparation.

Of monographic histories of special subjects, those of Louis Lewin on toxicology (1920), arrow-poisons (1923), and narcotics (1924), Erich Ebstein (physicians' letters, memoirs, and speeches, 1920–26), Richard Greef (revised history of spectacles, 1921), I. Münz (medieval Jewish physicians, 1922), F G. Crookshank (influenza, 1922), Andrea Corsini (medical charlatanry, 1922), Sir Charles Ballance (brain surgery, 1922), Lynn Thorndike (history of magic, 1923), D. Barduzzi (Italian medicine, 1923), R. C. Thompson (Assyrian medicine, 1923–24), Mukhopadhyaya (Ayurvedic medicine, 1923–26), Hubötter (Chinese medical literature, 1924), W. H. S. Jones (Hippocratic Oath, 1924), Meinsma (1924), and Nohl (1926) on the Black Death, F. Haurowitz (biochemistry, 1925), Charles Singer (anatomy, 1925), Fischer (therapeutics, 1925), G. Rashdall (medieval universities, 1925), Max Neuburger (Healing Power of Nature, 1926), Donald Campbell (Arabian medicine, 1926), Klebs and Sudhoff (pest tracts, 1926), August Bier (medical theories of the past, 1926–27), Sigerist (ancient medicine, 1927), Sticker (German medicine, 1927), Sudhoff (Kos und Knidos, 1927), R. Schiaffino (Uruguayan medicine, 1927), Wallis Budge (ancient herbals, 1928), and J. J. Haggerty (Canadian medicine, 1928) may be listed as illustrating the amount and variety of research work undertaken since the end of the World War. The anthologies of pediatric texts of Sudhoff (1925) and John Rührah (1925), Walter von Brunn's edition of Caspar Stromayr's *Practica* (1925), and the iconographic atlases of Edgar Goldschmid (history of pathology, 1925), Ernest Wickersheimer (Mundinus and Vigevano, 1926), A. Sonderegger (teratology, 1927), C. Proskauer (dentistry, 1926), O. Neustätter (orthopedics, 1926), Victor Madsen and Vilhelm Thomsen (Manchu anatomy, 1928) are valuable reference-tomes of a more sumptuous, keepsake *genre*. Of recent American contributions, those of A. F. Hess (scurvy, 1921), Walter A. Jayne (medical mythology, 1925), Abraham Flexner (medical education, 1925), R. B. Osgood (orthopedics, 1925), B. W. Weinberger (orthodontia, 1926), J. F. Fulton (muscular contraction, 1926), G. W. Corner (Salernitan anatomy, 1927), C. D. Leake (medical ethics, 1927), W. C. Alvarez (gastro-enterology, 1928), and E. R. Long (history of pathology, 1928) are worthy of especial note. George Sarton's massive prolegomena of the history of science, "from Homer to Omar" (1927), is a wonderful shipload of unique data and references, with an able steersman at the helm. Of recent medical biographies, Cushing's *Osler* takes the lead, with Karl Pearson's Galton, as permanent memorials of these benign figures. The autobiography of the late Professor Naunyn (1925) comes well up to the expectations aroused by his earlier fragment on German clinical teaching in the second half of the 19th century, and Wilhelm Haberling's *Johannes Müller* (1924) is a tribute to that great master well worthy of a place beside Roth's *Vesalius*. "Finch and Baines" by Archibald Malloch, the accomplished Librarian of the New York Academy of Medicine, was inspired by Osler and is notable for its iconography and its sidelights on English medicine in the 17th century. Dr. Le Roy Crummer (Omaha) has just edited an important unpublished MS. of the elder Heberden. Of medico-historical periodicals, the most recent is *Kyklos*, a year-book of the Leipzig Institute (1928). Under the editorial guidance of Dr. Francis R. Packard, the Annals of Medical History (New York) has just completed a decade of stimulating activity.

As stated in the first edition, this volume was originally conceived along four parallel lines—the graphic, the biographic, the bibliographic, and the cultural. Detailed exposition of facts, dates, and special subjects have been thrown into small type, with bibliographies in the footnotes, as being for reference and not to destroy the continuity of the narrative portion. Adherence to this plan through four editions has impressed the writer latterly with the fact that the limits of stress and strain will now have been reached with reference to the expository portion. Even with enlarged pages and the use of a smaller font of type in some places, it is doubtful to the publishers if the bindings would hold more material than is contained in the present volume. This will account for some necessary omissions, such as the history of the American College of Surgeons, the Royal Society of Medicine and other important medical societies, the intimate history of medical education, medical ethics and medical journalism, the story of the various subdivisions of public hygiene and similar details indicated in the chronology. The history of medicine and hygiene touches human activity on all sides, like a vast circle defined by multifarious tangents, and no single volume could include everything. But it is believed that enough has been presented in the text and bibliographies to enable anyone to repair such omissions by investigations of his own. In a most sympathetic review of the first edition the late Dr. James Gregory Mumford voiced the author's primary intention as follows:

"The story of medicine is vital and inspiring, no matter from what angle you approach it. It is closely interwoven with the story of peoples, of civilizations, and of the human mind. It deals with great men and small men—with philosophers and scientists, with monarchs and ecclesiastics, with scoundrels and humbugs. On the one hand, it springs from folk-ways, legends, credulity, and superstition; on the other from intelligence, culture, labor, valor, and truth. And always it seems to reflect the character and progress of the people with whom for the time it is lodged—be they reactionary or be they progressive. Whatever else it is, the history of medicine is never dull. It is certainly not a catalogue—an arid depositary of names and formulas."

As far as possible, however, it has been attempted to make the volume useful for reference purposes by following the Germanic plan of a close *rendement* of essential facts over a substratum of confirmatory footnotes, the mode of documentation employed by Sprengel and Haeser and even in our medical history of American participation in the World War. My best lessons in medical history have been learned, in fact, from the great German masters, and I should be a poor creature, indeed, if I did not here acknowledge, *zum letzten Mal*, my immense debt to them. It is doubtful if special progress in this subject could ever have been made without these serious, patient, accurate, faithful, and reliable guides.

As previously stated, this work is essentially a product of the Surgeon General's Library, hence of the Medical Department of the U. S. Army. I desire once more to thank the successive Librarians for their encouragement and their generosity in the loan of books and graphic material, and the present Librarian, Col. Percy M. Ashburn, M. C., for his acute and sagacious counsel. In the matter of general revision, including the correction of slips and blunders in the third edition, I am genuinely indebted to Geheimrat Sudhoff (Leipzig), with whom my correspondence has been extensive, to his successor, Professor Sigerist, to Dr. Charles Singer (London), whose generous aid in the matter of corrigenda has gone far beyond the limits of his valuable time, to Drs. W. W. Francis (Oxford), Oscar Clark (Lima), Wu Lien Teh (Peking), Edward B. Krumbhaar (Philadelphia), Ludvig Hektoen (Chicago), Esmond R. Long (Chicago), John F. Fulton (Cambridge), John Fallon (Worcester, Mass.), Joseph Collins (New York), Victor Robinson (New York), Walter C. Alvarez (Rochester, Minn.), the late Dr. Jacob Rosenbloom (Pittsburgh), Paul B. Hoeber (New York), and others impossible momentarily to recall. Mr. Felix Neumann, Assistant Librarian, S. G. O., has kindly placed at my disposal his wide command of reference resources. To the publishers my gratitude is once more due for their patience through the tediums and doldrums of resetting the text, and to Miss Christina Hilbrandt (Army Medical Library) I express my best thanks for her efficient co-operation in the management of the author and subject indexes, this time a bewildering excursus in *la science des noms*.

F. H. G.

ARMY MEDICAL LIBRARY,
WASHINGTON, D. C.,
January, 1929.

CONTENTS

"Science has no country."—Pasteur.

"Research begins as physics and ends as mathematics."—Lord Bacon.

"Medicine is science in the making."—Magendie.

"Science begets knowledge; opinion, ignorance."—Hippocrates.

"I also maintain that clear knowledge of natural science must be acquired, in the first instance, through mastery of medicine alone."—Hippocrates.

"Conscientious and careful physicians allocate causes of disease to natural laws, while the ablest men of science go back to medicine for their first principles."—Aristotle.

"I look back upon my medical studies as the school which taught me, in a more penetrating and convincing way than any other, the eternal principles of scientific work, principles so simple yet continually forgotten, so clear and yet ever shrouded by a deceptive veil."—Helmholtz.

"It is the customary fate of new truths to begin as heresies and to end as super-stitions."—Huxley.

"Truth is the daughter of Time and not of authority."—Leonardo, Bacon, Baglivi.

"Doctrinaire formula-worship, that is our real enemy."—Max Neuburger.

"The medical errors of one century constitute the popular faith of the next."—Alonzo Clark.

"The methods of quackery are merely a theft from the most ancient phases of folk-medicine."—Sudhoff.

"Medicine is as old as the human race, as old as the necessity for the removal of disease."—Haeser.

"Belief begins where science leaves off and ends where science begins."—Virchow.

"Science commits suicide when it adopts a creed."—Huxley.

"The duty of science is not to attack the objects of belief, but to stake out the limits of the knowable and to center consciousness within them."—Virchow.

"Science is the topography of ignorance."—O. W. Holmes.

"In the realm of error, the truth is only a point."—Marmontel.

"But like a man walking alone in the darkness, I resolved to proceed so slowly and carefully that, even if I did not get very far, I was certain not to fall."—Descartes.

"Man can learn nothing unless he proceeds from the known to the unknown."—Claude Bernard.

"Humanism is neither atheistic nor pantheistic, since it has but one formula for things unknowable, namely: I do not know."—Virchow.

"Science repulses the indefinite."—Claude Bernard.

"As long as vitalism and spiritualism are open questions, so long will the gateway of science be open to mysticism."—Virchow.

"If I had to define life in a word, it would be: Life is creation."—Claude Bernard.

14

"In all things relating to disease, credulity remains a permanent fact, uninfluenced by civilization or education."—OSLER.

"True science teaches us to doubt and, in ignorance, to refrain."—CLAUDE BERNARD.

"The man of science has learned to believe in justification, not by faith, but by verification."—HUXLEY.

"Observation is a passive science, experimentation an active science."—CLAUDE BERNARD.

"It is the mind which is really alive and sees things, yet it hardly sees anything without preliminary instruction."—CHARCOT.

"In science, the thing is to modify and change one's ideas as science advances." —CLAUDE BERNARD.

"Disease is from of old and nothing about it has changed. It is we who change, as we learn to recognize what was formerly imperceptible."—CHARCOT.

"A discovery is usually an unforeseen relation not confirmed in theory, for otherwise it would have been foreseen."—CLAUDE BERNARD.

"The success of a discovery depends upon the time of its appearance."—WEIR MITCHELL.

"If we are to speak of 'entities' in disease, these must not be the names, nor even our concepts, but the things—the thing Thompson and the thing Wilkinson in certain phases of their being."—ALLBUTT.

"How is it that, one fine morning, Duchenne discovered a disease which probably existed in the time of Hippocrates?"—CHARCOT.

"It is steadily forgotten that health is a diathesis as much as is scrofula or syphilis, and that each of these is a mode of growth."—ALLBUTT.

"Diseases are not even species, such as cats and toads, but abnormal, although not altogether irregular behaviors of animals and plants."—ALLBUTT.

"To know things well, one must know them in detail, and as this is infinite, our knowledge is necessarily superficial."—LaROCHEFOUCAULD.

"Science increases our power as it lessens our pride."—CLAUDE BERNARD.

"The education of most people ends upon graduation; that of the physician means a lifetime of incessant study."—MARX.

"Medicine absorbs the physician's whole being because it is concerned with the entire human organism."—GOETHE.

"In medicine, sins of commission are mortal, sins of omission venial."—TRONCHIN.

"From Hippocrates to Hunter, the treatment of disease was one long traffic in hypotheses."—OSLER.

"In science, a law is not a rule imposed from without, but an expression of an intrinsic process."—ALLBUTT.

"The laws of the lawgiver are impotent beside the laws of human nature as, to his disillusion, many a lawgiver has discovered."—ALLBUTT.

"The names of the prime-movers of science disappear gradually in a general fusion, and the more a science advances, the more impersonal and detached it becomes."—CLAUDE BERNARD.

"The doubter is a true man of science: he doubts only himself and his interpretations, but he believes in science."—CLAUDE BERNARD.

"It is with medicine as with mathematics: we should occupy our minds only with what we continue to know; what we once knew is of little consequence."—SAINTE-BEUVE.

"Medicine, likewise, because it deals with things, has always been for our serener circles a Cinderella, blooming maid as happily she has grown nevertheless."—ALLBUTT.

"An important phase of medicine is the ability to appraise the literature correctly."—HIPPOCRATES.

"Brevity in writing is the best insurance for its perusal."—VIRCHOW.

"The man of science appears to be the only man who has something to say just now, and the only man who does not know how to say it."—SIR JAMES BARRIE.

"The greatest men I have ever known have written their own papers."—ARCHIBALD MALLOCH.

"All knowledge attains its ethical value and its human significance only by the humane sense in which it is employed. Only a good man can be a great physician."—NOTHNAGEL.

"Even in populous districts, the practice of medicine is a lonely road which winds uphill all the way, and a man may easily go astray and never reach the Delectable Mountains, unless he early finds those shepherd guides of whom Bunyan tells, Knowledge, Experience, Watchful, and Sincere."—OSLER.

"I thought that all was right in the system of the universe—that consistent with our desires and passions was the shortness of our life and our being liable to suffering and disease—that without this we should have been inanimate, cold, and heartless creatures."—SIR CHARLES BELL.

"Medicine is a sacred calling, and he who makes it ridiculous is guilty of sacrilege."—SUDHOFF.

"For thousands of years medicine has united the aims and aspirations of the best and noblest of mankind. To depreciate its treasures is to discount all human endeavor and achievement at naught."—MARX.

"The future belongs to those who shall have done most for suffering humanity."—PASTEUR.

"Where there is love for humanity, there also is love for the art of medicine."—HIPPOCRATES.

"If there is any possible means of increasing the common wisdom and ability of mankind, it must be sought in medicine."—DESCARTES.

"Aims, methods, and persistency are common to the medical profession of all countries. On its flag is inscribed what should be the life rule of all nations: Fraternity and solidarity."—ABRAHAM JACOBI.

AN INTRODUCTION
TO THE
HISTORY OF MEDICINE

THE IDENTITY OF ALL FORMS OF ANCIENT AND PRIMITIVE MEDICINE

ONE of the best accredited doctrines of recent times is that of the unity or solidarity of folk-ways. The collective investigations of historians, ethnologists, archeologists, philologists, and sociologists reveal the singular fact that all phases of social anthropology which have to do with instinctive actions inevitably converge to a common point of similarity or identity. This is now fairly well established for ordinary reactions to environment, and is true of all customs of primitive peoples (as also of the cruder ethnic aspects of religions) which are concerned with the fundamental instincts of self-preservation and reproduction. It is possible, as we shall see, that many myths, inventions, and bizarre cultural practices, such as mummification, circumcision, or the couvade, may have been transported by migrations from one place to another (Elliot Smith). But the fact remains that, for those human actions which have been defined as instinctive, as based upon the innate necessity which is the mother of invention, "folklore is an essential unity."[1] The mind of savage man, in its pathetic efforts to cope with hostile forces, form religious and ethical systems for moral and spiritual guidance, or beautify the commoner aspects of life with romance and poetry, has unconsciously taken the same lines of least resistance, followed the same planes of cleavage. The civilized mind differs from the savage mind mainly in respect of a higher evolutionary development. In their reactions to folk-ways and settled custom, both exhibit the same inertia, fear of change, and aversion to the untried or unknowable. "To primitive and modern alike, ceremonial is a shock-absorber, a mitigating diversion from the change become inevitable" (Parsons[2]). Human races and racial customs have changed, in the sense of becoming more highly specialized. The heart of man remains the same.

---

[1] For a good summary of the matter, see the presidential address of Charlotte S. Burne in Folk-Lore, Lond., 1911, xxii, 14–41; also, her revision of "The Handbook of Folklore" (Pub. Folk-Lore Soc., No. lxxiii, Lond., 1914).

[2] Elsie Clews Parsons: Fear and Conventionality, New York, 1914; also Am. Anthrop., Lancaster, Pa., 1915, xvii, 409; 600.

It follows that, under different aspects of space and time, the essential traits of folk-medicine and ancient medicine have been alike in tendency, differing only in unimportant details. In the light of anthropology, this proposition may be taken as proved. Cuneiform, hieroglyphic, runic, birch-bark, and palm-leaf inscriptions all indicate that the folk-ways of early medicine, whether Accadian or Scandinavian, Slavic or Celtic, Roman or Polynesian, have been the same—in each case an affair of charms and spells, plant-lore and psychotherapy, to stave off the effects of supernatural agencies. Wherever this frame of mind persists, there is no possibility of advancement for medicine.

In relation to the origin of ethnic traits and practices, opinion is divided into two schools. The **convergence theory,** originated by Adolf Bastian in 1881,[1] affirms that the appearance of identical ethnic phenomena in different relations of space and time is due to the spontaneous development of certain "elemental ideas" (*Elementargedanken*), which are common to primitive man everywhere. The **convection (diffusion) theory,** originated by Friedrich Ratzel (1882),[2] asserts that no isolated action or primary "elemental thought" is possible to primitive races, but that each race has derived something from its neighbors in space or from its predecessors in time. Ratzel's theory of the geographic diffusion of ethnic culture has been vigorously defended by Felix von Luschan,[3] and separately maintained by Elliot Smith, in his doctrine of the convection of "heliolithic culture." The Bastian doctrine is strongly supported by the imposing array of facts which have been assembled in furtherance of the modern theory of evolution, viz., that the development of the individual is but an epitome of the development of the race. Left to itself in a favorable environment, it is conceivable that any savage tribe might evolve a culture all its own, for the regulation of food supply, sexual and social relations, adjustment to the unknown, manifesting itself as political economy, ethics, law, medicine, religion, and so on. The weak point in the convection theory is that it deals with accidentals and non-essentials, such as the constant recurrence of the self-same folk-tales and proverbs all over the earth, similarities in language, artistic forms, detached cultural practices, ethnic type (Hindu and Aryan, Malay and North American Indian), many (not all) of which may have been mechanically transmitted from one race or culture to another. Thus, the Africans of Benin and Cameroon learned to make armor and artistic devices in metal from North-European invaders; the Ganymede in the Vatican is strikingly reproduced in a Buddhist relief in a cloister near Sanghao; the cobra symbol is found alike in Indian, Egyptian, Scandinavian, and Aztec devices; the symbolism of the Symplegades is the same in Greek and Mayan art; but the *cherchez la femme* motive may well have originated scores of Trojan or other wars, and such episodes as those of Hercules, Œdipus, Siegfried, or Machaon are apt to occur spontaneously anywhere. Elliot Smith asserts that Americans uphold the convergence theory "as a kind of dogma" over against the diffusionist theory, but, as a matter of fact, there are strong elements of probability in both. Hence, neither can be erected into dogma.

Of the ultimate origin of folk-ways and ideas we know little or nothing. Innumerable hypotheses have been advanced, in each case the attempt of a civilized or educated mind to interpret the workings of the primitive mind from isolated instances and, in almost every case, the investigator has become obsessed by his particular theory to the extent of becoming a hobby-horse rider, in the sense of reading into savage folk-ways his own arbitrary view of them. Thus Fraser holds

---

[1] A. Bastian: Der Völkergedanke, Berlin, 1881.

[2] F. Ratzel: Anthropogeographie, Stuttgart, 1882.

[3] F. von Luschan: Zusammenhänge und Konvergenz. Mitt. d. anthrop. Gesellsch. in Wien, 1918, xlviii, 1–117.

that civilized and primitive minds differ in degree only; Levy-Brühl, that they differ in kind. But all anthropologists agree that the general origin of folk-ways and *mores* (religious or other) is *social*, concerned with the great question "how to live," which is different at different times, in different places, among different peoples. Of the mind of primitive man, we know that it is inferior to the civilized mind mainly in respect of education and development, that is, in the ability to perceive and assign the right causes for phenomena which gave us science, and in certain perceptions of "values" which gave us our standards of morality and taste. But in all these things the primitive mind everywhere has its own natural standards, which are worthy of deepest consideration.

Apart from any theories as to his origin or evolution, we may assume that prehistoric man was not different from what we often find primitive man to be—a savage sunk in his animal instincts. At this stage of his existence, he killed his food and fought his enemies with sticks and stones, raped his women, hid himself in caves, and was probably not unaware of certain hygienic precautions which are instinctive in lower animals. A dog licks its wounds, hides in holes if sick or injured, limps on three legs if maimed, tries to destroy parasites on its body, exercises, stretches, and warms in the sun, assumes a definite posture in sleeping, and seeks out certain herbs and grasses when sick.[1] It is not unreasonable to suppose that actions like these may have been as instinctive in a grown-up prehistoric man as they are in a primitive child of his race today. "Man has climbed up from some lower animal form," says John Burroughs, "but he has, as it were, pulled the ladder up after him." We do not know when or where, how or why, this occurred, but we do know the first rung of the ladder. In the Hall of Anthropology of the National Museum at Washington (or in any other good collection of this kind) there are to be seen innumerable specimens of a small object in chipped flint which is the symbol of prehistoric man's uplift, his first step in the direction of civilization. With this leaf-shaped flint in hand, he had a new means of protecting himself against enemies, procuring and preparing food, and of manufacturing other weapons and implements of the same kind or of more highly specialized kinds. Now the interesting point about these prehistoric flints is that they are to be found wherever traces of the existence of man are found, changing in shape during the successive interglacial and postglacial periods, but following his migrations over the surface of the earth. Here cropping up as spear or arrow-point, there as tool or ceremonial object, these primitive "celts," as they are called, have been excavated from the river-drifts of England, France, and North America, in the caverns of Devonshire and the Dordogne, in the plains of Egypt and Palestine, in the frozen tundra of Siberia and Alaska, in each case

---

[1] Usually *Triticum caninum*, *Cynosurus cristatus*, and *Agrestis canina* for emesis and purgation. Cats have a known fondness for *Valeriana officinalis* and *Nepeta cataria* (catmint).

bearing the same identical form. In the Early Stone Age (Paleolithic Period), up to the Solutrean Period, these chipped celts were little more than the result of a necessarily crude flaking cf oval or ovoid stones. From the time of arrival of the pre-Chellean flint-workers in Europe during the Second Interglacial Period, 100,000 years ago, each successive race had its peculiar technic of flint-chipping, its characteristic retouch, until the crude *coups de poing* of the Chelleans become the exquisite laurel-leaf points of Solutrean man. But in the Magdalenian period, the forms are again crude, and finally dwindle away into the faultier Azilian forms and the strange trapeziform shapes of the Tardenoisian microliths.[1] In the Later Stone Age (Neolithic Period), they were brought to a high point of specialization and polish, but in shape and intention they have remained the same throughout geologic space and time. Their employment in surgery by the ancient Egyptians, or in ritual circumcision by the Hebrews in the desert, goes to show the unusual veneration in which they were held among these peoples by reason of their great antiquity. In one of the most interesting of American contributions to archeology,[2] Professor William H. Holmes has demonstrated inductively (by working out the initial methods of chipping and flaking, himself) that even in remains of recent American Indians, such as those of the Piney Branch quarries in the District of Columbia, the process of shaping and specializing the leaf-shaped flints was probably not different from that employed by Paleolithic man or even in what seem to be the rude artefacts of Eolithic man. There is apparently no distinction in space and time in the flaking of prehistoric and primitive implements. Similarly, ethnologists have found that the traditions and superstitions of primitive peoples have a strong family likeness at all times and places.

The common point of convergence of all medical folk-lore is animism, *i. e.*, the notion that the world swarms with invisible spirits which are the efficient causes of disease and death. Primitive medicine is inseparable from primitive modes of religious belief. If we are to understand the attitude of the primitive mind toward the diagnosis and treatment of disease, we must recognize that medicine, in our sense, was only one phase of a set of magic or mystic processes designed to promote human well-being, such as averting the wrath of angered gods or evil spirits, fire-making, making rain, purifying streams or habitations, fertilizing soil, improving sexual potency or fecundity, preventing or removing blight of crops and epidemic diseases. These powers, originally united in one person, were he god, hero, king, sorcerer, priest, prophet, or physician, formed the savage's generic concept of "making medicine." A true medicine-maker, in the primitive sense, was the analogue of our

---

[1] See H. F. Osborn: Men of the Old Stone Age, New York, 1916, *passim*.

[2] W. H. Holmes: "Stone Implements of the Potomac-Chesapeake Tide-water Province," Rep. Bur. Ethnol., 1893–4, Wash., 1897, xv, 1–152. Also: Mem. Internat. Cong. Anthrop., Chicago, 1894, 120–139, 4 pl.

scientific experts, philanthropists, and "efficiency engineers," a general promoter of human prosperity.

In his attempts to interpret the ways of nature, savage man, untutored because inexperienced, first of all confused life with motion. Like Mime in Wagner's "Siegfried," he was puzzled if not awed by the rustling of leaves in the forest, the crash and flash of thunder and lightning, the flicker and play of sunlight and firelight, and he could see no causal relation between a natural object and its moving shadow, a sound and its echo, flowing water and the reflections on its surface. Winds, clouds, storms, earthquakes, or unusual sights and sounds in nature were to him the outward and visible signs of malevolent gods, demons, spirits, or other supernatural agencies. The natural was to him the supernatural, as it still is to many of us, but with this curious difference, that what we should qualify as supernatural was to him as natural as the light of day. In respect of religion primitive man was an essential pantheist. He therefore worshiped the sun, the moon, the stars, trees, rivers, springs, fire, winds, or even serpents, cats, dogs, apes, and oxen; and, as he came to set up carved stocks and stones to represent these, he passed from nature-worship to fetish-worship. At this stage he confused the symbol with the reality, the name with the thing it stood for, and imputed even to inanimate objects the occasional presence of an invisible power (*mana* or *physis*). In his artistic productions, Paleolithic man is usually animistic and ideographic, tends to vitalize inanimate objects, and achieves a startling realism in the portrayal of action and movement, while his later (Neolithic) art inclines to static, geometric pattern work and perfection of form.[1] Disease, in particular, he was prone to regard at first as an evil spirit or the work of such a spirit, to be placated or cajoled, as with other deities, by burnt offerings and sacrifice. A further association of ideas led our *primitif* to regard disease as something produced by a human enemy possessing supernatural powers, which he strove to ward off by appropriate spells and sorcery, similar to those employed by the enemy himself. Again, his own reflection in water, his shadow in the sunlight, what he saw in dreams, or in an occasional nightmare from gluttony, suggested the existence of a spirit-world apart from his daily life and of a soul or *alter ego* apart from his body. In this way he hit upon a third way of looking at disease as the work of offended spirits of the dead, whether of men, animals, or plants. These three views of disease are common beliefs of the lowest grades of human life. As Rivers says, the category of natural causes "can hardly be said to exist" among

---

[1] That there is a strong resemblance between some of the concepts of savage and paranoiac art is strikingly shown in the remarkable carvings of a paranoiac collected by G. Marro, Ann. de freniat., Turin, 1913, xxiii, 157–192, 6 pl. See also Hans Prinzhorn: Bildnerei der Geisteskrankheiten, 2 Aufl., Berlin, 1923. W. H. Holmes has shown that, in the savage, perfection of pattern forms and figures had to follow upon development of the metric and geometric arts, such as the shaping of pottery, textiles, technics, and architecture. (Rep. Bur. Ethnol., 1882–3, Wash., 1886, iv, 443–465.)

them. Savages, as a rule, cheerfully accept all three viewpoints. A lingering belief in human sorcery and the displeasure of the dead is always a trait of the peasant, and sometimes of his descendants in "civilized" communities. Among savages, such beliefs usually go hand in hand with shamanism—an intermediate stage between polytheism (pantheism) and monotheism—which apparently assumes a "Great Spirit," with lesser divinities and demons subordinated. With the beginnings of shamanism[1] we have everywhere the advent of the medicine man, the bilbo or witch-doctor, who assumes a solemn supervisory relation to disease and its cure, not unlike that of the priest to religion. The shaman handles disease almost entirely by psychotherapeutic manœuvers, which serve to awaken a co-responsive state of autosuggestion in his patients. Whether North American Indian or Asiatic Samoyed, he does his best to frighten away the demons of disease by assuming a terrifying aspect, covering himself with the skins of animals, so as to resemble an enormous beast walking on its hind legs, resorting to such demonstrations as shouting, raving, slapping his hands or shaking a rattle, and pretending (or endeavoring) to extract the active principle of the disease by sucking it through a hollow tube. To prevent future attacks, in other words, to keep the demon away for the future, he provides his patient with a special fetish or amulet to be worn or carried about his person. Furthermore, any fantastic thing he may elect to do or not to do, such as passing in or out of a door or stepping over an object with intention, he considers in the light of "making medicine." We may smile at these phases of shamanistic procedure, but, except for the noise, they are not essentially different from the mind-medicine or faith-healing of our own day. Both rely upon psychotherapy and suggestion and, for a sick savage, the fantastic clamor made about him might be conceivably as effective as the quieter methods of Christian Science to a modern nervous patient.

In opposition to the English anthropologists, Levy-Brühl[2] argues that primitive thinking is at once animistic and prelogical, i. e., incoherent, inconsistent, capricious, and not really susceptible to the logical arrangement and classification which Fraser has imposed upon its collective manifestations. Accepting the latter as generalized, labor-saving summaries got up for our convenience, we must always bear in mind that the individual savage shows the same incapacity for consecutive thought that is noticeable in the infantile, the mentally defective, and the insane. The sentiment of the children of nature is allied to what the young Italian said to the grave Goethe: *Perché pensa? Pensando s'invecchia* (with knowledge increaseth sorrow). Vegetative, instinctive (brainstem) people dislike to think, and even an idiot was once called a "natural."

---

[1] For the ritual of preparation and initiation of candidates into the four degrees of shamanism, see W. J. Hoffmann: Rep. Bur. Am. Ethnol., Wash., 1891, vii, 151–300.

[2] L. Levy-Brühl: Les fonctions mentales dans les sociétés inférieures, Paris, 1910.

Whatever interpretation we put upon savage medicine must, there-fore, be viewed with caution as something read into it by our own mentality and which may be as far removed from the thing in itself as the savage's own attempt to explain it to us. Thus, in Frazer's view, magic is a kind of primitive pseudo-science, which assumes that natural processes are rigid and invariable in operation and controllable by man; while religion implies belief in a superhuman power or powers controlling natural forces, capable of altering them, and to be propitiated or conciliated by submission, sacrifice, and prayer. But, as we have seen, one criterion of the savage mind is that to it only the supernatural exists. In more advanced phases, Melanesian magic implies gaining control of the *mana* (innate power) resident in exceptional invididuals protected by the barrier of taboo; Chinese magic, the materialization of malevolent agencies out of the void; Hindu magic, the power to destroy by mental absorption in the central reservoir of consciousness; medieval magic, "a lonely passion of the soul" which aimed to penetrate behind the veil of consciousness into forbidden spheres. The *mana* of the Melanesian, the *manitou* of the Algonquin, the *orenda* of the Huron, the *wakan* of the Sioux, are all virtually equivalent. Like Egyptian or Greek or Celtic or African magic, each is a vague precursor or primitive prototype of modern science, but some modalities of magic were rela-tively impious, as opposing the will of a god or gods, while others are independent of the idea of godhead. Magic, as Salomon Reinach said, is "the strategy of animism." To the primitive mind, steam-power, electricity, x-rays, the telephone, radio, and television are magic, as were false hair and false teeth to the wild Moro and, not so long ago, their inventors would have been persecuted and burned in Europe as sorcerers and atheists. Medicine could not begin to be medicine until it was dissociated from magic and religion. Primitive medicine stands midway between magic and religion, as an attempt to safeguard health by control of natural (supernatural) processes, by warding off evil in-fluences, or by propitiation of gods, and was often fused or confused with either. Even today, medicine sometimes partakes of magical and mystic (religious) as well as of scientific elements.

It is highly probable that, in all primitive societies, priest, magician, and medicine-man were one and the same, and that the powers ascribed to them ranked with courage and the sword as means of securing leadership or kingship. As these functions became specialized and differentiated, religion as such came to be the communal belief in and worship of some universal power or powers greater than man himself; magic, a special set of processes within the power of some isolated man, whereby he sought usually to wreak evil, in opposition to the will of the god or gods; and medicine, the attempt to direct and control those natural phenomena which produce disease and death in man (Rivers[1]). Thus religion, through the inhibitions which man put upon himself to attain to the godlike, became the origin of law and ethics; the secret practices of magic engendered alchemy (chemistry) and other precursors of natural science; astrology begat astronomy; while primitive medicine remained more or less stationary among all peoples, usually following in the wake of other sciences, until it could, in its turn, utilize advances made in physics

[1] See W. H. R. Rivers, Fitzpatrick Lectures, Lancet, Lond., 1916, i, 59; 117.

or chemistry. Black magic was concerned with producing drought, famine, disease, death, or other evils; white magic with averting these, or with such positive good as rain-making, fire-making, or promotion of vegetation. Primitive therapy, therefore, was a mode of white magic.

Primitive pathology ascribes disease to something projected into the body of the victim, something taken from it, or to the effect of sorcery upon some part of or some object connected with the body of the patient. The first category corresponds with our infectious and toxic diseases; the second, e. g., the predilection of the Australian savage for the adrenal fat of his enemies, with the diathetic (metabolic) and deficiency diseases. The third category Frazer defines as sympathetic magic (action at a distance[1]), including homeopathic or mimetic magic (action by or upon similar objects for good or evil) and contagious magic (magical effect of a thing which has once been in contact with a person or thing or has formed part of it). As part of this cult, the soul was regarded as "the animal inside the animal, the man inside the man," a mannikin, counterpart or double, sometimes a shadow or reflection,[2] absent from the body in sleep, sometimes a truant and a wanderer, capable of being extracted from the body by an enemy, or of being deposited in some safe place to secure immortality, or even of existing as a second self or "external soul" in various plants or animals, upon whose welfare the welfare of the individual depended.[3] The "perils of the soul," in primitive medicine, were averted by complex systems of totems and taboos. On Eddystone Island (Melanesia), nearly every disease is ascribed to eating the fruit of tabooed trees. In other parts of Melanesia, disease follows upon any infraction of totemic ordinances, such as killing or eating the totem (Rivers). Thus primitive medicine, magic, and religion are, at the start, inseparable from animism. A good example is afforded in Max Höfler's fine study of the prehistory of organotherapy.[4]

To the primitive, animals are supernatural beings to be feared and revered. To envelop the body with their skins, as among the ancient Gauls and Teutons or the Algonquin Indians, wards off evil influences (including disease). A girdle of wolf's hide (*Wolfsgürtel*) or a necklace of teeth is apotropaic. The skin of man or animal is the "external soul" (Fraser). Hercules wore a lion's skin because the lion was the totem of the Heraclidæ and Ajacidæ. The priests of Babylon conducted incantations in fish skins. In ancient Ireland, the sick patient awaited recovery clad in the skin of a sacrificial sheep. In like manner, particular parts of particular animals were regarded as infallible remedies for disease and usually eaten raw (omophagy). Among savages, to partake of the totem animal is a healing rite, at all other times taboo. The same thing is true of the *concessa animalia* of the ancient Teutons (Tacitus), the sacrificial and chthonian ritual of the Greeks and Romans up to the time of Porphyry (304 A. D.), or even the "Winchester goose" of 1621. Heart, liver, and brain (the ancient "triad of life") were particularly favored and blood was a super-remedy. Scribonius Largus (47 A. D.) even records the drinking of one's own blood as a therapeutic rite (*nam sunt et qui sanguinem ex vena sua missum bibunt*). These things were carried over into the earlier pharmacopœias even unto the 18th century. In the religious ritual, they became sacrificial cakes or sacrificial bread and wine. The cult was pure isotherapy, and in no sense associated with any intuitions about the endocrine organs.

Apart from animism and shamanism, the actual medical knowledge of primitive man, given his limitations, was far from contemptible. The function of the medicine-man was a limited one, and the art of healing never progressed very far so long as it was under the sway of belief in the supernatural. As the savage advanced a little further in the knowledge which is gained from experience, it followed that some

---

[1] Sir James G. Frazer: The Magic Art (The Golden Bough, pt. i), London, 1913, i, 52–219.

[2] Frazer: Taboo and the Perils of the Soul (Golden Bough, pt. ii), London, 1911.

[3] Frazer: Balder the Beautiful (Golden Bough, pt. vii), London, 1913, ii, 95–278.

[4] Höfler: Lehrbuch der Organotherapie (Wagner-Jauregg and Bayer), Leipzig, 1914, 1–26.

special talent for herb-doctoring, bone-setting, and rude surgery should be developed and employed as a special means of livelihood by certain individuals. Along with these nature-healers there went, of course, the inevitable "wise woman," who followed herb-therapy and midwifery, and such specialists soon perceived not only what substances are good or harmful as foods, but that a number of poisons are also remedies under various conditions. Indo-Germanic medicine, which Huxley has so truly styled the foster-mother of many sciences, really began with this crude food- and poison-lore of primitive peoples.

Early man regarded the poisoner with the same horror and loathing that we feel, because, as Thomas points out,[1] the use of poison involves the idea of death without the possibility of motor resistance, without giving the victim a fighting chance. When Ulysses applied to Ilus at Ephyra for a deadly arrow-poison, Ilus declined, "for he had in awe the immortal gods" (Odyssey, i, 260). At the ancient Greek festival of the Thargelia, given at Athens every May, two public outcasts, set apart for the purpose, were flogged with squills, wild fig-branches or *agnus castus*, and possibly stoned to death or flung into the sea. The scapegoat, in this case, was called the Pharmakos, originally a sorcerer or poisoner, while φάρμακον meant something used by a sorcerer, whether a charm, an enchanted potion, or a drug.[2] It is plain that the original pharmacologist was eyed with suspicion.

Primitive man's knowledge of medicinal simples was exactly like the drug phase of our modern therapeutics—extensive, if not intensive—and where he made mistakes, it was (as in our own case) due to the cause which Kant assigns for all human error—the inveteracy of the *post hoc, propter hoc* tendency in the human mind. Like many physicians today, he tried to treat the disease rather than the patient, not realizing (as we have just begun to realize) that the dynamic effect of a drug upon the patient's body depends as much upon the delicate chemical adjustments of that body as upon the composition of the drug itself. Whenever many different remedies are proposed for a disease, it usually means that we know very little about treating the disease, which is also true of a drug when it is vaunted as a panacea or cure-all for many diseases. "In listening to the praises of these panaceas," said Peter Krukenberg, the old Halle clinician, "we seem actually to be standing before the booth of a mountebank."[3] We are not much better off than early man in this respect. Thus, the hieratic writings of the Egyptian papyri reveal an unusually extensive materia medica, the excellence of which is vouched for in the Homeric poems, and which can today be duplicated, in extent at least, in the materia medica of old civilizations like China or Japan, or even in our own bulky pharmacopeias. The ancient Egyptians, Chinese, and Aztecs had botanic gardens (Hill). We find that savages in widely separated countries easily get to know the most fatal arrow-poisons—curare, ouabain, veratrin, boundou—as well as the virtues of drugs like opium, hashish, hemp, coca, cinchona, eucalyptus, sarsaparilla, tobacco, acacia, kousso, copaiba,

[1] W. I. Thomas: Sex and Society, Chicago, 1907, 163–167.
[2] See Morley Roberts: The Pharmakos, Folk-Lore, Lond., 1916, xxvii, 218–224.
[3] Cited by Baas.

guaiac, jalap, podophyllin, or quassia. Abel and Macht have shown
that the ancient European belief in the venomous nature of the toad
and the power of its dried skin to cure dropsy is explained by the two
alkaloids, bufagin and epinephrin, which they isolated from the tropical
Bufo agua. Bufagin ($C_{18}H_{24}O_4$) has a marked diuretic action.[1] Safford
has shown that the various narcotic snuffs used by the Indians of the
West Indies and South America are all products of *Piptadenia peregrina*.[2]
Not to go further than our own country, we find North American Indians aware that arbutus is "good" for rheumatism; lobelia for coughs
and colds; wild sage-tea, goldenseal, flowering dogwood, and prickly
ash-berries for fevers; elder, wild cherry, and sumac for colds and
quinsies; wild ginger, ginseng, and euphorbia for digestive disorders; inhalations of pennyroyal for headache; sassafras or violet leaves for
wounds and felons; and the roots of sassafras and sarsaparilla for
"cooling and purifying the blood." In 1535–36 the Iroquois around
Quebec, as Jacques Cartier relates, treated scurvy in his crew very
successfully with an infusion of the bark and leaves of the hemlock
spruce; while the French at Onondaga, in 1657, found the sassafras leaves,
recommended by the same tribe, "marvellous" for closing wounds of all
kinds.[3] The *Materia Medica Americana* (1780) of the old Anspach-
Bayreuth surgeon Schoepf, who came over with the Hessian troops
during the war of the Revolution, shows that the Anglo-Saxon settlers
in the New World had already learned many wrinkles in herb-therapy
from the red men, in addition to the very rich medical folk-lore which
they undoubtedly brought with them from Old England. Some of this
had been, in turn, acquired from early MSS. of the elder Pliny
(Singer). The plant-lore of rural England included a knowledge of the
virtues of camomile-, sage-, and dandelion-teas as laxatives; of mar-
joram and primrose root for headache; of wormwood as a tonic; of
valerian for the "nerves"; of agrimony and parsley for jaundice; of
meadow-saffron (colchicum) for gout; of fennel, eye-bright (euphrasy),
and rue for bad eyesight; of male fern and peach leaves for worms; of
tansy as a vermifuge and abortifacient; of horehound, marshmallow, or
candied elecampane for coughs and colds; of foxglove as "the opium of
the heart"; and of such "vulnerary plants" as bryony, agrimony, hare's
ears, moonwort, alehoof, and goldenrod for the treatment of wounds.
English poetry and folk-lore are full of references to thyme and mar-
joram, rosemary and rue, mistletoe and ash, as well as to poisons like
hemlock, leopard's bane (aconite), the deadly nightshade (belladonna),
"the juice of cursed hebenon" (yew), and henbane (hyoscyamus),

---

[1] Abel and Macht: J. Pharm. Exper. Therap., Balt., 1911–12, iii, 319–377.

[2] W. E. Safford: Jour. Wash. Acad. Sc., 1916, vi, 547–562.

[3] See Yager: "Medicine in the Forest," Oneonta, N. Y., 1910. Yager notes
the infrequency of panaceas and gunshot prescriptions among the North American
Indians; each remedy was administered by itself for a given condition. For the
theory and formulæ of Cherokee medicine, see J. Mooney: Bur. Am. Ethnol. Rep.,
Wash., 1891, vii, 319–369.

which Aretæus regarded as a cause of insanity and to which Shakespeare refers in the same spirit as

> . . . the insane root
> That takes the reason prisoner.

Asphodel or dittany is mentioned in the Homeric poems as a balm against the pain of newly inflicted wounds. The same tradition, derived from Pliny and Apuleius (*Herbarium*), is still current among the country folk of Lancashire, Ireland, and the moors of Scotland with reference to the daffodil, which was thought to be identical with asphodel.[1] Kipling has summed up the whole matter in a charming verse—

> Alexanders and Marigold,
>   Eyebright, Orris and Elecampane,
> Basil, Rocket, Valerian, Rue,
>   (Almost singing themselves they run),
> Vervain, Dittany, Call-me-to-you—
>   Cowslip, Melilot, Rose of the Sun.
> Anything green that grew out of the mould
> Was an excellent herb to our fathers of old.

In the use of natural or physical means against disease, it is plain that primitive man, in spite of his ill-ventilated habitations, keeps healthy through his hardy life in the open air, has advantages which his civilized brother often seeks or finds only on compulsion. The Indian[2] sensed, for example, the importance of keeping the skin, bowels, and kidneys open, and, to this end, the geyser, the warm spring, and the sweat-oven were his natural substitutes for a Turkish bath. Emesis or catharsis, followed by a vapor bath and a cold plunge, set off by a dose of willow-bark decoction (salicin), was the North American Indian's successful therapeutic scheme in the case of intermittent and remittent fevers. A vapor bath and cimicifuga were his mainstays against rheumatism. Like the ancient Babylonians, he had his fixed periods for ritual emesis and catharsis (*e. g.*, the green-corn feast), much as our forefathers used zodiacal calendars for blood-letting. Massage was long known and practised by the Indians, Japanese, Malays, and East Indians. In the opinion of Rivers,[3] Polynesian massage is apparently a true rational therapeutic measure, while Melanesian massage, imported into Melanesia by Polynesian castaways, acquires the status of a superimposed magic rite. Hypnotism originated among the Hindus; inoculation against smallpox among the Hindus, Persians, and Chinese. Lady Mary Wortley Montagu got her idea of variolation from the East, and it is still employed among the

---

[1] Singer points out that the medieval peoples of northwestern Europe, through their devotion to Pliny, confused their flora with the pictures of plants of southern Europe. The Latin words in English botany, crocus, dandelion, hyacinth, plantain, etc., all derive from Pliny.

[2] For a full account of the medicine of the 20th century Indian, see A. Hrdlička Bur. Am. Ethnol., Bull. No. 34, Wash., 1908, 220–253.

[3] W. H. R. Rivers: Massage in Melanesia: Tr. xvii. Internat. Cong. Med., 1913, Lond., 1914, Sect. xxiii, 39–42.

North and Central African tribes and races (Arnold Klebs[1]). The early Japanese employed the moxa as the Chinese did acupuncture. The Chinese of the Mongol dynasty (1260[2]) probably learned of the the use of spectacles from India *via* Turkestan. Snow-spectacles have been employed by polar tribes.

Surgery became a science in recent times, not so much through individual skill or specialization of instruments, as through the introduction of such new factors as anesthesia, antisepsis, Röentgenology, and safeguards against shock. Primitive surgery included all the rudiments of the art. The earliest surgical instrument was, in all probability, not the specialized leaf-shaped flint or "celt," already referred to, but rather some fragment, unusually sharpened as to edge and point by accidental flaking,[3] as in the obsidian knives of Peru. By means of these sharpened flints or of fishes' teeth, blood was let, abscesses emptied, tissues scarified, skulls trephined, and, at a later period, ritual operations like circumcision were performed, as we have seen, with the primitive celts themselves. Decompressive trephining for epilepsy or other cerebral disorders goes back to prehistoric times. The finds show that it was repeated as often as five times upon the same person, the bits of skull excised (*rondelles*) being used as amulets. It was common among neolithic Gauls and Bohemians, and has been practised in recent times by Polynesians, Kabyl tribes, Montenegrins, the Aymaras of Bolivia, and the Quichuas of Peru.[4] A remarkable variant of it is the ritual crosswise mutilation along the lines of the coronal and sagittal sutures, first noticed as a common practice among the Loyalty Islanders by an English missionary, Rev. Samuel Ella, in 1874,[5] and which Manouvrier found afterward in neolithic female crania from Seine-et-Oise and called the "sincipital T" (1895[6]). Trephining has been done on the skull with sharpened prehistoric flints in thirty-five to fifty minutes by Lucas-Championnière and Holländer.[7] Primitive man's wounds were dressed with moss or fresh leaves, ashes or natural balsams, and, when poisoned, treated by sucking or cauterization. Cupping

---

[1] Klebs: Johns Hopkins Hosp. Bull., Balt., 1913, xxiv, 70.

[2] B. Laufer: Mitt. z. Gesch. d. Med., Leipz., 1907, vi, 379–385.

[3] The writer is indebted to Prof. William H. Holmes for this important information.

[4] A. Bandelier: Ueber Trepanieren unter den heutigen Indianern Bolivias (Internat. Cong. Americanists, 1894). S. J. Mozans (Rev. J. A. Zahm), in his "Along the Andes and Down the Amazon" (New York, 1911), pp. 206, 207, is of opinion that the leaves of *Erythroxylon coca*, when chewed, have anesthetic properties, of which he gives a remarkable instance suggesting how easily the Peruvians may have accomplished trephining with the aid of a sharp piece of flint or obsidian.

[5] Ella: Med. Times & Gaz., Lond., 1874, i, 50.

[6] L. Manouvrier: Rev. mens. de l'École d'anthrop. de Paris, 1896, vi, 57; 1903, xiii, 431. Manouvrier thinks the sincipital T may have been identical with the crucial cauterizations of the skull recommended by Avicenna and others, if not a ritual mutilation. Grön regards it as a mode of judicial torture. Sudhoff identifies it with a derivative procedure employed by the Alexandrian surgeons for ocular catarrhs and mentioned by Celsus (vii, cap. xii, sect. 15).

[7] Lucas-Championnière: Trepanation néolithique, Paris, 1912.

was effected by means of animals' horns. The revulsive effects of some accidental wound or hemorrhage, or the natural and periodic process of menstruation suggested, no doubt, the advantages of blood-letting, which was to become a sort of therapeutic sheet-anchor through the ages. For couching a cataract or opening an abscess, even a sharp thorn sufficed. The Dayaks of Borneo employ a sharp root (*pinjampo*). In the more advanced phases of cultural development, pieces of hard wood may have been pointed and edged, like the flint knives. Neolithic saws of stone and bone exist, obviously imitated from the teeth of animals. With these Holländer has performed amputation in six or seven minutes.[1] The characteristic signs of amputation have been found in prehistoric bones. During the Bronze and Iron Ages, expert skill in metal work became accomplished fact, and surgical instrumentation was correspondingly improved. In the excavations of the Swiss Lake Dwellings, which were discovered in 1853,[2] the different cultural objects were found in successive layers, from the Stone Age (Neolithic or Alluvial Period, 3000–1500 B. C.) up to the Bronze and Iron Ages (1500–400 B. C.). The real beginnings of North-European culture are now held to be the metal implements and objects found at La Tène. The phrase "La Tène" symbolizes (for anthropologists) the starting-point of the cultural periods following upon the three Ice Ages, with their two interglacial periods, not because the Lake Dwelling finds are necessarily the earliest iron objects known, but because they are the most representative and characteristic. La Tène was preceded by the Eolithic, Paleolithic, Neolithic, and Bronze Ages, and the Iron (Halstatt) Age (700–400 B. C.). In the Bronze Age surgical saws and files were plentiful everywhere, from Egypt to Central Europe.[3] The La Tène finds, dating from about 500 B. C. to 100 A. D., are entirely distinct from Egyptian, Indian, or Greek culture, and include iron knives, needles, fibulæ, swords and lances, with bracelets, necklaces, and ear-rings of Etruscan or West Celtic pattern, and funeral urns containing human remains. These show that cremation was the rule among the La Tène people. Some time later, as, for instance, among the Gallo-Roman finds in France, we can trace the evolution of the jointed or articulated surgical instruments, like scissors, in which cutting was done by indirect action.[4] With improved metal instruments, such cosmetic operations as tattooing, infibulation, boring holes for ear-rings and nose-rings, or the Mica operation (external urethrotomy), as well as amputation and lithotomy, could be essayed. The ancient Hindus performed almost every major operation except ligation

[1] E. Holländer: Die chirurgische Säge. Arch. f. klin. Chir., Berl., 1915, cvi, 317–320.

[2] Lake-dwellings were first investigated by Ferdinand Keller in 1853–4, and (Irish Crannogs) by Sir William Wilde (1839–58).

[3] Holländer: Die chirurgische Säge. Arch. f. klin. Chir., Berl., 1915, cvi, 320–336.

[4] See M. Baudouin: Arch. prov. de chir., Paris, 1910, xix, 228–238.

of the arteries. Ovariotomy has been done by Indian and Australian natives, and Felkin witnessed a native Cesarean section in Uganda in 1878. Both operations are said to have been performed by German sowgelders in the 16th century.

The use of a soporific potion, as a substitute for anesthesia, goes back to remote antiquity, as symbolized in Genesis (II, 21): "And the Lord God caused a deep sleep to fall upon Adam, and he slept: and he took one of his ribs, and closed up the flesh instead thereof." From the soothing Egyptian nepenthe of the Odyssey which Helen casts into the wine for Telemachus, to the *samme de shinta* of the Talmud, the *bhang* of the Arabian Nights, or the "drowsy syrups" of Shakespeare's time, the soporific virtues of opium, Indian hemp (*Cannabis indica*), the mandrake (*Atropa mandragora*), henbane (*Hyoscyamus*), dewtry (*Datura stramonium*), hemlock (*Conium*), and lettuce (*Lactucarium*) appear to have been well known to the Orientals and the Greeks.[1] In the 13th and 14th centuries, a mixture of some of these ingredients (*oleum de lateribus*) was formally recommended for surgical anesthesia by the mediæval masters in the form of a *spongia somnifera* or *confectio soporis*. Again, the use of such natural antiseptics as extreme dryness, smoke (creosote), honey, niter, and wine was common to early man. In seeking an "artificial paradise" by means of narcotics and intoxicants like alcohol, opium, hashish, or mescal, priority certainly belongs to primitive man, to whom we also owe such private luxuries as tea, coffee, cocoa, and tobacco. Medicine is curiously indebted to the non-medical man for many of its innovations. As Oliver Wendell Holmes has said:

"It learned from a monk how to use antimony, from a Jesuit how to cure agues, from a friar how to cut for stone, from a soldier how to treat gout, from a sailor how to keep off scurvy, from a postmaster how to sound the Eustachian tube, from a

---

[1] Poppy and Indian hemp were probably known to the Egyptians and consequently to the Greeks; mandragora to the Egyptians, Babylonians, and Hebrews. Theophrastus and Dioscorides were the first to mention the aphrodisiac and soporific properties of *Atropa mandragora*. It is not clear whether the mandrakes which Rachel sought of Leah (Genesis xxx, 14–16) were for aphrodisiac purposes or to ease the pangs of childbirth. Dioscorides was the first to recommend mandragora wine for surgical anesthesia. His original recipe was tried out with success by Sir Benjamin Ward Richardson (Brit. For. Med.-Chir. Rev., Lond., 1874, liii. 244). The mandrake is also mentioned by Celsus, Pliny, Apuleius, Paul of Ægina, and Avicenna. The legends about the human shape of the root of the plant, its frightful shrieks when uprooted, and the necessity of employing a dog, hitched to it for this purpose (Josephus), are a common feature of early English and German folk-lore. Drugging with Indian hemp or henbane (*tabannuj*) was common among the ancient Hindus and the later Arabs, and Sir Richard Burton notes: "These have been used in surgery throughout the East for centuries before ether and chloroform became the fashion in the civilized West." (Arabian Nights, Denver edition, vol. iv, footnote to p. 71.) Hua, a Chinese physician, is said to have used hashish in surgery about 200 B. C. According to S. J. Mozans ("Along the Andes and Down the Amazon," New York, 1911, pp. 206, 207), the ancient Peruvian Incas probably utilized the anesthetic properties of the active principle of *Erythroxylon coca* in trephining. He cites a modern instance of a *coquero* (habitual chewer of coca leaves) who was run over by a car and experienced no apparent pain, although his foot had been taken off in the accident.

dairy-maid how to prevent smallpox, and from an old market-woman how to catch the itch-insect. It borrowed acupuncture and the moxa from the Japanese heathen, and was taught the use of lobelia by the American savage."[1]

In the field of obstetrics, we find the midwife to be one of the most ancient of professional figures. Engelmann's careful ethnic studies of posture in labor show the universal tendency of primitive and frontier women to assume attitudes best adapted to aid or hasten delivery.[2] The obstetric chair, first mentioned in the Bible and by the Greek writers, appears to be of great antiquity, and is still used by some races of the Far East.

The development of a rational, scientific concept of disease, not as a demon or "entity" inside the body, but as altered physiology (dis-ease), is essentially modern, and of very recent vintage. The most difficult problem which confronts the medical historian is: How did early man acquire correct logical thinking in regard to the treatment of disease?

It really got its stride among the active-minded Greeks. One of the best sources of evidence is the Hippocratic Tract on Ancient Medicine *(circa* 430–420 B. C.)[3] which sets forth how men came "to learn by themselves how their own sufferings came about and cease" and asserts that "medicine has long had all its means to hand, and has discovered both a principle and a method, through which the discoveries made during a long period are many and excellent." This method was acquired by discussion with "ordinary folk when they are sick or in pain" and turned upon the fact that "there would have been no need for medicine if sick men had profited by the same mode of living and regimen as the food, drink, and mode of living of men in health, and if there had been no other things for the sick better than these. . . . For many and terrible were the sufferings of men from strong and brutish living when they partook of crude foods, uncompounded and possessing great powers." The beginnings were therefore empirical observations on dietetics. Prehistoric and primitive man, like the infant, was apt to swallow anything that seemed edible, and one of his first taboos was upon poisonous substances. This is borne out by the Mosaic code, with its intelligent interdictions upon ungulates, tardigrades, smooth fish, reptiles and batrachians, unclean birds, water contaminated by dead animals (Leviticus xii, 3–43), "any thing that dieth of itself" (Lev. xi, 9) and suchlike. Hippocrates notes the advantages of restricted and slop diet in illness, the disadvantages of coarse cereals, of unseasonable abstinence or repletion, of taking lunch when used only to one or two meals daily. When he notes the "heaviness, yawning, drowsiness, thirst"· which follows the lunch, and the "flatulence, colic and diarrhea" following the dinner (if taken), we are already in the full current of primitive diagnosis and semeiology as far as early Greek medicine is concerned. The whole matter is beautifully summarized in the lucid paragraph from Celsus, as cited by Osler (Silliman Lectures):

"Some of the sick, on account of their eagerness, took food on the first day, some, on account of loathing, abstained; and the disease in those who refrained was more relieved. Some ate during a fever, some a little before it, others after it had subsided, and those who had waited to the end did best. For the same reason, some at the beginning of an illness used a full diet, others a spare, and the former were made worse. Occurring daily, such things impressed careful men, who noted what had best helped the sick, then began to prescribe them. In this way, medicine had its rise from the experience of the recovery of some, of the death of others, distinguishing the hurtful from the salutary things."

---

[1] O. W. Holmes: Medical Essays, Boston, 1883, 289. See also G. M Gould: "Medical Discoveries by the Non-Medical," Jour. Amer. Med. Assoc., Chicago, 1903, xl, 1477–1487.

[2] G. J. Engelmann: "Labor Among Primitive Peoples," St. Louis, 1882.

[3] Hippocrates (*ed.* W. H. S. Jones): London and New York, 1923, i, 13–63, *passim.*

In his analytical studies of the development of scientific medicine from pre-historic, folk and magic medicine, Hovorka postulates certain "laws of congruence, in virtue of which primitive or ancient man everywhere, in space and time, deduced identical remedies for certain diseases, proceeding (1) by "repetition and imitation," evolving and adopting effective remedies by the trying-out process; (2) by establishment of such therapeutic principles along well-trodden paths; (3) by promoting belief and confidence through devices of similarity or symbolism and through the suggestive effect of verbal and ocular magic. The fundamental phases of therapeutic reasoning are thus "the device of gaining time" until nature effects recovery or a fatal termination, "the inquiry into the cause" where accessible and "the flight into mysticism" when causes are inscrutable.[1]

We now come to a phase of primitive healing which is intimately connected with even the most recent aspects of the subject, namely, the potency of therapeutic superstitions and the actual cure of disease through the influence of the mind upon the body. This is a matter which can be approached in no derisive spirit, particularly in the light of quackery and its successes. The closer we look into the ways of primitive man, the more liable it is to take down our own conceit. The untutored savage, as we have seen, thinks that motion of any kind is equivalent to life. Wherein does he differ from the ultra-mechanistic physiologist who reverses the equation? Simply in this, that the mind of the savage is, as Black says,[2] like a looking-glass, reflecting everything and retaining nothing. As soon as an object passed from his observation, its image disappeared from his mental vision and he ceased to hug the fact of its existence, still less to reason about it. The primitive mind is, as Rowland scornfully said of "the ordinary cultivated or legal mind," essentially "discontinuous." The scientific mind at least aims, in its methods, at consecutive thought. The folk-mind, even today, has the inevitable tendency to mix up the *post hoc* with the *propter hoc* and to confuse accidentals with essentials. Almost any one who has lived in the country, for instance, will be familiar with various rural superstitions relating to warts—that killing or handling a toad may cause them, and that they can be removed by some one touching them with pebbles or muttering charms over them; or with the notion that stump water is good for freckles, or that bad eyesight can be remedied by the water into which the blacksmith has dipped his red-hot iron. In some parts of Holland, it is believed that when a boy carrying water-lilies in his hand falls down, it renders him liable to fits. Readers of Longfellow's "Evangeline" may recall the line which refers to malaria as

"Cured by wearing a spider hung around one's neck in a nutshell."

In Norfolk, England, this spider was tied up in a piece of muslin and pinned over the mantelpiece as a remedy for whooping-cough. In Donegal, a beetle in a bottle was regarded as a cure for the same dis-

---

[1] O. von Hovorka: Leitmotive und Elementarmethoden der allgemeinen Heilkunde, Mitt. d. anthrop. Gesellsch. in Wien, 1915, xxxv, 125–136. Also his Geist der Medizin, Wien and Leipzig, 1915.

[2] W. G. Black: Folk-Medicine, London, 1883, p. 207.

ease; in Suffolk, to dip the child, head downward, in a hole dug in a meadow; in northeast Lincolnshire, fried mice; in Yorkshire, owl-broth; in other parts of England, riding the child on a bear; in Scotland, anything that might be suggested by a man riding upon a piebald horse.[1] Compare these fallacies, inept as they seem, with what has happened so often in the history of therapeutics. A patient's cure follows seemingly upon the administration of some new-fangled remedy or drug. Immediately, a causal relation is established and the discoverer rushes into print with the glad tidings. Statistics begin to mount up, until presently the correlation curve acquires such an insignificant slope that nothing positive can be affirmed of the remedy whatever. It is then speedily consigned to the limbo of forgotten things.[2] Not so with folk-remedies. The superstition becomes, as the derivation implies, something standing over; and for a very important reason, namely, that in some cases "Nature cures the disease while the remedy amuses the patient"; in others a cure is, in all probability, brought about by the effect of the mind upon the body. In general, we have to remember that the average human mind everywhere is more characterized by inertia and rock-ribbed conservatism than by originality, alertness, free-play, or forward movement. In the normal human being, who is healthy and happy because he is "a good animal," the whole body participates when, as Leigh Hunt wittily said, "he thinks he's thinking"; in other words, what passes as impersonal thought is only an expression of subconscious feeling. But as Clodd says, "Feeling travels along the line of least resistance, while thought, or the challenge by inquiry, with its assumption that there may be two sides to a question, must pursue a path obstructed by the dominance of taboo and custom, by the force of imitation and by the strength of prejudice, passion and fear."[3] In this regard, he quotes Turgot: "It is not error which opposes the progress of truth; it is indolence, obstinacy, the spirit of routine, every thing which favors inaction." It is for this reason that science itself is frequently seen to be passing, as Mencken has described it, not from truth to truth, but from error to error. The creative mind, which demands boundless freedom, and the bureaucratic mind, which functions in boxed categories, are ever at swords' points. The primitive mind, with its taboos and totems, its childish inconsequence, is equidistant from either and has some vague semblance to both.

Black, a leading English authority on medical folk-lore, has made a careful and exhaustive classification of the different superstitions

---

[1] Black: Op. cit., *passim.*

[2] J. C. Bateson cites a recorded case of a Turkish upholsterer who, during the delirium of typhus fever, drank from a pail of pickled cabbage and recovered, whereupon the Turkish doctors declared cabbage-juice a specific for the disease. The next patient dying under this régime, however, they modified the dogma by saying that cabbage-juice is good for typhus provided the patient be an upholsterer. Dietet. & Hyg. Gaz., N. Y., 1911, xxvii, pp. 297, 298.

[3] E. Clodd: Magic in Names, London, 1920, 77.

to which average suffering humanity is liable.[1] They include ideas as to the possible transference of disease, sympathetic relationships, the possibility of new-birth or regeneration, the effects of such accidental specific factors as color, number, solar and lunar influences, magic writings, rings, precious stones, parts of the lower animals, and charms connected with the names of the saints, the lore of plants, the evil eye, birth, death, and the grave. To look into these is to see clearly that "wonder is of the soul." As the savage "sees God in clouds, or hears him in the wind," so our ancestors saw disease not as a quality or condition of the patient, but as something material and positive inside his body—a view held even by Paracelsus. This idea engendered the notion that disease can be transferred from one body to another, as where Pliny, in his Natural History, claims that abdominal pain can be transferred to a dog or a duck. Touching warts with pebbles, healing snake-bite by clapping the bleeding entrails of a bisected fowl to the wound (natural absorption), or the negro superstition of pegging a hank of the patient's hair into a tree in order to transfer chills and fever to the tree or its owner, are well-known forms of this curious belief. Sir Kenelm Digby proposed the following remedy for fever and ague: "Pare the patient's nails; put the parings in a little bag, and hang the bag around the neck of a live eel, and place him in a tub of water. The eel will die, the patient will recover."[2] Among the lower and criminal classes of both England and America helpless infants and ignorant, if innocent women, are frequently exposed to venereal infection, through the notion that it may be gotten rid of by "giving it away."

In medical mythology the doctrine of transference of disease derives from the idea of purification (cathar is) or lustration. The scapegoat was usually a god, or a folk-appointed surrogate in the shape of a person, animal, or inanimate object, upon which the sins of the people might be unloaded. Among the Aztecs a human being was annually sacrificed in place of Vitzliputzli or other gods. At the festival of Xipe, the Flayed God, the Mexicans killed all prisoners taken in war, who were flayed beforehand, the skins being worn by those consecrated to the cult. In the Roman Saturnalia, Saturn was personated by a man-scapegoat, who was afterward put to death. In the Greek Thargelia, as we have seen, there were two scapegoats (φαρμάκοι[3]). Ancient sacrifice was sometimes honorific (hostia honoraria), a gift to the god; sometimes cathartic or piacular (hostia piacularis), to conciliate the wrath of the good or evil powers, in which case human sacrifice was usually demanded; sometimes mystical or sacramental, in which the god was conceived to be slain or eaten by his worshipers (Robertson Smith). In honorific sacrifice, the god and his worshipers shared the sacrifice as commensals or totem-companions, of the same totem-kin, and the victim was sometimes an animal representing a hostile totem, sometimes one sacred to the god. In piacular sacrifice, a totem animal or plant could be substituted for the human victim. In mystic sacrifice, the god was represented by a similar animal or plant, to partake of which was to enter into communion with him.[4] With this obscure set of cults, widely different in different peoples, is connected the consecration of sacrificial plants or parts of sacrificial animals as therapeutic agencies.[5] The Katharmata or rejects of sacrifice, eaten by the wor-

---

[1] Black: Op. cit., pp. 34–177.

[2] Cited by Holmes, "Medical Essays," Boston and New York, 1883, 381.

[3] Frazer: The Scapegoat (Golden Bough, pt. 6), Lond., 1913, 252; 275; 306.

[4] N. W. Thomas: Encycl. Britan., 11 ed., Cambridge, 1911, xxiii, 980–984.

[5] M. Höfler: Wald- und Baumkult (Munich, 1892); Die volksmedizinische Organotherapie, Stuttgart, 1908; Janus, Amst., 1912, xvii, 3; 76; 190.

shipers, were literally "made sacred" by the rite.   To this day the custom of "eating the god" (theophagy) persists in the belief of European peasants that medicinal herbs are materialized benevolent spirits.   In nearly all European countries the plants culled at Midsummer (St. John's) Eve acquired transient magical or medicinal virtues.[1]

Closely connected with this idea of transference was the old tradition of a sympathy existing between parts of bodies separated in space (Frazer's "sympathetic magic"), amusingly illustrated in Sir Kenelm Digby's weapon-salve, which was applied to the weapon instead of the wound, and in the same worthy's

> "Strange hermetic powder
> That wounds nine miles point blank would solder,
> By skilful chemist with great cost
> Extracted from a rotten post."

The idea of material regeneration or new-birth is of Hindu (Aryan) origin and sprang from the primitive worship of the generative power of nature, the cult of the lingam and the yoni, the Hellenized form of which is strikingly elaborated in Lucretius (IV–V).   A cloven tree or a hole in a rock was regarded as symbolic of the sacred yoni, and children (even adults), were supposed to be freed from scrofula, spinal deformity, or other infirmities when passed through it.   Traces of the Saxon form of this superstition survive in the "holed stone" near Lanyon, Cornwall, through which scrofulous children were passed naked three times; in the "Deil's Needle"[2] in the bed of the River Dee (Aberdeenshire) which was held to make barren women fertile if they crept through it; and in the Crick Stone in Morva (Cornwall), passage through which was esteemed a cure for any one with a "crick in the back." It was White of Selborne[3] who described the most recent form of this folk-belief in sympathetic magic, which consists in passing a child afflicted with hernia through a cleft in an ash-tree.   In 1804, such a tree stood at the edge of Shirley Heath, on the road to Birmingham.[4] As late as 1895–6, ash trees were described as existing for this purpose in Suffolk and Richmond Park;[5] there was once a similar tree in Burlington County, New Jersey.   The Scotch custom of passing a consumptive child through a wreath of woodbine, the English trait of crawling under a bramble bush for rheumatism, and the "eye of the needle tree" on the island of Innisfallen (Killarney), squeezing through which insures long life and safe delivery to women with child, are variants of this superstition (Black).   Frazer regards the practice as a phase of sympathetic magic, associated with the idea that the "external soul" (the life of a person), is bound up with the life of a tree or plant.[6]

---

[1] Frazer: Balder the Beautiful (Golden Bough, pt. 7), London, 1913, ii, 45–75.

[2] D. Rorie: Caledon. Med. Jour., Glasgow, 1911, viii, 410–415, with photograph of the "Deil's Needle."

[3] Gilbert White: Natural History of Selborne, 1789, 202 (cited by Black).

[4] Gentleman's Mag., Lond., 1804, 909.   Cited by Frazer.

[5] Folk-Lore, Lond., 1896, vii, p. 303; 1898, ix, p. 330, with photos.

[6] Frazer: Balder the Beautiful (Golden Bough, pt. 7), London, 1913 ii, 159–195.

In folk-lore and common usage, each primary color has associations all its own. "True blue," "a streak of yellow," "seeing red," "a green old age," "born to the purple," "the Black Death," "white-souled," are all truthful expressions of human feeling in this regard. Color is a factor of great moment in folk-healing; in particular, red, which the Chinese and New Zealanders regard as hateful to evil spirits, and other peoples vaguely associate with inflammation as a heat-producer. Red silken bands, necklaces of coral beads, red pills and red fire, as well as the red coral ring and bells with which the baby cuts its teeth, have all had their superstitious associations, and the virtues of the familiar red flannel cloth worn around the neck for sore throat were supposed to reside "not in the flannel but in the red color."[1] Finsen's red-light treatment, to prevent pitting in smallpox, was once an ancient folk-belief, known to the Japanese, and employed by Gilbertus Anglicus, Bernard de Gordon, and by John of Gaddesden in the case of the son of Edward II. According to Valescus of Taranta, the rationale of the red-light treatment was the ancient "doctrine of signatures," in virtue of which a remedy was applied on account of some fancied resemblance, in shape or color, to the disease. The red cloth hangings around the smallpox patient were supposed to lower his temperature by drawing the red blood outward.

The idea that certain numerals may be sacred or malignant is of Accadian origin, connected with Chaldean and Babylonian astrology, and familiar to us in the Horatian *"nec Babylonios tentaris numeros."* Of mystic numbers (usually odd), three or a multiple of three is the most popular for luck, good or bad; seven or one of its multiples for supernatural powers. Hesiod (*Works and Days*, 765–828) says that the first, fourth and seventh days of the month are "holy days," the eighth ($4 + 4$) and the ninth (3×3) "specially good for the works of man"; the twelfth (3×4) is better than the eleventh; the fifth "unkindly and terrible," because on a fifth "the Erinnyes assisted at the birth of Horcus." The tenth is a favorable for a boy to be born, the fourth for a girl; the ninth of the first month "is a good day on which to beget or be born, both for a male and a female: it is never an wholly evil day." It was not for nothing that there were three Fates, three Furies, nine Muses, twelve months, twelve signs of the zodiac, twelve hours around the clock, seven days to the week, and so on. Three handfuls of earth are always dropped on the coffin at burial. Palmists, fortune-tellers, and others of their kind work assiduously (as their signs read) "from nine to nine," and gamblers usually bet on odd numbers. In Scotland and Portugal, the seventh son of a seventh son is often regarded with horror or veneration, as one possessed of second sight and other uncanny attributes. Cato the Censor treated sick oxen with three grains of salt, three leaves of laurel, of rue, and so on, for three consecutive days, during which both beeves and old fogy fasted; such folk-

---

[1] Black: Folk-Medicine, London, 1883, 111.

remedies as the West Sussex recipe for ague—"eat fasting seven sage leaves for seven mornings fasting"—are common enough. Valescus de Taranta arranged his huge therapeutic *Philonium* in seven books, out of a serious veneration for the solemn number seven, which was the theme of a pseudo-Hippocratic tract.[1] In Chinese medicine, five is the sacred number. A reasonable aspect of number-lore in medical literature is the Hippocratic doctrine of crises and critical days[2] (*dies nefasti*) which probably derived from the teaching of Pythagoras, who had assimilated it from Chaldean folk-tradition. Here the folk-lore of numbers has a germ of scientific truth in that there is a certain periodicity in some of the phenomena of disease. The curves of rape, murder, and general "running amok" (including wars) rise in hot weather. That certain infectious diseases recur at definite periods gave rise to the doctrine of the *genius epidemicus* or epidemic constitutions. The known periodicity of epidemic diseases from year to year justified the old Chaldaic superstition of the "evil year" (*malus annus*), which, in the Middle Ages was associated with a certain serpiginous or bullous eruption in man and animals (*Malum malannum*[3]). Another superstition deriving from Chaldean astrology was the belief that the heavenly bodies influence disease. The sun, moon, stars, and planets were regarded as sentient, animated beings, exerting a profound influence upon human weal and woe and, even into the 17th century, European mankind resorted to horoscopes (*judicia astrorum*) before attempting any enterprise of moment, in particular to determine the proper time for blood-letting emesis, and purgation. Health, strength, and sexual power were supposed to vary with the waxing and waning of the moon. Moonshine was supposed to be potent alike in causing lunacy, conferring beauty, or curing warts and diseases.[4] Menstruation was connected with the lunar cycles. The full moon was a libido symbol (White[5]). To let blood when the moon and tides were at full (*dies Ægyptiaci*) was adjudged bad practice in the Middle Ages. The lunar influence may be further sensed in the common superstition that death occurs, as in the case of Shakespeare's Falstaff or of Barkis (David Copperfield), at the turning of the tide. Darwin thought that the tidal periodicity of physiological phenomena in vertebrates might be explained by their descent from "an animal allied to the existing tidal ascidians."[6] Arrhenius, in his study of the influences of cosmic phenomena upon the organism, has compared the curves of nativity, mortality, menstruation, and epileptic attacks with periodic maxima and

---

[1] See, also, Aulus Gellius: Noctes Atticæ, iii, 10.

[2] For a historical study of the doctrine of critical days, see Sudhoff: Wien. med. Wochenschr., 1902, lii, 210; 272; 321; 371. Also, R. Steele: Dies Ægyptiaci, Proc. Roy. Soc. Med., Lond., 1919, xii, Sect. Hist. Med., 108–121.

[3] Höfler: Janus, Amst., 1909, xiv, 512–526.

[4] Frazer: Adonis (Golden Bough, pt. iv), London, 1914, ii, 140–150.

[5] W. A. White: Psychoanalyt. Rev., N. Y., 1913–14, i, 241–256. Cf. the fooleries in Middleton's "A Chaste Maid in Cheapside" (end of Act I, sc. 2).

[6] Darwin: Descent of Man, London, 1871, i, 212, footnote.

minima of the electrical condition of the air.[1] Comparable with the notion that "the stars incline but do not compel" is the idea, already mentioned, that disease is a scourge or punishment inflicted by gods or demons alike and remediable only through divine or diabolic intervention. The mischievous powers, whose ideas of good and evil were apparently so interchangeable, could be propitiated or conciliated only by sacrifice, which, as Jakob Grimm pointed out, had the double purpose (like the graft given to politicians) of keeping the powers in a good humor or of restoring good humor when necessary. "To coerce the spiritual powers, or to square them and get them on our side," says William James, "was, during enormous tracts of time, the one great object in our dealings with the natural world."[2] The Greek myth of the arrows of far-darting Apollo, Bhowani, the cholera goddess of the Hindus, the many medical divinities of the Romans, the Indian and Samoyed lore of "magic bullets" (a *motif* in "Der Freischütz"), the passage in the Book of Job in which the patriach attributes his sufferings to "the arrows of the Almighty," Martin Luther's conviction that "pestilence, fever, and other severe diseases are naught else than the devil's work," Cotton Mather's definition of sickness as *Flagellum Dei pro peccatis mundi*, the medieval figurations of death as a reaper (the *Schnitter Tod* of German folk-song), the folk-superstition that erysipelas (or "wild fire") originates from fairy malice, all illustrate the strength of this deep-rooted belief, which survived in the many sermons and prayers delivered in time of pestilence throughout the 17th and 18th centuries and even crops up in our day under various guises. In process of time, medical polytheism merged into monotheism. The Egyptian Phtah became Allah; the Chaldean Ea, the Sumerian Adapa and Gula, the Babylonian Marduk, the Chthonian deities of the Greeks, the complex Roman scheme of household gods, the Druidic Belen, the Mexican Ixtlilton, all became unified through the syncretic process common to all folk-lore, and even the separate functions of the demons of disease, from Babylon to medieval Europe, were eventually absorbed by the Devil.[3] Of a piece with this theory of disease was the benign or malign power which was supposed to attach to certain personalities. A child born on Easter Eve could cure tertian or quartan fever. Persons born "with a caul" were supposed to be clairvoyant. The power to heal scrofula by Royal Touch was part and parcel of the divine right of kings. How Vespasian cured blindness by his spittle, and lameness by the tread of his foot, is related by Tacitus (*Historia*, iv, 81) and Suetonius (*Vespasian*, vii). In the West of Ireland the blood of the Walshes, Keoghs, and Cahills is held to be an infallible remedy for erysipelas or toothache.[4] The medical lore of holy men, their special days, the diseases they presided over, the holy wells and other things

---

[1] Arrhenius: Skandin. Arch. f. Physiol., Leipz., 1898, i, 367–416.

[2] W. James: Gifford Lectures, New York, 1902. Cited by Osborn.

[3] See W. A. Jayne: The Healing Gods of Ancient Civilizations, New Haven, 1925.

[4] Black: "Folk-Lore," London, 1883, p. 140.

blessed by them, form a special field in itself. The saints were supposed, as usual, to have the power both of inflicting and healing diseases, most of which were, however, associated with the names of several saints. Thus the names of St. Guy, St. Vitus, and St. With are eponymic for chorea; St. Avertin, St. John, and St. Valentine stood sponsors for epilepsy; St. Hubert of Ardennes, the patron of huntsmen, cared for hydrophobia, while St. Anthony, St. Benedict, St. Martial, and St. Genevieve presided over ergotism. Kerler[1] has compiled a bulky volume made up of these indices of patron saints of medicine alone. Sacred bits of pastry (*Heilbrōte*), deriving, as Höfler shows, from the ancient sacrificial cakes, were dedicated to these saints and eaten to ward off particular diseases.[2]

A remarkable example of belief in the malevolence of personality is the superstition of the Evil Eye, which causes Orientals to wear a crescent of horns over the forehead, as a safeguard, and Levantines to cross their fingers or protrude the thumb between the index and middle finger (*mano fica*).

This belief, as Seligmann has shown, has existed from the earliest times, and is common to all human races. Mentioned in the Assyro-Babylonian incantations, declared a capital crime in the tables of the Roman Decemvirs (450 B. C.), this power of inflicting evil has been ascribed variously to whole races or religious sects, to dogs, wolves, and animals of the cat family, to reptiles and mythical creatures, like the basilisk, to statues and inanimate objects, to gods, demons, spirits and all supernatural beings. In the Purana legend, Siva destroys a whole town with one withering glance, as Wotan destroys Hunding in "Die Walküre." Lord Byron, Napoleon III, Queen Maria Amelia of Portugal, the Popes Pius IX and Leo XIII, and the composer Offenbach were all feared for this hypnotic power. According to the Roman writers, the evil eye was nystagmic, strabismic, dicoric or otherwise abnormal or diseased. Ovid (*Amores*, viii, 15–16) attributes a double pupil to the sorceress Dipea:

"Oculis quoque pupilla duplex
Fulminat, et geminum lumen in orbe manet,"

and says that eyes which gaze upon the diseased will suffer themselves—

"Dum spectant oculi laesos, laeduntur et ipsi."

Persius (ii, 34) attributed evil power to inflamed or reddened eyes (*urentes oculi*).

There is a strong human prejudice against disconcerting, intensive, or forbidding appearances of the eye, as, indeed, for any abnormity, whether it be the *fascinatio* of the ancient Romans, the strabismic *regard louche* of the French writers, the *jettatura* of the Corsican, the *mal-occhio* of the Italian, the filmy glance of some gypsies, the "steady, ambiguous look" which Arthur Symons ascribes to Orientals, or the stony stare of the blue-eyed northern races which a line of Tennyson's likens to the effect of the Gorgon's head. We dislike a stare. The phrase, *Sie fixieren mich, mein Herr!* has caused many a duel in Ger-

---

[1] D. H. Kerler: "Die Patronate der Heiligen," Ulm, 1905. For saints on medals, with their attributes, see A. M. Pachinger: Arch. f. Gesch. d. Med., Leipzig, 1909–10, iii, 227–268, 3 pl.

[2] M. Höfler: Janus, Amst., 1902, vii, 189; 233; 301.

[3] For an exhaustive study of this fascinating subject, see S. Seligmann, Der böse Blick, 2 v., Berlin, 1910.

many. We have a natural aversion for a person having but one eye, because, as Charles Dickens neatly said, "popular prejudice is in favor of two." Particolored eyes or eyes each of a different color are nowise reassuring. The blind are sometimes known to develop dubious tendencies along sexual and other lines. It is easy to see, from facts of this kind, how the notion of the Evil Eye came to be ingrained in the beliefs of the Eastern and Levantine races, the Celts, and the African Negro.

An essential part of the theory of divine or personal influence is the doctrine of amulets and talismans and, of course, the appropriate charms and spells that go with them. The amulet (from the Arabic *hamalet*, a pendant) was an object usually hung or worn about the patient's body as a safeguard against disease or other misfortune. The cult is often followed by those who believe that success or failure, luck or misfortune are personal matters. Amulets include a motley array of strange and incongruous objects, such as the bits of crania excised in prehistoric trephining, objects of nephrite, Egyptian scarabs, the grigris of African savages, the voodoo fetishes of Hayti and Louisiana, teeth from the mouths of corpses, bones and other parts of the lower animals, the

Finger of birth-strangled babe,
Ditch-delivered by a drab

of the Weird Sisters in Macbeth, rings made of coffin-nails, widows' wedding-rings, rings made from pennies collected by beggars at a church porch and changed for a silver coin from the offertory, "sacrament shillings" collected on Easter Sunday, and the ikons and scapularies blessed by the dignitaries of the church. Tylor has shown that the brass objects on harness were originally Roman amulets. In the interesting exhibit of folk-medicine in the National Museum at Washington,[1] a buckeye or horse-chestnut (*Æsculus flavus*), an Irish potato, a rabbit's foot, a leather strap previously worn by a horse, and a carbon from an arc light are shown as sovereign charms against rheumatism. As Dr. Oliver Wendell Holmes used to point out, in his quizzical way, a belief in the efficacy of some of these anti-rheumatics is by no means confined to the European peasant and the negro. Other amulets in the Washington exhibit are the patella of a sheep and a ring made out of a coffin-nail (dug up out of a graveyard) for cramps and epilepsy, a peony root to be carried in the pocket against insanity, and rare and precious stones for all and sundry diseases.

The folk-lore of stones is of great antiquity. The oldest prescription in existence—that discovered in Egypt by W. Max Müller—displayed in the Museum of Natural History in New York, calls for the exhibition of a green stone as a fumigation against hysteria. Robert

---

[1] Visitors in Washington who are interested in folk-medicine and the cultural aspects of medical history will do well to see this unique collection, prepared by the late Rear-Admiral James M. Flint, Surgeon, U. S. N.

Fletcher has shown[1] that "scopelism," the ancient Arabic custom of piling up stones in a field, either to prevent its tillage or as a menace of death to the owner, is to be found everywhere as a symbol of the hatred of Cain for Abel, of the outlaw for the worker, of the barbarian for civilization. The lore relating to mad-stones, snake-stones, eye-stones, and wart-stones is considerable. Bezoars (enteroliths or other concretions from the bodies of animals) were supposed to prevent melancholia and all kinds of poisoning, including snake-bite. In England and Scotland, holed stones (fairy mill-stones, pixy's grindstones) and elf-bolts (flint arrow-heads) were sometimes handsomely mounted and worn about the person for protection. Hildburgh's extensive studies of Spanish amulets reveal a highly developed folk-cult against the evil eye and other malevolent influences. Every horse, mule, or donkey is belled, as also infants' toys and horns; claws, beads, and other objects are usually mounted in silver and help out the quaint Spanish and gypsy scheme of personal ornamentation.[2] Precious stones came to be esteemed, in the first instance, no doubt, for their rarity, but equally for their supposed potency against disease. From the engraved stones in the High-Priest's breast-plate, representing the Twelve Tribes of Israel, to the birth-stones and month-stones of our own day, there is a continuity of belief in the power of these precious objects. Many women dread to wear an opal; there is a supposed fatality about pearls, and the diamond now, as of yore, will "preserve peace" and "prevent storms" in a household. M. Josse, in Molière's *L'Amour Médecin*, archly opines that nothing is so well calculated to restore a drooping young lady to health as "a handsome set of diamonds, rubies, or emeralds."

Talismans (from the Arabic *talasim*) wore amulets or other charms which were carefully guarded but not necessarily worn about the person. It is highly probable that the magical authority attaching to the ownership of these precious objects gave them an enlarged purchasing power, and was thus the origin or (as in the obolus given to Charon), at least a symbol of money and wealth, in the sense of stored up (potential) energy.[3] Talismans were often written charms or "characts," such as the Hebrew phylacteries, or verses from the Bible, Talmud, Koran, or Iliad. If worn about the body, they were called "periapts." When the Indians saw Catlin, the explorer, reading the *New York Commercial Advertiser*, they thought it was "a medicine cloth for sore eyes."[4] In the category of spoken charms must be included all prayers, incantations, conjurations, and exorcisms used to drive away disease, as well as mystic words like ABRACADABRA,[5] SICYCUMA, Erra Pater,

---

[1] R. Fletcher: American Anthropologist, Wash., 1897, x, pp. 201–213.

[2] W. L. Hildburgh: Folk-Lore, Lond., 1906, xvii, 454; 1913, xxiv, 63; 1914, xxv, 206; 1916, xxvi, 404.

[3] M. Mauss: Compt. rend. Inst. franç. d'anthrop., Par., 1914, ii, 14–20. A. Reinach: *Ibid.*, 24–27.

[4] Black: Op. cit., p. 49.   [5] First mentioned by Quintus Serenus Sammonicus.

Hax Pax Max, and the like.[1] Thus Cato the Censor, who hated Greek medicine, endeavored to treat dislocations by repeating the following bit of gibberish: *"Huat hanat ista pista sista domiabo damnaustra et luxato."* Jakob Grimm found a charm of Marcellus Empiricus against dust in the eyes to be an ancient Celtic verse (Neuburger). Charles Singer cites many Greek sentences degraded by syncretism into Byzantine and British charms, notably the passage in the Greek liturgy of St. Chrysostom:

στῶμεν καλῶς. στῶμεν μετὰ φόβου,
Let us stand seemly, let us stand in awe,

which became a charm for intractable hemorrhage (written on the part affected, or worn as a periapt), and is still used by Macedonian peasants.[2] The charms of the Byzantine period imposed a very heavy onus of responsibility upon the several saints.

The magic charm or mystic power which attaches to *names* is strikingly illustrated by the fact that through the whole course of civilization the mere name is commonly mistaken for the thing it represents.

Since consecutive thought itself is a function of language, the savage, whose mental processes remain inchoate and chaotic until he has acquired speech, regards a name not as a mere label, but as the very essence of what it stands for. To learn the name of a person was to acquire power over him. To disclose one's name was always dangerous. Gods and kings acquired sundry names, one of which was never uttered. A fundamental principle of magic was that to disclose a charm or spell destroyed its efficacy. Hence the taboos on "taking in vain" the names of gods, kings, or priest (the "god-box" of the Canton Chinese). About 1642 blasphemies against the Scotch clergy were regarded as an infraction of the Third Commandment. The *nie sollst du mich befragen* in Wagner's Lohengrin has been abundantly ridiculed, but it is one of the fundamental ideas of primitive magic. Tacitus records that only soldiers with lucky names (*fausta nomina*) participated in the dedication of the shrine on the Capitol. American Indians consulted the medicine man before giving a child a name, which the Singhalese determined by astrology. Something of this ritual feeling survives in the Christian ceremonial of baptism. Hindu parents, who have lost an infant, give the next baby an opprobrious name, while the Chinese give the newborn a disgusting name or (if a boy) a female name and primitives in Borneo, Lapland, and modern Greece change a sick child's name[3] to avert the envious malice of evil powers. Diseases were called by flattering names to propitiate the malignant forces behind them. The names of the dead are avoided lest they discover the whereabouts of the living and hunt them down. *De mortuis nil.* And thus it happens that the healing or disease-conveying *mana* attaching to charms, spells, prayers, curses, mantras, talismans, or inscribed amulets are inevitably bound up with superstitions confusing words and names with the actual, imaginary, unknown. or unknowable things they are supposed to represent. Creeds survive, as Clodd observes, until found out and exploded by science, but the rites or ritual feeling attaching to them "survive all dogmas." "Man felt before he reasoned. . . . As a creature of emotion, he has an immeasurable past; as a creature of reason, he is only of yesterday."

In surveying these different superstitions, one point becomes of especial moment. It is highly improbable that any of the remedies mentioned actually cured disease, but there is abundant evidence of the most trustworthy kind that there have been sick people who got well

---

[1] Black: Op. cit., pp. 167, 168.

[2] C. Singer: Early English Magic and Medicine, London, 1920, 31.

[3] E. Clodd: Magic in Names, London, 1920, *passim*.

with the aid of nothing else. How did they get well? Short of accepting the existence of supernatural forces, we can only fall back upon such
vague explanations as "the healing power of nature," the tendency of
nature to throw off the *materies morbi* or to bring unstable chemical
states to equilibrium, the latter being the most plausible. But, in
many neuroses or in neurotic individuals, there is indubitable evidence
of the effect of the mind upon the body, and in such cases it is possible
that a sensory impression may so influence the vasomotor centers or
the internal secretions of the ductless glands as to bring about definite
chemical changes in the blood, glands, or other tissues, which, in some
cases, might constitute a "cure." We know that the reverse is possible, for example, in such occurrences as the whitening of the hair from
intense grief, worry or fear, or the production of convulsions in a suckling infant whose mother has been exposed to anger, fright, or other
violent emotions before nursing it. As Loeb strongly puts it, "Since
Pawlow and his pupils have succeeded in causing the secretion of saliva
in the dog by means of optic and acoustic signals, it no longer seems
strange to us that what the philosopher terms an 'idea' is a process
which can cause chemical changes in the body."[1] Billings compares
the sensation obtained by placing the hand on a cold object in a dark
room with the way in which the blood "runs cold" when one realizes
that this object is a corpse.[2] Crile's important studies of surgical shock
show the strong analogy existing between the phenomena produced
by shock, the extreme passion of fear, and the symptom-complex of
Graves' disease, particularly as to the pouring out of the thyroid secretions and the destruction of the Purkinje cells in the brain. W. B. Cannon shows that in fear, rage, anger, or any emotions which prepare
the animal for fight or flight, the digestive and sexual functions are
immediately inhibited, the adrenal secretion is rapidly poured into the
blood, mobilizing sugar from the hepatic glycogen up to the point of
glycosuria, counteracting the effects of muscular fatigue, and hastening
the coagulation time of the blood, thus giving the organism a heightened
capacity for offence, defence, flight, and repair of injured tissues.[3] A
man in a fighting or frightened mood is a ductless-gland phenomenon.
The pathological effect of ideas upon the sacral autonomic is seen in the
phenomena of sexual perversion. Extreme mental irritation or depression may superinduce dyspepsia, jaundice, chlorosis, or general
decline. Fright has produced cardiac palpitation, and heart-failure may
result from a shock due to a set-back in business. Rage may induce
anything from precordial spasm up to angina pectoris, as in the case
of John Hunter. The outward manifestations of hysteria are innumerable; and it is well known that it is bad for any person to go under
a surgical operation with the idea that he or she will not recover. A

---

[1] J. Loeb: "The Mechanistic Conception of Life," Chicago, 1912, p. 62.

[2] J. S. Billings: Boston Med. and Surg. Jour., 1888, cxviii, p. 59.

[3] W. B. Cannon: Bodily Changes in Pain, Hunger, Fear, and Rage. New
York, 1915.

number of cases are on record of persons mentally depressed but not otherwise unwell, who have realized the imminence of their own death and predicted it with certainty. An impressive instance was given from personal recollection by Billings, in his Lowell Institute lectures on the history of medicine (1887[1]). An officer of unusually strong and active physique, and in the best of health, had sustained a slight flesh wound at the battle of Gettysburg. Becoming depressed in mind at the start he declared he would die, which he did on the fourth day. The postmortem showed that every organ was healthy and normal and the wound itself so trivial as to be a negligible factor. Crile's whole philosophy of "anoci-association" in surgery turns upon these mysterious mental influences, the combating of which constitutes the essence of psychotherapy. People who have become dyspeptic, bilious, or melancholy from worry or hope deferred, green-sick girls and women grown hysteric from disappointment in love, usually brighten up on receipt of good news. Babinski's dismemberment of hysteria identifies its phenomena solely with those capable of being produced in the hypnotic state. In treating the different neuroses, Charcot was guided almost entirely by his favorite maxim (from Coleridge): "The best inspirer of hope is the best physician," an aphorism which contains the germ of the Freudian theory of psychoanalysis—to "minister to the mind diseased" by removing the splinter of worry or misery from the brain, in order to restore the patient to a cheerful state of mental equilibrium. This fact has been utilized by all "nature healers" and faith-curists with varying degrees of success, and it is the secret of all charlatans, from Apollonius of Tyana, Valentine Greatrakes, Cagliostro, "Spot" Ward, Joanna Stevens, Mesmer, James Graham, John St. John Long, and the Zouave Jacob, down to the days of Dowieism and Eddyism. It is also the secret of the influence of religion upon mankind, and here the priest or pastor becomes, in the truest sense, *ein Arzt der Seele*. In practical medicine, the principle now has a definite footing as psychotherapy. Psychotherapy cannot knit a fractured bone, antagonize the action of poisons or heal a specific infection, but in various bodily ills, especially of the nervous system, its use is far more efficient and respectable than that of many a drug which is claimed to be a specific in an unimaginable number of disorders.

In fine, the lesson of the unity of primitive medicine, which is only a corollary to the general proposition of the unity of folk-lore, is that certain beliefs and superstitions have become ingrained in humanity through space and time, and can be eradicated only through the kind of public enlightenment which teaches that prevention is better than cure. The tendency of humanity to seek medical assistance in time of sickness or injury has been likened to the emotional element in religion, both being based upon "a deep-lying instinct in human nature that relief from suffering is an obtainable goal."[2] As the supernatural ele-

---

[1] J. S. Billings: Boston Med. and Surg. Jour., 1888, cxviii, p. 57.

[2] B. M. Randolph: Wash. Med. Ann., 1912, xi, p. 152.

ment in religion appeals to humanity in its moments of dependence and weakness, so for the weary and heavy-laden, the down-trodden of the earth in the past, medical superstitions were simply a phase of what Stevenson calls "ancestral feelings." This explains the ascendency of quackery. In order to deceive their patients, as Morris holds, it was necessary for the elder quacks to deceive themselves, just as no one can perpetrate an effective ghost story who does not apparently believe it. Fool and rogue being, as Carlyle says, only opposite sides of the same medal, the modern charlatan exploits suggestion, sensation, and mystery objectively and with intention, relying upon Rabelais' arch device for effective lying: *Il faut mentir par nombre impair*.

Thus the history of medicine is also the history of human fallibility and error. The history of the advancement of medical science, however, is the history of the discovery of a number of important fundamental principles leading to new views of disease, to the invention of new instruments, procedures, and devices, and to the formulation of public hygienic laws, all converging to the great ideal of preventive or social medicine; and this was accomplished by the arduous labor of a few devoted workers in science. The development of science has never been continuous, nor even progressive, but rather like the tangled, tortuous line which Laurence Sterne drew to represent the course of his whimsical narrative of Tristram Shandy. Ideas of the greatest scientific moment have been throttled at birth or veered into a blind alley through some current theologic prepossessions, or deprived of their chance of fruition through human indifference, narrow-mindedness, or other accidental circumstances. It is no exaggeration to say that science owes most to the shining individualism of a few chosen spirits. Apart from this, "the success of a discovery depends upon the time of its appearance" (Weir Mitchell).

Buckle maintained that ignorance and low-grade minds are the cause of fanaticism and superstition and, since his equation is reversible, we may consider this proposition true if we apply it to certain fanatical leaders of mankind, savage or civilized, who, as "moulders of public opinion," have retarded human progress. Chamfort said that there are centuries in which public opinion is the most imbecile of all opinions, but this reproach cannot be saddled entirely upon "the complaining millions of men." History teaches everywhere that permanent ignorance and superstition are the results of the oppression of mankind by fanatical overmen. In medicine, this is sometimes ludicrously true. "There is nothing men will not do," says Holmes, "there is nothing they have not done to recover their health and save their lives. They have submitted to be half-drowned in water, and half-choked with gases, to be buried up to their chins in earth, to be seared with hot irons like galley-slaves, to be crimped with knives like codfish, to have needles thrust into their flesh, and bonfires kindled on their skin, to swallow all sorts of abominations, and to pay for all this, as if to be singed and scalded were a costly privilege, as if blisters were a blessing and leeches a luxury.　What more can be asked to prove their honesty and sincerity?"[1]　Yet, while lack of public enlightenment in certain periods produces the stationary or discontinuous mind, there are signs that the modern organized advancement of science may bring forth rich fruit for the medicine of the future through the social co-operation of the mass of mankind with the medical profession.　As the ancient Greeks hung upon the teachings of Empedocles and Hippocrates, as modern humanity responded beautifully to the ideas of Jenner, Pasteur, and Lister, so there has been at no time a greater interest in the advancement of medicine and public health, as manifested in periodicals and newspapers, than in our own.　The awakening of the people to looking after their own interests in regard to the organization and administration of public hygiene is, no doubt, the hope of the preventive medicine of the future.　Man's religion is based upon fear of the unknown or unknowable (*Primum in orbe fecit Deos timor*).　He possesses apparently but a limited number of original or worthwhile ideas, which occur and recur, with monotonous regularity, through the ages.　The rest of his thinking is, in reality, subconscious feeling, whence it follows that he is usually timorous and inert as to changing his folk-ways and, in doubt, harks back to them "with the greatest possible resolution."　Man, as Matthew Arnold observed, is prone to lie "in the unclean straw of his intellectual habits."　Even under the best conditions, it is therefore possible and probable that many highly intelligent and highly educated persons will continue to hug their whims and superstitions, consult quacks, and be otherwise amenable to psychotherapy, absent treatment, and "action at a distance."　"To folk-medicine," says Allbutt, "doubt is unknown; it brings the peace of security."

---

[1] O. W. Holmes: "Medical Essays," Boston, 1883, pp. 378, 379.

PREHISTORIC PHASES

WHETHER the human race is descended from several distinct anthropoid species, or from a single ancestor, common to man and the anthropoid apes, is lost in the dark backward and abysm of time. The prehistory of man begins with the origins of anthropoid life in the Oligocene, the transformations of ape-men into men in the Pleiocene, the extinction of the great mammals, and the dawn of the Old Stone Age culture in the Pleistocene. There is no evidence of the existence of man before the Ice Age and whether flint implements were actually chipped in the Eolithic Period is not positively known; but the fact that all subsequent remains are found embedded in successive layers of strata points to a gradual and inevitable cultural development.

In the late Pleiocene or early Pleistocene (first interglacial period) appeared the ape-man (*Pithecanthropus erectus*, 500,000 B. C.), whose remains were excavated by Dubois at Trinil River, Java (1891). In the Middle Pleistocene (second interglacial period) came the Heidelberg man (*Palæoanthropus*, 1907). He was followed in the late Pleistocene (third interglacial period) by Piltdown man (*Eoanthropus Dawsoni*, 1911); a little later (in Africa) by the gorilla-like Rhodesian man (1921); at the close of the glacial period (about 120,000 B. C.) by Neanderthal man (Gibraltar, 1848; Neanderthal, 1856). About 20,000 B. C. came Crô-Magnon man (*Homo sapiens* 1868), and about 20,000 B. C., the subvariety of Crô-Magnon known as Predmost man (1880).

More than 350 skeletal and cranial remains, excavated within the last seventy-five years, have been allocated to these six main groups. As Tilney shows,[1] the bony conformation is of little moment by comparison with the reconstructions of the actual prehistoric brain which have been made from endocranial casts. These reveal a progressive increase in size, particularly of the frontal, parietal and occipital lobes, indicating that Dawn Man (*Pithecanthropus*) even 500,000 years ago, had already deserted his arboreal habitat, had abandoned his all-four status to attain to the erect posture, set free his fingers for manual dexterity and his toes for walking, expanded his visual and auditory perceptions, and even acquired speech and personality by association and competition with his fellows. The great step forward was the setting free of the hand and foot as he abandoned the arboreal status of the smaller monkeys, in consequence of increased height and weight, so that definite centers for biped locomotion, manipulation, increased visual and auditory perception, speech and associative memory were set up in the fore-brain, while the brain-stem, the locus of the animal instincts, began to dwindle by comparison with the extra-growth of the frontal lobes. The marks of the beast, the receding forehead, the ponderous supraorbital ridge, the wide orbits, broad flat nose, heavy simian jaw, fang-like teeth, long arms, and vaulted back, were still there; but, by 25,000 B. C., Crô-Magnon man, the "Paleolithic Greek,"

---

[1] F. Tilney: The Brain from Ape to Man, New York, 1928.

had already acquired a rude nobility of stature and countenance, had learned to make weapons, tools and clothes, to domesticate cattle, to bridle horses, and to cultivate wild wheat. He buried his dead in sepulchres, trephined the skull, used cranial amulets and other personal adornments, knew how to dance and, in the Aurignacian period, was a skilled painter and sculptor. Whether Dawn Man were simian or human, all craniologic evidence seems to prove that he was more closely akin to the higher (anthropoid) apes than they are to the lower, a kinship which is borne out by the medico-legal (precipitin) test of blood-grouping and blood-relationship. At the same time, the gap between Paleolithic and Neolithic man is much greater than that between Later Stone Age man and the peoples of Egypt and Mesopotamia. In the Mousterian (Neanderthal) period,[1] prehistoric man was probably more ape-like then the Australian savage. In the Aurignacian (early Crô-Magnon) period (25,000–20,000 B. C.) he was taller, cleaner limbed, and bigger brained than we are—the mighty, mammoth-hunting "giant" of Genesis (vi, 4), long-headed, broad-faced, with well-hung chin, a dexterous warrior, huntsman, and artist. In the Solutrean period (20,000–15,000 B. C.) there were types like the Bushmen; in the Magdalenian (15,000–10,000 B. C.) there were people who resembled the Mongolians and the Esquimaux. Solutrean and Magdalenian skulls, found in the Grimaldi caves (1871–84), and at Chancelade (1888), are of negroid and mongoloid type respectively. This seems slightly in favor of Virchow's contention that humanity is of diverse origin. Even within the Crô Magnon race, there were fossil men, who, like the three sons of Noah (Genesis, ix, 18–27), corresponded with Linnæus' classification of man as white, yellow, and black. Yet these types were of one species, as being fertile with one another and like one another structurally, yet as different from the higher apes as chimpanzee, gorilla, and orang are alike but different from the lower apes. All anatomical evidence points to the monophyletic origin of man; all polyphyletic arguments are based upon hazy conjectures from the scant and scattered remains of fossil men. What then constitutes difference of race? Huxley said: "Race is pigmentation," in other words, some chemical difference of endocrine assertion (Keith). There is no essential difference in basic structure, skeletal, visceral or organic, only considerable unlikeness in constitutional peculiarities of physical habitus and facies, which are again endocrine. Admitting that Pithecanthropus, and the higher apes stemmed from a common ancestor in the Oligocene, yet had there been no definite parting of the ways some time, somehow, and somewhere, we should be where the higher apes are or they where

---

[1] The terms Acheulean, Mousterian, Solutrean, Magdalenian were introduced by Gabriel de Mortillet to indicate the successive stages in the specialization of flint and other prehistoric implements found at St. Acheul, Le Moustier, Solutré, and La Madeleine, to which have since been added the pre-Chellean (Mesvin), Chellean (Chelles-sur-Marne), Aurignacian (Aurignac), and Azilian (Mas d'Azil). They are now used in a purely arbitrary way to indicate cranial and skeletal remains found in sites corresponding, in order of geologic time, with these localities.

we are. As Dorsey observes, man himself "never was a gorilla, a chimpanzee, an orang, or a gibbon." In a highly ingenious argument, Crookshank[1] allocates the præcox type of Aryan or Semite as a throwback to the chimpanzee, the Mongol and the Mongolian idiot to the orang, the African Negro to the gorilla, but it would probably be more nearly exact to regard each and all as products or victims of endocrine assertion.

What was the relation of prehistoric man to medicine? As far as records go, he began, curiously enough, with human and comparative anatomy, as evidenced by innumerable carvings, statuettes and line engravings of man and animals on stone and bone, as well as polychrome mural paintings, which abound in all caves of the Old Stone Age (Paleolithic Period). The earliest known representation of the human figure, the Venus of Willendorf, found by Szombathy (1908[2]) in the loess of the Middle Aurignacian Period (22,000 B. C.), is a limestone statuette of a Paleolithic woman, $4\frac{1}{2}$ inches high, which conveys all the implications of endocrine obesity, and is thus a definite contribution to constitutional (external) anatomy. This particular type, an index of the sedentary, overfed life of woman in the prehistoric caves, is presented in all Paleolithic sculptures of the female body, through the Neolithic figurines discovered in the Maltese caves (Singer and Zammit), down to occasional bas-relief carvings of Egypt (Queen of Punt), or the processional female figures on Assyro-Babylonian bas-reliefs, or even such a belated estray as the obese girl of Careño de Miranda in the Prado. Figurations of the prehistoric male, on the other hand, have the inevitable straight flanks, narrow hips, and serviceable musculature of the athletic warrior-huntsman (limestone bas-relief at Laussel). Cave representations of animals are often identifiable as to species, and convey a startling semblance of life and motion, such as is ordinarily compassed only by instantaneous photography or the movies.[3] This externalized or constitutional anatomy, at once physiological and pathological, continued to be the most vital and going phase, even through the greater period of Greek sculpture, and down to the time of Leonardo da Vinci and Vesalius. Even in recent times, primitives in Peru have conveyed the external aspects of disease and deformity in sculpture without realizing it.

What were the primary reactions of prehistoric man to agonizing wounds, fatal hemorrhage, terrifying diseases, suffocation, or violent death? From the medical folk-lore of the ancient (primitive) Germans, they have been assimilated by Sudhoff[4] to the panicky reactions of

---

[1] F. G. Crookshank: The Mongol in Our Midst, New York, 1925.

[2] Szombathy: Kor.-Bl. d. deutsch. Gesellsch. f. Anthrop., Braunschweig, 1909, xi, 87.

[3] Herbert Kühn (Ztschr. f. Ethnol., Berlin, 1927, lviii, 349–367) groups Paleolithic art as Franco-Cantabrian, characterized by a triumph of feeling for perspective over flat representation; East-Spanish, notable for realization of movement; and North African, remarkable for a firm grasp of contour.

[4] Sudhoff: Skizzen, Leipzig, 1921, 63–72.

4

animals when frightened or puzzled by things obviously dangerous but beyond their ken; albeit cave-man, annoyed or harassed by a fracture, a dislocation, an ordinary wound or ailment, was doubtless fain, like animals, to crawl to shelter and quietude, as does the Filipino in the *Hinterland*. But Sudhoff's intuitive perception of the graver contretemps is at once profound, penetrating, and true to human nature:

"Whether life came to a close at the end of a mysteriously long-drawn-out illness, or whether the joyous human was annihilated with terrifying suddenness, in either case, there arose, in opposition to the horror, the urgent question: 'What and whence this dreadful thing that assails us.' . . . Ever and anon, the suspicion is awakened in early man that departed souls play their parts in the cohorts of disease entities, souls of our kin and of our enemies. With the Teutons, also, the souls of the departed join the great army of demons. Sometimes the disease demons appear in the actual world under the manifold aspects of the diseases themselves, such as stringy wormy things creeping under the skin or as worms in wounds and in the cavities and secretions of the body. With the Teutons, the incarnation of the wriggling worm as a disease demon is very general. . . . Pathogenic parasites and disease demons are closely related."

Equally impressive are the "helpful healing proverbs," "life-runes of prolonged efficiency," "helpful staves and preventive runes," and "staves of curative power," derived from Odin the Wise as white magic against the demon hosts, such as the wound-spell of Gawain after applying a bandage: *Zer wunden wunden segen* ("Of wounds to wounds a blessing") or *verstand! du bluotrinna* ("stop! thou bleeding!"), or "thy stinging, thy swelling, thy torturing, thy raging, thy stinking, thy festering, thy running shall cease!" Such conjurations, Sudhoff says, were magic practised by the individual against individual demons, but bloody sacrifice by the tribal priest was an apotropaic rite of the whole tribe against the entire horde of disease demons, and there were also general incantations against the sheer possibility of disease, "whatever elf may have been involved." In Assyro-Babylonian magic, these incantations against disease-demons[1] fairly pulsate with the spirit of mental perturbation and protest against undecipherable calamity, in the rhythmus of some heaven-storming crescendo of Beethoven or Tchaikowsky.

Prehistoric trephining was performed, in the way already described, by Neolithic man 10,000 years ago, usually for headache, probably for epilepsy, insanity and, what he most feared, blindness (Sudhoff). The philosophy of cerebral decompression was to release or drive out the demon, as indicated by the innumerable circular, perforated cranial amulets (*rondelles*), fashioned either from fragments of the skull of the trepanned or acquired in surgical practice on dead subjects. Crosswise cauterization of the skull (the sincipital T of Manouvrier) was a common Neolithic practice in Northern France, and has been found in a pre-Columbian skull from Peru. Amputation of the fingers, another superstitious rite, goes back to the late Paleolithic (Aurignacian) Period, perhaps 25,000 years ago. Over 200 silhouettes of this kind have

[1] F. Lenormant: Chaldean Magic, London, 1878, *passim*. A. H. Sayce: Hibbert Lectures, London, 1898, 441–540.

been found on the walls of Paleolithic caverns in Spain and elsewhere. The earliest known diseases to which prehistoric man was exposed were probably those which affected and, perhaps, helped to exterminate, the Mesozoic reptiles and the later fossil mammals, viz., necrosis, exostoses, and other bony lesions, the arthritides, including rheumatoid arthritis and spondylitis deformans, and diseases of the teeth.   The femur of the Javanese Pithecanthropus shows marked exostoses; the skull of Pilt-down man (*Eoanthropus*), signs of acromegaly or of osteitis deformans. The left ulna of the original Neanderthal skeleton is fractured and, in the opinion of Virchow, the left humerous is rhachitic.   The spine of Heidelberg man (7000 B. C.) shows signs of Pott's disease, which is also common in later Egyptian mummies.   Human paleopathology thus goes back to the late Pleiocene (500,000 B. C.), while osteomyelitis in fossil reptiles is already found in the topmost strata of the Paleozoic, which the physician-geologist Murchison called Permian.

Bacteria probably functioned from the earliest times as rock-builders, by de-position of lime extracted from sea-water.   In the Cambrian coal-beds they began to swarm, in the Permian they became pathogenic.   Recent knowledge of diseases of fossil animals is largely the work of Roy L. Moodie (1916–27).[1]   Lesions in fossil bones were first studied by E. J. C. Esper (1774) and P. C. Schmerling (1835), more particularly by the physicians William Cleft (1823), P. F. von Walther (1825), A. F. J. C. Mayer (1854), and Virchow (1870–95), later by J. M. Clarke (1908–21) and R. L. Moodie (1916–27).   Pathogenic parasitism was evolved from easy going commensalism and symbiosis in the Cambrian period.   In course of time, "familiar-ity bred contempt and advantage-taking."   Worms began to bore into crinoids, even as the sponge justifies its name by boring into the oyster.[2]   Osteomyelitis and caries began to attack the reptiles, armored amphibians, and fishes of the Permian.   The oldest known fractures occur in Permian reptiles of Texas.   The earliest known bony tumor (hemangioma) was found in a Mesozoic dinosaur of Wyoming.   A crocodile of the Oxford Jurassic shows necrosis with metastases.   The aquatic mosasaurs and plesiosaurs of the Kansan Cretaceous show osteoperiostitis, osteoma, arthritides, and dental caries; a fracture of the humerus in a horned dinosaur re-sulted in a subperiosteal abscess with several liters of pus.   In this period there is a definite correlation between focal infection (pyorrhea) and arthritis (spondylitis) deformans.   With the rise of the higher mammals in the Eocene, rheumatoid arthritis is a common lesion up to the cave-bears of the Pleistocene.   Actinomycosis is prob-able in the jaw of a three-toed horse of the South Dakotan Miocene and a rhinoceros of the Pleiocene.   Fossil tsetse-flies (*Glossina*) in the Colorado Oligocene suggest the possibility of nagana in early Tertiary ungulates.

In Neolithic man, the cave-gout (*Höhlengicht*) of Virchow (arthritis deformans) is as common in Egyptian mummies as in the skeletons of the primeval Teutonic forests or the cave-bears of the Pleistocene. In consequence of the environmental effects of the damp walls of caves or contact with the damp ground, this disease afflicted early man with appalling frequency, until the lake-dwellings and floored habitations enabled him to rise above his low estate, just as prehistoric disposal of the dead by exposure, burial, incineration, entombment, and floating sepulchres followed upon transition from the nomadic to the pastoral stage, the domestic use of fire, the development of building and of navigation by boat.   In later skeletal remains of subjects of the Incas

---

[1] R. L. Moodie: Palæopathology, Chicago, 1923.
[2] J. H. Bradley: Forum, N. Y., 1927, lxxviii, 551–555.

in the highlands of Peru, arthritis deformans disappears, but reappears among the earlier North American Indians. Osteoporosis and uta (cutaneous Leishmaniasis) in Peruvian remains have been regarded as syphilitic, but neither bony lesions nor the Carabelli tubercle afford convincing evidence of the existence of prehistoric syphilis. Peruvian pottery conveys striking representations of uta, goundou, verruga Peruviana, achondroplasia, and spinal deformities. North American Indian remains of the pre-Columbian period reveal the usual impact of inflammation upon the bones (osteitis) and joints (arthritides), and some of the pottery again depicts Pott's disease and spinal deformities. Of lesions of the soft parts in Neolithic man, the only satisfactory evidence comes from the paleopathology of ancient Egypt.

EGYPTIAN MEDICINE

THE oldest historic phase of medicine known to us is that of ancient Egypt. In the last twenty years, excavations of archeologists, particularly at Badari in the Fayum, afford a fairly complete purview of the culture of the predynastic (prehistoric) period, with its delicately flaked implements of chipped flint, its pottery, glazed beads, and objects of stone and bone, of which a flint knife with carved ivory handle (from Gebel-el-Araq) is perhaps the most striking. Consideration of the finds from the Old Kingdom (3400–2440 B. C.), the Middle Kingdom (2440–1580 B. C.) and the New Empire (1580–1200 B. C.) reveals the continuous development of a highly specialized and eventually sophisticated civilization, with a sensible organization of society into learned, military, and industrial classes.

The whole story of man's rise from the prehistoric status is there, from the rude beginnings of metallurgy, carpentry, masonry, architecture, ship-building, cabinet-making, agriculture, warfare and art, to the wonderful jewelry, the tapestry, furniture, oil-cups, candles, razors, manicure sets, private secretaries, steam-baths, and other creature comforts and luxuries of the tombs of the New Empire. Excavations of the great temples and pyramids reveal arrangements for the collection of rain-water and for the disposal of sewage by a system of copper pipes. The pottery comprises all the graceful shapes that became known to the Greeks. The rugged representations of the human face and form in the earlier sculpture reveal the same keen capacity for observation of surface anatomy which we find in prehistoric remains; the representations of animals are easily identifiable as to species. In the decadent period (New Empire), painting, outline drawing and modelling *en profil* are highly sophisticated. All human figures are represented as gazing directly forward. In such profile pictures as the "Four Races of Man" or the tumbling acrobatic girl, absolute purity and precision of line was attained. Among the 640 cultural objects listed in Sudhoff's Dresden Catalogue (1911[1]) are: a dining table set for the dead (2000 B. C.); a papyric drawing of a woman prinking herself with cosmetics before a mirror; bathing in common (19th dynasty); a queen in labor on an obstetric chair, attended by four midwives (18th dynasty); statues of physicians; apotropaic amulets against vermin and pathogenic worms; interment of a dead child in its bed; complaint of a Greek woman to Ptolemy that she had been parboiled in her bath by a careless attendant (220 B. C.); circumcision (4000 B. C.), and a plaque recording a suit for recovery of costs of clitoridectomy (163 B. C.). Egypt was regarded as the aboriginal home of prostitution. Sudhoff finds even traces of the *Animierkneipe* (a dubious distinction). Toward the Ptolemaic period, Egyptian civilization had acquired the gamy, "sleepy pear" flavor of decadence. Egyptian medicine actually improves in worth as we move backward in time and, as in all ancient cultures, much was Orphic, Delphic, conveyed by indirection (Hans Much).

It is probable that many phases of Egyptian culture were spread, even to the New World, by the mechanical process of convection, as Elliot Smith maintains.

This so-called heliolithic culture included sun-worship and its symbols; the building of megalithic monuments and the rearing of gigantic stone images; the practice of mummification, or embalming the dead, even among the North American

---

[1] Sudhoff: Internationale Hygiene Ausstellung, Dresden, 1911, Histor. Abteil., 34–41.

Indians (H. C. Yarrow), the practices of tattooing (Miss Buckland), piercing the ears (Park Harrison), massage (W. H. R. Rivers), circumcision, etc., may have influenced the early Minoan civilization of Crete after 2800 B. C. After 900 B. C. the Phœnician navigators may have been the middlemen, while the giant craft of Malaysia and Polynesia may have carried it from the mainland of Asia to the Americas.[1]

Our main sources of Egyptian medicine are the medical papyri, but antedating even these are the well-splinted fractures of the 5th dynasty (2750–2625 B. C.) and certain pictures, engraved on the doorposts of a tomb in the burial ground near Memphis and regarded by their discoverer, W. Max Müller, as the earliest known pictures of surgical operations (2500 B. C.[2]). Although we have reasons for believing that the Egyptians never carried surgery to the extent of opening the body, yet here are clear and unmistakable representations of circumcision and possibly of surgery of the extremities and neck, the attitudes and the hieroglyphics indicating that the patients are undergoing great pain. Apart from this, there is no evidence of surgery except in the splints found on the limbs of mummies of all periods. As conveyed in the extant papyri, Egyptian anatomy and physiology were, apparently, of the most rudimentary character.

The medicine chest of an Egyptian queen of the 11th dynasty (2500 B. C.[3]), containing vases, spoons, dried drugs and roots, is an unusually important find. There is also an inscription on a tomb near the pyramids of Sakarah, which localizes it as the grave of a highly esteemed practitioner who served the 5th dynasty of Pharaohs about 2700 B. C. There are many statuettes of the earliest known physician, Im-hotep ("He who cometh in peace"), a medical demigod, the Æsculapius of King Zoser's reign[4] (3d dynasty 2980–2900 B. C.), who was afterward worshiped at Memphis and had a temple erected in his honor upon the island of Philæ. He was the earliest known physician. A papyric fragment of the 2d century A. D., recently published by the Egyptian Exploration Fund, shows that he was worshiped even in the time of Mycerinus.[5] A statue of the physician Iwte of the 19th dynasty (1320–1170 B. C.), is in the Imperial Museum at Leyden.[6]

Besides the hieroglyphics, which were usually engraved or painted on stone, like the picture-writing of American or Australian savages, the Egyptian employed certain cursive script (hieratic and demotic), usually etched upon thin sheets of the papyrus leaf.

---

[1] G. Elliot Smith: The Migrations of Early Culture, Manchester, 1915. For the debt of Minoan Crete to Egypt, see Sir A. Evans: Huxley Memorial Lecture, London, 1925.

[2] W. Max Müller: Egyptological Researches, Washington, Carnegie Institution, 1906. See also J. J. Walsh: Jour. Amer. Med. Assoc., Chicago, 1907, xlix, pp. 1593–1595.

[3] For a picture of the same, see Jour. Amer. Med. Assoc., 1905, xlv, 1932.

[4] Kurt Sethe: Imhotep, der Asklepios der Aegypter. Leipzig, 1902. J. B. Hurry: Imhotep, Oxford, 1926.

[5] Lancet, Lond., 1915, ii, 1204.

[6] A. Fonahn: Arch. f. Gesch. d. Med., Leipz., 1908–9, 375–378, pl. vi.

The principal papyri are the Papyrus Ebers, translated by H. Joachim (1890), the Westcar (Lesser Berlin) Papyrus, translated by Adolf Erman (1890), the Kahun papyri of the Petrie collection, translated by F. L. Griffiths (1893), the Brugsch (Greater Berlin) Papyrus (1300 B. C.) and the badly preserved London Papyrus, both translated by Walter Wreszinski (1909, 1910), and the Hearst (Philadelphia) Papyrus, containing about half the text of the Papyrus Ebers. The Edwin Smith Papyrus (1600 B. C.), translated by J. H. Breasted, is mainly surgical. The Gardiner Papyrus is gynecological. The oldest papyri are the gynecological and veterinary scripts of the Petrie Collection from Kahun (1893), which date back to the Middle Kingdom (2160–1788 B. C.).

The most valuable medical papyrus in respect of actual content is that acquired by Edwin Smith (1822–1906) at Thebes in 1862 and presented by his daughter to the New York Historical Society. As described by Breasted,[1] the Edwin Smith Papyrus (1600 B. C.) is a roll over 15 feet (4.68 meters) long, written on both sides, comprising twenty-two columns or pages (nearly 500 lines) of cursive script. The seventeen columns of the front comprise 48 cases in clinical surgery, covering injuries from the head to the chest and spine, with a logical, methodical arrangement in each case, viz., descriptive title (provisional diagnosis), examination, semeiology, diagnosis, prognosis, treatment, and glosses on archaic terms employed.

The 27 head injuries include cranial fractures, gashes in the skull by sword strokes, fractures, and injuries of the nose, the lower jaw, the temporal bone. The remaining 21 injuries cover the throat, the cervical, and dorsal vertebræ, and the breasts. The sword gashes (the *hedra* of Hippocrates) and the fatal comminuted sword fractures correspond with the actual findings in Nubian mummies by Elliot Smith and Wood Jones. Feeble pulse and fever are noted in hopeless head injuries. The coronoid process and condyle of the ramus (*'am 'et*) of the mandible are likened to the claw of the *'am'e* bird and the frontal sinus is described as "the region between the eyebrows." Deafness in fracture of the temporal bone (*gema*) is noted also fever in a knife wound of the gullet. In dislocation (*wenekk*) of the cervical vertebræ, there is paralysis of the arms, legs, and sphincters, with bad prognosis. In crushing injuries of the neck, the scribe notes deafness, loss of speech, brachial and crural palsies. In subcutaneous cranial fractures, decompression at the seat of contusion is unconditional, but whether the trephine was employed is not known. The glosses are in the language of the Middle Kingdom, thus allocating the text to the Old Kingdom. The five columns on the back are mere incantations against pestilential winds and for rejuvenation of old men, and, like the Brugsch magic papyri, probably belong to the New Kingdom, when Egyptian medicine had reverted to the primitive type. As Breasted observes, the 17 columns on the front are undoubtedly the torso of some great surgical treatise. The resemblances to the Hippocratic surgical treatises suggest, even more than Lüring's findings (Strassburg Diss., 1888), the possibility of a long foreground to Greek medicine.

The next most important of the medical papyri is that obtained by Georg Ebers at Thebes in 1872, which dates back to about 1550 B. C. It consists of 110 pages or columns of hieratic (cursive) script, a total of 2289 lines, the text in black letter, the rubrics in red. Ebers himself supposed it to be one of the lost sacred or Hermetic Books of Thoth (Hermes Trismegistus), the moon god, who, like Apollo in Greece, was the special deity of medicine.[2] This assumption has not stood the test of time,

---

[1] J. H. Breasted: Bull. Soc. Med. Hist., Chicago, 1923, iii, 58–78.

[2] Hermes Trismegistus was first mentioned in a papyrus of the 3d century A. D. from Hermopolis. K. Wessely: Mitt. a. d. Samml. Erzh. Rainer, 1892, v, 133. Cited by Sudhoff.

and the Ebers Papyrus, with its marginal notes and comments, is now regarded as a simple compilation,[1] albeit a veritable *édition de luxe*, as if prepared for some great temple. The fact that it is written in several dialects indicates that it is an encyclopedia, made up of several treatises. It begins with a number of incantations against disease and then proceeds to list a large number of diseases in detail, with some 875 recipes, and 47 diagnosed cases. The most interesting parts are the extensive sections on the eye and ear, including a notation of the Egyptian trachoma observed by Larrey in 1802, and the descriptions of the ĀAĀ disease, the UHA disease and the Uχedu (painful swelling), all three of which have been thought by Joachim to be identical with different stages of the hookworm infection (*Chlorosis Ægyptiaca*[2]). In addition to the hookworm, Filaria, Tænia, Ascaris, and other parasites are mentioned and prescribed for. Arthritis deformans is specified as "hardening in the limbs," with prescriptions "to make the joints limber."[3]   The large number of remedies and prescriptions cited in the Papyrus suggests a highly specialized therapeusis, even in the 16th century B. C., but it cannot be claimed, as many seem to contend, that the 700 odd remedies indicate any special advancement in the art of healing. The prescriptions, the weights and measures, are very modern, but, as in our own period, the swarms of specific remedies suggest decadence. We do not find a few well-selected drugs, as opium, hellebore, hyoscyamus, used, as Hippocrates employed them, with skill and discrimination. In the late period Egyptian therapy must have been, of necessity, haphazard, since, as we shall see, each Egyptian physician was a narrow specialist, confining himself to one disease or to diseases affecting one part of the body only. Many minerals and vegetable simples are mentioned, from the salts of lead and copper to squills, colchicum, gentian, castor oil, and opium and, as in pharmacopeias of the 17th and 18th centuries, these were compounded of such ingredients as the blood, excreta, fats, and visceral parts of birds, mammals, and reptiles. Intelligent use of inunction is claimed for a popular Egyptian pomade for baldness, consisting of equal parts of the fats of the lion, hippopotamus, crocodile, goose, serpent, and ibex. Another consisted simply of equal parts of writing ink and cerebrospinal fluid. An ointment for the eye consisted of a trituration of antimony in

---

[1] The hieratic writing of the Ebers Papyrus had first to be rendered into hieroglyphics, by a method devised at the Orientalists' Congress in 1874. One of the first to attempt to decipher the hieroglyphics on the Rosetta Stone (1799) was the English physician, Thomas Young. The difficult task was finally accomplished by J. F. Champollion (1818–28), and carried further by Richard Lepsius (1810–84), Heinrich Brugsch (1827–94), who published a "Hieratic-Demotic Dictionary" (1867–82), Joseph Chabas (1817–82), Gaston Maspero, and others.

[2] Joachim, Papyros Ebers, Berlin, 1890. Edwin Pfister, however, thinks that the āaā disease of the Ebers and Brugsch papyri was bilharziosis, since its hieroglyph is a phallus. See Sudhoff's Arch., 1912–13, vi, pp. 12–20. Paul Richter (*Ibid.*, 1908–9, ii, 73–83) maintains that to the Egyptians *uhedu* stood for a disease, while to moderns it only signifies a symptom (inflammation).

[3] Joachim: Op. cit., 130–134; 137–151.

goose-fat. Another for conjunctivitis employs a copper salt. A poultice for suppuration consisted of equal parts of a meal of dates and wheat chaff, bicarbonate of soda, and seeds of endives. The cult of amulets attained an unparalleled vogue in Egypt.[1] There is a small pediatric section in the Ebers papyrus, mainly of prognostic and therapeutic import. Egyptian gynecology and obstetrics have been studied in the five principal papyri by Felix Reinhard.[2]

The most interesting part of the Ebers Papyrus is the last section of all, which treats of tumors. Here, as in the description of the $\overline{A}A\overline{A}$ disease, we find some approach to the accurate clinical pictures of Hippocrates. Some ethical precepts of the ancient Egyptian physicians are very much like the Hippocratic Oath in sentiment and expression, and this alone would suggest that pre-Hippocratic medicine in Greece owed much to Egyptian medicine. There is, however, one marked point of divergence, namely, that later Egyptian medicine was entirely in the hands of priests, while Greek medicine, even at the time of the Trojan War, would seem to be entirely independent of priestly domination. Surgery, in particular, was practised by Homer's warrior kings. Homer (Odyssey, IV, 220–223) says of Egyptian medicine: "There the fruitful earth brings forth many drugs, many excellent when mingled, and many fatal. There, every physician is skilled above all other men, for truly they are of the race of Pæon." Our principal authorities for the state of Egyptian medicine during the 5th century B. C. are Herodotus and Diodorus Siculus. From Herodotus we learn of the hygienic customs of the Egyptians, the gods of their worship, their ideas about medicine, and their methods of embalming dead bodies. "The art of medicine," says Herodotus, "is thus divided among them: Each physician applies himself to one disease only, and not more. All places abound in physicians; some physicians are for the eyes, others for the head, others for the teeth, others for the intestines, and others for internal disorders."[3] Medical practice was rigidly prescribed by the Hermetic Books of Thoth. If a patient's death resulted from any deviation from this set line of treatment, it was regarded as a capital crime. Aristotle, writing one century later, says, in his Politics, that physicians were allowed to alter the treatment after the fourth day i: the patient did not improve.[4] The simple dress and frequent baths o: the Egyptians were what is suitable in a subtropical climate, and no: unlike those of the Greeks. "They purge themselves every month three days in succession," says Herodotus, "seeking to preserve healtl by emetics and clysters; for they suppose that all diseases to whicl men are subject proceed from the food they use. And, indeed, in othe: respects, the Egyptians, next to the Libyans, are the most healthy people in the world, as I think, on account of the seasons, because the

---

[1] W. M. Flinders Petrie: Amulets, London, 1914.

[2] F. Reinhard: Arch. f. Gesch. d. Med., Leipzig, 1915–16, ix, 315; 1916–17 x, 124.

[3] Herodotus: ii, 84.   [4] Aristotle: Politics, iii, 15.

are not liable to change."[1] This view of the old historian does not
harmonize with the great frequency of rheumatoid arthritis in the
Egyptian mummies, which was probably due to exposure on damp
ground during the inundations of the Nile. The account of Egyptian
embalming in Herodotus is, in the light of all recent investigations,
authentic and accurate[2] and it shows that the Egyptians already knew
the antiseptic virtues of extreme dryness and of certain chemicals, like
nitre and common salt.

The brain was first drawn out through the nostrils by an iron hook and the
skull cleared of the rest by rinsing with drugs. The abdomen was then incised
with a sharp flint knife, eviscerated, cleansed with wine and aromatics, filled with
myrrh, cassia, and spices and the wound sewed up. The body was then steeped for
seventy days in sodium chloride or bicarbonate (natron), and afterward washed and
enveloped completely in linen bandages smeared together with gum. The relatives
put it in a wooden coffin, shaped like a man, which was deposited in the burial
chamber along with four Canopic jars containing the viscera. As with our North
American Indians, the departed spirit was furnished with food, drink, and other
appointments and conveniences, and there was a special ritual or Book of the Dead,
which every Egyptian learned by heart, as a sort of Baedeker to the other world.[3]
According to Diodorus Siculus, the *paraschistes*, who made the initial incision with
the flint knife, was held in such aversion that he was driven away with curses, pelted
with stones, and otherwise roughly handled if caught. On the other hand, the
taricheutes, who eviscerated the body and prepared it for the tomb, was revered as
belonging to the priestly class. But this was probably only a perfunctory piece
of ritualism. Sudhoff has published interesting plates[4] representing the characteristic stone knives and iron hooks used by the Egyptian embalmers, and Comrie,[5]
describes what are probably the earliest known surgical instruments of the ancient
Egyptians (about 1500 B. C.), consisting of three saber-shaped copper knives with
hooked or incurvated handles, found in a tomb near Thebes. They are characteristic specimens of the Bronze Age. Elliot Smith and Wood Jones have described
the use of splints of palm fiber in mending fractures. The results of healing are
surprisingly good, with little shortening.[6]

The **paleopathology** of Egypt was first investigated by Fouquet in
1889. In 1907, the Egyptian government instituted an archeological
survey of that part of Nubia which would be subsequently flooded by
the raising of the Assuan dam. The anthropological and pathological
phases of the investigation were entrusted to G. Elliot Smith with the
assistance of F. Wood Jones and others.[7]

The bulletins of this inquiry, with fine atlases of plates covering mummies of
all periods, from the pre-Dynastic to the Byzantine, show that syphilis, cancer, and
rickets were unknown, that rheumatoid arthritis, essentially an environmental and
not a racial affection, was "*par excellence* the bone disease of the ancient Egyptian

---

[1] Herodotus: ii, 77.

[2] *Ibid.:* ii, 86.

[3] For a full account of this complex matter, see Sir. E. A. Wallis Budge: The
Mummy, 2d ed., London, 1925.

[4] Sudhoff: Arch. f. Gesch. d. Med., Leipz., 1911, v, pp. 161–171, 2 pl.

[5] Comrie: Arch. f. Gesch. d. Med., Leipz., 1909, iii, pp. 269–272, 1 pl.

[6] Brit. Med. Jour.. Lond., 1908, i, 732–737.

[7] Egypt. *Ministry of Finance. Survey Department.* The Archæological Survey of Nubia. Bulletins, Nos. 1–7, Cairo, 1907–11. Reports for 1907–8, Vol. II,
on the human remains, by G. Elliot Smith and F. Wood Jones, with Atlas, Cairo, 1910.

and Nubian," that the teeth of the pre-Dynastic people were uniformly good, as might be inferred from the coarse, husky food found in the intestines, and that deposits of tartar and caries, as also true gout (yielding uric-acid reactions) became more common in the New Empire, when luxurious habits were formed. There was no caries in the milk dentition of children of the pre-Dynastic period, and when caries did appear, it was followed by abscess formation spreading to the alveoli, showing that the Egyptians had not the slightest rudiments of dentistry. Evidences of mastoid disease, adhesions in appendicitis, pleural adhesions, fusion of the atlas to the occiput from spondylitis deformans, necrosis of bones, cranial ulceration in females from carrying water-jars, and fatal sword-cuts of the skull were found. Of fractures, those in the cranium and forearm (at a uniform site near the wrist) were most common, and probably caused by fending blows aimed at the skull with the *Naboot*. Fractures of the femur were more common than today, but no fractures of the patella were found, and few below the knee-joint, the immunity probably resulting from locomotion with bared feet and the absence of slippery pavements and curbstones. Similarly, the small number of fractures in the hand and wrist suggest freedom from violence by machinery.

Elliot Smith and Sir Marc Armand Ruffer (1859–1917) have described a genuine case of spinal tuberculosis (Pott's disease) with psoas abscess in a mummy of the twenty-first dynasty (*circa* 1000 B. C.[1]). The histological examinations of Sir Marc Armand Ruffer demonstrated spondylitis deformans (2980 B. C.–300 A. D.), dental caries and alveolar abscess (2000–550 B. C.), arteriosclerosis (1580–527 B. C.), calcification of the aorta (1215 B. C.), schistosomiasis (1250–1000 B. C.), Bouchard's nodes (525 B. C.), ague cake, gall-stones and an eruption resembling smallpox in a mummy of the 20th dynasty (1200–1100 B. C.[2]). Infantile paralysis is apparently represented in a stela of the 18th dynasty (1580 B. C.) in the Carlsberg Glyptothek at Copenhagen.[3] Many ancient Egyptian statuettes in bronze or varnished earth, representing the gods Bes and Phtah, are accurate figurations of achondroplasia (Charcot[4]). The Museum at Bulaq contains a bronze statuette of a hump-backed Egyptian boy, suggesting rickets or spondylitis deformans (Meige[5]).

The main interest of Egyptian medicine lies in its proximity and relationship to Greek medicine. The references in Homer to the skill of the Egyptian physicians in compounding drugs bring to mind the fact that the word "chemistry" itself is derived from *chemi* (the "Black Land"), the ancient name of Egypt, whence the science was called the "Black Art." Doubtless the ancient Greeks learned as much of medicine as of chemistry from these wise elders across the sea, who told Solon that his people were "mere children, talkative and vain, knowing nothing of the past"; who were so skilled in metallurgy, dyeing, distillation, preparing leather, making glass, soap, alloys, and amalgams, and who, even in Homer's time, knew more anatomy and therapeutics than the Hellenes. But Egyptian medicine, like Egyptian art, was fated to go backward as the centuries advanced. Long before the Alexandrian period, Egyptian civilization had become absolutely stationary in character and, in the Alexandrian period, Egypt's physicians were going to school to Greece. As the Egyptian gods—the dog- or ibis-headed Thoth (the Egyptian Hermes), the cat-headed Pacht, their

---

[1] G. Elliot Smith & M. A. Ruffer: "Pott'sche Krankheit an einer ägyptischen Mumie," Giessen, 1910.

[2] Ruffer: Studies in the Palæopathology of Egypt, Chicago, 1921, *passim*.

[3] O. Hamburger: Bull. Soc. franç. d'hist. de méd., Par., 1911, xi, 407–412.

[4] Charcot: Les difformes et les malades dans l'art. Paris, 1889, 12–26. F. Ballod: Prolegomena zur Geschichte der zwerghaften Götter in Ægypten. Munich dissertation (Moscow, 1913).

[5] H. Meige: Trav. d. Neurol. Chir. (Chipault), Paris, 1911, ii, 101–105.

deity of parturition, the beak-nosed Horus, the horned Chnum, the veiled Neith at Sais—remained forever the same, while the Greek mythology was a continuous and consistent evolution of deific figures of permanent beauty and human interest, so Greek medicine was destined to go beyond Egyptian or Oriental medicine as surely as Greek poetry, sculpture, and architecture surpassed the efforts of those peoples in the same kind.

SUMERIAN AND ORIENTAL MEDICINE

In the book of Genesis we read that Nimrod was "a mighty hunter before the Lord," and that "the beginning of his kingdom was Babel and Erech, and Accad and Calneh in the land of Shinar." The plain of Shinar (Sumer) was the southern portion of Mesopotamia, the "land between the two rivers." This fertile valley of the Tigris and the Euphrates comprised: At the extreme north, Assyria (Assur); below it, Accad (upper Shinar); further south, Sumer; and at the southernmost part, between the mouths of the rivers, Chaldea. Babylon (Babel) and Nineveh were on the eastern banks of the Euphrates and Tigris respectively, in the fertile alluvial plain called Eden (Babylonia). On the west bank of the Tigris was the Assyrian capital, Assur. When prehistoric man discovered that wild wheat and barley could be cultivated,[1] he gave up his nomadic existence for husbandry. These fertile plains, known to Herodotus (I, 193) for their enormous wheat-yield, became the seat of endless wars. The vast agricultural area was first dominated by the Semitic Accadians; then by the Sumerian monarchs, who styled themselves "Kings of Sumer and Accad"; then the Semites regained their ascendancy under Hamurabi as King of Babylon (1958–1916 B. C.); then Babylon fell successively before the Assyrians, Chaldeans, Persians, and the Greeks under Alexander the Great (331 B. C.). Before the advent of the Semitic Accadians (Babylonians), it is supposed that an original non-Semitic or Sumerian race existed, about 4000–3000 B. C., who laid the foundations of modern civilization by the invention of pictorial writing and the development of astronomy. Others assume that the cursive script of the Sumerians, which, like Hebrew and Arabic, runs from right to left, was in the first instance only a sort of cipher-code used by the dominant Semitic race. In any case Mesopotamia was the starting-point of Oriental civilization, of which the Babylonians were undoubtedly the principal founders. They were skilled in mathematics and astronomy, originated the decimal system of notation, weights and measures, made the divisions of time into twelve months in the year, seven days in the week, sixty minutes and seconds in the hour and minute respectively, and divided the circle, as we do, into 360 degrees. They invented the cuneiform inscriptions, reading from left to right, they knew much about military tactics and the art of war, and were skilled in music, architecture, pottery, glass-blowing, weaving, and carpet-making.

It is said that astronomy is the oldest of the sciences, and in all early civilizations we find it applied to the practical affairs of life as

---

[1] The primitive wild wheat of Egypt and Babylon, figured in a carving on a tomb of Zer, has been identified as Emmer wheat (*Triticum dicoccum*). Our bread wheat (*T. vulgare*) grows only in cool northern climates. The wild barley of prehistoric man was probably *Hordeum spontaneum*.

astrology. This trait, symbolized in the Sumerian boundary stone with its zodiacal signs (1185 B. C.), is the essence of Assyro-Babylonian medicine. Wars, epidemics, famines, successions of monarchs, and other affairs of public or private life, were closely studied in relation to the precession of the equinoxes, eclipses, comets, changes of the moon and stars, and other meteorologic and astronomic events, and from these fatalistic coincidences arose the idea that certain numerals are lucky or unlucky. Thus astrology and the interpretation of omens merged into prognosis and, as with all early civilizations, the first Babylonian physician was a priest or the first priest a physician. Inspection of the viscera, an essential part of augury, led to inspection of the urine and, among the Babylonians, soothsaying was concentrated upon the liver, terra-cotta models of which, about 3000 years old, have been found, divided into squares and studded with prophetic inscriptions. In Ezekiel (xxi, 21) we read: "For the king of Babylon stood at the parting of the ways, at the head of the two ways to use divination: he made his arrows bright, he consulted with images, he looked in the liver." Neuburger points out how the priestly interest in omens might have led to the collection and collocation of clinical observations, such as facial expression, the appearances of the urine, the saliva, the blood drawn in blood-letting, and other signs which were used as indices or tokens of recovery or death; and he goes on to say that the next step in the direction of scientific advancement would be the elimination of the supernatural from the matter.[1] This step, unfortunately, is and has been the hardest one to take in medical reasoning, but, as shown by recent medical texts,[2] the Assyro-Babylonians eventually got beyond it and attained to a vague semeiology, classification, and purposeful therapy of diseases not unlike the data in the Ebers papyrus. For the most part, however, the Babylonian physicians regarded disease as the work of demons, which swarmed in the earth, air and water, and against which long litanies or incantations were recited.

In 1849, Sir Henry Layard, during his excavations of the mound Kouyunjik, opposite Mosul, the site of Nineveh, discovered the great library of some 30,000 clay tablets gathered by King Assurbanipal of Assyria (668–626 B. C.), which is now in the British Museum. From some 800 medical tablets in this archival collection, which probably numbered 100,000, our knowledge of Assyro-Babylonian medicine is mainly derived. In Morris Jastrow's reading[3] of these, shifting the blame for anything to demons (our disease germs) was the Assyrian concept of etiology; diagnosis was probably based upon simple inspection of the patient, helped out by associative memory and terminology; prognosis (iatromancy) was divination or augury from liver inspection (hepatoscopy), birth omens, disease-omens, and astrological signs and portents; therapy was exorcism by a special ritual, of which the exhibition of herbal remedies was a part; incantation was prophylaxis. The physician was more prophet than priest. From hepatoscopy the Babylonians learned the structure of the liver, and their clay models are better specimens of anatomical

---

[1] Neuburger: Geschichte der Medizin, Stuttgart, 1906, i, 31.

[2] E. Ebeling: Arch. f. Gesch. d. Med., Leipz., 1920–21, xiii, 1, 129; 1921–22, xiv, 26; 65. F. Küchler: Beiträge zur Kenntnis der assyrisch-babylonischen Medizin, Leipzig, 1904. Thompson: Assyrian Medical Texts, London, 1926. Assyrian Herbal, London, 1926.

[3] M. Jastrow: Proc. Roy. Soc. Med., Sect. Hist. Med., Lond., 1914, vii, 109–176.

illustration than the five-lobed medieval figurations. Similar models of the liver have been found on ancient Hittite sites in Asia Minor, and Etruscan livers in bronze, dating from the 3d century B. C., have been found near Piacenza. The liver, as the source of blood, was regarded as the seat of the soul and, as the god identified himself with the sacrificial animal, to inspect the liver was to see into the soul of the animal and the mind of the god. The birth-omens, which have been specially studied by Dennefeld and Jastrow,[1] led to the pseudosciences of physiognomy and palmistry and stimulated the study of fetal and adult abnormities. All possible phases of parturition and abnormities of the fœtus (*Monstra*) were regarded as signs and tokens of the individual's future fate, as being the attendant phenomena of a new life issuing from another. An abnormally large organ (*monstrum per excessum*), or an abnormity on the right side, was a token of future power and success, probably from association of the right-sided liver or the right hand with the idea of power. An abnormally small organ (*monstrum per defectum*), or a defect on the left side, pointed to weakness, disease, and failure. The birth-omens indicated whether the individual was to be superman or underling. The rites of exorcism and the litanies to drive away diseases influenced Egyptian, Hindu, and Chinese medicine and these were carried over into late Syrian medicine, and thence to Islam and Medieval Christianity. Over a hundred drugs were known, and two general classes of these, *shammu* and *abnu*, represent, Jastrow believes, organic and inorganic substances respectively. The filthier remedies (*Dreckapotheke*) were probably designed to disgust the demon inside the body. Rumination, acid stomach, rheumatism, neuralgia, and cardiac diseases are described in the clay tablets. Liver diseases and eye diseases form the centric feature of Babylonian as of Arabic pathology, but in the *sualu* or "mucus-series" (Küchler, 1904) we have already some foreshadowing of the humoral pathology (Oefele), while in Thompson's *Assyrian Texts* (1926[2]) we find a clean-cut arrangement of diseases of the head and eyes, as in the Smith and Ebers papyri, with well-defined clinical concepts, such as gonorrhea (*musû*), day and night blindness (*sin-lurmâ*), paralytic stroke (*misittû*) falling sickness (*makatu*), scabies (*ikkitu*), pediculosis (*rišutu*), and the comparison of foamy urine to beer or veast (*suršummu*). Sudhoff[3] interprets the concepts *bennu* and *sibtu* as epilepsy and contagion (seizure by demons). In the Middle Ages, epileptic seizure came to be regarded as a contagion.

The beginnings of the practice of medicine among the **Babylonians** have been described by Herodotus (I, 80) as follows: "They bring out their sick to the market place, for they have no physicians; then those who pass by the sick person confer with him about the disease, to discover whether they have themselves been afflicted with the same disease as the sick person, or have seen others so afflicted; thus the passers-by confer with him, and advise him to have recourse to the same treatment as that by which they escaped a similar disease, or as they have known to cure others. And they are not allowed to pass by a sick person in silence, without inquiring the nature of his distemper." With the Babylonians, as Montaigne quaintly observes, "the whole people was the physician." They eventually reached the stage at which, like the Egyptians, they had a special doctor for every disease. We learn from the Code Hammurabi (2250 B. C.) that the medical profession in Babylon had advanced far enough in public esteem to be rewarded with adequate fees, carefully prescribed and regulated by law. Thus, ten shekels in silver was the statutory fee for treating a wound or

[1] M. Jastrow: Babylonian-Assyrian Birth-Omens, Giessen, 1913. L. Dennefeld: Babylonisch-assyrische Geburts-Omina, Leipzig, 1914. Jastrow: Aspects of Belief and Practice in Babylonia and Assyria, New York, 1911, ch. iii.

[2] R. C. Thompson: Proc. Roy. Soc. Med. (Sect. Hist. Med.), Lond., 1923–4, xvii, 1; 1925–6, xix, 29.

[3] Sudhoff: Arch. f. Gesch. d. Med., Leipz., 1910–11, iv, 353; 1912–13, vi, 454.

opening an abscess of the eye with a bronze lancet, if the patient happened to be a "gentleman"; if he were a poor man or a servant, the fee was five or two shekels, respectively. If the doctor caused the patient to lose his life or his eye, he had his hands cut off in the case of the gentleman, or had to render value for value in the case of a slave. It is clear from all this that Babylonian physicians owned and treated slaves and couched even for cataract. Here as everywhere, it was surgery that made the first step in the right direction. Internal medicine was mainly concerned with endeavoring to cast out the demons of disease. Jastrow cites a number of pediatric epistles, from the physician Arad-Nanâ to the king Assurbanipal (668–626 B. C.), on ailments of his little son, in each of which Nineb, the god of healing, and his consort Gula are invoked. Lists of animals, insects, and plants are found in the cuneiform inscriptions. Different varieties of flies, bugs, and lice were noted. The wide-spread theory that a worm is the cause of toothache was of Babylonian origin. A votive object found at Susa (Persia) bears a conjuration against mosquitos. A cylinder seal in Pierpont Morgan's collection bears the "Fly Symbol" emblematic of Nergal, the Mesopotamian god of disease and death.[1] The Assyro-Babylonians protected themselves from the fierce sunlight with parasols, from insect pests with fly-flaps, wore Semitic plaids wound about the body terrace-wise, went in for boxing and other manly exercises, employed inflated bladders as water wings, knew how to brew beer and to fertilize the date-palm, regulated wet-nursing, buried their dead in slipper-shaped coffins and fan-shaped tombs. They had a highly organized military service with an efficient cavalry arm, often employed, as their imposing bas-reliefs indicate, in the destruction of predatory wild animals. A carved limestone pillar of the Sumerian period (2920 B. C.), known as the Stele of the Vultures, shows policing the battlefield with the aid of vultures, assemblage of the wounded, and burial in huge common trenches.[2] The outstanding achievement of the Assyro-Babylonians in public hygiene was their perception of the *transmissibility of leprosy*, which took the practical line of expulsion of lepers from the community. "Nevermore shall he know the ways of his abiding place" was the formula proclaiming outlawry. "transmitted to us," as Sudhoff says, "upon the stone landmarks of Babylon over 3500 years ago." Excavations of the huge Babylonian drains, of which models were exhibited at the Dresden Exposition (1911) and at the Gesolei at Düsseldorf (1926[3]), show that they understood the proper disposal of sewage. A stone privy in the palace of Sargon at Chorsabad (1300 B. C.) has been excavated.

Persian medicine is, like Indian medicine, a phase or offshoot of

---

[1] J. Offord: Sc. Progress, Lond., 1916, x, 572.

[2] Sudhoff: Dresden Catalogue, 1911, 20–28.

[3] The Gesolei at Düsseldorf exhibited models of water-closets from Babylon, Nineveh, Knossos, Tell-el-Amerna (1400 B. C.), Cairo (640 B. C.), Priene, Pompeii, Puteoli (45 seats), Timgad (28 seats), and Rome.

Aryan tradition, and is part of the cult of Zoroaster (1000 B. C.), as conveyed in the Zendavesta (the Bible of the Parsee) and the Vendidad (Book of the Law). Entering the Iranian plateau, the Persian conquerors did not disturb the Sumerian and Semitic cultures, as shown by the trilingual inscriptions; and ancient Persian medicine, as distinguished from Oriental phases of medicine in Persia, is mainly of interest for its likeness to or influence upon Jewish medicine.

The main features are cult-cleanliness, particularly ritual uncleanness in menstruating women; the idea that contact with a corpse is unclean, which, as Neuburger says, did much to hinder the progress of medicine; disease as possession by the devil (Ahriman); medicine and surgery as deriving from God (Ahrumazda); fire-worship; pollution of streams by bathing, spitting or urination as sacrilege; casting of corpses to the elements on high places (even now a Parsee practice) lest burial pollute the sanctity of earth; incantations against evil demons (*drug*), and the extraordinary meting out of distances in rites of purification, which Sticker has so graphically described. Incest, sexual vice and perversions were punishable offences against religion, as in Leviticus. Magic was white or black, accordingly as a good or bad demon was invoked. According to the Vendidad, the competence of a medical candidate was to be ascertained by practising upon heretics. If all three died, in succession, he was regarded as unfit, and the loss of another patient became premeditated murder. If all three recovered, he was admitted to practice. The same test was applied to surgical skill. As Sticker points out[1] many traits of Avesta medicine, such as the sacredness of domestic animals, the hostility toward strangers (heretics), the barbarous way of disposing of the dead, the ritual meting out of distances, the constant ablutions, signalize it as the medicine of a nomadic people passing into the pastoral stage. The nomadic rites of purification, e. g., sprinkling with cow's urine, were of religious rather than of hygienic significance. As Laufer has shown,[2] many Chinese drugs and plants were of Iranian provenance.

Closely connected with Sumerian-Semitic medicine in point of time is the medicine of the Jewish people, in relation to the Assyrian captivity (722 B. C.) and the Babylonian captivity (604 B. C.). The principal sources of our knowledge of **Jewish medicine** are the Bible and the Talmud, the first throwing only such light upon the subject as we should expect to find in the details of a legendary historic narrative. In the Old Testament, disease is an expression of the wrath of God, to be removed only by moral reform, prayers, and sacrifice; and it is God who confers both health and disease: "I will put none of these diseases upon thee, which I have brought upon the Egyptians: for I am the Lord that healeth thee" (Exodus xv, 26). The priests acted as hygienic police in relation to contagious diseases, but there is not a single reference in the Bible to priests acting as physicians. The latter were a class apart, of whom we read, for example, that Joseph "commanded his servants the physicians to embalm his father" (Gen. L, 2), that King Asa consulted physicians instead of the Lord and "slept with his fathers" for his pains (II Chron. xvi, 12, 13), or that if two men fight and one of them be injured to the extent of having to keep his bed, the other "shall pay for the loss of his time, and shall cause him to be thoroughly healed" (Exodus xxi, 19). The Prophets, on the other hand, frequently performed miracles, as where both Elijah and Elisha

---

[1] G. Sticker: Sudhoff-Festschrift (Essays), Zürich, 1924, 8–23.

[2] B. Laufer: Sino-iranica, Chicago, 1919.

5

raised children from the dead. The "healing" of the waters of Jordan by Elisha (II Kings ii, 22) is a good example of the ancient, primitive concept of "making medicine," as also the references to the use of hyssop as an agent of catharsis, purification, or lustration (Psalms li, 7; Exodus xi, 22; Leviticus xiv, 4–7, 49–52), and the ritual of transferring leprosy to a bird (Leviticus xiv, 1–8). A striking example of the relation between the Divine wrath and the efficacy of prayer is to be found in the case of Hezekiah, who, "sick unto death" and told by the Lord to set his house in order, turned his face to the wall; his prayers were answered by the prophet Isaiah who, at the Divine instance, ordered that a lump of figs be applied to the afflicted part, with the result that Hezekiah recovered (II Kings xx, 1–8). Besides the physicians and the high priests, who acted as public health officers, there were also professional pharmacists (Exodus xxx, 25; Nehemiah iii, 8) and professional midwives, who are mentioned in the cases of Rachel, of Tamar, and particularly in the striking reference to the ancient Oriental usage of the obstetric chair in labor (Exodus i, 16), where Pharaoh commands the midwives to slay all Jewish infants of the male sex, "when ye do the office of a midwife to the Hebrew women, and see them upon the stools." Maternal impressions form the subject of Genesis xxx, 29–43, in which Jacob retaliates upon Laban for the deception which the latter practised upon him about Leah and Rachel, by outwitting him in a method of raising speckled and spotted livestock hardly explicable by Mendel's law. The sign-language of crooks is indicated in Proverbs vi, 13. Dreams are rightly regarded as "visions of the head," that is, emanations of the brain (Daniel iv, 5, 13; vii, 1). The use of the primitive chipped flint in ritual circumcision is referred to in the book of Exodus (iv, 25), where Zipporah, the wife of Moses, "took a sharp stone and cut off the foreskin of her son." In Joshua (v, 2), God commanded Joshua, the successor of Moses, to make sharp knives and circumcise the children of Israel born after the Exodus from Egypt. This is the only surgical procedure mentioned in the Bible, but the use of the roller-bandage in fractures is referred to in Ezekiel (xxx, 22) as follows: "Son of man, I have broken the arm of Pharaoh king of Egypt; and, lo, it shall not be bound up to be healed, to put a roller to bind it, to make it strong to hold the sword." Wounds[1] were dressed, as among all ancient peoples, with oil, wine, and balsams. In Deuteronomy, Moses lays down a careful dietetic regimen (xiv, 3–21) and excellent rules of military hygiene, in relation to the policing of camps (xxiii, 9–14). The census or "numbering of the people" by Moses is described in Numbers i, 1–49; xxvi, 1–65, and by Joab, at the instance of David, in I Chronicles (xxi, 3–7). Among the remarkable notations in the Old Testament are left-handedness (Judges xx, 16); acromegaly, with supernumerary digits, in the case of the son of Goliath (II Samuel xxi, 20; I Chronicles xx, 6); uniovular

---

[1] The preparation of ointments by the apothecary is referred to in Exodus xxx, 25, and their therapeutic indications in Isaiah i, 6.

twins (Gen. xxxviii, 27); cardiac shock in precipitate labor (I Samuel iv, 19); epilepsy (Numbers xxiv, 4); the effects of inebriety (Proverbs xxiii, 20–35); fatal apoplexy from drunkenness (I Samuel xxv, 36), and heatstroke (II Kings iv, 18–20; Judith vii, 2–3). Of the different communicable diseases mentioned in the Bible, the most important are leprosy, the "issue," and the several plagues visited upon Israel, notably the plague of Baal Peor, in which twenty-four thousand perished (Numbers xxv, 9). Yet these diseases are so vaguely outlined that it is impossible to identify them with any latter-day equivalents. Modern dermatologists contend, for instance, that Biblical leprosy (zaraath[1]), of which Naaman was healed by dipping himself "seven times in Jordan," and which was transferred (in the folk-lore sense) to Gehazi, so that "he went out from his presence a leper as white as snow," was, in reality, psoriasis. On the other hand, Iwan Bloch and others maintain that the venereal plagues mentioned in the Bible (Baal-peor and the rest) are not the same as present-day lues or gonorrhea.[2] Plague after quail-eating is mentioned in Numbers (xi, 31–33). Highly significant is the episode of Ahaziah (II Kings i, 2), who, when ill, sent to Beelzebub at Ekron to learn if he might recover, for, according to Josephus, this god is to be equated with the Greek Zeus Apomuios, the "averter of flies." The fiery serpents mentioned in Numbers (xxi, 7) may have been the dracunculus, and Castellani holds that the disease with "emerods" in I Samuel (v, 6; vi, 4–5) was bubonic plague, because the "mice died and marred the land."[3]

The principal interest in these Biblical diseases lies in the remarkable efforts made to prevent them. The ancient Hebrews were, in fact, the founders of prophylaxis, and the high priests were true medical police. They had a definite code of ritual hygiene and cult-cleanliness, gradually enlarged from contact and inter-relation with different civilizations. The book of Leviticus contains the sternest mandates in regard to touching unclean objects, the proper food to be eaten, the purifying of women after childbirth, the hygiene of the menstrual periods, the abomination of sexual perversions, and the prevention of contagious diseases. In the remarkable chapters on the diagnosis and

---

[1] Described in Leviticus xiii, 1–46. For an elaborate exegesis of the Mosaic doctrine of *contagio per contactum*, see G. Sticker: Sudhoff Festschrift, Zürich, 1924, 23–42.

[2] Medical scholars, who speculate about these uncertain details in such dogmatic fashion, fail to consider the point, well known to mathematicians and physicists, that the inherent probability of any occurrence tends the closer to zero the further we get away from it, and that the effect of any event tends to "die out asymptomatically" in indefinite or infinite time. Æsculapius was very much of a reality to Homer, Hippocrates, and Celsus. To us he is well-nigh a myth. Bloch forgets that the logical opposite of the "morbus Americanus" theory of syphilis, which he advances with such fanatical zeal, is just as likely to be true as the theory itself.

[3] The rodents appear in Poussin's painting "The Plague of the Philistines" (Janus, Amst., 1898, iii, 138). It is noticeable that the evidence of the association of mice with the plague is stronger in the Septuagint than in the Vulgate (see L. Aschoff, Janus, Amst., 1900, v, 611–613). In the Revised Version the *nati sunt mures* is absent, but verse 8 of I Samuel v suggests the inguinal bubo of plague.

prevention of leprosy, gonorrhea, and leukorrhea (Leviticus XIII–XV), the most definite common-sense directions are given in regard to segregation, disinfection (even to the point of scraping the walls of the house, or destroying it completely), and the old Mosaic rite of incineration of the patient's garments and other fomites. In the Middle Ages, these precepts from Leviticus, derived, in the first instance, from Assyro-Babylonian practice, were still in force against leprosy, and the principle of isolation of patients and suspects was extended to plague, syphilis, phthisis, scabies, erysipelas, anthrax, trachoma and epilepsy (Sudhoff). Who but does not admire the rigorous Hebrew regulation of sexual hygiene which, however severe, enforced exogamy, put a ban upon perversions, and invested the figure of a good and virtuous woman with that peculiar halo of respect which has been preserved by all highly civilized nations down to the present time?[1] The institution of the Sabbath day gave tired workaday humanity a sort of permanent splint to rest upon.[2] In short, the chief glory of Biblical medicine lies, as Neuburger rightly says, in the institution of social hygiene as a science. How highly the physician was esteemed by the Hebrews of a later time may be gathered from the impressive language of Jesus, son of Sirach (180 B. C.):

1. Honour a physician according to thy need of him with the honours
   due unto him:
   For verily the Lord hath created him.
2. For from the Most High cometh healing:
   And from the King he shall receive a gift.
3. The skill of the physician shall lift up his head:
   And in the sight of great men he shall be admired.

The writings of Flavius Josephus (born 37 A. D.), as investigated by Max Neuburger,[3] differ frequently from the Biblical narrative in medical details. Physicians are more frequently mentioned, and their definite independent status is plain. Visitation of epidemic diseases is more frequent, and the third plague of Egypt is defined as pediculosis, that of Baal Peor as pest, that of the Philistines as dysentery. The precepts of Jewish hygiene, particularly the Mosaic rules for the isolation and purification of lepers, are given with drastic force. Saul's melancholia is defined as demonomania with ecstasy. Apoplexy may be inferred in the cases of Nabal and Alkimos. David is described as feigning insanity before the King of Gath. In the later narratives, psychiatric details are frequently given, particularly in the case of Herod.

In contradistinction to the written Mosaic law in the five books of the Pentateuch (Torah), the Talmud[4] consists of the law as transmitted by verbal tradition (Mishna), with its several interpretations and com-

---

[1] It is worthy of note that the Mosaic mandates against bestiality, sexual inversion, etc., in Exodus (XXI, XXII) and Leviticus (XVIII) are the beginnings of medical jurisprudence.

[2] The number-lore of Babylonian astrologers predicated that seventh days or multiples of seventh days were unlucky (*dies atra*), hence days of suspended business and enforced inactivity. Even if the "rest" accruing from this process was an epiphenomenon, we are none the less grateful for the accidental advantage gained.

[3] M. Neuburger: Die Medizin im Flavius Josephus. Reichenhall, 1920.

[4] From the famous Venice press of Daniel Bomberg, who learned Hebrew from Abraham de Balmes, physician to Cardinal Grimaldi, came the *editio princeps* of the Rabbinic Bible (1516), the Babylonian Talmud (15 vols., 1520–23) and the Palestinian Talmud (1522–3).

mentaries (Gemara). This mass of knowledge began to accumulate after the Babylonian Captivity, about 536 B. C., and is embodied in the Palestinian Talmud (370–390 A. D.) and the Babylonian Talmud (352–427 A. D.), the latter being the ordinary source of reference. The Babylonian Talmud is essentially a law book, dating from the 2d century A. D., and the information about Jewish medicine conveyed in it is, in consequence, of a more definite and detailed character than we should expect to find in the half-legendary narrative of the Bible. Its most interesting feature is the light it throws upon later Jewish anatomy and surgery, and upon the knowledge of postmortem appearances which the Hebrews gained through the inspection of meat for food. Anatomy of any kind before the time of Vesalius was a thing of shreds and patches, and Jewish anatomy was no exception to the rule. Only a very few of the parts of the body are mentioned in the Bible, and these references are as vague and general as those in the Iliad. In the Talmud the number of bones in the skeleton is variously estimated at 248 or 252, and of these, one, the bone Luz, which was supposed to lie somewhere between the base of the skull and the coccyx, was regarded as the indestructible nucleus from which the body is to be raised from the dead at the Resurrection. This myth, which modern rabbinical authority holds to have originated from the ancient Egyptian rite of "burying the spinal column of Osiris," was exploded by Vesalius in a striking passage in the "Fabrica."[1] The Talmud displays considerable knowledge of the esophagus, larynx, trachea, the membranes of the brain, and the generative organs. The pancreas is called the "finger of the liver," and structures like the spleen, kidneys, and spinal cord are frequently mentioned but not described. The blood is held to be the vital principle, identical with the soul, and the heart is essential to life. Respiration is likened to burning. The effect of the saliva upon food and the churning movements of the stomach are noted, and the liver is believed to elaborate the blood. Among the Hebrews, the flesh of diseased or injured animals was always considered unfit for food, and the autopsies, made upon slaughtered animals to determine what was *kosher* and *trepha*, threw a light upon pathologic appearances which the ancient Greeks never gained. Hyperemia, caseous degeneration and tumors of the lungs were noted, as also atrophy and abscess of the kidneys, and cirrhosis and necrosis of the liver. Tropical dysentery, pallid anemia, dropsy, intestinal worms, phthiriasis, and scorbutic stomatitis were described. Jaundice and biliary disorders were commonplaces in Jewish and Mohammedan medicine. Diphtheria, known as *askara* (ἐσχάρα) or *serunke* (σύναγχη, cynanche), was so much feared by the Hebrews that the first case located in a community was immediately heralded by a warning blast of the shofar, although the instrument was ordinarily sounded only after the occurrence of the third case of an infectious disease (Preuss). There are no Hebrew words for

---

[1] See F. H. Garrison: New York Med. Jour., 1911, xcii, 149–151.

"cough" or "phthisis," to which the arid plains of Palestine were of old inimical. Talmudic surgery included the usual "wound-surgery," with treatment by sutures and bandages, applications of wine and oil, and the device of freshening the edges of old wounds to secure more perfect union. Venesection, leeching, and cupping were common and, before attempting the major operations, a sleeping draught (*samme de shinta*) was administered. The earliest known reference to hemophilia is, perhaps, the dispensation in the Babylonian Talmud (Jebamoth, 64b), which interdicts circumcision if fatal in two successive children, as indicating a family of bleeders.[1] Cesarean section, excision of the spleen, amputations, trephining, and the operation for imperforate anus in infants were known, as also the use of the speculum and the uterine sound. Fractures and dislocations were discussed, and crutches, artificial limbs and artificial teeth employed.[2] Careful rules for the hygiene and nutrition of newborn children are given. There is no evidence of specialized medical education among the Jews until the Alexandrian period, and individual Jewish physicians did not attain any particular prominence until the Middle Ages and, more especially, in the modern period.

As the Hebrews attained the highest eminence among Oriental peoples in hygiene, so the **ancient Hindus** excelled all other nations of their time in operative surgery. In the earliest Sanskrit documents, the Rig Veda (1500 B. C.) and the Atharva-Veda,[3] medicine is wholly theurgic, and treatment consists of the usual versified spells and incantations against the demons of disease or their human agents, the witches and wizards. In the Brahminical period (800 B. C.–1000 A. D.), medicine was entirely in the hands of the Brahmin priests and scholars, and the center of medical education was at Benares. In an Indian rock-inscription, king Asoka (*circa* 226 B. C.) records the erection of hospitals by him, and Cingalese records indicate the existence of hospitals in Ceylon in 437 and 137 B. C. Indian and Ceylonese hospitals existed as late as 368 A. D. The three leading texts of Brahminical medicine are the Charaka Samhita, a compendium made by Charaka (2d century A. D.) from an earlier work of Agnivéra, based upon the lectures of his master Atreya (6th century B. C.[4]), the Susruta (5th century A. D.) and the Vagbhata (7th century A. D.). Of these, the most remarkable is Susruta, whose work, bearing the same name, is the great storehouse of Aryan surgery.[5] Indian medicine was particularly weak

---

[1] See Joseph Klapersak: Leipzig diss., 1926, 5–6.

[2] For further information about Biblical and Talmudic medicine, see Julius Preuss, Biblisch-Talmudische Medizin, Berlin, 1911, and the article by Dr. Charles D. Spivak in the Jewish Encyclopedia, N. Y., 1904, viii, pp. 409–414.

[3] Atharva-Veda Samhita: Translated by William D. Whitney. Revised by C. R. Lanman (Harvard Oriental Series, v. 7–8), Cambridge, 1905.

[4] Charaka's text was completed by Dridhabala. See A. F. R. Hoernle: Arch. f. Gesch. d. Med., Leipz., 1907–8, i, 29–40.

[5] Translated into Latin by F. Hessler, 3 vols., Erlangen, 1844. Translated into English by Kaviraj Kunja Lal Bhishagratna, 3 vols., Calcutta, 1907–16.

in its anatomy, which consisted of purely fanciful numerations of un-imaginable parts of the body, *e. g.*, 360 bones, 800 ligaments, 500 muscles, 300 veins, and so on. Hindu physiology presupposes that the vital processes are activated by means of the air (below the navel), the bile (between the navel and the heart) and the phlegm (above the heart), from which are derived the seven proximal principles, chyle, blood, flesh, fat, bone, marrow, and semen. Health consists in a normal quantitative relationship of these primary constituents, disease in a derangement of their proper proportions. Diseases are again minutely subdivided, the Suśruta enumerating as many as 1120, which are classed in two grand divisions (natural and supernatural). Diagnosis was carefully made, and included inspection, palpation, auscultation, and the use of the special senses. Semeiology and prognosis combined acute observation with the usual folk-superstitions. As examples, witness the Suśruta's very recognizable description of malarial fever, which is attributed to mosquitos, or the passage in the Bhâgavata Purana which warns people to desert their houses "when rats fall from the roofs above, jump about and die," presumably from plague. Essential diabetes mellitus was recognized as *Madhumeha* or "honey-urine" (Jolly), and the symptoms of thirst, foul breath, and languor were noted (W. Eb-stein). Evidences of variolation (inoculation against smallpox) have been found in the Sanskrit text *Sacteya*, attributed to Dhanwantari.[1] In therapeutics, a proper diet and regimen were carefully detailed, and baths, enemata, emetics, inhalations, gargles, blood-letting, and urethral and vaginal injections employed. The Hindu system of respiratory gymnastics is highly praised by Hans Much.[2] In Marco Polo's travels there is a description of a kind of mosquito-netting used on the Coro-mandel Coast to keep away flies and vermin.[3] The materia medica of India was particularly rich. Suśruta mentions 760 medicinal plants, of which nard, cinnamon, pepper, cardamom, spices, and sugar were native. Especial attention was paid to aphrodisiacs and poisons, par-ticularly antidotes for the bites of venomous snakes and other animals. Jolly mentions some 13 alcoholic drinks. The soporific effects of hyoscyamus and *Cannabis indica* were known, and their employment in surgical anesthesia was, according to Burton, of great antiquity. The Bower MS., a Sanskrit document on birch-bark, found by a native in the ruins of Mingai (Turkestan), and purchased by Lieutenant Bower in 1890 (edited by Hoernle), contains a remarkable dithyramb in praise of garlic (*Allium sativum*[4]). In the obstetric chapter of the Suśruta, there is an admirable section on infant hygiene and nutrition, unexcelled by anything before the time of Aulus Gellius or Soranus of Ephesus. The purgative effect of honey (sugar diarrhea) in the newborn infant

---

[1] Madras Courier. Jan. 2, 1919. Cited by E. von Schrötter: Ztschr. f. ärztl. Fortbild., Berl., 1919, xvi, 244.

[2] H. Much: Hippocrates der Grosse, Stuttgart, 1927, 41.

[3] H. Schröder: Arch. f. Schiffs- u. Tropen-Hyg., Leipz., 1917, xxi, 350.

[4] L. Aschoff: Janus, Amst., 1900, v, 493–501.

was known. The surgical arm of treatment in India reached, as we have said, the highest point of development attained in antiquity. The Su ruta describes about 121 different surgical instruments, including scalpels, lancets, saws, scissors, needles, hooks, probes, directors, sounds, forceps, trocars, catheters, syringes, bougies, and a rectal speculum.[1] These were properly handled and jointed, the blade instruments sharp enough to cut a hair and kept clean by wrapping in flannel in a box. The Hindus apparently knew every important operative procedure except the use of the ligature. They amputated limbs, checking hemorrhage by cauterization, boiling oil, or pressure. They treated fractures and dislocations by a special splint made of withes of bamboo, which was subsequently adopted in the British Army as the "patent rattan cane splint." They performed lithotomy (without the staff), Cesarean section, excision of tumors, and the removal of omental hernia through the scrotum. Their mode of couching for cataract[2] has survived to the present day, and they were especially strong in skin-grafting and other phases of plastic surgery. The method of rhinoplasty was probably learned from them in the first instance by the itinerant Arabian surgeons, and so transmitted through private families, like the Norsini, from generation to generation even to the time of Tagliacozzi. The Hindus were especially clever in their method of teaching surgery. Realizing the importance of rapid, dexterous incision in operations without anesthesia, they had the student begin by practising upon plants. The hollow stalks of water-lilies or the veins of large leaves were punctured and lanced, as well as the blood-vessels of dead animals. Gourds, cucumbers and other soft fruits, or leather bags filled with water, were tapped or incised in lieu of hydrocele or any other disorder of a hollow cavity. Flexible models were used for bandaging, and amputations and the plastic operations were practised upon dead animals. In so teaching the student to acquire ease and surety in operating by "going through the motions," the Hindus were pioneers of many recent wrinkles on the didactic side of experimental surgery.[3]

The Hindus probably borrowed something from Greek medicine and a few drugs used by Greek physicians were of Indian origin. It is certain that, at the time of Alexander's Indian expedition (327 B. C.), Hindu physicians and surgeons enjoyed a well-deserved reputation for superior knowledge and skill. Some writers even maintain that

---

[1] See Girindranath Mukhopadhyana: The Surgical Instruments of the Hindus, 2 vols., Calcutta, 1914. Also, Sir Bhagvat Sinh Jee: "A Short History of Aryan Medical Science," London, 1896, 176–186, with pictures of surgical instruments and other apparatus, on plates 1–10.

[2] See R. H. Elliott: "The Indian Operation of Couching for Cataract," London, 1917.

[3] Readers of Captain Marryat's novels may recall how the apothecary, Mr. Cophagus, taught venesection to the fatherless Japhet by making him, "in the first instance, puncture very scientifically all the larger veins of a cabbage leaf, until, well satisfied with the delicacy of my hand and the precision of my hand, he wound up his instructions by permitting me to breathe a vein in his own arm." Marryat, Japhet in Search of a Father, ch. iv.

Aristotle, who lived about this time, got some of his ideas from the East.

With the Mohammedan conquest, Indian medicine passed under the sway of the Arabic domination, and its influence declined. But Vedic medicine still flourishes in India, and the proposition has even been made that its schools be endowed by government. It is interesting to note, however, that the three Englishmen who did most to put hypnotism upon a permanent basis in practical therapeutics—Braid, Esdaile, and Elliotson—undoubtedly got their ideas, and some of their experience, from contact with India.

Until recently **Chinese medicine** has been what our own medicine might be had we been guided by medieval ideas down to the present time, that is, absolutely stationary. Its literature consists of a large number of works, few of which are of the slightest scientific importance. They are usually characterized by reverence for authority, petrified formalism, and a pedantic excess of detail.

Ancient Chinese medicine is purely legendary. The emperor Shen Nung (2737 B. C.), the putative father and founder, is said to have originated the Chinese materia medica by experimenting with poisons and classifying medical plants. To him is attributed the *Pentsao* (Great Herbal), and to emperor Huang-ti (2697 B. C.), the *Neiching* (Canon of Medicine). The great literary source of Chinese medicine, however, is perhaps not earlier than the Han dynasty. The making of medicinal decoctions is attributed to I Yin, a famous prime minister of the Shang dynasty (1176–1123 B. C.). The *Pentsao* and *Neiching* were done in lacquer upon strips of bamboo or palm-leaves. The tadpole characters, derived from the ancient device of making knots in strings, were arranged vertically, to accommodate themselves to the narrow bamboo surface. These tadpole ideograms, the analogue of the Egyptian picture-writings, were later modified and done with pen and paper. The ideogram for "physician" (pronounced *i*) contains, like the Egyptian hieroglyph, an arrow or lancet in the upper half and a drug- or bleeding-glass in the lower. The historical period begins in the middle of the Chow dynasty (1123–256 B. C.), the period of Lao-tse, Confucius and Mencius, the principal medical text of which is the *Nan Ching*, a treatise on the arterial and visceral systems, which gives the weights of the different organs. In this period it is said that state medical examinations were introduced, the work of each doctor being appraised at the end of every year and his salary fixed accordingly. In the Chow period lived Pien Ch'iao (6th-5th century B. C.), who originated the Chinese pulse-lore. But it was in the Han dynasty (202 B. C.–263 A. D.) that Chinese medicine began to advance through the work of Tsang Kung (170 B. C.), who was the first to record clinical cases, Chang Chung-Ching (195 A. D.), author of treatises on dietetics and fevers (*Shang-han-lun*), and Hua To, the most famous surgeon of China, who is said to have employed *Cannabis indica* for anesthesia. In 68 A. D., Buddhism was introduced by Ming Ti, and thereafter, in the inevitable conflict between Buddhists and Taoists, both took up medical magic (charms and incantations) as a sop to popular favor. Desire for long life (*shou*) led the Taoists to the search for the Golden Pill (*chin tan*) or *aurum potabile* (elixir of life), whence alchemy became a cult of long duration. The most famous of the alchemists was Keh Hung (281–360 A. D.), who flourished in the Tsin dynasty (263–420) and whose Handbook of Emergencies is said to contain an authentic account of smallpox. In the Tsin period, Huang Fu wrote the classical treatise on acupuncture (*Chia-i-ching*). The Tang dynasty (618–906) is characterized by huge medical encyclopedias in many volumes, the Sung dynasty (906–1280) by paper books and by special monographs on particular diseases, the Yuan dynasty (1280–1367) by controversial writing, the Ming dynasty (1367–1644) by the use of wooden block types and the publication of the great Synopsis of Ancient Herbals (1590) of Li Shi Chen. A remarkable work of the Sung Dynasty is the *Hsi Yüan Lu* (1241–43) or Instructions to Coroners, a compilation giving minute directions for the examination of a corpse before or after burial, the signs of wounds, blows, strangulation, suicide, poisoning, with directions for resuscitation and antidotes for poisons.[1] It was the official text of forensic medicine for hundreds of years. In the Ming dynasty (1368 A. D.), Chang Chi Ping wrote a similar treatise (*Leiching*), and in the Ching dynasty, the Emperor Chien Lung edited an Encyclopedia of Chinese medicine (1644 A. D.), and Sheng Tung wrote a book on osteology. Chinese anatomy is mainly splanchnology, angiology and physical anthropometry. As with all early peoples, there is a strong predilection for number-lore. There are two cosmic principles, the celestial Yan (light, heat, life) and the earthly Yin (darkness, cold, death). Life consists in the interaction of a male and female principle, equilibrium between which constitutes health, and imbalance, disease. These principles are then distributed to the different parts of the body, e. g., the hand receives the great female principle of the lung and the young male principle of the "three burning spaces," i. e., the thorax, abdomen, and pelvis. The principles contain air and blood in varying quantities, e. g., "the great male principle has much blood and little air." The function of organs is to store up, that of viscera to break down and eliminate. In the *Neiching* (*circa* 1000 B. C.) the liver stores the blood, which contains the soul; the heart stores the pulse (spirit); the spleen the nutrition (thought); the lungs, the breath (energy); the kidneys the germ principle (will). These five organs control all parts of the body, e. g., the lungs produce the skin and hair, form the kidneys and control the heart, which produces the blood, forms the spleen, and controls the kidneys. The six viscera (stomach, colon and duodenum, gall-bladder, bladder, and three burning spaces) and the five organs are similarly interrelated in a sort of hierarchical physiology, the heart being king and director, the lungs his executors, the liver his general, the gall-bladder his attorney general, the spleen his granary officer who creates the five tastes, the three burning spaces (filled with fat) the sewage system, draining into the bladder. The *Neiching* gives valuable measurements of the bones and alimentary tract. Physical anthropometry is clearly of Chinese origin. In the Ching period, regional anatomy was much improved by Feng Chiao Chang (1644 A. D.). In the later Ching period (1796–1821), Wang Chin Jen made 24 good pictures of the organs and viscera. Angiology and osteology were cultivated as topographic aids to acupuncture (2697 B. C.), cauterization and osteopathy. Along the 12 pairs of traveling vessels, there are 365 needling or puncture points for the evacuation of the pulse (air); also 365 capillary vessels, 365 muscular junctions, 365 bones, 365 articulations. The cranium in some systems consists of only one bone, in others of 8 in the male sex, 6 in the female; the lung has 8 lobes, the liver 7. There is good evidence that osteology was studied from the skeletons in uncovered graves, and that dissection was performed, usually upon the bodies of executed criminals.[2]

Chinese anatomy and physiology are thus dominated by the *Neiching*, with its strange antinomies of a fantastic number-lore and an exact physical anthropometry, its fabulous hierarchy of feudal and intersocial relations between the organs and viscera. Each organ is related to a color, taste, season, and time of the day, has a parent and friends and enemies. The heart is the son of the liver, the son of the heart is the stomach, its friend the spleen, its enemy the kidney; red is its color, summer its season; it receives at mid-day (Welch). Other things being equal, the fantastic number-lore of Chinese physiology is no more contemptible than the numerical system of Galen, which occupied the attention of European physicians for no less than 1700 years. But with such inadequate knowledge of human structure and function there could be very little surgery, particularly among a people whose religious convictions were against the drawing of blood or the mutilation of the body. Castration is the only operation they perform and,

---

[1] H. A. Giles: Proc. Roy. Soc. Med., Lond., 1923–24, xvii, Sect. Hist. Med., 59–107.

[2] For the above details I am indebted to the clear, terse, and ship-shape presentation of Dr. E. T. Hsieh, in Anat. Rec., Phila., 1920–21, xx, 97–127.

while they use dry cupping and massage, they do not resort to venesection, but substitute the moxa and acupuncture. The moxa, probably introduced into Chinese and European practice from Egypt, consists of little combustible cones which are applied all over the body
and ignited. Acupuncture is the pricking of the body with needles,
coarse or fine, which are sometimes twisted in the stretched skin. Both
procedures are employed for purposes of counterirritation in gouty
and rheumatic disorders. Practice in acupuncture is attained by punc-
turing the strategic holes of election on bronze images over pieces of
paper (Cowdry). The Chinese were wonderfully clever at massage, and
were the first to employ the blind as masseurs. They were early acquainted with identification by finger-prints (dactyloscopy). Chinese
pathology is characterized by an excessive amount of detail; for example, 10,000 varieties of fevers or 14 kinds of dysentery. In diagnosis
they attach great importance to the pulse, the varieties of which are
minutely subdivided and investigated by touching different parts of
the radial artery of either hand with the fingers, after the fashion of
striking the keys of a piano. In this way six sets of pulse-data are
elicited, which are connected with the different organs and their diseases. Michael Boym, a Jesuit missionary in China, first wrote on
Chinese pulse-lore (1666), giving plates representing their peculiar mode
of feeling the pulse. His work was resurrected and published by the
physician-botanist, Andreas Cleyer (1686). In his own compilation
(1682), Cleyer gives wood-cuts illustrating the Chinese doctrine of the
pulse and the semeiology of the tongue, also thirty plates of Chinese
anatomy, and other phases of medical sinology. The Chinese materia
medica is unusually extensive. It includes such well-known drugs as
ginseng, rhubarb, pomegranate root, aconite, opium, arsenic, sulphur,
and mercury (for inunction and fumigation in syphilis), and many disgusting remedies, such as the parts or excreta of animals. Millions of
dollars are spent annually on drugs. At a famous drug-store in Peking,
300 years old, it is said that $1000 worth of native drugs are sold daily
(Cowdry). Syphilis in China is said to go back to the Ming dynasty,
and references to gonorrhea are attributed to Huang-ti.[1] The *Hsi
Yüan Lu* contains many empirical observations on poisons (Wu Lien-
Teh). The ancient Chinese knew of preventive inoculation against
smallpox, which they probably got from India. Annual statistical records of disease were already established in the *Chon Li* (1105 B. C.).
The *I Chin Ching* is a well-known manual of physical culture, with
illustrations. The plan of eating only cooked food, the sensible costume of cotton and silk, the characteristic adaptation of their architecture to climate, all show the good common sense of the Chinese in
personal hygiene. But the persistence of ancestor worship, the demon
theory of disease and similar cults for centuries, in other words, the
tendency to live by memory rather than reason, to hug the past rather

---

[1] See Keizo Dohi: Beiträge zur Geschichte der Syphilis, Tokyo, 1923.

than to face the future, engenders fatalism and inertia, so that China has been described as a "fertile land of poverty." Where there is no organized regulation of food supply, famine, as in Bolshevik Russia, is ever imminent. The three religions of China counsel inaction and meditation, indeed, public opinion in the East is, as Cowdry affirms, a narcotic rather than a stimulant, whence the general indifference to modern science. The infectious diseases are not all of them notifiable, so that scarlatina and smallpox sweep away thousands. During the Manchurian epidemic of plague (1910–11), strategic centers were established along the main railway lines in North China and have availed to keep the disease out in the last five years. This is also true of the systematic rat-proofing of houses in Shanghai.[1]

Following the International Plague Conference at Mukden (1911), the Manchurian Plague Prevention Service was established in 1912. Pneumonic plague appeared in North China in 1918 and, from the million-dollar fund loaned by the group banks, a central Epidemic Bureau was established in The Temple of Heaven (1919). During the epidemic of 1920–21, so efficient was the cordon that only 9000 lives were lost (Wu Lien Teh).

Modern medicine has been developed in China through the hospitals and medical schools established by the foreign missionaries, through similar institutions established by the governments of Great Britain (Hong Kong), Germany (Shanghai, Tsingtau), France (Canton), Japan (Peking, Shanghai, Hangkow, Mukden), by the China Medical Board of the Rockefeller Foundation (Peking), and by the Chinese government. There are now 26 medical schools in China, the best of which are the Peking Union Medical College (Rockefeller Foundation), the Medical Department of the University of Hong Kong, the Japanese Medical School at Mukden and the Army and Navy Medical Schools at Peking and Tientsin respectively.[2]

Vaccination was introduced into Canton by Dr. Pearson, of the East India Company (1806). The originator of medical missions in China was Dr. Peter Parker (1804–88), a Yale graduate, who founded the Ophthalmic Hospital at Canton (1835) and made the unique collection of Chinese surgical paintings now in Yale.[3] Later came the Shantung Road Hospital (Shanghai), founded by Dr. William Lockhart, of London (1846); the Alice Memorial Hospital (Hong Kong), established by Ho-Kai, the first Chinese to study medicine in England; the Chinese Red Cross Hospital (Shanghai), founded by Shen Fun Ho (1901); the Central Hospital (Peking) and North Eastern Hospital at Mukden (1924), both founded and completed by Wu Lien Teh. The Peiyang Medical College (Tientsin) was established by Li Hung Chang. During 1888–98, the Hong Kong College of Medicine was managed by James Cantlie. President Charles W. Eliot, in a tour of China, stated that the most urgent need was medical education. To him was mainly due the foundation of the Harvard Medical School of China, the equipment of which was taken over in 1916 by the Rockefeller Foundation, along with the medical establishment of the University of Nanking. In 1916, the cornerstone of the Hunan-Yale Medical School was laid. The Chinese government has a National Medical College at Peking, the schools of military and naval medicine mentioned, and five provincial schools. The Japanese Medical School at Mukden, while actually owned by the South Manchuria Railway, is under strict governmental control, has a full-time staff, and publishes annual researches. The Rockefeller Foundation has spent seven million dollars on the Peking Union Medical College alone (1920). This establishment, with its splendid buildings, is destined to be the nucleus of advanced medical teaching in China. The deficiencies in Chinese medicine being mainly due to adherence to the stationary and fantastic scheme of Chinese anatomy, the sensible course has been taken of laying a firm foundation for instruction in this basic discipline. Progress is slow, owing to the preponderance of lecture hours in most of the schools, the difficulty in obtaining material for dissection, and the impression which

---

[1] Wu Lien Teh: Nat. Med. Jour., China, Shanghai, 1916, ii, 32–36.

[2] E. V. Cowdry: Anat. Rec., Phila., 1920–21, xx, 97–127.

[3] C. J. Bartlett: Jour. Amer. Med. Assoc., Chicago, 1916, lxvii, 407–411.

seems to prevail in the provincial schools that what is to be taught is practice of medicine and surgery and not the fundamental sciences upon which modern medicine is based. There is, further, the *intransigeance* and distrust of the native population, lack of funds on the part of the government, and a conviction of forty centuries' standing that medicine is a poor, fifth-rate occupation. Student attendance is slender, the matriculating classes at the 26 medical schools not being more than 600 annually for a population of millions. The National Medical Association of China, founded by Wu Lien Teh and others, had its first meetings in Shanghai on February 7–12, 1916 and has as its literary organ the *National Medical Journal of China* (1916). The Anatomical and Anthropological Association of China held its first meeting at Peking on February 26, 1920.[1]

The Japanese are noted for their remarkable power of assimilating the culture of other nations, and, before they came in contact with European civilization, their medicine was simply an extension of Chinese medicine. Up till 96 B. C., **Japanese medicine** was passing through the mythical phases common to all forms of early medicine.[2] Disease was supposed to be caused by divine influence (*Kamino-no-ke*), by devils and evil spirits, or by spirits of the dead. Two deities, with particularly long names, presided over healing, which was further helped out by prayers and incantations, and at a later period, by internal remedies, venesection, and mineral baths. The period 96 B. C.–709 A. D. marks the ascendancy of Chinese medicine, which was introduced by way of Corea. The practitioners and teachers were priests. Pupils were sent to China at government expense. By 702 A. D. there were native medical schools, with seven-year courses in internal medicine and shorter periods for the other branches. The students were made *ishi* (doctors) after passing a final examination in the presence of the Minister, and women were occasionally trained as midwives. During the succeeding periods (710–1333), called the "Nara," "Heian," and so on, after the names of the different capitals of Japan, the influence of the Chinese priest-healers was still dominant, with some advances in surgical procedure, such as suturing intestinal wounds with mulberry fiber, or couching a cataract with needles. In 758, a hospital for the indigent sick was erected by Empress Komyo. The oldest Japanese medical book, the Ishinho, written by Yasuhori Tambu in 982, describes these surgical novelties, and also records the existence of lying-in hospitals and isolation houses for smallpox patients. During the medieval period, personal observations of clinical cases were recorded. The moxa, acupunture, and many of the Chinese herbal or mineral remedies were in vogue, and massage was delegated to the blind as a suitable occupation. A striking phase of the ancient Japanese approach to therapeutics was their use of red hangings in the treatment of smallpox, the remedy afterward employed by John of Gaddesden and Finsen. The first Portuguese ship touched Japan in 1542, and with the arrival of St. Francis Xavier in 1549 begins the rise of European influences. The physicians who came with him and with the later missionaries—

---

[1] Cowdry: *Op. cit.*

[2] Most of these details are taken from Y. Fujikawa's "Geschichte der Medizin in Japan," Tokyo, 1911. See, also, Léon Ardouin's "Aperçu," Paris, 1884.

there was a Catholic church at Kyoto in 1568—treated the sick gratuitously, did surgical work, founded hospitals, and planted botanic
gardens. After the expulsion of the missionaries, two of their Japanese
pupils settled at Sakai and founded a school. The Dutch traders came
in 1597 and their ship's surgeons also exerted some influence. A translation of Ambroïse Paré's works was made in the 17th century, but
the importation of European books was forbidden until the year 1700,
after which time translations of Boerhaave, Van Swieten, Heister, and
other writers began to appear. Dutch influences became paramount
in 1771, when dissection showed the anatomical likeness of Dutch and
Japanese bodies. Vaccination was introduced by Mohnike in 1848.
The medical school founded by the Dutch physicians at Yeddo in 1857
passed into the hands of the government in 1860, and became in time
the present University of Tokyo. The modern or Meiji period of
Japanese medicine begins with the year of revolution, 1868. Its distinctive feature is the rise of Germanic influences. Of 80 scientific
bureaus, 54 were started since 1872, notably the laboratories of
hygiene at Tokyo (1874) and Osaka (1875). The universities and
medical academies, the state examinations, the medical societies and
medical journals, are all copied after German models, and the ablest
Japanese medical men of today—Shiga, Kitasato, Noguchi, Hata—have
received their education and training in Germany. This influence has
persisted, even since the outbreak of the pan-European war. German
is still the language of science in Japan, and religious ceremonies are
still held at the little shinto shrine dedicated to the memory of Koch.

To sum up what is due to Oriental medicine, the Babylonians had
some intuition of the nature and prevention of communicable diseases;
the Jews originated medical jurisprudence and public hygiene, and
ordained a weekly day of rest; the Chinese introduced anthropometry,
finger-prints, massage (osteopathy), acupuncture, the moxa, and many
drugs; and the Hindus demonstrated that skill in operative surgery,
which has been a permanent possession of the Aryan race ever since.

GREEK MEDICINE

I. Before Hippocrates

The Greeks were a *Sammelvolk*, a composite people, and their diverse elements—Ionian, Thessalian, Arcadian, Achaian, Æolian, Dorian—gave them the self-willed independence, the restless individuality of a mountaineer and sea-faring race, traits which were at once the secret of their greatness and their downfall. The physical geography of insular and peninsular Greece, with its deep coastwise indentations and abrupt mountain walls, isolated the whole country and its separate states in a way that made at once for intense local patriotism, and at the same time gave the cultural advantages of abundant maritime intercourse with other nations, while such grandeur in external nature could only inspire the loftiest freedom of mind and spirit. Yet this very freedom of thought prevented Greece from becoming a nation in the end, for her people were too diverse in racial strain, pulled too many different ways, to become permanently united. Greek history is the history of city-states "too wilful to combine."[1]

In the time of Grote, Greek history began with the first Olympiad (776 B. C.). Today, the origins of Greek civilization go back to at least 3400 B. C., and are found outside the Greek peninsula. Schliemann uncovered the plains of Troy in 1870–73, and unveiled the Ægean civilization of Mycenæ and Tiryns (1600–1200 B. C.) in 1876–84. The Minoan civilization of Crete, which goes back to Neolithic man, was revealed in the excavations of Sir Arthur Evans in 1894–1908. These investigations[2] go to show that Crete, "a kind of half-way house between two continents," independently of the Eurasian and Eurafrican cultures, was the starting point of European civilization.

In the early Minoan culture (3400–2000 B. C.), contemporaneous with the early dynasties of Egypt, the excavations lie over Neolithic strata which go back to 9000 B. C. Polished stone axes, finely burnished pottery, steatopygous female figures of clay, with pronounced breasts, like those of Aurignacian woman are among the findings, with perhaps evidences of the worship of the *Magna Mater*, or Great Mother of the Matriarchate, with the divine child-husband. In the Middle Minoan Period (2000–1850 B. C.), corresponding with the twelfth Egyptian dynasty, polychrome decorations, fine faience, and painted sherds abound. Some specimens were found by Flinders Petrie among twelfth dynasty remains at Kahun in the Fayum. The late Minoan Period (1850–1400 B. C.), corresponding with the Hyksos period and the New Empire in Egypt, is best represented by the palaces excavated at Knossos and Hagia Triada. The Knossian palace (the Cretan Labyrinth) is a stately, many-storied structure, with winding corridors and subterranean passages, elaborate domestic arrangements and the best sanitation, including ingenious devices for ventilation, water-ways for drainage, cannon-shaped terra-cotta piping, and latrines

---

[1] Sir T. Clifford Allbutt: "Science and Mediæval Thought," London, 1901, p. 21.

[2] See Sir A. Evans: Reports of Excavations, 1900–1908, in Ann. Brit. School, Athens, 1900–1908, *passim*. Also his "Prehistoric Tombs of Knossos" (1906), and Science, N. Y., 1916, n. s., xliv, 399; 448.

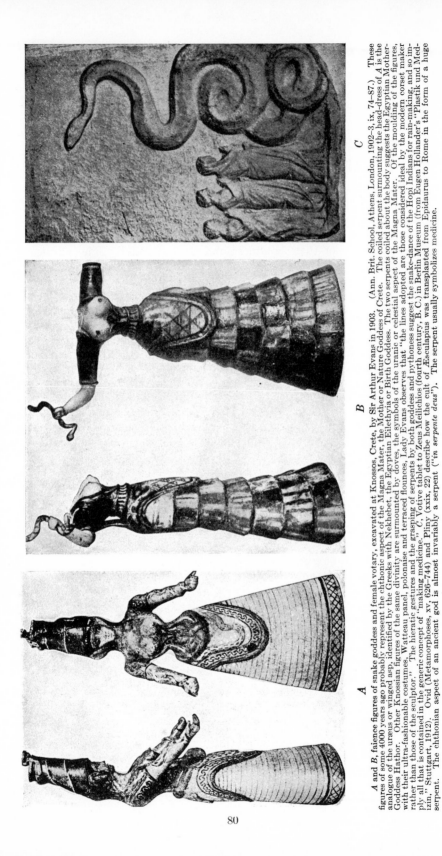

A   *B*   *C*

A and *B*, faience figures of snake goddess and female votary, excavated at Knossos, Crete, by Sir Arthur Evans in 1903. (Ann. Brit. School, Athens, London, 1902–3, ix, 74–87.) These figures of some 4000 years ago probably represent the chthonic aspect of the Magna Mater, the Mother or Nature Goddess of Crete. The coiled serpent surmounting the head-dress of *A* is the analogue of the ureus or winged asp, identified by the Greeks with Nekhebet, the Egyptian Eileithyia or Birth Goddess. The two serpents coiled about the body suggests the Egyptian Mother-Goddess Hathor. Other Knossian figures of the same divinity are surmounted by doves, the symbols of the uranic or celestial aspect of the Magna Mater. Of the moulding of the figures, with their ultra-fashionable costumes, Watteau panel, polonaise and terraced flounces, Lady Evans observes that "the lines adopted are those considered ideal by the modern corset maker rather than those of the sculptor." The hieratic gestures and the grasping of serpents by both goddess and pythoness suggest the snake-dance of the Hopi Indians for rain-making, and so imply all that is contained in the generic concept of "making medicine." *C*, Votive tablet to Zeus Meilichios (fourth century, B.C.) in Berlin Museum (from Eugen Hollander's "Plastik und Medizin," Stuttgart, 1912). Ovid (Metamorphoses, xv, 626–744) and Pliny (xxix, 22) describe how the cult of Æsculapius was transplanted from Epidaurus to Rome in the form of a huge serpent. The chthonian aspect of an ancient god is almost invariably a serpent ("*in serpente deus*"). The serpent usually symbolizes medicine.

which, in construction, excel anything of the kind before the 19th century.[1] The corridors, landings, and porticos are decorated with animated wall-paintings, representing groups of court ladies in curiously modern jackets, fashionable robes, with terraced flounces, and gloves. Naturalistic faience images of the Mother Goddess and her female votaries represent her chthonic (earthly) aspect, with serpents, a tightly-waisted figure, the neolithic bell-shaped gown, of approved modern cut. A late Minoan model of the forearm from Knossos (1500 B. C.) compares favorably, as to muscular contour, with the dissected preparation of the part (Singer).

In the Ægean or Mycenæan culture revealed by Schliemann, there is the same skill in ceramics and sculpture, fresco-painting and ornamentation, the same massive architecture, as in the Lion's Gate at Mycenæ. The aniconic stage of worship of trees and pillars is succeeded by the cult of the Great Mother, with the chthonic snakes or uranic doves. Shaft-burial of the dead, in cysts sunk in rock, was succeeded by beehive tombs. The Mycenæan culture is probably synchronous with the Pelasgian. The post-Mycenæan culture of the Homeric period shows Minoan influences. In place of the round shield and armor of the Homeric Greeks, the Minoan and Mycenæan peoples used shields covering the whole body. Their ornaments are of the Bronze Age. The Homeric Greeks used iron weapons and cremated their dead. Their Olympian Gods are not found in the Minoan and Mycenæan cultures.

Of the early achievements of the historic Greeks, the Hellenes, Thucydides himself says, at the beginning of his history, that "they were no great things." He points out that ancient Hellas had no settled population, wars and factions keeping the people in a state of constant migration, so that "the richest soils were always the most subject to change of masters." Under conditions like these, a restless, athletic, warlike, and sea-faring people was developed, whose chief interests were the active lives they led and the influence exerted upon their affairs by the gods of their worship.

As Walter Pater notes, in his studies of Dionysus and "Hippolytus Veiled," it is a common error to suppose that the ancient Greeks everywhere worshiped the same Pantheon of gods. In point of fact, as being a divided people, the Hellenes of the mountains, the coast, the valleys, farms, and riversides had each a separate religion of their own, the whole forming, of course, an essential polytheism, in that every little clan or village community worshiped its special god, at the same time paying a vague general reverence to the greater gods. Thus, Demeter was the special divinity of those who lived on farms and among cornfields, Dionysus of those who cultivated vineyards, Poseidon of those who dwelt by the sea, Pallas Athene of the Athenians, while the lesser gods had each a particular locality where their worship was a cult. "Like a network over the land of gracious poetic tradition," says Pater, "the local religions had been never wholly superseded by the worship of the great national temples."[2] Thus we find, at the start, that there were many tutelary divinities of medicine among the Greeks, with overlapping or interchangeable functions in different localities. The Greeks, as Pater says, had not a religion, but *religions*, "a theology with no central authority, no link on historic time, liable from the first to an unobserved transformation." Artemis (Diana), Demeter (Ceres),

---

[1] T. H. M. Clarke: Prehistoric Sanitation in Crete, Brit. Med. Jour., Lond., 1903, ii, 597–599.

[2] Pater: "Hippolytus Veiled," in his: Greek Studies, London, 1895, 162.

6

Hermes (Mercury), Hera (Juno), Poseidon (Neptune), Dionysus (Bacchus) were, all of them, patron gods and goddesses of the healing art, and were able, at need, to produce disease themselves. In the Hippocratic treatise "On the Sacred Disease," we read of epileptics that

"if they imitate a goat, or grind their teeth, or if their right side be convulsed, they say that the mother of the gods (Cybele) is the cause. If they speak in a sharper, shriller tone, they liken this state to a horse and say that Poseidon is the cause. . . . But if foam be emitted by the mouth and the patient kick with his feet, Ares (Mars) gets the blame. But terrors which happen during the night, and fevers, and delirium, and jumpings out of bed, and frightful apparitions, and fleeing away— all these they hold to be the plots of Hecate, and the invasions of the Heroes, and use purifications and incantations, and, as appears to me, make the divinity to be most wicked and impious."

Thus, as appears from the deprecating Hippocratic allusion to Hecate, there existed, apart from the cult of the Olympian gods a darker, obscurer cult, namely, the medical magic associated with the ritual of propitiating the so-called chthonian deities of the earth and the underworld. This was again not a general belief, but confined to distinct localities, vaguely including the cults of the celestial gods in their ancient chthonic aspect, the cave gods, deified heroes, heroized physicians (*Heroi Iatroi*), and the perturbed spirits of the dead. The sacrificial rites were conducted in the witching hours before dawn and the deities invoked were never addressed directly by name, but *pleno titulo*, with flattering appellations. The references to chthonic deities in the Greek authors are therefore obscure. In the Greek Pantheon, the greater χθόνιοι are identical with Frazer's "Spirits of the Corn and the Wild." Hades (Aidoneus, Pluto), also styled Zeus Katachthonius, Demeter chthonia (the Corn Mother) and Persephone (Kore), goddess of death and the "poppied sleep" Hermes Psychopompos of the golden wand and sandals, the conductor of souls to Hades (Odyssey XXIV, 1), Cerberus, Hecate, the Erinnyes and all other malevolent spirits, were associated with this cult, and coördinate with it was the ritual of propitiating or invoking the departed spirits of the dead.[1] Apart from the purely religious ritual of the χθόνιοι and the cult of the dead, there arose an esoteric ritual therapy, derived from the circumstance that these dark powers controlled not only fruitfulness of the earth and in man, but could inflict or avert disease, insanity, or death. Infernal deities, thirsting for the blood of human sacrifice, they were feared for their power of wreaking evil in the shape of insanity, epilepsy, hysteria, and other major neuroses. This archaic neurology is implicit in all the Greek poets, dramatists, and philosophers. Thus Plato (Phædrus, 244) speaks of insanity as due to "ancient wrath," which Rohde interprets as the anger of the unburied dead. Pre-Hippocratic medicine was entirely prognostic and prophylactic. Prophylactic medicine was threefold: (1) Apotropaic, designed to *avert* disease by ritual sacrifice; (2) Hilastic, designed to *abort* disease by rites of propitiation or atonement; (3) Cathartic, designed to *expel* disease from the body by rites of lustration (purification). Disease, once in the body, was regarded as a miasm, contamination or taboo, cast upon the soul by angered infernal gods and spirits. The chthonian animals and plants, sacred to these deities, and employed in lieu of human sacrifice to propitiate them, came to have associative remedial functions, whether for purification from the stigma or as connected with the rite of communion or "eating the god," in the form of the parts of animals,[2] sacrificial cakes or incense plants dedicated to their worship. The ashes and rejects of sacrifice (*katharmata*) formed a kind of sacred pharmacopœia, sometimes distributed among the worshipers and eaten by them, as in the Ascle ieia. Of the innumerable medicinal simples and animal remedies recommended by Galen, Dioscorides, and Pliny, it is obvious that but few have any pharmacologic rationale in the laboratory sense. Nearly all have mythologic (*chthonian*) associations. Some simples are even described by Dioscorides and Pliny as the "blood" of different gods and chthonian animals. But even as the drug (φάρμακον) was sacred in a good and a bad sense, through its relation to the chthonian idea of atonement or catharsis by means of a sacrificial scapegoat (φαρμακός), so this empirical therapy became detached from

---

[1] Rohde: Psyche, 3. Aufl., Tübingen & Leipzig, 1903, i, 204–278, *passim*.

[2] Frazer: "The homeopathic magic of a flesh diet," Spirits of the Corn and the Wild, 1912, ii, 138–168.

the priestly therapy of the temples, and its secret practitioners came to be regarded as magicians. The careful study of Max Höfler shows that the modern theory of animal remedies did not originate with the Greeks, but with the doctrine of signatures (*Similia similibus*). From an analysis and tabulation of 1254 ancient organotherapeutic prescriptions, Höfler finds that, except in the case of the liver, spleen, and heart (all worthless), parts of the animal body were never employed exclusively to heal diseases of the same parts, but in the most varied and capricious way, depending upon the tenets of the chthonian cult.[1] Ancient Greek organotherapy was "homeopathic magic" in the folkloristic sense, but by no means isotherapy in the sense of "like cures like."

The chief god of healing in the Greek Pantheon was Apollo, commonly called Alexikakos (the averter of ills), whose far-darting arrows visited plagues and epidemics upon mankind and who could, at need, avert them. He was also the god of purity and well-being in youth and, as Homer relates, the physician to the Olympian gods, whose wounds or diseases he cured by means of the root of the peony. Hence his name "Pæan," and the epithet "sons of Pæan," as applied to physicians. Legend relates that a knowledge of medicine was communicated by Apollo and his sister Artemis to the Centaur Chiron, the son of Saturn. As one skilled in music and surgery and especially versed in ancient lore, Chiron was entrusted with the rearing and education of the heroes Jason, Hercules, Achilles and, in particular, Æsculapius, the son of Apollo by the nymph Coronis. As Pindar sings, in his third Pythian ode, Æsculapius became so proficient in the healing art that Pluto accused him of diminishing the number of shades in Hades. He was then destroyed by a thunderbolt of Zeus, and so became an ob-

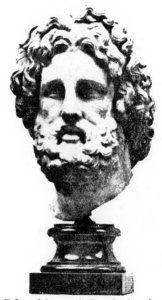

Colossal bust of Æsculapius in the British Museum.

ject of worship. His followers made up an organized guild of physicians, the Asclepiads. The temples of his cult were the famous Asclepieia, of which the most celebrated were those at Cos, Epidaurus, Cnidus, and Pergamus. These temples, commonly situated on wooded hills or mountain sides, near mineral springs, became popular sanitaria, managed by trained priests and, in intention, not unlike the health-resorts of modern times. The patients were received by the physician-priests, who stirred their imaginations by recounting the deeds of Æsculapius, the success of the temple treatment and the remedies employed. After appropriate prayers and sacrifice, the patient was further purified by a bath from the mineral spring, with massage, inunction, and the like.

---

[1] M. Höfler: Die volksmedizinische Organotherapie, Stuttgart, 1908.

After the sacrifice of a cock or a ram before the image of the god, he was inducted into the special rite of "incubation" or temple-sleep. This consisted in lying down to sleep in the sanctuary where, during the night, the priest, in the guise of the god, presented himself before the patient to administer medical advice, if he happened to be awake. If he slept, as was usually the case, the advice came in a dream, which was interpreted afterward by the priests, who then prescribed catharsis, emesis, blood-letting or whatever remedies seemed appropriate. If the treatment was successful and the patient cured, he then presented a thank-offering to the god, usually a model of the diseased part in wax, silver, or gold, while a votive tablet giving the history of his case and its treatment was suspended in the temple.

The whole rite of incubation has been facetiously described in the "Plutus" of Aristophanes, and in more elevated and dignified style in the third chapter of Walter Pater's "Marius the Epicurean." The votive tablets in the Asclepieia at Cos and Cnidus became the permanent clinical records of the Coan and Cnidian Schools of Medicine, of the first of which Hippocrates himself was perhaps a pupil. The Greek traveler Pausanias noticed six of these votive columns when he visited the temple at Epidaurus about 150 A. D. Two of them were excavated in recent times by Cavvadias. Engraved upon these last are about thirty clinical cases, giving the names of the patients, their bodily ills, and what was done for them. The details of symptoms and treatment are very meager. In most cases it sufficed if the god anointed the patient in his sleep, or if one of the sacred dogs or snakes in the temple licked the diseased part. One patient came with four fingers of his hand paralyzed, another was blind on one eye, another had carried a spear-point in his jaw for six years, another had an ulcer of the stomach, another empyema, another was infested with vermin. All were reported as cured.[1] These fragmentary case-histories, none of them conveying any medical information of positive value, are sometimes supposed, on very slender evidence, to have been the starting-point of early Grecian descriptions of disease.

Many antique images in marble or terra cotta exist, representing different parts of the body. These may be ex voto objects, for suspension in the temples, or simple plastic figurations of normal anatomy. Those representing coils of intestines (in the Schliemann collection, Athens; or the Museo dei Termi, Rome), the chest, with ribs (Vatican), or the *situs viscerum* (Vatican), are life-like enough to be simple examples of anatomic illustration in three dimensions, with or without didactic intention.[2] The votive objects in the temples were merely indices of the parts of the body affected, and seldom, if ever, represented the actual disease or deformity (Sudhoff).

Among the legendary children of Æsculapius, by his wife, Epione, were his daughters Hygieia and Panacea, who assisted in the temple rites and fed the sacred snakes. With the ancient Greeks, as with the Egyptians, Cretans, and Hindus, the serpent was venerated as the companion of many gods or the favorite chthonian shape in which they sometimes appeared, e. g., Zeus Meilichios. In his uranic aspect,

---

[1] For further details, see E. T. Withington, "Medical History," London, 1894, Appendix ii, 370–397.

[2] See E. Holländer: Plastik und Medizin, Stuttgart, 1912.

Æsculapius is commonly represented as a handsome Jove-like figure, the accessories being the sacred snake entwined around a rod, a miniature Omphalos, like that of the temple of Apollo at Delphi (a plastic expression of his iatromantic gift), and a grotesque, childish figure (like a tinyhooded monk or *Münchener Kindl*) called Telesphorus, the god of convalescence.[1] Of the sons of Æsculapius, two, Machaon and Podalirius, are mentioned in Homer's Catalogue of the Ships as leaders, commanding thirty vessels, and "good physicians both." In a manner, they were the first military and naval surgeons. Æsculapius is himself referred to in the Iliad as a real chieftain of Thessaly who learned medicine from the centaur Chiron, from whose teaching, again, Achilles was able to impart his knowledge of the healing art to his friend Patroclus. Machaon and Podalirius are often referred to in Homer's narrative as men skilled in extracting weapons, binding up wounds, and applying soothing drugs. In the fourth Iliad, Machaon is summoned to remove an arrow which was driven through the belt of Menelaus, King of Sparta. He arrives to find a circle of warriors gathered about the hero.

"Instantly thereupon he extracted the arrow from the well-fitted belt. But while it was being extracted the sharp barbs were broken. Then he loosed the variegated belt and the girdle beneath, and the plated belt which brass-workers had forged. But when he perceived the wound, where the bitter shaft had fallen, having sucked out the blood, he skilfully sprinkled on it soothing remedies, which benevolent Chiron had formerly given to his father."

In the eleventh Iliad, Idomeneus refers to Machaon as follows: "O Neleian Nestor, great glory of the Greeks, come, ascend thy chariot and let Machaon mount beside thee; and direct thy solid-hoofed horses with all speed towards the ships, for a medical man is the equal of many others, both to cut out arrows, and to apply mild remedies." At the end of the same book, Eurypylus, wounded by an arrow in the thigh, calls upon Patroclus to remove it. He is borne to a tent, and there, Patroclus, "laying him at length, cut out with a knife the bitter, sharp arrow from his thigh, and washed the black blood from it with warm water. Then he applied a bitter, pain-assuaging root, rubbing it between his hands, which checked all his pains; the wound indeed dried up, and the bleeding ceased." In the thirteenth Iliad, Helenus, son of Priam, is smitten through the hand by the brass spear of Menelaus, and we have a glimpse of the "great-hearted Agenor" extracting it and binding the wounded hand, "sling-wise in well-twisted sheep's wool, which his attendant carried for the shepherd of the people."

---

[1] Telesphorus appears in the statues of Æsculapius in the Villa Borghese and Palazzo Massimo (Rome), in the ivory placque in the Liverpool Museum, and in coins of Apamea and Nicæa. Images have even been found in England. In certain Eastern coins he is transformed into a cupping glass of mushroom shape. See L. Schenk: De Telesphoro deo (Göttingen dissertation, 1888). E. Holländer: Plastik und Medizin, Stuttgart, 1912, 125–140. H. Barnes: Proc. Roy. Soc. Med., Lond., vii, Sect. Hist. Med., 71.

Homeric scenes of this kind are frequently depicted on antique vases (Daremberg) particularly on the "bowl of Sosias" (500 B. C.), a specimen of Greek ceramics in the Antiquarium of the Berlin Museum, representing Achilles in the act of applying a two-roller bandage (somewhat faultily) to the wounded arm of Patroclus. In the eighth Iliad (lines 81–86) there is a striking picture of the rotatory movements made by a horse which had been wounded in the cerebellum by an arrow. In such details as the transfixion of the bladder by a spear driven through the buttocks and emerging at the symphysis pubis (V, 65), exposure of the pericardium in an epigastric wound (XVI, 481) preservation of speech in a neck wound missing the trachea (XXII, 328), and instant death from a wound at the junction of the skull and the spine (XX, 481–485). Homer, as Allbutt says, "records each stab with anatomical precision." The effect of Leonardo's experiment of needling the heart is indicated as follows: "And the spear was fixed in his heart, which, palpitating, shook even the extremity of the weapon" (XIII, 430–444). The tenth Iliad (lines 25–31) contains, Cardamatis thinks, a reference to autumnal malarial fevers (the *epiala* of Theognis), which he attributes to the stagnant marshes and the destruction of forests in the Bronze Age.[1] As indicated by the epidemic attacking "mules, swift dogs, and men,"[2] and attributed to the arrows of Apollo (Iliad I, 43), the Greeks were really "blind to the fact of contagion" (Sudhoff). That women sometimes rendered medical aid we gather from the references in the Iliad to "yellow-haired Agamede, who well understood as many drugs as the wide earth nourishes," or, in the Odyssey (IV, 221), to the soporific which Helen casts into the wine, a drug "which Polydamna, the wife of Thon, had given her, a woman of Egypt." In the Odyssey, a healer of diseases is said to be as welcome at a feast as a prophet, a builder of ships, or even a godlike minstrel. From these specimens of the war-surgery of the Iliad it is plain that the surgeon's art was held in high esteem by the ancient Greeks, and that chieftains of high rank did not disdain to follow it.

Frölich counted 147 records of war wounds in the Iliad, of which 106 were spear wounds with 80 per cent. mortality, 17 sword thrusts with total mortality, 12 arrow wounds with 42 per cent. mortality, 12 wounds from slings with 66⅔ per cent. mortality. The total mortality was 114 or 77.6 per cent. and of these fatal cases, 31 were head wounds, 13 in the neck, 67 in the chest, 10 and 11 in the upper and lower extremities respectively. This is what might be expected in wounds from *armes blanches*, with no aseptic treatment or operative intervention.[3]

The anatomic terms used by Homer are, according to Malgaigne and Daremberg, more or less identical with those employed by Hippocrates. There is no observation of disease, but Delpech thought the description of Thersites (second Iliad) a typical picture of rickets. The

[1] J. P. Cardamatis: Arch. f. Schiffs- u. Tropen-Hyg., Leipz., 1915, xix, 305 *et seq.*

[2] Identified with the dysentery of Gallipoli (1915) by F. H. Edgeworth: Bristol Med.-Chir. Jour., 1916, xxxiv, 115.

[3] H. Frölich: Die Militärmedicin Homers, Stuttgart, 1879, 58–60.

scientific disposal of the dead by cremation was a common practice of the Homeric Greeks.[1]

There is no mention of the Asclepieia in the Homeric poems, which date back to at least 1000 B. C., but we may assume that, even then, laic physicians and surgeons were independent of priests, although perhaps associated with the latter in time of peace. Apart from such "priests" and the medical men proper, the healing art was studied by the philosophers, and practised in some details by the "gymnasts," who bathed and anointed the body and tried to treat wounds and injuries, and even internal diseases. Greek medicine, as Osler has said, "had a triple relationship with science, with gymnastics, and with theology," and before the time of Hippocrates it was regarded simply as a branch of philosophy.

Greek philosophy before the age of Pericles was of Ionian origin, and was derived from Egypt and the East. Huxley regarded the growth of the Ionian philosophy in the 8th to 6th centuries B. C. as "only one of the several sporadic indications of some powerful mental ferment over the whole of the area comprised between the Ægean and Northern Hindustan." This ferment, in the view of Zelia Nuttall and Elliot Smith,[2] was the spread of a complex Eurasian and Eurafrican culture by the Phœnician navigators. It is significant that along the 35th parallel of North latitude we find, almost simultaneously in point of time, Zoroaster, Confucius, Buddha, Thales, and Pythagoras (Wright[3]). The earliest of the Ionian philosophers was Thales of Miletus (639–544 B. C.), who had studied under the Egyptian priests, made a successful prediction of an eclipse (583 B. C.), and taught that water is the primary element from which all else is derived. He was followed by Anaximander of Miletus (611 B. C.), who first mapped the heavens, Anaximenes of Miletus (570–500 B. C.), and Heraclitus of Ephesus (*circa* 556–460 B. C.), who, in succession, assumed that indivisible matter (earth), air, or fire respectively, are the primordial elements. These four elements, earth, air, fire, water, were assumed by Anaxagoras of Clazomenæ (500–428 B. C.) to be made up of as many parts or "seed" as there are varieties of sensible or perceptible matter. These categories were thrown into striking relief in the teaching of Empedocles of Agrigentum in Sicily (504–443 B. C.), the picturesque hero of Matthew Arnold's poem, who as philosopher, physician, poet, traveled through the Greek cities, clad in a purple robe, gold-cinctured, laurel-crowned, long haired severe of mien and, on account of his medical skill, held by the people to be endowed with supernatural powers. One of his poetic fragments shows the unusual reverence in which the Greek physician was held at this time:

[1] H. Frölich: Janus, Amst., 1897–8, ii, 248–251.

[2] Nuttall: Archæol. and Ethnol. Papers, Peabody Mus. Harvard Univ., Cambridge, 1901, ii, 526. Elliot Smith: Bull. John Rylands Library, Manchester, 1916, iii, 61.

[3] J. Wright: Scient. Monthly, N. Y., 1920, xi, 131.

> Ye friends, who in the mighty city dwell
> Along the yellow Acragas, hard by
> The Acropolis, ye stewards of good works,
> The stranger's refuge venerable and kind,
> All hail, O friends! But unto ye I walk
> As god immortal now, no more as man,
> On all sides honored fittingly and well,
> Crowned both with fillets, and with flowering wreaths
> When with my throngs of men and women I come
> To thriving cities I am sought by prayers,
> And thousands follow me that they may ask
> The path to weal and vantage, craving some
> For oracles, whilst others seek to hear
> A healing word 'gainst many a foul disease
> That all too long hath pierced with grievous pains.[1]

Empedocles introduced into philosophy the doctrine of the elements, earth, air, fire, water, as "the four-fold root of all things."

The human body is supposed to be made up of these primordial substances, health resulting from their balance, disease from imbalance. He held that nothing can be created or destroyed, and that there is only transformation, which is the modern theory of conservation of energy. Everything originates from the attraction of the four elements and is destroyed by their repulsion, and he applies the same idea, under the forms of love and hate, to the moral world. Development is due to the union of dissimilar elements, decay to the return of like to like, air to air, fire to fire, earth to earth.

Empedocles is said to have raised Pantheia from a trance, to have checked an epidemic of malarial fever by draining swampy lands and to have improved the climatic condition of his native town by blocking a cleft in a mountain side. Legend relates that he ended his life by throwing himself into the crater of Mount Etna. His pupil Pausanias is said by Plutarch to have used fire in checking an epidemic.

The Italian School of Philosophers was founded by **Pythagoras** of Samos (580–489 B. C.) at Crotona. Pythagoras was a good geometer and discovered the *pons asinorum* (Euclid, I, 47). He had studied in Egypt, whence he probably acquired his doctrine of the mystic power of numbers.

He held that unity being perfection and representing God, the number 12 represents the whole material universe, of which the factors 3 and 4 represent the worlds, the spheres, and the primordial elements. With the latter are connected the 4 elements. The monad (1) denotes the active or vital principle in nature, the dyad (2) the passive principle or matter, the triad (3) the world, formed by the union of the two former, and the tetrad (4), the perfection of eternally flowing nature. Heaven is made up of 10 celestial spheres (9 of which are visible), the fixed stars, the 7 planets and the earth. The distances of the celestial spheres from the earth correspond with the proportion of sounds in the musical scale.

Pythagoras was the first to investigate the mathematical physics of sound. In passing a blacksmith's shop, one day, he noticed that, when the smith's hammers were struck in rapid succession upon the anvil, the chords elicited (the octave, thirds and fifths) were all harmonious; the chord of the fourth was not. Going into the shop, he found this to be due to the differences in weights of individual hammers. Upon this hint, he stretched four strings of the same material, length and thickness by means of weights equal to the weights of the four hammers respectively. Upon

---

[1] From the interesting translations of the poetic fragments of Empedocles, by William Ellery Leonard in the Monist, Chicago, 1907, xvii, p. 468.

striking these strings, he got the chords which he had heard in the smithy. By subdividing the strings with other weights, he was able to construct the musical scale. This was the earliest recorded experiment in physics, and the scale was, after his death, engraved on brass, and set up in the temple of Juno at Samos. Pythagoras reasoned that the celestial spheres might produce sounds by striking upon the surrounding ether, and these sounds would vary with the velocity of impact and the relative distance. The distances of the spheres from the earth correspond, as we have seen, to the proportion of sounds in the scale, and as the heavenly bodies move according to fixed laws, the sounds produced by them must be harmonious. This is the doctrine of the "harmony of the spheres."

The Chaldean number-lore of Pythagoras exerted a profound influence upon the Hippocratic doctrine of crises and critical days, which assigned fixed periods to the resolution of different diseases. More than to anything else, the Greek physicians aspired to the scientific power of prediction. In pathology, the plastic significance of the number four was combined, in the teaching of Plato and Aristotle, with the doctrine of the four elements, as follows:

Corresponding with the 4 elements, earth, air, fire, and water, were the qualities dry, cold, hot, and moist, according to the scheme:

$$\text{hot} + \text{dry} = \text{fire}; \qquad \text{cold} + \text{dry} = \text{earth}.$$
$$\text{hot} + \text{moist} = \text{air}; \qquad \text{cold} + \text{moist} = \text{water}.$$

By reversing these equations, the four elements fire, air, earth, and water could be resolved into their qualitative components. Long before Aristotle, probably before Hippocrates, it was held that, corresponding to the four elements of Empedocles, fire, air, water, earth, and the four qualities, hot, cold, moist, dry, are the four humors of the body, viz., blood, phlegm, yellow bile, and black bile. These three sets of elements, qualities and humors could then be brought, by permutation and combination, into a complex system of arrangements, based upon the following scheme:

$$\text{hot} + \text{moist} = \text{blood}; \qquad \text{cold} + \text{moist} = \text{phlegm};$$
$$\text{hot} + \text{dry} = \text{yellow bile}; \qquad \text{cold} + \text{dry} = \text{black bile}.$$

In relation to the qualitative aspects of disease, and of the physiologic action of drugs the doctrine of the four humors was a vague foreshadowing of the endocrine and general biochemical aspects of human physiology. The whole arrangement made up the "humoral pathology" which regarded health and disease as the proper adjustment or imbalance respectively of the different components mentioned. The scheme was further elaborated by Galen (*Methodus medendi*) and the Arabian physicians, in that remedies and their compounds were classified in numerical scales according to the "degrees" or relative proportions of their several qualities. Thus, the Arabian pharmacists held that sugar is cold in the first degree, warm in the second degree, dry in the second degree, and moist in the first degree; cardamoms are warm in the first degree, cold by one-half a degree, dry in the first degree, and so forth. In Galen's system, the Pythagorean doctrine of numbers was applied to every aspect of medicine.[1]

In Egypt, Pythagoras learned the doctrine of transmigration of souls or metempsychosis. He is credited with being the first to advance the idea that the brain is the central organ of the higher activities, a proposition upheld by Alcmæon, Hippocrates, and Galen, denied by Aristotle, and long afterward put to experimental proof by Flourens and Goltz.

After Pythagoras, the most important of the Greek Philosophers, with the exception of Plato and Aristotle, was his pupil, the almost mythical **Alcmæon** of Crotona (*circa* 500 B. C.), who anticipated

---

[1] E. T. Withington: Medical History, London, 1894, 386–390.

Empedocles in the doctrine that health is the equipoise (*isonomia*) disease, the preponderance (*monarchia*) of heat, cold, moisture, dryness, acidity, sweetness, etc.; probably knew of the doctrine of atoms and pores; discovered the optic nerves and the Eustachian tubes; knew that the head of the fetus is the first part to be developed, and stated that the brain is the central organ of the higher activities and the origin of the nerves. Democritus of Abdera (460–360 B. C.) first stated the atomic theory, that everything in nature, including the body and the soul, is made up of atoms of different shapes and sizes, the movements of which are the cause of life and mental activity.[1]

During the Heroic Age, and at the time of the Trojan War, the dominant people in the Peloponnesus were the athletic, simple-minded Achaians, whose high regard for surgery and the surgeon was in striking contrast with the attitude of the ancient Romans. In later times Greek civilization was made up of two main elements, the Ionian (Attic) and the Doric (Spartan). The composite, imaginative, artistic peoples of Ionia and the islands were interested in everything, and at once brave and warlike, keen and business-like, serious and high-minded or, at need, flippant and ironical. As we see them in the comedies of Aristophanes, Lucian's dialogues and the idyls of Theocritus, the city-bred Greeks were a gay, quick-minded, supremely talkative people, adoring intelligence for itself, fonder of speculation than of material facts, keen at taking an advantage, and cheerfully complaisant as to their neighbors' morals. Yet they were the same people who could listen with reverent attention to the dramas of Æschylus and Sophocles. In striking contrast were the Dorians or Spartans, who were essentially robust, unimaginative warriors, severe in such morals as they had and, like the Homeric Greeks and the ancient Romans, cultivated the body rather than the mind, as an essential part of their scheme of military government. Under the harsh laws of Lycurgus, eugenic procreation was compulsory. Crippled and deformed infants were exposed or thrown into the Eurotas. As with all military peoples, the Spartans were narrowly jealous, suspicious or contemptuous of achievement or prosperity in other nations. Both Ionians and Spartans were extremely curious about the future and, like all people of early civilizations, attached enormous importance to oracles, presages, and omens. Thus, prognosis became the essential feature of Greek medicine. Among the Spartans, the surgeons were held in the same high regard as among the Homeric heroes. Lycurgus classed them as non-combatant officials. Among the Attic or Ionian Greeks, the medical profession, as we approach the Age of Pericles, is found to be more highly specialized. In the first place, general practitioners began, toward the later period, to receive stipulated fees for their services instead of the usual thank-offerings of the temples and, further, city and district (public) physi-

---

[1] For an interesting examination of the views of these philosophers, see the papers of Jonathan Wright in Scient. Monthly, N. Y., 1920, xi, 127–140; and New York Med. Jour., 1918–28, *passim*.

cians came to be appointed at an annual salary which, for the times, was quite high—in the case of Democedes at Athens (*circa* 525 B. C.) about $2000. These public physicians existed from Homer's time, are mentioned by Herodotus and Diodorus, and were well-known in Athens from the Periclean Age down to the 1st century A. D., as evidenced in Aristophanes, and many Greek inscriptions. After this time, they became known as *archiatroi*, whence the Roman *archiater* and the German *"Arzt."* In Thessaly, the land of horses, there was a public veterinarian (*Hippiatros*[1]). There were also military and naval surgeons among the Athenians, as among the Spartans. Xenophon records that there were eight army surgeons with the expedition of the Ten Thousand at the end of the 5th century; describes the review and enumeration of troops, including the slight sick reports, at Cerasus (V, 3); refers to snow-blindness, and gangrene from frostbite (IV, 5); and mentions the use of silver kettles for boiling water.[2] There were again midwives, professional lithotomists, druggists and veterinarians, and finally a special class, the *rhizotomi* or root gatherers, who wandered through the fields and forests collecting vegetable simples. The physician's office was called the *Iatreion*, and was used indifferently as a dispensary, consulting room, and operating theater. In the larger cities there were public *Iatreia*, supported by special taxes.

Medical instruction was not organized and was in effect private, either under some renowned physician or received from the adherents of the different schools. On finishing his course, the graduate simply took the physician's oath of the particular medical clan or sect to which he belonged.

Such human anatomy as the Greek physicians and surgeons learned was identical with the sculptor's knowledge of the subject, which the artist acquired through constant familiarity with the appearance of the nude body in action, either during the athletic contests celebrated by Pindar or in the palæstra. "It was here," says Waldstein, "with hundreds of nude youths, not only wrestling, jumping, and running, but endeavoring by systematic practice to remedy any defect or abnormality in any one limb or organ, that the artist, day by day, studied his anatomy of the human figure without the need of entering the dissecting room."[3] What Pater calls "the age of athletic prizemen" was also the great age of Greek sculpture, and in nothing is the discriminating power of Greek intelligence more beautifully and nobly shown than in the masterpieces of the great artists of this period. From the crude ikon, with no differentiation of eyes or limbs, there were gradually fashioned, "like the red outline of beginning Adam," first such rudimentary figures as the Apollo of Tenedos, then such supreme triumphs of anatomical figuration as the Doryophorus of Praxiteles, the Apoxy-

---

[1] R. Pohl: De Græcorum medicis publicis, Janus, Amst., 1905, x, 491–494.

[2] Th. Beck: Cor.-Bl. f. schweiz-Aerzte, Basel, 1905, xxxiv, 24.

[3] See Charles Waldstein: "The Argive Heræum," Boston, 1902, pp. 400, 401.

omenos of Lysippus, the Nike of Paionios, and such studies of violent muscular action as the Borghese Warrior (Lysippus), the Farnese Bull and the Laocoon (Rhodian school). As to the remarkable capacity of the Greek sculptors for close observation, Waldstein notes that the pectineus muscle, hidden at the base of Scarpa's triangle, but highly developed in the stress of Greek athletics, appears in some of their statues, although it has escaped the attention of modern artistic anatomists.[1] The same talent for acute observation is apparent in the lifelike representations of squid and oxen by the Cretan artists; of animals and plants on Greek coins; of the mane, paws and dentition of lions; the beak and claws of the sea-eagle (*Haliaetus albicilla*); of the contour, fins and dorsal spines of such identifiable sea fishes as *Sargus vulgaris* or *Crenilabrus Mediterraneus*, on Greek vases[2]; or of horses' heads on the Parthenon (440 B. C.). As Singer observes, "The very name for a painter in Greek (*zoographos*) recalls the attention paid to living forms." Here, indeed, were the beginnings of Greek biology.[3]

The medical lore in the Greek poets and writers between Homer and Hippocrates is considerable and has been collated, classified as to anatomy, physiology, pathology, military medicine and medical education by Charles Daremberg[4]; but much of this vast territory needs further exploration in the light of recent medicine.

In respect of education and personal hygiene, the Greeks cultivated that ideal of a harmonious development of all the individual faculties which was set aside or lost sight of during the Middle Ages, but has been steadily coming more and more to the front in later times. With such training, it is not strange that the Hellenes of the 5th century attained a degree of civilization and a supremacy in philosophy, lyrical and dramatic poetry, sculpture and architecture, which has not been equaled by any people who came after them. And this culminating period was also the Age of Hippocrates.

II. THE CLASSIC PERIOD (460–136 B. C.)

European medicine begins properly in the Age of Pericles and its scientific advancement centers in the figure of **Hippocrates** (460–370 B. C.), who gave to Greek medicine its scientific spirit and its ethical ideals. A contemporary of Sophocles and Euripides, Aristophanes and Pindar, Socrates and Plato, Herodotus and Thucydides, Phidias and Polygnotus, he lived at a time when the Athenian democracy had attained its highest point of development. Never, before or since, had so many men of genius appeared within the same narrow limits of space and time.

The ancient biographers of Hippocrates were Suidas, Tzetzes and Soranus. According to Soranus, Hippocrates was born on the island of

---

[1] See Waldstein: Op. cit., 186, pp. xxx and xxxiv.

[2] J. Morin: Le dessin des animaux en Grèce d'après les vases peints, Paris, 1911. Cited by Singer.

[3] See Singer: Greek Biology and Greek Medicine, Oxford, 1922, 5–18.

[4] C. Daremberg: État de la médecine entre Homère et Hippocrate, Paris, 1869.

Cos, at the beginning of the eightieth Olympiad, of an Asclepiad family.[1] He received his first medical instruction from his father, studied at Athens, and acquired extensive experience by travel and practice among the cities of Thrace, Thessaly, and Macedonia. The date of his death is unknown, his age being variously estimated as anywhere from 85 to 109 years. The eminence of Hippocrates is three-fold: he dissociated medicine from theurgy and philosophy,[2] crystallized the loose knowledge of the Coan and Cnidian Schools into systematic science, and gave physicians the highest moral inspiration they have. No future facts which may be dug up about cuneiform or papyric medicine will quite impair the value of the great advance thus made in synthetic science.

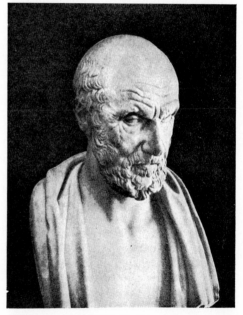

Hippocrates (460–370 B. C.). (Greek marble bust in the British Museum.)

Before the Age of Pericles, the Greek physician was either an associate of priests in times of peace or a surgeon in time of war. As the Greek mind was essentially plastic, so, in anatomy, his knowledge was mainly the sculptor's knowledge of visible or palpable parts and, for this reason, his clinical knowledge of internal diseases was confined to externalities also. Even as

The Grecian gods were like the Greeks,
As keen-eyed, cold and fair,

so the early Hellenic physician remained essentially a surgeon rather than a clinician in his attitude toward his patients, considering only the surface indications. In cold, dry enumeration of symptoms, the Coan and Cnidian tablets and sentences, like the Egyptian papyri, might have been scientific, if the physicians of the time had known how to group and coördinate symptoms and consequently to interpret them. All this was changed

---

[1] He is mentioned as an Asclepiad, who trained medical students for fees by Plato (*Protagoras*, 311 B; *Phœdrus* 270 C–E) and as "Hippocrates the Great" by Aristotle (*Politics*, VII, 4). In the view of Wilamovitz, Hippocrates is "a name without writings." By "Hippocrates," however, we mean the great mind behind the greater texts, which evince first hand study of actual conditions rather than mere summation of past knowledge.

[2] "Primus quidem ex omnibus memoria dignus, ab studio sapientiæ disciplinam hanc separavit." Celsus, De re medica, Proœmium.

with the advent of Hippocrates. All that a man of genius could do for internal medicine, with no other instrument of precision than his own open mind and keen senses, he accomplished, and, with these reservations, his best descriptions of disease are models of their kind today. To him medicine owes the art of clinical inspection and observation, and he is, above all, the exemplar of that flexible, critical, well-poised attitude of mind, ever on the lookout for sources of error, which is the very essence of the scientific spirit. As Allbutt points out,[1] Hippocrates taught the Coan physicians that, in relation to an internal malady like empyema or malarial fever, the basis of all real knowledge lies in the inductive *tribe meta logou*, that "reasoned rubbing in," which, better than the mere haphazard notation of symptoms, consists in going over them again and again, until the real values in the clinical picture begin to stand out of themselves.[2] Thus, instead of attributing disease to the gods or other fantastic imaginations, like his predecessors, Hippocrates virtually founded that bedside method which has been the distinctive talent of all true clinicians, from Sydenham and Heberden to Charcot and Osler. Huchard says that the revival of the Hippocratic methods in the 17th century and their triumphant vindication by the concerted scientific movement of the 19th, is the whole history of internal medicine. The central Hippocratic doctrine, the humoral pathology, which, as we have seen, attributes all disease to disorders of the fluids of the body, has, in its original form, long since been discarded, although some phases of it still survive in the modern theory of serodiagnosis and serotherapy. It is the method of Hippocrates—his use of the mind and senses as diagnostic instruments, together with his transparent honesty and his elevated conception of the dignity of the physician's calling, his high seriousness and deep respect for his patients—that makes him, by common consent, the "Father of Medicine" and the greatest of all physicians.

Claude Bernard said that observation is a passive science, experimentation an active science. Hippocrates was not acquainted with experiment, but no physician ever profited more by experience. Although Asclepiades called this observational method "a meditation upon death," the work of Hippocrates must be judged by its results. He described the "bilious, malarial, hemoglobinuric" fevers of Thessaly and Thrace very much as the modern Greek writers, Cardamatis, Kanellis, and the rest, have found them today, indeed, Jones points out that this part of the Canon was the basic text on malarial fevers up to 1840, when they ceased to be a real menace to Northern Europe up to the Russian Revolution of 1917. It has been remarked that the Hippocratic pictures of phthisis, puerperal septicemia, epilepsy, epidemic parotitis, the quotidian, tertian, and quartan varieties of remittent fever, and some other diseases might, with a few changes and additions,

---

[1] Sir T. C. Allbutt: "The Historical Relations of Medicine and Surgery," London, 1905, 6–13.

[2] See Dr. Howard Kelly's Hunterian Oration (1928).

take their place in any modern text-book. Most of the clinical histories in the Hippocratic Corpus have been provided with a diagnosis-tag by Littré. The diseases actually specified are the respiratory affections, the malarial fevers, diarrhea, dysentery, melancholia and mania. Hippocrates described anthrax as πῦρ ἄγριον (*ignis agrestis*[1]), the "Persian fire" of Avicenna, which Galen wrongly interpreted as erysipelas.[2]

The neurological data in the books of Epidemic Diseases include notations of paralysis on the opposite side of the lesion in wounds of the head (VII, 36), brachial palsies associated with epidemic cough (II, 2, §8; IV, 50), epidemic winter paralysis (I, 8) and the truly modern observation that epilepsy is incompatible with quartan fever and will disappear after malarial infection (VI, 6, §5). The correlation between parapl gia, epistaxis, and influenzal fevers is noted Lathyrism is described as impotency in the legs from a monotone diet of peas (II, Sect. IV, 3).

A bad prognosis is declared when muscular atrophy supervenes upon paralysis of a limb (Prorrhetics, 39). Insanity is classified as phrenitis (febrile delirium), mania (acute non-febrile insanity), and melancholia (mental depression). Tabes meant wasting, usually from excessive venery, as in the line of Persius:

"Virtutem videant intabescantque relictâ."

Crookshank and Wright assume that the "lethargy" of Hippocrates, Cælius Aurelianus, and other writers may have been encephalitis lethargica.

Of 42 clinical cases in Hippocrates—almost the only records of the kind for the next 1700 years—25 (60 per cent.) are reported, with characteristic sincerity, as fatal and, unlike Galen, the author has nothing whatever to say about his own clever diagnoses and remarkable cures, or of blunders on the part of his fellow practitioners. "I have written this down deliberately," says Hippocrates in one passage, "believing it is valuable to learn of unsuccessful experiments and to know the causes of their failure."[3] "He seems," says Billings, "to have written mainly for the purpose of telling what he himself knew, and this motive—rare among all writers—is especially rare among writers on medicine."[4] Through Hippocrates, it was the chief glory of Greek medicine to have introduced that spontaneous, first-hand study of nature, with a definitely honest intention, which is the motor power of modern science. After the Hippocratic period, the practice of taking clinical case-histories died out, for Galen's cases were written only to puff his own reputation and, apart from a few Arabian case-histories, there was nothing of value up to the postmortems of Benivieni and Vesalius.

In the view of classical philologists, Hippocrates is "a name without writings." The works attributed to the Hippocratic school are, in fact, a Canon or scriptural body of doctrine and, as Jones infers, probably the remains of the library of the school at Cos. From the internal evidence of style, he allocates the following dates to certain works,[5] viz.,

---

[1] Epidem., vii, 20.

[2] P. Richter: Arch. f. Gesch. d. Med., Leipz., 1912–13, vi, 281–297.

[3] Cited by Osler in his Silliman Lectures, New Haven, 1921.

[4] J. S. Billings: "History of Surgery," New York, 1895, p. 24.

[5] For a chronologic schema of the Hippocratic writings (Petersen-Littré) see Landsberg: Janus, Gotha, 1853, ii, 107–110.

Sevens (Pythagorean) 480 B. C.; *Prorrhetics*, 440 B. C.; *Breaths* (Diogenes of Apollonia), 436 B. C.; *Ancient Medicine*, 430–420 B. C.; *Prognostics* and *Aphorisms*, 415 B. C.; *Coan Prenotions*, 410 B. C.; *Nutriment* (Heraclitean), 400 B. C.; *Precepts* (Epicurean), 400 B. C.; *Physician*, 350–300 B. C.; *Decorum*, later than 300 B. C. Somewhere in the probable period of *Ancient Medicine*, the *Prognostics* and the *Aphorisms* (430–400 B. C.), *i. e.*, in the prime of Hippocrates' life, fall the greater treatises now usually regarded as genuine, viz., *Epidemic Diseases*, I–III; *Regimen in Acute Diseases; Airs, Waters, and Places; Fractures; Joints (Dislocations)* and *Wounds of the Head*. The excursus, on *Airs, Waters and Places*, is at once the first book ever written on medical geography, climatology, and anthropology, if we except the contemporary narrative of Herodotus, with whom Hippocrates is often in such striking accord. In like manner, the discourse on *Ancient Medicine* takes us into the presumable origins of rational diagnosis and therapy out of reasoned dietetics. The Oath, the earliest and most impressive document in medical ethics, is not usually regarded as a genuine Hippocratic writing. As Jones points out, it is a composite production, containing both an oath to uphold a high ethical standard in practice and an indenture in which the candidate agrees to share his livelihood with his teacher, to help him financially where necessary, and to teach student signatories of the oath, like his own children. The sentences interdicting the use of the pessary in abortion and of the knife in stone are in the original pagan (Urbinas MS.) reading of the Oath. The Christianized version (Ambrosian MS.) forbids abortion by any process.[1] Yet both the *Oath* and the *Law* are so much in keeping with the ethical spirit of the great Coan that they are usually included in the Hippocratic Canon. The Oath has been administered to medical graduates in many European universities for centuries. To a modern reader, the best of the *Aphorisms* seem like the short-hand notes of a keen mind at the bedside, intent on establishing a true relation between generals and particulars, accidentals and essentials. While many of them go straight to the mark, others are strongly suggestive of the kind of inadequate information which was probably conveyed in the Coan and Cnidian sentences. Of the tracts on prognosis, the first book of the *Prorrhetics* is the oldest of the Hippocratic writings, the *Coan Prenotions* the latest. The Prognostics were written independently, with some knowledge of Prorrhetics I. The dignity of the Greek physician was based more upon his supposed ability to predict clinical and epidemiological happenings than upon his power to control them. To this end Hippocrates instituted, for the first time, a careful, systematic, and thorough-going examination of the patient's

---

[1] The oath is described as genuinely Hippocratic by Erotian (*circa* 50 A. D.) and is mentioned by Scribonius Largus (43 A. D.), but it is astonishing that Galen never refers to it. Jones cites a flagrant violation of the abortion clause in the Canon itself (Littré, VII, 490). See Jones: Hippocrates, London, 1923, i, 291–297, and his "The Doctor's Oath," Cambridge, 1924.

condition, including the facial appearance, pulse, temperature, respiration, excreta, sputum, localized pains, and movements of the body. He even notes the ominous symptom of picking at the coverlid in fevers. He introduced the doctrines of the four humors (humoral pathology), coction of food in the stomach, healing by first intention; and divided diseases into acute and chronic, endemic and epidemic. The treatise on *Nutrition* (*Peritrophes, circa* 400 B. C.) contains the first mention of the pulse in Greek medicine and of the peculiar theory of the circulation (arteries from the heart, veins from the liver) which persisted up to the time of Harvey (Singer). The books on *Epidemic Diseases*—classical studies on the external causes of epidemics—contain the remarkable case-histories and clinical pictures to which we have referred. Not the least among these is the famous *facies Hippocratica*, that wonderful thumb-nail sketch of the signs of approaching dissolution,[1] some touches of which are given in Shakespeare's account of Falstaff's death

The anatomical treatises on the heart (*circa* 400 B. C.), on the muscles (*circa* 390 B. C.) contain arrangements of the parts of the body in systems of sevens, with descriptions of the cardiac valves, the ventricles and the great vessels, and of the organs of special sense. The treatise on generation (*circa* 380 B. C.) records incubations of hen's eggs for embryological study, comparisons between vegetable, animal, and human embryology, and discussions of pangenesis, survival of the strongest and the inheritance of acquired characters—in short the beginnings of pre-Aristotelian biology (Singer).

While there is much in the surgical writings of Hippocrates that is faulty, incomplete, or not in accordance with modern practice, they are the only thing of value on the subject before the time of Celsus. The treatises on *Fractures, Dislocations,* and *Wounds of the Head* may be thought of as modern works in the same sense in which Matthew Arnold regarded Thucydides as a modern writer, illustrating the wonderful capacity of Greek intelligence for separating essentials from accidentals, "the tendency to observe facts with a critical spirit; to search for their law, not to wander among them at random; to judge by the rule of reason, not by the impulse of prejudice or caprice."[2] In the view of Malgaigne, Littré, Petrequin, Allbutt, and Jones, these treatises, given the limitations under which they were written, are not surpassed by any similar works of recent times. In *Wounds of the Head,* Hippocrates argued for decompressive trephining, even in contusions, but advised simple expectant treatment in an open depressed fracture. Dislocations of the shoulder, he says, are "rarely inwards or outwards, but frequently and chiefly downwards." His methods of reduction are practically those of modern times. He was particularly strong in his account of congenital dislocations, and in reducing and bandaging fractures. He was the first to notice that[3] gibbous spine

---

[1] Prognosis, §2.
[2] Matthew Arnold: "Essays in Criticism," third series, Boston, 1910, p. 48.
[3] Dislocations, §41; Aphorisms, vi, 46.

7

(Pott's disease) often coexists with tubercle of the lungs, and was familiar with club-foot. In his treatise on dislocations (§47), he describes the Calot treatment of spinal deformity by *redressement forcé*. He was acquainted with fracture of the clavicle and dislocation of its acromial end, and knew how to treat both conditions. *Iatreion* (The Surgical Clinic), a tract on bandaging, was abridged from the treatise on *Fractures*, and *Mochlicon* (Reduction Apparatus) from *"Joints,"* probably by apprentices of 400–350 B. C. (Jones). In *Wounds* Hippocrates says that they should never be irrigated except with clean water or wine, the dry state being nearest to the healthy, the wet to the diseased. The aseptic advantages of extreme dryness were utilized in the avoidance of greasy dressings and in the effort to bring the fresh edges of the wound into close apposition, sometimes by the use of astringents.[1] Hippocrates recognizes that "rest and immobilization are of capital importance," and to keep still is even a better splint than bandaging. He describes the symptoms of suppuration, and says that, in such cases, medicated dressings, if applied at all, should be "not upon the wound itself, but around it." If water was used for irrigation, it had either to be very pure or else boiled, and the hands and nails of the operator were to be cleansed. Hippocrates gives the first description of healing by first and second intention. In his description of the operating-room, he lays stress upon good illumination, posture of the patient, and the presence of capable assistants. He refers to trephining and paracentesis, but apparently knew nothing of amputation. In his directions for trephining in head injuries he notes that a wound of the left temporal region will cause convulsions on the right side and *vice versa*. The Hippocratic aphorism that diseases not curable by iron are curable by fire, which caused no end of surgical bungling and malpractice down to the time of Paré, is really pre-Hippocratic, being already mentioned in the Agamemnon of Æschylus. It has been traced by Baas to the ancient Hindus. In clinical diagnosis, Hippocrates was the first to note the "succussion sound," obtained by shaking the patient on a rigid seat, the ear being applied to the chest. Gee also comments on a "friction râle," and a pleural sound like that of new leather.[2] Cheyne-Stokes respiration ("like that of a person recollecting himself") is noted in the cases of Philiscus and the wife of Dealces.[3]

In therapeutics, Hippocrates believed simply in assisting nature, and although he knew the use of many drugs, his scheme of treatment was usually confined to such plain expedients as fresh air, good diet, purgation, blood-letting, tisans[4] of barley gruel, barley water, hydromel

[1] While the dry treatment of wounds was undoubtedly aseptic, as far as it went, Sudhoff warns us against the erroneous tendency of Anagnostakis and others to regard Hippocratic wound surgery as "antiseptic" in the modern sense.

[2] DeMorbis, I, 6; 15: II, 47; 59; 61: III, 7; 16.

[3] Epid. Dis., i, Sect. 3, §13, Case 1: III, Sect. 3, §17, Case 15. Cited by Finlayson.

[4] During the Middle Ages, and indeed into the 18th century, a tisan was called "hippocras" (Singer).

(honey and water), oxymel (honey and vinegar), massage, and hydrotherapy. In Greek medicine, black hellebore (*Helleborus niger*) was the universal purge; white hellebore (*Veratrum album*) the universal emetic.

Thus, the Hippocratic or **Coan School** aimed at prognosis by means of a general semeiology of known diseases, with very generalized therapy. It centered on the patient, his individual reaction to the disease, and envisaged symptoms and syndromes as merely episodic in its total history, yet often indicative of its remote or final phases (the *general pathology* of the Germans). The patient was the real thing, the disease not an entity (the savage's indwelling demon) but a fluctuating condition of the patient's body, a battle between the *materies morbi* and the natural self-healing tendency (*physis*) of the body. In like manner, treatment was centered upon assisting the patient, through his particular *physis* (nature), to react, in his own peculiar, individual way, against the disease, which was regarded as an imbalance of the four humors. In disease, forces or morbid principles from without brought the humors into a raw condition (*apepsia*), with resulting symptoms. By the natural reaction of the body (*physis*), the apeptic humors were brought into a state of coction (*pepsis*), expressing itself as fever, inflammation or pus. Recovery resulted from elimination of the concocted humors and morbid material (*crisis*), or by the slower process of increased secretion or excretion (*lysis*). The patient's reaction, in each case, was individual and peculiar to himself. The base-line semeiology was used merely as a convenient fiction (conceptual short-hand) like a fashion-plate or a general equation in mathematics. The **Cnidian School**, on the other hand, centered on the disease rather than the patient, aimed at exact diagnosis and classification (*special pathology*), with specific therapy: but, as Hippocrates himself observes it erred by excess of detail. As in the International Causes of Death it mistook and labelled mere symptoms for individualized diseases. Its actual therapy was limited to purges, milk, and whey. The chief physician of this school was Euryphon, the reputed author of the Cnidian Sentences (Galen). Coan medicine is the medicine of the greater physicians, who, like Charcot, saw the patient's condition as "only an accident" in the total, serial history of the disease, the symptoms of which might be distributed among the members of a family or community (in space) or through successive generations of people (in time). Cnidian medicine, the medicine of library classifiers, of the pathological s ecimen of Broussais' "diseas° s rved on a plat ," is largely the medicine of our own period of ultra-refined diagnosis and highly specialized therapy.

In literary style, Hippocrates is like the best Greek writers of the classic period—clear, precise, and simple. The tract on ancient medicine is the first script on medical history. The Law, the Oath, and the opening chapters of the discourse *On the Sacred Disease* are the loftiest utterances of Greek medicine and, whether due to Hippocrates or not, they are informed with the spirit of his ethical teaching. Behind the sensible phenomena of nature he surmised the existence of some tremendous power (*enormon*), which sets things going. The argument of the "Sacred Disease," which ridicules the supposedly divine origin of epilepsy, was the highest reach of free thought for centuries, and had it been heeded, would have done away forever with the foolish idea that human ills are caused by gods or demons.

The usual portraits of Hippocrates represent an old, bearded man of venerable aspect. They are in no sense "counterfeit presentments," but only traditional. In the *Clouds* of Aristophanes, there is a satirical reference to physicians as lazy, long-haired, foppish individuals with rings and carefully polished nails, which is supposed to have been, incidentally, a slap at the Father of Medicine. It is highly probable that physicians of the Periclean Age wore their hair and beards as much

like the figures of Jove or Æsculapius as possible, and were otherwise
not lacking in the self-sufficiency which characterized the Greeks of the
period. Some of the supposed portraits of Hippocrates are, perhaps,
only variants of the bust of Æsculapius as rendered into marble by
Praxiteles (in the British Museum), or as seen in statuettes from the
shrine of Epidaurus or on the Greek coins of Cos, Pergamus, and
Epidaurus, representing him enthroned.

The most important editions of Hippocrates are:

1. The folio Latin text of the *Opera Omnia*, translated and edited by Fabius
Calvus, the friend and patron of Raphael, and published at Rome under the auspices
of Pope Clement VII in 1525. This was the first complete edition of Hippocrates
to be printed.

2. The folio *editio princeps* of the Greek text, published in the following year
(1526) by Aldus at Venice.

3. The Basel *Opera Omnia*, edited by Janus Cornarius and printed by Froben
(1538), highly prized on account of its textual and critical accuracy.

4. The Greek text and Latin translation of Hieronymus Mercurialis, printed
by the house of Giunta at Venice in 1538.

5. The invaluable *Œconomia Hippocratis* (1588) of Anutius Foesius, which is
also found in the Geneva edition (1675) of his Latin translation (Frankfurt, 1595),
along with the glossaries of Erotian and Galen, and the notes of his Greek text
of 1595.

6. The ten-volume edition of Émile Littré (Paris, 1839–61), containing the
Greek text, a French translation (all the readings known having been carefully
collated with critical notes), a biographic introduction, special introductions to each
separate treatise, and diagnosis tags to most of the diseases described. It was
the work of twenty-two years of continuous labor.

The earlier commentators were Herophilus, his pupil Bacchius, Heraclides of
Tarentum, Galen, and Erotian (Glossary). The first Greek text of the Aphorisms
was edited by François Rabelais, and published at Lyons, in 1532. The parallel
Greek and Latin texts of J. A. van der Linden (Leyden, 1665), and C. G. Kühn
(3 v., Leipzig, 1825–7) are highly esteemed. The critical edition of F. Z. Ermerins
(Utrecht, 1859–64) is regarded by Jones as the most stimulating and useful, although
"as a philologist, he was very deficient." In this regard, the Teubner text of Johann
Ilberg and Hugo Kühlewein (Leipzig, 1894–1902) is the most authoritative in respect
of collation and emendation of readings from the known MSS. Of commentators of
separate texts Jones gives the palm to Gompertz, Wilamovitz-Möllendorf, and Adam-
antius Coray. The English translation of the Scotch scholar Francis Adams (London,
1849) is limited to the so-called genuine works of Hippocrates. This is likely to be
superseded by the bilingual of Jones and Withington (Loeb Classical Library, 4 v.,
London, 1923–27), which contains, in addition to the authentic writings, such remarkably instructive tracts as the *Precepts, Nutriment, Breaths, Decorum,* and *Dentition*. Jones' general introduction and the illuminating special prefaces to the separate
treatises afford a new view of the Hippocratic Canon. The edition is thus invaluable to English readers. Very handy for practical use is the *Œuvres choisies* of
Charles Daremberg (Paris, 1834). A German translation is that of R. Fuchs (3 v.,
Munich, 1895–1908). The surgical writings have been edited, with splendid commentaries, by J. E. Petrequin (2 v., Paris, 1877–8). The standard concordances of
Hippocrates are the glosses of Erotian (Paris, 1564; best edition, Leipzig, 1777),
the *Œconomia Hippocratis* of Anutius Foesius (Frankfort, 1588) and the index
(vol. X) of Littré (1861). To understand the relation of Hippocrates to modern
medicine, the bilingual anthology of Theodor Beck (Hippocrates' Erkenntnisse,
Jena, 1907) is highly recommended for beginners by Sudhoff. The treatise called
περὶ τέχνης in the *corpus Hippocraticum* has been translated by Theodor Gomperz
as "Die Apologie der Heilkunst" (Leipzig, 1910), and is attributed by him to a
sophist of the 5th century, probably of the school of Protagoras.

Hippocrates voiced the spirit of an entire epoch, and after his time
there was a great gap in the continuity of Greek medicine. In succeeding centuries, the open-minded, receptive spirit of his teaching became

merged into the case-hardened formalism of dogmatists like Praxagoras, who cared more for rigid doctrine than for investigation. The dogmatists divided medical science into five branches: physiology, etiology (pathology), hygiene, semeiology, and therapeutics. Of these, the later Empirics retained only the practical branches of semeiology and therapeutics, with its subdivisions of dietetics, pharmacology, surgery, and sometimes hygiene.

The greatest scientific name after Hippocrates is that of "the master of those who know," the Asclepiad **Aristotle** (384–322 B. C.) of Stagira, who gave to medicine the beginnings of botany, zoölogy, comparative anatomy, embryology, teratology and physiology, and the use of formal logic as an instrument of precision. He taught anatomy by the dissection of animals, and by the use of "anatomical diagrams" ("paradigms, diagraphs, schemata") which were "represented on the walls of his Lyceum."[1] Aristotle was a pupil of Plato, whose *Timæus* imposed some very fantastic theories upon physiological reasoning for centuries, but he easily surpassed his master in direct observation of external nature. He was, in fact, the greatest biologist, not only of antiquity, but for the 2000 or more years preceding the advent of such men as Linnæus or Cuvier. Aristotle describes some 500 kinds of animals, mostly from the island of Lesbos (Mitylene) and the northeastern shores of the Ægean. As soon as he gets away from the Ægean basin, his descriptions are apt to be fantastic or fictitious. His most important works are the *Historia animalium,* the treatises on Generation, on the Parts of Animals, and his book on the soul.

Aristotle is at his weakest in physics and physiology, in which he is mainly speculative. He is at his best in logic, ethics, embryology, and natural history. He studied the development of the chick day by day, noted the punctum saliens and the beat of the fetal heart, the vitelline and allantoic veins, the enveloping membrane, and the possibility of superfetation. He regarded the semen as the formative, activating agent or "soul," the female element as the passive soil to be fertilized or moulded as the potter's clay, a view of things which is borne out to some extent by Loeb's experiments on parthenogenesis. He named the aorta, and announced the doctrine of the primacy of the heart, as the source of "innate heat," the seat of sensation and thought, a view which held its own in the *pectora cæca* of Virgil and even in Harvey. Contrary to the view of Alcmæon, that the brain feels and thinks, Aristotle regarded it as a gland secreting cold humors to prevent overheating of the body by the fiery heart (*via* the lungs). His criterion of living things was the possession of soul (*psyche*), vegetative in plants, sensitive in animals, rational in man. Inanimate things were apsychic. He classifies animals as *Enaima* or sanguineous (vertebrates) and *Anaima* or bloodless (invertebrates), then as to their reproductive status (viviparous, oviparous, gemmulous, spontaneous generation), then by further dichotomies, some of which, such as his distinction between bony and cartilaginous (Selachian) fishes, reveal shrewd powers of observation. The same essential keenness of perception is evident in his distinction between species (*eidos*) as a class having attributes common to all its members, and *genus* as a general similarity in size, shape or externalities; as also in his notation of carbon monoxide poisoning, or his account of reproduction in the dogfish (*Mustelus lævis*) and the

---

[1] Aristotle: Die generatione animalium, i, 7. Historia animalium, i, 14, 17, 24; ii, 13; iii, 1. Cited by Choulant. The diagrams of the male genito-urinary system (mammalian) and the mammalian uterus have been reconstructed by Singer, from Aristotle's own description, in The Evolution of Anatomy, London and New York, 1925, 19–20.

cephalopoda which were verified long after by Johannes Müller (1842) and Racovitza (1894[1]). He was the first to use the term "anthropologist," but in the sense of a vain, self-important person, the logical opposite of the "high-minded man" of his Nichomachean *Ethics*. His "entelechies," which he regarded as intermediaries between the soul and the body, have been revived, as a substitute for "vital principles," by the morphologist Driesch.

Aristotle left his library and botanic garden to his friend and pupil, **Theophrastus** of Eresos (370–286 B. C.), who was also a physician, and was called the "protobotanist" because he did for the vegetable kingdom what Hippocrates had previously done for surgery and clinical medicine, in that he collated the loose plant-lore of the woodmen, farmers, and rhizotomists into a systematic treatise. The earliest Greek herbal, that of Diocles of Carystos (350 B. C.) exists only in fragments studied by Max Wellmann (1901–13), and G. A. Gerhard (1913). The *De Historia Plantarum* of Theophrastus contains descriptions of some 500 different plants. The ninth book, the earliest surviving "herbal," is, however, not Theophrastian, but a compilation, probably from later Alexandrian sources (250 B. C.).

In his first chapter[2] Theophrastus divides plants variously into trees, shrubs, undershrubs, and herbs; wild and cultivated flowering and flowerless fruit-bearing and fruitless, terrestrial, aquatic, marshy and marine; and even attempts some classification by root, leaf, seed flower, and fruit; but attains to no definite arrangement or nomenclature. Such classifications as he made, however, were not improved upon until the time of Valerius Cordus (*Historia plantarum*, 1561). Theophrastus described all the external organs of plants in sequence from root to fruit. He studied the development of seeds, differentiated between dicotyledons and monocotyledons, and before Goethe recognized the flower as a metamorphosed leaf, although ignorant of its sexual nature. He regarded fruit as virtually a congeries of seeds (carpus) invested by a husk (pericarp). He established relations between the structure, habits, and functions of plants and their geographical distribution. His ninth chapter summarizes all that was known in his time of medicinal properties of plants, from the nepenthe and moly of Homer to the arrow poisons of African tribes. The principal MSS. of Theophrastus are the Urbinas (Vatican) and Paris Codices. The most important editions of Theophrastus are the two Aldines of 1495–8 (Greek) and 1504 (Latin), the Latin version of Gaza (1483), Stapel's Greek and Latin text of 1644 and the 5-volume edition of J. G. Schneider (Leipzig, 1818–21), supplemented by the textual commentaries of Sprengel (1822) and Wimmer (1842). The handy bilingual of Sir Arthur Hort (Loeb's Classical Library, 1896) is most convenient for English readers.

Menon, another pupil of Aristotle, made the earliest contribution to medical history after Hippocrates in his *Iatrika*, which was mentioned by Galen and excerpted in a papyrus (*Anonymus Londinensis*) edited by Diels (*Supplementum Aristotelicum*, III, Berlin, 1893).

With the founding of **Alexandria** (331 B. C.), Greek science and culture were firmly implanted in the ancient civilization of Egypt. Alexandria, with its great university and library, with such leaders as

---

[1] For a full account of Aristotle's work in biology, see Singer: Studies in the History and Method of Science, Oxford, 1921, ii, 13–56. Greek Biology and Greek Medicine, Oxford, 1922, 18–54. Also the translations of Aristotle's Parts of Animals by W. Ogle (London, 1882), his *De anima* by R. D. Hicks (Cambridge, 1907) and his *Historia Animalium* by D'A. W. Thompson (Oxford, 1910). For the medicine of the Aristotelian school, see H. Diels: Preuss. Jahrb., Berl., 1893, lxxiv, 412–429.

[2] E. L. Greene: "Landmarks of Botanical History," Washington, Smithsonian Inst., 1909, 52–142. C. Singer: Studies, Oxford, 1921, ii, 79–98.

Ptolemy and Euclid, Hero and Strato, thus became the means of preserving the Greek texts and of spreading Greek doctrine to the East.

Our knowledge of the two great Alexandrian anatomists, **Herophilus** and **Erasistratus** (4th century B. C.), the originators of dissecting, is not based upon any textual record of their writings, but was pieced together out of Galen, by the scholarship of Marx, Hieronymus,[1] and Finlayson. Herophilus was, in Sudhoff's phrase, the Father of Scientific Anatomy. Erasistratus was the first experimental physiologist. Both Herophilus and Erasistratus made important investigations of the nervous system, showing the relations of the larger nerves to the brain and spinal cord, and distinguishing sensory and motor nerves, with which they sometimes confused the tendons. Both followed Praxagoras in regarding the blood-vessels as filled with air. Both are credited with a vague reference to the lacteal vessels. Both were charged, by Celsus and Tertullian, with human vivisection. Herophilus of Chalcedon, a pupil of Praxagoras, differentiated the cerebrum and cerebellum, described the torcular Herophili, the meninges, and the fourth ventricle of the brain, including the calamus scriptorius; also the hyoid bone, the parotid and submaxillary glands, the pulmonary artery, which he called the arterial vein, the duodenum, the ovary, the cornua uteri, the seminal vesicles, and the prostate gland, and in the eye, the retina, vitreous and ciliary body. He counted the pulse with a water-clock,[2] and made an elaborate analysis of its rate and rhythm. Erasistratus (*circa* 310–250 B. C.) of Iulis (Keos), a pupil of Chrysippus, described the aortic and pulmonary valves, the chordæ tendinæ of the heart, and the capillary ramifications of arteries and veins, which he conceived of as provided with *synanastomoses* (adjacent mouths). He saw the heart clearly as a pump and was close upon the mystery of the circulation, but conceived it backwards, from the liver by the arteries to the heart and thence to the lungs by the veins. Digestion he regarded, not as coction (*pepsis*), but as a purely mechanical process. He had some notion of metabolism and devised the first crude respiration calorimeter, a jar in which he kept fowls, weighing them and their excreta, after feeding and completed digestion.[3] Erasistratus conceived of *pneuma* as outside air, sublimated into spirit after leaving the lung. He knew of monoxide poisoning. His main cause of disease was hyperemia (*plethora*), by which he explained the pathology of angina, pleurisy, and dropsy. He treated stricture with an S-shaped catheter of his invention. A well known aphorism of Herophilus has been cleverly paraphrased by the poet Gay:

> "Nor Love nor Honor, Wealth nor Power
> Can give the heart a cheerful hour,
> When Health is lost."

---

[1] K. F. H. Marx: Herophilus, Carlsruhe, 1838. J. F. Hieronymus: Jena diss., 1790.

[2] H. Schöne: Festschr. z. 49 Versamml. deutscher Philologen, Basel, 1907, 448–472.

[3] Diels: Anonymus Londinensis, Berlin, 1893, ch. 33, 44. Cited by Heidel.

The Alexandrian surgeon Hegetor (100 B. C.) discussed the anatomical relations of dislocation at the hip-joint and first described the
ligamentum teres (Singer).

Considerable light is thrown upon the Hellenic medical culture
grafted upon Egypt in the Alexandrian period—the dietetics, materia
medica, pathology, regulation of wet-nursing, public baths, the surviving "etiquette" of circumcision and embalming, the temples of Serapis
and Isis (Serapieia, Isieia, corresponding to the Greek Asclepieia)—in
Karl Sudhoff's splendid study of Alexandrian medicine in the Oxy-
rhyncus and other Greek papyri.[1]

In the 3d century B. C., Alexandrian medicine was introduced into
Mesopotamia, and in this way Syria acquired the main body of Hippocratic doctrine *via* Egypt, while retaining many of the astrologic
features of Assyro-Babylonian medicine. This dual system was studied
by Syrian physicians for over a thousand years. In evidence of this
transition, we have the Syriac version of the Hippocratic aphorisms,
edited by Pognon,[2] and a Syriac translation of Galen's *De locis affectis*
(Wallis Budge[3]). Syria became the stepping-stone or first station between Oriental, Græco-Alexandrian and medieval medicine. In the
early Middle Ages, medical translations from the Greek texts were
usually made backwards, first into Syriac, then into Arabic or Hebrew,
then into Latin.

The tendencies of the school of Empirics, which sprang from the
Alexandrian school in the 2d century before Christ, culminated in
an actual development of quasi-experimental pharmacology and toxicology at the hands of physicians and wary dilettante rulers, of whom
Mithridates, King of Pontus (120–63 B. C.), achieved a reputation in
the art of giving and taking poisons. He is said to have immunized
himself against poisoning by means of the blood of ducks fed upon toxic
principles, and he aspired to make a universal antidote (alexipharmacy).[4]
These "mithridates" and "theriacs," as they were called, engaged the
talents of pharmacists up to the beginning of the 18th century and, in
a manner, Mithridates may be regarded as the originator of the idea
of polyvalent drugs and sera. The principal relics of this empirical
poison-lore are the treatise on poisonous animals by Apollodorus of
Alexandria and two hexameter poems of Nikander[5] on poisonous animals (*Theriaca*), and antidotes for poisons (*Alexipharmaca*), which
have been preserved in the two Aldine editions of 1499 and 1523, and
in the French versification of these poems by Jacques Grevin (Plantin

---

[1] K. Sudhoff: Studien z. Gesch. d. Med. (Puschmann-Stiftung), Nos. 5, 6,
Leipzig, 1909.

[2] H. Pognon: Une version Syriaque des aphorismes d'Hippocrate, 2 parts,
Leipzig, 1903.

[3] Syrian anatomy (etc.) or "The Book of Medicines," ed. E. A. Wallis Budge.
2 v., Oxford, 1913.

[4] Th. Reinach: Mithridate Eupator, Paris, 1890, 283–285.

[5] Singer (Studies, Oxford, 1921, ii, 63, pl. ix) mentions a particularly interesting
MS. of Nikander containing illustrations of plants.

edition, Antwerp, 1568). In the reign of Mithridates flourished the botanist **Crateuas,** who wrote a herbal (*Rhizotomikon*), some of the illustrations of which may have found their way into the famous Julia Anicia (Constantinople) codex of Dioscorides (512 A. D.), now in St. Mark's Library at Venice. One picture, indeed, represents Epinoia (Intelligence) holding a mandrake, which Dioscorides describes, while Crateuas paints it. He was, thus, the earliest known illustrator of plants.[1]

III. The Græco-Roman Period (156 B. C.–576 A. D.)

In the early history of Rome, the primitive, dark, small autochthonous Ligurian strain was mastered and overcome by warriors from the North, the "close-fisted Umbrian" and the "sombre, Puritanical Sabine," to which Catullus (xxxix, 10) adds another dominant element, the "obese Etruscan," an Oriental race whose ceremonies and divinations "may have been witnessed by Abraham himself on his entry into Hebron" (Allbutt[2]). The Southern half of Italy and Sicily were not conquered by the Northern invaders, but remained "Magna Græcia" from the 6th century B. C. to the 10th century A. D., and from Magna Græcia came one of the streams of cultural influences which helped to form the School of Salerno.

After the destruction of Corinth (146 B. C.), Greek medicine may be said to have migrated to Rome. Before the Greek invasion, the Romans, as the elder Pliny tells us, "got on for 600 years without doctors," relying mainly on medicinal herbs and domestic simples, votive objects set up in temples, superstitious rites, and religious observances. To the Romans of the Empire, the Greek of any description was the *Græculus esuriens* of Juvenal. The proud Roman citizen, who had a household god for nearly every disease or physiologic function known to him,[3] a domestic herbal medicine of his own,[4] looked askance upon the itinerant Greek physician, despising him as a mercenary for accepting compensation for his services, and otherwise distrusting him as a possible poisoner or assassin (Pliny, xxix, 7). Archagathus, who came to Rome in the year of the city 535 (220 B. C.), the first Greek physician to practice there, came to be known as "Carnifex" for his cruelty in surgery (Pliny, xxix, 6). It is further recorded that the intrigues of the physicians Vettius Valens and Eudemus with Messalina and Livia, royal ladies both, the non-existence of laws to punish malpractice, poisoning and fraudulent manipulation of wills (by hired

---

[1] For a restoration of the *Rhizotomikon* of Crateuas, see C. Singer: Jour. Hellenic Studies, London, 1927, xlvii, 5–18. For the remains of Crateuas, see Max Wellmann's Dioscorides, Berlin, 1914, iii, 144.

[2] Sir T. C. Allbutt: Brit. Med. Jour., Lond., 1909, ii, 1451.

[3] These Roman gods were worshiped under fanciful but appropriate names, as Febris, Scabies, Angeronia, Fluonia, Uterina, Cloacina, Mephitis, Dea Salus, and the like.

[4] The favorite household remedy of the elder Cato was the cabbage.

physicians), and the enormous number of snakes kept in private houses in pursuance of the Æsculapian cult,[1] did little to make medicine respectable in the eyes of the austere Roman, who did not relish the intrusion of foreign ideas (Pliny, xxix, 5–8, 22). Apart from the writings of a private *littérateur* like Celsus, the principal Roman contribution to medicine was the splendid sanitary engineering of architects like Vitruvius. As Cos and Alexandria were the starting-points of Greek medicine, early and late, so the most eminent physicians in Rome came from Asia Minor, from the Schools of Pergamus, Ephesus, Tralles and Miletus (Wellmann). Greek medicine was finally established on a respectable footing in Rome through the personality, tact, and superior ability of **Asclepiades** of Bithynia (124 B. C.), who stood apart from the Dogmatists and the Empirics, and whose fragments are presented in Gumpert's Greek text (Weimar, 1794[2]). Asclepiades was a formal opponent of the Hippocratic idea that morbid conditions are due to a disturbance of the humors of the body (Humoralism). He attributed disease to constricted or relaxed conditions of its solid particles (Solidism). This is the so-called doctrine of the *strictum et laxum,* which was derived from the atomic theory of Democritus, and has been revived at different times under such various guises as the Brunonian theory of sthenic and asthenic states, Friedrich Hoffmann's idea of tonic and atonic conditions, Broussais' theory of irritation as a cause of disease, and Rasori's doctrine of stimulus and contrastimulus. As a logical consequence of his antagonism to Hippocrates, Asclepiades founded his therapeutic scheme on the efficiency of systematic interference as opposed to the healing power of nature; but in practice he was a real Asclepiad, wisely falling back upon the Coan régime of fresh air, light, appropriate diet, hydrotherapy, massage, clysters, local applications, and sparing internal medication. Asclepiades was the pioneer in the humane treatment of mental disorders, indeed, as Friedreich observes, "first taught us how to treat the insane." In differentiating between the Hippocratic febrile phrenitis (toxic or infectious psychoses) and afebrile mania, he notes that the frenzied patient has hallucinations (sees what is not present), the maniacal patient delusions (wrong conclusions from actuality). He therefore discarded the antique practice of keeping mental sufferers in the dark, by letting in broad daylight, since hallucinations are exaggerated in the dark (Jelliffe). For treatment, he employed occupation therapy, exercises in promoting memory and fixing attention, music and wine to promote sleep. Asclepiades was also the first to mention tracheotomy. His influence for good was that of a superior personality but died with him. His pupils and adherents, Themison and others, exaggerated his doctrines

---

[1] In 293 B. C., the cult of Æsculapius was introduced into Rome in the form of a huge serpent from Epidaurus, representing the god in his chthonian aspect (see Ovid, Metamorphoses, B., xv, 626–744).

[2] For a list of the writings of Asclepiades, see M. Wellmann, in Pauly-Wissowa: Real. Encyclop., 1896, iv, 1632.

into a formal "Methodism,"[1] while the followers of the Stoic philosophers endeavored to found a system of medicine based upon the physical action and status of the vital air or *pneuma*, which, taken in by the lungs to cool the inner heat engendered by the heart, is carried to the latter, while the blood is derived from the liver. The Hellenic Renaissance in Rome was thus characterized by three different ways of looking at disease as disturbances of the liquid, solid, or gaseous constituents of the body, viz., Humoralism, Solidism, and Pneumatism. In all this welter of theorizing, six names stand out above the rest—Celsus, Dioscorides, Rufus, Soranus, Galen, and Antyllus, and most of these were, in reality, free-lances, that is, "Eclectics." The Pneumatic School, founded by Athenæus of Attalia, and continued by his pupil, Claudius Agathinus of Sparta, the teacher of Archigenes and Leonidas, was the most important departure. The Syrian Archigenes of Apamea (*circa* 54–117 A. D.) is held by Max Wellmann to be the source of the text of Aretæus and of much in Aetius.[2] The medical literature of the 2d century A. D.—Galen, Soranus, Heliodorus, Antyllus, Aretæus, as also the great collective works of the Byzantines—was made up of excerpts and paraphrases; and this tendency persisted through the Middle Ages up to the Renaissance.

Although Roman medicine was almost entirely in Greek hands, the best account of it we have goes by the name of Aurelius Cornelius **Celsus,** who lived in the reign of Tiberius Cæsar. Celsus was inferentially, not a physician, but a private gentleman of the noble family of the Cornelii who, like Cato and Varro, compiled or, more probably, translated encyclopedic treatises on medicine, agriculture, and other subjects for the benefit of the Admirable Crichtons of his own station in life. Celsus wrote on medicine in the same spirit in which Virgil treated of veterinary matters in the third book of the Georgics, and it is presumable that in accordance with Roman usage, he rendered medical assistance gratis, very much as the mistress of an old English estate or Southern plantation played Lady Bountiful among her friends and dependents. Classed by Pliny among the men of letters (*auctores*) rather than the *medici*, Celsus was ignored by the Roman practitioners of his day, and slighted as "mediocre" (*mediocri vir ingenio*) by Quintilian. His name is mentioned only four times by the medieval commentators; but with the Revival of Learning, he had his revenge, in that his work (*De re medicina*) was one of the first medical books to be printed (1478), afterward passing through more separate editions than almost any other scientific treatise. This was due largely to the

---

[1] Allbutt says that the Methodists and the Empirics were, in some sort, a continuation of the Coan and Cnidian schools, the former considering the whole patient and his environment, the latter the locality of the disease and its local treatment. The Cnidians and the Empirics merely listed symptoms without coördinating them and were, in consequence, only haphazard therapeutists. Allbutt, Brit. Med. Jour., Lond., 1909, ii, 1449; 1515; 1598.

[2] Wellmann: Die pneumatische Schule bis auf Archigenes. Berlin, 1895. For a detailed account of the doctrines of the Pneumatic School, see pages 131–231.

purity and precison of his literary style. His elegant Latinity assured him the title of *Cicero medicorum*. Celsus is the oldest medical document after the Hippocratic writings, and, of the 72 medical authors mentioned by him, only the work of Hippocrates himself has come down to us relatively intact. The *De re medicina* consists of eight books, the first four of which deal with diseases treated by diet and regimen, the last four describing those amenable to drugs and surgery. The third book contains, among other things, the first use of the term "insanity" (*Insania*) and the first adumbration of heart disease (*Cardiacus*), which became the canon of subsequent knowledge in antiquity.[1] The fourth book contains the four classical signs of inflammation (Ch. 10). The fifth book begins with a classified list of drugs, followed by a chapter on weights and measures, pharmaceutic methods, and prescriptions, very much like a modern hand-book of therapeutics. Celsus was the first to recommend nutritive enemata. The sixth book treats of skin[2] and venereal diseases as well as those of the eye, ear, nose, throat, and mouth. The seventh book is surgical, and contains one of the first accounts of the use of the ligature, and a classic description of lateral lithotomy. Under the Romans, surgery (including obstetrics and ophthalmology) attained a degree of perfection which it was not to reach again before the time of Ambroise Paré. Surgical instrumentation, in particular, was highly specialized. Over two hundred different surgical instruments were found at Pompeii. Herniotomy and plastic surgery were known, as well as the operations for cataract, version, and Cesarean section. Sufficient reason for all this may be found in the constant contact of the Romans with gladiatorial and military surgery, and the fact that the dissection of executed criminals was sometimes allowed. Hippocrates said that "war is the only proper school for the surgeon." Celsus is also very effective on the different malarial fevers of Italy and their treatment, on gout, and on the treatment of different kinds of insanity. With a flash of intuition, he infers the return of the blood-current to its starting-point (*sanguis cursus revocetur*). He was the first important writer on medical history. His Proæmium establishes the status of Hippocrates, Herophilus, Erasistratus, and other great names of the past in the spirit of one who might himself have said

> I write as others wrote
> On Sunium's height.

The close and careful investigation of the sources of Celsus by Max Wellmann[3] suggests, by confrontation and comparison of many parallel passages, that this great

[1] For a full account of the ancient conception of cardiac diseases, see Landsberg: Janus, Bresl., 1847, ii, 53–124.

[2] Of the forty skin diseases described by Celsus, alopecia areata is still remembered as "area Celsi."

[3] Wellmann: A. Cornelius Celsus: Eine Quellenuntersuchung, Berlin, 1913. Arch. f. Gesch. d. med., Leipz., 1924–5, xvi, 209–213; Ann. Med. Hist., N. Y., 1926, viii, 203–207.

text is probably a compilation, perhaps a translation, deriving mainly from the genuine Hippocratic writings, from the fragment on fistula by Asclepiades' pupil, the surgeon Meges, from the pharmacologic and therapeutic writings of Heraclides of Tarentum (including his exegesis of Hippocrates), and from Asclepiades himself and his school. In Wellmann's view, the presumable Greek source of Celsus would then be some medical handbook for the laity, written before 20 A. D. by Tiberius Claudius Menecrates, a body-physician to Tiberius Cæsar (14–37 A. D.). Of the 105 different editions of Celsus extant, the most interesting are the Florentine *editio princeps* (1478), the Milan imprint of 1481, the Venetian imprint of 1524 (the rarest and costliest of all), the Aldine of 1525, and the handsome Elzevir of 1657. The handiest modern editions are Daremberg's Teubner (Leipzig, 1859) and the bilinguals of Alexander Lee (1831) and A. Vedrènes (1876), which is prefaced by the lucid and scholarly essay of Paul Broca (1865). The authoritative modern edition is the Teubner of Friedrich Marx (1915).

The three leading Greek surgeons of the period contemporary with Celsus were the Pneumatists Heliodorus, Archigenes (both mentioned in Juvenal and the latter contemporaneous with Celsus), Antyllus, contemporaneous with Galen, all of whom have come down to us in the compilations of the Byzantine writers. **Heliodorus,** who antedated Celsus, gave the first account of ligation and torsion of blood-vessels, and was one of the first to treat stricture by internal urethrotomy. He also described head injuries, the operative treatment of hernia, circular and flap amputations. The latter procedure was fully described by **Archigenes** of Apamea, and both surgeons employed ligatures which, in Galen's time, were to be bought at a special shop in the Via Sacra. **Antyllus,** long before Daviel, mentions the removal of cataract by extraction and suction, but his name and fame are permanently associated with his well-known method of treating aneurysms by applying two ligatures and cutting down between them, which held the field until the time of John Hunter.

Pedacius **Dioscorides,** the originator of the materia medica, was a Greek army surgeon in the service of Nero (54–68 A. D.), and utilized his opportunities of travel in the study of plants. His work is the authoritative source on the materia medica of antiquity, of which he describes about 600 plants and plant-principles, over a hundred more than Theophrastus. About 149 of these were already known to Hippocrates,[1] and no less than 90 are still in use today.[2] As Theophrastus was the first scientific botanist, so Dioscorides was the first to write on medical botany as an applied science. His first book deals with aromatic, oily, gummy, or resinous plant-products; the second with animal products of dietetic and medicinal value, and with cereals and garden herbs; the third and fourth, with the other medicinal plants. His classification was qualitative, as in a materia medica, rather than botanical, but, like Theophrastus, he recognized natural families of plants before Linnæus, Adanson, and Jussieu. His descriptions were followed "word by word" for sixteen centuries, and his book was more attentively studied than any other botanical work, with the possible exception of

---

[1] See Rudolf Mock: Tübingen diss., 1909.
[2] See Rudolf Schmid: Tübingen diss., 1919.

Bauhin's *Pinax* (1623[1]).   Up to the beginning of the 17th century the best books on medical botany were virtual commentaries on the treatise of Dioscorides, the historic source of most of our herbal therapy, even of the famous medieval substitutes for anesthesia.   Mandragora wine (*oinos mandragorites*) is prescribed internally by Dioscorides as a draught for insomnia or pain, and in three places (IV, 76) he recommends it explicitly in surgical operations or cauterization.

The most important codex of Dioscorides is the 9th century MS. in the Bibliothèque Nationale, Paris (gr. 2179), which is beautifully illustrated and is basic for establishing the text, as going back to an early tradition.   The alphabetized codices include the Constantinopolitan or Vienna Codex (prepared for the Byzantine princess Julia Anicia before 512 A. D.; reprinted in photographic facsimile, Leyden, 1906) and the Neapolitan, both illustrated and now in the St. Mark's Library (Venice). The Cheltenham (Phillipps) MS. (21,975), of the 10th century, is now in the Pierpont Morgan Library (New York).   The "Latin Dioscorides" translated in the time of Cassiodorus (490–585 A. D.) for the use of the monks at Squillace, comprises two variants, the Lombard Dioscorides,[2] a 9th century MS. in Beneventan script (Munich MS. 337), and a Dioscorides vulgaris (Singer) in a palimpsest of 600 at Vienna (Latin MS. 16), printed at Colle, near Siena, by Johann von Medemblich in 1478 (Hain, 6258) and at Leyden (1512).   After Dioscorides, the only Greek herbal of consequence was the De simplicibus of Galen (180 A. D.).   The most interesting editions of Dioscorides are the Aldine of 1499 (Greek text), the Stephanus of 1516 (Latin translation of Ruellius), the rare bilingual text of Cologne (1529), and the Latin text and commentary of Mattioli (Venice, 1554), which passed through many editions and translations, including the rare Italian (Venice, 1554) and the two Czech versions (Prague, 1562, 1596).   The Græco-Latin text of Kurt Sprengel (Leipzig, 1829–30), the definitive Greek text of Max Wellmann (3 vols., 1906–14), and the German translation, with marginalia, by J. Berendes (Stuttgart, 1902) are all valuable.   The spurious Latin *Dyascorides de herbis femininis* is a 6th century hodge-podge from the Latin Dioscorides, pseudo-Apuleius and Pliny, found in a 9th century MS. at Rome (Barberini MS. 160[3]), and vaguely known as "pseudo-Dioscorides."[4]

Aretæus the Cappadocian, who also lived either under Domitian or Hadrian (2d to 3d century A. D.) comes nearer than any other Greek to the spirit and method of Hippocrates, and is on this account more readily appreciated by modern readers.   In opposition to the view of Klose, Max Wellmann claims, from careful comparison of texts, that Aretæus derives in part from Archigenes, but he is, at any rate, our most important source for the teachings of the Pneumatic School.[5]   As a clinician, Aretæus ranks next to the Father of Medicine in the graphic accuracy and fidelity of his pictures of disease, of which he has given the classic accounts of pneumonia, pleurisy with empyema,

---

[1] E. L. Greene: "Landmarks of Botanical History," Wash., 1909, 151–155. Max Wellmann: Die Schrift des Dioscorides, Berlin, 1914, and Hermes, Berlin, 1889, xxiv, 530–569.

[2] For authentic text of the Lombard (Munich) Dioscorides, see Romanische Forschungen (K. Vollmoller), Erlangen, 1882–97, i, 50; x, 181, 301; xi, 1.

[3] For text of De herbis feminis, see Hermes, Berlin, 1896, xxxi, pp. 578 et seq.

[4] H. Stadler: Janus, Amst., 1899, iv, 548–550.

[5] See Wellmann: Die pneumatische Schule, Berlin, 1895, 22–64.   The relation between Aretæus and Archigenes was first noted by Sprengel.   C. W. Klose (Janus, Gotha, 1851, i, 105; 217) maintained that Aretæus preceded Archigenes and was copied by him, but Wellmann's view seems the more probable.   For the many attempts to fix the lifetime of Aretæus, see Klose, p. 109.

uiabetes, tetanus, elephantiasis, diphtheria (ulcera Syriaca), the aura in epilepsy, the first clear differentiation between cerebral and spinal paralysis, indicating the decussation of the pyramids, and a very full account of the different kinds of insanity. He notes the transition in adults from melancholia (a black-bile condition with fixed ideas) to acute maniacal excitement, in other words, the intermittent character of circular (manic-depressive) insanity, as contrasted with the hopeless, settled, incurable status of senile (involutional) melancholia. Aretæus is easily the most attractive medical author of his time. He was essentially a stylist, and the character of his Ionic Greek is held to indicate a late period. His work is preserved in the faulty Greek text of 1554, in Wigan's valued Clarendon Press edition (Oxford, 1723), the Leipzig text of Kühn (1828), and the Greek text with English translation by Francis Adams (London, 1858).

Another great eclectic was **Rufus of Ephesus**, who lived in the reign of Trajan (98–117 A. D.), and whose literary remains and fragments have been preserved in the Paris text of 1554, and the bilingual of Daremberg (Paris, 1879).

He wrote a little work on anatomy in which he described the crystalline lens, the membranes of the eye, the optic chiasm, and the oviduct in the sheep. He was the first to describe the liver as porcine (five-lobed), a blunder which was perpetrated up to Vesalius. Rufus wrote an excellent tract on the pulse, noting that pulse, heart-beat and systole are synchronous. He also gave the first descriptions of traumatic erysipelas, epithelioma, and bubonic plague (derived from Alexandrian sources). His treatise on gout was translated into Latin (6th century A. D.). He added many new compounds to the materia medica, of which his *hiera*, a purgative containing colocynth, became celebrated. Rufus was a good surgeon and described all the known methods of hemostasis, "digital compression, styptics, the cautery, torsion, and the ligature" (Osler).

Soranus of Ephesus of the 2d century A. D., a follower of the Methodist school of Asclepiades, is our leading authority on the gynecology, obstetrics, and pediatrics of antiquity. His treatise on midwifery and diseases of women, preserved in Dietz's Greek text (Königsberg, 1838[1]), was the original of such famous works as Röslin's *Rosengarten* (1513), and Raynalde's *Byrthe of Mankynde* (1545). Most of the supposed innovations in these books, such as the obstetric chair or podalic version, have been traced back to Soranus. Deriving from Soranus is the obstetric treatise of Moschion (6th century A. D.), edited by Caspar Wolff (Gynæcia, Basel, 1566), and F. O. Dewez (Vienna, 1793), and containing drawings of the female genitalia and of the *fœtus in utero*, which may go back to classical antiquity. After Soranus, there were no real additions to obstetrics before the time of Paré, some 1500 years later. The pediatric section in Soranus is the finest contribution to the subject in antiquity, containing the most rational precepts as to infant hygiene and nutrition, with separate

---

[1] Later editions of Soranus by Ermerins (1869), Valentine Rose (1882), and one in preparation by Joh. Ilberg. German translation by H. Lüneberg (München, 1894). French version by F. J. Herrgott (Nancy, 1895). See also J. Ilberg: Abhandl. d. philol.-hist. Kl. d. sächs. Gesellsch. d. Wissensch., Leipz., 1910, xxviii, 1–122.

chapters on infantile diseases, including a recognizable account of rickets.

The Natural History of **Pliny the Elder** (23–79 A. D.), of which Books XX–XXXII deal exclusively with medicine, is a vast compilation of all that was known in his time of geography, meteorology, anthropology, botany, zoölogy, and mineralogy, and is interesting for its many curious facts about plants and drugs, its sidelights on Roman medicine,[1] and its author's many slaps at physicians. It was the one book of classical antiquity which was read steadily throughout the Dark Ages, as evidenced by the hundred or more extant manuscripts. After the invention of printing, it passed through more than 80 editions.

It contains the original references to many unique things, such as scurvy (*stomacace*), Druidical medicine, superfetation, and atavism (*ipse avum regeneravit æthiopum*), the case of Marcus Curius Dentatus, who was born with teeth, the artificial iron hand of Marcus Sergius, the great-grandfather of Catiline,[2] Mithridates' experiments with poisons, the narcotic properties of mandragora juice, or Nero's use of an emerald as a mirror (*Nero princeps gladiatorum pugnas spectabat in smaragdo*), which, some writers think, may have been an actual eyeglass. Books XX–XXV comprise a vast herbal, derived mainly from Theophrastus[3] and which exerted a profound influence upon Anglo-Saxon medical plant-lore (Singer). The botanical errors of Pliny remained unchallenged until the time of Nicholas Leonicenus (1492).

The ancient period closes with the name of the greatest Greek physician after Hippocrates, **Galen**[4] (131–201 A. D.), the founder of experimental physiology. Born an architect's son at Pergamus, Galen's youth and old age were those of a peripatetic. His life was one long *Wanderjahr*. At Rome, where he commenced practice in 164 A. D., he soon attained the leadership of his profession, but retired early to devote himself to study, travel, and teaching. Compared with Hippocrates, Galen seems like the versatile, many-sided man of talent as contrasted with the man of true genius. He was the most skilled practioner of his time, but left no good accounts of clinical cases, only miraculous cures. He usually got his patients well, and to this end instituted an elaborated system of polypharmacy,[5] the memory of which survives in our language in the term "galenicals," as applied to vegetable simples.[6] Galen's place in science is very high, but his roving disposition undoubtedly did much to develop that cocksure attitude of mind, which made his writings the fountain-head of ready-made theory and "polypragmatism."

---

[1] Summarized in the Medicina Plinii, edited by Pighinucci (Rome, 1509). See V. Rose: Hermes, Berlin, 1874, viii, 19–66.

[2] See Sudhoff: Mitt. z. Gesch. d. Med., Leipz., 1916, xv, 1–5.

[3] J. G. Sprengel: Marburg diss., 1890.

[4] From the 15th century on, the erroneous form "Claudius Galen" has been much employed. Klebs (Prosopographia imperii Romani, 1897, i, 374–380), shows it to be a misreading of Cl[arissimus] Galen (Sudhoff).

[5] Asclepiades, Allbutt says, tended to dissipate the specific in the universal (physiologic therapeutics); Galen, proceeding from a theoretic monotheism, tended to lose the universal in the particular (polypharmacy).

[6] The *De simplicibus* of Galen (*circa* 180 B. C.) was the only Greek herbal of importance after Dioscorides, and was cribbed extensively in the *Synagoge* of Oribasius (Singer).

He had an answer ready for every problem, a reason to assign for every phenomenon. He elaborated a system of pathology, which combined the humoral ideas of Hippocrates with the Pythagorean theory of the four elements and his own conception of a spirit or *"pneuma"* penetrating all the parts. Referring all pathologic phenomena back to these postulates, Galen, with fatal facility and ingenuity, proceeded to explain everything in the light of pure theory, thus substituting a pragmatical system of medical philosophy for the plain notation and interpretation of facts as taught by Hippocrates. The effect of this dogmatism and infallibility upon after-time was appalling; for while Galen's monotheism and piety appealed to the Moslems, his assumption of omniscience was specially adapted to appease the mental indolence and flatter the complacency of those who were swayed entirely by reverence for authority. Up to the time of Vesalius, European medicine was one vast *argumentum ad hominem* in which everything relating to anatomy and physiology, as well as disease, was referred back to Galen as a final authority, from whom there could be no appeal. After his death, European medicine remained at a dead level for nearly fourteen centuries.

Galenic physiology and pathology was based upon an abstruse and artificial combination of humoralism and Pythagorean number lore, viz., the doctrine of naturals (7), non-naturals (6), and contranaturals (3) which dominated Arabic and medieval medicine for centuries. The subjoined arrangement is from Joannitius (Withington[1]).

The seven naturals are the elements (4), the qualities (9), the humors (4), the members (4), the faculties (3), the operations (2), the spirits (3), to which were sometimes added the ages (4), the colors (2), the figures (5), and the sexes (2). The elements (4) are fire, air, earth, and water, the 9 qualities are hot, cold, moist, and dry, the qualities of fire (hot and dry), air (hot and moist), earth (cold and dry), and water (cold and moist), the ninth quality being a fairly equal distribution of heat, cold, moisture, and dryness in the body. The 4 humors are blood (hot and moist), phlegm (cold and moist), yellow bile (hot and dry), black bile (cold and dry). The 4 members are the fundamental (brain, heart, liver), the subservient (nerves, arteries, veins), the specific (bone, membranes, muscles), the dependent (stomach, kidneys, intestines). The 3 faculties are natural, spiritual, and animal. The animal faculties comprise cerebration *via* imagination (forebrain), cogitation (midbrain), and memory (hind-brain), also voluntary motion and sensation. Operations include the simple, viz., hunger (heat and dryness), digestion (heat and moisture), retention (coldness and dryness), and expulsion, (coldness and moisture), and the compound (due to appetites and sensations). The 3 spirits are the natural (from the liver to the body by the veins), the vital (from the heart by the arteries), and the animal (from the brain by the nerves). The ages are youth (hot and moist), manhood (hot and dry), age (cold and dry), and senility (cold and moist). Colors (2) are red, white, yellow, and black, due to balance or excess of the humors, and those due to external temperature (heat and cold). Figures (5) are fat, thin, synthetic (cold and dry), squalid (cold and moist), and equable (balanced). Sexes are male and female. The 6 non-naturals (things not innate) are air, food, and drink, rest and exercise, sleep and waking, excretions and retentions (coitus), and mental affections. The 3 contranaturals (things against nature) are diseases, their causes and sequels. Galen divides diseases into three classes, viz., (a) those affecting similar parts or simple tissues (muscles, nerves); (b) organic (affecting compound tissues); and (c) general or humoral, *i. e.*, dyscrasias (imbalance of the humors). Organic diseases comprise malformations and abnormities of size, position, and number (presence or absence). Causes of disease are (a) procatartic or exciting; (b) proegumenic or predisposing, and synectic or coincident. Symptoms follow the disease "as the shadow follows the

---

[1] See E. T. Withington: Medical History, London, 1894, 98; 386.

8

substance," and are altered functions, vitiated qualities (*vide supra*) or results of both (morbid excretions and retentions). Signs show what the disease is (diagnostic, pathognomonic) or how it will end (prognostic). Fevers are three, viz., (1) ephemeral, in the spirits; (2) putrid, in the putrefying humors; (3) hectic, in the solids. Putrid fevers are four, viz., (1) synochal or continued (in the blood); (2) tertian (in the yellow bile); (3) quotidian (in the phlegm); (4) quartan (in the black bile). Inflammations are four, viz., (1) phlegmon (from blood); (2) erysipelas (from yellow bile); (3) edema, tumor (from coagulated phlegm); (4) cancer (from black bile). Therapeutics are either general, as dealing with the management of the six non-naturals, or specific, as dealing with diseases of similar parts or of organs and wounds. It is plain that this elaborate scheme of things is virtually a phase of Cnidian medicine which has left its mark upon text-books of practice up to very recent times.

Galen was the most voluminous of all the ancient writers, and the greatest of the theorists and systematists. His works are a gigantic encyclopedia of the knowledge of his time, including 9 books on anatomy (*Encheiresis*), 17 on physiology (*De usu partium*), 6 on pathology (*De locis affectis*), 16 essays on the pulse, the Megatechne (*Ars magna*) or therapeutics (14 books), the Microtechne (*Ars parva*) or "practice," 3 books on the temperaments, and 30 books on pharmacy. He differentiated pneumonia from pleurisy, was the first to mention aneurysm,[1] separating the traumatic from the dilated form, described the different forms of phthisis, mentioning its infectious nature and proposing a full milk diet and climatotherapy (sea voyages and dry elevated places) for treatment; he understood the diathetic relation between calculus and gout, and his prescriptions indicate a most intelligent use of opium, hyoscyamus, hellebore and colocynth, hartshorn, turpentine, alcohol (wine), sugar diet (honey), grape-juice, barley-water, and cold compresses. He introduced the doctrine of the four temperaments, and set the pace for a fantastic pulse-lore or *ars sphygmica*, which was still in vogue in the 18th century. He traveled far to learn all he could about the native remedies of different regions, and even paid two special vists to the isle of Lemnos in order to investigate the therapeutic value of its sacred sealed earth (*terra sigillata*[2]).

As an anatomist, Galen left many excellent descriptions, especially of the motor and locomotor systems, but his work was faulty and inaccurate, as being based largely on the dissection of apes and swine. He studied osteology in the ape (*Macacus ecaudatus*) and from stray human skeletons, such as that of the robber he once found on a lonely mountainside. His myology was based mainly upon the study of the musculature of the Barbary ape (*Macacus inuus*), but he clearly understood the difference between origin and insertion and knew most of the muscles and their functions, although he had little nomenclature.[3] His splanchnology was defective and erroneous; his neurology is the best feature of his anatomical work. From his dissections of the brains of oxen, he distinguished the dura mater and pia mater, the corpus cal-

[1] "Methodus Medendi," lib. v, f. 63 (Linacre's translation of 1519).

[2] C. J. S. Thompson: Terra sigillata, Tr. XVII. Internat. Med. Cong., 1913 Lond., 1914, sect. xxiii, 433–444.

[3] J. S. Milne: Galen's knowledge of muscular anatomy, *ibid.*, 389–400.

losum, the third and fourth ventricles with the iter (Sylvian aqueduct), the fornix, corpora quadrigemina, vermiform process, calamus scriptorius, hypophysis, and infundibulum. Of the twelve cerebral nerves, he knew seven pairs,[1] also the sympathetic ganglia, which he described as the reinforcers of the nerves. His treatise on anatomical "administration" (*Encheiresis*) was the first treatise on dissection,[2] and authoritative through the centuries. His contributions to the science were accepted as finalities up to the time of Vesalius. But if Galen's anatomy failed in the long run, through the fact that it was simian, canine, bovine, porcine, rather than human, and because he subordinated accurate description of structures to speculation about their functions, he was the first and foremost contributor to **experimental physiology**[3] before Harvey, and the first experimental neurologist. He was the first to describe the cranial nerves and the sympathetic system, made the first experimental sections of the spinal cord, producing hemiplegia; produced aphonia by cutting the recurrent laryngeal nerve, and gave the first valid explanation of the mechanism of respiration. His notations of experimental paralyses, produced by section of the spinal cord[4] at different levels, were copied by Oribasius.[5] He showed that the arteries contain blood (by performing the Antyllus operation), and demonstrated the motor power of the heart by showing that the blood pulsates between the heart and a ligated artery, but not beyond it. Like Erasistratus, he inferred that the capillaries are provided with adjacent mouths (*synanastomoses*). He also showed that an excised heart will beat outside the body, a common incident at the sacrificial rites, and good evidence that its beat does not depend upon the nervous system. In like manner, he inferred, from experiments with excised muscle, that its contractions may be independent of volition or nerve-supply at need, likened contraction to clinical tetanus, introduced the concept *tonus* as "active posture" (Sherrington), and had some notion of reciprocal action of antagonistic muscles (Fulton). In these matters Galen gave to medicine that method of putting questions to nature and of arranging things so that nature may answer them, which we call experiment. Here, he fully deserves the encomium of Guy de Chauliac, that he was "greatest in experimental demonstration." Daremberg once repeated all of Galen's experiments in the Jardin des Plantes. In his physiologic speculations about his findings, Galen spoiled his work by his mania for teleology, which he got from Aristotle's reading of nature. His bump of reverence was inordinately developed and, al-

---

[1] For Galen's knowledge of the cerebral nerves, see Th. Beck, Arch. f. Gesch. Med., Leipz., 1909–10, iii, 110–114.

[2] For Galen's technique in dissection and vivisection, see Friedrich Ullrich, Leipzig diss. (Inst. f. Gesch. d. Med.), 1919.

[3] For an analysis of Galen's physiological achievement see Th. Meyer-Steineg: Arch. f. Gesch. d. Med., Leipz., 1911–12, v, 172; 417.

[4] Galen: Encheiresis, viii, 9 (Kühn, ii, 696–698). De symptomatum causis, i, 5 (Kühn, vii, 111).

[5] Oribasius, xxiv, 3 (Daremberg, iii, 290–294).

though he was right in his primary assumption that structure follows function, his enthusiasm led him into the strangest and most arbitrary hypotheses, based *a priori* upon his centric idea that every thing in nature shows an element of design and the goodness of the Creator. Modern biologists see the living creature and its life-history as the resultant of the parallelogram of two forces, the reaction of the innate heredity against the outer environment. They reason that differences in structure are the resultant of adaptation to the stress and strain of environment. But Galen, as Neuburger puts it, made his whole physiological theory "a skilful and well-instructed special pleading for the cause of design in nature," whereby he lost himself in *a priori* speculations "to explain nature's execution before even her mechanism had been demonstrated." He never really sought *how* an organ functions, but in blind obeisance to Aristotle ("Nature makes nothing in vain") he reiterated the transcendental *why*, which Kant and Claude Bernard pronounced to be forever insoluble. Yet in spite of this subjective teleology, Galen's experiments on the physiology of the nervous, respiratory, and circulatory systems were the only real knowledge for seventeen centuries.[1]

There are three Galenic superstitions which, through their plausible character, have had a great deal to do with preventing the advancement of medical science. First, the doctrine of Vitalism, which maintained that the blood is endued with "natural spirits" in the liver, with "vital spirits" in the left ventricle of the heart, and that the vital spirits are converted into "animal spirits" in the brain, the whole organism being animated by a "pneuma." Modifications of this theory, however attractive, have driven physiology into many a delusive blind alley, even up to the time of Driesch. Second, the notion that the blood, in its transit through the body, passes from the right to the left ventricle by means of certain imaginary invisible pores in the interventricular septum, prevented theorists from having real insight into the circulation until the time of Harvey.[2] Third, the idea that "coction" or suppuration is an essential part of the healing of wounds led to those Arabist notions of "healing by second intention," setons and laudable pus, which, although combated by Mondeville, Paracelsus and Paré, were not entirely overthrown before the advent of Lister.

Of the many editions of Galen's works, the most important are the Aldine Greek text of 1525 (five volumes), the Basel edition of 1538, with the initial letter by Holbein, and the nine different editions of the Latin text published by the house

[1] A possible exception to this statement would be the few physiologic experiments made by Vesalius which, however, passed unnoticed in his time.

[2] Galen regarded the arterial blood (charged with "vital" spirits) and the venous blood (charged with "natural" spirits) as ebbing and flowing, back and forth, through their respective channels, but having no connection with each other except through the interventricular pores. In like manner the "animal (psychical) spirits" were supposed to course back and forth through the hollow nerves, which became solid after death. For a good account of this archaic physiology, see Sir Michael Foster, "Lectures on the History of Physiology," Cambridge, 1901, pp. 12, 13.

of Giunta at Venice between the years 1541 and 1625. Of Latin translations, Conrad Gesner's (Basel, 1562), with the biographic illustrations on the title page, and those of Linacre, are perhaps the most famous. The best and most readable are the Giunta and the Froben. Among the modern editions, the most useful for ready reference is the 20-volume Greek and Latin text of Kühn (Leipzig, 1821–33[1]), with a valuable index supplementing the wonderful concordance made by Brassavola (1551). Very handy is Daremberg's anthology in two volumes (Paris, 1854–6). Galen's seven books of anatomy, an Arabic MS. of the 9th century A. D., with German translation and commentary by Max Simon (Leipzig, 1906) is very valuable. The most famous single treatise of Galen is his monograph on the physiologic and teleo-logic aspects of the different parts of the human body (*De usu partium*), the proto-type of all subsequent "Bridgewater treatises." The treatise on the physiology of muscle (*De motu musculorum*) was Latinized by Leonicenus (1509–20), edited by Linacre and published by Pynson (London, 1522) and Simon Colinæus (Paris, 1528). The Corpus medicorum Græcorum (Leipzig and Berlin), a series of Teubner texts published under the auspices of the collective scientific academies of Europe, will include all the Greek writers. The standard source for the minor Greek and Græco-Latin writers is Valentin Rose's *Anecdota græca et græco latina* (Berlin, 1864–70).

Of the condition of medicine under the Romans considerable is known but little need be said. Much of Roman medicine is found in the secular writers, particularly the poets, dramatists, satirists, and epigrammatists, and in the inscriptions.

Of the Latin writers, Plautus and Terence are remarkable for sidelights on obstetrics and popular medicine; Lucretius for anatomy, physiology, dietetics, hygiene, climatology, and the famous account of the plague at Athens which ter-minates his sixth book; Virgil for veterinary medicine; Horace, Juvenal, and Persius for satirical sidelights on diseases and drugs of the time, personal hygiene, criminal abortion, insanity; Ovid, Catullus, Tibullus, and Propertius for innumerable details about sexual vices, venereal diseases, aphrodisiacs, and cosmetics; Martial and Petronius for sexual perversions; Cicero and the younger Pliny for internal medicine; Lucan for vivid accounts of war wounds and bites of poisonous serpents; Livy for Roman medico-military administration; Tacitus for the anthropology of ancient Germany; Suetonius for the vices and mental disorders of the Cæsars. Horace, an intimate of the physician Antonius Musa, gives semeiologic details with classic concision. Ovid, in his account of the plague of Ægina, is a better epidemiologist than Thucydides or Lucretius. Virgil, most learned in medicine, described anthrax in sheep, and indicates the knowledge of contagion from herd to herd.

"Nec mala vicini pecoris contagia laedent."

Mosquito netting (*conopeum*) is mentioned by Horace and Juvenal. Aulus Gellius is quite modern in his exposition of infant hygiene and nutrition. Medicine in the Latin poets has been carefully studied by Prosper Menière[2] and Edmond Dupouy.[3] Birkholtz made an anthology of medical excerpts from Cicero (1806[4]); Jelliffe has studied the Roman psychiaters of the Augustan period; but the whole field, so rich in details for medical historians, has been but little explored.

Rome was ever a hard, cold-blooded task-mistress, with a callous policy of "duties without rights" for the army and the people, who were governed by force, fear, hunger, impoverishment, and worked to the stage of exhaustion which destroys inventive genius. The later

---

[1] For a valuable tabulation of Galen's citations from the older writers (ed. Kühn), see J. Zimmermann's Berlin dissertation (1902).

[2] P. Menière: Études médicales sur les poètes latines, Paris, 1858.

[3] E. Dupouy: Médecine et mœurs de l'ancienne Rome, 2 éd., Paris, 1892.

[4] Birkholtz: Cicero medicus, Leipzig, 1806.

Empire was a virtual bureaucracy in which, as in pre-war Petrograd, everyone was a functionary. Only the well-to-do had a home (*domus*). In the city, most of the people lived huddled together in huge, rambling, jerry-built tenements (*insulæ*), which sometimes collapsed of their own weight. Exhaustion-psychoses were common and a general exhaustion-neurosis is noted by recent historians as one of the causes of the downfall. Underneath the elaborate formalities of a highly artificial veneer of culture, Wells notes a childish delight in cruelty, as if "the misshapen, hairy paw" of Neanderthal man were thrust at us by a morning caller, along with the mental infantilism which favored augury, ignored geography, was inept in chronology, and snubbed science and medicine. Before the 2d century A. D., the Romans employed medical slaves (*servi medici*), or relied upon their household medical gods, with an occasional dilettante interest in healing on their own account. But even after Asclepiades, Galen and Soranus had made the status of medicine respectable, the Roman Quirites continued to regard the profession as beneath them. Under Augustus Cæsar, however, physicians acquired the equestrian dignity of the knightly class (*equites*), and the army had a well-organized medical corps. In arrangement and appointments, the military hospitals excavated at Novæsium, near Bonn (1887–1901) and Carnuntum, on the Danube (1904), both of the 1st century A. D., surpass anything else of the kind in antiquity. These, and all other construction and public works, such as the building of forts, canals, sewers, water-courses, the dredging of harbors and the drainage of swamps, were done by soldiers of the Roman army.[1]

Some Romans, early and late, practised or wrote upon medicine, such as Scribonius Largus, author of *Compositiones Medicorum* (47 A. D.), a compilation of drugs and prescriptions, who also left an important expectorant mixture for phthisis and first suggested the use of the electric ray-fish in headaches; Cælius Aurelianus, the 5th century neurologist, who gives the most sensible and humane treatment of insanity in antiquity, prescribed sun-baths for chronic affections, and paraphrased a lost work of Soranus of Ephesus on practice; Quintus Serenus Samonicus, who wrote a didactic poem on popular medicine in the 3d century A. D. (taken from Pliny); Sextus Placitus Papyriensis, who wrote a book on animal medicine (4th century); Vindicianus Afer, who wrote anatomic treatises and a formulary in the same period; Cassius Felix, some time regarded as the original source of Celsus (Wellmann), and Theodorus Priscianus, court physician to Gratian.

Besides the "medici" proper, there were the herb gatherers (*rhizotomi*), the drug-peddlers (*pharmacopolæ*), the salve-dealers (*unguentarii*), the army surgeons (*medici cohortis, medici legionis*), and the *archiatri* or body physicians to the emperors, some of whom were also public or communal (*archiatri populares*). There were also the less reputable *iatroliptæ* or bath attendants, *medicæ* or female healers, *sagæ* or wise-women, *obstetricæ*, or midwives, the professional poisoners (*pharmacopæi*), and the depraved characters who sold philters and abortifacients. A very dubious and much satirized class were the eye

[1] Marquardt and Mommsen: Handbuch der römischen Alterthümer. 2. Aufl., Leipzig, 1884, v, 568–573.

specialists or oculists (*medici ocularii*) who, each of them, sold a special eye-salve stamped with his own private seal, usually compounded of salts of zinc and other metals. Nearly 200 of these seals have been found. The house of the Vettii, excavated at Pompeii, has a mural painting, representing cupids and psyches as "*unguentarii*" in the act of expressing, heating, testing, and selling olive oil (Peters). Many evidences of Roman medicine have been found in Britain.[1]

A special feature of Roman medicine was the cultivation of warm public baths (*thermæ*) and of mineral springs.

General hydrotherapy was introduced by Asclepiades, and no less than 1800 public baths had been founded during the period 334 B. C.–180 A. D. (Haeser). The baths of Caracalla and Diocletian had marble accommodations for 1600 and 3000 persons respectively, the water being supplied from the great aqueducts. The establishments for cold bathing (*frigidaria*) often had a swimming-pool (*piscina*) attached, and the warm baths (*tepidaria, calidaria*) were sometimes heated both as to the water and to the air of the room. **Central heating** of habitations by piping from hollow chambers under the floor (*hypocausta*), introduced by Sergius Orata (100 B. C.) was described by Vitruvius (50 B. C.), became common practice in the houses of the wealthy about 10 A. D., and even extended to Britain.[2] Specimens have been excavated under the *caldarum* (sweating room) of the old and new baths at Pompeii, in the baths of Caracalla (Herculaneum) and the palace and *thermæ* at Treves (*circa* 286–388 A. D.). The principal natural springs were the thermæ at Baiæ near Naples, Thermopylæ in Greece (especially patronized by the Emperor Hadrian), and, in the Roman Colonies, Aix les Bains (*Aquæ Gratinæ Allobrogum*), Aix in Provence (*Aquæ Sextiæ*), Bagnères de Bigorre (*Vicus Aquensis*), Baden in Switzerland (*Thermopolis*), Baden near Vienna (*Aquæ Pannonicæ*), Baden-Baden (*Civitas Aquensis*), Aix la Chapelle (*Aquisgranum*), and Wiesbaden (*Aquæ Mattiacenses*[3]). Military hospitals (*valetudinaria*) are mentioned by Hyginus, and have been excavated at Neuss (*Castrum Novæsium*) and Carnuntum (near Vienna).

The Etruscans were wonderfully skilled in dentistry. Martial mentions false teeth. Some remarkable specimens of Etruscan bridgework are preserved in the museum of Corneto and have been described by Guerini and Walsh.[4]

The Roman rite of lustration, or purification of a town-site, field, or body of people within an area, by a repeated processional around it, was intimately connected with the enumeration of troops before and after battle, and the quinquennial **census** of Rome. The Roman census, as conducted by the censors, was probably a matter of military necessity.[5]

The special talent of the Romans was for military science, and the making and administration of laws. Their hygienic achievements, such as cremation, town-planning, the sensible, well-ventilated houses, central heating, the paved streets and macadamized roads, the great aqueducts, sewers, drains and public baths, the solicitude for pure food

---

[1] See H. Barnes: Proc. Roy. Soc. Med. (Sect. Hist. Med.), Lond., 1913–14, vii, 71–87.

[2] O. Krell: Altrömische Heizungen, Munich, 1901. W. Berman (R. Meikleham): History and Art of Warming, 2 v., London, 1845.

[3] Haeser: "Lehrb. d. Gesch. d. Med." 3. Aufl., Leipz., 1875, i, 494.

[4] Guerini: "History of Dentistry," New York, 1909, 67–76, and J. J. Walsh, "Modern Progress and History," New York, 1912, 79–103. For ancient dental forceps, see Sudhoff: Arch. f. Gesch. d. Med., Leipz., 1908–9, ii, 55–69, 3 pl.

[5] "Lustrum nominatum tempus quinquenniale a luendo, id est solvendo; quod quinto quoque anno vectegalia et ultro tributa per censores persolvebantur," Varro: De lingua Latina, vi, 11. Cited by W. W. Fowler in Anthropology and the Classics, Oxford, 1908, 173.

as part of the cult of Vesta and Juturna, were of far greater consequence than their native literary contributions to medicine. Yet even here, as Sudhoff says, they often produced hygienic results without medical intention, things of hygienic value but of non-medical origin.[1] Roman medicine, at best, can only be regarded as an offshoot or subvariety of Greek medicine.

[1] Karl Sudhoff: Deutsche Revue, Stuttg., Oct., 1911, 40–50.

THE BYZANTINE PERIOD (476–732 A. D.)

The Western Roman Empire lasted 500 years. The Eastern Empire lasted over 1000 years (395–1453 A. D.).

The downfall of the Western Empire was mainly due to the degeneration of the Roman stock through mixture with weaker and inferior races. The soldiers who had never known defeat became an easy prey to the invading barbarians of the North, informed with the rugged and primitive virtues which they themselves had once possessed. In the days of the Republic, the Roman had matched the Spartan as a virile soldier and law giver, essentially simple in mind and morals. In a state of society "where wealth accumulates and men decay," he could not hold his own with the flexible, wily Greek of later times, nor with the subtle, fatalistic Oriental, both of them more agile in mind and more dexterous in action than he. Like the Normans in Sicily, or those English colonists in Ireland, who became proverbially *Hibernis ipsis Hiberniores*, he fell under that strange law by which the conqueror, in the end, assimilates himself to the conquered people. By process of race-inmixture, the Romans of the 5th century A. D. had acquired the "serene impartiality" of spirit which Professor Huxley attributes to the mongrel races, and some think that the malarial fevers which had begun to devastate the Italian peninsula had as much to do with weakening their fiber as the luxuries and dissipations to which they were continually exposed.[1] Degeneration of mind and body, with consequent relaxation of morals, led to mysticism and that respect for the authority of magic and the supernatural which was to pave the way for the bigotry, dogmatism, and mental inertia of the Middle Ages. Under these conditions, the physician became more and more of a mercenary parasite and vendor of quack medicines. Long before the downfall of Rome the magician, the thaumaturgist, the professional poisoner, and the courtezan who peddled drugs—

> Ambubaiarum collegia, pharmocopolæ,
> Mendici, mimæ, balatrones, hoc genus omne,

were familiar figures. In the Eastern Empire, the decomposition of intelligence was even more pronounced, and today the adjective "Byzantine" connotes little more than luxury, effemination, and sloth. The effect of the imposition of Roman administrative machinery upon a population, ultimately Greek in cast, was to keep science stationary until it finally went into retrogression. The traditions of Roman law and military science were rigorously maintained, and the general level of civilization was higher than that of any other European state during the Middle Ages. But beyond that point, Byzantium was a *città morte*.

---

[1] In particular, W. H. S. Jones: Malaria and Greek history, Manchester, 1909. His view is vigorously opposed by J. P. Cardamatis (Arch. f. Schiffs- u. Tropen-Hyg., Leipzig, 1915, xix, 273, 301).

Through the conflict of Pagan and Christian modes of thought, almost all of the intellectual energy of the period was dissipated in religious controversy, while medicine had become an affair of salves and poultices, talismans and pentagrams, with a mumbling of incantations and spells very like the backwoods pranks of Tom Sawyer and Huckleberry Finn, or some of the vagaries of Christian Science. There were doubtless good people, then as now, but they did not come to the front, and there is pith in Gibbon's sarcasm about two pious characters of the period: "We know his vices and are ignorant of her virtues." This supine cast of mind and morals is well reflected in the Byzantine mysticism of Wagner's Parsifal; and the figure of Kundry, the sorcerer's minion, who brings nostrums from the far East to alleviate the sufferings of Anfortas, may serve as a sort of type and symbol of Byzantine medicine. In spite of all that has been written by Curtis, Finlay, Zinkeisen, and others, little more can be claimed for Byzantium than is contained in the sentence of Allbutt: "The chief monuments of learning were stored in Byzantium until Western Europe was fit to take care of them."[1] The solitary thing the Eastern Empire did for European medicine was to preserve something of the language, culture, and literary texts of Greece. Concerning this point, Hirschberg says conclusively that Byzantium had no medieval period, but simply went on "marking time" in the past. The habit of compilation established by the later Greek and Roman writers remained a set custom in Eastern and Western Europe, even beyond the Renaissance period. Byzantine medicine still flourishes in the monasteries on Mount Athos in late 19th-century MSS. (Singer).

Although the Byzantine power lasted over a thousand years (395–1453 A. D.), medical history is concerned chiefly with the names of four industrious compilers who were prominent physicians in the first three centuries of its existence. Of these, the courtier **Oribasius** (325–403 A. D.), a friend and physician-in-ordinary to Julian the Apostate and sometimes quæstor of Constantinople, is chiefly remarkable as a torch-bearer of knowledge rather than as an original writer, but his compilations are highly valued by scholars in that he always gives his authorities and, as far as is known, quotes them exactly. Medicine is indebted to him for a remarkable anthology of the works of his predecessors, many of whom (the surgeons Archigenes, Hileodorus, Antyllus, for instance) might otherwise have been lost to posterity. Galen in particular he expounded with loving care, and did much to establish him in his central position of authority during the Dark Ages. Like Galen, Oribasius took all knowledge for his province. His great *Synagoge* or Encyclopedia of Medicine (Paris, 1556) comprised indeed over seventy volumes, dealing with all aspects of the subject. Much of this has been lost, but its author epitomized his knowledge in the little *Synopsis* which he made for the use of his son. In the Dark Ages, his

---

[1] Allbutt: Science and Mediæval Thought, London, 1901, 65. See also his Finlayson lecture in Glasgow Med. Jour., 1913, lxxx, 321, 422.

Euporista was the popular treatise on medicine, and had the rare merit of avoiding any current superstitions and inculcating sound therapeutic doctrine. Oribasius gives a very clean-cut semeiology of lesions at different levels of the spinal cord (Galen). In his memorable paragraph on the stupefying effects of intimidation of intelligent children by beating and browbeating at the hands of incompetent schoolmasters, he may be regarded as the founder of pedagogics. The student of medical history will read Oribasius to best advantage in Daremberg's splendid six-volume bilingual (Paris, 1851–76[1]).

Aëtius of Amida, who lived in the 6th century A. D., was also a royal physician (to Justinian I, 527–65) and *comes absequii* (lord high chamberlain) at the court of Byzantium. He left an extensive compilation, usually called the *Tetrabiblion*, which is a principal authority for what we know of the work of Rufus of Ephesus and Leonides in surgery, Soranus and Philumenus in gynecology and obstetrics. The first eight books were published at Venice in 1534. The hitherto unprinted books IX–XVI are to be edited by Max Wellmann. Aëtius gives a description of epidemic diphtheria not unlike that of Aretæus, mentioning paralysis of the palate as a sequel, and his work contains the best account of diseases of the eye, ear, nose, throat, and teeth in the literature of antiquity. He has also interesting chapters on goiter and hydrophobia. Much of Aëtius, as Max Wellmann has shown, is taken from Archigenes through Philumenus. His accounts of elephantiasis, ileus, the varieties of headache, pneumonia, pleurisy, epilepsy, and the treatment of these conditions, are far more accurate than those of Aretæus, whose work may also derive from the same common source. In surgery, Aëtius supplies many lost passages in Oribasius, and describes modes of procedure (tonsillotomy, urethrotomy, treatment of hemorrhoids) not found elsewhere. To him is due the first description of ligation of the brachial artery above the sac for aneurysm, which was later done by Guillemeau (1594) and Anel (1710), to become in time the Hunterian method (1786) (Osler[2]). Aëtius recommended many salves and plasters, and is supposed to have been a Christian by reason of the charms and spells he proposes for their preparation. Thus, in preparing a plaster, he says, one should intone repeatedly, "The God of Abraham, the God of Isaac, the God of Jacob, give virtue to this medicament." To remove a bone stuck in the throat, one should cry out in a loud voice: "As Jesus Christ drew Lazarus from the grave, and Jonah out of the whale, thus Blasius, the martyr and servant of God, commands 'Bone come up or go down.'"

Alexander of Tralles (525–605), a much traveled practitioner who finally settled in Rome, was brother of the architect of St. Sophia at

---

[1] The earlier editions of Oribasius are the Greek text of the *Synagoge* (Paris, 1556), the Latin Aldine of the *Synopsis* (Venice, 1554), the Latin *Euporista* (Basel, 1529) and the Latin *Opera omnia* (Basel, 1557).

[2] Osler: Lancet, London, 1915, i, 950. Osler says that the original description of Aëtius was wrongly attributed by Sprengel to Philagrius.

Constantinople. He was the only one of the Byzantine compilers who displayed any special originality. Although a follower of Galen, his *Practica* (first printed at Lyons in 1504[1]) contains some descriptions of disease and some prescriptions which seem to be his own, notably those containing burnt substances. His accounts of insanity, gout, and the dysenteric and choleraic disorders are above the average. He has a highly original chapter on intestinal worms and vermifuges, is said to have been the first to mention rhubarb, and first recommended colchicum (hermodactyl) in gout. Like Galen, he recommends a full milk diet, change of air, and sea voyages for phthisis, but his other prescriptions are often disfigured by the obtrusion of the usual Byzantine charms.

Paul of Ægina (625–690), the last of the Greek eclectics and compilers, was the author of an *Epitome* of medicine in seven books, first printed by the Aldine press at Venice in 1528 and 1553, later in the modern text (with French translation) of René Briau (Paris, 1855), and Englished for the Sydenham Society by Francis Adams (London, 1834–47[2]). Although Paul was a physician of high repute, we may judge how low medicine had sunk in the 7th century by his apologetic statements as to lack of originality on his part. He frankly admits that the ancients had said all that could be said on the subject, and that he is only a humble scribe. Paul was, however, a very capable surgeon, and the sixth book of his Epitome was the standard work on the subject up to the time of Albucasis who, indeed, drew upon it for most of his information. Paul gives original descriptions of lithotomy, trephining, tonsillotomy, paracentesis and amputation of the breast, but stopped short of opening the chest for empyema. In describing herniotomy he recommends removal of the testicles, a mutilation which was perpetuated by the Arabians, and continued to be the vogue with the outcast medieval surgeons until far into the 16th century. Paul gives the fullest account we have of the eye surgery and military surgery of antiquity. He mentions the frequency of naval physicians in his time. The Pauline pediatrics and obstetrics summarize all that was known of these subjects from classical antiquity up to the Renaissance. Paul omits all reference to podalic version and, as his authority was upheld by the Arabians, the procedure disappears from literature until the time of Röslin and Paré.

Among the minor writers of the Byzantine period, we may mention Publius **Vegetius** Renatus, a horse trader and farrier of the 5th century A. D., whose *Ars Veterinaria*, published at Basel in 1528, contains the first authentic account of glanders; and Theophilus Protospatharius, physician and captain of the guard to the Emperor Heraclius (603–41), and a contemporary of Paul of Ægina. He left an original description of the palmaris brevis muscle and the olfactory nerve,

---

[1] The best edition of Alexander Trallianus is that of Theodor Puschmann (2 vols.), Vienna, 1878–9, with German translation and biographic introduction.

[2] This is Adams' *opus magnum*. A valuable German translation, with commentary, by J. Berendes, was published in Janus, Amst., 1908–13, *passim*, and at Leyden (E. J. Brill, 1914).

and wrote a treatise on the urine[1] which for centuries upheld the Galenic doctrine that urine is a filtrate of the blood, secreted in the portal vein and vena cava. The same view was maintained unchanged in the 13th century by Johannes Actuarius, the last of the Byzantine writers, whose elaborate treatise on the urine made the notion authoritative with the absurd "water-casters" of a later time. He is memorable as the first to use a graduated glass for examining the urine, although the markings upon it were not quantitative but qualitative, indicating the possible position of the different scums, precipitates and sediments.

During the Byzantine period, an interesting contribution to clinical medicine was made by the Fathers of the Christian Church, namely, the description of the earlier epidemics of smallpox and diphtheria.

Eusebius described a Syrian epidemic in 302 A. D. Another was described by Gregory of Tours in 581, and the term "variola" was first employed by Marius, Bishop of Avenches, in 570. It is said that the disease was also described in the Irish monastery records of 675 A. D. as *Bolgagh* and *Galar Breac*. The Chronicle of St. Denis (580) mentions diphtheria as *esquinancie*. Baronius described Roman epidemics of 856 and 1004, and Cedrenus records a Byzantine epidemic of 1039 as *cynanche* (Hirsch). **Nemesius,** Bishop of Emesa (Syria), who lived in the 4th–5th centuries, A. D. wrote a book on *The Nature of Man*, which is remarkable for its sound physiology, particularly of the nervous system. It was Latinized by Alphanus, Archbishop of Salerno, and was a very influential text in the Middle Ages. Jeanselme gives a careful and circumstantial account of gout, epilepsy, and alcoholism at the court of Byzantium,[2] derived from the local historians and patristic writers. The symptoms of gout were very well described, causes were located, and there was extensive treatment, but the term "arthritis" connoted both gout and chronic rheumatism until the 17th century.

In 1495, a valuable illustrated collection of surgical MSS., made by the Byzantine physician Niketas (900 A. D.), was purchased in Crete by Janos Laskaris for Lorenzo de Medici, was subsequently acquired by Cardinal Nicolas Rudolfi, and is now one of the treasures of the Laurentian Library at Florence (Codex lxxiv, 7). This contains 30 full-sized plates illustrating the commentary of **Apollonius of Kitium** on the Hippocratic treatise on dislocations ($\pi\epsilon\rho\grave{\iota}$ $\check{\alpha}\rho\theta\rho\omega\nu$[3]) and 63 smaller cuts scattered through the pages of Soranus' treatise on bandaging. The Apollonian pictures, which are also to be found in Codex 3632 of the University Library at Bologna, are pen-and-brush drawings in dark brown tone representing the various manipulations and apparatus employed in reducing dislocations, the figures in each case being surmounted by an archway of ornate Byzantine design. Their origins, Sudhoff thinks, go back to Alexandria or Cyprus, where Apollonius wrote his commentary *circa* 81–58 B. C. They were undoubtedly transmitted directly from antiquity,[4] and, therefore, represent the genuine Hippocratic tradition of surgical practice as transmitted through later Greek channels to Byzantium. The two sets of pictures were reproduced in freehand style by the Renaissance artists Jan Santorinos and Francesco Primaticcio, and these reproductions were used by Guido Guidi to illustrate his surgical collections (Paris, 1544[5]). The treatise of Apollonius has since been reprinted, with the illustrations, by Hermann Schöne (1896[6]). The 200 designs used by Guido Guidi have been reproduced by Henri Omont.[7]

---

[1] Edited by W. A. Greenhill (Oxford, 1842).

[2] E. Jeanselme: Bull. Soc. fran;. d'hist. de méd., Par., 1920, xiv, 137; 1924, xviii, 225, 289.

[3] Edited by F. R. Dietz (Königsberg, 1834) and C. G. Kühn (Leipzig, 1838).

[4] Sudhoff: Beiträge zur Geschichte der Chirurgie im Mittelalter, Leipzig, 1914, 4–7.

[5] The pictures are to be found in Guido Guidi's *Chiurgia e greco in latinum conversa* (Paris, 1544), in vol. iii of his *Ars Medicinalis* (Venice, 1611), in his *Opera omnia* (Frankfort, 1668), and in Conrad Gesner's collection *De chirurgia scriptores optimi*, Zürich, 1555, 321–358 (Sudhoff).

[6] Apollonius von Kitium: Illustrierter Kommentar zur der Hippokratischen Schrift $\pi\epsilon\rho\grave{\iota}$ $\check{\alpha}\rho\theta\rho\omega\nu$, hrsg. von H. Schöne, Leipzig, 1896.

[7] Bibliothèque nationale. Département des manuscrits. Collection de chirurgiens grecs (MS. latin, 6866). Ed. H. Omont, Paris (s. d.).

THE MOHAMMEDAN AND JEWISH PERIODS
(732–1096 A. D.)

By the swords of Mohammed and his emirs, the wild outlaw clans of the Asian and African deserts were converted into nations capable of acting as military and social units; but it was not until long after his death, when the mighty empire which he founded was subdivided into caliphates, that the sciences and arts were permitted to develop. During the period of conquest and conversion, the fanatical, fatalistic zeal of the Moslems tended naturally toward the destruction and persecution of the things of the mind. The word *Islam* means resigned submission to the will of God. The popularity of the given names Iskander, Ibrahim, Ismaïl, Miriam, evidences the close contact of Mohammedan with Greek and Jewish culture. While the principal service of Islam to medicine was the preservation of Greek culture, yet the Saracens themselves were the originators not only of algebra, chemistry, and geology, but of many of the so-called improvements or refinements of civilization, such as street-lamps, window-panes, fireworks, stringed instruments, cultivated fruits, perfumes, spices, and that "often-changed and often-washed undergarment of linen or cotton which still passes among ladies under its old Arabic name."[1] The power of Islamic culture is still sensed in such words as admiral, alcohol, alfalfa or arsenal, and from the astronomer al-Kwarizmi who introduced the Arabic numerals came "algorism" (arithmetic). In the intellectual sphere, the monotheism and the dialectic tendencies of Galen and Aristotle appealed strongly to the Mohammedans. Galen's polypharmacy in particular appealed to these natural chemists, and his haphazard polypragmatism was molded by them into iron-clad dogma. The Oriental idea that it is sinful to touch the dead body with the hands did little to advance anatomy or surgery. The general trend of Oriental religious fatalism was toward contemplative brooding and resigned submission to authority. Such eagerness or free-play of the mind as the Moslems possessed was expended in hair-splitting subtleties. Thus the intellectual tendencies of the Middle Ages were determined for them in advance; indeed, can we trust the statements of men so different as Sir Henry Layard, Sir Henry Maine, and the ophthalmologist Hirschberg, the great mass of the people in the East detest all reforms and scientific inquiry to this day. We call the medical authors of the Mohammedan period "Arabic" on account of the language in which they wrote, but, in reality, most of them were Persian or Spanish born, and many of them were Jewish. The medical litera-

---

[1] Draper: "History of the Intellectual Development of Europe," New York, 1876, ii, pp. 33, 34. The Alhambra, like the Cretan palace at Knossos, contains a specimen of the sanitary invention known in Europe as W. C.

ture of the period is thus Arabian rather than Arabic, and was derived directly from Greece.

The Mohammedan physicians themselves owed their medical knowledge, in the first instance, to a persecuted sect of Christians. Nestorius, a priest who had been made patriarch of Constantinople in 428, taught the heretical doctrine that Mary should not be styled the "Mother of God" but the "Mother of Christ." In consequence, he and his followers were driven into the desert and, like the Jews after them, took up the study of medicine because of religious and social ostracism. The

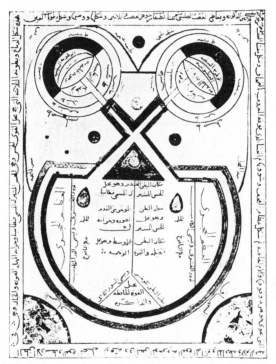

Schema of the brain, crossing of the optic nerves and cross-section of the eyes, showing lens, vitreous, retina, conjunctiva, cornea, and tunics. From MS. 924 in the New Mosque at Constantinople (Pansier, Hirschberg, Sudhoff).

Nestorian heretics gained control of the school at Edessa in Mesopotamia with its two large hospitals, and made it a remarkable institution for teaching medicine, but were driven out by the orthodox Bishop Cyrus in 489. Fleeing to Persia, where their theologic notions were not opposed, they established the famous school at Gondisapor, which was the true starting-point of Mohammedan medicine.

The Eastern or Bagdad Caliphate (749–1258) was under the sway of the Abbasides, who were friends of learning and science and included such liberal-minded rulers as the caliphs Al-Mansur (754–775), Harun al-Rashid (786–802) and Al-Meiamun (813–833). These monarchs encouraged the collection and copying of Greek manuscripts, so that the earlier centuries of the Mohammedan period were occupied in translating the works of Hippocrates, Galen, Dioscorides, and other Greek classics into Arabic. The principal Arabic translators in the 8th and 9th centuries were Johannes **Mesuë** the elder (777–837), called Janus Damascenus, a Christian who became director of the hospital at Bagdad, and the Nestorian teacher Honain ben Isaac or **Johannitius** (809–873), whom Withington calls "The Erasmus of the Arabic Renaissance." Johannitius had an adventurous career, translated Hippoc-

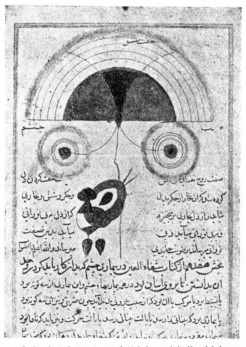

Arabic schema of the head, eyes, and "sight-spirit," which proceeded from the brain to envelop the object of vision and carry it back to the crystalline humor. (From a Persian MS. of the 17th century.)　Meyerhof and Prüfer (Sudhoff's Archiv, 1912, vi, 26).

rates, Galen, Oribasius, and Paul of Ægina, and was in his day the leading medical spirit of Bagdad. He wrote a commentary on Galen's Microtechne (*Isagoge in Artem parvum*), and the oldest treatise in Arabic on eye diseases (Hirschberg[1]). The ten sections have been translated by M. Meyerhof and C. Prüfer of Cairo, with an interpreta-

---

[1] Arch. f. Gesch. d. Med., Leipzig, 1910–11, iv, 163–190, 1 pl; 1912–13, vi, 21–33. This work is not to be confused with the *Monitorium oculariorum* of Haly ben Isa (Jesu Hali), an 11th century writing which became the classic text-book on ophthalmology in later Islam and is still authoritative (Hirschberg). The medieval Latin translation of this work is valueless and unintelligible. The best modern translation is that of Hirschberg and Lippert (Leipzig, 1907).

tion of Honain's theory of vision, and interesting plates representing the "schematic eye" (Cairene MS.) and the Galenic "sight-spirit" (*Sehgeist*), which was supposed to proceed from the brain *via* the nerves to envelop the object seen, proceeding thence to the crystalline humor to complete the act of vision.

The greatest physicians of the Eastern Caliphate were the three Persians: Rhazes, Haly Abbas, and Avicenna.

Rhazes (860–932), a great clinician, ranks with Hippocrates, Aretæus, and Sydenham as one of the original portrayers of disease. His description of smallpox and measles is the first authentic account in literature, a classic text, preserved in the original Arabic with parallel Latin translation in Channing's edition (London, 1766). Although smallpox had been vaguely described as early as the 6th century by some of the church fathers, and by the 7th century chronicler Aaron (cited in the Continent of Rhazes), the account of Rhazes is so vivid and complete that it is almost modern. His great encyclopedia of medicine, the *El Hawi* or *Continens*, which Haller preferred to any other Arabic treatise, is preserved in the Latin translation completed by Ferragut on February 13, 1279 (Brescia, 1486). Made up of an enormous mass of extracts from many sources, together with original clinical histories and experiments in therapeutics, it reveals Rhazes as a Galenist in theory, but a true follower of Hippocrates in the simplicity of his practice. The Brescia *editio princeps* of 1486 is incidentally the largest and heaviest of all the incunabula. The ninth book of Rhazes, which was revised by Vesalius and commentated by Gatinaria, was the source of therapeutic knowledge until long after the Renaissance.

Haly ben Abbas, a Persian mage who died in 994, was the author of the *Almaleki* (*Liber regius* or "Royal Book"), a work which was the canonical treatise on medicine for a hundred years, when it was superseded by the *Canon* of Avicenna. It was translated into Latin about 1070–80 by Constantinus Africanus under the title *Pantegni*,[1] and later by Stephen of Antioch (1127[2]). This translation contains a description of smallpox and "Persian fire" (malignant anthrax), also the Latin term for smallpox (variola[3]). The anatomical section (*Pars practica*, II, III) was the sole source of knowledge, at Salerno and elsewhere, during the century 1070–1170.

Ibn Sina or **Avicenna** (980–1037), called "the Prince of Physicians," a convivial Omarian spirit, eminently successful in practice as court

---

[1] Printed in full in *Opera Ysaac* (Lyons, 1515) and (*Pars theorica* only) in *Opera Constantini* (Basel, 1536–9).

[2] *Alias* Stephen of Pisa. For Antioch, Singer suggests Anticaria or Antiguerra in Andalusia. This translation was printed as *Liber regalis* at Venice (1492) and Lyons (1523). The Arabic original was printed in Egypt in 1877 (Sudhoff).

[3] The term "variola" was first employed in the Chronicle of Bishop Marius of Avenches, viz.: "Anno 570, Hoc anno morbus validus cum profluvio ventris et variola Italiam Galliamque valde afflixit, et animalia bubula per loca suprascripta maxime interierunt." Gregory of Tours, Historia Francorum, in M. Bouquet: Recueil des historiens des Gaules, Paris, 1739, ii, 18. Cited by Paul Richter, Arch. f. Gesch. d. Med., Leipz., 1911–12, v, 325.

9

physician and vizier to different caliphs, was one who trod the primrose path at ease and died in the prime of life from the effect of its pleasures. He was physician in chief to the celebrated hospital at Bagdad, and is said to have written over one hundred works on different subjects, only a few of which have been preserved. His wonderful description of the origin of mountains (cited by Draper and Withington) fully entitles him to be called the "Father of Geology," and it is interesting to note that two physicians, widely separated in space and time—Avicenna and Fracastorius—are the only writers who contributed anything of value to this science for centuries. Avicenna is said to have been the first to describe the preparation and properties of sulphuric acid and alcohol. His *Canon*,[1] which Haller styled a "methodic inanity," is a huge, unwieldy storehouse of learning, in which the author attempts to codify the whole medical knowledge of his time and to square its facts with the systems of Galen and Aristotle. Written in meticulous style (the Arabian mania for classification), this gigantic tome became a fountain-head of authority in the Middle Ages, for Avicenna's elaborated train of reasoning, a miracle of syllogism in its way, appealed particularly to the medieval mind and, indeed, set the pace for its movement in many directions. Arnold of Villanova defined Avicenna as a professional scribbler who had stupefied European physicians by his misinterpretation of Galen (Neuburger). In fairness to Avicenna, it is proper to say that his clinical records, which he intended as an appendix to the Canon, were irrecoverably lost, and only the Arabic text of the latter, published at Rome in 1593, and at Bulak in 1877, survives. That Avicenna must have been a clever practitioner we should naturally infer from his great reputation. For example, the striking plates in the Giunta edition of 1595[2] suggest that he must have known and practised the Hippocratic method of treating spinal deformities by forcible reduction (reintroduced by Calot in 1896). His recommendation of wine as the best dressing for wounds was very popular in medieval practice. Avicenna also described the guinea-worm (*Vena medinensis*[3]); anthrax as "Persian fire" (Canon, Bulak ed. 1294, 1877, III, 118), gave a good account of diabetes, and is said to have noticed the sweetish taste of diabetic urine.[4] The Latin texts of Avicenna were enormously popular in the Middle Ages, but upon the whole, the influence of the "Canon" upon medieval medicine was bad, in that it confirmed physi-

---

[1] The principal Latin editions of the Canon are the Milan imprint of 1473, the Paduan of 1476 and 1497, the Venetian of 1482, 1486, 1490, 1491, 1494, and 1500, the Giuntas of 1527, 1544, 1555, 1582, 1595, and 1608. The commentaries *in toto* were printed in five giant volumes by the Giunti at Venice in 1523.

[2] Most of these plates probably derive from the great Florentine codex of Apollonius of Kitium.

[3] Avicenna, Canon, sect. III, tract. II, cap. XXI.

[4] Dinquizzi: Bull. Acad. de méd., Paris, 1913, lxx, 631. Erich Ebstein (Ztschr. f. Urol., Leipzig, 1915, ix, 243) shows that the *Viaticum peregrinantes* of Ibn-el-Ischezzar (–1004) contains a remarkable account of diabetes (*De passione diabetica*) in which the thirst, polyuria, canine appetite, etc., are noted, but not the sweetish urine.

cians in the pernicious idea that ratiocination is better than first-hand investigation. It also set back the progress of surgery by inculcating the novel doctrine that the surgical art is an inferior and separate branch of medicine and by substituting the use of the cautery for the knife.

The anatomical treatises in Rhazes, Haly Abbas, and Avicenna have been edited by de Koning (1903[1]).

Useibia (1203–69), of Damascus, the first historian of Arabic medicine, wrote a series of biographies of ancient physicians, the Arabic text of which was edited by August Müller (Königsberg, 1884). It was the main source of the histories of Wüstenfeld and L. Leclerc.[2]

Other prominent medical figures of the Eastern Caliphate were the Jewish physician and neo-Platonist philosopher, Isaac Israeli (ben Solomon), of Kaironan, called **Isaac Judæus** (855–955), who wrote a book on uroscopy and a treatise upon dietetics (*De diæta*, Padua, 1487), which became deservedly popular in Europe; Ibn al Haitham or Alhazan (996–1038), of Bassora, whose Thesaurus of Optics (Basel, 1572) contains the first note of ocular refraction (*omnis visio fit refracte*) and of the fact that a segment of a glass ball will magnify objects (Greeff); and the Arabian traveler **Abdollatif** (1161–1231), who visited Egypt at Saladin's instance and, while there, had opportunities for studying human skeletons which convinced him that Galen's osteology must be wrong in many important respects.

The Western or Cordovan Caliphate (655–1236) attained highest prosperity under the Spanish or Ommiade dynasty (755–1036). Its leading medical authors were the clinician Avenzoar, the surgeon Albucasis, and the physician-philosophers Averroës and Moses Maimonides.

Abulkasim, called **Albucasis** (1013–1106), born in the Andalusian town Zahra, near Cordova, was author of a great medicochirurgical treatise called the *Altasrif* (or "Collection"), of which the surgical part[3] survives in Channing's Arabic text and translation (Oxford, Clarendon Press, 1778). It contains illustrations of surgical and dental instruments (interpolated in the Venetian surgical anthology of 1500) and was the leading text-book on surgery in the Middle Ages up to the time of Saliceto. It consists of three books, founded upon the work of Paul of Ægina. The first book deals with the use of the actual cautery (the special feature of Arabian surgery) and gives descriptions and figurations of the peculiar instruments used; the second book contains full descriptions of lithotomy, lithotrity, amputations for gangrene, and the treatment of wounds; the third book deals with fractures and dislocations, including fracture of the pelvis and a mention of paralysis in fracture of the spine. Albucasis was apparently the

---

[1] P. de Koning: Trois traités d'anatomie arabe, Leyden, 1903.

[2] German translation (Book VII) by Wally Hamed (Berlin diss.. 19ˑ0; partly translated into French by B. R. Sanguinetti (Journal asiatique, Paris, 1854–6).

[3] A Latin translation of the medical part was published at Augsburg in 1519.

first to write on the treatment of deformities of the mouth and dental arches, and he mentions the obstetric posture which is now known as the "Walcher position."[1] In Gurlt's time, the illustrations of surgical (including dental) instruments in Albucasis counted as the earliest known, but many earlier have since been discovered in medieval manuscripts by Sudhoff and others. The Oriental horror of touching the dead body with hands or knife was the sufficient reason why these pictures from the antique were not often reproduced in the Arabic MSS. of the Persian Mohammedans, nor in the Latin MSS.

The greatest of the Moslem physicians of the Western Caliphate was the Cordovan **Avenzoar,** who died at Seville in 1162. He was one of the few men of his time who had courage to tilt against Galenism, and by his description of the itch-mite (*Acarus scabiei*) he may be accounted the first parasitologist after Alexander of Tralles. He also described serous pericarditis, mediastinal abscess, pharyngeal paralysis, and inflammation of the middle ear, and he recommended the use of goat's milk in phthisis and tracheotomy. His *Teisir* or "Rectification of Health" is preserved in a Latin translation from the Hebrew (1280), published at Venice in 1490.

His pupil, **Averroës,** also Cordovan-born (1126–1198), and a Spanish Moslem, was more noted as a philosopher and free thinker than as a physician. His *Kitab-al-Kullyat* transliterated as *Colliget*[2] (Book of Universals), was an attempt to found a system of medicine upon the customary neo-Platonic modification of Aristotle's philosophy. Averroës advanced the Pantheistic doctrines of an eternally changing, self-renewing world (emergent evolution) and of the absorption of the soul or nature of man into universal nature at death. This virtual denial of creation and of personal immortality caused Averroës to be persecuted in his own lifetime, and his followers to be anathematized during the Middle Ages. It was largely through Averroës that Islamic philosophy came to be regarded as "Aristotle seen through neo-Platonic spectacles," but he was influenced also by Jewish thought and, in turn, exerted a profound influence upon later Jewish thinkers. Renan made an elaborate study of his work in *Averroës et l'averroisme* (1852).

The Rabbi Moses ben Maimon, called **Moses Maimonides** (1135–1204), also of Cordova, was court-physician to Saladin, and the great liberalizer of his people, in the sense of including science and philosophy as phases of Jewish culture, which had hitherto been restricted to the Talmud. His treatise on personal hygiene (*Tractatus de Regimine Sanitatis*) was written for Saladin's private use. It contains some admirable precepts of diet and regimen, including a rhubarb and tamarind pill, and

---

[1] "Tum decumbat mulier in collum suum, pendeantque deorsum pedes ejus, illa vero in lectum decumbat, etc.," cited by Dr. Herbert Spencer in Lancet, Lond., 1912, i, p. 1568. Mercurio, in La Comare (1596), also described the hanging position of Walcher.

[2] Translated into Latin by the Jew Bonacosa at Padua in 1265. Published at Venice in 1482 and 1553 (standard edition of Jacob Mantino).

its first edition, the Florentine of 1478, is esteemed as one of the rarest books. His tract on poisons was much cited by medieval writers. It was translated into Latin by Armeng and Blasii in 1305, into French in 1865, and into German by Steinschneider in 1873.[1] His *Guide for the Perplexed* attempts to harmonize the Jewish sacred canon with Aristotle.[2]

Such able chemists as the Arabians could not fail of being good pharmacologists. Their descriptions of the materia medica and of the preparation of drugs became standard authority throughout the Middle Ages. Even to this day what Osler calls "the heavy hand of the Arabian" is sensed in the enormous bulk of our own pharmacopeias. The oldest memorial of Arabic medicine is a MS. on toxicology, by the Persian Geber ibn Hajan (*circa* 750–760), which derives definitely from Greek sources. Dioscorides (Greek text) was, in fact, translated into Arabic at Bagdad (854) and Cordova (951), again from a 13th century Syriac version of Bar Hebræus, and "has influenced the whole practice of medicine among Arabic-speaking peoples" to date (Singer). The principal storehouse of the Arabian materia medica is the *Jami* of Ibn Baitar, a huge 13th century compilation, describing some 1400 drugs, of which about 300 are said to be new. The *Grabadin*, or apothecary's manual (*Antidotarium*), of the eponymous or pseudonymous **Mesue** junior, now called "pseudo-Mesue," a mysterious Latin compilation of the 10th or 11th century, of which the Arabic originals have never been found, was the most popular compendium of drugs in medieval Europe, and was used everywhere in their preparation. The Mesue treatise on purgatives divides the latter into laxative (tamarinds, figs, prunes, cassia), mild (wormwood, senna, aloes, rhubarb) and drastic (jalap, scammony, colocynth). The esteem in which these works were held is shown by the fact that a Latin translation of both was one of the first medical books to be printed (Venice, 1471). It passed through more than 30 editions up to 1581, and has influenced all later pharmacopeias. The popular drug-list attributed to Serapion junior was translated into Latin by Simon Cordo and Abraham ben Shemtob in 1290. The most important Persian work on pharmacology is the materia medica (*circa* 970) of **Abu Mansur,**[3] containing descriptions of 585 drugs, of which 466 are vegetable, 75 mineral, and 44 animal. The Arabic writings on toxicology up to the end of the 12th century have been exhaustively considered by Steinschneider (1871[4]). A Persian manu-

---

[1] M. Steinschneider: Arch. f. path. Anat., [etc.], Berl., 1873, lvii, 63–120.

[2] See Singer's diagrams of the structure of the universe, as conceived by Aristotle, Maimonides and Dante, in The Legacy of Israel, London, 1927, 195; 199. Aristotle's 56 Intelligences revolving the heavenly bodies become Biblical and Talmudic angels.

[3] Epitomized in Latin by R. Seligmann from a MS. of 1055 (Vienna, 1830–33), and translated into German under the direction of Rudolf Kobert (Histor. Stud. a. d. pharm. Inst. d. Univ. Dorpat, 3. Heft, Halle, 1893).

[4] M. Steinschneider: Arch. f. path. Anat., [etc.], Berl., 1871, 411, 340; 467. For the influence of Dioscorides on Oriental medicine, see his articles in Virchow's Archiv., Berl., 1891, cxxiv, 480, and Ztschr. f. Kunde d. Morgenl., Wien, Vienna, 1896–1900, xi–xiii, *passim.*

script of the 11th century by Ismail of Jurjani contains probably the most complete directions of the period for examining the urine. There is much of value on climatology and medical geography in the Arabic writers.[1]

Cultural Aspects of Mohammedan Medicine.—In Sir Richard Burton's translation of the Arabian Nights,[2] there is a tale of a spendthrift heir who has squandered all his substance save a beautiful slave-girl of extraordinary talents, who, realizing her master's plight, urges him to bring her before the Caliph Harun al-Rashid to be sold for a sum large enough to cover his losses. On seeing her, the Caliph decides to test the extent of her knowledge, and has specialists put her through a lengthy cross-examination which, incidentally, furnishes us a good documentation of the social aspects of Arabian medicine. As the fair slave exploits her extensive knowledge of Mohammedan theology, law, philosophy, medicine, astronomy, astrology, music, chess-playing, and other arts and sciences, we perceive that these accomplishments were also an essential part of the Arabian physician's training, and at the same time, that a certain acquaintance with the Galenical system of medicine was a feature of the cultural equipment of any well-educated Mohammedan of the period. The Arabians derived their knowledge of Greek medicine from the Nestorian monks, many practical details from the Jews, and their astrologic lore from Egypt and the far East. So the slave girl follows the Talmud in regard to the number of the bones (249), gives an exact account of the four humors, and details at length the effects of different conjunctions of the planets. Diagnosis of internal disease is founded upon six canons: (1) The patient's actions; (2) his excreta; (3) the nature of the pain; (4) its site; (5) swelling; (6) the effluvia of the body; and further information is elicited by "the feel of the hands," whether firm or flabby, hot or cool, moist or dry, or by such indications as "yellowness of the whites of the eye" (jaundice) or "bending of the back" (lung disease). The symptoms of yellow bile are a sallow complexion, dryness of the throat, a bitter taste, loss of appetite, and rapid pulse; those of black bile, "false appetite and great mental disquiet and cark and care," terminating in melancholia.[3] Medicinal draughts are best taken "when the sap runs in the wood and the grape thickens in the cluster and the two auspicious planets, Jupiter and Venus, are in the ascendant." Cupping is most effective at the wane of the moon, with the weather at set-fair, preferably the 17th of the month and on a Tuesday. This, or something like it, was about the character of Mohammedan practice toward the end of the 14th century, the period assigned for the composition of the Arabian Nights, and we may reasonably infer that it is also fairly repre-

---

[1] E. Wiedemann: Arch. f. Gesch. d. Naturw., Leipz., 1914–15, v, 56–68.

[2] Denver edition, 1899, vol. v, pp. 189–245 ("Abu al-Husn and his Slave-girl Tawaddud"), the medical portion being on pp. 218–226.

[3] Maurice Girardeau (Paris Dissertation No. 107, 1910) shows that the cholemic diathesis was perhaps the most prominent feature of Arabic pathology.

sentative of the best period of Moslem medicine as handed down by tradition. According to Hirschberg's dictum, the peoples of Islam have not attained to modernity, but rely upon the same medical authorities which they employed in the Middle Ages.[1] In the past, the Arabian physician, whose professional importance was gauged by the height of his turban and the richness and length of his sleeves, was usually an astrologer and a magician, who regarded the heart as "the prince of the body," the lungs as the fan of the heart, the liver as the guard of the heart and the seat of the soul, the pit of the stomach as the seat of pleasure and the gall-bladder as the seat of courage. From the Arabic medical texts, we know that their authors upheld the Galenic pulse-lore, affected to arrive at inaccessible data, such as the sex of the child in pregnancy by inspection of the urine (uroscopy), wrote charms in cups with "purgative ink" to mystify their patients, indeed, resorted to all manner of sensational trade-tricks and surprises in order to impose their authority. Like some of our modern spiritualists and similar fakers, the Arab physician hired confederates, who found out about the patient's condition in advance or even feigned to be patients themselves in order to puff his reputation.[2] They abstained from dissecting out of religious conviction, left operative surgery and venesection to the wandering specialists, and the care of women's diseases and obstetric cases to midwives; were constantly squabbling among themselves, stipulated their fees in advance, and tried to collect at least half if the case took an unfavorable turn or did not improve. Some of the fees they received were phenomenal. Gabriel Batischua, a favorite of Harun al-Rashid, got about $1500 per annum "for bleeding and purging the Commander of the Faithful," besides a regular monthly salary of about $2500 and a New Year's purse of $6250. He estimated his total fortune in fees at $10,000,000, and on being recalled from banishment to heal Al-Meiamun, he received $125,000, which Withington regards as the largest fee on record. Abu Nasr, according to the same authority, received more than $60,000 for curing one of the Caliphs of stone. Nearly all the prominent physicians of the period aimed to curry favor with the reigning potentates, or to supplant rival colleagues in their good graces. The Caliphs themselves, after the Mohammedan passion for conquest had been sated, became loyal supporters of science, and were instrumental in founding hospitals, libraries, and schools. Even private collections of books were sometimes of extraordinary extent, and all Greek, Egyptian, Indian, and Jewish culture that did not conflict with the creed of Islam was rapidly assimilated.

---

[1] J. Hirschberg: Geschichte der Augenheilkunde, 2. Aufl., Leipz., 1908, ii, 2, footnote. He gives several examples, e. g., a Druse in Syria who in 1860 treated eye diseases from the ten centuries older canon of Honain and Haly ben Isaac. A Cairene book of eye-magic of 1859 contains an illustration of 1296 A. D., etc.

[2] The tricks of these people were legion, and formed the subject of a lucubration of Rhazes. See, in particular, M. Steinschneider: Wissenschaft und Charlatanerie unter den Arabern im neunten Jahrhundert. Virchow's Arch., Berlin, 1866, xxxvi, 570; xxxvii, 560.

As early as 707 A. D., the Caliph El Welid had founded a hospital at Damascus. Another was established at Cairo (874), two at Bagdad (918), another at Misr (Egypt) (957), two others in the same city in 925 and 977. In course of time, dispensaries and infirmaries existed in all the important cities of the Eastern Caliphate, and about 1160 a Jewish traveler found as many as 60 of these institutions in Bagdad alone.

The largest and best appointed of the Mohammedan hospitals were those founded at Damascus (1160) and Cairo (1276). In the Damascus hospital, treatment was given and drugs dispensed free of charge for three centuries. As late as 1427, it was said its fires had never been put out since its opening. The great Al-Mansur hospital at Cairo (1283[1]) was a huge quadrangular structure with fountains playing in the four courtyards, separate wards for important diseases, wards for women and convalescents, lecture rooms, an extensive library, outpatient clinics, diet kitchens, an orphan asylum, and a chapel. It employed male and female nurses, had an income of about $100,000, and disbursed a suitable sum to each convalescent on his departure, so that he might not have to go to work at once. The patients were nourished upon a rich and attractive diet, and the sleepless were provided with soft music or, as in the Arabian Nights, with accomplished tellers of tales. The Cordovan Caliphate was equally well off in the number, if not the extent, of its hospitals. The Bagdad Caliphate was especially noted for its ophthalmic dispensaries and lunatic asylums. The Arabians were far ahead of their European contemporaries in kindly treatment of the insane. Medical instruction was given either at the great hospitals at Bagdad, Damascus and Cairo, or as a special course at the academies which existed in all the cities. Of these, the Hall of Wisdom at Cairo was the most famous. The principal courses were clinical medicine, pharmacology, and therapeutics. Anatomy and surgery were neglected, but chemistry was held in special esteem. Arabian medicine was, in fact, the parent of alchemy, the founder of which was Jabu or Geber (702–765), the discoverer of nitric acid and aqua regia and the describer of distillation, filtration, sublimation, water-baths, and other essentials of chemical procedure. Alchemy was combined with astrology in this wise: The ancient Chaldaic Pantheism, the doctrine of an *anima mundi*, or "soul of the world," with indwelling spirits in all things, was applied to whatever could be extracted from substances by fire, as "spirit" of wine, "spirit" of nitre, or the various essences and quintessences; while to the seven planets (the sun, the moon, Mars, Mercury, Jupiter, Saturn, Venus) corresponded the seven days of the week and the seven known metals (gold, silver, iron, quicksilver, tin, lead and copper). As these metals were supposed to be generated in the bowels of the earth, the special aim of alchemy was to find the fecundating or germinal substance, under appropriate planetary influences. Thus Geber's parable of a medicine, which could heal any of six lepers, was regarded by Boerhaave as nothing more than an allegory of the philosopher's stone for transmuting the six baser planetary metals

---

[1] Wüstenfeld: Janus, Breslau, 1846, i, 28–39.

into gold. Hand in hand with this idea of transmutation of metals went the notion of a polyvalent "elixir of life," which could cure all diseases and confer immortal youth, and which was supposed to be of the nature of a "potable gold" (*aurum potabile*). The search for potable gold led to the discovery of aqua regia and the strong acids by Geber and Rhazes, and the quest of the elixir was the starting point of chemical pharmaceutics. Even as late as the 16th century, we find Paracelsus upholding Geber's idea that everything is made of mercury, sulphur and salt, and that as "the sun rules the heart, the moon the brain, Jupiter the liver, Saturn the spleen, Mercury the lungs, Mars the bile, Venus the kidneys," so the seven planetary metals and their compounds were specifics for the diseases of these organs under the will of the stars. Arabian chemistry probably survived beyond the decadence of Arabian medicine, for Leo Africanus, a traveler of the 15th century, mentions a chemical society which existed at Fez at that time. From their constant contact with strange lands and peoples, the Arabian pharmacists or "*sandalani*" were the exploiters if not the introducers of a vast number of new drugs; in particular, senna, camphor, sandalwood, rhubarb, musk, myrrh, cassia, tamarind, nutmeg, cloves, cubebs, aconite, ambergris and mercury. They were also the originators of syrups, juleps, alcohol, aldehydes (all Arabic terms), and the inventors of flavoring extracts made of rosewater, orange and lemon peel, tragacanth, and other attractive ingredients. The use of hashish (*Cannabis indica*) and bhang (either Indian hemp or hyoscyamus) to produce drug-intoxication (*tabannuj*) or deep sleep was common, and the unseemly behavior of addicts of these drugs is described in the Arabian Nights.[1] King Omar casts the Princess Abrizah into a heavy slumber with "a piece of concentrated bhang, if an elephant smelt it he would sleep from year to year."[2] In another tale, the thief Ahmad Kamakim drugs the guards "with hemp fumes."[3] Thus the possibilities of anesthesia by inhalation were known to the Arabians, as well as to Dioscorides and the medieval surgeons, and presumably the original knowledge came from India, since the Egyptians did but little surgery. The Arabian apothecary shops were regularly inspected by a syndic (*Muhtasib*) who threatened the merchants with humiliating corporal punishments if they adulterated drugs (Guigues[4]). The effect of Arabian chemistry and pharmacy upon European medicine lasted long after the Mohammedan power itself had waned and, with the simples of Dioscorides and Pliny, their additions to the materia medica made up the better part of the European pharmacopeias for centuries.

Closely connected with Mohammedan medical culture is the influence of the Jews upon European medicine. Following the Diaspora or

---

[1] Burton's Arabian Nights (Denver edition), iii, 91–93, Suppl., iv, 19; 189.

[2] *Op. cit.*, ii, 122–124.

[3] *Op. cit.*, iv, 71.

[4] Guigues: Bull. d. sc. pharm., Paris, 1916, xxiii, 107–118. An interesting list of the substances used to adulterate various standard drugs is given.

dispersal of the Jews outside Palestine, they were subjected to persecution by the Romans and the later Christians, on account of their obstinate fidelity to their religion. Such well-known instances as the ghetto, the marano, the auto-de-fé, the suppression of the Waad (1764), are phases of an alienation to which they were not subjected by the Mohammedans. Under the Arabian domination, Jewish physicians were prominent figures at the courts of the caliphs, and a common belief in a stern monotheism created a strong bond of sympathy between Moslem and Hebrew. Another point of contact was the fact that the Hebrew and Mohammedan physicians, with their peculiar analytic cast of mind, their intensive modes of thought and their appreciation of "values," soon acquired a right materialistic way of looking at concrete things. Thus, while medical men under Christianity were still trifling with charms, amulets, saintly relics, the Cabala, and other superstitions, Jewish and Mohammedan physicians were beginning to look upon these things with a certain secret contempt.

During the Middle Ages and long after, the lot of the Jewish physician in Europe was to be used and abused. In the 10th and 11th centuries, he was, as Billings says, "a sort of contraband luxury,"[1] resorted to and protected by prince and prelate alike, on account of his superior scientific knowledge, but hardly countenanced for any other reason. Raymond Lully, who proposed to convert them wholesale by *force majeure*, said that every monastery had its Jewish physician. In 1267 the Council of Vienna forbade the Jews to practise among Christians. Under the Western Caliphate, Jewish physicians were prominent figures in Spain until they were banished the country in 1492. The School of Salerno utilized them as teachers, until it had developed enough home-grown talent to get along without them. The same thing was true of Montpellier, which was closed to the Jews in 1301. There were many at Avignon up to the 15th century.[2] The interdictions put upon Jewish physicians by Popes Paul IV (1555–9) and Pius V (1566–72) were lifted by Gregory XIII in 1584.[3] Although the different emperors continued to retain Jews as their body physicians, yet, up to the time of the French Revolution, they were not allowed to study at the European universities and being, moreover, excluded from the liberal professions, played little part in medicine during this period. At the outset of the modern industrial movement, they were admitted to the rights of citizenship all over Europe and given the freedom of the universities. The effect of this liberal policy was to bring forth a great array of brilliant talent which contributed very materially to the development of medicine in all its branches, as witness the work of Henle, Cohnheim,

---

[1] J. S. Billings: "The History and Literature of Surgery" (Dennis's System of Surgery, New York, 1895, vol. i, p. 38). For the Jewish physicians of the Middle Ages, see M. Steinschneider in Hebräische Bibliographie, Frankfurt a. M., 1914, and I. Münz: Die jüdischen Aerzte in Mittelalter, Frankfurt a. M., 1922.

[2] For a list of Jewish physicians at Avignon, see P. Pansier, Janus, Amst., 1910, xv, 421–451.

[3] A copy of this document is in the Surgeon General's Library.

Weigert, Traube, Stricker, and Pick in pathology; Senator, Hayem, and Boas in internal medicine; Romberg, Moll and Freud in neurology; von Hebra, Kaposi, Neumann, von Zeissl, and Unna in dermatology; Caspar, Lesser, Ottolenghi, and Lombroso in forensic medicine; Hirsch, Marx, Pagel, Magnus, and Neuburger in medical history and, in the science of infection, Metchnikoff, Fränkel, Friedländer, Marmorek, Haffkine, Neisser, and Paul Ehrlich,[1] to mention only a few well-known names.

[1] For a more complete list of modern Jewish physicians, see F. T. Haneman's article in the Jewish Encyclopædia, New York, 1904, viii, 421, 422.

THE MEDIEVAL PERIOD (1096–1438)

THE Middle Ages, the period of feudalism and ecclesiasticism, are commonly decried for servile obeisance to authority, with its attending evils of bigotry, pedantry, and cruelty. We regard any one who seeks to suppress the truth by overbearing or underhanded methods as "medieval-minded," and we think of special privileges, vested interests, unearned increments, *Faustrecht*, and other phases of Rob Roy's "simple plan," as smacking of feudalism. Yet, in the Middle Ages, there was true "consent of the governed." Even before the downfall of the Western Roman Empire, Greek science was practically dead, and Greek philosophy (neo-Platonism) had proved a total failure. The downfall of Rome left Europe practically nationless, at the mercy of wandering barbarians, her peoples *terræ filii*, adscripts of the glebe, "the indifferent children of the earth" of Shakespeare's line.[1] The social history of Europe for several centuries was the upbuilding of organized nations from loose tribal groups.[2] The larger groups became nations, the smaller groups remained tribal units or congeries of tribes. In Allbutt's view the medieval period was taken up with the organization of social groups of this kind "upon a provisional theory of life." In the welter of race-inmixture and race-absorption which ensued, the greatest need of European humanity was for a spiritual uplift, for regeneration and renewal of character rather than for intellectual development. We may glean some notion of the paralyzing effect of the downfall of the Western Empire upon human activity from some of the more immediate effects of the recent World War. To understand the impulses which drove the hermits to the desert and founded the monasteries, one can read Gibbon, Lecky, Montalembert, Gregorovius, Froude on the break-up of Roman society, Turgenieff's wonderful evocation of a Cæsarean triumph, or Flaubert's miracle-play of The Temptation of St. Anthony. Matthew Arnold, with his fine historic sense, summed all this up in stirring verses:

> On that hard Pagan world disgust
> And secret loathing fell.
> Deep weariness and sated lust
> Made human life a hell.
>
> She veiled her eagles, snapp'd her sword,
> And laid her sceptre down;
> Her stately purple she abhorr'd,
> And her imperial crown.
>
> She broke her flutes, she stopp'd her sports,
> Her artists could not please;
> She tore her books, she shut her courts,
> She fled her palaces.

---

[1] Cited by Hemmeter.

[2] As an example of the loose tribal aggregations of the Middle Ages, Singer cites an edict of Catania, Sicily (1168) to the effect that the local Latin, Greek, Saracen, and Jewish groups were each to be governed by its own laws. (Legacy of Israel, London, 1927, footnote to p. 175.)

Thus, the Christian Church, with its spiritual appeal, its attractive symbolism, its splendid organization and its consolidation with Feudalism in protecting Europe from Moslem invasion, could not but triumph. The Crusades aroused the feeling of nationhood. The organization of citizens against the robber barons awakened civic consciousness. In the great struggle between collectivism and individualism which began from that hour, intellectual independence was bound to go to the wall if it came into conflict with Church or State. In the Middle Ages, there was immense concern lest "the centrifugal forces of society overcome the centripetal."[1] The growth of the Christian virtue of compassion toward weakness and suffering, and the more elevated and enlarged conception of the position and mission of women which grew out of it, led to new departures in medicine along untried paths, particularly in nursing the sick and in erecting hospitals everywhere for their care. Only idle bigotry could affirm that Pope and Emperor did not do a great deal for medicine in the advancement of good medical legislation, in the chartering and upbuilding of the medieval universities, in the great hospital movement of the Middle Ages and in the encouragement of individual medical talent in many cases. Yet, as Allbutt has shown, the strife of intellects during the Ages of Faith was manifested in a way that tended to the absolute suppression of experimental science or even of the actual verification of premises. The Greek philosophers, as we have seen, held opinions the most disparate without any special strife among themselves and, above all, with a certain definite immunity from persecution. To those who can appreciate the fine individualism of the Greeks, the sentiment of the English poet will not seem exaggerated:

"Greece, where only man whose manhood was as godhead ever trod,
Bears the blind world witness yet of light wherewith her feet are shod:
Freedom, armed of Greece, was always very man and very God."

The medieval thinkers were all under the ban of authority, and for the strangest, yet most potent, of reasons. From the earliest times, human ideas as to the meaning of life and the forces behind the material world have usually progressed along two distinct, often parallel, lines, viz., a tendency to deify and worship the objects or forces of external nature, culminating logically in either Pantheism or Buddhistic Pessimism; and the rude fetishism of the savage, which passed through the successive stages of idolatry, hero-worship, ancestor-worship, polytheism, shamanism, finally merging into the pure monotheism of Israel, Christianity, and Islam. Christian Theism assumes that God is a spirit, omnipresent and immanent in nature yet different from it, accessible to prayer, and capable, at need, of divine intervention in human affairs. Pantheism simply identifies God with nature and natural forces. Now, in medieval times, the opposition between Theism and Pantheism took the form of

---

[1] The phrase is used as a criterion of good and bad government in Roosevelt's Romanes lecture on "Biological Analogies in History," Oxford, 1910, p. 23.

a dispute between "Realists" and "Nominalists," which, says Allbutt (paraphrasing the language of John of Salisbury), "engaged more of the time and passions of men than for the house of Cæsar to conquer and govern the world."[1] To the medieval logician, "Realism" meant just the opposite of our modern concept of a knowledge of material things. The Realist assumed, with Plato, that the idea is as actual as the thing itself and creative of it, the form as real as the matter or substance and anterior to it, whence it follows that all things proceed from the will of God. The Nominalist, on the other hand, affirmed that the form or idea is only a name or abstract conception, existing in the mind of the observer alone, and that God, therefore, exists impersonally in each and every object of the material world. To medieval theologians, such an approach to Pantheism could be no less than infidelity and unbelief, since it tended to dissolve the dogmas of faith and was subversive of the ideas of divine revelation and personal immortality, the hope held out to the Christian. To medieval physicians, such a manifesto of free-thought as the Hippocratic treatise "On the sacred disease" would have been abhorrent, but Galen, with his devout monotheism, his careful Bridgewater teleology, became an object of almost veneration. Aristotle, in his Logic and Metaphysics, never made an absolutely clear distinction between the supposed reality of idea and substance, yet public and private reading of his scientific works was forbidden by a provincial Synod at Paris in 1210, and the prohibition was repeated and extended to his Metaphysics (or rather to what Averroës had read into it) by the Papal legate in 1215. Not until the decree of Gregory IX (1231) did they regain favor, to appear in the Arts Course (Paris) in 1255, and later to be regarded as an almost infallible authority.[2] The more scientific writings of Aristotle were never studied in the critical, inquiring way in which the Greeks would have regarded such things. Ptolemy said that "He who would serve the cause of truth in science must be, above all, a free thinker," yet his geocentric system of astronomy came to be defended by the Church as if an article of faith. The natural histories of Pliny and the Physics of Aristotle were accepted by medieval authorities as beyond cavil. The biological works of Aristotle, although commentated by Albertus Magnus, were never studied or understood, but merely parodied in the queer "Herbals" and "Bestiaries" (or Beast-Books) of the time. All reasoning was formal and deductive. Until the Renaissance, there was neither induction nor experiment. Grown-up men, both Christian and Moslem, accepted such a nonsensical farrago of obscure reasoning as the *Timæus* of Plato for sound physiologic doctrine. Nature herself was never questioned for her secrets and, as Allbutt puts it, "Logic, which for us is but a drill and, like all drills, a little out of fashion, was for the Middle Ages a means of discovery, nay, the very source of

---

[1] For a full account of the subject, see Allbutt's Harveian oration, "Science and Mediæval Thought" (1901).

[2] C. H. Haskins: Harvard Stud. Class. Philol., Boston, 1909, xx, 86.

truth. . . . The dialectically irresistible was the true."[1] In the *Golden Legend* of Longfellow, medieval physicians and medical students are represented as frittering away their time in endless discussions about the nature of universals, the relation between the idea and matter, and other dialectic subtleties. The Nominalist of advanced and dogmatic type was even liable to persecution. Without going further into the lengthy disputes between Nominalists and Realists, it may be said that their adjustments of cause and effect have been traced through the ages in the *pneuma* of Galen, the *archæus* of Paracelsus, the animism of Van Helmont and Stahl, the "thought and extension" of Descartes and Spinoza, the *noumenon* and *phenomenon* of Kant, the "being and becoming" of Hegel, the "will and idea" of Schopenhauer, and in such modern concepts as natural law and natural phenomenon, type and individual, force and matter, statics and dynamics, vital principles and "the fortuitous concurrence of physicochemical forces." In our own day, the controversy has become merged into the opposition between Vitalism and Materialism. In the Middle Ages, the enormous expenditure of mental energy over this sterile, insoluble problem fortified the top-heavy feudalized scholastic in an ill-concealed contempt for all manual arts and crafts, especially for anatomy and surgery. Hence the surprising ignorance of Hippocrates in medieval times. "Had Galen's works been lost," says Withington, "there can be little doubt that the dark age of medicine would have been darker and more prolonged than it was, for the medieval practitioner could no more have appreciated the higher and freer teaching of the physician of Cos than he could have understood those grand words, 'It seemed good to the Demos,' which Hippocrates saw inscribed at the head of every decree, and heard proclaimed in every assembly."[2]

Through the Galenic dialectics, which led the medieval physicians to ask "why" rather than "how," to assign arbitrary reasons for phenomena without grasping, or even investigating their real nature, the medicine of the Middle Ages fell under the bondage of words, mistook the symbol for the thing, was forward in mechanical inventions, in military surgery and public sanitation, but decidedly backward in anatomy, physiology, pathology and internal medicine.

The fundamental error of medieval medical science, as originally pointed out by Guy de Chauliac, and elucidated by Allbutt,[3] was in the divorce of medicine from surgery. Greek intelligence, as personified in Hippocrates, saw internal medicine in terms of surgery and saw surgery not only as a mode of therapy, but as "the very right arm of internal medicine," since, in diagnosis, the outward and visible signs of internal malady (the only indices the Greek surgeon had) were also the main data of the clinician. Beginning with Avicenna, medieval medical

---

[1] Allbutt: *Op. cit.*, pp. 50, 51.

[2] Withington: Medical History, London, 1894, 104.

[3] Allbutt: "The Historical Relations of Medicine and Surgery," London & New York, 1905.

authority pushed Galen's dictum, "surgery is only a mode of treatment," to the extreme limit of treating the surgeon himself as a lackey and an inferior. The Arabian commentators of Galen, and the medieval Arabists who copied them, were obsessed with the idea, peculiar to Oriental religions, that it is unclean or unholy to touch the human body with the hands. As this tenet gained ground, scholastic and monastic minds became, as we have said, gradually penetrated with the conviction that redecraft is superior to handcraft, culminating in the famous edict of the Council of Tours, "*Ecclesia abhorret a sanguine*" (1163). The general practice of surgery, including most of the major operations, was, in the end, relegated to barbers, bath-keepers, sow-gelders, and wayfaring mountebanks. The surgeon himself came to be regarded in such a menial light that, even in Prussia, up to the time of Frederick the Great, it remained one of the duties of the army surgeon to shave the officers of the line. Again, the heresy imposed by the Arabist commentators of Galen, that "coction" (suppuration) and "laudable pus" are essential to the healing of wounds, made operative surgery a perilous and meddlesome undertaking, all the more danger-ous, indeed, in that the surgeon, whether scholar or mountebank, stood in jeopardy of life or limb if he operated unsuccessfully on any of the feudal lords of earth. The greatest surgeons of the time shrewdly ad-vised their professional brethren, therefore, to avoid or evade the operative treatment of difficult or incurable cases. When they at-tempted the major operations, their custom was to require a written guarantee that no harm should come to them in the event of a fatal termination. To lift the surgical art to its modern scientific (aseptic) status required the genius and personal influence of the three greatest surgeons of all time—Ambroïse Paré, John Hunter, and Lord Lister. The principal interest of the medieval period, therefore, lies not in its internal medicine, for there was precious little of it, but in the gradual development of surgery from the ground up by faithful, sometimes obscure followers of the craft, who (in France at least) were kept ostracized and short-coated by the edicts of the clerical bigots of St. Côme—the *chirurgiens de longue robe*. Quarrels between St. Côme, the Paris Faculty, and the barbers were continuous, but ended in the admission of the barbers to the practice of minor surgery in 1372.

The history of medieval medicine is mainly the history of the Latinization and subsequent Arabization of the West. Neuburger di-vides it into four periods, viz., the Monastic or Latinizing period (5th–10th centuries); the Salernitan (11th–12th centuries); the tempo-rary enlightenment of the 13th century, in which the Arabist culture was grafted upon that of the West; and the pre-Renaissance period (14th century), in which this culture became dominant. Both the Latin and Arabic cultures came from Greece.

With the downfall of Rome came the **Dark Ages** during which Western Europe passed into a tedious period of material waste and intellectual decadence.

The transition was not catastrophic, but gradual. The Germanic conquest entailed the loss of thousands of lives, the devastation of great tracts of country, the desolation of many cities, and the destruction of innumerable landmarks of art and culture, while the East still possessed a far-flung network of marts of commerce, covering three-fourths of the earth's surface, and so maintained its culture. In contrast with the imposing financial system of the Orient, the West, through slackening of trade, the splitting up of countries into small, separate states, and the falling back of its peoples upon agriculture as a last resort, acquired petty, parochial forms of economics, hole-and-corner modes of finance, and a general peasant complexion, which afforded little incentive toward a finer conduct of life. Nations were gradually built up, but, in the process, culture and free thought were inhibited. While the Moslem conquerors imposed the Arabic language and culture upon the conquered, the Germanic conquerors came under the sway of the Latinized culture of Christendom. In western Europe, Latin became the official language of Church and State. Pliny was the most popular writer. Only Latin translations of the Greek authors were read. By 600 A. D. the Vulgate of St. Jerome (337–420) had replaced all other Latin translations of the Bible (Singer). Science and learning sought refuge in the bosom of the Church, and no less than Cassiodorus, "the last of the Romans," pointed the way (Neuburger).

Thus began the period of **Monastic medicine,** in which, along with a praiseworthy zeal for preserving the remains of ancient literature and the traditions of a rational praxis, there grew up a cult of faith-healing or theurgic therapy, an implicit belief in the miraculous healing power of the saints and of holy relics. Supernatural aid came to be more esteemed as the medical art showed itself to be powerless, particularly in the time of the great epidemics. Western medicine, unlike that of Byzantium and Islam, went into eclipse and its practice, as Neuburger affirms, became as rudimentary and stereotyped as that of primitive man.

Under the beneficent reign of Theodoric the Great (493–526), there was an inter-period of peace, with material prosperity and due regard for art and science. An interesting relic of this early Ostrogothic period is the dietetic epistle of the Greek physician **Anthimus,** which is full of sound, sensible precepts, throwing much light upon the food-staples and kitchen practices of the time. Among other Latin remains of the Dark Ages are versions of Dioscorides, Hippocrates on airs, waters, and places,[1] certain works of Galen and Oribasius, a book of Paul of Ægina,[2] and the Swiss formularies collected by Sigerist and Jörimann.[3] The trend of the Ostrogothic period, indeed the principal task then set for medieval medicine, was by way of translating, compiling and paraphrasing from the ancients, a trend already established by the later Romans and the Byzantine writers. In this matter, Boëthius (circa 480–524) was the great exemplar. In the 6th century, the gradual passage of science into the hands of the clergy was accomplished, in the face of desolating wars between the Ostrogoths and Byzantines, the incursion and establishment of the Lombards in Italy (568–774), and devastating epidemics, like the plague of Justinian (543). Science and culture went to the wall, the schools of secular learning crumbled and disappeared, religious zeal and fanatical asceticism became the order of the day. Crushed by the Lombards, left in the lurch by Byzantium, the Latin population turned to the Church for protection. Glorified by the nimbus of ancient Rome, the Church thus became a real territorial power, able to practice genuine statecraft and to protect Western civilization. "The Benedictines became the Nestorians of the West" (Neuburger). In the Forum Pacis, where physicians once assembled and Galen dwelt, Pope Felix IV (526–530) set up the Basilica of SS. Cosmas and Damian, the patron saints of medicine. In the same year in which Justinian closed the School of Philosophy at Athens (529),

---

[1] Edited by G. Gundermann, Bonn, 1911.

[2] Edited by J. L. Heiberg, Leipzig, 1912.

[3] Frühmittelalterliche Receptarien, ed. Julius Jörimann, Zürich, 1925.

St. Benedict of Nursia (480–544) founded, on the site of an ancient temple of Apollo, the cloister of the Benedictine order at **Monte Cassino,** in the Campagna.   In 540 **Cassiodorus** (490–575) of Squillace (Calabria), after serving Theodoric and his grandson Athalaric as an official, retired to Squillace to found a monastery after the Benedictine pattern, where he devoted the remaining thirty-five years of his life to learning.   He turned the attention of the monks to the value of the older writings. Literary studies were assiduously cultivated and vows to nurse the sick were taken as the prime duty of the order, in accordance with the exhortation of St. Benedict (*Infirmorum cura ante omnia adhibenda est, ut sicut re vera Christo, ita eis serviatur*). The cloisters of Monte Cassino, Benevente, and Squillace had valuable collections of medical manuscripts, written in a peculiar Latin script,[1] the Beneventan.   To Cassiodorus, indeed, is due the preservation of the ancient Latin writings.   The *Commentarium medicinale* of Benedetto Crespi, Archbishop of Milan (681), a didactic hexameter poem dealing with the herbal treatment of 26 diseases after the fashion of Serenus Samonicus, is a relic of this period.   Another consists of two treatises on diseases and their remedies by Bertharius (857–884), the learned abbot of Monte Cassino.   The Lombard conquerors soon began to favor science, and names of laic physicians are preserved in the *Codex lombardus* and elsewhere.   In accordance with the precepts of Cassiodorus, the aim of the time was to make a summation of all medical knowledge (*summa medicinæ*), gleaned from the Greek and Latin authors. Serenus Samonicus, pseudo-Apuleius, pseudo-Pliny, and Cælius Aurelianus in therapeutics, and in obstetrics the pseudo-Soranic midwifery-book of Muscio, were most favored in these compilations.   Various works of Hippocrates, Galen, Rufus, Oribasius, Alexander Trallianus, and Dioscorides were translated into Latin (5th and 8th centuries) and, in the process of compilation, a number of spurious writings attributed to pseudo-authors were foisted off.   The medical part of Pliny, mixed up and seasoned with excerpts from Cælius Aurelianus, Apuleius, and Vindician, became our "pseudo-Pliny."   Many a summary, masquerading under the names of Dioscorides or Oribasius, was a mere hodge-podge from different sources.   Most of the medieval herbals were a mixture of the spurious pseudo-Apuleius (4th century, A. D.[2]), the Latin Dioscorides subsequently printed at Colle (1478) and the pseudo-Dioscorides (*De herbis feminiis*).   Of this character, too, were the pseudonymous epistles attributed to Hippocrates, in particular the Dynamidia (*De virtutibus herbarum*), the *De cibis*, the epistle to Ptolemy (*De hominis fabrica*), and the *Capsula eburnea*.   This "ivory capsule," a tract on the prognosis of skin affections, alleged to have been found by Cæsar in the tomb of Hippocrates, was first printed in a Milan incunable of 1481, reprinted in Wittwer's *Archiv* (1790), and has been carefully studied in all the MS. readings by Sudhoff (1916[3]).   The compilation known as the Lombard Dioscorides, drawn from Dioscorides, pseudo-Apuleius and Pliny, describes 71 herbs and their properties.   The basic MS., with beautiful illustrations, is of the 9th century and was prepared at Monte Cassino, but the original text is probably of the Gothic period (493–555).   Under the Visigoths in Spain (507–711), the activities of the medical profession were crushed by a Draconic code of laws. With the conversion of the Visigoths to Christianity (586), monastic medicine took its usual course.   Cloisters and church foundations even had their own physicians. A laparotomy for retained fetus in ectopic pregnancy is attributed to Bishop Paul, of Merida, where Bishop Masona founded a large hospital about 580.   The most learned man of his time was Bishop **Isidore of Seville** (*circa* 570–636), author of an *Etymologia* or encyclopedia of origins and etymologies, the fourth book of which contains a survey of medicine, but with many false and far-fetched derivations of medical terms.

Under the Merovingian monarchs (*les rois fainéants*) in France (486–741), Latin influences prevailed, but the dynasty has little to its credit save a string of bloody civil wars, and physicians had a hard time of it.   Gregory of Tours (538–593) records that the Frankish physicians had some skill in surgery and were sometimes in request as forensic experts in trials, but even those in attendance on royalty were humiliated or put to death if they failed to cure.   The people were given over to a belief in wonder-cures by strolling surgeons, to holy relics and exorcism.   In

---

[1] E. A. Lowe: The Beneventan Script, Oxford, 1914, with list of South Italian (Beneventan) medical MSS. on pp. 18–19.

[2] The Latin *Herbarium* of pseudo-Apuleius, first printed at Rome (1481), has been recently edited by Ernest Howald and H. E. Sigerist.

[3] Sudhoff: Arch. f. Gesch. d. Med., Leipz., 1915–16, ix, 79; 200.

time of epidemics, they came in great crowds to pass nightly vigils in the churches, an analogue of the temple-sleep. With such crude, bungling surgery as obtained, little wonder that Gregory counselled prayer and endurance of pain. With the advent of Charlemagne (768–814) as Emperor of the West (800), medicine came into better times. The cultural soil was prepared by the wandering Irish and Anglo-Saxon monks, who travelled from Bangor and Iona to the continent, and founded the monasteries of Bobbio and St. Gall. Cloister schools were founded at Fulda by the English Boniface, at Tours by the English Alcuin (735–804), at Chartres by Fulbert (1006–1028), to become famous centers of learning. Charlemagne had a physic-garden. From the Ecclesiastical History of the Venerable Bede (674–735), we gather that medicine was not neglected by English monks. He tells of a cure of aphasia by methodic exercises, and left a treatise on blood-letting.

The encyclopedic *Physica* of the Abbot of Fulda and Archbishop of Mainz, **Hrabanus Maurus** (776–856), Alcuin's favorite pupil and the *primus præceptor Germaniæ*, treats of medicine in the 6th, 7th, and 18th books and gives a German-Latin glossary of anatomic terms. In the 9th century, medicine was taught as part of *Physica*, which included arithmetic, astronomy, mechanics, geometry, and music, whence the physician was styled *physicus*. The *Hortulus* of Walafrid Strabo of Suabia (809–849), the best pupil of Hrabanus, describes, in 44 pleasant hexameters,[1] the plants in the garden of the cloister at Reichenau, of which he was abbot. Anglo-Saxon literature took its start in the reign of Alfred the Great (871–901), and held its own until the middle of the 12th century. The principal medical writings of the period are the *Leech-Book* of Bald, the *Lacnunga*, a book of Anglo-Celtic magic and translations of Apuleius and Sextus Placitus. The medieval penchant for allegory is exemplified in the Byzantine or Smyrna **Physiologus** (11th century) a popular purview of the virtues and vices in the form of twelve real or fantastic animals, which was translated into all languages and although pure allegory in itself became the original of "Beast-Books" or Bestiaries. Under the Carolingian monarchs, Jewish physicians were much favored in France. In lower Italy, Sabbatai ben Abraham, called **Donnolo** (913–965) was a famous practitioner and his *Antidotarium*,[2] a formulary of some 120 remedies, is the oldest known Hebrew medical work written in Europe. The oldest medical work in Spanish is a treatise on fevers by Isaac, a Jewish physician of the 11th century. Perhaps the oldest Hebrew medical text written in Asia is a book of remedies by Asaf Judæus, a Mesopotamian physician of the 7th century.[3]

Medicine in the 11th and 12th centuries was lifted to a much higher level by the **School of Salerno** which, as Neuburger says, aroused the healing art from the decreptitude of half a millenium, infused new life into things, and guarded as a Palladium the best traditions of ancient practice. Its origins are obscure. We only know that it came into existence in "a most mysterious way." That it was an ecclesiastical foundation is regarded by most historians as an agreeable *fable convenue*, for the whole character of the school was that of an isolated laical institution, a *civitas Hippocratica*, in the midst of purely clerical foundations, and there is significant silence about Salerno in the ecclesiastical chronicles. But the city itself was a bishopric; after 974, an archbishopric, where the Benedictines had a cloister and a hospital (820); and the friendliest relations are said to have existed between the clergy and the Salernitan physicians. The little seaside town of Salerno,

---

[1] Composed in 827. Published at Vienna, 1510. Edited by Sudhoff, Leipzig, 1927. Englished by R. S. Lambert as "Hortulus or The Little Garden," London, 1924.

[2] Edited by Steinschneider, Berlin, 1868.

[3] L. Venetianer: Asaf Judæus, Strassburg, 1916–17. Toznanski (Hebräische Bibliographie, 1916, 24) holds that Asaf lived in a much later period than the 7th century. (See I. Münz: Die jüdischen Aerzte im Mittelalter, Frankfurt a. M., 1922.)

near Naples, was mentioned by Horace (Epistles, I, xv) and was known to the Romans as an ideal health resort. The medical teachings and traditions of its famous school, the first independent medical school of the time, came upon the dreary stagnation of the Dark Ages, with something of the invigorating freshness of the sea. Its anatomy was based upon that of swine, its physiology and pathology were Galenic, its diagnosis mainly pulse- and urine-lore, but diseases were studied first-hand, in a straightforward, spontaneous, engaging manner, therapy was rational, with an effective scheme of dietetics, Salernitan surgery was new and original, obstetrics and nursing were cultivated by talented women. The Salernitan masters, as Neuburger observes, were the first medieval physicians to cultivate medicine as an independent branch of science. Whatever of Salernitan medical culture was Hellenistic was attributable to the fact that Sicily and what Singer calls "the shin and toe of Italy" (Magna Græcia) were still part of the Eastern Empire, and were entirely uninfluenced by Latin culture from the 7th century B. C. to the 10th century A. D. Here Greek was the spoken, albeit seldom the written language, up to the 15th century. From Magna Græcia, Byzantium, and Toledo came the three main streams of Greek culture which went to the formation of the Hellenic tradition. In Singer's view, the other contributory influences were the Monastic, deriving from St. Benedict's storehouses of learning, which had now spread all over Southern Italy; the Jewish, of which there were flourishing centers, surviving in spite of persecution, at Rome, Milan, Genoa, Palermo, Messina, and elsewhere; and the Arabic, dating from the conquest of Sicily and Southern Italy by the Moslem power (827–884), and culminating in the advent of Constantine of Africa at Salerno (1072). Thus, the legend that the School of Salerno was founded by "Four Masters," a Greek, a Latin, a Jew and a Saracen, may symbolize (Singer infers[1]) the four cultural influences which went to its making, in the period of racial conflict and inmixture in which it arose. But the best of it was Greek, and its spirit was transmitted to the great Schools of Bologna and Padua. The oldest documents of Salernitan medicine are compilations in barbarous Latin from the later Roman authors and pseudo-authors, and date from the first half of the 11th century.

Of these, the *Passionarius*, a handbook of special pathology and therapeutics, associated with the name of Galen and attributed to the Lombard Warimpotus or Gariopontus (died *circa* 1050), is in the opinion of Sudhoff not a genuine Salernitan writing, but a compilation from Byzantine sources, dating back to the 8th or 9th century. The Latin translation of Nemesius by Alphanus, Bishop of Salerno (*circa* 1050), the *Practica* of Petrocellus, an Anglo-Saxon version of the same in Cockayne's Leechdoms, and the poem *Speculum hominis* (*circa* 1050) are the only other Salernitan relics before the time of Constantinus Africanus.

Arabic medical doctrine was introduced at Salerno and fastened upon Western European culture until the 17th century by **Constantinus Africanus** (*circa* 1020–1087). The advent of Constantine at Salerno is

---

[1] C. and D. Singer: Sudhoff-Festschrift, Zürich, 1924, 121–138.

the *terminus a quo* of what Sudhoff calls High or Middle Salerno (1072–1224), the period of its greatest literary activity, in which, following the Norman conquest of the town in 1076, it became something approaching a university. The decline of Salerno (Late Salernitan period) dates from 1224 onward.

A native of Carthage, Constantine gained a close knowledge of Oriental languages by extensive travel and, returning to his native city, is said to have been persecuted as a magician. Fleeing to Italy, he lived for some time at Salerno, but whether he taught there is uncertain. About 1072, we find Constantinus in the cloisters at Monte Cassino, where he ended his days in his literary work. This consisted mainly of Latin translations of the *Liber regius* of Haly Abbas (*Pantegni*); the *Dietetics, Elements, Fevers,* and *Wines* of Isaac Judæus; the Arabicized versions of the *Aphorisms, Prognostics,* and *Regimen* of Hippocrates; the *Megatechne, Microtechne, De locis affectis,* and lesser treatises of Galen. Constantine was not remarkably proficient either in knowledge of Latin or of medicine, but he knew Arabic well and, with such resources as he had, proceeded to foist upon the Salernitan public sundry rough Latin paraphrases of the works of these Greek, Arabic, and Jewish writers as his own, subsequently polished by his pupil Atto. The influence of Constantine as a Latinizer of the Arabist culture[1] was far-reaching, as Sudhoff says, "a symptom of a great historic process," namely, the imposition of Mohammedan modes of thought upon Western European medicine from the 12th to the 17th centuries. Johannes Afflacius (*circa* 1040–1100), a Saracen pupil of Constantine, was the probable author of the *Liber aureus,* attributed to his master, and of a Salernitan tract, *De febribus et urinis,* which contains a device for cooling the sick-room by dripping water from a perforated vessel. Taddeo Alderotti later bore witness that these translations of Constantine were very faulty performances (*nam ille insanus monacus in transferrendo peccavit quantitate et qualitate[2]*).

Independent treatises on practice of medicine, notable for clarity of conception and concision of style were written severally by Magister Bartholomæus, Copho junior, Johannes Platearius junior, and by Archimathæus,[3] who also wrote an important tract on hodegetics (*De instructione medici*) or the etiquette of the physician's approach to the bedside (*De adventu medici ad aegrotum*). The most remarkable contribution of the Salernitan school to internal medicine is the *Tractatus de aegritudinum curatione,* the first example of an encyclopedic text-book of medicine, written by many authors, and no doubt designed for posterity as the *Summa medicinalis* of Salerno. It became the standard school book of internal medicine in the first half of the 12th century. As in each *Practica* listed above, it treats of local diseases *seriatim,* from top to toe (*a capite ad calcem*).

Among the earliest of the 12th century contributions to natural history was the compilation called *Macer Floridus* (1161), a didactic hexameter poem on the therapeutic virtues of 77 simples, attributed to Odo of Meudon, which was highly popular and frequently translated,[4] and was the original of the oldest Scandinavian medical writing, the Danish *Lægebog* of Henrik Harpestreng. The *Lapidarius* or stone-book of Bishop Marbod of Rennes (died 1123) deals with the medical and magic virtues of 60 precious stones.

Many Salernitan productions are contained in the "Breslau Codex" (*circa* 1160–70[5]) discovered by Henschel in 1837, containing 35 treatises reproduced, in part, in the collections of Salvatore De Renzi

---

[1] For the Arabic sources of Constantine, see M. Steinschneider: Virchow's Arch., Berlin, 1866, xxvii, 351–410.

[2] Preface to "Expositiones in arduum aphorismorum Ipocratis." Cited by Neuburger.

[3] For Archimathæus, see Hans Erchenbrecher, Leipzig diss., 1919.

[4] Edited by Ludwig Choulant, Leipzig, 1832.

[5] For a revised and classified table of contents of the Breslau Codex, see Friedrich Hartmann: Die Litteratur von Früh- und Hochsalerno, Leipzig diss., 1919. Also, Sudhoff: Arch. f. Gesch. d. Med., Leipz., 1920, xii, 101–148.

(1853–6) and Piero Giacosa (1901). The extant MSS. have been carefully collated by Sudhoff and his pupils. The total output of Salerno numbers 100 texts, by some thirty or forty authors. The famous *Regimen* (*Sanitatis*) *Salernitanum* or *Flos medicinæ* (1260–1300), a poem in leonine (double rhymed) hexameters, was first printed in Latin in 1484.

The date of origin of the *Flos* is unknown, but Sudhoff holds that its probable prototype was a pseudo-Aristotelian epistle to Alexander the Great (*De regimine sanitatis*), Latinized by John of Toledo (Joannes Hispanus), a baptized Jew, about 1130. This tract, dedicated to a Spanish princess, had a wide circulation and was followed by a similar dietetic epistle, addressed to Frederick II himself by his court philosopher, Magister Theodorus. In Arnold of Villanova's time, the Salernitan *Regimen*, which probably did not appear before 1260, consisted of 362 verses, which the additions and interpolations of De Renzi and others have expanded to 3520. Thus the famous Salernitan text owes its origin to Toledan sources, was probably not known either to Frederick II or Gilles de Corbeil, and consequently was not circulated until long after 1101,[1] the spurious date assigned for its composition in Warton's *History of English Poetry*.

The regimen consists of a string of very sensible dietetic and hygienic precepts, dedicated, in the several imprints, to the King of England (*Anglorum Regi*), in most of the manuscripts to the King of France (*Francorum Regi*). It passed through some 240 separate editions, including Irish, Bohemian, Provençal, and Hebrew.[2]

Of the "Ladies of Salerno," Abella wrote *De natura seminis hominis* and *De atra bile*, while **Trotula**, whom the 13th century trouvère Rutebœuf styled "Dame Trot" (*Madame Trotte de Salerne*) is credited with a gynecologic and cosmetic treatise (*De passionibus mulierum*). As Malgaigne and Sudhoff show, Trotula is not a person but the title of a book, which asserts that Trotula was a nickname common to all Salernitan midwives (*communiter Trotula vocata*). According to Daremberg and De Renzi, it is the name of an authoress, whom some suppose to have been of the Ruggiero family and the wife of the elder Platearius.

The *Antidotarium* of **Nicolaus Salernitanus**[3] was the first formulary and one of the first medical books to be printed (in the superb typography of Nicholas Jensen, Venice, 1471). It consists of 139 complex prescriptions in alphabetical order, contains many new Eastern drugs, also the original formula for the "anesthetic sponge" (*spongia somnifera*) and a table of weights and measures. The 12th century Antidotarium of Matthæus Platearius, known as *"Circa instans,"* which derives from the Latin Dioscorides, was the original of the first French herbal (*Le grant herbier*), and also exists in an Italian translation.

For a century (1070–1170), almost the sole source of anatomical knowledge was Constantine's translation of the Almaleki (II, 2, 3) of Haly Abbas (1080). The principal texts were:

---

[1] See Sudhoff: Arch. f. Gesch. d. Med., Leipzig, 1914–15, viii, 377; 1915–16, ix, 1; also, Pagel-Sudhoff, 173, and the Leipzig dissertation of Johannes Brinkmann: "Die apokryphen Gesundheitsregeln," [etc.]. 1915.

[2] An attractive English versification (bilingual text) is that of Dr. John Ordronaux (Philadelphia, 1870).

[3] Sometimes called Nicolaus Præpositus (*i. e.*, Præses of the faculty), but now to be differentiated from Nicole Prevost. See Wickersheimer, Bull. Soc. franç. d'hist. de méd., Paris, 1911, x, 388–397.

1. The so-called first Salernitan demonstrat'on probably of Matthæus Platearius (Sudhoff) *i. e.*, the pseudo-Galenic *Ars parva* or *Anatomia Cophonis*, a brief tract on the dissection of the pig sometimes attributed to **Copho**, a supposititious teacher at Salerno, but first printed in the second Latin edition (*Secunda impressio*) of Galen (Venice, 1502), and later in the *Divi Mesue Vita* (Lyons, 1531), the *Anatomia* of Dryander (1537) and the *Zoötomia* of Severino (1645). It was already known at Salerno in the first decade of the 12th century and, in the view of Sudhoff, is undoubtedly pre-Constantinian. 2. The Constantinian version of Haly Abbas (*supra*). 3. The second Salernitan *demonstratio anatomica*, also of the pig, discovered by Henschel (*Breslau Codex*) in 1846, revised by Benedict (1920) and translated by Corner (1927). It is based upon Constantinian material and of date *circa* 1170. 4. The *Anatomia Mauri*, or "third Salernitan demonstratio ľ" (1150–70) edited by Ploss (1921) and Sudhoff (1922). 5. The *Anatomia* of Ricardus Anglicus (died 1252), written about 1210, as part of his *Micrologus*, transcribed by Haeser, edited by Florian (1875) and Schwarz (1907), and collated from 4 MSS. for the first time by Sudhoff (1927), is also based on Constantine, but is not of Salernitan, but of English provenance. 6. The *Anatomia Magistri Nicolai Physici* edited by Redeker (1917), is probably an amplification of 5 by a pupil (Sudhoff). 7. The text called *Anatomia vivorum*, translated by Corner from a 13th century MS. (284) at Chartres, listed by Pansier (1909) derived largely from Gerard of Cremona's translation of Avicenna (1170–87) and falsely attributed to Aristotle, Galen, and Ricardus Anglicus (Töply, 1902), is common to 15th cen ury MSS. and all collective (printed) editions of Galen from 1502 on. It is post-Constantinian, in no sense Galenic, and of date *circa* 1225 (Corner[1]). 8. A ' fourth Salernitan demonstratioľ" recently printed by Sudhoff (1928) from the Pommersfeld parchment Codex 178 (2462), *circa* 1300–1310, and ascribed by him to Urso.

The principal Salernitan treatises on uroscopy were those of Johannes Afflacius, Johannes Platearius, the younger Archimathæus, Maurus and Urso.

Gilles de Corbeil (Ægidius Corboliensis), Canon of Paris and physician to Philippe Auguste of France (1165–1213), wrote two poems on the pulse and the urine,[2] based upon the Byzantine treatises of Theophilus Protospatharius, also a poem on the composition of medicines and a satire on the clergy (*Hierapigra ad purgandos prelatos*). He laments the decline of Salerno after it had been sacked by **Henry VI** (1194). After this terrible event, according to Ægidius, the Salernitan professors degenerated into beardless striplings who cared only for books of prescriptions. In the 13th century, the medical authority of Salerno was gradually impinged upon by the great rival schools of Naples, Palermo, and Montpellier. Its fame and influence became more and more of a vanishing fraction, until the great school was finally abolished by Napoleon on November 29, 1811.

The *Physica* of **St. Hildegard** (1099–1179), Abbess of Rupertsberg, near Bingen, describes the healing powers of the known plants, minerals and animals, giving the German names by preference, contains precepts for the hygiene of pregnancy and puerperium and rules for suppressing sexual desire. It is interesting for its sidelights upon the medicine, botany, and gardening of 12th-century Germany. Her little tract on clinical medicine (*Causae et curae*), a medley with many interpolations, has recently been edited by P. Kaiser (Leipzig, 1903). St. Hildegard's "Visions" (*Scivias*), wonderfully beautiful specimens of the medieval art of illumination, not

---

[1] See G. W. Corner: Anatomical Texts of the Earlier Middle Ages, Washington (Carnegie Inst.), 1927, to be checked by H. H. Beusing: Leipzig diss., 1912, and Sudhoff: Arch. f. Gesch. d. Med., Leipz., 1914–16, vii, 414; 1922, xiv, 56; 1927, xix, 209; 1928. xx, 33; Janus, Amst., 1924, xxviii, 397; 1927, xxxi, 294; Arch. f. Gesch. d. Math., [etc.]. Leipz., 1927, x, 1; 136.

[2] Printed at Padua (1484) and Venice (1494). Edited by L. Choulant as "Carmina medica," Leipzig, 1826.

unlike similar drawings by William Blake, are a revelation of her religious life. Charles Singer suggests that these visions may have had a primary physical basis, in that the shimmering, radiating figures resemble the stars, colored spots, and fortification spectra associated with the scotoma scintillans of migraine.[1]

The principal outcome of the School of Salerno was the work of two surgeons, **Roger** (Ruggiero Frugardi) of Palermo and **Roland** (Rolando Capelluti) of Parma, whose writings were independent of the influence of Constantinus Africanus or other Arabist sources (Gurlt). Roger's *Practica*, written about 1170 (Sudhoff), re-edited by his pupil Roland about 1230–40 (Sudhoff[2]) and commented upon by the "Four Masters" a little later, was never separately printed, but exists apart in manuscript, although Daremberg published a unique edition of the famous commentary (*Glossulæ quatuor magistrorum*) in 1854. Roger's work became a standard text-book at Salerno, where he himself had been a student and teacher. He knew of cancer and (possibly) syphilis, described a case of hernia of the lungs, prescribed ashes of sponge and seaweed (iodine) for goiter or scrofula, employed the significant mercurial salves for chronic dermal and parasitic affections, introduced the seton and suture of the intestines over a hollow tube,[3] taught the use of styptics, sutures and ligatures in hemorrhage, and the healing of wounds by second intention (laudable pus).

Roger, Roland, and the Four Masters were succeeded by the 12th century surgeon Jamerius,[4] by **Hugh** of Lucca (Ugo Borgognoni), who is quoted by Theodoric, but left no extant record of his own work behind him; by Bruno of Longoburg, an advocate of dry (aseptic) wound treatment, whose *Chirurgia magna* (completed at Padua in 1252) is the first treatise of the time in which Arabic authors are drawn upon; and by Hugh's son or disciple, Teodorico Borgognoni (1205-1296), or **Theodoric**, Bishop of Cervia, whose treatise (completed in 1266) is preserved in the surgical anthology (*Cyrurgia*) of 1498 and 1499. Theodoric was reviled by Guy de Chauliac as a copyist and plagiarist, probably because, like Hugh before him, he contradicted the pseudo-Galenist dogma of coction, laudable pus, or healing by second intention, and stood out in his day as a sturdy pioneer of a simple, expectant, dry treatment (rational asepsis): "For it is not necessary, as Roger and Roland have written, as many of their disciples teach, and as all modern surgeons profess," he says, "that pus should be generated in wounds. No error can be greater than this. Such a practice is indeed to hinder nature, to prolong the disease, and to prevent the conglutination and

---

[1] C. Singer: Studies in the History of Science, Oxford, 1917, i, 1–55.

[2] Printed in the Venetian encyclopedic collections (entitled "Cyrurgia"), of date 1498 and 1499, in the Juntine of 1546, and in De Renzi's collections. The close investigations of Sudhoff and his pupils show that the Rolandina is nowise an independent work, the new material being mainly glosses from the various MSS. of the Rogerina. See Waldemar Linge: Leipzig diss., 1919.

[3] In the glosses of the Four Masters a quill is used.

[4] First printed from a Munich MS. by Pagel as "Chirurgia Jamati" (Berlin, 1909). See also the Berlin dissertation of Artur Saland (1895).

consolidation of the wound" (Book II, ch. 27). This simple statement, as Allbutt points out, makes Theodoric one of the most original surgeons of all time, for only Mondeville and Paracelsus upheld these principles before Lord Lister and von Bergmann. In the long interregnum "the advocates of suppuration won all along the line." Hugh and Theodoric are also memorable for the inunction cure by the mercurial salve (*unguentum sarracenicum*), the sparing use of the cautery, and for setting the limitations of treatment with apparatus in fractures and dislocations. Their names are also associated with the **medieval substitutes for anesthesia,** the origins of which, however, go back to the remote past, probably to Alexandria.

Surgical sleeping draughts are mentioned by the Church Fathers St. Hilary of Poitiers (*De trinitate*, x, 14) and Origen. Salernitan reference to the "soporific sponge" occurs as an interpolation in the beautiful Jensen *Antidotarium* of Nicholas of Salerno (Venice, 1471, fol. 32 *verso*[1]), but Sigerist has found the identical recipe in a Bamberg Antidotarium of the 9th century and Sudhoff in a Monte Cassino Codex (lxix, 6) of the same period.[2] It is not found in the MS. codices of Nicolaus and is obviously pre-Salernitan, probably of Alexandrian provenance out of Dioscorides (iv 76). The sponge was steeped in a mixture of opium, hyoscyamus, mulberry juice, lettuce, hemlock, mandragora and ivy, dried and, when moistened, "inhaled" (probably swallowed) by the patient, who was subsequently awakened by applying fennel-juice to the nostrils. Cataplasms for local anesthesia are to be found in the *Antidotarium* of Nicholas (Oleum mandragoratum, fol. 22 *verso*), in the *Practica* of Copho, in the *Tractatus de aegritudinum curatione* and even in Gaddesden and Varignana. The recipe of the spongia somnifera occurs also in Hugh and Theodoric (*confectio somnifera*), Gilbertus Anglicus (1200), Pfolspeundt (1460), Guy de Chauliac, and the low-German *Gothaer Arzneibuch*. The old Dioscoridean sleeping potion was taken up by Avicenna, Serapion, Jocelyn of Furness (1177–99), Isidore of Seville, Thomas of Cantimpré, Conrad of Megenburg, Jerome Bock, Jerome of Brunswick (who substituted belladonna), Matteo Silvatico, and Brassavola. The fact that this narcotic potion was usually administered as a draught *per os* is indicated in Boccaccio (iii, 8; iv, 10), Macchiavelli (Il Mandragola), Du Bartas, Marlowe, Middleton and Shakespeare (Romeo and Juliet, IV, i, 3). Through the Middle Ages, mandragora was the soporific *par excellence*, preferable to opium and hemlock, because it was not, like these, "cold in the fourth degree," but in the third. John Donne (*Pseudomartyr*, 1610) says its "operation is between sleep and poison." Its dubious effects are indicated in Marlowe's Jew of Malta (Act V, sc. i):

> "I drank of poppy and cold mandrake juice
> And being asleep, belike they thought me dead."

The ablest Italian surgeon of the 13th century was Guglielmo Salicetti, called **Saliceto** or Salicet (*circa* 1210–1277), a man well educated in hospital and on the battlefield, as also in respect of university training. He was professor at Bologna (*circa* 1268), later city physician at Verona and, during 1269–75, prepared his *Cyrurgia*[3] (first printed

---

[1] See Husemann: Deutsch. Ztschr. f. Chir., Leipzig, 1895. xlii, 577–596, who is, however, otherwise misleading and has been corrected by Held (Nicolaus Salernitanus, Leipzig diss., 1916), and W. von Brünn (Sudhoff's Arch., Leipz., 1920–21, xii, 93–95). Sudhoff (Beitr. z. Gesch. d. Chir., Leipz., 1918, ii, 482–487) gives an account of sundry MSS. of 1300 in which many other drugs used in medieval anesthesia (*ars somnifera*) are listed.

[2] Sudhoff: Arch. f. Gesch. d. Med., Leipz., 1921–22, xiii, 127. This modest little note illustrates the danger of trusting implicitly to the incunabula, when the unwritten history of medieval medicine is buried in the vast array of unprinted MSS.

[3] Completed June 7–8, 1275.

at Piacenza in 1476[1]) for the benefit of his son, whom he brought up to the profession of medicine. Although far shorter than his treatise on internal medicine, the Surgery stands out as a great landmark or sea-mark in the history of the craft, and for the following reasons[2]: Saliceto did not separate surgical diagnosis from internal medicine and kept a good record of case histories, which he held to be the foundation of his subject. Book IV of his treatise contains the first known treatise on regional or surgical anatomy (Sudhoff). He restored the use of the knife, which Arabian practice had set aside in favor of the cautery, but says not a word of the dry, aseptic wound treatment recommended and practised by Hugh and Theodoric in Bologna. He shows how to suture divided nerves, to diagnose bleeding from an artery by the spurt of blood, and specifies contralateral paralysis as a sequel of head injuries (Hippocrates), for which he recommends a thick compress to prevent the injurious admission of air. Crepitus (*sonitus ossis fracti*) is empha-sized as a diagnostic sign of fractures; arrow wounds are described in graphic fashion, and a furrier's suture is prescribed for intestinal wounds. He was the first after Roger to assign venereal contagion (*coitus cum fœda meretrice*) as the real cause of chancre, bubo, and phagedenic ulcers, and even recommends a prophylactic *ablutio cum aqua frigida et roratio loci cum aceto* (Neuburger). In his treatise on practice, Saliceto left a classic description of dropsy due to contracted kidney (*"durities in renibus"*[3]) a remarkable account of melancholia, and valuable contributions to gynecology. The sound surgical principles of Saliceto were ably up-held by his pupil, **Lanfranchi** of Milan, who became involved in the squabbles of the Guelphs and Ghibellines and was driven out of his native town by the Visconti. At Lyons, he wrote his *Chirurgia parva*. Arriving in Paris in 1295, he found himself, as a married man, shut out from teaching at the university, where the professors were celibate clerics. He therefore became associated with the College de Saint Côme, organized before 1260 by Jean Pitard,[4] surgeon to Philip the Fair (1306–28). Here, by his straightforward style of lecturing and his use of bedside instruction, Lanfranc became the virtual founder of French surgery. He died in 1315. In his *Chirurgia magna*, completed

---

[1] Translated into French, by Nicole Prévost (Lyons, 1492) and again with commentaries, by Paul Pifteau (Toulouse, 1898). Saliceto's treatise on practice (*Summa conservationis et curationis*) was first printed at Piacenza (*circa* 1475–6), and his *De salute corporis* at Leipzig (1495). His merits as a physician have been studied in the Berlin dissertations which Pagel set for his pupils, H. Grunow (1895), E. Loewy (1897), W. Herkner (1897) and O. Basch (1898). For his treatise on anatomy, see F. O. Schaarschmidt, Leipzig diss., 1919.

[2] See Gurlt, i, 754–765; Neuburger, ii, 380–384, and Allbutt: "The Historical Relations of Medicine and Surgery," London, 1905, 32–33.

[3] Saliceto: "Liber . . . in scientia medicinali," Placentiæ, 1476, ch. 140. See also, Haeser, "Zur Geschichte der Brightschen Krankheit," Janus, Breslau, 1848, iii, 371, which gives interesting references to nephritis by the Arabic writers Serapion and Rhazes.

[4] For a surgical manual by Pitard, from MS. in Lüneberg (Latin) and Paris (old French) see Sudhoff: Arch. f. Gesch. d. Med., Leipz., 1908–9, ii, 189–278.

in 1296 and dedicated to Philip the Fair (Venice, 1490[1]), he made a resolute and valiant stand against the medieval schism between surgery and medicine which had existed since Avicenna's time, stating his conviction that the surgeon should also be an internist in a neat syllogism: *"Omnis practicus est theoricus: omnis cyrurgicus est practicus: ergo omnis cyrurgicus est theoricus."* He was the first to describe concussion of the brain, and his chapter on the symptoms of fracture of the skull is accounted a classic. Depressed fragments and irritation of the dura are his only indications for trephining. He also differentiated between venous and arterial hemorrhage, and between cancer and hypertrophy of the female breast. Such procedures as intubation of the esophagus, reunion of divided nerves, and neurotomy for tetanus are among his innovations. Unlike Saliceto, Lanfranc was a cauterist and averse to the knife. He therefore avoided trephining, cataract extraction, or lithotomy, and treated hernia with trusses only; but did not hesitate to operate for empyema and wounds of the intestines, treating hemorrhage by styptics, digital compression, torsion, or even the ligature. He gives careful directions for venesection, lamenting that this procedure should be the province of the barbers. On the dry conglutinative treatment of wounds he is again silent. His ethical advice to the surgeon is quaint and characteristic, and although he looked upon Paris as an earthly paradise, he held the French surgery of his day in sovereign contempt. The work of Saliceto and Lanfranc, coincident with the development of the great medieval universities—Paris (1110), Bologna (1113), Oxford (1167), Montpellier (1181), Padua (1222), Naples (1224)—and the brilliant false dawn of culture and liberalism in the 13th century,[2] did much to further the growth of surgical talent in France, England, and Flanders. Of the old Italian families delle Preci and da Norsia were the Preciani and the Norsini, whole generations of itinerant surgeons, who practised herniotomy, lithotomy, urethrotomy, and cataract extraction as a family secret.

Contemporary with Lanfranc was his loyal follower, **Henri de Mondeville** (1260–1320), a hardy and original thinker, endowed with great powers of wit and sarcasm, who made a valiant last stand for the principle of avoiding suppuration by simple cleanliness as originally taught by Hippocrates, and which Mondeville got from Theodoric. Before 1301 he was one of the four body surgeons of Philip the Fair, and in 1304 he delivered lectures on anatomy at the University of Montpellier. The surgical treatise of Mondeville, begun in 1306 and left a torso (1316), was first edited and printed from the several manu-

---

[1] Also printed in the surgical anthologies of 1498–9. There was a French translation by G. Yvoire (Lyons, 1490), an old English version (Old English Text Society, 1894), and another (*Chirurgia parva*) in black letter by John Halle (London, 1565). A Spanish translation of the *Chirurgia parva* in black letter was printed at Seville in 1495 by "tres alemanes compañeros." It was translated into German by Otho Brunfels (Strassburg, 1528).

[2] For this *Aufklärung*, which unfortunately did not last long, see J. J. Walsh, "The Thirteenth, Greatest of Centuries," New York, 1912.

scripts by Pagel in 1892, and later translated into French by Nicaise (Paris, 1893[1]). This treatise, like that of Saliceto, contains a chapter on anatomy, with 13 illustrations *en miniature*.[2] It abounds in directions of the rarest common sense for the aseptic treatment of wounds, and in shrewd practical advice to the surgeon as to the conduct of his professional life. In opposition to the salve-surgery of the Galenists, Mondeville advises simply to wash the wound clean and put nothing whatever into it, since "wounds dry much better before suppuration than after it." Wine and other "wound-drinks" were given to strengthen the patient,[3] in opposition to the routine practice of cutting down his diet. For hemorrhage Henri recommends styptics, digital compression, acupressure, and torsion of the isolated vessel by means of a sliding-noose ligature. Guy says that Henri's teachers were Parisian scholastics and, in truth, his pages abound in verbose maunderings, but he was capable of such biting utterances as these: "God did not exhaust all His creative power in making Galen."—"Many more surgeons know how to cause suppuration than to heal a wound."—"Keep up your patient's spirits by music of viols and ten-stringed psaltery, or by forged letters describing the death of his enemies, or by telling him that he has been elected to a bishopric, if a churchman."—"Never dine with a patient who is in your debt, but get your dinner at an inn, otherwise he will deduct his hospitality from your fee." Henri's rapacity in the matter of fees shows how hard they were to get in the Middle Ages,[4] and he himself was obviously the type of surgeon who had to succeed by dint of hard knocks. Like the heroes of Smollett, as described by Sir Walter Scott, his cynical spirit seemed to delight in things "attended with disgrace, mental pain, and bodily mischief to others," yet it is hard to say offhand whether this was the fruit of harsh experience or the expression of supreme irony.

A man of far different type was **Guy de Chauliac** (1300–68), the most eminent authority on surgery in the 14th and 15th centuries. A country boy from Auvergne, Guy managed, through friends, to take holy orders and to get an excellent medical education at Toulouse, Montpellier, and Paris, with a special course in anatomy at Bologna.[5] He thus became the most erudite surgeon of his time, and in due course, settled down at Avignon as physician and "commensal chaplain" to Popes Clement VI, Innocent VI, and Urban V. He died on July 25,

---

[1] A fragmentary old French version of 1314 has been published by A. Bos (Paris, Société des anciens textes français, 1897–9); another MS. of 1478 is in the University Library of Upsala.

[2] Mondeville's anatomy was reprinted from a Berlin MS. by Pagel (1889).

[3] See A. Raubach: Ueber die Wundtränke in der mittelalterlichen Chirurgie, Berlin dissertation, 1898.

[4] The Salernitan *Dum dolet, accipe* was the rule, as indicated by John of Salisbury (Neuburger, ii, 325). See also, C. Vieillard: Le pacte médical au moyen âge, Bull. Soc. franç. d'hist. de méd., Paris, 1904, iii, 482–496.

[5] Guy learned his anatomy from Mondino's pupil, Niccolò Bertuccio, and also owed much to the translation of Galen's *De usu partium* by Niccolò de Regio (1317–45).

1368. Guy was a writer of rare learning, endowed with a fine critical and historic sense. In the *Capitulum singulare* of his great work he stands out as the only medical historian of consequence between Celsus and Champier.[1] As an operator, he set great store by the study of human anatomy and, although he hesitated to cut for stone, was one of the first to take the operations for hernia and cataract out of the hands of the strolling montebanks.

He believed in cutting out cancer at an early stage with the knife, but employed the actual cautery in the fungous variety as well as in caries, anthrax, and similar lesions. Ulcers he treated by means of an investing collar or guard of sheet lead. He suspended fractures in a sling bandage, or (if in the thigh) by means of weight and pulley. Guy also gives an interesting summary of the dentistry of the period.[2] He throws a great light upon the operative procedure of his time by his description of Theodoric's narcotic or soporific inhalation. This, the medieval substitute for anesthesia, as above described, was even in vogue in the 17th century, as evidenced in the well-worn citation from Thomas Middleton's tragedy of *Women Beware Women* (Act IV, sc. i):

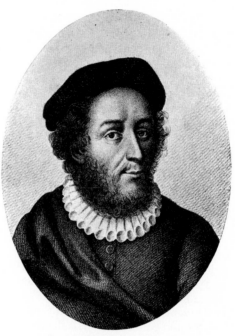

Guy de Chauliac (1300–70).

> I'll imitate the pities of old surgeons
> To this lost limb, who, ere they show their art,
> Cast one asleep, then cut the diseased part.

In spite of his wide experience, Guy de Chauliac was on the whole a reactionary in the important matter of the treatment of wounds, and threw back the progress of surgery for some six centuries by giving his personal weight to the doctrine that the healing of a wound must be accomplished by the surgeon's interference—salves, plasters and

---

[1] Guy's *chapitre singulier* on the history of medicine was edited separately by Jean Canappe, and printed by Étienne Dolet (Lyons, 1542). The value of this chapter was first emphasized by Symphorien Champier in *Le Guidon en francoys*, Lyons, 1503 (E. C. Streeter).

[2] For which, see V. Guerini's "History of Dentistry," Phila., 1909, 142–149; J. J. Walsh: "Old-Time Makers of Medicine," New York, 1912, 319–323.

other meddling—rather than by the healing power of nature. As an ethical teacher, Guy holds up a far nobler ideal to the surgeon than Henri: his mode of expression reveals the gentleman and the scholar. During the epidemics of plague at Avignon in 1348 and 1360, he stuck manfully to his post as a healer of the sick, while other physicians fled the locality. His most important work is the *Inventarium et Collectorium (Chirurgia magna)*, written in 1363, and first published in French translation at Lyons in 1478.[1] This book passed through many editions, translations, and abridgments (*les fleurs du grand Guidon*). In the abridged form, it became the *vade mecum* or *"guidon"* of surgical practice even beyond the 16th century.[2]

Guy's most distinguished pupil was Pietro d'Argelata (died 1423), a professor at Bologna, whose *Cirurgia* was printed at Venice in 1480. The chapter on the custody of the dead body tells how he embalmed the corpse of Alexander V. D'Argelata taught the dry treatment of wounds, but powdered them; was skilled in dentistry, used sutures and drainage-tubes in wounds, trephined the skull, incised the linea alba in post-mortem Cesarean section, and sometimes operated for hernia, stone, and fistula in ano. The latter operation attained a high degree of perfection in the hands of John of Arderne (1306–90 [?]), the earliest of the English surgeons. Arderne was a well educated man, who got his training by an adventurous career as army surgeon in the Hundred Years War. His surgical writings were widely read in England for nearly 200 years, as evidenced by the many illustrated MSS., some of which were copied as late as the 16th century (Singer). He wrote treatises on *passio iliaca* (appendicitis or intestinal obstruction) and gout; and an essay on clysters (1370), advocating an instrument of his own invention. He employed irrigation in renal and intestinal colic, cystitis, and gonorrhea. His illustrated treatise on fistula in ano (1376), edited by D'Arcy Power (1910), describes a well authenticated surgical operation for a condition which most of his predecessors had abandoned as incurable. Getting his patient into the lithotomy position, Arderne boldly incised the outer wall of the fistula in all its branches instead of fretting it by probes and ligatures; hemorrhage was checked with sponges, and all corrosive or irritating after-treatment of the wound avoided. This asepsis, akin to Mondeville's, is a reflex of Arderne's training as a Norman surgeon. The Saxon leech crops out in his lean-

---

[1] La pratique en chirurgie du maistre Guidon de Chauliac, Lyon, Barthelemy Buyer, 1478. The Latin text (Chirurgia) was first printed at Venice (1490); a Venetian text in *lingua franca* (in 1480); a good Latin text by Laurent Joubert, chancellor of Montpellier (Lyons, 1578); also a French text (Rouen, 1615), and glossary by his son (1585). The best modern edition is that of Edouard Nicaise (Paris, 1890). Many commentaries and abridgments were made by Symphorien Champier (1503–37), Louis Verduc (1731) and others. English, German, and Spanish versions exist. The black-letter *Questyonary* of Robert Wyer (London, 1541) is a beautiful impression. A rare English MS. owned by E. C. Streeter is described by him in Proc. Charaka Club, N. Y., 1916, iv, 107–111, 2 pl.

[2] For a thoroughgoing exegesis of the surgical content of the *Inventarium*, see W. von Brünn in Sudhoff's Arch., Leipz., 1920–21, xii, 85; 1921–22, xiii, 65.

ing toward astrology, charms, and wort-cunning. "Nothing pleased him more than a charm" (Power).

Giovanni **Arcolani** (died 1484), or **Arculanus,** a professor of medicine and surgery at Bologna (1422–1427) and Padua, whose treatise on surgery (*Practica*) was published at Venice (1483), is memorable as one of the leading pioneers of **dentistry** and the surgery of the mouth. The surgical sections contain figurations of the instruments used,[1] including aural syringes and flexible catheters. He describes the filling of hollow teeth with gold-leaf, and gives a remarkable account of the mental symptoms of alcoholism. Otherwise he is but a typical expositor of Avicenna and Arabian surgery.

The *Chirurgia* of Leonardo da Bertapaglia (died 1460) is again only an arrangement of the fourth book of Avicenna's *Canon*, full of Arabian polypharmacy, with strong leanings toward astrology.

The Flemish surgeon Jean **Yperman** (1295–1351), whose *Chirurgie* was printed from the Flemish manuscript by Carolus (Ghent, 1854), by Broeckx (Antwerp, 1863[2]), and latterly in a splendid definitive edition by van Leersum (1912[3]), was a pupil of Lanfranc's and worthily upheld his master's teaching, especially in regard to ligation and torsion of arteries. During the 14th century he was the great authority on surgery in the Low Countries.

He gives good accounts of trephining, arrow-wounds (with a special wound-drink), healing of harelip by means of freshened edges and special sutures, artificial feeding by a silver tube, and enlargement of the opening in reposition of prolapsed viscera. The chapter on leprosy stresses the anesthesia, and the possibility of infection by sexual intercourse. Of the Royal Touch for scrofula, he slyly notes that curable cases will get well without it (Neuburger).

Hand in hand with the medieval development of surgery, there necessarily went some effort to improve the status of human **anatomy.** Dissecting, at first rigorously proscribed by law and sentiment, became more and more a matter of course, following the decree of Emperor Frederick II in 1240. Payne has divided medieval anatomic teaching into three periods: First, the Salernitan (800–1200), in which instruction was based upon the dissection of animals as set forth in the *Anatomia Porci* of Copho; second, the Arabist period (13th century), in which such dissections were superseded by books and lectures.

The only texts of the period extant are the *Anatomia* in the *Micrologus* of Richard of Wendover (died 1252), an anomymous *Anatomia vivorum*, included in all the earlier *Opera omnia* of Galen, an amplification of the latter, known as *anatomia Nicolai*, and the anatomical treatise which Henri de Mondeville prefixed to his surgery (1306–16). The 13 miniature paintings which Henri employed have been reproduced and described by Sudhoff from a French MS of 1314, also a number of crude pen-drawings from MSS. at Berlin and Erfurt.[4] These tiny pictures are, perhaps, the earliest anatomical illustrations of the time, and establish sundry traditional norms, *e. g.*, the muscular and visceral schemata, which were slavishly

---

[1] Neuburger, *op. cit.*, ii, 508. J. J. Walsh: Old-Time Makers of Medicine, New York, 1911, and his Modern Progress and History, New York, 1912, 116–118.

[2] A *Traité de médecine pratique du maître Jehan Yperman* was also edited and published by Broeckx (Antwerp, 1867).

[3] Van Leersum: De Cyrurgie van Meester Jan Yperman, Leyden, 1912.

[4] Sudhoff: Anatomie im Mittelalter (Stud. z. Gesch. d. Med., Leipz., 1908, Heft 4), 82–89, pl. xxiv.

followed for a long time. Better executed are the 18 colored figures from the *Anatomia* of Guido de Vigevano (1345), which Wickersheimer reproduced from MS. 569 in the Musée Condé (Chantilly[1]). The anatomy in these drawings, intended to illustrate the technic of dissecting, is extremely diagrammatic. In most of these MSS., the skeleton has the spectral aspect (*Lemurengestalt*) familiar in the many figurations of the Dance of Death, suggesting a dried disemboweled preparation with the bones shining through the skin; the stomach is inverted, giving the visceral schema the appearance of a bagpipe. The spinal column looks like a Malay creese.

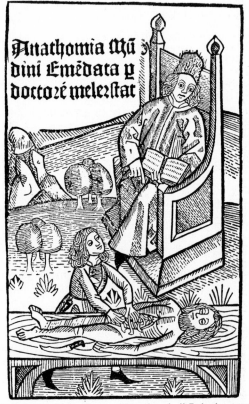

Title-page of Mundinus: "Anathomia," Leipzig, 1493.

The interest of the third period centers in the revival of human dissecting by Mondino de Luzzi (*circa* 1275–90), called **Mundinus** of Bologna, whose *Anothomia* was completed in 1316 and first published at Padua in 1487, and later at Leipzig in 1493 by Martin Pollich von Mellerstadt. In intention, this work was really a little horn-book of dissecting[2] rather than a formal treatise on gross anatomy.

Mundinus' scheme of dissection begins with the abdominal cavity, as containing the perishable viscera. In this section, he incidentally describes abdominal para-

---

[1] Wickersheimer: Arch. f. Gesch. d. Med., Leipz., 1913–14, vii, 1–25, 5 pl.; also, reprinted by Wickersheimer in an *édition de luxe*: Anatomies de Mondino dei Luzzi et de Guido de Vigevano, Paris, E. Droz, 1926.

[2] Otherwise a general medical manual (*quoddam opus in medicina*).

centesis, radical cure of hernia and lithotomy, gives the differential diagnosis between renal and intestinal colic, and records his postmortems on two female cadavers (January, March, 1315) to ascertain the relative size of the uterus in virgins and multiparæ. He then passes to the chest and neck, giving a lengthy description of the heart, and concludes with the opening of the skull. In speaking of the ear, he says we might understand the temporal bone better if it were cleaned by boiling, only this is sinful (*sed propter peccatum dimittere consuevi*) (Neuburger).

Although full of Galenical errors in regard to the structure of the human frame, preserving the old fictive anatomy of the Arabists, with the Arabic terms, this work was the most popular text-book during the period 1470–1530.[1] After the invention of printing, it became a kind of student's compend, and passed through 39 separate editions and translations (Mortimer Frank). Mundinus' work at Bologna was continued by his pupil Niccolò Bertuccio (died 1347), who taught Guy de Chauliac. After this time, dissecting gained a firmer foothold as a mode of instruction.

Gentile da Foligno gave a public dissection at Padua in 1341. In 1286 a physician of Cremona opened a corpse to find out the cause of death during a pestilence then raging. The first recorded postmortem was conducted on a case of suspected poisoning by Bartolomeo da Varignana at Bologna in 1302. In 1348 necropsies were conducted at Siena and were authorized at Montpellier about 1376–7. Public dissections were decreed at the University of Montpellier in 1366, at Venice (1368), at Florence (1388), at Lerida (1391), at Vienna (1404), at Bologna (1405), at Padua (1429), at Prague (1460), at Paris (1478), and at Tübingen (1485[2]). An anatomic theater was erected at Padua in 1445, and, at the Paris Faculty, four dissections annually had been required from the latter half of the 15th century on.

Even before the advent of Vesalius, the great painters of the Renaissance were making dissections in the hospitals at Florence (Santo Spirito), Milan, and Rome; but apart from these artists, whose paintings really advanced anatomy without didactic intention, dissecting, as Neuburger remarks, was mainly a showy, ornamental feature of medieval instruction. In regard to the bull *De sepulturis* of Pope Boniface VIII (1300), which many suppose to have put a damper upon anatomic research, it is shown by Neuburger and Walsh that it was, in intention at least, a simple mandate to prevent the bodies of dead Crusaders from being boiled and dismembered before returning them to their relatives.[3]

In the 13th century the Arabist culture was securely grafted upon European medicine by means of Latin translations, and **internal medicine** in this period had strong scholastic leanings. Its votaries were men of the type of the foremost intellectual leaders of the 13th century, such as Roger Bacon or Albertus Magnus. The medieval lawyers and logicians did good service in sharpening men's minds and teaching them how to use dialectics as an instrument or weapon, but science

---

[1] Before the invention of printing, Galen's manual of dissecting (*De juvamentis membrorum*) was commoner in Latin, French, and English MSS. (Singer).

[2] See F. Baker: Johns Hopkins Hosp. Bull., Balt., 1909, xx, footnote to p. 331.

[3] Neuburger: *Op. cit.*, ii, 432. For Latin text, see Walsh: The Popes and Science, New York, 1908, 413, and English translation: Med. Library and Histor. Jour., 1906, iv, 265. See also Ernst von Rudloff: Ueber das Conservieren von Leichen im Mittelalter, Freiburg diss., 1921.

itself could not advance as long as the pitfalls of syllogism were preferred to inductive demonstration of fact. We call the medieval writers on practice of medicine "Arabists" on account of their unswerving fidelity to Galenic dogma as transmuted through Mohammedan sources. The great center of this **translating movement** was Toledo, which, after falling into the hands of the Christians in 1085, was sought by all and sundry for its rich stores of Arabic manuscripts. In this work of transmitting Greek culture from the Arabic into Latin, the learned Jews, as Steinschneider has so exhaustively shown, were the natural intermediaries. Arabic was spoken by Spanish Jews up to the 13th century, and was known to learned Spanish Jews long after. Latin medical translations from the Arabic are associated with Toledo. Most of the Hebrew translations from the Arabic came later from Provence.

Gerard of Cremona (1114–87), who came from Italy to Toledo to learn Arabic and remained there all his life, was the principal interpreter of this Toledan treasure-hoard. He translated Rhazes, Serapion, Isaac Judæus, Albucasis, and the Canon of Avicenna. Marcus of Toledo translated some of Galen and the Isagoge of Johannitius. At the instance of Charles of Anjou, the Salernitan Jew Ferragut ben Salem, of Girgenti, translated Rhazes in Sicily (1279) and the *Tacuinum sanitatis* at Naples (1296). John of Toledo (Joannes Hispanus) profoundly influenced Salerno by his Latin version of the hygienic epistle of pseudo-Aristotle (1130). In this work of transplantation of Arabist doctrine the Jews, the natural intermediaries between East and West, played the most considerable part. The so-called "translators," ignorant of Arabic, usually had some learned Jew turn the text orally into colloquial Spanish, to be rendered into barbarous Latin *currente calamo* by a Mozarab (native Christian) of Vicar-of-Bray type. Through medical, as well as linguistic, ignorance, the technical terms were simply transferred without translation, the sense of the text was frequently distorted, and the many contractions made it otherwise unintelligible.[1] This great mass of Arabist doctrine was now attacked by the scholastic physicians, who were either commentators in the orthodox sense, "aggregators," *i. e.*, compilers of the best things in their authors; "conciliators," *i. e.*, those who sought to settle and reconcile the contradictions in Hellenist and Arabist doctrine by dialectics; or "concorders," *i. e.*, arrangers and harmonizers of the outstanding ideas and sentences of an author in regular order.[2] The chief merit of all these medieval compilers was in their feeling for orderly arrangement. There was little independent thought. The influence of the Arabic authors imported by Constantine was already noticeable in such early 13th-century physicians as Ricardus Anglicus, Gualtherus Agulinus, Petrus Hispanus, Gilbertus Anglicus and **Jean de St. Amand,** Canon of Tournay, who wrote a commentary on the *Antidotarium* of Nicholas the Salernitan; a *Revocativum memoriæ*, a labor-saving compend, designed to spare students sleepless nights over their Galen and Avicenna, and consisting of a Concordance of these authors arranged by catchwords, an abbreviated key to the contents of the Hippocratic and Galenic writings; and the *Areolæ*, a condensed materia medica, which enjoyed great popularity in the schools. The founder of medical dialectics (and the real founder of the **Bolognese school**) was **Taddeo Alderotti** (1223–1303), called Thaddeus of Florence, a writer of dry scholia and good consilia, who began to teach logical or scholastic medicine at Bologna in 1260, and was a thrifty, much-envied practitioner. Not only did he encourage Latin translation directly from Greek medical texts, but he was a prime mover in advancing the technic of postmortem examinations and consequently of dissecting. No less than Mundinus, Mondeville, and Varignana were his pupils (Singer). In his *Schriftstellerei*, Thaddeus introduced the practice of swamping a text in a veritable inunda-

---

[1] M. Steinschneider: Die hebräischen Uebersetzungen des Mittelalters und die Juden als Dolmetscher, Berlin, 1893. Die arabische Literatur der Juden, Frankfurt, 1902. Die europäischen Uebersetzungen aus dem Arabischen, Vienna, 1904–5. Also, Neuburger, *op. cit.*, 329–337, and Singer in The Legacy of Israel, London, 1927, 204–206.

[2] Pagel-Sudhoff (Berlin, 1915), 181.

tion of commentary. He early noted the faulty translations made by Constantine, and clung to the original Greek sources, but his own skill in logic-chopping suggests his training in the Canon of Avicenna. The scholastic method attained its highest development at once in Bologna, which was then the great center of legal casuistry and forensic triumphs.[1]

The *Conciliator differentiarum* (Venice, 1471) of the heretic **Peter of Abano** (1250–1315), the great "Lombard," who as the title of his work implies, tried to reconcile the views of the Arabists and Grecians, marks the rise of the rival **school of Padua** as a center of medical dialectics, of which Thaddeus and Peter were the patterns for a century.[2]

The *Liber Pandectæ Medicinæ* of **Matthæus Sylvaticus** (died 1342), of Mantua, one of the first medical incunabula to be printed (Strassburg, 1470 [?]) illustrates the conciliating tendency. The most prominent of the Arabists, however, were associated with the rise of the **medical school at Montpellier**. Founded about 738, this famous school, like that of Salerno, was charmingly situated near the sea, not far from mineral baths. As early as 1137, Bishop Adelbert of Mainz visited the school to listen to its medical lecturers. St. Bernard refers to the visit of the Archbishop of Lyons in his letter (1153), and its influence in France has survived to this day. A prominent early representative of the Arabist learnings was the Majorcan alchemist **Raymond Lully** (1235–1315) who, in addition to the philosopher's stone, sought the *aurum potabile* (liquid gold) as a sovereign elixir against disease. Having entered the order of the Minorites, he learned Arabic through his desire to convert the Moslems of North Africa and, in this way, became acquainted with Arabian chemistry and brought some of its ideas into Europe. To convert heretics, he invented a logical machine, in which premises inserted came out as orthodox conclusions, as in a hopper. A man of more adventurous type was the Catalan **Arnold of Villanova** (1235–1311), who was a doctor of theology, law, philosophy, and medicine, and counsellor or consultant to Peter III of Aragon. A follower of the Arabian chemists, he also sought an universal elixir of life, and was one of the earliest European writers on alchemy. These tendencies, along with his theologic heresies, caused him to be anathematized after his death. Arnold is credited with the introduction of tinctures and of brandy (*aurum potabile*) into the pharmacopeia, and in many ways he was a sort of refined Paracelsus, a man full of strange contradictions. He translated Avicenna on the heart and probably Avenzoar on diet. He was a pioneer in the classification of diseases and opposed the abuse of dialectics, the tendency of the Parisian scholastics to lose themselves in universal and ignore particulars, as well as their footless therapeutic empiricism, which lost itself in particulars and ignored general principles.

He was a copious, elegant, uncritical writer, who, according to Symphorien Champier, declined to revise any copy, once he had penned it. His "Breviary of Practice" (Milan, 1483), one of the best of the medieval handbooks, contains much independent observation, and many citations from now unknown physicians. Arnold's greatest work is the *Parabolæ*, a set of 345 pithy aphorisms, dedicated to Philip the Fair (1300), and containing much original thought. His commentary on the Regimen Sanitatis, is not to be confused with the Regimen itself, sometimes ascribed to him nor with the other commentary attributable to Magnino of Milan.[3] The best modern studies of Arnold are those of Hauréau, on the textual side, and Paul Diepgen, on the medical side.[4]

Other prominent pupils of **Montpellier** were the surgeons Guy de Chauliac, Arderne, and Mondeville; Valescus de Taranta (1382–1417), physician to Charles VI

---

[1] Neuburger, *op. cit.*, 375.

[2] Peter's *Conciliator* consists of 210 moot-points to be resolved by dispute, e. g., "Utrum nervi oriantur a cerebro necne?" "Utrum medicina sit scientia, necne," "An ossa sentiant," etc., which became the fashion for students' dissertations and disputations even beyond the 17th century.

[3] Neuburger (ii, 391) attributes Arnold's commentary to Magninus Mediolanensis.

[4] Hauréau, in "Histoire littéraire de France," 1881. xxviii, 26–126, 487. Diepgen: Arch. f. Gesch. d. Med., Leipz., 1909–10, iii, 115, 188, 369; 1911–12, v, 88; 1912–13, vi, 380

of France, whose *Tractatus de peste* was one of the earliest incunabula (1470 [?]); Johannes de Tornamira, physician to Popes Gregory IX and Clement VII, for many years chancellor of Montpellier and remembered by his *Introductorium* (Lyons, 1490), a popular text-book on practice in the 14th and 15th centuries; Peter of Spain (1277), called Petrus Hispanus, physician to Pope Gregory X and afterward himself Pope John XXI, whose *Thesaurus Pauperum* was the most popular of the medieval formularies; and the leading representatives of Anglo-Norman medicine, Bernard de Gordon, Richard of Wendover (the anatomist), Gilbertus Anglicus, and John of Gaddesden.

Before the advent of the Norman conquerors, **English medicine** was entirely in the hands of the Saxon leeches, whose practice was made up of charms, spells and herb-doctoring, and whose folk-medicine survives in *Beowulf*, the *Leech-Book* of Bald (*circa* 900–950), the *Lacnunga* (1100), *Perididaxeon* (1250), and other Anglo-Saxon "leechdoms."[1] This lay-magic is syncretic, a blend of Græco-Latin, Mozarabic, Indo-Germanic, Celtic, Byzantine (Smyrna *Physiologus*), and native Anglo-Saxon elements. The plant-lore derives mainly from Pliny and the decorative illustrations of plants are mainly servile copies from South Italian sources, with a remarkable upthrust of naturalism in a MS. of 1120 from Bury St. Edmunds (Bodley MS. 130).[2] The Normans raised the social and intellectual status of the Anglo-Saxon physicians by having them educated abroad as clerics.

Bernard de Gordon, inferentially a Scotchman, did not practice in England, but was a teacher at Montpellier from 1285 to 1307. His *Lilium Medicinæ*, which exists in several rare manuscripts and was first published at Venice (1496), is a characteristic Arabist text-book of the practice of medicine, nowise classic, and typical of the Middle Ages in scholastic subtlety and rigid adherence to dogma. The subject matter is well arranged; acute fever (bubonic plague), phthisis, epilepsy, scabies, *ignis sacer*, anthrax, trachoma, and leprosy are described as contagious, and the book is notable as containing the first description of a modern truss and the first mention of spectacles as *oculus berellinus*.[3] The *Compendium medicinæ* (London, 1510) of **Gilbertus Anglicus** (died 1250), the leading exponent of Anglo-Norman medicine, is very much like Gordon's Lily in style, arrangement of contents and modes of thought. The author avows his preference for the simple expectant treatment of Hippocrates, but hesitates to employ it for fear of seeming an oddfish.[4] The most important feature of his work is an original account of leprosy, which became the basis of medieval information upon the subject. Gilbert was the first to refer to smallpox as a contagious disease, a view afterward contradicted even by Sydenham. The book concludes with hygienic directions for travelers and seafarers, a literary species, which, like the hygienic regimina written for great overlords and ladies, was to become fashionable in time.[5] **John of Gaddesden** [?]–1361), a prebendary of St. Paul's, whom some think the original of Chaucer's Doctor of Physic, was physician to King Edward II of England and a fellow and professor at Merton College, Oxford. His *Rosa Anglica*,[6] compiled in 1314, and printed

---

[1] See Oswald Cockayne: Leechdoms, Wortcunning and Starcraft of Early England. 3 vols. London, 1864–6.

[2] C. Singer: Early English Magic and Medicine, Oxford, 1920.

[3] For the other writings of Bernard de Gordon, see R. von Töply, Mitth. z. Gesch. d. Med., Leipz., 1907, vi, 94; Sudhoff: Arch. f. Gesch. d. Med., Leipz., 1916–17, x, 162–188.

[4] Neuburger, ii, 369.

[5] See Sudhoff (Arch. f. Gesch. d. Med., Leipz., 1910–11, iv, 263–281) on the oldest known regimen (*circa* 1227), and Pagel-Sudhoff, p. 185.

[6] The medieval *Rosa mundi*, the main ingredient of syrup of roses, is still grown in England as "cottage maid."

at Pavia in 1492,[1] contains an early reference to the red-light[2] (Finsen) treatment of smallpox, which was already known to Gilbertus Anglicus and Bernard de Gordon; but it is otherwise mainly a farrago of Arabist quackeries and countryside superstitions. Guy de Chauliac called it "a vapid rose, devoid of fragrance," and Haller referred to its author as "an empiric, full of superstition, obviously untrained, a lover and eulogist of quack medicines, greedy of gain, an expert in kitchen-lore." John Mirfeld, a monkish physician who worked in the cloisters of St. Bartholomew in the second half of the 14th century, wrote a glossary and a breviary to the treatise of Bartholomæus Anglicus. Among the popular writings of the early 15th century were the many herb-books and formularies in Middle-High and Middle-Low German, Middle English, Danish, and Icelandic, the *Meinauer Naturlehre*, and the Welsh *Meddygon Myddfai*.[3] The *Danske Laegebog*[4] of Henrik Harpestreng (died 1244), canon of Roeskilde, consists of two herb books, deriving mainly from Macer Floridus, and a stone-book, which derives from Marbod. A treatise on purgatives by Harpestreng was edited by J. W. S. Johnsson in 1914. Sudhoff has published a valuable catalogue of all the medical texts of the Middle Ages printed in the Germanic languages, including Norse, Anglo-Saxon, and Middle English.[5]

The most eminent naturalist of the 13th century was the Dominican monk, Albert von Bollstädt (1193–1280), called **Albertus Magnus,** who was successively a teacher at Paris and Cologne, and later Bishop of Ratisbon (1260–1263), ending his days in Cologne. He was the Aristotle of his period; indeed, he said that the object of his *Physica* was to furnish the brethren of his order with an Aristotelian Book of Nature. His *De vegetabilibus*[6] was based upon his own botanical observations and contains some therapeutic material. His best work is his huge book on animals (*De animalibus*),[7] based upon Aristotle as transmitted by Michael Scott, and also replete with original observations. He assisted Frederick II in his work on falconry. The often reprinted work on cosmetics (*De secretis mulierum*), which usually goes by his name, was in reality a compilation made by his pupil, Henry of Saxony. Albertus Magnus did not write on medical practice, a subject forbidden the Dominicans. His pupil, Thomas Aquinas, discussed physiologic questions in his theologic writings and advanced the dubious animistic doctrine of *qualitates occultæ*. Albertus Magnus was followed by such encyclopedists as the Dominican, Vincent de Beauvais (*Speculum majus*, 1473–5); the Franciscan, Bartholomæus Anglicus (*De proprietatibus rerum*, written 1240, Englished by John of Trevisa [1398], printed by Wynkyn de Worde [1495]); the Dominican, Thomas de Cantipré (1204–80), whose *De naturis rerum* was the original of the *Buch der Natur* (1350) of Conrad von Megenberg (1309–74), and the *Tesoro* of Dante's teacher, Brunetto Latini. All these tomes contain medical matter.

The greatest experimenter of the 13th century was the English Franciscan **Roger Bacon** (1214–94), called *Doctor mirabilis*, who was a comparative philologist, mathematician, astronomer, physicist, physical geographer, chemist, and physician.

He reformed the calendar, did much for the theory of lenses and vision, anticipated spectacles, the telescope, gunpowder, diving bells, locomotives and flying machines, and was a forerunner of inductive and experimental science. Medicine he regarded as a means of prolonging life through alchemy (chemistry) and he approved of astrology and other modes of superstition on account of their psycho-

---

[1] The later editions were those of Venice (1502), Pavia (1517), and Augsburg (1595). See G. Dock, Janus, Amst., 1907, xii, 425–435.

[2] Neuburger, ii, 369; 502. H. P. Cholmeley: John of Gaddesden and the Rosa Medicinæ, Oxford, 1912, 41. Compare Gilbert's "Compendium Medicinæ," Lyons, 1510, fol. 348, *verso*, col. I, with Gaddesden (fol. 51 recto, col. II).

[3] Translated by John Pughe, edited by John Williams at Ithel, Llandovery, 1861. See also the critical edition by P. Diverres, Paris (*le Dault*), 1913.

[4] Edited by C. Molbech, 1861.

[5] Sudhoff: Arch. f. Gesch. d. Med., Leipz., 1909–10, iii, 273–305.

[6] Edited by C. Jensen, Berlin, 1867.

[7] Edited by H. Stadler, 2 vols., Munich, 1916.

therapeutic effect.[1] His principal contributions to medical literature are his astrological tracts on critical days.

In connection with the earlier history of **medical dictionaries** three writers on
medical plants and simples deserve especial mention, viz., Giacomo **de Dondi**
(1298–1359), whose *Aggregator de medicinis simplicibus,* printed at S'rassburg *circa*
1470–80 by Adolf Rusch (the "R" printer[2]), is one of the earliest known medical
incunabula,[3] Simone **de Cordo** (died 1330), whose *Synonyma medicinæ* (1473) was
the first dictionary of drugs and simples, under the Greek, Latin, and Arabic names,
and the above-mentioned **Matteo Silvatico,** whose *Pandects,* also printed by Rusch
at Strassburg (*circa* 1470–1473) and followed by some 12 subsequent editions (1474–
1541) is a similar glossary of Arabic, Greek, and Latin medical terms, giving also
botanic descriptions and therapeutic indications. These three books did for the
Arabic botanic terms what Hyrtl later did for the anatomic and are, in fact,
encyclopedic dictionaries of medicine.

The **pre-Renaissance medicine** of the 14th and early 15th centuries
was characterized by the attempt to cast the Arabist tradition into a
rigid mold by means of Aristotelian dialectics and assimilation to the
Aristotelian philosophy. The result was that the Galenic doctrine, after
translation and re-translation through the Arabic, Syrian, and Hebrew
glosses, was badly distorted and wrenched away from its original meaning. The "spell of Aristotle" was over all. The scholiast and the
dialectician ruled supreme, until more advanced spirits became rank
sophists or skeptics, thus preparing the ground for the true Revival
of Learning. The medical literature of the 14th century was entirely
receptive and passive, consisting of compilations, commentaries, glosses,
glossaries, concordances, breviaries of practice (often called after the
Lily and the Rose), and casuistic writings or *Consilia.* In this period
flourished Mundinus, Guy, Mondeville, Arderne, Yperman, and Argelata.

A salient feature of clinical medicine in the 14th and 15th centuries
was the writing of **"Consilia"** or medical-case books, consisting of
clinical records from the practice of well known physicians and letters

---

[1] For a full account of Roger Bacon's work in science, see the "Commemo-
rative Essays," edited for his seventh centenary by A. G. Little (Oxford, 1914),
with an account of his work in medicine by E. T. Withington.

[2] The fact that the "R" printer was Adolf Rusch, and not his employer Mentelin,
was settled by the distinguished Göttingen philologist Karl Dziatzko, in his essay
"Der Drucker mit dem bizarren R" (Samml. bibliothekswissensch. Arbeiten, Halle,
1904, Heft 17, 13–24). Rusch, it seems, married Mentelin's daughter, Salome, and
eventually took over his business. The much disputed "R" is in reality a monogram
of the initial letters of Rusch's name, which he was in the habit of inserting here and
there in the books printed by him, as a sign of his handiwork during the days of his
apprenticeship.

[3] The question, "What is the earliest printed medical book of size?" is still
unsettled. The Gutenberg *Laxierkalender* of 1457 of course antedates everything
else, but it is only a sheet of paper. Mlle. Pellechet assigns the date 1467 to Johann
Gerson's three tracts on self-abuse, printed by Ulrich Zell at Cologne. The *Opus
universum* of Hrabanus Maurus, printed by Rusch at Strassburg, July 20, 1467, contains a chapter *De medicina et morbis* (Osl'r). The date "1468" has been claimed
for Roland of Parma's pest-tract, and 1469 for Giammateo Ferrari da Grado's
Practica (Pt. 1). The question cannot be finally decided until all the known medical
incunabula have been catalogued, collated and compared as to fonts of type, filigranes (water-marks), majuscules (initial letters), and the internal evidence of biographic and other data. This important task is in the hands of Dr. Arnold C.
Klebs, who in his catalogue of pest-tracts (1926), has already assigned dates and
printers to many undated incunabula.

of advice written by them to imaginary patients or else to real pupils or country doctors, who had appealed to their superior knowledge as consultants.

The earliest writer in this *genre* was Taddeo Alderotti, whose Consilia still "slumber in the manuscripts" (Sudhoff). The practice was kept up by nearly all the scholastic physicians of the Bolognese and Paduan schools. The most important Consilia were those written by the Paduan professors Gentile da Foligno (who was a victim of the Black Death in 1348 and was the first to observe gall-stones), Hugo Senensis (gastric vertigo, nasopharyngeal polyp), Antonio Cermisone (foot-baths, turpentine in sciatica), Baverius de Baveriis (caries of the temporal bone, paralysis with aphasia, iron in chlorosis) and Bartolommeo Montagnana (1470), a descendant of a long line of physicians, author of an early book on balneology (1497), an anatomist who had dissected as many as 14 bodies, and a surgeon who described strangulated hernia, operated for lacrimal fistula and extracted decayed teeth. These Consilia, of which Montagnana gives some 305, usually run over the patient's physical condition and disease, winding up with seasonable advice as to what to eat, what drugs to take and what things to avoid. Being personal histories, they have not the classic flavor of the clinical delineations of Hippocrates and Aretæus, and are of interest mainly as unique or rare notations and as showing that physicians had already begun to keep careful records of their daily practice. The custom was kept up in the later periods, *e. g.*, by Johann Lange (1554) who described chlorosis, by John Locke who sent Consilia to Sydenham, and in the medical cases discussed in the correspondence of Bretonneau with his pupils Velpeau and Trousseau.

Of the scholastic writers on internal medicine, Guglielmo Corvi of Brescia (1250–1326) whose *Practica* was called *Aggregator Brixiensis*, Dino del Garbo and his son Tommaso, Torrigiano di Torrigiani, Niccolò Bertuccio the teacher of Guy, Pietro di Tussignano, the surgeon Giovanni Arcolani, and Giovanni da Parma (*Practicella[1]*) belonged to the **School of Bologna.** The rival **School of Padua,** which followed the Averroistic leanings of Pietro d'Abano, numbered among its masters Gentile da Foligno (died 1348), famous for his Consilia; Giacomo de Dondi (1298–1359) and his son Giovanni; Marsilio de Santa Sophia and his nephew Galeazzo; Giacomo della Torre called Jacobus Foroliviensis; and Matteo Silvatico of Mantua, author of the famous *Pandectæ;* Francesco di Piedimonte, whose *Supplementum Mesuæ* was one of the best text-books of the time on special pathology and therapeutics, expressing the final union of Salernitan and Arabic medicine; and Niccolò Falcucci (died *circa* 1412), called Nicolaus Florentinus, author of a vast repertory called *Sermones medicinales* (1484), which summarizes the whole of medieval medicine teeming with original citations from all the known authorities.

Before the invention of printing there had accumulated a huge quantity of medical literature in manuscript, the investigation of which has been mainly the work of Professor Karl Sudhoff and the Institute of Medical History at Leipzig. This literature includes many hitherto unprinted texts and text-books of the medieval physicians and surgeons, calendars, and schemata for blood-letting and purgation, "death-prognoses" setting forth the signs of dissolution (*signa mortis*), Lepraschau-*briefe* or medicolegal *expertises* as to the civil status of supposititious lepers, business announcements of vagrant physicians, municipal ordinances against quackery, old German MSS. on farriery (*Rossarzneibücher*), consilia and even warnings against the abuse of alcohol.

The **Montpellier School** includes the names of Guy, Jean de Tournemire, Jean Jasme (Johannes Jacobi), and many other famous chancellors and Papal physicians. The leading medical writers of the early 15th century were Ugo Benzi, called Hugo Senensis (died 1439), a great medical philosopher, commentator and consiliary, who taught in all the famous Italian schools; Antonio Cermisone, Antonio Guainerio, Savonarola, Bartolommeo Montagnana of Padua, Arculano, Argelata, Marco Gatinaria; and Giammateo Ferrari da Grado (died 1472), professor of medicine at Pavia, whose *Practica* (printed 1469–71) and *Consilia* contain much original observation, *e. g.*, of writer's cramp, facial paralysis, hemoptysis in dysmenorrhea, sterility from displacement of the uterus, and the use of the pessary and the truss

---

[1] M. A. Mehner: Leipzig diss., 1918, gives a list of the vegetable simples used in this *Practicella*.

in uterine prolapse and hernia, respectively. In France, the Portuguese Valescus de Taranta, a leading teacher and practitioner at Montpellier, wrote a famous tract on pest (1473–4) and a therapeutic *Philonium* (1490) which was often reprinted. Jacques Despars (Jacobus de Partibus), at Paris, was a commentator of Avicenna, Mesuë, and Alexander Trallianus.

Cultural and Social Aspects of Medieval Medicine.—During the Dark Ages (476–1000), Western European civilization was in a chaotic, formless state, the turbulent fermentation of barbaric or decadent peoples vaguely striving to resolve themselves into new nations. Feudalism put nationhood on its feet, while the Church was the only foster-mother that science could find.[1] In the Dark Ages the clergy were the only class who had any pretense to education and, before the time of the School of Salerno, medicine was entirely in the hands of Jewish and Arabian physicians.[2] The rest were simply vagrant quacks or stationary humbugs, whose practice was discountenanced by the Church on the ground that faith, prayers, and fasting were better than pagan amulets, while the sick were advised to emulate the saints in their capacity for endurance of suffering (Gregory of Tours). With the rise of the School of Salerno, European medicine began to look up a little but, as soon as monks and clerics began to practise medicine, it was found that the seeking of medical fees to the detriment of regular duties; the sight of many aspects of the sick which might offend modesty; the possibility of being the cause of a patient's death, and other happenings were somewhat inconsistent with the original intention of holy orders. And so we find the Church instituting that long series of edicts, which, in the first instance, were aimed not so much at medicine as at its malpractice by monks.[3] These were the decrees of the councils of Clermont (1130), Rheims (1131), the Second Lateran (1139), Montpellier (1162), Tours (1163), Paris (1212), the Fourth Lateran (1215), and Le Mans (1247[4]). The general effect was, unfortunately, not only to stop the monks from practising, but to extend the special odium of these decrees to the whole medical profession. As Allbutt says: "If Papal bulls conferred privileges, they usually implied or imposed restrictions." The famous maxim of the Council of Tours (*Ecclesia abhorret a sanguine*), for example, went wide of its supposed intention

---

[1] How carefully the clergy collected medical literature is evidenced by the remarkable bequest of medical books to the cathedral library at Hildesheim, as listed in the will of Bishop Bruno (1161). See Neuburger, ii, 321–322.

[2] In spite of the Decretum Gratiani, excluding Jewish physicians from practising among Christians, Archbishop Bruno of Trèves (1102–24) was attended by the learned Joshua, Moses of Liège was consulted by the clergy in 1138 and, in the 12th century, medical practice at Prague was entirely in the hands of the Jews (Neuburger, ii, 325–333).

[3] The earliest of these, that of Clermont (1130), refers specifically to the "*neglecta animarum cura*," the "*detestanda pecunia*," and the "*impudicus oculus*." Even in 877 the synod of Ratisbon had decreed that "*Leges et physicum non studeant sacerdotes*" (Neuburger).

[4] Sprengel gives the sources of these decrees, viz., G. D. Mansi: Sacrorum consiliorum nova et amplissima collectio, Florence, 1759–98, xxi, col. 459, 528, 1160; xxii, col. 1010; xxiii, col. 756.

since, in casting discredit upon the sometimes murderous vagabond surgeon, the weight of its authority made the surgeon of better type still an inferior to the average practitioner, even in Protestant Germany to the end of the 18th century. Worse still, the bigots of the Paris Faculty went much further than the Papal See in widening the gap between surgery and medicine. The Roman Pontiffs themselves were, some of them, liberal-minded men of the world, who did not hesitate talented Jewish physicians at need and, in later times, did much to foster the arts and sciences, in Italy at least. John XXI and Paul II were physicians. "Around the Papal Chair," says Allbutt, "the velvet of the hand of the Church was thicker than the iron. In the air of Rome or of Avignon the grim rigor of Paris was marvelously softened." While great harm was done to medicine by the Papal decrees which degraded the surgeon's status, we should not forget that, up to the time of the crusades, all Europe outside of Italy was in a state of barbarism and that the status of surgery in these countries was lower than it was among the Greeks at the time of the Trojan War. A few shreds of technical knowledge may have drifted over from far Byzantium, but the evidence of the Niebelungenlied, the Anglo-Saxon Leech-Books, and the Norse Sagas all point to the same conclusion, viz., that the care of the sick and wounded was first in the hands of women and later intrusted to a class of men who, in war-time, were no doubt in great request but, in times of peace, ranked on a level with menials.

Druidical medicine in Britain was entirely priestly.

The Druids were a corporation of magicians, and of these, the Seer (*vates*) assumed iatromantic functions, with augury (inspection of sacrificial entrails) for prognosis; magic, and wort-cunning for therapy. Mistletoe (all-heal) was the panacea; the six herbs, lycopodium, pulsatilla, trifolium, primula, hyoscyamus, and verbena, were highly esteemed; artemisia, betony, bryonia, centauria, belladonna, hellebore, and mandragora were some of them, acquired from Pliny. Druidesses were also prominent in sorcery, second-sight and herb-therapy.[1] The Anglo-Saxon leechdoms tell the old story of charms, spells, and simples. Blood-letting, purging, and drugging were regulated by the moon's age. The 9th century *Phlebotomia* attributed to the Venerable Bede reckoned the period April 8th to May 25th as lucky (*dies fausta*), while certain days in the interim, when the moon and tides were at full, were regarded as unlucky or Egyptian days (*dies Ægyptiaci*), a late Roman superstition mentioned by St. Augustine, and probably of Babylonian origin.[2] Ancient **Irish medicine** has many signs of Oriental provenance, particularly in the austere regulations of medical practice and quackery in the Brehon Laws, which suggest the Code Hammurabi. A strange MS. attributed to Roger Bacon, written either in Gaelic or cipher and full of remarkably naturalistic figurations of pregnancy *en miniature*, suggests some kind of esoteric or mesmeric magic, like that of the Hindu fakirs.[3]

In Tacitus (Germania, VII), it is said that the wounded Teutons sought their wives and mothers, who, like the professional blood-suckers of the 18th century, applied their lips to the wounds (*ad matres, ad conjuges vulnera ferunt, nec illae numerari et exigere plagas pavent*). The

---

[1] Neuburger, ii, 234–236.

[2] J. F. Payne: English Medicine in the Anglo-Saxon Times, Oxford, 1904.

[3] In the possession of Mr. Wilfred M. de Voynich. In Singer's view, it is of the period *circa* 1580, and perhaps written by John Dee.

reverence of the ancient Germans for the intuitive powers of woman was the origin of *weise Frauen,* who practised herbal medicine.

Of these, the seeresses Veleda and Aurinia were revered as divinities (Tacitus). In the epic of "Gudrun" (l. 529) mention is also made of "wild women" (*wilde Weiber*), who knew of healing herbs. Demon-lore, magic, charms, and amulets made up the rest of **early German medicine.**[1] As among the Greeks, the wrath of the gods was appeased by bloody sacrifice, the demons dispelled by exorcism, the therapeutic properties ascribed to certain plants, parts of animals, and the votive (usually heart-shaped) pastry used in sacrifice were based upon their sacral associations with the gods in their chthonian or earthly aspect. From this cult arose a sacred pharmacopeia and a "sacrificial anatomy" (*Opferanatomie*), the technical terms of which were long a part of the vocabulary of German huntsmen, and eventually made up the culinary anatomy of the slaughter-pen and the kitchen (Höfler[2]). The vernacular names of diseases were derived in the same way, directly from the bodily effects or from demoniac etiology.[3] To ward off the demons of disease, the *gode* or sacrificial priest was assisted by the aboriginal medicine-man, the *lêkeis* or *lâhki,* the equivalent of the Anglo-Saxon *laeca* (*leech*). Shepherds, herdsmen, and smiths, as being natural veterinarians, also became renowned as healers, bonesetters, and masseurs (*Streicher*) in isolated localities.

In Russia, medicine was originally in the hands of the *volkhava* or wolf-men, who, like the Druids and wise women, culled medicinal herbs and resorted to charms and spells. The earliest relic of Russian medicine is a vase of Greek pattern excavated at Koul-Oba, representing a Scythian chieftain in consultation with a volkhava, a Scythian warrior examining another's teeth and a surgeon bandaging an injured leg. This unique vase epitomizes medieval medicine and surgery up to the time of the School of Salerno.[4] After the introduction of Christianity in the 10th century, Russian medicine passed into the hands of the priesthood, the wolf-men gave place to the monks of Mount Athos, and the Russian Church, like the Roman, put severe interdictions upon sorcery and magic. Thus religion, at the start, tended to improve the status of medicine, but speedily, if unintentionally, degraded it when it found its own medical ministrants falling into evil ways. Even the special nurses or *parabolani,*[5] whom the Church employed to seek out the sick and convey them to places of shelter and safety, were soon shorn of their powers as they became uppish, quarrelsome, and overbearing. Even before this time, however, the Visigothic Code (5th–7th centuries) put the same severe **restrictions upon medical practice** which we find in the Code Hammurabi.

Before taking up a case, the physician, under the Visigothic Code, had to make a contract and give pledges and, if his patient died, he got no fee. If he injured a nobleman in venesection he had to pay 100 solidi (about \$225); if the

---

[1] Neuburger, *op. cit.,* ii, 236–240.

[2] M. Höfler: "Wald- und Baumkult," Munich, 1892; also "Die volksmedizinische Organotherapie," Stuttgart, 1908.

[3] See Max Höfler's learned "Deutsches Krankheitsnamenbuch," Munich, 1899.

[4] For a photograph of the Koul-Oba vase, see "Nouvelle Iconographie de la Salpêtrière," Paris, 1901, xiv, plate No. 72, opposite page 528.

[5] First mentioned, A. D. 416, in the Codex (de legationibus) of Emperor Theodosius (lib. xvi, tit. ii, 42–43), but already known as *Parapemponti,* in St. Basil's account of his hospital at Cæsarea (370–379). See C. F. Heusinger, Janus, Breslau, 1847, ii, 500–525, which corrects the errors made by Sprengel.

nobleman died, the physician was turned over to the relatives of the deceased, to be dealt with as they pleased.   If he killed or injured a slave, he had to replace him by one of equal value.   He was forbidden to bleed a married woman in the absence of her relatives, for fear of the commission of adultery, and he could not visit a prisoner lest he defeat the ends of justice by furnishing him with poison.   On the other hand, it is stated that no one might cast a physician into prison without a hearing, except in case of murder, and that the statutory fee for instructing medical students should be 12 solidi ($27) each.   The other *"Leges barbarorum"* were equally severe. Under the Bavarian Code (Lex Bajuvarum, vii, 19), the administration of an abortifacient entailed a fine of one solidus in the culprit's family, even unto the seventh generation.[1]

From these regulations, made by the secular arm of authority, and designed to protect the public as well as the physician, it may be gathered that, with medicine in such an unorganized condition, something more than the guardianship of Church and State was necessary to elevate the status of the healing art; and this was accomplished by improved medical legislation, by the foundation of the great medieval universities, and by the subsequent formation of "guilds" among the physicians themselves.   Under the legal restrictions of medieval times the surgeon worked daily and hourly in jeopardy of life or limb.[2] Marileif, Chilperic's body physician, was flogged, shorn of his possessions, and made a serf.   In 580, Guntram, King of Burgundy, had two physicians executed upon the tomb of his queen, Austrichildes, because she had died of plague in spite of their treatment.   In 1337, a strolling eye surgeon was thrown in the Oder because he failed to cure John of Bohemia of his blindness.   In 1464, Matthias, King of Hungary, issued a proclamation that whoever cured him of an arrow wound should be richly rewarded, but, failing that, should be put to death.   These barbarities point their own moral, for the strolling medieval montebanks, in couching a cataract, sometimes put out an eye, mangled the viscera in "cutting" for stone, and, in attempting to effect a "radical cure" for hernia, as Baas says, not infrequently excised "the radix of humanity itself."[3]   Allbutt mentions a striking instance of a medieval incisor who, in ligating an artery, paralyzed his patient's arm by crushing the musculospiral nerve and was afterward pursued with curses by his miserable victim whenever he dared show himself in the street. In like manner, Delpech, Pozzi, and other modern surgeons were assassinated by patients, who held them responsible for various mischances.   If the Church "abhorred the shedding of blood," therefore, it is fair to suppose that, in the first instance, its aversion had the same human significance as the well-founded horror of hospitals and surgical

---

[1] Neuburger, ii, 258.

[2] For a careful study of this subject, see Sir John Tweedy: Tr. Med. Leg. Soc., London, 1911, viii, pp. 1–8.   Even among recent North American Indians, a medicine-man who has failed to cure in a succession of cases is believed to have lost his curative powers, as among the ancient Persians, and may be put to death.   (See A. Hrdlička: Bur. Am. Ethnol., Bull. No. 34, Washington, 1908, 234.)

[3] The strolling herniotomists held castration to be necessary, believing that the intestines and testicles were inclosed in the same sac, which must be removed in its entirety to obviate relapses and faulty healing of the peritoneum.

operations which existed in the minds of the laity up to the end of the 19th century.

A striking illustration of the medieval neglect of surgery is to be found in the late appearance of **artificial limbs,** which were known to Herodotus and Pliny.

In the Middle Ages, there was an enormous loss of limbs, due to the mutilating effects of anesthetic leprosy and ergotism, to wounds from cannon-shot (introduced at Crécy in 1346) and half-pound gunshot (Perugia, 1364), and to gruesome judicial punishments. The stumps were commonly bound up in splints. Crutches and wooden legs, afterward so familiar in the works of Callot and Brueghel, are mentioned in the *Acta sanctorum* and other medieval chronicles and frequently appear in the sacred frescoes of the time. The iron hand is first seen in a picture of 1400. Goetz von Berlichingen, after losing his right hand by musket-shot at Landshut in 1504, had several hands made, movable in the joints, with flexible fingers, capable of closure. One of these still exists and was exhibited at Berlin in 1916.[1]

As the physicians looked down upon the surgeons, so the surgeons of higher education, who in the Middle Ages could be counted on the fingers, looked down upon the barbers, who were originally trained for the purpose of bleeding and shaving the monks.

In the 13th century the **Collège de Saint Côme** was organized as a Paris guild (*circa* 1210). The members were divided into the clerical barber-surgeons or surgeons of the long robe, and the lay barbers or surgeons of the short robe and, in 1311, 1352, and 1364, royal decrees were issued, forbidding the latter to practise surgery without being duly examined by the former. In 1372, Charles V decreed that the barbers should be allowed to treat wounds and not be interfered with by their long-robed confrères. The same thing happened in England, where the master-surgeons formed a separate guild in 1368, recognized women physicians in 1389,[2] combined with the physicians about 1421,[3] while the "Mystery of the Barbers of London" obtained a separate charter from Edward IV on February 24, 1462, which was enrolled by the Court of Common Council in 1463.

In this way, barber-surgery (the surgery of the common people) became "wound-surgery," that is, was restricted to blood-letting and the healing of wounds. The barbers (*barbitonsores*) themselves owed their later business largely to the fact that, after the monks were forbidden to wear beards (1092), smooth chins and shaving became the fashion. In Germany the barber was often a bath keeper (*balneator*), who, in addition to bleeding, cupping and leeching, gave enemas, picked lint, and extracted teeth. His examination or *Meisterstück* consisted in sharpening a knife or in preparing certain salves and plasters.

Throughout the Middle Ages, there were some vague attempts to formulate the principles of **medical jurisprudence.**

The earliest of these, as Cumston points out, are found in the laws of the Germanic and Slavic tribes, the Salic law, the Capitularies of Charlemagne (9th century), the Assizes of the Crusaders and, in the 13th century and after, the law of Emperor

---

[1] Holländer: Berl. klin. Wchnschr., 1916, liii, 355.

[2] For Jacoba and other women physicians. see Eileen Power: Proc. Roy. Soc. Med., Lond., 1921–2, xv, sect. Hist. Med., 20–22.

[3] South (Memorials of the Craft of Surgery in England, London, 1886, 53) says that the date of this conjoint faculty of physicians and surgeons fell somewhere between May, 1421 and May, 1423.

Frederick, the Decretals of the Popes and general canon laws. The procedure in such cases was often of the crudest kind, the tests being by ordeal, torture, *de facto* verification of impotence, and "cruentation," or the spontaneous bleeding of a corpse in the presence of the true murderer. The expert opinions given were usually in the nature of hair-splitting casuistry, but Cousin and Cumston[1] give a number of cases from French legal procedure of the 14th century in which surgeons were commonly consulted in cases of wounds, homicide, rape, and the like.

In the year 1140, Roger II of Sicily issued an edict forbidding any one to practise medicine without proper examination, under pain of imprisonment and the sale of his belongings at auction. This important law was followed by an ordinance of larger scope issued by Roger's grandson, the generous and liberal-minded Hohenstauffen Emperor, **Frederick II** in 1224.[2]

Frederick's edict required that a candidate for license to practise must be properly examined in public by the masters at Salerno, the license being issued by the Emperor himself or his representative; failure to comply with the statute being again punishable by a year's imprisonment and forfeiture of property. The examination was based upon the genuine books of Hippocrates, Galen, and Avicenna and, before taking it, the candidate must have studied logic for three years, medicine and surgery for five years, and have practised for one year under some experienced physician. The candidate in surgery had to give evidence that he had studied the art for at least a year, in particular, anatomy. The physician was required to treat the poor for nothing; to visit his patients twice a day and once a night, if necessary; to avoid collusion with apothecaries, and to inform upon them if they adulterated or substituted drugs. The medical fee was fixed at half a tarenus (about 35 cents) for office practice or for patients residing in the city; four tareni ($3.00) for out-of-town visits, the physician paying his expenses, or three tareni ($2.25), if the patient paid them. For a successful operation for anal fistula, John of Arderne required 100 shillings, at least; £40 from the well-to-do; £40, with robes and a life annuity of 100 shillings annually, from the wealthy. Nicholas Colnet, physician to Henry V at Agincourt, was guaranteed twelvepence a day by indentures. Thomas Morstede, the king's surgeon, got the same with the usual allowance of 100 marks (£66 13s. 4d.) a quarter (Power). The purchasing power of money in this period is said to have been fifteen or twenty times what it is at present. The ordinary laborer's pay in England was a penny a day as against 8 to 10 shillings now. The sale of poisons, magic potions, and aphrodisiac philters was punishable by death if any person lost his life thereby. Food, drugs, and apothecaries' mixtures were examined at stated intervals by inspectors; and timely regulations were made in municipal hygiene and rural hygiene, such as for the proper depth of graves or the suitable disposal of refuse.

Given the time at which it was issued, it would be hard to improve upon the plain scope and intention of this law, which was followed by similar ordinances for Spain (1283) and Germany (1347), and was again confirmed by Joanna of Naples (1365[3]). Frederick's edict did much to elevate the status of the respectable physician and correspondingly to diminish the number of quacks. Another circumstance which brought physicians to the front as *medici publici* was the fact that they

---

[1] André Cousin: "Essai sur les origines de la médecine légale," Paris, diss. No. 252, 1905. C. G. Cumston: Jour. Am. Inst. Crim. Law, Chicago, 1913, iii, 855–865.

[2] Translated by J. J. Walsh, in his "The Popes and Science," New York, 1908, 420–423.

[3] Sudhoff states that the alleged ordinance for city physicians of 1426, attributed to Kaiser Sigmund (1410–37), is probably mythical, although he has discovered a city ordinance of 1439, which he reproduces in Mitt. z. Gesch. d. Med., Leipz., 1912, xi, 126, 127.

were required to determine the possible existence of leprosy in suspected persons (*Lepraschau*) in order to ascertain the civil status of the latter.[1] The improvement of the medical profession was also furthered by the introduction of a new element—the rise and growth of the great **medieval universities,** which usually began as a high-school or "*studium generale,*" *i. e.*, migration or assemblage of students in some locality.

The earliest of these were at Paris (1110), Bologna (1158), Oxford (1167) and Montpellier (1181), Cambridge (1209), Padua (1222), Naples (1224) Toulouse (1233), Salamanca (1243), Siena (1246–8), Piacenza (1248), Seville (1254), Lisbon (1290), Lerida (1300), Rome (1303), Perugia (1308), Co mbra (1308–9), Palermo (1312), Florence (1320–49), Grenoble (1339), Pisa (1343), Valencia (1345–50) Valladolid (1346), Pavia (1361), Ferrara (1391), Turin (1404), and Louvain (1426), and Ba celona (1450) followed. The 14th and 15th centuries witnessed also the rise of the principal German and Slavic universities, in particular Prague (1348), Cracow (1364), Vienna (1365), Erfurt (1379), Heidelberg (1386), Würzburg (1402), Leipzig (1409), Rostock (1419), Greifswald (1456), Freiburg im Breisgau (1457), Basel (1460), Budapest (1465), Ingolstadt (1472), and Tübingen (1477); of the Scandinavian, Upsala (1477) and Copenhagen (1478), and in Scotland, St. Andrew's (1411), Glasgow (1451), and Aberdeen (1494). After the general dispersal of students over the Continent and England to form "studios," like those at Salerno (medicine), Bologna (law), and Paris (theology), three **types of universities** or privileged corporations of students, as distinguished from the public high-school (*studium generale*) and private school (*studium particulare*), became established. The great law-school of Bologna became the type of civic university in which the rector was elected by the students, as at Padua and Siena. The University of Paris, the center of medieval theology and philosophy (Abelard), was the type of the ecclesiastical foundation, like Montpellier, Oxford, and Cambridge, in which the students and masters combined as a closed corporation under a chancellor, with the votes in the hands of the masters. The studium of Naples represented the state University, like Salamanca or Lisbon, founded by a monarch with Papal recognition as "*studia generalia respectu regni.*" The medical school at Montpellier formed a separate corporation, apart from the schools of law and the arts (Neuburger). All these were soon thronged with great concourses of students and, during the 13th century, especially at Paris, the learned university teachers were recruited mostly from the Franciscans or Gray Friars (founded 1209 by St. Francis of Assisi) and the Dominicans or Black Friars (founded 1215 by St. Dominic). It was through the influence of the medieval universities that the physician came to be regarded, in the end, as a member of a "learned profession." The *trivium* (grammar, rhetoric, dialectics) and *quadrivium* (arithmetic, geometry, astronomy, music), made up the "seven liberal arts," first introduced at Bishop Fulbert's cathedral school at Chartres. Apart from these, medicine was taught as a branch of philosophy (*Physica*), as set forth in Aristotle, Averroës, and the other Arabic writers. Before the revival of learning and the invention of printing, the Greek writers were seldom read in the original or even in a straight translation, but "doubly disguised and half buried in glosses which not only overlaid the text but often supplanted it."[2] The favorite text-books were the *Isagoge* of Johannitius, Avicenna (i, iv), Rhazes' *Liber medicinalis* (ix), Galen's *Ars parva* and the *Aphorisms, Prognostics,* and *Dietetics* of Hippocrates. Most of these were contained in the well-known "Articella." The Cambridge Statutes of 1396 required the student to hear Johannitius, Philaretus *De pulsibus,* Theophilus *De urinis,* the *Antidotarium* of Nicolaus Salernitanus and some book of Isaac Judæus once, and the works of Galen, with glosses and commentaries twice, with cursory reading of some book on medical praxis.[3] The curriculum at Tübingen in the 14th century, as given by Haeser, comprised, in the first year, the first Canon of Avicenna

---

[1] MS. forensic protocols on suspected lepers (*Lepraschaubriefe*), of dates, 1357, 1380, 1397, and later, have been discovered and published by Wickersheimer and Sudhoff (Arch. f. Gesch. d. Med., Leipz., 1908–9, ii, 434; 1910–11, iv, 370).

[2] Allbutt: Science and Medieval Thought, London, 1901, 69.

[3] Brit. Med. Jour., London, 1920, i, 371.

and the ninth book of Rhazes, as expounded by Jacob of Forlì and Arculanus; in the second year, the *Ars parva* of Galen with the commentary of Torrigiani, and the fourth canon of Avicenna; in the third year, the Aphorisms of Hippocrates and (again) Avicenna, with suitable commentaries. The courses and text-books were usually determined by papal bulls, and the libraries of the medieval universities were small in extent, seldom exceeding a hundred or more volumes. The house-inventory of Ugolino da Montecatino, who died at Florence in 1415. gives a catalogue of his medical library, which may be typical for medieval Italy.[1] The interesting catalogue of the medical section of the library of the cloister at Alt-Zelle (founded 1162) has been published by Leon Rosenblum, one of Sudhoff's pupils.[2] The professors' salaries usually ranged from $35 to $50 per annum. The term "doctor of medicine" was first applied to the Salernitan graduates by Gilles de Corbeil, in the 12th century, and the graduation ceremonies were commonly modeled after the Salernitan pattern. The candidate was first required to defend four theses from Aristotle, Hippocrates, Galen, and a modern writer then to take an oath, the conditions of which corresponded, in the main, with the decree of Emperor Frederick. He then received "a ring, a wreath of laurel and ivy, a book first closed and then opened, the kiss of peace" and the rank of "Doctor in Philosophy and Medicine."[3] John Locke describes very much the same thing at Montpellier in 1675, and the custom of the modern German universities is along similar lines.

From monastic institutions came the European **botanic gardens** (*hortus*) and **physic-gardens** (*herbulares*).

These oblong enclosures were originally cultivated to protect physicians and apothecaries from the drug-sellers, who attempted to monopolize the business by encouraging popular superstitions about plants. The *hortus medicus* of the monastic infirmary at St. Gall, built by Abbot Gozbert in 830, was carefully planned, with special plots for 16 plants, but never executed.[4]

Medical ethics and **medical etiquette** were regulated in detail[5] by sets of stereotyped rules, the earliest of which is the *Formula comitis archiatrorum* of Theodoric (5th century A. D.). Medical deontology and hodegetics, the *savoir faire* of the practitioner, were little sciences in the Middle Ages. In the Salernitan treatises of Archimathæus, the physician is instructed to approach the bedside *humili vultu*, with the same humble mien and wall-eyed expression which we find in so many of the old miniature paintings. His remarks at table were to be punctuated by continued inquiries about the patient's condition, which he should always regard as grave, in order that either a favorable or a fatal termination might redound to his credit as wonder-working therapeutist or shrewd prognostician. He should not diminish his professional status by ogling the patient's wife, daughter, or maid-servants. Illusory treatment by harmless remedies was permissible, since otherwise the patient's mind might be ruffled by not getting his

---

[1] W. Bombe and K. Sudhoff: Arch. f. Gesch. d. Med., Leipz., 1911–12, v, 225–239. For the 26 medical books in the library of Bishop Bruno of Hildesheim (1161), see Sudhoff: *Ibid.*, 1916–17, x, 348–356, and for a 14th century inventory of medical MSS., *Ibid.*, 1918–19, xi, 212–215.

[2] Leon Rosenblum: Leipzig diss., 1918.

[3] Before 1592, the degree at Salerno was Master or Doctor of Arts and Medicine. For three facsimile Salernitan diplomas of 1573, 1640, and 1665, see P. Capparoni: Riv. di storia crit. di sc. med. e nat., 1916, vii, 65–74, 3 pl.

[4] For plan (from Ann. Ord. St. Benedicti, ii, 571), see E. T. Withington's Medical History, London, 1894, opposite p. 1.

[5] Neuburger: Geschichte der Medizin, ii, 448–455.

money's worth, while a normal recovery by the healing powers of nature might injure the physician's therapeutic reputation.[1] A later authority suggests that, if a convalescent show signs of ingratitude in the matter of payment, he might be temporarily sickened by some harmless dosing.

Gaddesden says that he kept his best remedies a secret, apart from the vulgar, lest knowledge of the same cheapen the physician's status. Mondeville, Saliceto, Lanfranc, and Arderne are all skeptical and caustic about the ingratitude of the public in the payment of just dues.[2] Guy and Arnold of Villanova upheld the noblest ideals. Perhaps the best medieval tracts on medical etiquette are the *De cautelis medicorum habendis* of Alberto de Zancariis, formerly attributed to Arnold,[3] and the *Cautele medicorum* (1495) of the anatomist Gabriele Zerbi, of Verona. Medicine and quackery were freely satirized on the stage in the medieval farces and moralities, such as *Maistre Pathelin*.[4]

The chief glory of medieval medicine was undoubtedly in the organization of **hospitals and sick-nursing**,[5] which had its origin in the teachings of Christ. For while the germ of the hospital idea may have existed in the ancient Babylonian custom of bringing the sick into the market-place for consultation, as it were and, while the Iatreia and Asclepieia of the Greeks and the military hospitals of the Romans may have served this purpose to some extent, the spirit of antiquity toward sickness and misfortune was not one of compassion, and the credit of ministering to human suffering on an extended scale belongs to Christianity. The Arabian hospitals, large and liberal as were their endowments and capacity, came long after the beginning of the Christian era, and the Mohammedans probably got the idea from India or from the Christians. The Asclepieia and other pagan temples were closed by the decree of Constantine (A. D. 335) and, very soon after, the movement of founding and building the Christian hospitals went forward, in which Helena, the mother of Constantine, is said to have played an active part. These were probably small at first, the wealthier Christians taking care of the sick in Valetudinaria, but by the accession of Julian the Apostate (361) the movement was in full swing. In 369 the celebrated Basilias at Cæsarea (Cappadocia) was founded by St. Basil, consisting of a large number of buildings, with houses for physicians and nurses, workshops and industrial schools. It was followed by a charity hospital of 300 beds for the plague-stricken at Edessa, which was founded by St. Ephraim in 375. A hospital was founded at Alexandria by St. John the Almsgiver in 610, and, during the Byzantine period, other large

---

[1] *Ibid.*, 293–295.

[2] See D'Arcy Power's introduction to Arderne (Early English Text Society, No. 139), pp. xix–xxvii.

[3] See the inaugural dissertation of Manuel Morris, Leipzig, 1914.

[4] Maurice Boutarel: Paris dissertation, 1918, No. 142. For a delightful presentation of this medieval feeling, see Anatole France's medical farce, "*La comédie de celui qui épousa une femme muette.*"

[5] In the preparation of this section I have been much indebted to the interesting article by Dr. James J. Walsh in the Catholic Encyclopædia, *sub voce* "Hospitals," and to Sudhoff's "Aus der Geschichte des Krankenhauswesens" (Jena, 1913).

hospitals arose at Ephesus, Constantinople, and elsewhere. These eventually became specialized, according to Christian ideas of the obligation of charity and hospitality, as: Nosocomia or claustral hospitals, for the reception and care of the sick alone; Brephotrophia, for foundlings; Orphanotrophia, for orphans; Ptochia, for the helpless poor; Gerontochia, for the aged; and Xenodochia, for poor and infirm pilgrims. At the beginning of the 5th century, hospitals began to spring up in the Western Empire. The first nosocomium in Western Europe was founded by Fabiola about 400, "to gather in the sick from the streets and to nurse the wretched sufferers, wasted with poverty and disease" (St. Jerome).

Other nosocomia were founded in Rome by Belisarius, in the Via Lata, and by Pelagius; and, further west, by Cæsarius at Arles (542), by Childebert I at Lyons (542[1]), and by Bishop Masona at Merida (580). The Hôtel Dieu is said to have been founded between 641 and 691 by St. Landry, Bishop of Paris, and was first mentioned in 829. A Milanese hospital was founded in 777 and the first foundling asylum by Archbishop Datheus at Milan in 787. St. Albans Hospital in England dates from the year 794. In the early Middle Ages, infirmaries and hospices grew up alongside the cloisters. The ideal plan of St. Gall (820) included a hospital, with a room for grave cases, dwelling-houses for physicians, bath-rooms for cupping and bleeding, and a pharmacy.[2] The mountain xenodochia or hospices of Mont Cenis (825) and the Great St. Bernard (962) are still in existence.

After the death of Charlemagne, the larger hospitals began to decline through subdivision or loss of revenue and, in this period, we find the monasteries, such as those of the Benedictine order at Cluny, Fulda and elsewhere, provided with private infirmaries and "eleemosynary hospitals." About the same time arose the various Catholic hospital orders and fraternities for looking after the sick, of which the earliest were the Parabolani who, according to Gibbon, were first organized at Alexandria during the plague of Gallienus (A. D. 253–268). Parabolani sought out the sick, not unlike the monks of St. Bernard today, but soon exceeded their authority and were gradually suppressed. The term "sorority" probably comes from Soror, who founded the hospital Santa Maria della Scala at Siena in 898. Other religious orders which sprang up about the time of the Crusades were the Alexians, the Antonines, and the Beguins; the Hospitallers, comprising the followers of St. Elizabeth of Hungary, who founded two hospitals at Eisenach with a third on the Wartburg; the Sisters of St. Catherine; the order of St. John of Jerusalem, which was founded when the Crusaders reached the Holy City in 1099; and the Teutonic Order, which was started in a field hospital outside the walls of Acre and was approved by Clement III in 1191. The Teutonic Knights vowed themselves to care for the sick and to build a hospital wherever their order was introduced, and played a great part in Germany in medieval times, but eventually died out from lack of funds in the 15th century. Similarly, the Order

---

[1] Founded as a xenodochium under laic authority; given over to the clergy in 1308.

[2] F. Keller: Bauriss des Klosters St. Gallen, Zürich, 1844. Cited by Neuburger.

12

of St. John of Jerusalem became merged into a purely military order, and declined in the 13th century.   Parallel with the specialization of nursing orders during the Crusades, however, there went the great medieval hospital movement initiated by Pope Innocent III in 1198, which has received the just encomium of Virchow.   In 1145, Guy of Montpellier opened a hospital in honor of the Holy Ghost, which was approved by the Pope (1198), who himself built the hospital at Rome called "Santo Spirito in Sassia" in 1204.   The example of the Pontiff was soon followed all over Europe, with the result that nearly every city had its Hospital of the Holy Ghost, and it became the ambition of many a prince or landgrave to found a *"xenodochium pauperum, debilium et infirmorum."*   Virchow, in his essay on the hospitals of the Middle Ages,[1] gives a remarkable catalogue of these institutions in 155 German cities.   Many were, of course, merely first-aid and nursing stations of the charitable order of Teutonic Knights, but Virchow's list shows the definite social character of the movement.   In Rome, says Walsh, there were four city hospitals in the 11th century, six in the 12th, ten in the 13th.   Another circumstance which vastly aided the city hospital movement was the immense spread of **leprosy** in the Middle Ages.   Already known to the ancient Hebrews, Greeks and Romans, this disease began to appear in Northern Europe in the 6th and 7th centuries A. D., and its spread in connection with the Crusades was appalling.   It reached its full height in the 13th century.   The leper, wandering abroad, an outcast from human society, condemned to civil death by medical inspection (*Lepraschau*), living apart in huts in the open field, giving warning of his approach by horn or bell, became a common figure and the subject of frequent reference in the chronicles and romances of the period, such as *Der arme Heinrich* of Hartmann von Aue,[2] the *Frauendienst* of Ulrich von Lichtenstein,[3] the *Grandes Chroniques de France*,[4] or the unforgettable passage in the *Lüneburger Chronik*, which Heine paraphrased:

> Living corpses, they wandered to and fro, muffled from head to foot; a hood drawn over the face, and carrying in the hand a bell, the Lazarus-bell, as it was called, through which they were to give timely warning of their approach, so that every one could get out of the way in time.[5]

Leper hospitals were already mentioned by Gregory of Tours (*circa* 560).   As leprosy spread far and wide, the advantage of these retreats

---

[1] R. Virchow: Ges. Abhandl. a. d. Gebiete d. öffentlichen Medicin u. d. Seuchenlehre, Berl., 1879, ii, 1–130.

[2] In this poetical romance of the 13th century, "poor Henry," the hero, journeys to Montpellier and Salerno to be cured of leprosy.

[3] The *Frauendienst* affords a ludicrous sidelight on the excesses of chivalry. The leper-episode represents the henpecked hero as consorting with lepers to gratify the caprices of his exacting "lady."

[4] Swinburne's poem of *The Leper*, filled with the fantastic *Frauendienst* spirit of the Middle Ages, is based upon an episode in this chronicle, although the alleged citation in old French at the end of the poem was written by the poet himself.

[5] Heinrich Heine: "Geständnisse" (Sämmtl. Werke, Cotta ed., Leipz., x, 241, 242).

for purposes of segregation became apparent, and they turned out to be a potent factor in the eventual stamping out of the disease. The number of these lazar-houses (leprodochia or leprosoria), as they were then called, was extraordinary. There were some 220 in England and Scotland and 2000 in France alone.[1] Virchow, in his wonderful study of leprosy in the Middle Ages, has listed and described, with his usual patient fidelity, an amazing number of these leper hospitals in all the Germanic cities of the 13th and 14th centuries.[2] Although in all the medieval hospitals nursing and seclusion was the rule, with absolute neglect of treatment, it is clear, from Virchow's thoroughgoing narrative, that the building of the leprosoria represented a great social and hygienic movement, a wave of genuine prophylaxis as well as of human charity. Billings characterizes the true spirit of the hospital movement of the Middle Ages as follows:

When the medieval priest established in each great city of France a Hôtel Dieu, a place for God's hospitality, it was in the interests of charity as he understood it, including both the helping of the sick poor and the affording to those who were neither sick nor poor an opportunity and a stimulus to help their fellow men; and doubtless the cause of humanity and religion was advanced more by the effect on the givers than on the receivers.[3]

About the beginning of the 13th century, the hospitals began to pass, without friction and by mutual agreement, from the hands of the ecclesiastic authorities into those of the municipality. By this time there were many splendid city hospitals, like the Hôtel Dieu or the Santo Spirito. Hospital construction had attained its height in the 15th century.

Prominent English hospitals of the medieval period were the Hospital St. Gregory, founded by Archbishop Lanfranc in 1084; St. Bartholomew's, founded in 1137 by Rahere, a jester, who joined a religious order and obtained a grant of land from Henry I about 1123; the Holy Cross Hospital at Winchester, founded 1132; and St. Thomas's Hospital, founded by Peter, Bishop of Winchester, in 1215 and rebuilt in 1693.

Few reflect that the great struggles for commercial supremacy and sea power, beginning with the Middle Ages, and lasting for nine centuries (during which time the centers of trade shifted successively from Venice to Lisbon, Amsterdam, and London), were largely concerned with the enormous profits derived from the **drug-trade,** and associated with the fact that drugs were the lightest, most compact, and most lucrative of all cargoes.

The rise of the naval power of the Venetian Republic (820–1517) began with the lucrative Mediterranean transport service necessitated by the Crusades (1096–1272). The influences of Arabic pharmacy, and actual contact of the Crusaders

[1] See P. H. Denifle: La desolation des églises, monastères et hôpitaux pendant la guerre de cent ans. Paris, 1897.

[2] R. Virchow: "Zur Geschichte des Aussatzes und der Spitäler," Arch. f. path. Anat. (etc.), Berl., 1860, xviii, 138, 273; xix, 43; 1861, xx, 166.

[3] J. S. Billings: "Description of the Johns Hopkins Hospital," Baltimore, 1890, p. 48. See also Dorothy-Louise Mackay: Les hôpitaux et la charité à Paris an XIIIe siecle, Paris diss., 1923.

with their Moslem foes, greatly enhanced the value of far-Eastern drugs. The records of the custom-house at the port of Acre (1191–1291), and the later narrative of Marino Sanuto, show a lively traffic in aloes, benzoin, camphor, cinnamon, cloves, cubebs, ginger, mace, musk, nard, nutmegs, opium, pepper, and rhubarb (Tschirch). Balsams, spices, dyes, resins, rare woods, and drugs had much to do with the struggles of the Venetians with the Genoese and the Turks, culminating in the battle of Lepanto (1571). The defeat of the Genoese in the sea-fight off Chioggia (1380) marks the height of Venetian supremacy. The fall of Constantinople (1453) marred much of the Eastern and Egyptian trade, and the high cost of pepper and other condiments gave an incentive to the Portuguese navigators. When Vasco da Gama doubled the Cape and sailed into Calicut (May 20, 1498), the doom of Venetian commerce was sealed. Priuli, in his diary, records the gloom which fell upon the Rialto when it became known that Portuguese carricks, laden with spices, were in the harbor of Lisbon. For the next hundred years, the center of the drug trade was to be in the Portuguese capital.[1]

In studying the cultural phases of medicine, there is no documentation so effective or instructive as the graphic, and for a period so remote and well-nigh inaccessible to modern comprehension as the Middle Ages, the great cathedrals, with their stained glass windows, the liturgies, Books of Hours and illuminated missals, the chansons and epics, the miracle plays and moralities furnish us the shortest path to such comprehension. Perhaps the best available sidelights upon earlier medieval medicine are afforded in the **miniature paintings** which illuminate certain manuscript codices of the Salernitan masters, compiled and edited by Piero Giacosa in 1901.[2] One of these, an illustration to the Turin Codex of Pliny's Natural History, represents an imposing interior, showing three physicians with features of unmistakably Jewish cast, clad in flowing Oriental robes and turbans, in professional attendance upon some great personage. One of them is feeling the patient's pulse, the other two stand in grave consultation, while their horses champ outside; while within, long-haired pages in doublet and hose remain in waiting or converse among themselves. Another miniature on the same page shows a number of monks in a magic circle, exorcising the devil. This theurgic therapy of medieval times, with its centric feature of a devil for each disease and a particular saint to cast him out, was a crude form of the doctrine of specificity. In the many pictures of exorcism collected by Charcot and Richer,[3] from 5th century mosaics and miniatures or set paintings, engravings, and frescoes by Giotto, Francesco Vanni, Mezzasti, Rubens, and other medieval and post-medieval artists, the devil is always represented in full sight, in the act of escaping from the mouth of the energumen. A cut from the Bolognese Codex of the Canon of Avicenna shows the medieval physi-

---

[1] See Tschirch: Pharmakognosie, Leipzig, 1910, i, 695–702; and A. W. Linton: Jour. Amer. Pharm. Assoc., Phila., 1916, v, 250–255.

[2] Piero Giacosa: "Magistri Salernitani nondum editi," one vol. and atlas, Turin, Fratelli Bocca, 1901. A recent Italian album of similar type is, G. Carbonelli and R. Ravalini: "Comenti sopra alcune miniature e pitture italiane a soggetto medico," Rome, F. Centenari, 1918. It is made up of miniatures from the Urbino codices in the Vatican, the Paris, Vienna, and Casanatense codices of the *Tacuinum sanitatis*, etc.

[3] J. M. Charcot and P. Richer: Les démoniaques dans l'art, Paris, 1887.

cian, in gown and biretta, lecturing to his students, as on the title page of the Mellerstadt Mundinus. A superb miniature, from the Turin Codex of the *El Hawi* of Rhazes, shows a Salernitan master inspecting urine in a glass, while a humble-looking patient of rustic mien stands uncovered before him, holding the urine basket in his hand. The contrast between the professional gravity of the doctor's face and the pathetic solemnity of his mute, enduring patient is one of the cleverest things in medieval art. Uroscopy or water-casting was, in fact, a favorite theme of the painter and wood-engraver down to the beginning of the 18th century, and the accessories in these representations are nearly always the same. The urinal became the emblem of medical practice in the Middle Ages, and was even used in some places as a sign-board device (Neuburger). The urine was always contained in a characteristic flask of Erlenmeyer shape, sometimes graduated, and this flask was carried in an osier basket with lid and handle, looking very like a modern champagne bucket. The physician, of whatever period, is always represented as inspecting the urine in a most judicial way, often holding it up to the light in such wise that there will be no reflection or refraction from the sun's rays. Some medieval pictures represent the physician as disdaining to touch the Erlenmeyer urinal with his hands. In the Ketham Fasciculus of 1493, for instance, two Venetian pages hold up the urine in glasses, while the doctors, in gowns and skull-caps, inspect it and comment upon it. An effective miniature from Avicenna, in Giacosa's collection, shows a physician in office consultation with a number of patients, each of whom stands with his osier basket in his hands, while the practitioner descants upon the properties of each individual specimen of urine. Sometimes the urine was carried to the physician or wise-woman by a messenger, the diagnosis being thus made at a distance. As may be imagined, offhand diagnoses of this kind were a favorite imposture of the strolling quacks, who reaped a rich harvest from the deception. Another miniature, in the Bolognese Codex of Avicenna, shows us the front of an apothecary's shop, with the apprentices braying drugs in mortars, a physician riding by on horseback, the medicine jars upon the shelves being labeled with Arabic inscriptions. The cuts around the border represent a cold bath in a running torrent of water, another bath of a quasi-social character taken by several persons together in one of the piscines or circular bathing pools, with further representations of cupping, blood-letting, and the exploration of a chest wound. The most striking cuts in Giacosa's collection, however, are the rude pen drawings from the Codex of Roland's Surgery in the Biblioteca Casanatense, representing different episodes in the surgeon's experience, such as the diagnosis of a fracture, the reduction of a dislocation, the inspection, widening, or suturing of a wound, the withdrawal of an arrow, the setting of a fracture of the jaw and so on. These pictures, crude as they are, will decidedly enhance any one's opinion of the Salernitan surgeons, and must be seen to be appreciated. The splendid series of manuscript pictures published by Sudhoff in his recent study of **medieval surgery** (1914[1]) afford us a unique visualization of all phases of surgical practice in the 11th–15th centuries.

In these, chosen variously from the Sloane and Harleian MSS. (British Museum), the Ashmole and Rawlinson MSS. (Oxford) and the Marcian Codex (Venice), we see surgeons cutting for hemorrhoids, fistula, and stricture, removing nasal polyps, opening abscesses, trephining, removing arrows, bandaging, cupping, letting blood, and applying the cautery, with innumerable scenes of consultation, and schematic manikins for cauterization, cupping, venesection, and zodiacal prognosis. The second part contains many illustrations of surgical instruments, and an exhaustive exegesis of hitherto unprinted Latin and German texts, which will require a complete recasting of the literary history of medieval surgery by future historians. This is by far the most considerable contribution to the history and graphics of medieval surgery since the time of Gurlt's masterpiece.

Of the costume and personal appearance of the 14th century surgeon we get a faint, far-away impression from the illuminated picture of John of Arderne in the Sloane MS., representing the blond-bearded Saxon surgeon in gown, cloak and cap, seated in a throne-like chair, in the act of demonstrating his mode of procedure in fistula; or from the miniature frontispiece in Nicaise's edition of Mondeville (1314), representing that sharp-featured, gray-haired master, tall and slim, in a purple gown of clerical cut, black skull-cap, red stockings and slippered feet, reading lectures with uplifted forefinger. Thirteenth century practice is well depicted in the Ashmole MS. 399 in the Bodleian (Singer[2]). Sudhoff has reproduced a vast number of consultation scenes from the Sloane (1977), Leyden, and other medieval MSS. representing all phases of bedside and consultation practice.[3] The Latin MS. Codex of Galen at Dresden (Db 92–93), which is assigned to the second half of the 15th century, contains beautiful miniatures illustrating the blue, ermine-bordered mantle of the medieval physician of rank, details of uroscopy, venesection, rectal irrigation, preparation of drugs, bedside scenes, with clinical and anatomic demonstrations, showing that the living nude body was sometimes boldly used for didactic purposes in anatomic and obstetric teaching. These are by far the best of the medical miniatures in point of artistic merit.[4] Gilles de Corbeil satirized the fine raiment and outward display of the medical celebrities in the 12th century. Petrarch ridiculed the 14th century physicians for their rings on the fingers, tall horses, golden spurs, gorgeous clothes and pompous airs, a far cry from a passage in Saxo Grammaticus (I, 9), which describes King Gram (disguised as a Danish physician of the 12th century) as "dressed in the dirtiest rags he could

[1] K. Sudhoff: Beiträge zur Geschichte der Chirurgie im Mittelalter (Studien, Heft 10–12), Leipzig, 1914–18.

[2] C. Singer: Proc. Roy. Soc. Med. (Hist. Sect.), Lond., 1915, ix, 29–42.

[3] Sudhoff: Arch. f. Gesch. d. Med., Leipz., 1915–16, ix, 10, 293, 11 pl.; 1916–17, x, 71, 105, 10 pl.

[4] The pictures in the two-volume codex have all been handsomely reproduced by E. C. van Leersum and W. Martin in "Miniaturen der lateinischen Galenos-Handschrift," Leyden, 1910. This unique MS. was first noticed by Choulant.

find and sitting among the lowest menials in the hall" (Withington). A curious obsequiousness, the head cocked, in servile fashion, on one side, is noticeable in many of the medieval delineations of physicians and surgeons. The faces in all these pictures have the facile, wall-eyed expression which is found even in the paintings of such masters as Giotto, Cimabue and Lucas Cranach, and which seem to suggest that there was no self-revelation in the workings of the medieval mind. The methods of the medieval artists were unmistakably objective, as in Holbein's portraits, or the life-like representations of the nude by Jan van Eyck (St. Bavo altar at Ghent) and Pollajuolo. In this connection, let mention be made of the memorable "Stultitia" of Giotto in the Chapel of the Madonna dell'Arena at Padua, Ghirlandajo's picture of rhinophyma in the Louvre, and another representation of the same disease by the younger Holbein in the Prado. Leprosy is depicted in a German MS. (circa 1000) and in a colored miniature of the Leyden Codex of Theodoric. In the beautiful triptych in the Church of San Lazzaro at Capo di Faro, Sicily (1150), which was transferred to the Albergo dei Poveri (Genoa) and restored in 1851, Lazarus is represented as a leper.[1] Turold, a dwarf, is represented in the Bayeux Tapestry. A carved figure of a woman, high up on one of the flying buttresses of the north side of Rheims Cathedral (13th century), is described as strikingly acromegalic (Leonard Mark[2]). In such paintings as Stephen Lochner's Virgin (1447), and the Adoration of the Child (1470), both in the Cologne-Richartz Museum; Michael Wolhgemut's Nativity (Marienkirche, Zwickau, 1479), Bernhard Strigel's Holy Family (Germanic Museum, Nuremberg, 1485), and Hans Bergmaier's Virgin and Child (Nuremberg, 1500), the square head, protuberant abdomen, bow-legs, Harrison's groove and other stigmata of infantile rickets are strikingly shown (Foote[3]). Charcot found the facies of glossolabial hemispasm in a mascaron of the Santa Maria Formosa at Venice.

In the 15th century there were numbers of pictures painted to represent scenes in the lying-in chamber. These, contrary to modern custom and sentiment, are usually thronged with figures plying various avocations about the sick-room, and some of them frankly represent the act and moment of delivery. In the foreground of each, there is the inevitable nursemaid in the act of washing the newborn infant, and from some of these pictures we gather the curious fact that, in the Middle Ages, the sensitive naked foot was used as a sort of clinical thermometer. In a fresco of Luini's, in the Brera Gallery at Milan, the nursemaid is dipping her hand into the basin to ascertain if the water is too hot or too cold for the infant. In most of the pictures, however, a wooden tub is used, and in those representing the "Birth

---

[1] Portigliotti: L'Illustrazione med. ital., Genoa, 1923, v, 141–146.

[2] L. Mark: Lancet, Lond., 1914, ii, 1413.

[3] J. A. Foote: Amer. Jour. Dis. Child., Chicago, 1927, xxxiv, 443–452.

of the Virgin," by the elder Holbein (Augsburg Gallery), Bernhard Strigel (Berlin Gallery), and Bartholomäus Zeitblom (Augsburg and Sigmaringen Galleries), particularly in a *Wochenstube* of an unknown Tyrolese artist in the Ferdinandeum at Innsbruck, the nursemaid is represented, like the Highland laundresses in *Waverley*, with "kilted kirtle," her bare feet testing the temperature of the water in the tub. The different methods of investing an infant in its swaddling clothes are strikingly shown in the bas-relief *bambini* in glazed clay by Andrea della Robbia in the loggia of the Spedale degli Innocenti at Florence.[1]

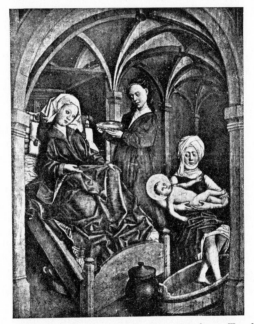

The Human Foot as a Thermometer. (Painting by a Tyrolese artist in the Ferdinandeum at Innsbruck.) From Dr. Robert Müllerheim's "Die Wochenstube in der Kunst" (Stuttgart, 1904).

Another important fact, thrown into relief by the 15th century pictures, is that the use of **spectacles** had by this time become quite common. They were introduced about 1270–80 by the glass-workers of Venice.

The discovery of spectacle-lenses[2] has been variously attributed to the Chinese, to the Romans, and to Roger Bacon. The only authentic reference is Pliny's statement that Nero looked at the gladiators through an emerald (*smaragd*), which Lessing discussed at great length in his "Antiquarian Letters," and which, at best, can be construed only as a sort of eye-shield or lorgnette. The truth is that the

[1] See Witkowski: *Histoire des accouchements*, Paris, 1887; and Robert Müllerheim: *Die Wochenstube in der Kunst*, Stuttgart, 1904.

[2] R. Greeff: Die Erfindung der Augengläser, Berlin, 1921.

ancients, as Cicero, Cornelius Nepos, and Suetonius owned, were resigned, after fifty, to having MSS. read to them by slaves. In the Middle Ages, the Arabians alone made any advances in optics. In his Treasury of Optics, Ibn al Haitham or Alhazan (996–1038) notes refraction and the magnification of objects through a segment of a glass sphere, which Roger Bacon later proposed as a reading glass for weak-eyed and elderly people. Roger Bacon's book was sent to the Pope in 1267. Then, in the State Archives of Venice (1300–1301), edicts began to appear forbidding the manufacture of spectacles (ogli) out of any other than crystal glass. Venice and adjacent Murano were, indeed, the centers for finished glassware of all kinds. In a chronicle of the cloister of St. Catharine at Pisa (1305), it is stated that a monk, Alessandro della Spina, could manufacture spectacles. In the Palatine (113) and Riccardi (1268) Codices at Florence there is a sermon of Fra Giordano da Rivolto (1305) which affirms that spectacles had been invented less than twenty years before. Greeff fixes this date as circa 1270–80. The attribution of the invention to Salvino

d'Armato degli Armati (1285) of Florence (died 1317) is shown by Greeff to be a solemn supercherie of the 17th century. Spectacles are mentioned in many wills of 1372–1524 (Heymann), also by Dante (Inferno, 33), Petrarca (1364), Charles d'Orléans (lunettes) and late 13th century Minnesänger (Greeff). They are first depicted in a fresco by Tommaso di Modena in the capitol hall near the Church of San Niccolò at Treviso (1352). As Greeff observes, most of the representations are anachronisms, for it was well after the invention of printing and the appearance of the incunabula, that spectacles came into common use. Bernard de Gordon first referred to them, about 1305, as oculus berellinus, because they were originally made from a smoky stone (berillus), whence the German Brillen (Parillen) and the French besicles (bericles). Arnold of Villanova terms them vitrea vocata conspicilia, and Guy de Chauliac, in his Chirurgia Magna (1363), recommends them, if collyria fail. During the 14th and 15th centuries, spectacles consisted of convex lenses in heavy unsightly frames, which were sold at an uncommonly high price. They figure as a detail in Friedrich Herlin's decorations on the altar of St. Jacob's Church at Rothenburg an der Tauber (1466); Jan van Eyck's Madonna at Bruges in the

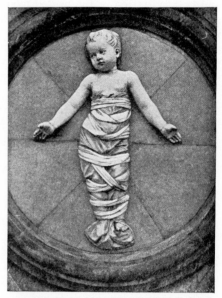

Bas-relief of Bambino in glazed clay in the Foundling Asylum at Florence, by Andrea della Robbia (1437–1525), showing method of swaddling infants. From Dr. Robert Müllerheim's "Die Wochenstube in der Kunst" (Stuttgart, 1904).

hand of the donor Georg van der Pale; in Dürer's painting of the Christ child in the temple (1500), and the elder Holbein's Martyrdom of St. Bartholomew (1503), both in the Dresden Gallery; in Joerg Syrlin's wood-carving of St. Luke on the choir-bench from the Benedictine abbey of Weingarten, Württemberg (National Gallery, Munich); in Ghirlandajo's Saint Jerome in the church of Ognissanti at Florence; in Martin Schöngauer's engraving of the Death of Mary; in a colored picture in a manuscript in the University Library at Prague, representing the investiture of the Elector of Brandenburg (1417); in a wood-engraving of 1461 (University Library, Munich); in the wood-cut of the book-worm in Sebastian Brand's Narrenschiff (1494); and in the painted title-page of a MS. of 1496 (Codex Pal. Germ., 126), in the University Library at Heidelberg. In the Prague MS., they give the wearer the appearance of a Chinese mandarin. The earliest known pairs of spectacles, consisting of two large circular lenses connected by a nose-bridge of pince nez pattern, one pair the property of the Renaissance humanist Willibald Pirkheimer (1470–1530), are now on exhibition in

Nuremberg Museum and the Wartburg.[1] The earliest books on spectacles were the *Uso de los antoios* of Benito Daça de Valdes (Seville, 1623), a French version of which was printed by G. Albertotti in 1892, and *L'occhiale all'occhio* by Carlo Antonio Manzini (Bologna, 1660). The first is illustrated, has tables for sight-testing, and recommends spectacles in those operated for cataract.

During the Middle Ages European humanity was plagued with **epidemic diseases** as never before or since, and these were variously attributed to comets and other astral influences, to storms, the failure of crops, famines, the sinking of mountains, the effects of drought or inundation, swarms of insects, poisoning of wells by the Jews, and other absurd causes. The real predisposing factors were the crowded condition and bad sanitation of the walled medieval towns; the squalor, misrule, and gross immorality occasioned by the many wars; the fact that Europe was overrun by wandering soldiers, students, and other vagabond characters; and the general superstition, ignorance, and uncleanliness of the masses, who, even in their bath-houses, were crowded together in one common compartment, sometimes with the sexes commingled.

In the Middle Ages it was customary to regard **eight diseases** as contagious, in accordance with the pseudo-Salernitan verse cited by Bernard de Gordon (1307), the idea of which derives from Aristotle's *Problemata* (Sticker) and Rhazes (Singer):

> Febris acuta, ptisis, pedicon, scabies, sacer ignis,
> Antrax, lippa, lepra nobis contagia praestant.

In an ordinance of the city of Basel (1350), in the *Pest Regiment* of Hans Wircker (1450), and in the *Tractatulus de regimine sanitatis* of Siegmund Abich of Prague (1484[2]) these eight diseases correspond with the above as bubonic plague, phthisis, epilepsy, scabies, erysipelas, anthrax, trachoma, leprosy (Sudhoff). Patients afflicted with these maladies were not permitted to enter cities, or were isolated, if inside cities, or driven from them, and not permitted to sell articles of food and drink. Of these eight diseases, scabies and lepra were ofttimes syphilis. The notion of epilepsy as contagious sprang, Sudhoff thinks, from the ancient Assyro-Babylonian concept of seizure by demons (*sibtu*), the ἐπαφή (*contagium*) of the Greek papyri of 77–350 A. D., as applied to the "sacred disease" (ἱερά νόσος) of the Hippocratic Canon. The idea of contagion in nervous diseases acquired considerable momentum from such neurotic manifestations of crowd psychology as epidemic chorea (later known variously as St. Vitus's Dance, *danse de St. Guy* and the Dancing Mania), the Children's Crusade, the processions of Flagellants and, with some reservations, the major Crusades themselves.

The earliest of the great medieval pandemics were the leprosy, Saint Anthony's fire or ergotism (857[3]), scurvy (1218[4]), the "Dancing Mania" (epidemic chorea),

---

[1] R. Greeff: *Die ältesten uns erhaltenen Brillen*, in Arch. f. Augenh., Wiesbaden, 1912, lxxii, 44–51. Ztschr. f. ophthal. Optik, Berl., 1913–14, i, ii, 46, 77; and A. von Pflugk: *Ibid.*, 1927, xiv, 138–145.

[2] Peter Ochs: Geschichte der Stadt und Landschaft Basel, Basel, 1792, 452–453. Cited by Sudhoff (Wien. med. Wochenschr., 1913, lxiii, 3077–3081, and Arch. f. Gesch. d. Med., Leipz., 1912–13, vi, 454; 1914–15, viii, 188; 220). In a 14th century pest-tract of Magister Henricus of Prague, unearthed by Sudhoff (Arch. f. Gesch. d. Med., Leipzig, 1913–14, vii, 81–89), the eight diseases *"qui transeunt de hominibus in homines"* are reduced to five, viz., fevers, pest, leprosy, epilepsy, and catarrhs (influenza or phthisis).

[3] Mezeray, in his History of France, describes the epidemic of 944 and 1090, to the latter of which he gave the name St. Anthony's fire.

[4] First described by Jacques de Vitry as ravaging the army of the Crusaders before Damietta (Collect. Guizot, liv, iii, § 351) and by Joinville in his Histoire de St.-Loys, Paris, 1617, 121.

sweating sickness, which was probably a modality of influenza, and plica Polonica (1287); the most formidable were the Black Death and syphilis. Of these, leprosy, scurvy, and influenza were either introduced or spread by the Crusades. Influenza, in particular, was regarded as a cosmic, telluric or celestial "influence" (*influentia coeli*), whence its name, which first appears in Buoninsegni's History of Florence (1580), with reference to an epidemic of 1357; and is later applied by Sozomeno to a Tuscan epidemic of 1387. The term *coqueluche* was used by Mezeray with reference to a Parisian epidemic of 1414 (Crookshank). Chorea (dancing mania) was probably the result of physical degeneracy plus fanatical religious enthusiasm, and acquired the name of St. Vitus's Dance from the processions of dancing patients in the Strassburg epidemic of 1418, who proceeded in this wise to the chapel of St. Vitus in Zabern for treatment. Plica Polonica, the unsightly disease of matted hair, was introduced into Poland by the Mongol invasion (1287). In a passage in the Codex Lat. 25060 of the City Library of Munich (pp. 54–55), exhumed by Sudhoff, a diphtheria epidemic of 1492 is described by the Nuremberg city physician Hartmann Schedel.[1] Ergotism, variously known as *ignis sacer, ignis infernalis,* or St. Anthony's fire,[2] was often as not erysipelas, but usually a characteristic disease of the Middle Ages, due to the formation of the fungus *Claviceps purpurea* in spurshaped masses upon rye, the common bread-staple of the poorer classes. The first allusion to it occurs in the Annals of the Convent at Xanten, near the Rhine, of date about 857. Even in this brief paragraph, reference is already made to its gangrenous character, and the eventual dropping off of the limbs from mortification. Later French epidemics occurred in 944, 957, 1039, 1089, 1096, and 1129, which were described, in the chronicles of the time, by Frodoard, Felibien, and Siegbert. The disease usually began with sensations of extreme coldness in the affected part, followed by intense burning pains; or else a crop of blisters broke out, the limb becoming livid, foul, and putrescent, and eventually dropping off: in either case after causing great suffering in the unfortunate victim. Recovery commonly followed the loss of a limb and, by some cruel sport of fate, patients sometimes survived after losing all four limbs. When the gangrene attacked the viscera, however, it was speedily fatal. In the different chronicles, true ergotism was undoubtedly confused with erysipelas, gangrene and bubonic plague. The so-called *mal des ardents* was probably the plague. The convulsive form of ergotism, which Crookshank believes to have been a mode of influenza, did not appear until a later period. The correlation of famine and (typhus) fever had already been noted in the Anglo-Saxon Chronicle (1087). Stow's *Survey of London* notes the deaths of the jailers of Newgate and Ludgate and of 64 prisoners doubtless from lice-transmitted typhus.[3]

During the 9th–12th centuries, there were many prayers, conjurations, charms, and amulets against a strange periodic affection which, from its recurrence in "evil years," was called *Malum Malannum*. It was a serpiginous carbuncular or gangrenous eruption, often affecting the jaws of man or animals, and possibly identical with glanders or anthrax.[4]

The **Black Death,** which caused the unprecedented mortality of one-fourth of the population of the earth (over sixty millions of human beings), appeared in Europe about 1348, after devastating Asia and Africa. From a focus in the Crimea, it spread, *via* Turkey, Greece, and Italy, northward and westward over the whole of Europe, again attacking it from a second focus by way of lower Austria. It broke out anew, at intervals, up to the end of the 17th century. Sweeping everything before it, this terrible plague brought panic and confusion

---

[1] Sudhoff: Arch. f. Gesch. d. Med., Leipz., 1912–13, vi, 121–126.

[2] The name St. Anthony's Fire was first used by the French historian Mezeray, in speaking of the epidemic of 1090. The Order of St. Anthony for the care of the sufferers was founded in 1093. St. Martial, St. Genevieve, and St. Benedict were also regarded as patron saints of ergotism, for which, see Edvard Ehlers: Ignis sacer, Kjøbenhavn, 1895; L'ergotisme, Paris, 1896. R. Fletcher: Bristol Med.-Chir. Jour., Dec., 1912, 295–315.

[3] MacArthur: Tr. Roy. Soc. Trop. Med., Lond., 1927, xx, 490–491.

[4] See M. Höfler: Janus, Amst., 1909, xix, 512–526.

in its train and broke down all restrictions of morality, decency, and humanity. Parents, children and lifelong friends forsook one another, every one striving to save only himself and to come off with a whole skin. Some took to vessels in the open sea, only to find that the pestilence was hot upon them; some prayed and fasted in sanctuaries, others gave themselves up to unbridled indulgence or, as in the Decameron of Boccaccio, one of the most graphic accounts of the plague of 1348, fled the country to idle away their time in some safe retreat; others lapsed into sullen indifference and despair. The dead were hurled pell-mell into huge pits, hastily dug for the purpose, and putrefying bodies lay about everywhere in the houses and streets. "Shrift there was none; churches and chapels were open, but neither priests nor penitents entered—all went to the charnelhouse. The sexton and the physician were cast into the same deep and wide grave; the testator and his heirs and executors were hurled from the same cart into the same hole together."[1] In short, the Black Death, with its dark stains upon the skin, its hemorrhages and gangrenous destruction of the lungs, its paralyzing effect upon mind and body, was, in the grim phrase of the Italians, the *mortalega grande* ("the great mortality"), a veritable sign and symbol of the King of Terrors. The axillary and inguinal, with the pulmonary lesions, would make it identical with modern Oriental plague. It was ably described by Guy de Chauliac ("*transgressio de mortalitate*"), Boccaccio, and Simon de Covino. The epidemic of 1382 was described in close detail in the *De peste* of Chalin de Vinario. The epidemic had at least one good effect, that it led the Venetian Republic to appoint three guardians of public health (1348), to exclude infected and suspected ships (1374), and to make the first *quarantine* of infected areas (1403), so called because travelers from the Levant were isolated in a detention hospital for 40 days (*quaranta giorni*). This 40 days' quarantine was first practised by Marseilles (1383). Ragusa first practised detention for a month (1377). The *trentina* gradually became a *quarantina*. The first lazaretto or detention station was established at Pisa, near the church of San Lazzaro, in 1464.[2] In other cities there were plague ordinances and private personal directions (*Pestschriften*), pesthouses and other hygienic improvements.

One of the earliest of the **pest-tracts** was the versified Regimen (1357) of Jean Jasme (Johannes Jacobi), which is preceded by the earliest Spanish tract on the pest, in a Catalan MS. of 1348 at Lerida, and has been shown by Klebs and Droz to be identical with the tract ascribed to Knut, Bishop of Vesterås (1461), and some other versions. Another is that of John of Burgundy or Johannes ad Barbam (1365), who was identical with Sir John Mandeville. This MS. of Bearded John, which was widely duplicated, translated and copied, is astrologic in tendency. Recently, the 130 known incunabula on the pest have been carefully collated and studied by A. C. Klebs and Sudhoff (1926), who has also edited and printed the extant MSS. of 1348–1498. Of the 281 MSS. of pest-tracts studied by Sudhoff, 141 were of German

---

[1] Cited from an old writer of the period by Fletcher, Johns Hopkins Hosp. Bull., 1898, ix, 176.

[2] D. Barduzzi: Riv. di storia crit. d. sc. med., Siena, 1919, x, 167.

provenance, 77 Italian, 21 French, 9 Spanish, 9 English, and 7 Swiss. Plague is held to be the effect of miasms or corrupt vapors upon the humoral complexion of the patient, the pestilence entering as an evil emanation through the pores of the skin and traveling thence to the heart, the liver, and the brain. To combat this, bathing was interdicted, lest the pores of the skin be opened, light diet, acid fruits and drinks, and especially liberal potations of vinegar, were recommended, the air of rooms was purified by burning juniper branches or throwing powders on live coals for the patients' inhalation; aromatic drugs were exhibited internally and carried in the hand, mixed with resin or amber (*pomum ambre*). If the disease supervened, phlebotomy was the therapeutic sheet-anchor. Blood was let from the superficial vein corresponding to the particular part affected and its emunctory or excretory channel. As time went on, vinegar acquired a prominent status in the pest-tracts as an antiseptic measure.[1]

The other great scourge of the Middle Ages was **syphilis,** which was supposed to have first appeared in epidemic form at the siege of Naples in 1495, and to have been communicated to the French invaders by the Spanish occupants, who got it (authorities conjecture) from Columbus's sailors, a visitation from the New World. That sporadic syphilis existed in antiquity and even in prehistoric times is quite within the range of probability. The supposed Neapolitan epidemic of 1495–96 Sudhoff holds to have been an outbreak of typhoid or paratyphoid infection.[2] If Columbian in origin, malignant syphilis was perhaps the usual result of the contact of civilized and primitive races, as in the "Black Lion" of the Peninsular Wars, or the syphilis of Mexico, Japan, and the South Seas. Syphilis is first mentioned in the following works, printed in facsimile by Professor Karl Sudhoff (1912[3]):

1. The Edict against Blasphemers (*Gotteslästereredikt*) of Emperor Maximilian I, issued August 7, 1495.
2. The *Vaticinium* or "astrological vision" of the Frisian poet-physician Theodoricus Ulsenius (Dietrich Uelzen), printed at Nuremberg August 1, 1496, with a colored print of a syphilitic by Albrecht Dürer. (Reprinted at Augsburg by Johann Froschauer, 1496.)
3. The *Eulogium,* a poem by Sebastian Brant, printed in September, 1496, by Joh. Bergmann von Olpe at Basel.
4. The *Tractatus de pestilentiali Scorra* (Augsburg, Hans Schauer, October 18, 1496), and *Ein hübscher Tractat von dem Ursprung des Bösen Franzos* (Augsburg, Hans Schauer, December 17, 1496), the first of these reprinted three times at Nuremberg, Cologne, and Leipzig (1496), and the latter once at Nuremberg, early in 1497.
5. The *Enarratio Satyrica*, a poem of the Veronese patrician Giorgio Sommariva, printed at Venice in December, 1496.

---

[1] D. W. Singer: Proc. Roy. Soc. Med., Sect. Hist. Med., London, 1916, ix, 159–212. Sudhoff: Pestschriften aus den ersten 150 Jahren nach der Epidemie des "schwarzen Todes" 1348 (Arch. f. Gesch. d. Med., Leipz., 1910–25, iv–vxii, *passim*). A. C. Klebs & E. Droz: Remèdes contre la peste, Paris, 1925. Klebs & Sudhoff: Die ersten gedruckten Pestschriften, München, 1926.

[2] In confirmation of this, G. Sticker cites a camp epidemic of typhoid at Louvain and Nymwegen in 1635, described by Diemerbroeck (Obs. et curat. med., xxiv) as "vulgariter *febris gallica*, a multis etiam *morbus gallicus* appellabatur" (Mitt. z. Gesch. d. Med., Leipz., 1916, xv, 77).

[3] Karl Sudhoff: Graphische und typographische Erstlinge der Syphilis-literatur, Leipzig, 1912. This work, translated by C. Singer, is essential for comprehension of recent views of the subject as controlled by first-hand investigation (with typographic and photographic reproduction) of the original texts and documents. See also Sudhoff: "Aus der Frühgeschichte der Syphilis" (Stud. z. Gesch. d. Med., Heft 9), Leipzig, 1912.

6. The *Concilium breve contra malas pustulas* of Konrad Schellig (Schelling), physician to the Elector Palatine (printed at Heidelberg in 1496).

7. Four prayers, one to St. Minus (Nuremberg, 1496), one to St. Dionysius (Nuremberg, 1496), one printed at Vienna, 1497, and one in low German of uncertain date.

8. A letter from Barcelona (1495) by Nicolò Scillacio of Messina, printed in his *Opuscula*, March 9, 1496, at Pavia showing that, in June, 1495, syphilis had broken out at Barcelona, simultaneously with the Naples epidemic, and was thought to have come from France (*qui nuper ex Gallia defluxit in alias nationes*).

All these tracts tend to show, Sudhoff thinks, that syphilis was known in Europe before the siege of Naples, since the name of the disease had already so many different synonyms and its general semeiology seems to have been definitely outlined as early as 1495.

It is also discussed at length before the year 1501 in various tracts by Joseph Grünpeck (1496), Caspare Torrella (1497), Niccolò Leoniceno (1497), Johannes Widmann (1497), Corradino Gillino (1497), Bartolommeo Montagnana (1498), Bartholomæus Steber (1498), Natale Montesauro (1498), Antonio Scanaroli (1498), Simon Pistor (1500), Martin Pollich (1500), and Gasparo Torella (1500[1]).

The first reference to the supposed West Indian origin of syphilis is contained in a work of Diaz de Isla (*Tractado contra el mal serpentino*[2]), written about 1510, and published in 1539 and 1542, in which the disease is said to be described as an absolutely new and unheard-of affection in Barcelona, brought from Hayti by Columbus's sailors in April, 1493. Isla is one of the rarest of books, and, if we may trust current accounts, its author had treated sailors in Columbus' fleet for syphilis before they landed at Palos. Also it is said that both Monardes and Montejo speak of the disease as then prevalent in nearby Seville, where a special hospital was built for syphilitics. The *Lucubratiuncula* of Leonhard Schmaus (1518) also refers to the West Indian origin of the disease on the authority of sea-captains of the period. In favor of the West Indian hypothesis, Hutchinson contended that, if transmissible syphilis existed in Europe before 1492, it would have been mentioned in Chaucer and Boccaccio, while it was found in Hayti and San Domingo after Columbus' second voyage. Virchow maintained that the *caries sicca* of prehistoric and pre-Columbian skulls was not true syphilis but either identical with the arthritis deformans (*Höhlengicht*) of old cave-bears, or else caused by plants and insects, which would eliminate the question of prehistoric syphilis in Europe. Medieval syphilis was first known as *mal franzoso, morbus gallicus* or *mala napoletana*, after the suppositious siege of Naples (1495), where it is supposed to have been communicated to the French soldiers under Charles VIII by the Spanish immigrants. After it became epidemic, it was called the Spanish, Polish, German, or Turkish "pocks," from the anxiety of the different nations to shift the blame upon one another. Iwan Bloch has attempted to prove that the evidences of *mal franzoso* in the cases of King Wenzel, the chorister of Mainz (1473), and Peter Martyr's letter (1488) were either fabrications or forgeries. On the other hand, the exhaustive studies recently made by Karl Sudhoff show that, in the *Gotteslasteredikt* of Emperor Maximilian (August 7, 1495), mention is made of "*malum francicum*," but nothing is said about syphilis in relation to the siege of Naples. According to Guicciardini, there was no actual siege at Naples, since Charles VIII passed through the city without opposition on February 21, 1495. Furthermore, in moving homeward through Tuscany the troops were besieged at Novara early in July, and did not get away until October 10th, two months after the date of Maximilian's Edict (August 7th); yet the latter shows that the disease was well known in Germany in July, while the actual march of events makes it clear that it could not have been spread about by wandering soldiery until long after, as Sudhoff shows. Sudhoff also gives a large number of recipes for syphilis, indicating that, far from being helpless in the treatment of the disease, physicians at the end of the 14th century were already prescribing the mercurial inunctions, which had been used as far back as the 12th century for an

---

[1] For the texts of German tracts on syphilis between 1495 and 1510, see C. H. Fuchs: Die ältesten Schriftsteller über die Lustseuche in Deutschland (Göttingen, 1843). Ten tracts of 1495–8 have been collected by Sudhoff (Zehn Syphilis Drücke, Milan, 1924) and Englished by Singer (Monumenta medica, III, Florence 1925). For bibliography down to 1899, see J. K. Proksch: Die Litteratur über die venerischen Krankheiten, 4 v., Bonn, 1889–1900.

[2] For the text of Isla, see Janus, Amst., 1901, vi, 653; 1902, vii, 31.

indefinable class of skin eruptions, comprising leprosy, psoriasis, and eczema. A special group of such eruptions, as yielding to mercury, was, Sudhoff thinks, an endemic spirochetosis, in all probability syphilis.[1] Mercury is first referred to in the *Circa instans* of Matthæus Platearius (1140), but its external use was already known to the Arab physicians (Astruc[2]). Indeed, mercurial salves were recommended for dermal eruptions by all medieval surgeons, from Roger down. Theodoric gives very explicit directions for inunction of mercury, with precautions against salivation. The most interesting of these recipes are two which Sudhoff found in an old Italian manuscript at Copenhagen, dated 1465, the handwriting of which has been assigned by the directors of the State Archives in the Uffizi at Florence to the first quarter of the 15th century.[3] These recipes read (*16*) *Electuario optimo al mal franzoso* and (*77*) *Per fare siropi da male franzoso*, and contain ingredients identical with those employed in the vegetable electuaries (*Kräuterlatwergen*) of the early German and Italian writers on syphilis. Thus, from the internal evidence of handwriting in some of the Uffizi manuscripts, syphilis may have been endemic in Italy as early as 1429. The old Swiss archives show that *scabies Gallicana* or *grossa verola* was regarded as a new disease about 1431.[4] Giannozzo Manetti (1396–1459), in his life of Pope Nicholas V, refers to it as a *"novus et molestus rugadiarum morbus."* On July 25, 1463, a prostitute of Dijon testified in open court that she had kept off an unwelcome suitor by stating that she was sick with *le gros mal*. On March 25, 1493 (1494), the town crier of Paris was directed to order from the city all afflicted with "the greater pox" (*la grosse vérole*), under pain of being thrown into the Seine.[5] Sudhoff shows that the alleged 90 per cent. mortality of French troops at Naples is a nursery tale (*Ammenmärchen*), that the Naples epidemic itself was a typhoidal infection like most of the *febres pestilentiales*, and that the Nuremberg prohibition of public bathing in a common chamber or tank (November 15, 1496) was similar to those already issued years before against leprosy and plague. At the end of his interesting studies,[6] he quotes a prognostication made by Paul von Middelburg on the occasion of the conjunction of Jupiter, Mars, and Saturn in the sign of the scorpion (November 24, 1494), which announces the approach of a fearful venereal disease, to reach its height about 1492–1500, and gives, along with a lurid purview of sexual debauchery, a series of resulting symptoms which are strikingly like those of syphilis.

The end-result of Sudhoff's investigations is to the effect that from the 12th century on, medieval physicians were richly supplied with mercurial recipes against an anomalous group of chronic skin affections, which, from their very names—*scabies grossa*, *variola grossa*, *grosse vérole*, *scabies mala*, *böse Blattern*, *mal franzoso*—were most likely syphilitic.

Aside from the astrologic view of its causation, the lues was latterly attributed to the rains and inundations of the same period (Leonicenus), intercourse of a leper with a prostitute (Monardes and Paracelsus), poisoning of the wells by the Spanish viceroys of Naples (Fallopius), or to disguised human flesh eaten by the French for ordinary meat (Fioravanti). It is evident that the disease was not clearly understood at the start, but, after it became pandemic, its sexual origin was recognized and, as it spread northward and southward from Italy, its differ-

---

[1] It is interesting to note that Sydenham thought that syphilis was identical with West African yaws; that Castellani's *Treponema pertenue* is hardly distinguishable from Schaudinn's parasite, and that, for the former, "606" is a true *therapia sterilisans*.

[2] "Primi omnium medici Arabes ausi sunt mercurium exterius adhibere" (Astruc: De morb. ven. Venice, i, 156).

[3] Sudhoff: Mal franzoso in Italien, Giessen, 1912.

[4] J. H. Hotzinger: Historie ecclestiasticæ Novi Testamenti, Zürich, 1651–9, iv, 9.

[5] Ordonnances des rois de France de la troisième race, Paris, 1840, xx, 436. Cited by Schuster and Sudhoff.

[6] Sudhoff: Aus der Frühgeschichte der Syphilis, Leipzig, 1912, 159–168.

ent stages were more or less accurately described between the years 1494 and 1550. In the 16th century, the Chevalier Bayard called it "the disease of him who has it" (*le mal de celui qui l'a*). Mercury, which Galen had interdicted as a "cold" poison, became the routine remedy. The introduction of the inunction-cure and the sweating cure was, Sudhoff thinks, the starting-point of curative treatment of diseases in hospitals (*curabiles, ergo curandi*), which had hitherto been neglected. There were many sensible regulations of public stews, such as that of Henry II (1161), which even antedated Saliceto's attribution of chancre to intercourse with prostitutes. Meanwhile humanity of high and low degree had to learn the hard lesson that syphilis is "no respecter of persons." Like the omnipresent grim skeleton in Holbein's "Dance of Death," it laid hold of lords and commons, just or unjust, in the same impartial spirit. The illustrated books of a later time, Blankaart's, for instance, teem with pictures representing the miseries wrought by the lues and the inconveniences of the clumsy, if heroic, modes of treatment in vogue. The disease was necessarily spread far and wide by ignorance of the non-sexual modes of infection, and today, medieval syphilis is practically endemic among native Arabs.[1] Apart from wars and famine, and even up to Ehrlich's time, syphilis has held its own with tuberculosis and alcoholism as a prime factor in bringing about the degeneration of the human stock.

[1] G. Lacapère: Syphilis arabe, Paris, 1923. B. Douchan: Paris diss., 1926, No. 218.

THE PERIOD OF THE RENAISSANCE, THE REVIVAL OF LEARNING, AND THE REFORMATION (1453-1600)

In the transition of civilized mankind from medieval to modern conditions, many forces were operative, but undoubtedly the most potent for the growth of individualism and release from the ban of authority were the inventions of gunpowder (which gave the *coup de grace* to feudalism), and of printing,[1] the most potent agent in uplifting mankind by self-education. With the discovery of America, the doubling of the Cape of Good Hope by Vasco da Gama, Magellan's circumnavigation of the globe, the establishment of heliocentric astronomy by Copernicus, and the Reformation, free thought came into its own again, and the critical spirit grew apace. The effect of the revival of Greek culture, by the Byzantine scholars who poured into the Italian peninsula after the fall of Constantinople (1453), was to substitute the spontaneous receptive attitude of Plato and Hippocrates for the dialectics and logic-chopping of Aristotle and the Galenists. Among the neo-Platonists, Leonardo da Vinci and Nicholas Cusanus were eminent in physics. The physician Jean Fernel, an accomplished mathematician, made the first exact measurement of a degree of the meridian,[2] and Garcia Hernandez, a practitioner at Palos, favored the project of Columbus in opposition to the University of Salamanca. Natural perception in science (*sentire est scire*) was the device of Campanella. Petrarch attacked scholastocism, Pomponeo Pomponazzi, Giambattista della Porta, Marsilio Ficino, Johan Weyer, and Giovanni Pico rationalized magic and astrology and opposed witchcraft, while Cornelius Agrippa (Heinrich von Nettesheim), 1486-1535, progressed from occultism (*De occulta philosophia*) to refined skepticism (*De incertitudine et vanitate scientiarum*, 1530[3]). Prime movers in this change for medicine were the great printers of the Renaissance and the so-called "medical humanists." At the start the early printers were frowned down upon lest they injure the business in manuscript books, which had been organized by the Universities of Paris and Bologna at the end of the 12th century. The MSS. were now nearly twice as expensive as the printed volumes (Ballard). The sack of Mainz, by Adolph of Nassau (1462), scattered the German printers over Europe. The Gutenberg Bible was printed in 1454. Johann Mentelin at Strassburg (1460) and Albert Pfister at Bamberg (1461) were followed by Conrad Sweynheym and Arnold Pannarts, who are credited with the first books printed in Italy, the Subiaco Cicero and Lactantius (1465). Johann Speyer and Nicolas Jenson began to print at Venice in 1469. Other Italian presses were set up at Foligno

---

[1] The claims to the invention are divided between Laurens Janszoon Coster, of Haarlem (1440), and Johan Gutenberg, of Mainz (1450).

[2] Fernel: Cosmotheoria, 1528. The passage is translated by Chéreau in Union méd., Par., 1864, 2. s., xxi, 530–532.

[3] See Neuburger: Introduction to Puschmann's *Handbuch*.

13

and Trevi (1470), Bologna, Ferrara, Florence, Milan, Naples, Pavia, and Treviso (1471). William Caxton began to print in English about 1474–5, and later the printing-houses of the Aldi and Giunti in Venice, Stephanus and Colinæus in Paris, Herbst (Oporinus) and Froben in Basel, Wynkyn de Worde and Wyer in London, Plantin at Antwerp, Elzevir in Leyden vied with one another in the issue of stately folios and beautiful texts. Such editors and translators as Niccolò Leoniceno and Giovanni Manardi at Ferrara, Rabelais at Meudon, Günther of Andernach at Strassburg, Johann Hagenbut (Cornarus) at Marburg, Pietro Mattioli at Rome, and Anutius Foesius at Metz, did for Hippocrates what Linacre and Caius in England did for Galen. These Renaissance versions and editions are not only remarkable for unapproachable typography (those of Oporinus, Colinæus, and the early German printers in Spain bearing away the palm in this respect), but are usually furnished with good tables of contents and oftentimes with subject and author indices at the end, giving accurate paginations. The large heavy type and excellent nutgall ink were eminently suited for weak or aged eyes, as yet unused to spectacles, which were invented about 1280, but did not come into general use until after the invention of printing (Greeff). The philologic study of Greek medicine supplanted the labors of the medieval "aggregators" and "conciliators," who sought to compare and reconcile Hellenist and Arabist doctrine (Neuburger). Giovanni Malpeghino at Ravenna awakened the sense of correct Latinity and accuracy of expression. With the medical philologists came the critical, questioning spirit in medicine.

Of the **medical humanists,** Niccolò Leoniceno (**Leonicenus**) (1428–1524), professor of medicine at Padua, Bologna, and Ferrara, a friend of Politian and Linacre and, like them, an elegant Latinist, made a famous translation of the Aphorisms of Hippocrates and, toward the close of his life, had even begun, by request, an accurate Latin translation of the works of Galen. He also wrote one of the earliest of the Renaissance tracts on syphilis (1497[1]), but his chief service to science lay in the difficult task of correcting the botanical errors in the Natural History of Pliny. In Leonicenus' day, this was a feat of the rarest intellectual courage. Hermolaus Barbarus, an earlier commentator, had already corrected some 500 orthographic and grammatic blunders perpetrated by the copyists of Pliny's manuscripts, but to assert that Pliny himself could be fallible in his statements of fact savored of rankest heresy, for his writings, like those of Galen and Aristotle, were regarded as sacrosanct and unimpeachable. Accordingly, when Leonicenus, who was a good botanist, published his little tract on the errors of Pliny[2] (1492), a violent storm of controversy broke loose over his

---

[1] Libellus de epidemia, quam Itali morbum gallicum vocant vulgo brossulas, Venice, 1497 (Hain, 10019); another edition was published at Milan in 1497 (Hain, 10020), and a third, printed in Gothic type, without place or date (Hain, 10018), is the earliest and rarest of all.

[2] Leonicenus: De Plinii et aliorum in medicina erroribus, Ferrara, 1492.

head.   His friend Poliziano, Colinuccio, and other non-botanists, who cared more for the letter than for the import of the old Roman's text, blazed away at the luckless commentator in truly medieval style for daring to challenge the accuracy of "our Pliny."   Leonicenus stuck to his guns, however, with the important sequel that all true botanists of later times—Ruellius, Matthiolus, Cesalpinus, Cordus—accepted his emendations without cavil.   In this respect Leonicenus may be said to have cleared the ground for the German "Fathers of Botany."   Without the careful work of these botanist-commentators, there could have been no scientific description of the materia medica.

Thomas **Linacre** (1460–1524), physician to Henry VII and Henry VIII, studied in Italy and was graduated M. D. from Padua and Oxford. On account of his services to humanism he was called by Fuller the

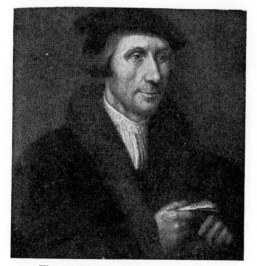

Thomas Linacre, M. D. (1460–1524).

"restorer of learning" in England.   He is remembered especially for his grammatic works (Payne thought him the original of Robert Browning's "Grammarian"), for his foundations of lectures on medicine at Oxford and Cambridge (1524), and for his Latin versions of Galen's treatises on hygiene (1517[1]), therapeutics (1519[2]), temperaments (1521[3]), natural faculties (1523[4]), the pulse (1523[5]), and semeiology (1524[6]).   These faithful and accurate translations had a wide circulation on the continent, and made it clear to the physicians that for centuries they

---

[1] Galen: De sanitate tuenda, Paris, 1517.

[2] Methodus medendi, Paris, 1519.

[3] De temperamentis, Cambridge, Siberch, 1521.

[4] De naturalibus facultatibus, London, Pynson, 1523.

[5] De pulsuum usu, London, Pynson, 1523.

[6] De symptomatum differentiis, London, Pynson, 1524.

had relied upon garbled and second-hand versions of their favorite author.

One of the earliest of the French humanists was Symphorien **Champier** (1472–1539), of Lyons, a medical graduate of Pavia (1515) and physician to Charles VIII, Louis XII, and the Duke of Lorraine.

Champier was one of the last of the conciliators of Greek and Arabist doctrine. His plan of bringing Hippocrates, Galen, Celsus, and Avicenna into a kind of symphonic relation with one another is visualized in the quaint wood engraving of a string quartet which prefaces his *Symphonia Platonis* (1516). In his *Hortus Gallicus* (1533), he was chauvinistic enough to affirm that the soil of France produces all remedies necessary for the treatment of disease, an extension of the old idea that "disease and remedy are found together." Champier wrote the earliest and best history of medicine in his time (1508[1]), the first medical dictionary after Simone de Cordo (1508[2]); also a *Rosa Gallica* (1514), a *Practica nova* (1517), and biographies of Arnold of Villanova (1520) and Mesuë (1523).

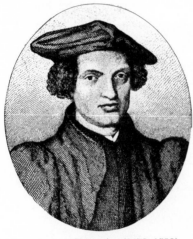

Symphorien Champier (1472–1539).

Francois **Rabelais** (1490–1553), who, like Linacre, was a priest as well as a physician, made one of the first Latin translations of the aphorisms of Hippocrates (Lyons, 1532), the original edition of which is much prized by bibliophiles.[3] Rabelais is best known, of course, by his immortal humorous works *"Gargantua"* and *"Pantagruel,"* which are not only filled with the strangest kind of medical erudition, but are exponents of Renaissance humanism in the broadest sense. The old medieval custom of stuffing the youthful mind with book-learning is keenly ridiculed, and the Greek ideal of education as a drawing out of all the faculties, including the physical and social, is upheld. Rabelais was the first to lecture on medicine at Montpellier with the Greek text before him.

Jean **Fernel** (1506–88), of Clermont (Oise), a Paris graduate of 1528–30, was the greatest French physician of the Renaissance. Well trained in mathematics and philosophy, he wasted his substance through his passion for astronomy, but eventually got down to practice and accumulated a great fortune. Having relieved the sterility of Catherine de Medici and the ill health of Diane de Poitiers, he feigned a pleurisy and other excuses to sidestep the dubious responsibility of royal physi-

---

[1] Champier: De claris medicinæ scriptoribus, Lyons, 1508. Another history of medicine was published by Marcellus Donatus in 1586.

[2] Champier: Vocabulorum medicinalium et terminorum difficilium explanatio, Lyons, 1508.

[3] Earlier Latin versions were published at Venice in 1495 (Hain, 8674) and at Nuremberg in 1496 (Hain, 8675).

cian, which was later forced upon him by Henri II. He attended the king on his campaigns up to the recapture of Calais (1588), and died soon after from grief over the loss of his wife. A man of melancholy nature and aspect, his face lighted up as he entered the sick-room, and no patient, however poor or humble, was ever turned away from his door.

A precise, orderly thinker and writer, who envisaged medicine from the analytical (Cnidian) viewpoint of the essential mathematician, Fernel made the best classification of diseases between Galen and Felix Platter. His *Medicina* (1554) is a concise, well-arranged summary of the four fundamental disciplines. The section *Pathologia* is the first explicit treatise on special pathology (*de partium morbis*) in that the semeiology of each disease is considered with reference to pathogenesis. Here gonorrhea is described as an independent affection of the bladder, apart from the chapter on lues, in which the various modes of contact transmission (*syphilis insontium*) are enumerated. As Crookshank has shown,[1] Fernel definitely correlated the respiratory and gastro-intestinal catarrhs of epidemic influenza with the paralytic, lethargic, and sensory manifestations, as Schiller had done with the German sweating sickness of 1528–30.[2] Fernel checked on many postmortem sections, notably those of tuberculosis (Bonet, 1553).[3] He corrected many Galenic errors, opposed intensive blood-letting, and sought the cause (virus) of a disease in the humors, the seat (lesion) in the solid parts, and the symptoms in the bodily functions.

Anutius **Foesius**, or Foes (1528–95), devoted forty years of a laborious and useful life as city physician in his native town of Metz, to his invaluable concordance of Hippocrates (*Œconomia Hippocratis*, 1588), and his well-known critical edition of the Greek text of the Coan master (1595).

In the group of medical philologists were also the botanist Leonhard Fuchs who was the bitterest opponent of Arabism, the clinician Johann Lange, John Kaye (1506–73), the Dr. **Caius** of the *Merry Wives of Windsor* and the historian of the sweating sickness (1552), his teacher, Giovanni Battista della Monte (Montanus) (1498–1552), of Padua, Geronimo Mercuriale (1530–1606), who made a critical exegesis (*Variae lectiones*) of difficult passages in the Greek and Latin authors, the lexicographer Jean de Gorris (1505–77), the Spaniard Francisco Valles and the Portuguese Luis de Lemos, who tested the genuineness of the Hippocratic writings.

Some time after the invention of printing, Germany entered the field of medicine with a remarkable array of semipopular treatises, most of them written, contrary to custom, in the vernacular—the language of the people. According to Sudhoff, the earliest printed document relating to medicine is the unique Purgation-Calendar (*Laxier-kalender*) of 1457, a half-sheet of paper, printed in the type of Gutenberg's 36-line Bible,[4] and contained in the Bibliothèque nationale

---

[1] "In intestina, alvi profluvium . . . in nervorum origines irruens, apoplexiam, paralysim, stuporem, tremorem; in sensuum organa, cæcitatem, surditatem, tennitum, odoratus privationem," Pathologia, lib. V, cap. iv. Cited by Crookshank: Influenza, Lond., 1922, 39.

[2] Schiller: De peste Britannica, Basel, 1531.

[3] From information kindly supplied by Dr. Esmond R. Long (Chicago) from his forthcoming history of pathology.

[4] For a facsimile of either, and a full account of all the calendar-incunabula, see Sudhoff's interesting "Lasstafelkunst in Drucken des 15. Jahrhunderts," in his Arch. f. Gesch. d. Med., Leipz., 1907–8, i, pp. 223 and 227, and p. 135 (opposite). The calendars of 1439 (Johann Nider von Gmünd) and 1448 contain nothing medical.

(Paris). A unique copy of a Calendar for Blood-Letting (*Aderlass-kalender*), printed at Mainz in 1462,[1] is one of the treasures of the Fürstenberg Library at Donaueschingen (Baden). These popular almanacs, consisting of loose leaves or broadsides, printed on one side only, show the hold which judicial astrology (the *Lasstafelkunst*) had taken upon the people. Some 46 were printed before 1481 and about 100 before 1501 (Haebler). In some of them a special figure, the "zodiac-man" (*Tierkreiszeichenmann*), familiar in drug-store almanacs of more recent date, indicates the parts of the body influenced by the different planetary conjunctions, the proper times and places for bleeding and purgation under each sign of the zodiac, with gloomy prognostications of the terrible diseases, wars, famines, and other pests which were to befall humanity under different ascendencies and conjunctions of the planets. Palmistry also attracted wide attention; the earliest publication on the subject was Johann Hartlieb's illustrated block-book, *Die Kunst Ciromantia* (Augsburg, *circa* 1470). The *Versehung des Leibs* (Nuremberg, 1489) contains the first book plate, a picture of a man with the *facies Hippocratica*. More scientific interest attaches to the remarkable incunable of Ulrich Ellenbog (–1499) on poisonous fumes and gases (1473) and the *Regiment der jungen Kinder* of Bartholomæus **Metlinger** (Augsburg, 1473), a little book on infant hygiene, which would be the first Renaissance contribution to **pediatrics** had it not been preceded by the *De ægritudinibus infantum* (Padua, 1472) of Paolo **Bagellardo**. A third tract by Cornelius **Roelants** of Mechlin (Louvain, *circa* 1483–4) exhumed by Sudhoff in an incunable in the University Library at Leipzig and the Hunterian Museum at Glasgow,[1] was plagiarized in the pediatric treatise of Sebastianus Austrius (1540).

The *Artzneibuch* of **Ortolff of Bavaria** (Nuremberg, 1477) was an important early German text of popular medicine, followed, about 1500, by Ortolff's quaint little *Frauenbüchlein*, or popular handbook for lying-in women. A few years later (in 1513) there appeared, at Worms, the *Rosegarten* of Eucharius **Röslin,** a work which bears about the same relation to Renaissance obstetrics that the *Anothomia* of Mundinus does to medieval anatomy. Although mainly a compilation from Soranus of Ephesus, as filtered through the manuscript codices of Moschion, it was still the only text-book in the field after a lapse of fourteen centuries. Three first editions were issued simultaneously, both extremely interesting for their quaint cuts (already faintly outlined in the Moschion codices), for the revival of podalic version as originally described by Soranus, and for the fact that Röslin's text was miserably plagiarized by Walther Reiff in 1545,[2] and also translated and reissued

---

[1] Sudhoff: Janus, Amst., 1909, xiv, 467–485 (with text). For the sources of the work, see Sudhoff: *Ibid.*, 1915, xx, 443–458.

[2] The plagiarist Reiff should not be confused with the Swiss obstetrician Jacob Rueff (1500–58), author of the "Trostbüchle" (Zürich, 1554), a midwifery of sterling character.

by William Raynalde as *The Byrthe of Mankynde*, London, 1545. The ordinance issued by the city of Ratisbon in 1555 for the direction of

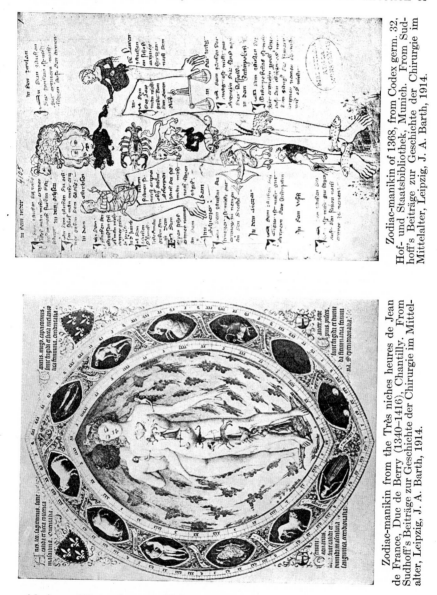

Zodiac-manikin of 1368, from Codex germ. 32, Hof- und Staatsbibliothek, Munich. From Sudhoff's Beiträge zur Geschichte der Chirurgie im Mittelalter, Leipzig, J. A. Barth, 1914.

Zodiac-manikin from the Très riches heures de Jean de France, Duc de Berry (1340–1416), Chantilly. From Sudhoff's Beiträge zur Geschichte der Chirurgie im Mittelalter, Leipzig, J. A. Barth, 1914.

midwives (*Regensburger Hebammenbuch*) has been proved by Felix Neumann[1] to be the earliest public document of this kind in the vernacular.

[1] F. Neumann: Arch. f. Gesch. d. Med., Leipz., 1911–12, v, 132–141.

A

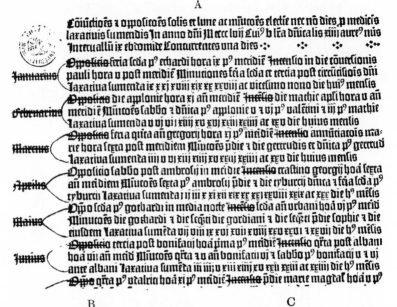

B   C

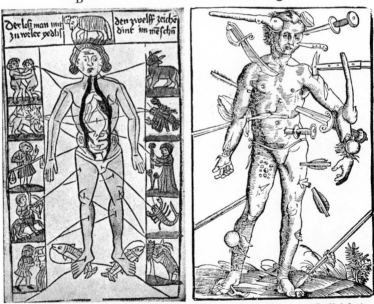

Specimens of the *Lasstafelkunst* (Horoscopic Medicine or Judicial Astrology). (By kind permission of Professor Karl Sudhoff, University of Leipzig.) A: Fragment of Purgation Calendar (*Laxierkalender*), printed with the types of Gutenberg's 36-line Bible (1457), and discovered by Professor Sudhoff in the Bibliothèque nationale, Paris. B: Blood-letting man (*Aderlassmann*), from the Calendar of Regiomontanus (1475), showing the points of election for blood-letting under the signs of the zodiac. C: Wound-man (*Wundenmann*), from Gersdorff's *Feldtbuch* (1517), showing the sites for ligation of the different arteries or for blood-letting. C is a later evolutionary form of the old zodiacal diagrams, which combined an exposition of planetary influences with schemata of the viscera (B).

Perhaps the earliest European text of **medical jurisprudence** of consequence is the "Constitutio Criminalis Carolina" (*Peinliche Gerichtsordnung*) issued by Emperior Charles V in 1533, as an extension of a similar ordinance issued by the Bishop of Bamberg in 1507. Interesting relics of the great medieval pandemics of syphilis and bubonic plague are preserved in the curious old tracts of Widman (1497), Steber (1498), Pollich (1501), Konrad Schellig (1502), Grünpeck (1503), Schmaus (1518), and Ulrich von Hutten (1519), and sweating sickness is the subject of a great mass of pamphlets, the best known of which is the little treatise of John Kaye or Caius (1552[1]). Matthaeus Friedrich, a pastor of Görenz, wrote the earliest tract on alcoholism (*Wider den Saufteuffel*, 1552). **Early German botany** had its beginnings in the *Herbarius Moguntinus*, the oldest herb-book with illustrations, printed by Peter Schöffer (Mainz, 1484), who also printed the *Hortus sanitatis*, an entirely different compilation from older writers, attributed to its editor, Johan (Wonnecke) von Kaub or Cube (Mainz, 1485), which was rendered into German as the *Gart der Gesundheit*.[2] This work contained some 500 engravings which, as Greene says, are "most wretched caricatures of plants," but it became popular enough to be the principal incentive for the work of the "German Fathers," Brunfels, Fuchs, Bock, and Valerius Cordus. It was followed by the greater *Hortus sanitatis* of Jacob Meidenbach (Mainz, 1491). In France, similar compilations, variously known as *Arbolayre* (*Herbolario*), translated from the German *Hortus sanitatis*, and *Le grant herbier*, were widely printed (Choulant). These incunabula were in turn the origins of many English "Herbals." The *Buch der Natur* of Conrad von Megenberg (Augsburg, 1475), an illustrated compilation which passed through six Augsburg editions before 1500, was the best known compendium of natural history.

Early German surgery begins with the *Bündth-Ertznei* of Heinrich von **Pfolspeundt,** a Bavarian army surgeon, whose work, written in 1460, remained long in manuscript, until it was discovered at Breslau and edited by Haeser and Middeldorpf (1868). Pfolspeundt was only a wound surgeon, had no skill in the major operations, which he left to the cutters or "incisors," and did not know how to treat fractures and dislocations; but he learned how to make artificial noses (by the Hindu method) from the wandering Italians. His military experience gave him a large practice in arrow wounds, and his book contains the first faint allusion to "powder-burns," and to the extraction of bullets by means of the sound.[3] He treated wounds by second intention, used the narcotic recommended by Nicholas of Salerno, and, like Mondeville and other surgeons of earlier times, gave his patients strengthening "wound-drinks." After Pfolspeundt came two Alsatian army surgeons, Hieronymus Brunschwig (*circa* 1450–1533) and Hans von Gersdorff,

---

[1] For the texts of the writers on sweating sickness, see C. G. Gruner's Scriptores de sudore anglico, edited by Haeser (Jena, 1847).

[2] For an account of the Hortus sanitatis, its history, origins, and variants, see L. Choulant's Graphische Inkunabeln, Leipz., 1858, 20–75; also J. F. Payne: Tr. Bibliog. Soc., Lond., 1901–2, vi, 63–126, and A. C. Klebs: Catalogue of Early Herbals, Lugano, 1925. Neither the *Herbarius Moguntiæ impressus* (1484) nor the German *Hortus sanitatis* (1485) is related to the *Herbarium* of [pseudo-] Apuleius Platonicus, printed at Rome in 1480, from a MS. at Monte Cassino, by Giovanni Filippo de Lignamine, physician to Pope Sixtus IV.

[3] Haeser and Middeldorpf at first asserted, in their commentary on Pfolspeundt (pp. xxii, xxvii), that there is no mention of gunshot wounds in the Bündth-Ertznei. This was afterward shown to be incorrect by H. Frœlich (Deutsche mil.-ärztl. Ztschr., Berl., 1874, vol. iii, pp. 592–594), who points out the "Item vor das büchsenpülüer auss den wünden" (Pfolspeundt, p. 10), and the following (p. 60): "Auch machstu solchs suchel [Sonde] wol von eissen machenn . . . mith dem hebstu die kleine gelödt oder *kugel* hiraus, die von buchsenn hinein geschossenn sein, und auch was sunst in den wunden ist."

called Schyllhans, both natives of Strassburg. The *Buch der Wund-Artzney* (Strassburg, 1497) of **Brunschwig** contains the first detailed account of gunshot wounds in medical literature. He regarded such wounds as poisoned, and thought the poison could be best removed by promoting suppuration, usually by means of the seton. As an army surgeon, Brunschwig did no major operations, confining himself to wounds, bone-setting, and amputation. In performing amputation, he applied the actual cautery or boiling oil to check hemorrhage from the stump. This book contains some of the earliest specimens of medical illustration

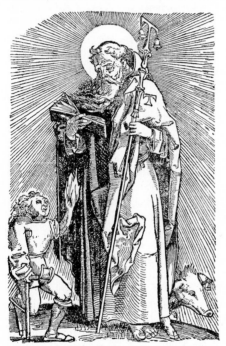

St. Anthony with a victim of ergotism. (From Hans von Gersdorff's Feldtbuch der Wundtartzney, Strassburg, 1540.)

by wood-cuts, rare and curious in their kind. The same thing is true of Gersdorff's Field-Book of Wound Surgery (*Feldtbuch der Wundartzney*), which was published at Strassburg in 1517. **Gersdorff** goes even more fully into gunshot wounds than Jerome of Brunswick. He did not regard them as poisonous, but probed for the bullet with special instruments and, like most surgeons of his time, poured hot oil into the wound. In amputating, he "Esmarched" the limb by means of a constricting band and, discarding the cautery, checked hemorrhage by a styptic of his own devising (containing lime, vitriol, alum, aloes, and nutgalls), inclosing the stump in "the bladder of a bull, ox, or hog," which may, in some cases, have been a good Listerian protective. Gersdorff's book contains some of the most instructive pictures of early surgical

procedure in existence; in particular, the first picture ever made of an amputation, and unique plates of leprosy and St. Anthony's fire. The wood-cut of the latter condition (*ignis sacer* or ergotism) represents the victim of the disease as hobbling upon a crutch and holding up a shriveled, gangrenous hand, bursting into flame, to excite the pity of Anthony, the patron-saint of the disease, who stands leaning upon his tau-cross, attended by his faithful swine. Another interesting picture book in the vernacular is the *Augendienst* (Dresden, 1583) of the court oculist, George **Bartisch** (1535–1606), the striking illustrations of which afford a complete purview of Renaissance eye-surgery. Among these may be mentioned the cuts showing the patient tied in a chair and ready for operation, the modes of procedure in cataract, and the perforated or stenopeic spectacles or visors (originally recommended by Paul of Ægina[1]) for strabismus. As Bartisch, originally an unlettered barber-surgeon, makes a great parade of learning and Latinity in his text (aside from its pompous title[2]), he is supposed to have employed a famulus or hired scribe to polish his book for him. None the less, this work did much to lift ophthalmology above what its author calls the "couchers and eye-destroyers" of his time. His treatise on lithotomy (1575) contains an interesting picture of the operation. The earliest printed book on the eye was the *De oculis, eorumque egritudinibus et curis* of Benvenuto (called Grassi or Graffeo) of Salerno (printed at Ferrara in 1475), which follows the ancients.

In the vernacular group may be mentioned the little eye-books of G. Vogtherr (Strassburg, 1538) and Walter Bailey (London, 1586), and the *Traité des maladies de l'œil* by Jacques Guillemeau (Paris, 1585), decidedly the best of the Renaissance books on ophthalmology. Even the English treatise of Richard Banister (1622) is only a translation of this work. The first medical book to be printed in England was called *A Passing Gode Lityll Boke Necessarye and Behovefull Agenst the Pestilence*, being a small quarto of twelve leaves, attributed to the press of William de Machlinia (London, *circa* 1485), translated from the *Tractatus contra pestilentiam* (1480), ascribed to Kanutus (Bengt Knutsson), Bishop of Vesterås, Sweden (1461), but which, as Sudhoff and latterly Arnold Klebs have shown, by parallel comparison of texts, was really written by the Papal physician Jean Jasme •(Johannes Jacobi) of Montpellier about 1357.[3] The English version was afterward reprinted by Wynkyn de Worde in 1510. Next came *The Governayle of Helthe*, printed at Caxton's press about 1491, followed by *The Judycyal of Urins* (1510), sometimes attributed to John of Arderne, and probably printed by Wynkyn de Worde. In 1516, Peter Treverus, a printer in Southwark, published *The Grete Herball* and, in 1521, Siberch of Cambridge printed Linacre's translation of Galen's *De temperamentis*, after which Pynson of London published other versions of Galen by the same scholar. The first work on anatomy to be printed in England was David Egar's little tract of 15 pages, entitled *In anatomicen introductio luculenta et brevis*. The first English anatomy printed in the vernacular was *The Englishman's Treasure* by Thomas Vicary (London, 1548[?]–1577[4]). The invention of shorthand by a physician is recorded in the *Characterie* (1588) of Timothy Bright (1551–1615), of which only one copy exists (in the Bodleian Library). It is supposed that Shakespeare got his knowledge of psychiatry from Bright's treatise on melancholy (1586).

The effect of these vernacular writings was to get men's minds away from scholasticism and turn them toward realities. This Renaissance tendency reached its highest development in the great medical leaders of the 16th century, Paracelsus, Vesalius, and Paré—three strong men of aggressive temperament, who, by shouldering past other men, literally "blazed the way," not only for the general advance of medicine, but for keen and liberal thinking in all its branches.

---

[1] For Paul's visor-mask see the Oporinus edition (Basel, 1546, lib. iii, cap. 22, 182). Stenopeic spectacles for squint were also known to Paré (1575). The term "stenopeic spectacles" was introduced by Donders (1854).

[2] 'Οφθαλμωδουλεία, das ist, Augendienst, Dresden, 1583.

[3] Sudhoff: Arch. f. Gesch. d. Med., Leipz., 1911–12, v, 56–58. A. C. Klebs and E. Droz: Remèdes contre la peste, Paris, 1925.

[4] J. F. Payne: Brit. Med. Jour., Lond., 1889, i, 1085.

Aureolus Theophrastus Bombastus von Hohenheim, or **Paracelsus** (1493–1541), precursor of chemical pharmacology and therapeutics, and the most original medical thinker of the 16th century, was, in spite of his bombastic assertion of rank and lineage,[1] a striking example of the very raw materials from which such aspirations are sometimes fashioned. His coarseness of fiber, though a better possession to him than vulgarity of spirit, often impeded his power to "think straight and see clear." A native of Einsiedeln, near Zürich, Switzerland, he had the truculent, independent spirit commonly ascribed to the man of mountaineer race, and was one of the few writers who ever advanced medicine by quarreling about it. Like the "roarers"

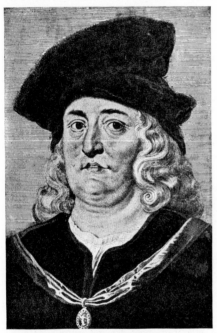

Paracelsus (1493–1541).

in Elizabethan comedy, or the *Zankbauer* in German farce, he tried to bully and browbeat his auditors and readers into accepting his views, and the writings which he dictated to his pupils are often a curious mixture of credulous fustian and swagger, set off by many successful guesses at truth and some remarkable intuitions. His humorous sallies, if he intended them as such, are usually of the lumpish kind that drift "from the obscene into the incomprehensible."[2] Paracelsus was the son of a learned physician, who had a fine library, and with whom he began to study medicine. He got his doctor's degree under Leonicenus at Ferrara (1515), and picked up an unusual knowledge of alchemy, astrology, and other occult sciences from the learned abbots and bishops of the country round, as also in the laboratory and mines owned by the Tyrolese alchemist, Sigismund Függer. Having the Swiss *Wanderlust*, he traveled all over Europe, collecting information from every source, and by his relations with barbers, executioners, bathkeepers, gypsies, midwives, and fortune-tellers, he learned a great deal about medical practice, and incidentally acquired an unusual knowledge of folk-medicine and a permanent taste for low company. Paracelsus thought and spoke in the language of the peo-

---

[1] The name "Paracelsus" is supposed to be either a free translation of "Hohenheim" or else an indication of his superiority to Celsus. He usually calls himself "Theophrastus ex Hohenheim eremita," *i. e.*, of Einsiedeln.

[2] George Moore.

ple, was "popular" as no other physician before him. When he appeared as a teacher at Freiburg and Strassburg (1525), his fame as a lucky practitioner preceded him. Appointed professor of medicine and city physician at Basel (1527), and imbued with a lifelong reverence for Hippocrates, implanted by his teacher, Leonicenus, he began his campaign of reform by publicly burning the works of Galen and Avicenna in a bonfire and lecturing in German out of his own experience. A year later (1528) he was already in violent conflict with the authorities about fees, and forced to leave the city. Resuming his wandering habits and practising all over Germany with varying success, he finally met his end from a wound in a tavern brawl at Salzburg (1541). As a pioneer in chemistry, Paracelsus was preceded by pseudo-Geber, the alchemists Albertus Magnus and Cornelius Agrippa, and followed by a swarm of chemiatrists, among them Johann Thölde, who wrote under the pseudonym of the mythical 15th century monk, Basil Valentine. Pseudo-Valentine is supposed to have given to chemistry hydrochloric acid, sugar of lead, the means of preparing ammonia and sulphuric acid and, in his "Triumphal Chariot of Antimony" (1604), fastened the latter metal upon medical practice for centuries.[1] Paracelsus took Geber's three chemical elements—combustible sulphur, volatile mercury, residual salt—and mixed them up with a species of theosophic lore, perhaps derived from the far East, where he is supposed to have traveled. Baas has compared reading Paracelsus to delving in a mine. We are in a strange world of mystic principles, macrocosms and microcosms, archæi and arcana, enlivened by gnomes, sylvans, sprites, and salamanders. Existence proceeds from God, all material things from the Yliaster (primordial substance), while the force in nature which sets things going (the vital principle) is the Archæus. The Archæus is the essence of life, contained in an invisible vehicle, the Mumia. In diseased conditions, this Mumia must be magnetically extracted from the patient's body and inoculated into a plant bearing the signature of the disease, so that it may attract the specific influence from the stars. Diseases, in Paracelsus' scheme of things, were caused by astral influences acting upon the "astral body" of man. Yet the author of all this high-flown verbiage, the actual Paracelsus, was a capable physician and surgeon, generous to the poor and, however despised and rejected, a man deserving of better human remembrance.

---

[1] For the Basil Valentine controversy, see Kopp (Die Alchemie, 1886), John Ferguson (Bibliotheca Chemica, 1906), Sudhoff's Bibliographia Paracelsica (Berlin, 1894), C. S. Pierce (Science, N. Y., 1898, n. s. viii, 169–176), and J. M. Stillmann (Pop. Sc. Monthly, N. Y., 1912, lxxxi, 591–600). These hold that the writings of pseudo-Valentine belong probably to the early 17th century literature. The picture of Basil Valentine in the Royal Cabinet of Etchings at Munich represents a monk, with retort and pentagram, looking very like the usual pictures of Paracelsus. The Currus triumphalis antimonii (1604) led all practitioners to prescribe antimony at the start in fevers. The vogue died out, but the drug was revived in 1657, when its exhibition cured Louis XIV of typhoid fever. Pseudo-Valentine refers to syphilis as the neue Krankheit der Kriegsleut, recommending a mixture of antimony, lead, and mercury against it.

For Paracelsus was neither the refined, supersubtle mystic of Browning's poem, nor yet the roistering, lying, tippling blackguard and quack-salver of tradition. His influence was far-reaching, and his real services were great.

While philosophy, alchemy, and astronomy were the pillars of his faith, his watchword in practice was "experimentation controlled by the authoritative litera-ture."[1] That he read his authors to some purpose is suggested by his statement that the only true physicians among the ancients were the Greeks. His pathology was mixed, but contained such good elements as the concept of disease as a dis-harmony of normal functions (life under altered conditions), *e. g.*, hereditary (in goiter), or as diathetic, in gout and stone. These diathetic diseases, he regarded as "tartaric" processes, caused by the precipitation of substances ordinarily voided from the body, the first attempt at a chemical etiology, and part of his general doctrine of calcifications and concretions. His five causes of disease (*entia*) were cosmic agencies (*ens astrorum*); pathologic poisons (*ens venene*), including auto-intoxications and contagia; natural causes (*ens naturale*) or predisposition to disease from organic defects; psychic causes (*ens spirituale*) and divine intervention (*ens deale*). His pupil, Peter Severinus, developed the idea of contagia (*ens venenata*) as animate pathology (*pathologia animata*).

Far in advance of his time, Paracelsus discarded Galenism and the four humors, and taught physicians to substitute chemical therapeutics for alchemy; he attacked witchcraft and the strolling mountebanks who butchered the body in lieu of surgical procedure; he opposed the silly uromancy and starcraft; he was the first to write on diathetic (tartaric) and miners' (occupational) diseases, and the first to establish a cor-relation between cretinism and endemic goiter; he was ahead of his time in noting the geographic differences of disease. Almost the only asepsist between Mondeville and Lister, he taught the unity of medi-cine and surgery, and that nature (the "natural balsam") heals wounds, and not officious meddling. He introduced mineral baths, and was one of the first to analyze them; he made opium (laudanum[2]), mercury, lead, sulphur, iron, arsenic, copper sulphate, and potassium sulphate (called the "*specificum purgans Paracelsi*") a part of the pharmacopeia, and regarded zinc as an elementary substance; he distinguished alum from ferrous sulphate, and demonstrated the iron content of water by means of gallic acid; with Croll and Valerius Cordus, he popularized tinctures and alcoholic extracts. His "doctrine of signatures" was re-vived by Rademacher and Hahnemann. His "arcana" were directed against the causes of disease rather than the symptoms (causal therapy), and, in comparing the action of these arcana, or intrinsic principles of drugs, to a spark, he grasped the idea of catalytic action; although his belief that remedies are not substantive but act through an immanent spiritual power or "quintessence" (active principle) was the occasion of much mysticism. As a theorist, Paracelsus believed in the descent of living organisms from the primordial ooze (*Urschleim*), and Baas credits him with anticipating Darwin in his observation that the strong war down and prey upon the weak—a fact, unfortunately, within the

---

[1] Experimenta ac ratio auctorum loco mihi suffragantur. Cited by Sudhoff.

[2] "Ich hab ein Arcanum, heiss ich Laudanum, ist über das alles, wo es zum Tod reichen will," Grosse Wundarznei, i, Tr. 3, cited by Haeser.

range of any beggar or footman. His comparison of apoplexy with lightning stroke, and his concept of atrophy as a drying out of the tissues show his contempt for anatomy. But none of these things can outweigh the influence which Paracelsus exerted on his time through his personality. In an age when heresy often meant death, he wasted no time in breaking butterflies upon wheels, but drove full tilt at many a superstition, risking his neck with all the recklessness of a border reiver. The importance attached to his name may be gathered from the line in Shakespeare's comedy which brackets it with that of Galen.[1] Paracelsus was great in respect of his own time. He does not seem particularly great in relation to our time. As with most of the old authors, his writings have been overlaid with much spurious matter and can be correctly interpreted only in the light of modern research.

The most exhaustive study yet made of Paracelsus and his writings is that of Professor Karl Sudhoff (1894–9), who is now editing the definitive edition of his collective writings (Leipzig, 1922–27).

The principal works of Paracelsus are the treatise on open wounds (1528), his *Chirurgia magna* (1536), his manual introducing the use of mercurials in syphilis (Frankfurt, 1553), the treatise *De gradibus* (Basel, 1568), which contains most of his innovations in chemical therapeutics, his monograph on miners' diseases (*Von der Bergsucht*, Dilingen 1567), and his booklet on mineral baths (Basel, 1576), recommending Gastein (*"Castyn"*), Töpplitz, Göppingen, and Plombières (*"Blumbers"*). The treatise on miners' diseases, the result of his observations in Fugger's mines in Tyrol, containing descriptions of miners' phthisis and the effects of choke-damp, was one of the few original contributions of the time to clinical medicine. Paracelsus knew of paralysis and disturbance of speech after head injuries.[2] In his chapter, *De generatione stultorum*,[3] he first notes the coincidence of cretinism and endemic goiter, a discovery also based upon original observations in the Salzburg region.

In the huge output of the **syphilographers**—Leonicenus (1497), Lacumarcino (1524–31[4]), Fracastorius (1530), Niccolò Massa (1532), Fernelius (1538), Fallopius (1564), and Luisinus (1566) there was some good clinical delineation. Leoniceno described syphilitic hemiplegia (1497), Massa the neuralgic manifestations (1532), Botallo cerebral blindness (1536) and Ferro the joint lesions (1537). Gruner gives a remarkable list of 191 semeiological varieties of syphilis described in the period.[5] The most remarkable clinical contributions are the original descriptions of typhus fever by Fracastorius (1546), of sweating sickness by Caius (1552), of varicella by Ingrassias (1553), of *tabardillo* (Spanish or Mexican typhus) by Francesco Bravo (1570), of whooping-cough (*"quinta"*) by Guillaume Baillou or Ballonius (1578), of chlorosis (*morbus virgineus*) in the epistles of Johann Lange (1554) and of the syndrome "mountain sickness" by the Jesuit traveler José d'Acosta (1590). Geronimo **Mercuriali** (1530–1606) wrote the first systematic treatise on skin diseases (1572), a famous illustrated treatise on medical gymnastics (1573), and one of the earlier books on diseases of children (1583). The first treatise on feigned diseases (*De iis qui morborum simulant deprehensis*), by Giambattista Silvatico, was published at Milan in 1595. The pediatric treatise of Sebastianus Austrius (1540) deserves mention,

---

[1] In "All's Well That Ends Well," Act II, sc. 3, where Lafeu refers to the King's case as incurable, "to be relinquished of the artists," and Parolles replies: "So I say, both of Galen and Paracelsus"—meaning, of course, that neither the Galenical nor the alchemical school of physicians could help him in any way.

[2] E. Ebstein: Deutsche Ztschr. f. Nervenheilk., Leipz., 1914, liii, 131.

[3] In his posthumous "Opera Omnia." Strassburg, 1603, ii, 174–182.

[4] E. C. Streeter has shown that the date 1505 assigned by Astruc for Lacumarcino's *De morbo gallico*. the best treatise on syphilis of its time, must be changed to 1524 or later (Tr. Internat. Cong. Med., 1913, Lond., 1914, sect. xxiii, 373–376). The Turin edition in the Surgeon General's Library bears the date 1532.

[5] C. G. Gruner: Morborum antiquitates, Breslau, 1774, 85–100.

as also the work of **Prospero Alpino** on Egyptian medicine (1591), and his unique treatise on medical prognosis (1601). *The Regiment of Life* (1546), by Thomas Phayre (1510?–60), a black-letter version of the Regimen sanitatis, contains the first English contribution to pediatrics (*The Boke of Children*). The first printed book on dietetics was that of Platina (1499). Savonarola is credited with the first incunable on balneology (1489). The earliest book on dentistry was the *Artzney-Büchlein* (Leipzig, 1530), reprinted as the *Zene Artzney* (Mainz, 1532). Of this 11 editions (1532–76) are known (Weinberger).

Guillaume de **Baillou** (1538–1616), a Paris graduate of 1570, whom Henri IV chose as physician to the Dauphin, and who first described whooping-cough (1578) and introduced the term "rheumatism," is regarded by Crookshank as "the first epidemiologist of modern times."

His works, all published after his death, include sets of *Consilia* (1635–49), treatises on gynecology (1643), gout and calculus (1643) and two books on epidemics and ephemeral diseases, with case-histories and postmortems (1640), which revive the old Hippocratic doctrine of "epidemic constitutions," *i. e.*, the external influences at work in the causation and spread of epidemics, foreshadowing much that was afterward taught by Sydenham.

Charles Singer points out[1] that some beginnings of tropical medicine were made in Oviedo's description of yaws as "bubas," afterward identified by André Thevet, in 1558, as "no other thing than the pocks which rageth and hath power over all Europe, specially among the Frenchmen." Oviedo and Thevet also mention the sandflea (*Pulex penetrans*). Singer draws attention to the first book on tropical medicine, by George Wateson, entitled *The Cures of the Diseased in Remote Regions* (London, 1598), the scope of the work being indicated by the versified table of contents:

> "The burning fever, calde the Calenture,
> The aking Tabardilla pestilent,
> The Espintas prickings which men do endure,
> *Cameras de sangre*, Fluxes violent,
> Th' *Erizipila*, swelling the Pacient,
> Th' *Tiñoso*, which we the Scurvey call,
> Are truly here described and cured all."

For a long time after Paracelsus **chemistry** still remained alchemy and, in the following century, became merged into the fantastic pseudoscience of the Rosicrucians. The arch-patron of alchemy in the 16th century was the Emperor Rudolph II of Germany (1576–1612), who devoted much of his fortune and the whole of his reign to the quest of potable gold, the philosopher's stone, and the elixir of life. In the spacious and gloomy chambers of his palace, the Hradschin at Prague, he held high court with alchemists, spritualists, judicial astrologers, clairvoyants, and other followers of psychic "science," and no reward was considered too great for any adventurer, however disreputable, who might manage to wheedle this fantastic monarch "of dark corners." The credulous Rudolph was continually the prey of all sorts of impudent knaves and sharp practitioners, upon whom he speedily revenged himself by imprisonment or execution if they failed to perform their promises.[2] Hither came the learned Cambridge scholar, John Dee, a solemn humbug, and his assistant, Edward Kelley, a sharp-witted im-

---

[1] Singer: Ann. Trop. Med. and Parasitol., Liverpool, 1912, vi, 87–101.

[2] For a full account of all this, see Henry Carrington Bolton's delightful book, "The Follies of Science at the Court of Rudolph II," Milwaukee, 1904.

postor, to make "projections" of the baser metals into gold, and, by crystal gazing in a shew-stone (now in the British Museum), to indulge the kind of self-hypnotism familiar today as "automatic writing." Kelley acted as "skryer," or clairvoyant, in the maneuver and both were richly rewarded. Dee escaped to England in the nick of time. Kelley remained to become a landed proprietor and *eques auratus* of the Bohemian Kingdom, but subsequently lost his life as a punishment for his brawls and impostures. To "Gold Alley," the charlatan street of Prague, came also Michael Sendivogius, "Count" Marco Bragadino, Gossenhauer, and Cornelius Drebbel, the perpetual motion man; and it was for the sake of alchemy that Rudolph brought Tycho Brahe and Kepler together, to the material adavntage of future astronomy. The foregatherings of Rudolph's physicians, Crato von Kraftheim, Oswald Croll, Guarinonius, Michael Maier, and the rest, made up the Rudolphine Academy of Medicine, of which an extraordinary session was once convened to hear Andreas Libau (Libavius) read an essay on the *aurum potabile*. This **Libavius** (1546–1616), a physician and teacher of Coburg, made a real start in chemistry. His *Alchymia* (Frankfurt, 1595) was the first systematic treatise on the science. He had, says Bolton, "a sumptuous laboratory, provided not only with every requisite for chemical experimentation, but also with means of entertaining visiting guests, including such luxuries as baths, inclosed corridors for exercise in inclement weather, and a well-stocked wine-cellar." Libavius discovered stannic chlorid, analyzed mineral waters with the balance (1597), wrote a city pharmacopeia (1606), and was one of the first to suggest the transfusion of blood (1615). His *Alchymia* is in two parts, the first dealing with the laboratory operations of chemistry, including instruments and furnaces; the latter half containing accurate and systematic descriptions of chemical substances. Of this half, no fewer than 80 pages are devoted to the philosopher's stone.

A typical follower of Paracelsus was the adventurous alchemist and swindler, Leonhard Thurnheysser zum Thurn (1531–95), of Basel, who started out as a goldsmith's apprentice, married at sixteen, and was soon embarked in a "gold-brick" imposture (selling tin coated with gold), for which he had to flee the city and take up a roving life. He traveled far and wide, became inspector of mines in Tyrol in 1558 and, after healing the wife of the Elector of Brandenburg of a desperate illness, became his body physician in 1578. In Berlin, he made so much money by pawnbroking, usury, and the sale of calendars, horoscopes, and secret remedies, that he was able to set up a private laboratory and printing office, with type-foundry attached. A scandalous law-suit with his third wife reduced him to beggary, and he died obscurely in a cloister at Cologne. His writings, full of mystical humbuggery, are without value, although much has been made of his discovery that mineral waters yield a certain residue upon evaporation.

Many physicians of this period were also mathematicians and authors of some of the earliest practical arithmetics (algorisms), notably those of Joh. Widman (1488), G. Valla (1501), Arnoldo de Villa Nova (1501), J. Fernelius (1528), Gemma Frisius (1540), Robert Recorde (1542), and M. Neander (1555[1]). Of this group the most picturesque figure was Geronimo **Cardano** (1501–76), whose roving life was filled with strange adventures. A medical graduate of Padua, he practised medicine and professed mathematics at Milan and was professor of medicine suc-

---

[1] D. E. Smith: Rara Arithmetica, Boston, 1908, *passim*.

cessively at Pavia and Bologna. Cardan made his mark with his treatise on arithmetic (1539) and his algebra (*Ars magna*, 1545), which contains his famous solution of
cubic equations, most of which was, however, stolen from Tartaglia. Although
excluded from the College of Physicians at Milan by his illegitimate birth, he gained
some practice by his cure of the child of the Milanese senator Sfondrato, and as the
medical adviser of the asthmatic Archbishop Hamilton of St. Andrew's. But he
was only a medical astrologer and empiric. His best work is his natural history
(*De subtilitate rerum*, 1550), which shows remarkable insight into biologic phenomena,
and is evolutionary in its tendency. It contains a device for **teaching the blind**
to read and write by the sense of touch (*quomodo cœcus scribere doceri potest*), which
is not very different from the modern invention of Braille (1829–36[1]). Jerome Cardan
also saw the possibility of **teaching the deaf** by signs. His *Metoposcopia* (1658) is
illustrated with 800 cuts of human faces, an astrologic physiognomy, based upon the
idea that the furrows in the forehead were influenced by the seven celestial bodies
and that horoscopes might be drawn from such data.

The idea of instructing the deaf was again taken up by Pedro Ponce de Leon
(1520–84), a Benedictine monk of Sahagun, Spain, who was the first, in his own
words, to teach the deaf "to speak, read, write, reckon, pray, serve at the altar,
know Christian doctrine, and confess with a loud voice." His written work on
the subject is lost, but his system was preserved in the treatise of Juan Pablo Bonet
(1620).

That the phenomena of hypnotism, autosuggestion and psychotherapy were well known in the 16th century is apparent from the
writings of Pomponazzi, Cornelius Agrippa, Cardan, Van Helmont, and
Kircher.[2]

After the time of Mundinus, a number of treatises and plates appeared, containing the first rude attempts at pictorial representation of
dissected parts. These are the so-called **"graphic incunabula"** of
anatomy and may conveniently take in all published illustrations of
the pre-Vesalian period. They are:

1. The 33 editions of Mundinus, printed between 1478 and 1580, including
those in Ketham.

2. The *Fasciculus medicinæ* (Venice, 1491) of Johannes de Ketham (Johann
von Kirchheim), a series of writings on uroscopy, venesection, surgery, etc., was the
first medical book to be illustrated with wood-cuts. It passed through six later
(Venetian) editions, viz., 1493 (Italian translation), 1495, 1500, 1513, 1522, 1522
(Italian translation), all containing the anatomy of Mundinus at the end.

3. The skeleton of Richard Helain, printed at Nuremberg in 1493.

4. An illustration of the abdominal muscles in the 1496 edition of the *Conciliator
differentiarum* of Peter of Abano.

5. The *Philosophiæ naturalis compendium* or *Compendiosa capitis physici
declaratio* (Leipzig, 1499) of the Leipzig jurist Johannes Peyligk (1474–1592?). This
work rapidly passed through seven subsequent editions. viz., 1503, 1509, 1510, 1513,
1515, 1516, 1518 (Sudhoff[3]).

6. The *Antropologium* (Leipzig, 1501) of the Leipzig professor Magnus Hundt
(1449–1519) contains one of the crude MS. schemata of phrenology, already published by Albertus Magnus (*Philosophia Naturalis*, 1490), allocating common sense,
imagination, ratiocination and memory to the frontal lobes, midbrain, and cerebellum, or to the four corresponding ventricles.

7. Gregor Reisch's *Margarita philosophica* (1503, 1504), containing a view of
the thoracic and abdominal viscera and the oldest schematic representation of

---

[1] H. Schelenz: Arch. f. Gesch. d. Naturwissensch., Leipzig, 1910–12, iii, 237.
About 1517, large letters cut in wood had been used by Francisco Lucas in Spain
and Rampazetto in Italy.

[2] See the Paris dissertation of Camille Rouzeaud (1918, No. 4), who styles the
period "le siècle de l'hypnotisme."

[3] Sudhoff: Arch. f. Gesch. d. Med., Leipz., 1915–16, ix, 309–314, 1 pl.; 1916–17,
x, 251.

the eye, which Sudhoff has traced to a pen drawing in a Leipzig codex of the 15th century.

8. The fugitive anatomic plates (*Fliegende Blätter*) of Johann Schott of Mainz (1517), Christian Wechel of Paris (1536), Heinrich Vogtherr of Strassburg (1539), and others.

9. The *Spiegl der Artzny* of Lorenz Fries (1519).

10. Giacomo Berengario da Carpi's commentary on Mundinus (1521); and his *Isagogæ breves* (Bonn, 1514).

11. The *Anatomiæ pars prior* (Marburg, 1536) of Johann Eichmann or Dryander (died 1560).

It has been shown, in the highly exhaustive researches of Karl Sudhoff,[1] that none of these earlier anatomic illustrations were based upon original observation or dissection, but that, for the most part, they are purely traditional, servile copies from manuscript sketches of the past, with little superadded touches here and there. The 9th century Breslau Codex 3714 and a 12th century Copenhagen MS. give the traditional pictures of the fetus in utero, as handed down from Moschion. The wood-cuts in Ketham's *Fasciculus* represent a circle of 21 urine glasses which Sudhoff has traced to a manuscript of 1400; sick-room and dissecting scenes, with groups of Venetian gentry in the costumes of the period; and a remarkable series of characteristic semi-squatting figures, indicating the sites of injury or disease and the most favorable localities for applying treatment, viz., the "zodiac-man" (*Tierkreiszeichenmann*), in which schemata of the viscera are often overlaid by the zodiacal figures; the "blood-letting man" (*Aderlassmann*), whose body is tattooed with marks indicating the best sites for venesection under the signs of the zodiac; the "planetman" (*Planetenmann*) of Western Europe, in which the planets or their symbols are substituted for the signs of the zodiac; the "sick-man" (*Krankheitsmann*), ringed about with names of diseases and vague indications as to their location in the body; the "wound-man" (*Wundenmann*), whose body is mauled and pierced all over by stones, arrows, swords and spears, the points of incision or lesion showing where the arteries are to be sought for in ligation; and the crouching pregnant woman (*Gravida*), exposing a crude diagrammatic view of the fetus in utero. These strange didactic pictures have all been interpreted by Sudhoff as sidelights on the almost stationary character of the medieval mind, standing out as rude indices of its workings in relation to the three great branches of internal medicine, surgery, and obstetrics.[2] They have all been located by him to manuscripts of earlier centuries, for instance, the blood-

---

[1] Karl Sudhoff: Tradition und Naturbeobachtung in den Illustrationen medizinischer Handschriften und Frühdrucke, vornehmlich des 15. Jahrhunderts, Leipzig, 1907; Ein Beitrag zur Geschichte der Anatomie im Mittelalter, Leipzig, 1908, his highly original studies of the prehistory of Ketham in the MS. sources, the schematic eye, the visceral schemata and the *Fünfbilderserie* (Arch. f. Gesch. d. Med., Leipz., 1907–16, *passim*); also, Walter Sudhoff's dissertation, "Die Lehre von den Hirnventrikeln in textlicher und graphischer Tradition des Altertums und Mittelalters" (Leipzig, 1913). For a good account of pre-Vesalian illustration in English, with reproductions of most of the figures, see Prof. William A. Locy's interesting essay in Jour. Morphol., Chicago, 1911, xxii, 945–987.

[2] Sudhoff: Arch. f. Gesch. d. Med., Leipz., 1907–8, i, 219, 351; 1908–9, ii, 84.

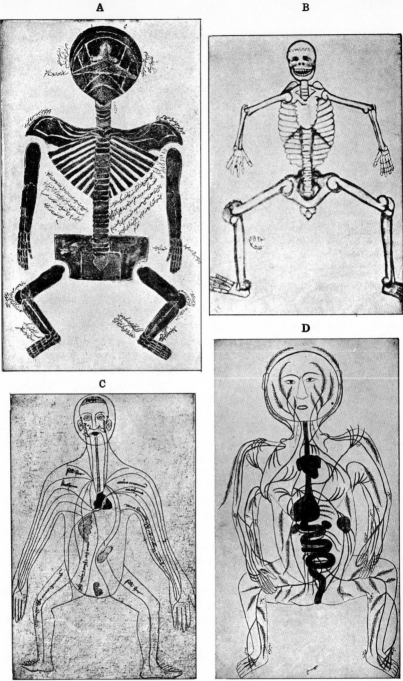

Drawings showing influence of tradition upon early anatomic illustration. (By kind permission of Professor Karl Sudhoff, University of Leipzig.) A: Skeleton from Persian MS. No. 2296, India Office, London. B: Skeleton in aquatint from Dresden MS. Codex 310 (A. D. 1323). C: Arterial system, from a fourteenth century MS. in the library of Prince von Lobkowicz (Raudnitz, Bohemia). D: Venous system, from Persian MS. No. 2296, India Office, London. Roth called attention to the traditional character of anatomic illustration in the pre-Vesalian period, but the development of the subject is almost entirely the work of Professor Sudhoff.

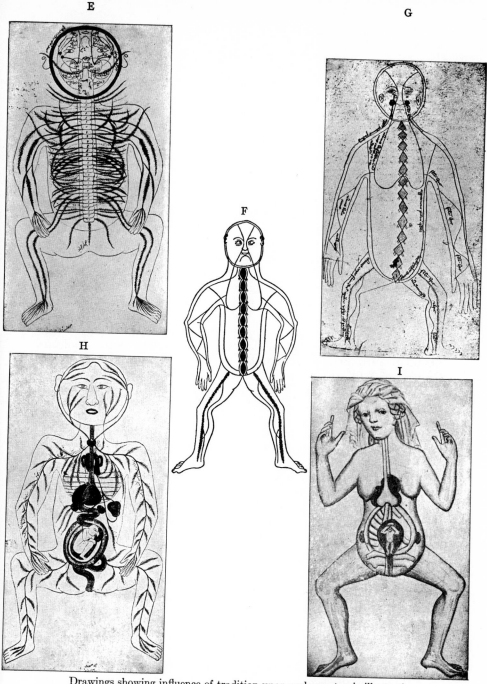

E

G

F

H

I

Drawings showing influence of tradition upon early anatomic illustration. (By kind permission of Professor Karl Sudhoff, University of Leipzig.) E: Nervous system, from Persian MS. No. 2296, India Office, London. F: Schema of the nervous system, from a MS. of 1152, discovered by Sir Victor Horsley in the Bodleian Library, Oxford. G: Nervous system, from a fourteenth century MS. in the library of Prince von Lobkowicz (Raudnitz, Bohemia). H: Arterial system of a pregnant woman, from Persian MS. No. 2296, India Office, London. I: Gravida, from a miniature painted about 1400 in Leipzig MS. Codex No. 1122. Compare G with the two centuries older F, and note the monotonous similarity in all these frog-like figures, which is common to Aztec, Thibetan, Persian, Provençal, and other anatomic MSS. of the time.

letting man of 1432 in the Munich library, or the figures in Persian MSS. of the Middle Ages. It was customary for the medieval illustrators to make a series of five schematic pictures (*Fünfbilderserie*), representing the osseous, nervous, muscular, venous, and arterial systems, to which the pregnant woman or a view of the generative organs of either sex was sometimes added. This series has been found by Sudhoff in German manuscripts from the cloisters at Prüfening (A. D. 1154) and Scheyern (1250), in a 13th century Provençal MS. at Basel, and even in Persian MSS. in the India office at London and the Bodleian Library at Oxford. The curious half-crouching posture, that of a reflex frog or a child's jumping-jack, is found even in the acupuncture manikins of ancient Chinese medicine (Hsieh). The medieval MS. drawings were plainly intended as crude mnemonic schemata, to refresh the memory of students, perhaps even for popular instruction. Some were purely diagrammatic, *e. g.*, the many MS. drawings of the schematic eye, described by Sudhoff,[1] the naïve gropings at localization of the functions of the brain[2]; the Arabic schema of crossing of the optic nerves from Constantinople,[3] which resembles an Oriental prayer-rug; or the 13th century schema of the uterus and adnexa in the Bodleian (Ashmore MS. 399), which has the same appearance.[4] In Ketham's Gravida of 1491, the parts of the body are labeled for the first time. This is also true of Richard Helain's skeleton of 1493, a good example of the fugitive anatomic plates which used to be exhibited in German barber-shops and bath-houses of the 15th and 16th centuries. This skeleton was copied by Grüninger in 1497, and by Johann Schott in 1517. As examples of pre-Berengarian anatomy, the cuts in Peyligk and Hundt look, in some of their details, like a child's scratching on a slate. Those in Peyligk have been traced by Sudhoff to a series of 18 manuscript figures in the Royal Libraries at Berlin and Erfurt, which were used by Henri de Mondeville to illustrate his anatomic lectures at Montpellier about 1304. The *Spiegl der Artzny* of Lorenz Fries has a much better executed engraving of the viscera (1517), attributed by Blumenbach to Johann Waechtlin, also to be found in Gersdorff's *Feldtbuch* (1517), and strikingly like the crude, earlier picture in Reisch's *Margarita philosophica* (1504). The marginal figurations of the brain and the tongue in Fries are excellent; five of the cross-sections of the brain were reproduced in Dryander's *Anatomia* (1536). Peter of Abano's *Conciliator* (1496) contains the first example of the "*Muskelmann*," *i. e.*, a full-length figure exhibiting its dissected muscles. In the works of Berengario da Carpi, who was the first to substitute drawing from nature for traditional schemata, this figure is represented as holding up the separate muscles for inspection. The same *motif* becomes the *écorché* or flayed figure in Vesalius. Berengario has a

[1] Sudhoff: Arch., f. Gesch. d. Med., Leipz., 1914–15, viii, 1–21, 2 pl.

[2] W. Sudhoff: *Ibid.*, 1913–14, vii, 149–205, 2 pl.

[3] See p. 122.

[4] Singer: Proc. Roy. Soc. Med. (Hist. Sect.), Lond., 1915, ix, 43–47, 2 pl.

tolerable skeleton, which is suspiciously like those of Helain, Grüninger, and Schott, and his picture of the pregnant woman in a reclining attitude, became afterward the theme of many variations by Stephanus and others, down to the time of Gautier d'Agoty's beautiful life-size panel in oils. These tentative efforts at representation, rare and curious as they are, pale almost into obscurity beside the cartoons, écorchés, and chalk drawings of the great artists of the period—Luca Signorelli, Michael Angelo, Raphael, Verocchio, and his pupil, Leonardo da Vinci. But, as shown by Streeter,[1] anatomy was advanced by the Florentine painters and aurifabers even before the time of Verocchio.

The temperamental 14th century Florentine was a "half-baked scientist." The early painters after Giotto aspired, like all *primitifs*, to realism and the representation of movement, to pass from the flat-land of the Italo-Byzantine mosaics into the tri-dimensional world of verisimilitude and motion. To this end, geometry, perspective, and the science of bodily proportion were arduously studied. The city itself was a "very paradise of little bank clerks," who wrote "solid works on mercantile arithmetic." All the great works on perspective and human proportion, except Dürer's, came from Florence. In realistic painting, Giotto's assistant and intimate, Stefano, called the *scimmia della natura*, became so successful that phlebotomists were said to stand before his canvases to study the branching of the veins. An interest in dissecting probably came about through the fact that the painters formed a sub-species of the Florentine "Guild of Physicians and Apothecaries," which Masaccio joined, first as an apothecary (1421), then as a painter (1423). At the apothecary-shop the painters bought their pigments and so came in closer contact with the physicians at the guild-functions. Thus dissecting, as to which the Florentine university statutes of 1387 give explicit directions, became a word of ambition with the artists, who soon got in the way of assisting at private dissections among their doctor friends, or of doing a little body-snatching on their own account. In Streeter's view, Leonardo, himself, is merely the end-result of this quest for uncompromising realism. Leonardo derives from Andrea del Castagno (1390–1457), through Domenico Veneziano, Alesso Baldonnetti (1427–99), and Andrea Verocchio (1435–88). Castagno, who dissected at Santa Maria Nuova, was called the Donatello of painting, on account of his skill in myologic detail and influenced Pollajuolo, who studied musculature by flaying the cadaver. "The Anatomy of the Miser's Heart," at Padua, by the sculptor Donatello, is a document in bronze of the interest taken in dissecting. Pollajuolo, Castagno, Mantegna, Leonardo, in a sneer of Ruskin's, "polluted their work with the science of the sepulchre." On the textual side, the continuum between Mundino and Leonardo is filled in part by the anatomists Gabriele **Zerbi** (1468–1505), of Verona, professor at Padua, who wrote an anatomic treatise (1502), first separated the organs into systems, was the first to treat of infantile anatomy and described the muscles of the stomach and the puncta lachrymalia; Alessandro **Benedetti** (1460–1525), his successor at Padua, founder of its anatomic theater (1490) and author of an *Anatomia* (1497); Alessandro **Achillini** (1463–1512), of Bologna, who discovered the malleus, incus, labyrinth, the ileocecal valve, and wrote an anatomy (1516); **Berengario da Carpi** (1470–1550); and Marc Antonio **della Torre** (1481–1512), professor at Padua and Pavia, who, according to Vasari, collaborated with Leonardo in a prospective anatomic treatise.

Leonardo da Vinci (1452–1519), the greatest artist and scientist of the Italian Renaissance, was the founder of iconographic and physiologic anatomy, although his chalk drawings (*circa* 1512) remained buried for over 200 years, when they were noted by William Hunter (1784) and Blumenbach (1788). During 1898–1916 all the known drawings of Leonardo have been handsomely and adequately reproduced, notably

---

[1] Streeter: Bull. Johns Hopkins Hosp., Balt., 1916, xxvii, 113–118.

those from the Royal Library at Windsor, the Ambrosian Library at Milan, and the Institut de France.[1]

Startlingly modern in their accuracy and display of physiologic knowledge, these impromptu sketches, made beside the dissected subject, reveal such acquaintance with muscular anatomy as was possible only to the Greek sculptors, and fully justify William Hunter's claim that their author was "the greatest anatomist of his epoch." Leonardo, like his forerunners, believed that a scientific knowledge of artistic anatomy—something quite different from the Greek sculptor's instinctive knowledge of the nude figure in action and repose—can be gained only at the dissecting table. Galenic anatomy he probably knew, possibly also Guy and Mundinus, but in his actual work he was his own best teacher. He made over 750 separate sketches, including not only delineations of muscles, but drawings of the heart, the lungs, the cervical, thoracic, abdominal and femoral blood-vessels, the bones and nerves, with deep dissections of the viscera and cross-sections of the brain in different planes, made long before those of Fries (1517). Remarkable are his studies of the bones, the skull, the spine, the valves, muscles and vessels of the heart, his discovery of the atrioventricular band in the right heart, his cross-sections of the brain and casts of its ventricles, his probable injections of the blood-vessels, his unique and accurate delineation of the statutory position of the fetus in utero, his studies of antagonistic muscles by tape models, his investigation of the hydrodynamics of the blood-current. Sometimes his notations of the origin and insertion of the muscles are too minute because, having no accurate nomenclature to guide him, he had to rely upon his own deductions from what he saw, which was, in any case, a great advance upon servile Galenism. He was the originator of cross-sectional an-

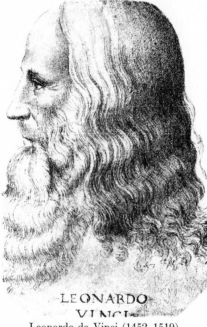

Leonardo da Vinci (1452–1519).

[1] I manoscritti di Leonardo da Vinci (ed. Sabachnikoff-Piumati), 2 v., Paris, Turin, 1898–1901. Quaderni d'anatomia (ed. Vangensten, Hopstock, and Fonahn), 6 v., Christiania, 1911–16. Notes et desseins, 12 v., Paris, E. Rouveyre, 1901. These have been closely studied by M. Holl (Arch. f. Anat., Leipz., 1913, 225; 1914, 37; 1915, 1), and A. C. Klebs (Bull. Med. Hist. Soc., Chicago, 1916, 66–83; Boston Med. and Surg. Jour., 1916, clxxv, 1, 45).

atomy. "With a few strokes of the pencil, he demonstrated morphological relations in a manner not approached before the time of Friedrich Merkel" (Sudhoff[1]). The marginal notes, which Leonardo has recorded in mirror-writing, perhaps lest others appropriate his ideas, suggest the cautious, secretive spirit of the time.[2]

Among the anatomic works of the pre-Vesalian period we should, of course, include Albrecht Dürer's treatise on human proportion (*De simmetria*, Nuremberg, 1532), which was the first application of anthropometry to esthetics, and is technically interesting as containing the first attempts to represent shades and shadows in wood-engraving by means of cross-hatching.

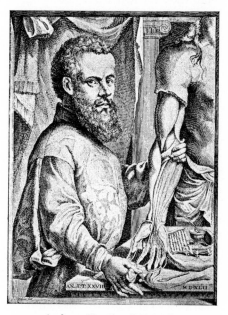

Andreas Vesalius (1514–64).

Thoroughly as the great artists of the Renaissance may have studied external anatomy, yet dissecting for teaching purposes was still hampered by the theologic idea of the sanctity of the human body and its resurrection. Moreover, as very little anatomic material could be obtained among a sparse and slowly growing population, people were naturally averse to the possible dissection of friends or relatives. The anatomy of the schools was still the anatomy of Galen. How far such teaching had progressed may be gathered from the quaint cut on the title-page of the Mellerstadt Mundinus (1493), in which the scholastic instructor, in long robe and biretta, wand in hand, gravely expounds Galen by the book from his pulpit-chair, while below the long-haired barber-servant[3] makes a desperate shift at demonstrating the viscera of the subject before him. The Faust who was to release the subject from these trammels and uphold the doctrine of the *visum et repertum* was Andreas **Vesalius**[4] (1514–64), the most commanding figure in European medicine after Galen and before Harvey. There were plenty

---

[1] Sudhoff: München. med. Wochenschr., 1919, lxvi, 1576.

[2] The possibility of right hemiplegia has also been suggested. That Leonardo's MS. may have been seen and studied by others is suggested by a copy of one of his drawings by Dürer and by the ambiguous skeletal figures in the Uffizi at Florence.

[3] It is possible that this may represent Alessandra Giliani, a talented girl of Persiceto, who assisted Mundinus in dissecting.

[4] Vesalius' family name was "Witing," later changed to "Wesel," where they once lived. Vesalius' coat of arms bore three weasels (*wesel*).

of dissectors and dissections before Vesalius, but he alone made anatomy what it is today—a living, working science. It was the effect
of his strong and engaging personality which made dissecting not only
viable, but respectable. His career is one of the most romantic in the
history of medicine. Flemish born, but of German extraction, a pupil
of that ardent and bigoted Galenist, Jacobus Sylvius, Vesalius in his
graduating thesis showed at first the conventional tendencies of the
scholiast; but his mind was too active, his spirit too keen and independent to feed long upon the dust of ages, and he soon established a
reputation for first-hand knowledge of the dissected human body, even
teaching himself the difficult art, so essential to surgeon and gynecologist, of recognizing the palpable structures by an educated sense of
touch. Five years' experience as public prosector at Padua, where he
taught students to dissect and inspect the parts *in situ,* culminated in
the magnificent *De Fabrica Humani Corporis* (1543), a work which
marks an epoch in breaking with the past and throwing overboard
Galenical tradition. The effect of a publication so radical on a superstitious and forelock-pulling age was immediate and self-evident.
Sylvius, his old teacher, turned against his brilliant pupil with acrimony
and coarse abuse, while his own pupil, Columbus, a man of questionable
honesty, sought to cast discredit and derision on him by sharp practice.
Others were inclined to "damn with faint praise," or joined in a con-
spiracy of silence and, as a last straw, he was subjected to subterranean
persecution at the instance of authority. Those things were not without their effect on Vesalius. His portrait suggests a doughty, swarthy,
shaggy, full-blooded nature, like some of Lucas Cranach's worthies—a
man ready to give no odds and take none, so long as his opponents
confronted him in the open; but nowise intended for the spiritual rôle
of a martyr. In a fit of indignation he burned his manuscripts, left
Padua, and accepted the lucrative post of court physician to Emperor
Charles V. He married, settled down, became a courtier, and gave up
anatomy so completely that, during the long, tedious years in Madrid,
"he could not get hold of so much as a dried skull, let alone the chance
of making a dissection." He paid the penalty of "the great refusal"
when his favorite pupil, Gabriele Falloppio, came to the front as a
worthy successor, and rumor began to make it clear that he himself
was fast becoming the shadow of a great name—

> Vesalius, who's Vesalius? This Fallopius
> It is who dragged the Galen-idol down.

On receiving the Fallopian *Observationes anatomicæ* in 1561, all the
aspirations of his youth revived, if we may trust his own burning,
enthusiastic words, language which fully justifies the implications of
Edith Wharton's poem:

> At least
> I repossess my past, am once again
> No courtier med'cining the whims of kings
> In muffled palace-chambers, but the free
> Friendless Vesalius, with his back against the wall,
> And all the world against him.

In the year 1563, Vesalius set out on a pilgrimage to Jerusalem, as a penance, some say, for an accidental human vivisection; more probably, the botanist Clusius thought, as a pretext for getting away from his tiresome surroundings. On his way back, in 1564, he received word of an invitation to resume his old chair at Padua, just vacated by the death of Fallopius. But his highest wish to "once more be able to study that true Bible, as we count it, of the human body and of the nature of man," was not to be realized. The sudden access of an obscure malady left Vesalius to die, solitary and unfriended, on the island of Zante.

The principal works of Vesalius include six anatomic plates (*Tabulæ anatomicæ*), printed at Venice in 1538, and reprinted in facsimile by Sir William Sterling Maxwell in 1874; the *Epitome* (Basel, 1540); an atlas compendium of the *Fabrica*, remarkable for the plates representing two handsome specimens of the human race, usually ascribed to Titian[1]; the epistle on the China root (1542[2]), which contains much acute criticism of Galen, and is especially valuable for the light it throws upon the life of Vesalius; finally the *Fabrica* itself, published in June, 1543, a superb example of the beautiful typography of his friend Oporinus (Herbst) of Basel. The *Fabrica* was sumptuously illustrated by Titian's pupil, Jan Kalkar, who was the first to attain what Choulant calls the true anatomic norm, that is, a picture at once scientifically exact and artistically beautiful, summing up, as in a composite photograph, the innumerable peculiarities and minor variations in structures encountered in dissection. The splendid wood-cuts representing majestic skeletons and flayed figures, dwarfing a background of landscape, set the fashion for over a century, and were copied or imitated by a long line of anatomic illustrators, such as Walther Ryff, Geminus, Tortebat,[3] Valverde di Hamusco, Dulaurens, Casserius, and Bidloo. In the second Basel edition of 1552–5, the beautiful typography of Oporinus appears in enlarged font, the faulty pagination and index of 1543 are corrected and improved, the text is revised and more scientific. Of the two editions, the second is, therefore, much the better worth having.

While written in Latin, the *Fabrica* is truly vernacular in the sweeping scorn and violence of its language in dealing with Galenical and other superstitions. Although it completely disposes of Galen's osteology and muscular anatomy for all time and, indeed, recreates the whole gross anatomy of the human body, it has never been translated. The dubious relations of the azygos vein, the rete mirabile of quadrupeds, the canine scalenus and simian rectus abdominis, the four- and five-lobed liver, the seven-segmented sternum, the double bile-duct, the horned uterus, the interventricular pores, the hypothetic sutures in the maxillaries, all these Galenic errors are roughly swept aside, along with the bone Luz, Adam's missing rib, the os cordis cervi as a remedy for heart disease, and other current superstitions. The edition of 1552–5 closes with a chapter on vivisection in which Vesalius verifies Galen's experimental sections of the spinal cord and recurrent laryngeal nerve, confirms his findings on the general functions of muscle and nerve, shows that artificial respiration will keep an animal alive after its chest has been opened, and that a quiescent heart may be resuscitated by the use of the bellows. In his chapter on the brain he appears, in theory at least, as a pioneer of experimental and comparative

[1] Titian's portrait of Vesalius is in the Pitti Palace at Florence.

[2] Translated into Dutch in Opusc. select. Neerlandica, Amst., 1915, iii.

[3] Tortebat was a pseudonym of Roger de Piles (Choulant).

psychology, rejecting the current view that the cerebration of brutes differs from that of man. He was also a pioneer in ethnic craniology, noting the globular shape of the skull in the Genoese, the Greeks, and the Turks, the flattened occiput and broad head (brachycephaly) in the "Germans" of his time, and the oblong skull of the Belgians.

He made many postmortems, noting the senile changes in the joints, the prolapse of the omentum in scrotal hernia, the rôle of the fossa navicularis urethræ in infection, the relations of splenic to hepatic disease, and the bad effects of corsets upon the viscera. As a clinician, he was the first to diagnose and describe aneurysm of the abdominal and thoracic aorta (1555[1]). In 1562 he performed a successful operation for empyema upon Don Carlos of Aragon, and was successful in two other cases of this procedure, as also in excisions of the cancerous breast.

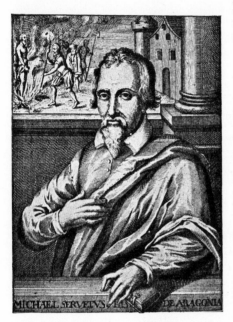

Michael Servetus (1509–53).

However scornful and truculent in his general onslaught against superstition, Vesalius displays the airy skepticism of a man of the world in dealing with these teleologic points so dear to medieval theologians. For instance, touching the Galenical crux that the blood passes through certain hypothetic pores in the ventricular septum, he says, "We are driven to wonder at the handiwork of the Almighty, by means of which the blood sweats from the right into the left ventricle through passages which escape the human vision."

What fate might have befallen him had he gone further is sensed in the case of the heretic Miguel Servede or **Servetus** (1509–53), whom Calvin caused to be burned at the stake for a mere juggling of verbiage, a theologic quibble. Servetus was one of the world's martyrs for "the crime of honest thought." His discovery that the blood in the pulmonary circulation passes into the heart, after having been mixed with air in the lungs is recorded in his book, the *Restitutio Christianismi* (1553), of which only copies at Paris and Vienna are known to exist. The rest were burned with him. A rare Nuremberg reprint was published in 1790.

The surpassing ability of Vesalius is seen not only in his establishment of anatomic norms for the description and figuration of the bones

---

[1] G. H. Velschius, Sylloge, Augsburg, 1667, pt. 4 (Rumber), pp. 46, 47, and Roth's Vesalius, p. 239. For another Consilium of Vesalius, see I. Schwarz: Sudhoff's Arch., Leipz., 1909–10, iii, 403–407.

and muscles, in his thorough descriptions of such parts as the eye, the ear, the accessory sinuses of the nose, the pituitary body,[1] or the pelvic cavity, but in his clean sweep of the whole subject. His ideas, sustained by his pupil Fallopius, were opposed not only by Sylvius and Columbus, but by an anatomist of equal rank with himself, Bartolommeo Eustachi (1524–74). **Eustachius** was professor at the Collegia della Sapienza in Rome, where, in 1552, he completed his *Tabulæ anatomicæ* (a set of superb plates drawn by himself) which remained unprinted in the Papal Library for 162 years. Finally, Pope Clement XI presented the engraved plates to his physician Lancisi, who, by the advice of

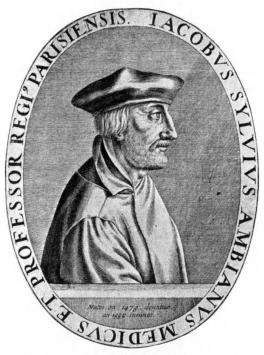

Jacques Dubois (Sylvius) (1478–1555).

Morgagni, published them with his own notes in 1714. They were the first anatomic plates on copper. The execution of these plates is dry and hard, but they are more accurate in delineation than those of Vesalius. Eustachius discovered the Eustachian tube, the thoracic duct, the suprarenal bodies[2] (1563), and the abducens nerve; described the origin of the optic nerves, the cochlea, the pulmonary veins, the muscles of the throat and neck, gave the first correct picture of the

---

[1] Vesalius called it the *glandula pituitam cerebri excipiens*, and thought it secreted the mucous discharges of the nose (Fabrica, lib. vii, cap. xi).

[2] *Glandulæ renibus incumbentes*, called *capsulæ renales* by Spigelius (1627) and *capsulæ suprarenales* by Riolanus (1628).

uterus, and wrote the best treatise of his time on the structure of the teeth (1563[1]), giving the nerve- and blood-supply. Although Eustachius declined to oppose Galenism, he was a natural genius in discovery.

Jacques Dubois (1478–1555), called **Sylvius,** Vesalius' teacher at Paris, was, in spite of his large following of pupils, a harsh, avaricious bigot, whose devotion to Galen was such that he declared Vesalius to be a madman (*vesanus*), and said, in reference to Galen's errors in human anatomy, that "Man had changed, but not for the better." Sylvius named the jugular, subclavian, renal, popliteal, and other blood-vessels, gave equally characteristic names to many of the muscles, which we still retain today and, in his *Isagoge* (Venice, 1556), was one of the first to mention the Sylvian aqueduct[2] and the valves in the veins.

The other opponent of Vesalius, Matteo Realdo Colombo (1516?–59), called **Columbus,** is sometimes spoken of as the discoverer of the pulmonary circulation, but the work in which his undoubtedly excellent account is contained (his *De re anatomica*) was published in 1559, at least six years after the burning of Servetus and his book, and there is some internal evidence indicating that Còlumbus may have plagiarized his facts from Servetus, as he certainly did in the case of Vesalius and Ingrassias (discovery of the stapes in the ear). Columbus begins his work with a title-page engraving, imitated from the frontispiece of the Fabrica, and, like Vesalius, winds up with a chapter on vivisection.[3] In prosecuting vivisection, he had the cleverness to substitute dogs for hogs, but while he professed a horror for human vivisections, he seems correspondingly callous in reference to the sufferings of the canine creatures which, as he constantly reminds us, he cut up in such numbers for the amusement of this or that exalted personage. Columbus showed by vivisection that the pulmonary veins contain blood, and while he held to the ancient theory of the cooling effect of respiration on the blood, he believed that, in the lungs, it is rendered "spirituous" by inmixture with air.

About 1541–2 Giambattista **Canano** (1515–79), of Ferrara, published some 26 copper-plates of the bones and muscles of the arm and fore-arm, from drawings by Girolamo da Carpi which, in realism and exactitude, surpassed anything between Leonardo and Vesalius; but having seen the unpublished wood-cuts of the *Fabrica*, the high-minded Ferrarese deliberately suppressed his own book, and only 11 copies are now extant (Klebs). This wonderful book has since been edited in facsimile reprint by Cushing and Streeter (Florence, 1925).

[1] Eustachius: Libellus de dentibus, Venice, 1563.

[2] The aqueduct between the third and fourth ventricles of the brain, attributed by various writers indifferently to Jacobus and Franciscus Sylvius, was described and figured by other anatomists long before the time of either. See F. Baker: Johns Hopkins Hosp. Bull., Balt., 1909, vol. xx, 329–339.

[3] For a translation of this chapter, see L. C. Boislinière: St. Louis Med. Rev., 1906, liv, 357–362.

Gabriele Falloppio (1523–62), or **Fallopius,** a loyal pupil of Vesalius, discovered and described the chorda tympani, the semicircular canals, the sphenoid sinus, the ovaries (Fallopian tubes), the round ligaments, the trigeminal, auditory, and glossopharyngeal nerves, and named the vagina and placenta. He was also a versatile writer on surgery, syphilis, mineral waters, and other subjects. Like Berengarius and Vesalius, he was falsely accused of vivisecting human beings in his ardors of research.[1] His pupil, Hieronymus **Fabricius ab Aquapendente** (1537–1619), was Harvey's teacher at Padua, and built at his own expense the fine anatomic theater in which Morgagni afterward worked. His studies of

the effect of ligatures and the valves in the veins (first noted by Erasistratus, Estienne, and Canano) influenced Harvey in his experiments to demonstrate the circulation of the blood. He wrote many important treatises on anatomy, embryology (*De formatu fœtu*, 1600), muscular mechanics (1618), and a surgical Pentateuch (1592). The names of the anatomists Costanzo Varolio (1543–75), or **Varolius,** physician to Pope Gregory XIII, Giulio Cesare Aranzio (1530–89), professor at Bologna, and Guido Guidi (died 1569), called **Vidius,** the organizer of the medical faculty of the Collège de France, have been eponymically preserved in the structures they discovered. Varolius, in particular, made some capital in-

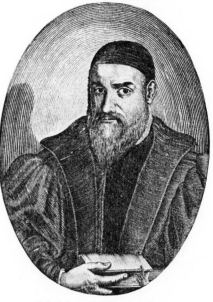

Gabriele Falloppio (1523–62).

vestigations of the nervous system, describing the crura cerebri, the commissure, and the pons. Volcher **Coiter** (1534–1600), of Groningen, a pupil of Fallopius, Eustachius, and Aldrovandi, investigated the formation and growth of bones (1566), the comparative osteology of animals (1575) and of children (1659), described the muscles of the nose and the eyelids, and experimented on decapitated (*decerebrated*) animals with remarkable intelligence.

Two striking landmarks of anatomic illustration came from France

---

[1] Berengarius himself explains (Commentaria, 1521, fol. 2 b) that what he calls *"anatomia in vivis"* was, in reality, the so-called *anatomia fortuita, i. e.,* the anatomic knowledge naturally gained by the surgeon in opening the body anywhere, the equivalent of Naunyn's "autopsies *in vivo.*" The prejudice of the ignorant and vulgar was excited by the superstitious horror of surgery, the cries of the patient, etc. See Choulant, Geschichte der anatomischen Abbildung, Leipzig, 1852, 28.

and Spain, viz., the folios of Stephanus (Paris, 1545[1]) and Juan Valverde de Hamusco (Rome, 1556[2]). Charles Estienne (-1564), or **Stephanus,** a pupil of Sylvius at Paris, and a prominent publisher of medical books during the Renaissance, was persecuted and imprisoned for heresy and died in prison. Estienne was the first to mention the valves of the veins as *apophyses membranarum.* His treatise also contains the first description of syringomyelia (1545[3]).

The anatomy of Thomas Vicary, published in 1577 and reprinted by Furnivall for the Early English Text Society in 1888, has been proved by the late Dr. J. F. Payne to be a transcript of a 14th century manuscript based upon the anatomy of Lanfranc, Guy, and Mondeville, and ist herefore valueless with reference to the Vesalian tradition. The book has a certain bibliographic interest of a' romantic character in that an edition, published in 1548, was once seen or heard of by somebody, but has never since been found.[4]

Through the work of Leonardo and Vesalius anatomy became the starting point of modern medicine. Osler saw the *Fabrica* as "The greatest book ever written, from which modern medicine dates." Physiology was no longer to be a teleological science, explaining hypothetical functions assumed *à priori,* but became, in Haller's phrase, "animated anatomy" (*anatomia animata*). When opening the body became commonplace, the closer study of pathological appearances became a necessity: a disease was now envisaged anatomically. The same *"anatomischer Gedanke"* is apparent in the development of histology, of cellular pathology, and of surgery as "anatomical therapy" (Sigerist).

The effect of Vesalius on **Renaissance surgery** is apparent in the life work of **Ambroïse Paré** (1510–90), who made the *Fabrica* popular and accessible to surgeons by writing an epitome of it in the vernacular. A rustic barber's apprentice when he came up from the provinces to Paris (1529) and afterward a dresser at the Hôtel Dieu, Paré became an army surgeon in 1537, and was incontinently thrown into the wars, where he soon made himself the greatest surgeon of his time by his courage, ability, and common sense. Snubbed by the College of St. Côme, and ridiculed as an upstart because he wrote in his native tongue, he made his way to the front on the field of battle. Like Vesalius and Paracelsus he did not hesitate to thrust aside ignorance or superstition if it stood in his way. Yet this greatest of army surgeons was so well beloved by his comrades that, one night when he slipped into Metz incognito, he was sought out and carried through the city by them in triumph. Brantôme and Sully record that he was

---

[1] Stephanus: De dissectione, Paris, 1545. As some of the plates in this work were signed as early as 1530–32, and are not unlike certain plates of Vesalius, the usual charge of plagiarism was revamped against Vesal, but this would seem to be sufficiently disproved by the appearance of Vesalius' six Venetian plates in 1538, seven years before Estienne's *De dissectione* was published (1545).

[2] Juan de Valverde de Hamusco: Historia de la composicion del cuerpo humano, Roma, 1556.

[3] Stephanus: De dissectione, 1545, iii, ch. 35.

[4] See Payne: Brit. Med. Jour., Lond., 1896, i, 200–203.

the only "Protestant" to be spared (by royal mandate) at St. Bartholomew.   In personality Paré stands between his surgical peers—the rude, outspoken Hunter and the refined, self-possessed Lister—as a man equally at home in the rigors of camp life or the slippery footing of courts.

Paré's greatest contribution to surgery hinges on the baneful effect of the pseudo-Hippocratic doctrine, that "diseases not curable by iron are curable by fire," upon the treatment of gunshot wounds, the new feature of Renaissance surgery.   Giovanni di Vigo (1460–1520), physician to Pope Julius II, had taught in his *Practica* (1514), like Brunschwig before him, that such wounds were poisoned burns and, therefore, should be treated with a first dressing of boiling oil.   How Paré's supply of boiling oil gave out one night in camp, and how he profited by

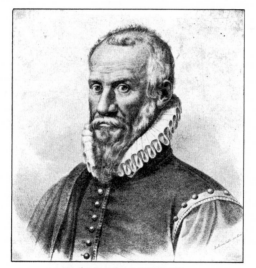

Ambroïse Paré (1510–90).

the experience to the extent of letting well enough alone in the future, is a well-known story.   Had it not been for his "fat of puppy-dogs," a lard or salve which, from some tenacity of superstition, he continued to apply, he would have been a true follower of Hugh, Theodoric, and Mondeville in the aseptic management of wounds.   As it is, his faith in the healing power of nature is summed up in the famous inscription on his statue, "*Je le pansay, Dieu le guarit.*"

Paré invented many new surgical instruments, made amputation what it is today by reintroducing the ligature, which had almost fallen into abeyance since the time of Celsus; was the first to popularize the use of the truss in hernia; did away with the strolling surgeons' trick of castrating the patient in herniotomy; introduced massage, artificial limbs, artificial eyes (of gold and silver), and staphyloplasty, and made the first exarticulation of the elbow-joint (1536).   He described fracture of the neck of the femur and strangury from hypertrophy of the prostate, and was the first to suggest syphilis as a cause of aneurysm.   As Howard A. Kelly

15

has pointed out,[1] he was probably also the first to see flies as transmitters of infectious disease. He described monoxide poisoning (1575). In obstetrics, he made podalic version viable and practicable, and had the courage to induce artificial labor in case of uterine hemorrhage. In dentistry, he introduced reimplantation of the teeth, and his little treatise on medical jurisprudence (1575) was the first work of consequence on the subject prior to the *Methodus testificandi* of Codronchi (1597).

Paré is a garrulous, gossipy, sometimes obscure writer and, like other medical celebrities of his day, by no means free from the "vanity of self-reference which accompanies great and even small reputations."[2] His many references to the ancients lead us to suppose that, like Bartisch, he employed a secretary or *pion* to embellish his writings for him, since it is most unlikely that he acquired his learning by actual study. His principal works are his treatise on gunshot wounds (1545[3]), his essay on podalic version (1550[4]), his great treatise on surgery (1564), and his discourse on the mummy and the unicorn (1582[5]), which successfully disposed of an ancient therapeutic superstition. A curious book is his treatise on monsters, terrestrial and marine (1573), embellished with pictures of many of the strange, hypothetic creatures which emanated from the brain of Aristotle.

The *Practica Copiosa* of Vigo (1514) had a success out of all proportion to its value, running through some 52 editions and innumerable translations, because it was almost the only book before Paré's time which dealt with the two great problems of Renaissance surgery—epidemic syphilis and wounds from firearms. Paré's campaign for a soothing treatment of gunshot wounds was very ably seconded by Bartolommeo Maggi (1516–52) of Bologna who, in 1551, demonstrated experimentally that such wounds could be neither burned nor poisoned. Another book which advanced this view was *An Excellent Treatise of Wounds made by Gonneshot* (London, 1563), by the English surgeon, Thomas Gale (1507–86?). The anatomist, Giacomo Berengario da Carpi, was another pioneer in the simple treatment of gunshot wounds. He describes two cases of excision of the uterus for prolapse: one performed by himself (1517), the other by his father and nephew.[6]

Two other Italian surgeons well deserving of mention are Mariano Santo de Barletta (1490–1550), a Neapolitan, who gave the original account of the "Marian operation" or median lithotomy (1535[7]); and Gasparo **Tagliacozzi** (1546–99), of Bologna, who in 1597[8] revived the operation of rhinoplasty which, during the 15th century, had been in the hands of a Sicilian family of plastic surgeons—the Brancas of Catania. For this innovation, Tagliacozzi was roundly abused by both Paré and Fallopius, and satirized during the following century in Butler's "Hudibras," while the ecclesiastics of his own time, we are told, were fain to regard such operations as meddling with the handiwork of God. Taglia-

---

[1] H. A. Kelly: Johns Hopkins Hosp. Bull., Balt., 1901, xii, 240–242.

[2] Rodomontades, as they were called, were the fashion of the period, and Brantôme wrote a whole book on the subject.

[3] Paré: La manière de traicter les playes (etc.), Paris, 1545.

[4] Paré: Briefve collection de l'administration anatomique (etc.), Paris, 1550.

[5] Paré: Discours, a savoir, de la mumie (etc.), Paris, 1582.

[6] Carpi: Commentaria, Bologna, 1521, f. ccxxv.

[7] Marianus Sanctus Barolitanus: De lapide renum, Venice, 1535.

[8] Tagliacozzi: De curtorum chirurgia per insitionem, Venice, 1597.

cozzi's remains were exhumed from the convent, where they reposed, to be buried in unconsecrated ground. In 1788 the Paris Faculty interdicted face-repairing altogether. In this way, plastic surgery fell into disrepute and disuse until the time of Dieffenbach. Like the Brancas were such itinerants· as the Norsini, who were skilful in hernia and lithotomy, and the Colots who cut for stone only. Out of this class was evolved the great Provençal surgeon **Pierre Franco** (*circa* 1500), a Huguenot, driven by the Waldensian · massacres into Switzerland, who did even more than Paré to put the operations for hernia, stone, and cataract upon a definite and dignified basis (1556–61[1]), and was the first to perform suprapubic cystotomy (1556). Another remarkable herniotomist and cataract-coucher, long forgotten, was Caspar **Stromayr** of Lindau, whose fascinating *Practica Copiosa* (1559), recently printed from the original MS. by Walter von Brunn (Berlin, 1925), is replete with wonderful full-page colored drawings, which afford the most complete and informing purview we have of surgical procedure in the 16th century. Felix **Würtz** (1518–75) was a follower of Paracelsus in the simple treatment of wounds, and a vigorous opponent of the common custom of thrusting "clouts and rags, balsam, oil, or salve" into them. His *Practica der Wundartzney* (Basel, 1563) was, like the *Traité des hernies* of Franco (Lyons, 1561), written in the vernacular, and was the fresh, straightforward work of a genuine child of nature. The almost forgotten Francisco **Diaz**, who was body physician to Philip II and whose surgical skill was praised in sonnets of Cervantes and Lope de Vega, published the first treatise on diseases of the kidney, bladder, and urethra (1588), and is, in effect, the founder of urology (Lejeune).

William **Clowes** (1540–1604) was probably the greatest of the English surgeons during the reign of Elizabeth. Experienced both in military and in naval medicine, he became consulting surgeon at St. Bartholomew's Hospital (1581), served as fleet surgeon against the Armada (1588), and was afterward made physician to the Queen. His works include a treatise on gunshot wounds (London, 1591[2]), and are pronounced by Norman Moore to be "the very best surgical writings of the Elizabethan age." As a satirist of the seamy side of medicine in his period, Clowes compares with Gideon Harvey and Butler in the 17th century or Smollett in the 18th.

The Scotch army surgeon, Peter **Lowe,** founded the Faculty of Physicians and Surgeons of Glasgow (1599), and made the first English translation of Hippocrates (1597). His *Whole Course of Chirurgerie* (1597) passed through four editions, and contains the first reference in English to ligation of the arteries in amputation. There were a number of Spanish surgeons in the 16th century, such as Francisco Arceo

---

[1] Pierre Franco: Petit traité (Lyons, 1556) and Traité des hernies, Lyons, 1561. Edited by E. Nicaise (Paris, 1895).

[2] Clowes: A proved practise for all young chirurgians concerning burnings with gunpowder and wounds made with gunshot (etc.), London, 1591.

(1493–1571) who followed Vigo in the treatment of wounds, or Dionisio Daça Chacon (1510–   ) who opposed him, but their works are only of bibliographic interest.

In the year 1500 Jacob Nufer, a sow-gelder, performed a successful Cesarean section upon his own wife—she lived to be 77 and bore other children—and this start in operative **gynecology** was succeeded by other Cesarean operations—those of Bain (1540), Dirlewang (1549), and so on, until we find François **Rousset** listing as many as 15 successful cases in his *L' Hysterotomotokie* (1580). Another sow-gelder performed double ovariotomy upon his own daughter, according to Johann Weyer (1515–88) the great Dutch opponent of the persecution of witches, who was himself an able physician and a surgeon enterprising enough to treat amenorrhea from imperforate hymen by incision of the membrane.

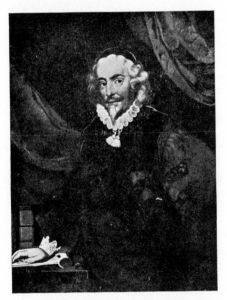

Peter Lowe (*circa* 1550–1612).

The growth of interest in diseases of women during the Renaissance period is seen in the huge *Gynæcia*, or encyclopedia of gynecology, issued by Caspar Wolf (1532–1601), of Zürich, in 1566, which was later enlarged by Caspar Bauhin (1550–1624), of Basel, in 1586. These two compilations of the best that had been written upon the subject were afterward reprinted in one volume by Israel Spach, of Strassburg, in 1597. Encyclopedic treatises on medicine by many authors, not unlike the "up-to-date" works written on the coöperative plan in our own time, were a special feature of Renaissance medicine, notably the Aldine *Medici Antiqui Omnes* (1547), the *Medicæ Artis Principes* of Stephanus (1567), the Venetian anthology of mineral waters, *De Balneis* (1553), the Gesner collection of surgical treatises (Zürich, 1555[1]), and the **medical dictionaries** of Symphorien Champier (1506), Lorenz Fries (1519), Henri Estienne, or Stephanus (1564), and Jean de Gorris or Gorræus (1564). With these may be classed the concordance of expressions from Erotian by Eustachius (1566), the *Variæ Lectiones* (1571) of Geronimo Mercuriali and the *Œconomia Hippocratis* of Anutius Fœsius (1588).

The eager, inquiring spirit of Renaissance humanity, greedy as a growing child for new knowledge, is sensed in the immense popularity of such a work as the *Hortus Sanitatis* (1491), with its quaint, colored wood-cuts of real or fanciful animals and plants. This picture book was so much sought after, in fact, that it was soon followed by a number of genuinely scientific treatises on botany and by extensive "Bestiaries," or animal-books, which described and figured the actual and

---

[1] De chirurgia scriptores optimi quique veteres et recentiores, 1555.

mythologic creatures which did or did not exist from the times of Aristotle and Pliny down.

Of the latter class, we may mention Ambroïse Paré's illustrated treatise on monsters (1573); the *Historia animalium* (Zürich, 1551–87) of Conrad Gesner (1516–65) and the many publications of Ulisse Aldrovandi (1522–1605) of Bologna. These rude beginnings of zoölogy, as Allbutt says, "mostly after Pliny's kind," were far inferior to the works of the **German Fathers .of Botany.**   The earliest of these, Otho **Brunfels** (1464–1534), of Mainz, originally a Carthusian novice, went over to Luther, graduated in medicine at Basel at the age of sixty-five, and was appointed city physician at Berne in 1533.   His *Herbarum Vivœ Icones* (Strassburg, 1530–36), which marks an epoch in the history of botanic illustration, consists of 135 careful figurations of plants executed by Hans Weydiz, the best wood-engraver of Strassburg in his day.   A German translation or "Counterfeit Herbal" followed (1532-37[1]).   Brunfels prepared the work at his own expense, to offset the wretched engravings of the Hortus Sanitatis.   In his text, he makes no attempt at original plant description, but simply follows Theophrastus, Dioscorides, Pliny and the other authorities up to his time.   His *Onomastikon* (1543) is a dictionary of simples. He was one of the first to publish a bibliographic list of eminent physicians and their writings (1530).   Next in order comes the Bavarian physician, Leonhard **Fuchs** (1501–66), who graduated at Ingolstadt (1524), and after many vicissitudes (he was also an adherent of Luther) held the chair of medicine at Tübingen for thirty-one years (1535–66), where he occupied his leisure in having artists figure plants which he afterward described.   His *De Historia Stirpium* (Basel, 1542), contains over 500 plates, superior to those in Brunfels' book, which had inspired it. It excited such an interest that it was followed, in 1544, by a new edition and, after 1545, by many small-sized popular reprints.   In purpose, it was entirely utilitarian, the work of a busy practitioner who wished to improve the actual knowledge of the materia medica, over and above advancing the science of botany.   Plant description, or phytography took its first fresh start since the days of Theophrastus in the work of Hieronymus **Bock** (1498–1554), called **Tragus,** a poor schoolmaster and gardener, born near Heidelberg, who paid the usual penalties of sympathizing with Luther, and finally died as pastor of a little Protestant church at Hornbach. Tragus loved plants for themselves and, in his *New Kreutterbuch* (1539), and in his *Kreutterbuch* of 1546, wrote down in the vernacular his fresh first-hand descriptions of what he saw.   A far greater than Tragus was **Valerius Cordus** (1515–44), the gifted Prussian youth, whose early death robbed science of one of its most promising names.   As the son of the physician-botanist, Euricius Cordus, he is known to medicine for his discovery of sulphuric ether (*oleum dulce vitrioli*) in 1540; but botanists revere him as the young Marcellus of their science.   Greene styles him "the inventor of phytography," and points out that the field-work and taxonomy of a well-equipped modern botanist were actually done "almost four centuries ago by a German boy in his teens."   His posthumous commentary on Dioscorides, edited with pious hand by Conrad Gesner (Strassburg, 1561), not only describes some 500 new species of plants (the ardent search for which eventually cost him his life) but recreates the species listed by Dioscorides in terms of modern botany.   The *Dispensatorium* of Cordus (Nuremberg, 1535) is of interest as the first real pharmacopeia to be published.[2]   It was more reprinted than any other work of its kind, passing through 35 editions and 8 translations.   It was preceded by the Venetian *Luminare majus* (1496) and the Florentine *Antidotarium* (1498), and followed by the three Basel dispensatories of Leonhard Fuchs (1555), Anutius Fœsius (1561) and J. J. Wecker (1595), also the city pharmacopeias of Mantua (1559), Antwerp (1561), Augsburg (1564), Cologne (1565) and Bergamo (1580[3]).

A remarkable Renaissance figure was Conrad **Gesner** (1516–65), of Zürich, whom Cuvier called "the German Pliny," on account of his equal attainment in botany, zoölogy, bibliography, and general erudition.   The son of a poor furrier, and in great want in his early days, he graduated in medicine at Basel (1541), and

---

[1] Brunfels: Contrefayt Kräuterbuch, Strassburg, 1532–7.

[2] E. L. Greene: "Landmarks of Botanical History," Smithsonian Misc. Collect., v, 54, Washington, 1909, pp. 169–314.

[3] Tschirch: "Die Pharmakopöe ein Spiegel ihrer Zeit," Janus, Amst., 1905, x, 281, 337, 393, 449, 505.

after a roving life as a practitioner in many European cities, he was at length appointed professor of natural history at Zürich (1555), was ennobled in 1564, and sacrificed his life to the plague in the following year. In spite of his struggles with poverty, sickness, and defective eyesight, he was a man of extraordinary industry. His *Bibliotheca universalis*, of which 20 volumes were published (1545–49), was the first example of good bibliography before Haller's time, and is in intention a catalogue, in Latin, Greek, and Hebrew, of all the writers who have ever lived. The medical part was unfortunately never completed. Gesner's *Historia Plantarum* (Paris, 1541) is a student's handbook of botany, giving the genera in alphabetic order—a sort of pocket dictionary of plants. He edited and published the works of Valerius Cordus (1561). His *Historia Animalium*, published in four folio volumes (1551–58) with a fifth volume on snakes (1587), was subsequently translated into German as the *Thierbuch*, and became one of the starting-points of modern zoölogy. It contains some 4500 folio pages, comprising a digest of about 250 authors, and illustrated with nearly 1000 wood-cuts, of which Gesner selected some of the best of the period, including Albert Dürer's rhinoceros. Gesner's index of purgatives was published by Froben in 1543.[1] He made some curious essays in other directions such as his *Mithridates*, an account of 130 different languages with the Lord's Prayer translated into 22 of them; and he is known to Alpine enthusiasts through his epistles on mountain climbing and his description of Mount Pilatus (1555). He was also the first to describe the canary-bird.

Caspar **Bauhin** (1550–1624) was professor of anatomy, botany, medicine, and Greek at Basel, and afterward city physician and rector of the university. His greatest work is the celebrated *"Pinax"* (1596), a wonderful index or compend of all the botanic literature up to his time which, it is said, has been more studied and commented upon by botanists than any other work except that of Dioscorides. Bauhin also wrote a *Theatrum Botanicum* which he left incomplete (1658), and a catalogue of the plants around Basel. His *Theatrum Anatomicum* (1592) is a valuable historic summary, as also his *Anatomica Historia* (1597). It contains an interesting account of the ancient Hebrew myth of the bone "Luz," in which the term appears for the first time outside the Rabbinical writings.

Pierre **Belon** (1517–64) or Bellonius, the author of a valued treatise on coniferous plants (1553), published a monograph on birds (1555), in which he compared the skeletons of birds and man in the same posture and "nearly as possible bone for bone." This was the first of those serial arrangements of homologies which Owen and Haeckel afterward made famous. In 1546–9 Belon traveled in Egypt, Greece, and the Orient to study the materia medica. He wrote an important little book on coniferous or resiniferous trees (1553[2]). The *Semplici* (Venice, 1561) of Luigi **Anguillara** is a botanical classic. The earliest English contributions to botany were the "Herbals" of Peter Treverus (1516), Richard Banckes (1525), Thomas Petyt (1541), William Middleton (1546), William Turner called the Father of English Botany (1551), and of the barber-surgeon John Gerard (1597[3]). The medicinal plants of the New World were described by Oviedo y Valdez, viceroy of Mexico (1525), and by Nicholas Monardes of Seville (1565). A rhymed *Promptuaire* of medicinal simples by Thibault Lespleigney (1537) was reprinted by Paul Dorveaux in 1899. Following the investigations of the optical properties of lenses by Leonardo da Vinci and Francesco Maurolyco, the magnifying glass came to be used in the drawings of minute objects in Georg Hoefnagel's *Archetypa* (Frankfurt, 1592), in Fabio Colonna's figures of lichens (1606), and in Thomas Mouffet's MS. on insects (1589), published in 1634 (Singer).

Besides the German Fathers of Botany, all of whom were medical men, we should mention a number of other prominent physician-botanists of the Renaissance period who did much to make the science what it is today. Of these, Jean de la Ruelle (1474–1537), or **Ruellius**, was physician to Francis I, but later became a canon and died in the cloister. Ruellius was an able botanist who had the courage to accept all of Leonicenus' corrections of Pliny, made the first Latin translation of Dioscorides with a good commentary, and in his *De Natura Stirpium* (Paris, 1536) was the first to give a full description of each plant, adding many new species and giving to each the popular French names, which he got by questioning the peasants

---

[1] Gesner: Enumeratio medicamentorum purgantium, Basel, 1543.

[2] Belon: De arboribus coniferis, Paris, 1553.

[3] Barlow: Proceedings of the Royal Society of Medicine, Sect. Hist. Med., Lond., 1913, vi, 108–149.

and mountaineers on his excursions.   Antonio Musa **Brassavola** (1500–55) of Ferrara, a pupil of Leonicenus, described over 200 different kinds of syphilis, is said to have performed tracheotomy, prepared an authoritative concordance of Galen (Venice, 1551[1]), and wrote a book of purges (1555), and a witty imaginary conversation entitled, "An Examination of Medicinal Simples" (*Examen omnium simplicium*, Rome, 1536), in which some new drugs are permanently introduced into the pharmacopœia.   This genial Renaissance idea of casting a botanical treatise into the form of a dialogue, had already been utilized by Euricius Cordus (1486–1535), the father of Valerius, in his *Botanologicon* (Cologne, 1534), in which he severely arraigns the German druggists of his time for falsely labeling their jars and receptacles with old Greek names which did not apply.   Pietro Andrea **Mattioli** (1501–77), of Siena, called the Brunfels of Italy, wrote a vernacular commentary on Dioscorides (Venice, 1544)—now exceedingly rare—in which, like Brunfels, he illustrated the plants, following Ruellius in giving a full description of each, and adding between 200 and 300 new species from southern Europe.   Rembert **Dodoens** (1517–85) of Malines, Belgium, physician to Maximilian II and Rudolph II, was, like Gesner and Bauhin, a polyhistorian, now best remembered as a botanist.   His *Cruydtboeck* (Antwerp, 1553), his treatise on purgatives (1554), and other works were afterward assembled in his *Stirpium historiæ* (1583), a huge tome containing 1341 illustrations, which was the original of Gerard's *Herball* of 1597.   In his posthumous treatise on practice (1616), he left an accurate account of the spasmodic form of ergotism.

Andrea **Cesalpino** (1524–1603), professor of medicine at Pisa, and physician to Pope Clement VIII, is regarded by the Italians as a discoverer of the circulation (1571–93) before Harvey (1616), and was honored by them with statues and a medical journal bearing his name. Cesalpinus had indeed grasped, as pure theory, the truth about the systemic and pulmonary circulations, viz., that the heart in systole sends blood into the aorta and pulmonary artery, and in diastole receives it back from the vena cava and pulmonary vein.   But his ideas were not supported by any convincing experiments and were thrown out in a purely controversial spirit, as an additional argument against Galenism.   They, therefore, had no influence upon his contemporaries and are to be entirely dissociated from Harvey's experimental demonstration, as bald theory from actual proof.   Cesalpinus was an ardent theologian, and his Pantheism got him into trouble with the Church. Although a rigid Aristotelian he was also an able naturalist, taught botany as well as medicine at Pisa, and was in charge of the Botanic Garden founded there in 1543.   Cesalpinus was called by Linnæus the first true systematist (*primus verus systematicus*) in botany.   He collected plants from all over Europe, was the first to classify them by their fruits, ranging some 1520 plants into 15 classes by this plan.   His great work, *De Plantis* (Florence, 1583), led to the distinction between systematic and applied (economic) botany.

Giovanni Battista **della Porta** (1536–1615) of Naples, who invented the camera obscura (1588), described the opera glass (1590), and was indeed one of the principal founders of optics, was also an opponent of witchcraft and, in his *De Humana Physiognomia* (Sorrento, 1586) was a forerunner of Lavater in estimating human character by the features, although he made the usual totemic error of assigning characteristic animal traits to individuals who looked like particular animals (Jastrow).

---

[1] Brassavola: Index refertissimus in omnes Galeni libros, Venice, 1551, 1557, 1625.

He believed in the doctrine of signatures. In botany, Porta was the first ecologist, grouping plants, in his *Phytognomonica* (1583), according to their geographic locale and distribution. He was a prolific writer of comedies. He went in for magic, and the Accademia de segrete, which he founded for this purpose in 1560, was suppressed by Pope Paul III.

The medical men we have just mentioned are, all of them, examples of the restless Renaissance spirit and, in the pioneering cast of mind, they are akin to the great pathbreakers of the period, Vesalius, Paracelsus, and Paré. There is yet another group of physicians, each remarkable for achievement along isolated and original lines. Of these, Pierre **Brissot** (1478–1522) stands out as a reformer in the practice of bloodletting. Up to the time of Brissot, physicians had accepted the Arabist teaching that bleeding should be "revulsive," that is, at a distance from the lesion. In 1514, Brissot, a professor of the Paris Faculty, deeply read in Greek medicine, made a stand for the original Hippocratic method of "derivative" bloodletting, that is, free venesection on the same side as and near to the lesion,[1] which he believed to be the most effective for the removal of peccant humors. This heresy engendered a storm which resulted in the banishment of Brissot by act of Parliament and a pronouncement of Charles V to the effect that such doctrine was as flagitious as Lutheranism. Clement VII and Vesalius were dragged into the controversy, which was brought to a sudden close by the fact that one of Charles V's relatives died from venesection by the Arabist method in an attack of pleurisy. The smug opponents of Hippocrates and Brissot were thus made ridiculous forever, although blood was still let in quantity until the time of Louis.

A gifted pathologist was the distinguished Florentine, Antonio **Benivieni** (–1502), who was an able surgeon and a remarkable pioneer in reporting postmortem sections, but regarded Galen as the last word in medicine. In his posthumous *De Abditis Causis Morborum*, published by the Giunti (1507), he appears as a founder of pathology before Morgagni. "Before Vesalius, before Eustachius," says Allbutt, "he opened the bodies of the dead as deliberately and clearsightedly as any pathologist in the spacious times of Baillie, Bright, and Addison," and Malgaigne described his book as "the only work on pathology which owes nothing to any one." But with all deference to authority so high, it may be doubted if Benivieni's slight performance (it consists of only 54 pages) can enter into comparison with the vast array of pathologic findings and descriptions of new diseases in Morgagni's majestic treatise. For such pioneer work as Benivieni's the time was hardly ripe, and the same thing is true of the speculations of that most original genius, **Fracastorius**. Girolamo Fracastoro (1484–1553), a Veronese of thick-set, hirsute appearance and jovial mien, who practised in the Lago di Garda region, was at once a physician, poet, physicist,

---

[1] The terms "derivative" and "revulsive" are sometimes employed indifferently to signify bleeding at a distance from, instead of at the site of, the lesion. The distinction is fanciful (Littré).

geologist, astronomer, and pathologist, and shares with Leonardo da Vinci the honor of being the first geologist to see fossil remains in the true light (1530). He was also the first scientist to refer to the magnetic poles of the earth (1543). His medical fame rests upon that most celebrated of medical poems, *Syphilis sive Morbus Gallicus* (Venice, 1530), which sums up the contemporary dietetic and therapeutic knowledge of the time, recognizes a venereal cause, and gave the disease its present name; and his treatise, *De Contagione* (1546), in which he states, with wonderful clairvoyance, the modern theory of infection by microörganisms (*seminaria contagionum*[1]) and describes (lib. III) an epidemic of foot-and-mouth disease (1514).

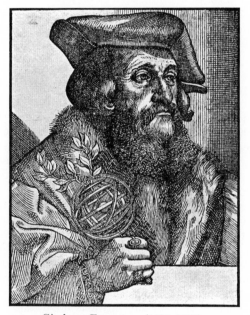

Girolamo Fracastoro (1484–1553).

Our account of Renaissance medicine may close with the works of two original characters who were not physicians: the Venetian, Luigi **Cornaro** (1467–1566), whose *Trattato della vita sobria* (Padua, 1558) is probably the best treatise on personal hygiene and the "simple life" in existence; and *The Metamorphosis of Ajax* (1596) of Sir John **Harington** (1561–1612), the witty, graceless godson of Queen Elizabeth, who was

---

[1] It is to be remembered, however, that Fracastorius nowhere refers to bacteria as living organisms (*contagia animata*), but describes them (in terms of physical chemistry) as something very like our modern "colloidal systems," although he regards them as capable of reproduction in appropriate media. As between Fracastorius and Athanasius Kircher, the decision of priority in regard to the germ theory will depend upon whether the arbiter is a materialist or a vitalist. In the *De Contagione*, Fracastorius also gives the first authentic account of typhus fever (1546), the "tabardillo" of contemporary Spanish and Mexican writers.

banished from her court for writing it. The work introduces an important and indispensable improvement in sanitary engineering, but the theme is handled entirely in the manner of Aristophanes, Rabelais, or the Zähdarm epitaph in *Sartor Resartus*, and the garrulous, whimsical old knight possibly got his invention from Oriental sources. Harington also made a quaint and amusing versification of the Salernitan *Regimen sanitatis* (1607[1]).

Carlo Ruini's treatise on the anatomy and diseases of the horse and their treatment (1598), sometimes attributed to Leonardo da Vinci,[2] is usually regarded as the foundation of modern veterinary medicine.

It is worth remembering that the first medical and surgical books to be published in the new world, such as the *Opera Medicinalia* of Francisco Bravo (1570), the *Summa y Recopilacion de Cirugia* of Alphonso Lopez de Hinojoso (1578; 2 ed., 1595), and the *Tractado Breve de Medicina* of Fray Augustin Farfán (1592) were printed in the city of Mexico.

CULTURAL AND SOCIAL ASPECTS OF RENAISSANCE MEDICINE

The invention of printing and the Revival of Learning, the discovery of America and the extension of travel and commerce, the heliocentric astronomy of the physician Copernicus, the beginnings of modern physics and chemistry, the struggle between masses and classes which began with Magna Charta (1215), the Reformation (1517), and the growth of vernacular literature, all combined to make the Renaissance a period of incessant intellectual ferment and activity. The Byzantine Greek scholars, who poured into Italy after the destruction of Constantinople, have been described as "sowers of dragon's teeth," and if we judge them by their effect upon the work of Paracelsus, Vesalius, and Paré, we may regard these Humanists as the true forerunners of modern medicine. The three great leaders of Renaissance medicine were all of them experimenters in the truest sense, but before the common medical mind could be penetrated with the advantages of experimentation over superstitious observances, it was necessary to clear the ground of the accumulated rubbish of the past, which could be accomplished only by searching, critical study of the medical authorities of antiquity. In the different universities, the courses of medical instruction and the text-books used—Avicenna's Canon, Galen's Ars parva, the Aphorisms of Hippocrates, Dioscorides—remained about the same,[3] but new and important features were gradually introduced, and the 16th century university training acquired a distinctive character of its own. Bologna, Padua, and Pisa had the most popular medical faculties, and after them Paris, Montpellier, and Basel; but the wide-spread

[1] Edited in a new edition by Francis R. Packard (New York, 1920).

[2] See Schmutzer: Arch. f. d. Gesch. d. Naturwissensch., Leipz., 1910–12, iii, 61–70.

[3] For lists of medical books used by Cracow physicians and students in the 16th century, see J. Lachs: Arch. f. Gesch. d. Med., Leipz., 1913–14, vii, 206–217.

interest in general culture soon led to the foundation of new universities at Valencia (1500), Wittenberg (1502), Santiago (1504), Toledo (1518), Marburg (1527), Granada (1531), Königsberg (1544), Jena (1558), Douai (Lille) (1561), Helmstädt (1575), Leyden (1575), Altdorf (1580), Edinburgh (1582), and Dublin (1591). Each of these Renaissance universities was a little democracy in that the students themselves elected the rector, the professors, and the officers, and had a voice in determining the courses of study. As a rule, the members of the faculty were chosen for only one year, and had to be renominated and reëlected for a further tenure of office. This peculiar arrangement kept the students and professors in continual movement from one university to another; a professor would sometimes give a *Gastspiel* of lectures in order to secure a good position, and even city physicians wandered from place to place after fulfilling their contracts. In Goethe's Faust, Mephistopheles introduces himself for the first time as a "wandering student" (*fahrender Scholastikus*). Characters of this rolling-stone order were a feature of the time. Many of these itinerant scholars were genuine vagabonds, so poor that they had to eke out a livelihood by begging like tramps, singing at doors like Christmas waits, attending to odd jobs or, their favorite expedient, stealing what they could lay their hands upon. The fagging and hazing among the different bodies of students were coarse beyond conception, license was unbridled, and many of them went frankly to the devil. Others, in the face of extreme poverty, led lives of noble self-denial for the advancement of learning and science. The absolute lack of medical periodicals and a slow and expensive postal service made it necessary for even the best to move from pillar to post in order to be in touch with new phases of thought. About 1543, Giambattista da Monte (1498–1552) introduced bedside teaching at Padua but, after Montanus' death, the practice lapsed (*circa* 1551), and was revived by Albertino Bottoni and Marco degli Oddi (1578) whose pupil, Jan van Heurne (1543–1601), carried the tradition to Leyden, where it was ultimately put upon a definite footing by his son Otto Heurne and Ewald Scrivelius (1636[1]).

The principal innovations in **medical teaching** were in the disciplines of anatomy and botany. Postmortem sections before students were tried upon defunct obstetric patients at Padua by Marco Oddi (1579), but these were soon done away with by popular prejudice. **Dissections**, however, became more frequent and were regarded in each case as a particular and expensive social function, for which a special papal indulgence was necessary. The cadaver was first made "respectable" by the reading of an official decree, and was then stamped with the seal of the university. Having been taken into the anatomic hall, it was next beheaded in deference to the then universal prejudice against opening the cranial cavity. The dissection was followed by such festivities as band music or even theatrical performances. All this led in time to the building of so-called anatomic theaters, notably those at Padua (1549), Montpellier (1551), and Basel (1588). In England the need for anatomic study led to the passing of the law of 1540 (32 Henry VIII, c. 42), authorizing the barbers and surgeons to use four bodies of executed criminals each year for "anathomyes," a provision which, however enlarged, remained substantially in force until the passing of the Anatomy Act of 1832. In 1564, John Caius obtained from Queen

---

[1] Pagel-Sudhoff: Geschichte der Medizin, 3 Aufl., Berlin, 1922, 238.

Elizabeth a formal grant of two bodies of criminals for dissections by the two holders of medical fellowships at Cambridge.[1] The extreme scarcity of anatomic material everywhere made it a special ambition of each teacher or practitioner to have a skeleton of his own. This, in due course, became the germinal idea of the splendid anatomic and pathologic museums of later times, from Ruysch to the Hunters and Dupuytren. Botanic teaching in the universities was forwarded by special outdoor excursions in the spring and autumn, to which the apothecaries were invited, and which were always followed by banquets and jollifications. The first chair of "simples" (*lectura simplicium*) was founded by Francesco Bonafede at the University of Padua in 1533, and about 1561 an *ostensio simplicium*, or demonstration of living plants, was added. Many universities had separate botanic gardens of their own, notably Pisa (1544), Padua (1545) of which Anguillara and Prospero Alpino were prefects, Zürich (1560), Bologna (1568), Leyden (1577), Leipzig (1579), Montpellier (1592), and Paris (1597) which, after 1635, was known as the Jardin des Plantes. These were again the originals of the great private collections and gardens of the 18th century. The salary of a university professor in the 16th century was a dependent variable and decidedly low in the northern countries. In Germany it ranged anywhere from $40 to about four or five times as much. The Linacre foundations at Oxford and Cambridge provided for two professorships at $60 each per annum and one at $30; but Vesalius got $1000 at Pisa. Toward the 17th century these sums had a purchasing value equal to about eight times the amount in modern money.[2] The salaries of city physicians and the **fees** charged by physicians in private practice were proportionately low. Power says that the average fee in Elizabethan England was a mark (13s. 4d.). City physicians in Germany got anywhere from $4.25 to $43, court physicians from $35 to $939. The physicians in ordinary of Henry VII, Henry VIII, and Queen Elizabeth all received about $200 annually. In Germany, a simple uroscopy cost about 3 cents; single visits anywhere from 8 to 50 cents according to the income of the patient; consultations $2.50 for each physician, or $1.25 if by letter. Johann May, the first to teach medicine at Tübingen (1477), got 30 florins for handling a medical case.[3] The most lucrative phase of practice was in the treatment of syphilis, in which physicians easily made small fortunes, even down to the time of Casanova's Memoirs. Kneeling before the statue of Charles VIII at St. Denis, Thierry de Hery said to a bystanding priest: "Charles VIII is a good enough saint for me: he put 30,000 francs in my pocket when he brought the pox into France." Surgeons were fairly well paid, the fee for a fracture for instance, being about $10.50. John of Arderne is said to have gotten 100 gold sols ($500) for his operation for fistula in ano. The apothecaries fared best of all, if we are to judge by a bill which was sent to Queen Elizabeth amounting to about $216 for one quarter.[4] Municipal apothecary shops in Germany, such as the old *Rathsapotheke* at Hannover (1566), were highly ornate structures.

Medical practice during the Renaissance period was bound up with superstition, herb-doctoring, and quackery. Petrarch ridiculed the doctors of his day for their subservience to the Arabs, their predilection for uromancy, their county-fair deceptions.[5] Poggio, the Florentine humanist, pilloried the profession in his *Liber facetiarum* (1470[6]). In the illustrations of the period the physician, whether in long robe or short fur-edged pelisse, is invariably represented as inspecting a urinal. He usually believed in astrology, and went in for the lore of amulets (*Pas-*

---

[1] Brit. Med. Jour., Lond., 1920, i, 370.

[2] J. J. Walsh: "Physicians' Fees Down the Ages," Internat. Clinics, Phila., 1910, 20 s., iv, p. 269.

[3] Med. Cor.-Bl. d. württemb. ärztl. Ver., Stuttg., 1914, lxxxiv, 609.

[4] The great center of the London drug trade in the Elizabethan era was Bucklersbury, immortalized in Falstaff's reference to "these lisping hawthorn buds, that come like women in men's apparel, and smell like Bucklersbury in simple time" (Merry Wives of Windsor, Act III, sc. 3).

[5] See Henschel: Janus, Bresl., 1846, i, 186–223.

[6] Roth: Vesalius, Berlin, 1892, 192.

sauer-Kunst) and the *Lasstafelkunst*, or the determination of the proper time for purging and blood-letting by the conjunction of the planets. Even a court physician was often an "astronomer royal," that is, a deviser of fortune-tellers' almanacs. The *Ludicrum Chiromanticum* (1661) of Johann Prætorius mentions some 77 publications of the 16th and 17th centuries, devoted to palmistry alone. The followers of Paracelsus believed in the "doctrine of signatures," in virtue of which the exhibition of a drug hinges upon some fanciful associative resemblance to the disease, as trefoil for heart disease, thistle for a stitch in the side, walnut shells for head injuries, bear's grease for baldness, topaz, the yellow celandine or turmeric for jaundice, powdered mummy for prolonging life, and so forth. We may judge of the true greatness of men like Vesalius, Leonicenus, Linacre, Fracastorius, and Benivieni by reflecting that they alone scorned to credit these things. In like manner only the surgeons of first rank—Paré, Gersdorff, Franco, Würtz, Tagliacozzi, Clowes, and Bartisch—were true surgeons. The unclassed horde of wandering cataract-couchers, lithotomists, herniotomists, and booth-surgeons generally were, in the words of William Clowes, "no better than runagates or vagabonds, . . . shameless in countenance, lewd in disposition, brutish in judgment and understanding," so disreputable, in fact, that special laws had to be passed to make the status of competent surgeons reputable—notably the edict of Charles V in 1548 which had to be renewed by Rudolph II in 1577.[1] The barber-surgeon who shaved a criminal condemned to death, or dressed the wounds of any one tortured on the rack, was regarded as himself a felon. Quackery was rampant everywhere, and in the vigorous language of the English surgeon just quoted, was practised by "tinkers, tooth-drawers, peddlers, ostlers, carters, porters, horse-gelders and horse-leeches, idiots, apple-squires, broom-men, bawds, witches, conjurers, soothsayers and sow-gelders, rogues, rat-catchers, runagates, and proctors of spittle-houses." Another class of impostors were the tramps of the period who, in spite of Henry VIII's statue against "sturdy and valiant beggars," tried to impose upon the charity of the hospitals, which in those days gave temporary shelter to all the poor. Robert Copland (1508–47), the old English printer, who was also a poet, wrote an amusing versified dialogue between himself and the porter of St. Bartholomew's, called *The Hye Way to the Spyttel House*, which throws considerable light upon the poor law, and free dispensary problems of the 16th century.[2]

Perhaps the worst phase of Renaissance medical practice was its **obstetrics**. We know little of medieval obstetrics, but we may gauge the extent of its degradation by what happened in the 16th century. In normal labor, a woman had an even chance if she did not succumb to puerperal fever or eclampsia. In difficult labor, she was usually

---

[1] For examination questions put to a German candidate in surgery in 1580, see J. W. S. Johnsson, Janus, Amst., 1910, xv, 129–142.

[2] See Lancet, Lond., 1909, ii, 1020.

butchered to death if attended by a Sairey Gamp of the time or one of the vagabond "surgeons." As a rule, only midwives attended women in labor. In 1580, a law was passed in Germany to prevent shepherds and herdsmen from attending obstetric cases. The Renaissance pictures, like the medieval data, show that the lying-in room was crowded with people bustling in every direction, giving the general impression, as Baas truly says, of "all sorts of female fussiness."[1] The obstetric abuses were remedied to some extent by city ordinances governing midwives, notably those of Ratisbon (1555), Frankfurt on the Main (by Adam Lonicerus, 1573), and Passau (1595).

In this period, infants were commonly breast-fed, but **wet-nursing,** although opposed by Phayre (1546) and others, grew apace, and baby-farming became a notorious evil. The high rate of **infantile mortality** was due to the low status of public, domestic, and personal hygiene, which was held in less regard than in the Middle Ages. The cities had no drainage, and dwelling-houses, with their floors strewn with rushes and their cesspools as described by Erasmus, were sinks of filth and infection.[2] Froude, at the beginning of his History of England, notes that the growth of the population was very slow, almost stationary, the result of high infantile mortality and the effect of wars and epidemics upon the adult population.

Certain criminal **laws** issued by the Bishop of Bamberg in 1507 and by the Elector of Brandenburg in 1516, led to the formulation (in 1521 and 1529) of the celebrated C.C.C. (*Constitutio Criminalis Carolina*), or *Peinliche Gerichtsordnung* of Charles V, published in 1533, which authorized the judge of a court to summon physicians or midwives as expert witnesses in such medicolegal cases as homicide, infanticide, criminal abortion, malpractice, and the like, but in deference to current superstitions, postmortem examinations were not authorized. The first judicial postmortem in France was made by Ambroïse Paré in 1562,[3] after which time the practice became common. Special laws were passed in regard to the sale of food, adulteration of drugs, alcoholic liquors,[4] street-cleaning, occupations, the plague, and other phases of municipal hygiene; but nothing was done to alleviate the condition of the insane, who were chained, beaten, starved, and otherwise maltreated, and frequently died of cold. In 1547 the monastery of St. Mary of Bethlehem at London (founded in 1246) was converted into a hospital for the insane, popularly known as "Bedlam," and in a few years was amply justifying its reputation as conveyed in this term.

A special feature of Renaissance legislation in France and England was the improvement of the status of the **barber-surgeons.** In 1505, the Paris Faculty took the barber-surgeons under its wing, in order to

---

[1] For a recent study of the lying-in room in the various periods, see A. Martin, Arch. f. Gesch. d. Med., 1916–17, x, 209–250, 2 pl.

[2] Forsyth: Proc. Roy. Soc. Med., Lond., 1910–11, iv, pt. 1, Sect. Dis. Child., 112–116.

[3] It was preceded by the Bolognese postmortem of Bartolomeo da Varignana in 1302.

[4] Sebastian Brant, in his *Narrenschiff* (1494), lashes the adulteration of wine, sausages, sugar, and saffron. Wine was adulterated by artificial coloring, sweetenng, and treatment with plaster-of-Paris.

spite the surgeons proper, of whom it was jealous. A few years later, these "surgeons of the long robe," having failed to become a separate faculty, decided to make the best of a bad bargain by coming under the sway of the physicians. In England, in 1462, the numerous and prosperous Guild of Barbers became the Company of Barbers under Edward IV; the surgeons obtained a special charter in 1492; and in 1540, under Henry VIII, this Barber Company was united with the small and exclusive Guild of Surgeons to form the United Barber-Surgeon Company, with the anatomist, Thomas Vicary as its first Master. A celebrated painting of the younger Holbein represents Henry VIII—huge, bluff, and disdainful—in the act of handing the statute to Vicary, in company with fourteen other surgeons on their knees before the monarch, who does not condescend even to look at them. This picture, one of the best of Holbein's works, not only gives a superb portrait of Henry VIII, but is probably the best representation in existence of the costume and appearance of the 16th century surgeon. In 1546, the king also founded the Regius Professorship of Medicine at Cambridge. A picture in the Hunterian Library at Glasgow[1] represents Dr. John Banister (1533–1610) as delivering the "Visceral Lecture" at the Barber-Surgeon's Hall (London) in 1581. A dissected cadaver is exposed, above the lecturer is an opened copy of Columbus, farther above are the armorial bearings of the United Barber-Surgeon's Company, while the skeleton at the left is supported and crowned with its colors, familiar in the candy-stick red and white of the barbers' pole.

The English act of 1511 (3. Henry VIII, cap. iii) decreed that no one should practice medicine or surgery in London, or seven miles around and about it, without being first examined, approved and admitted by four doctors of physic or expert surgeons, acting under the Bishop of London or the Dean of St. Paul's. Beyond the seven miles precinct, the applicant must be approved by similar bodies under the bishop of the diocese or his vicar general. On September 23, 1518, at the behest of Thomas Linacre and other physicians, Henry VIII organized these licensed practitioners into a College Perpetual of doctors and grave men, authorized to practise within the seven miles precinct. This charter was confirmed by the acts of 1522 (14.–15. Henry VIII, cap. 5) and 1553 (I Mary, St. 2, v, cap. 9) and the institution became the "College or Commonalty of the Faculty of Physick of London." In 1851 (21.–22. Victoria, cap. 90) it became the **Royal College of Physicians** of England which title was confirmed in 1860 (23–24. Victoria, cap. 66). The bilingual "Statutes" of this college constitute one of the earliest and most important examples of a **local code of ethics**.[2] In 1542–3, on account of the greed of surgeons "minding their own lucres," and disdaining to help the poor, Acts 34 and 35, Henry VIII, cap. 8, were enacted, permitting common persons having knowledge of herbal and folk-medicine to minister to the indigent, thus affording a loophole for unqualified practitioners, like the *Kurierfreiheit* of modern Germany.

During the Renaissance period, considerable advance was made in the theory and practice of **military medicine**. Field hospitals (*ambulancias*) were introduced by Queen Isabella of Spain at the siege of Malaga (August 19, 1487), and were revived by her grandson, Charles V, at the siege of Metz (1552), where Ambroïse Paré, the greatest military surgeon of the time, was the central figure. At this time, army surgeons were only in attendance upon their patrons, the great captains and nobles,

[1] D'Arcy Power: Proc. Roy. Soc. Med. (Sect. Hist. Med.), Lond., 1912–13, vi, 18–35.

[2] The Paris Faculty had similar statutes from 1452, those of Piacenza were printed in 1569, and many other local ethical codes followed these.

and returned to their civilian practice at the end of a campaign; but a decree of Coligny (1550) had assigned a surgeon to care for the sick and wounded of each company of infantry. Meanwhile, real military organization and discipline had been established in the armies of Maximilian I. The regulations for the sanitary dispositions of his *Landesknechte*, as given by Leonhard Fronsperger (1555) are, indeed, the foundation of the present medical regulations of the German army (Frölich). The directions for the disposal of the wounded and the minute assignment of duties to the chief physician in the field are quite modern, as are also the careful administrative preparations made for a besieged town by the Duke of Guise (Salignac). In the German army, the sick and wounded were sent to the baggage train, put under canvas, treated by the surgeon or barber and nursed by female camp-followers, the whole arrangement being under the administration of a hospital superintendent (*Spitalmeister*). In Guise's forces, cases of communicable disease were isolated, the pioneers, under the provost, looked after the sanitation of Metz, the surgeon-barbers were given money to carry on their functions, and the sick and wounded were at once sent to hospital. When the siege was raised, Guise and Alva established a mutual Red Cross agreement, which the Spanish again observed at the siege of Therouanne (1553), after which time prisoners and wounded enemies were not commonly massacred. After the capture of Havre (1563), the Queen Mother planned an *Invalides* or retreat for infirm and aged soldiers which, however, did not become an accomplished fact until 1676. Yet in spite of such remarkable administration, the losses were frightful and the importation of prisoners into Metz started an epidemic of typhus, which spread to the adjoining villages.[1]

Of the many **epidemic diseases** which had beset Europe in the Middle Ages, three, the sweating sickness, leprosy, and epidemic chorea, had well-nigh disappeared by the middle of the 16th century. In France, Italy, Spain, England, Denmark, and Switzerland, leprosy was so well stamped out that the lazar-houses were abolished, but the disease still continued to be epidemic through the 17th century in Germany, Scotland, and the Low Countries, and in Sweden and Norway it lasted until the 18th century. The most formidable epidemics of the 16th century were the plague and syphilis.

Between the years 1500–68, the ravages of the **plague** were particularly severe in Germany, Italy, and France and, in the sixth decade, spread all over Europe. After this time it broke out at intervals in different places in 1564, 1568, 1574, and 1591. All through the century, a vast number of *Pestschriften* were published. The most important were the public documents recognizing the contagious nature of the plague and proposing various methods of isolation and disinfection. Wittenberg and some of the other cities commemorated the different epidemics by striking off special coins, or pest-dollars (*Wittenberger Pesttaler*). The obverse of these commonly represented Moses' fiery serpent set upon a pole, with the inscription "Who looketh upon the serpent shall live" (Numbers xxi, 8, 9); the reverse represented Christ crucified, with the inscription, "He that believeth on me hath everlasting life" (St. John vi, 47). There were also comet medals (1558), and medals commemorating years of famine, of which the most remarkable celebrated the "Annona," or right of the Papacy to limit the price of corn. Famine medals of this kind were struck off in honor of Popes Julius II (1505–8), Pius IV (1560–75), Gregory XIII (1576–91), and Clement VIII (1599). Wittenberg pest-dollars and the "*zenechton*," arsenic-paste sewed up in dog-skin, were worn over the heart as amulets against the plague.

Syphilis was less malignant in character than in the 15th century, and this was perhaps due to a number of really efficient remedies which were a vast improvement upon the mild vegetable concoctions of the

---

[1] C. L. Heizmann: Ann. Med. History, N. Y., 1917–18, i, 281–287. The basic texts are: L. Fronsperger: Vom Kayserlichen Kriegsgerichten (1566); Salignac: Le siège de Metz (Paris, 1553), and the Apologia et voyages of Paré.

earlier period.   Mercury had become the great sheet-anchor, whether
for internal or external use, although opinion was pretty well divided
as to its ultimate value.   Leonicenus, Montagnana, and the German
writers generally opposed its use; Fracastorius and Benivieni gave it
the seal of their approval.   Thierry de Hery (died 1559), in his treatise
of 1552,[1] recommended either guaiac internally or mercury by fumigation or inunction, preferably the latter.   Paré's treatise on syphilis is
taken almost *verbatim* from this work.   A special feature of the anti-
syphilitic medication of the century was the introduction of new drugs
from the Western Hemisphere.   As alchemy introduced antimony, mercury, and sugar of lead, so the discovery of America brought in guaiac
(introduced in 1508–17), the root of *China smilax* (1525), exploited by
Vesalius, sarsaparilla (1536), and sassafras.   An old copper-plate of
1570, after Stradanus,[2] shows a sick room interior, with all the stages of
preparing the guaiac infusion, from chipping the huge logs to administration to the syphilitic patient.   Gonorrhea became common about
1520.   One remarkable effect of the venereal diseases was the suppression
of common public baths for either sex or both sexes.   In the Germanic
countries, these bathing establishments were a special feature of city
life, and, as depicted by the various Renaissance artists, their status
was peculiar.   Many of them were frequented indiscriminately by men
and women alike, all of whom sat and bathed together in one huge
common vat or tank.   Dürer's wood-cut of 1496 (*Die Badstube*) represents a group of naked men in a common bath-vat, some of whom are
playing musical instruments, others conversing, while a third is draining a stoup of wine.   This *motif* of wine bibbing and general pleasaunce
was frequently utilized by the lesser masters, Hans Sebald Beham,
Aldegrever, Hans Baldung Grien, Hans Bock, whose pictures show the
commingling of nude men and women, with scenes of feasting, cupping,
and venesection in the bath.   A favorite theme of Lucas Cranach and
Beham was the so-called *Jungbrunnen*, or "Fountain of Youth," which
represents a number of decrepit old women trundled in wheel-barrows
to one side of a huge bath-tank, in which they are supposed to be re-
juvenated; on the other side, they are promptly man-handled by a
number of amiable youths, who hurry these reinvigorated dames up
the bank to appropriate tents.   These roguish pictures of the old
German *Kleinmeister* really point a moral.   It was soon found that a
general mixing of able-bodied men and women in a state of nature in
common bathing pools could lead in the end only to general laxity of
morals, and such places could not long be frequented by decent people.
Laws were passed segregating the sexes, but the advent of leprosy,
plague, and syphilis demonstrated, over and above this, that the idea
of a common bath-tank was bad in itself, since the latter became a
simple medium of infection.   As examples of medical illustration in

---

[1] de Hery: La méthode curatoire de la maladie vénérienne, Paris, 1552.

[2] Reproduced in H. Peters, Der Arzt, Leipzig, 1900, p. 101.

16

Renaissance art, we should mention Dürer's celebrated wood-cut of a syphilitic (1496[1]); also the picture which he sent to his physician representing himself nude, with the legend, "Where the yellow spot is and my finger points, there am I sick within"; Raphael's cartoon of St. Peter and the lame man (South Kensington Museum); Orcagna's grisly procession of lepers in his "Triumph of Death" (Pisa); the elder Holbein's picture of St. Elizabeth ministering to three lepers (Munich); Matthias Grünewald's representation of bubonic plague (Colmar Gallery, 1515), and Francesco Carotto's St. Roch in the Verona Gallery (1528), showing the typical inguinal bubo. The Venetians, Paolo Veronese and Carpaccio, painted many dwarfs (Charcot). In the Uffizi Gallery at Florence, there is a remarkable painting of Ferdinand I of Spain by Lucas van Leyden (1524), in which the artist has given the characteristic *facies* of adenoid vegetations, without apparently knowing the existence of the condition in his subject. This is also true of the portrait of the acromegalic giant in the Ambras Schloss in Tyrol (1553). The prognathism of the Hapsburgs and the Medici, which is now regarded as a mode of malocclusion, appears in different portraits of these worthies. Divergent strabismus is apparent in Raphael's portrait of Tommaso Inghirami in the Pitti Palace (Florence). The clownism and opisthotonos of the major phase of hysteria are apparent in the frescoes of Andrea del Sarto (Annunziata, Florence), of Domenichino in the Convent of Grotta Ferrata and Raphael's Transfiguration (Vatican, 1520). The different gaits of paralytics and poliomyelitics are shown in the Procession of Cripples by Hieronymus Bosch. Feeling the pulse is represented in a frieze by Giovanni della Robbia in the Ospedale de Ceppo at Pistoia. Dentistry is symbolized in G. Spagna's fresco of its patroness, Saint Apollonia (holding an extracted tooth in a forceps) in the church of San Giacomo, near Spoleto (1526), a subject which was essayed in the charming picture by Carlo Dolci (1616–86), latterly in the Corsini Gallery at Rome. The pictures of women by the younger Holbein and other artists of the German and Italian Renaissance revel in the representation of full-bodied ideals, and particularly in the glorification of pregnancy as the chief end of womankind (Holländer).

Of **epidemic diseases,** smallpox and measles began to appear in the northern countries, notably in Germany (1493) and Sweden (1578). In 1572, there was an epidemic of lead-poisoning (called *colica Pictonum*) in the south of France which resembled the "Devonshire colic" of the 18th century, in that its probable cause was the use of lead in the cider and wine-presses. Scurvy, which appeared as early as 1218, and was first described by Jacques de Vitry and Joinville (1250), and later in the narrative of Vasco da Gama's voyage (1498), became quite common along the coast of northern Germany, Holland, and the Scandinavian countries, as described by Euricius Cordus (1534), George Agricola (1539), and other writers. It was also described by the poet Camoens in the fifth canto of his Lusiad (1558). Yellow fever is said to have exterminated the population of Ysabella, San Domingo, in 1493. Typhus fever was epidemic in Italy in 1505 and 1524–30, and was described by Fracastorius (1533[2]) and Francisco Bravo (1570[3]). As "gaol fever," it devastated

---

[1] Encircled by 110 Latin lines by Theodoricus Ulsenius and printed at Nuremberg.　　　　[2] Fracastorius: De morbis contagiosis, 1533, cap. vi.
　　[3] Francisco Bravo: Opera medicinalia, Mexico, 1570.

the court-rooms of the famous Black Assizes of Cambridge (1522), Oxford (1577), and Exeter (1589) by obvious lice transmission from the prisoners on trial. At Oxford, the mortality was 510; while the Exeter outbreak spread all over Devonshire. The louse infestation was no respecter of persons, as indicated by the long-handled curry-combs which the Tudor ladies employed to scratch their backs (MacArthur). In Spain, after the siege of Granada (1489), where it broke out among the Castilian troops, typhus was called *el tabardiglo* (a little cloak).   The Aztec disease *matlaza-huatl*, or *cocoliztli*, already known in Mexico in 1570–76,[1] was shown to be a table-land disease identical with tabardillo, by Stamm, in 1861.[2]   A Tabardillo Congress was held in Mexico on January 14–21, 1919.   The so-called Hungarian disease (*morbus Hungaricus*), which spread all over Europe in 1501 and in 1505–87, was frequently epidemic in Italy and France, is now regarded as, in all probability, typhus fever.   Another disease of obscure origin and character was a sort of pneu-motyphus or pleurotyphus, which was epidemic in Italy, France, Switzerland, Holland, and Germany between the years 1521 and 1598.   An epidemic in the cloister at Bergen on the Danube, in 1527, was described in the letters of a nun, Sabina, sister of Willibald Pirckheimer.[3]   **Diphtheria,** which had already been described by Schedel in 1492, was six times epidemic in Spain during the period 1581–1638, and by 1618 had spread to Italy.   It was described as *garrotillo* by Casales (1611), Fontecha (1611), Villa Real (1611), Nuñez Herrera (1615), Juan Soto (1616), Francisco de Figueroa (Lima, 1616), Lorenzo de San Millán (Zaragosa, 1616), Gerardo Sola (Seville, 1618), Jeronimo Gil Piña (Zaragosa, 1636), Nicolas Gutierrez de Angulo (1638), and Pedro Miguel de Heredia (1665[4]).   It was called after the Spanish mode of strangulation, familiar in the etchings of Goya; or, in the words of Herrera, *Sofoca la patiente à manera del garrota*.   The fullest accounts are those of Gil Pina (1636) and Heredia (1665), which were followed by the treatise of Juan Antonio Pascual (Valencia, 1784), covering 300 cases and the historical study of Fernandez Navarrete (1764–71).   In Codex 11548 of the Vienna Hofbibliothek (fol. 278 verso), it is described as a "new disease" (*nawe krannzkheyt*[5]).   Ergotism, in the gangrenous form, was prevalent in Spain in 1581 and 1590.   In Germany a form variously convulsive, spasmodic, stuporous or paralytic, preceded by the usual tingling, burning sensations, and known as the *Kriebelkrankheit*, appeared and was endemic in the years 1581, 1587, 1592, and 1595–6.   In 1597, the Medical Faculty of Marburg issued a pronouncement upon the 1595 epidemic, declaring its cause to be the use of bread made from spurred rye.   Crookshank regards *Kriebel-krankheit* as an epidemic influenzal encephalomyelitis.   The epidemics of sweating sickness (*sudor Anglicus*) which prevailed in 1528–9 were probably influenza.   The epidemic of 1580 was the first to be recognized definitely as influenza which, in the view of Crookshank, was also at the bottom of the manifestations known as *Hauptweh* in Germany (1504–5, 1543–5, 1580), *coqueluche* (1510, 1551, 1580) and *trousse galant* (1544–6) in France, *mal mazzuco* (1504–5, 1529) and *mal del castrone* (1580, 1597) in Italy.   In 1578, the popular term *coqueluche* was transferred to whooping-cough, which was described by Baillou in that year as *quinta*.   In the opinion of Crook-shank,[6] the epidemic agues of Le Paulmier (1578) were not malarial, but influenzal (*épidemies aiguës*).   To illustrate the changeable character of the influenzas in this period, he gives an apposite citation from Rabelais (1542): *Les catarrhes descen-dront ceste année du cerveau es membres inferieurs*.

In the 16th century the Eastern **drug-trade,** the quest for

"Cassia, sandal-buds and stripes
Of labdanum, and aloe-balls"

fell into the hands of the Portuguese navigators.

---

[1] N. León: ?Qué era el matlazahuatl y que el cocoliztli [etc.], Mexico, 1919. Also, A. von Humboldt: Reise in die Aequinoctial-Gegenden von Amerika, cited by Haeser.   [2] Stamm: Nosophthorie, Berlin, 1861, cited by Haeser.

[3] E. Reicke: Arch. f. Gesch. d. Med., Leipz., 1911–12, v, 418–424.

[4] For an account of these books, see Joaquin de Villalba: Epidemiologica española, Madrid, 1802; J. Sarabia y Parto· Pediatria español., Madrid, 1927, xvi, 1–9.

[5] Sudhoff: Arch. f. Gesch. d. Med., Leipz., 1912–13, vi, 127.

[6] F. G. Crookshank: Influenza, London, 1922, 36, 72.

The story of their explorations is told in Hakluyt and Purchas' *Pilgrimes*. The Lusiad of Camoens tells of Vasco da Gama's voyage around the Cape to India, which destroyed the commercial power of Venice. Ormuz and Goa were taken by Albuquerque; footholds were obtained in Ceylon for cinnamon, in Sumatra for ginger and benzoin; in Banda and Amboyna for nutmegs and mace; in the Moluccas for cloves; in Timor for sandalwood; in Cochin China for aloes and pepper. Malacca was made a customs station and caravan trade was established in China, the source of camphor, cinnabar, musk and Smilax china, while rhubarb was obtained from Persia. The profits of this trade were enormous. Two ducats' worth of cloves from the Moluccas fetched 1680 ducats in London. The Spaniards also made communication with the Moluccas, but their spheres of influence were destined to be the Philippines, Mexico, and Peru. Manila was founded by them in 1566. Oviedo and Monardes described the plants of the West Indies and Peru. The revolt of the Netherlands against Philip II (1568–1648) brought the Dutch into the drug marts, but the period of their ascendancy was to be the 17th century.[1]

Hospital construction approached perfection in the 15th century, the greatest technical care being devoted to these structures, as in the hospital at Milan, which was opened in 1445, but not completed until 1456. A painting of Andrea del Sarto's at Florence represents the interior of a woman's hospital, probably for lying-in purposes. The fact that an isolation hospital and home for epileptics was founded at the cloister of St. Valentine at Rufach (Upper Alsace), in 1486, indicates that the disease was still regarded as contagious, in accordance with the old pseudo-Salernitan verse (Sudhoff[2]). Before the Reformation there were 77 hospitals in Scotland alone, but, after that period, hospitals connected with religious institutions began to die out in the northern countries. The lazar-houses also began to diminish in number, as leprosy was gradually stamped out. Three famous English institutions of the period were the Hospital of St. Mary of Bethlehem, which was converted from a monastery into an insane asylum ("Bedlam") in 1547; Bridewell, anciently a palace, which became a penitentiary and house of correction for vagabonds and loose women in 1553; and Christ's Hospital, formerly the Grey Friars Monastery, which was chartered in 1553 as a charity for fatherless and motherless children, and became the famous school of the "Blue Coat Boys," at which Charles Lamb and Coleridge were educated.

---

[1] See Tschirch: Pharmakognosie, Leipzig, 1910, i, 2. Abth., 716–772; and A. W. Linton: Jour. Am. Pharm. Assoc., Phila., 1916, v, 366, 471.

[2] Sudhoff: Arch. f. Gesch. d. Med., Leipz., 1912–13, vi, 449, 455.

THE SEVENTEENTH CENTURY; THE AGE OF INDIVIDUAL SCIENTIFIC ENDEAVOR

THE 17th century, the age of Shakespeare and Milton, Velasquez and Rembrandt, Bach and Purcell, Cervantes and Molière, Newton and Leibnitz, Bacon and Descartes, Spinoza and Locke, was preëminently a period of intense individualism, intellectual and spiritual. What happened to men like Servetus and Sir Thomas More, Bruno and Dolet, Spinoza and Uriel Acosta, Galileo and Copernicus, did but lessen the dominion of the professional theologian, whether Catholic, Protestant, or Jewish. The great philosophers of the time, Spinoza, Bacon, Descartes, Locke, were all of them concerned with different aspects of natural science, and the scientific labors of physicians themselves were strongly individualized. Yet with the decline of collectivism there necessarily went a corresponding decline in the things which had thrived under its régime, in particular, organized nursing, charitable care of the sick, and well-managed hospitals to this end.

In the 17th century the German people, decimated and torn asunder by the ravages of the Thirty Years' War, could do little for medicine, as Baas laments, and the highest distinction in this field was attained by England, Italy, and Holland. The age of the Armada and the Great Rebellion of 1642 was the most glorious period of English history, the age "of her greatest golden-mouthed sons," from Shakespeare, Milton, and the great line of Elizabethan dramatists, to Bacon and Locke, Raleigh and Sidney, Vaughan and More, Herrick and Crashaw, Boyle and Wren. In this age also flourished some of the greatest English mathematicians and astronomers, Newton and Wallis, Halley and Flamsteed, Briggs and Napier. The very beginning of the century (1600) is memorable for the appearance of an epoch-making work in the history of physics—the *De magnete*[1] of William **Gilbert** (1540–1603), who was physician to Queen Elizabeth and James I, and left his books and instruments to the Royal College of Physicians, where they were destroyed by the Great Fire of 1666.

---

[1] This work ranks beside Newton's *Principia* in that it threw overboard the current Arabian Nights' superstitions attributing the deflection of the compass needle to "magnetic mountains" or magnetic influences from the stars, and the ancient sailors' belief that garlic destroys a magnet's power. After a thorough-going investigation of the properties of the lodestone, Gilbert establishes the theorem that the earth itself is a gigantic spherical magnet, a proposition which has been the starting-point of all subsequent works on terrestrial magnetic variations, magnetic storms, and of the charting of the earth's magnetic fields by Halley, Gauss, and Sabine. The florid encomium of Dryden,

> Gilbert shall live till lodestones cease to draw,

is certainly true of human chronology, if not of geologic or sidereal time. Gilbert is also memorable for the discovery of frictional electricity, to which he gave its name from the amber (ἤλεκτρον) employed.

The greatest name in 17th century medicine is that of William Harvey (1578–1657), of Folkestone in Kent, who studied at Padua (1599–1603) as a pupil of Fabricius and Casserius, and whose work has exerted a profounder influence upon modern medicine than that of any other man save Vesalius. The world has "heard great argument" concerning the merits and status of the *De Motu Cordis*, but the following simple facts seem irrefutable and unassailable. The observation that the blood is in motion may have occurred to the first primitive man who ever cut open a live animal or saw a wounded artery. The idea that this motion is along a definite path may well have been entertained by any ancient Egyptian or Greek, as well as by some hypothetic native of Muscovy or Illyria in Harvey's day. Galen's false concept about the pores in the ventricular septum diverted all speculation into the wrong channel for fourteen centuries, and even Servetus, who came nearest the truth, could only see that some (not all) of the blood takes a circuit through the lungs. In the drawings which Vesalius had made, indicating the close proximity of the terminal twigs of arteries and veins,[1] the truth about the circulation was literally staring in the face of any observer who had eyes to see or wit to discover it. Even Erasistratus and Galen had ascribed synanastomoses to the capillaries, while the *sanguis cursus revocetur* of Celsus is as prophetic of the circulation as the *motu girando* of Leonardo. Yet anatomists continued to see everything in the light of the Galenic idea of shuttlewise ebb and flow between the closed arterial and venous systems. Cesalpinus, at best, made only a clever guess. Columbus, although he saw that the blood undergoes change in the lungs, in all likelihood appropriated the ideas of Servetus. But Harvey, who knew the whole history and literature of the subject, first made a careful review of existing theories, showing their inadequacy, and then proceeded, by experimental vivisection, ligation, and perfusion, to an inductive proof that the heart acts as a muscular force-pump in propelling the blood along,

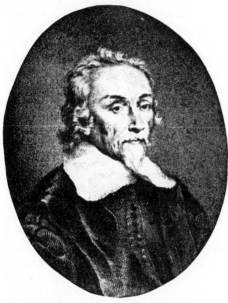

William Harvey (1578–1657).

---

[1] Vesalius: Fabrica, Basel, 1543, pp. 262, 268, 295, 305, 311, and plate opposite 312. See W. A. Locy: Biology and its Makers, New York, 1908, 49–50.

and that the blood's motion is continual, continuous, and in a cycle or circle. This was the starting-point of purely mechanical explanations of vital phenomena. The *crux* of Harvey's argument—that the actual quantity and velocity of the blood, as computed by him, make it physically impossible for it to do otherwise than return to the heart by the venous route—was the first application of the idea of measurement in any biologic investigation and, had he chosen to express this discovery in the language of algebra (by using the symbol of inequality), it would long since have taken its proper place as an application of mathematical physics to medicine. The importance of Harvey's work, then, is not so much the discovery of the circulation of the blood as its quantitative or mathematical demonstration. With this start, physiology became a dynamic science.

In asserting that the heart is a muscular force-pump, Harvey may have given credence to the "myogenic" theory of its autonomy (Galen), which, in any case, was soon displaced by Borelli's idea that the heartbeat has a neurogenic origin, the two views remaining in dispute to this day. In endeavoring to locate the motor power of the muscle itself, in his attempts to explain the function of the blood and the lungs, Harvey fell into a phase of medieval mysticism, derived from Aristotle's doctrine of the primacy of the heart,[1] as the seat of the soul (intelligence), which survives in the *pectora cœca* of Virgil and innumerable English usages.[2]

Aristotle had taught that the heart is the central abode of life, the mind, and the soul, the hearth from which emanates generative animal heat, something different from sterile, elemental fire, and that from the heart the blood and blood-vessels are derived. Harvey transferred this primacy to the blood, to which the heart is only of use as a pump to keep it in motion. He based this view upon his observation that in the primitive streak of the future embryo chick, the blood apparently exists before the pulse as a "leaping point," which, in cold eggs, warmed by pressure of a finger, "renews its pristine dance as though come back from Hades." The fibrillation of the auricle in a dying or quiescent heart he mistook for evidence that the blood is the last part of the body to die, although he had been the first to revive a quiescent heart by perfusion (wetting it with saliva). That the body is, in a sense, the expression of the soul, that the soul of man is, in Sherrington's phrase, the proper integration of his whole being, that "the soul is not in the body but the body in the soul," it was not given Harvey to see; for the "soul" of Aristotle and the ancients (ψυχή, *anima*) was a vague concept, existing in three kinds, the nutritive, the sensory, the intellectual. Following his master, Harvey, like Descartes, revived the ancient belief of Critias that "the soul is in the blood." The soul is not, as with Aristotle, associated with the innate generative heat, "analogous to the element of the stars," but the blood itself becomes the "innate warmth or first-born psychical heat," whence the circulation is the analogue of the circular motions of the heavenly bodies. The cause of the ventricular heart-beat is attributed to the distention of the ventricle through the contraction of the auricle, but the distention of the auricle must hark back to the Aristotelian ebullition of the hot blood; and although Harvey knew, with Galen, of the contractile power of muscle, and that the excised empty heart will beat outside the body, he could not explain the simultaneous contraction of both auricles. The doctrine of the heart as an automatic mechanism through contractile impulses passing from muscle-cell to muscle-cell, was to be the work of Gaskell and Engelmann. Finally, where Hippocrates had taught that something derived from the inspired air enters the heart and is distributed thence to the body,

[1] J. G. Curtis: "Harvey's Views on the Circulation," New York, 1915.

[2] For which, see Murray's New English Dictionary, Oxford, 1901, v, 159–167.

and Columbus had inferred that spirituous blood is concocted in the lungs by mixing with air, Harvey adhered to the old doctrine that the function of respiration was to cool the hot blood. He later saw that the fetus does not need this refrigeration, and finally gave up the problem as a "knotty subject." Thus Harvey, in his speculations, sided with the philosophers (Aristotle) rather than the physicians (Galen), which retarded the development of the true physiology of respiration for a long time.

The discovery of the circulation itself was the most momentous event in medical history since Galen's time. While it was opposed by the pedantic Riolanus,[1] Gassendi, Wormius, and others, it was soon supported by some of the ablest spirits of the period, including Rolfink, Sylvius de le Boë, Bartholinus, Ent, and Pecquet. Jan de Wale (1604–49), or **Walæus**, in particular, showed that incisions on either side of a ligature applied to an elevated blood-vessel cause the blood to ooze or to spurt, according to the direction in which it is flowing, thus affording a convincing proof of Harvey's discovery according to the laws of hydrodynamics (1640[2]).

The status of Harvey's other treatise, *De generatione animalium* (1651), is important in the history of embryology and a matter of frequent dispute. Some writers have tended to make Harvey's merits overshadow the just claims of men like Malpighi and von Baer. Of all pronouncements made, that of Huxley still seems the soundest and the best. In his demonstration of the circulation, Harvey was brought to a standstill at one point only, viz., the capillary anastomosis between arteries and veins, which, having no microscope, he could not see. In his investigation of the embryo, the minute and patient work of years was driven into an *impasse* for the same reason, while the manuscripts, containing his drawings and other results of experimental investigation of the embryo, were destroyed by the Parliamentary troopers who invaded his chambers in Whitehall in 1642. Long before Wolff and von Baer, Harvey maintained, as pure theory, the doctrine of "epigenesis"—that the organism does not exist encased or preformed in the ovum, but is evolved from it by gradual building up and aggregation of its parts; yet, through his inability to see microscopically, his idea of fecundation was totally wrong, for he believed the fertilization of the ovum to be something "incorporeal—as iron touched by the magnet is endowed with its own powers." By such mysticism, the famous dictum, *"Omne vivum ex ovo,"*[3] becomes self-contradictory, since it denies the continuity of the germ-plasm. Its true importance in Harvey's hands, was that it subverted the ancient concept that life is engendered out of corruption (or putrefaction)—an idea still familiar in the burial service.[4]

---

[1] Huxley styled Riolanus "a tympanitic Philistine, who would have been none the worse for a few sharp incisions."

[2] Walæus: Epistolæ duæ, 1640 [*In:* T. Bartholinus, Anatomia, Leyden, 1541, pp. 538–541 (plate)].

[3] First stated by Francesco Redi in the form, *"omne vivum ex vivo."*

[4] For a further discussion of this subject, see the admirable essay of W. K. Brooks in Bull. Johns Hopkins Hosp., Baltimore, 1897, viii, 167–174.

Besides the *De motu cordis* (Frankfurt, 1628[1]) and the treatise on generation (1651), we should mention the facsimile reprint of the MS. notes for the *"Praelectiones anatomicæ"* of the Lumleian foundation (1616), which shows that Harvey had completed his demonstration of the circulation and was lecturing on it at least twelve years before he printed it.

Harvey, as described by Aubrey, was of short stature, with bright black eyes and raven hair, "complexion like the wainscot," quick, alert, choleric, often fingering the handle of his dagger. The resemblance of his finely domed head to Shakespeare's is a matter of comment. Like many experimenters, he was but an indifferent practitioner. Yet he was no closet recluse, but highly honored in the worldly affairs of his day, as witness his publicity as Lumleian lecturer, his long association with Charles I, his assistance at the postmortem of "old Parr," or his merciful intervention in the affair, of the "late Lancashire witches." Although not a votary of the muse, he was, in the finest sense, a master of Dryden's "other harmony of prose." Read, for instance, his impressionistic account of the Bass Rock in a good English translation. It is a pen-picture which many a modern *prosateur* would be proud to sign. Having survived long enough to live down opposition and see his discovery accepted, Harvey prepared for approaching death with the cool self-possession of his race, meeting the end with a quiet resolution at the age of seventy-nine. While he was not ostentatious in piety, his will, with its liberal legacy to the poor of his native town, reveals the ideal English gentleman, tenderly solicitious of all his intimates, from Sir Charles Scarborough down to his humblest body servant.

Although Harvey's publication of his discovery caused an immediate falling off in his practice, its effect upon medical science was as definite and far reaching as that of the Fabrica. The 17th century was the great age of specialized anatomic research, and was notable for a long array of individual discoveries and investigations, nearly every one of which had a physiologic significance. Earliest among the achievements of the **post-Vesalian anatomists** was the clearing up of the old Galenical error that the veins and lymphatics of the intestines carried chyle to the liver.

This was dispelled by the discovery of the lacteal vessels in 1622[2] by Gasparo **Aselli** (1581–1626), who thought they went to the liver, the mistake being corrected by the discovery of the thoracic duct and receptaculum chyli by Jean **Pecquet** (1622–74[3]), and of the intestinal lymphatics and their connection with the thoracic duct (1651) by the Swede, Olof **Rudbeck**[4] (1630–1702). The latter discovery was disputed as to priority by the Dane, Thomas **Bartholinus** (1616–80[5]), in 1653, and

---

[1] Harvey's probable reason for printing the "Exercitatio" at Frankfurt a. M. was that this city was the center of the continental book-trade until after the Thirty Years' War, and that here, every semester, a book market was held at which all the new books of the world might be seen and which the leading London stationers attended (William Stirling).

[2] G. Aselli: De lactibus, Milan, 1627. This tract is illustrated by a variegated woodcut print in dull red, the first colored anatomic engraving of consequence.

[3] J. Pecquet: Experimenta nova anatomica, Paris, 1651.

[4] O. Rudbeck: Nova exercitatio anatomica exhibens ductus hepaticos aquosos et vasa glandularum serosa, Westeras, 1653.

[5] Th. Bartholinus: De lacteis thoracicis, Copenhagen, 1652.

by Jolyff, an Englishman, who did not publish his claims. Next came the finding of the pancreatic duct in Vesling's dissecting-room at Padua by his prosector, Georg Wirsung (1642[1]), to be followed, in order of time, by such important English discoveries as the antrum of **Highmore** (1651[2]), **Glisson's** capsule (1654[3]), **Wharton's** duct (1656[4]), the circle of **Willis** (1664[5]), Richard **Lower's** treatise on the heart as a muscle (1669[6]), Clopton **Havers'** discovery of the Haversian canals (1691[7]), and **Cowper's** glands (1694[8]). Italy won distinction in **Malpighi's** discovery of the capillary anastomosis in the lungs (1661[9]), which supplied the missing link in Harvey's demonstration; in Lorenzo **Bellini's** work on the structure of the kidneys (1662[10]), and in Antonio **Pacchioni's** description of the so-called Pacchionian bodies (1697[11]). Germany is memorable through Conrad Victor **Schneider's** classic treatise on the membranes of the nose (*De catarrhis*, 1660), **Meibom's** demonstration of the conjunctival glands (1666[12]), **Kerckring's** demonstration of the intestinal valvulæ conniventes (1670[13]), **Brunner's** discovery of the duodenal glands (1682[14]), and Holland by **Ruysch's** innovations in anatomic injecting (1665), and his many discoveries, e. g., the valves in the lymphatics (1665[15]); de **Graaf's** authentic account of the ovary and Graafian follicles (1672[16]), and **Nuck's** glands and ducts (1685[17]). Bishop Stensen (Nicholaus **Steno**) (1638–86), of Denmark, discovered the parotid duct (1662[18]) and Johann Conrad **Peyer** (1653–1712), of Switzerland, described the lymphoid follicles in the small intestine (1677[19]) which have such an important rôle in typhoid fever. In France, Joseph Guichard **Duverney** (1648–1730), professor of anatomy in Paris, made some important investigations of the inner structure of the ear which led him to write the first treatise on otology (1683); and Raymond **Vieussens** (1641–1716), professor at Montpellier, made various studies on the anatomy of the nervous system (*Neurologia universalis*, 1685), the position, structure, and pathology of the heart (1706–15) and the structure of the ear. Vieussens first correctly described the structure of the left ventricle, the course of the coronary vessels, the valve in the large coronary vein, and the *centrum ovale* in the brain. In his many autopsies he noted the significance of pericardial adhesions, and the relation of heart disease to asthma and hydrothorax (1672–6). He noted the diagnostic features of pericardial effusion and first described aortic insufficiency (1695) and mitral stenosis (1705), giving the character of the pulse and the pathologic features. He also discovered the fermentative effect of saliva and claimed priority in the discovery of an acid in the blood.

As the anatomic woodcut attained its height in the *Fabrica* of Vesalius, so the 17th century was the great age of copperplate engraving. Anatomic illustration reached a high point of perfection in the

[1] Recorded on a single rare copper plate of 1642..

[2] N. Highmore: Corporis humani disquisitio anatomica, The Hague, 1651.

[3] F. Glisson: De hepate, London, 1654.

[4] T. Wharton: Adenographia, London, 1656.

[5] T. Willis: Cerebri anatome, London, 1664.

[6] R. Lower: Tractatus de corde, London, 1669.

[7] C. Havers: Osteologia nova, London, 1691.

[8] W. Cowper: Glandularum quarundam . . . descriptio, London, 1702.

[9] M. Malpighi: De pulmonibus, Bologna, 1661.

[10] L. Bellini: De structura renum, Florence, 1662.

[11] A. Pacchioni: Diss. epistolaris de glandulis conglobatis duræ meningis humanæ, Rome, 1705.

[12] H. Meibom: De vasis palpebrarum, Helmstädt, 1666.

[13] Th. Kerckring: Spicilegium anatomicum, Amsterdam, 1670.

[14] J. C. Brunner: Glandulæ duodeni, Frankfort, 1687.

[15] F. Ruysch: Dilucidatio valvularum, The Hague, 1665.

[16] R. de Graaf: De mulierum organis generatione inservientibus, Leyden, 1672.

[17] A. Nuck: De ductu salivali novo, Leyden, 1685.

[18] N. Steno: Observationes anatomicæ, Leyden, 1662.

[19] J. C. Peyer: De glandulis intestinorum, Schaffhausen, 1677.

striking plates in such works as Govert **Bidloo**'s *Anatomia* (Amsterdam, 1685), Bernardino **Genga**'s *Anatomia* (Rome, 1691), the *Traité de la figure humaine*, of the painter Peter Paul **Rubens** (1577–1640), which was published over a century after his death (1773), the *Thesauri anatomici decem* (Amsterdam, 1701–16) of Frederik **Ruysch** (1638–1731), or the *Catoptron microcosmicum* (1613) of Johann **Remmelin** (1583–   ), of Ulm, one of the earliest anatomic atlases with superimposed plates.[1] A wonderful union of scientific accuracy with artistic perfection was attained in the *Tabulæ anatomicæ* (1627) of Giulio Casserio (1561–1616), or **Casserius**, one of Harvey's teachers at Padua, whose "eviscerated beauties," as Dr. Holmes has styled them, are as attractive in appearance as their dissected parts were held to be instructive to the student. These Correggio-like plates of Casserius were incorporated in the atlas (1627) of Adrian van Spieghel (1578–1625), or **Spigelius**, who wrote the letter-press around them and, in this way, is usually credited with the exquisite workmanship of the illustrations. Spieghel's name is associated with the Spigelian lobe of the liver. The 105 plates in Bidloo's Anatomy, of 1685, were actually plagiarized by William **Cowper** (1666–1709), whose *Anatomy of Human Bodies* (Oxford, 1698) is original only as to the text, and nine perfunctory plates supplied by Cowper himself.[2] For whimsical originality and exquisite delicacy of detail, the plates drawn by Frederik Ruysch (1638–1731[3]) deserve a special mention. Skeletons posed in quaintest attitudes, with appropriate mottoes of the *memento mori* variety attached, surrounded by strange reptiles, stuffed monsters, dried plants, and deep-sea creatures, constituted the favorite decorative scheme of the old Dutch anatomist, whose mortuary humors have been sublimated in Leopardi's dialogue.[4]

A very important outcome of Harvey's demonstration of the circulation was the art of **anatomic injection** which was advanced by Swammerdam, de Graaf, and Ruysch. Berengario da Carpi had filled the blood-vessels with tepid water, Stephanus with air, Eustachius with colored fluids, Malpighi and Glisson with ink, and Willis discovered the circle of Willis by injecting the brain with "*aqua crocata.*" Swammerdam aimed to get a preparation which could be injected warm and solidify afterward. He first tried suet but, in 1677, hit upon wax. In 1668, de Graaf introduced an improved syringe (*De usu syphonis*), and injected the spermatic vessels with mercury. In 1680, Swammerdam became convinced of the impiety of anatomy, and joined a fanatical religious sect. Before doing so, however, he published his method abroad, sending a preparation to the Royal Society in 1672, and especially training Ruysch to its use. The latter introduced the new feature of applying the microscope in the injection of the finer vessels. The process was subsequently

---

[1] Wrongly attributed by Baas to the publisher, Stephan Michelspacher. The idea of representing anatomic relations by superimposed pictures was already a feature of the Renaissance "*Fliegende Blätter*," was suggested by Vesalius, and utilized in L. Thurnheysser's *Confirmatio* (1567) and Bartisch's *Augendienst* (1583) (Choulant).

[2] Bidloo scolds about this in his "Gulielmus Cowper, criminis literarii citatus" (Leyden, 1700).

[3] Ruysch: Thesauri anatomici, Amsterdam, 1701–16.

[4] Giacomo Leopardi: "Dialogo di Federico Ruysch e delle sue mummie," in his collective works.

improved by Monro *primus*, Lieberkühn, Prochaska, Gerlach, and others, up to the time of Hyrtl's wonderful injections in two, three, and four different colors.[1]

The first crude attempt at **comparative anatomy** was made by Marco Aurelio Severino (1580–1656), whose *Zootomia Democritæ* (1645) antedates Malpighi, Leeuwenhoek, and Swammerdam. The woodcuts show the viscera of birds, fishes, and mammals, with some phases of their development, and slight as are the comparative features, the book is the only thing of its kind before the 18th century.

A remarkable comparative anatomist of the 17th century was Edward **Tyson** (1650–1708), of the University of Cambridge, who graduated there in 1678, and lectured on anatomy to the Barber-Surgeons up to 1699. Tyson was the first to publish elaborate monographs on the structure of the lower animals. His memoirs on the anatomy of the porpoise (1680), the rattlesnake (1683), and his dissections of such animal parasites as Lumbricus latus, Lumbricus teres (Ascaris lumbricoides), and Lumbricus hydropicus (hydatids), were a great advance on the *Anatomia porci* of Copho, the first adventure in this kind. The structures in the prepuce known as Tyson's glands are named after him, but his most important contribution to science is his *Orang-Outang, sive Homo Sylvestris* (1699), the first work of consequence in **comparative morphology**. In this book, Tyson compares the anatomy of man with that of monkeys, and between the two he placed what he thought was a typical pygmy—in reality, a chimpanzee—the skeleton of which is now in the South Kensington Museum of Natural History. This was the origin of the "missing-link" idea, which so many confuse with true Darwinism. Tyson's work concludes with a terminal essay setting forth that the satyrs, ægipans, cynocephali, and other mythical creatures of the ancients "are all either apes or monkeys, and not men, as formerly pretended."[2] This hypothesis was accepted by Buffon, and the existence of ape-like or pygmy races of men was doubted until Quatrefages (1887[3]) and Kollmann (1894[4]) proved that they have existed and do exist in space and time.

An important contribution to craniology was the idea of "cephalometric lines," conceived by the anatomist Spieghel, and which, says Meigs,[5] "may perhaps be regarded as constituting the earliest scientific attempt at cranial measurements." These *"lineæ cephalometricæ,"* when equal to each other in length, were Spieghel's criterion of a normally proportioned skull. Meigs observes that "in ascending the zoölogic scale these lines approximate equality just in proportion as the head measured approaches the human form."

The *Anthropometria* (1654) of Johann Sigismund Elsholtz (1623–88) is, as far as it goes, an illustrated scientific treatise following the lines laid down by Dürer.

The invention of the microscope[6] opened out a new departure for medicine in the direction of the invisible world, as Galileo's telescope had given a glimpse of the infinite vast in astronomy. The earliest of the **microscopists** was the learned Jesuit priest, Athanasius **Kircher** (1602–80), of Fulda, who was a mathematicisn, physicist, optician, Orientalist, musician, and virtuoso, as well as a medical man, and who was probably the first to employ the microscope in investigating the causes of disease. In his *Scrutinium pestis* (Rome, 1658), he not only details seven experiments upon the nature of putrefaction, showing how maggots and other living creatures are developed in decaying matter, but found that the blood of plague patients was filled with a countless brood of "worms," not perceptible to the naked eye, but to

---

[1] W. W. Keen: Early History of Practical Anatomy, Philadelphia, 1874, *passim*.

[2] See A. C. Haddon: History of Anthropology, New York & London, 1910, 15–16.

[3] A. Quatrefages: Les Pygmées, Paris, 1887.

[4] J. Kollmann: Pygmäen in Europa, 1894.

[5] J. A. Meigs: N. Am. Med.-Chir. Rev., 1861, v, 840, cited by Haddon.

[6] The early history of the microscope is somewhat complex and indefinite. An excellent account of it is that of Charles Singer: Proc. Roy. Soc. Med. (Sect. Hist. Med.), Lond., 1913–14, vii, 247–279.

be seen in all putrefying matter through the microscope. While Kircher's "worms," as Friedrich Loeffler[1] claimed, were probably nothing more than pus-cells and rouleaux of red blood-corpuscles, since he could not possibly have seen the *Bacillus pestis* with a 32-power microscope, yet it is quite within the range of possibility for him to have seen the larger microörganisms, and he was undoubtedly the first to state in explicit terms the doctrine of a *contagium animatum* as the cause of infectious disease. In his *Physiologia Kircheriana*, he was also the first to record an experiment in hypnotism or provoked catalepsy in animals (1680[2]). Another early worker with the microscope was Robert **Hooke** (1635–1703), a mechanical genius who anticipated many modern discoveries and inventions, and who laid claim to all that were thinkable in the period in which he lived. Hooke's *Micrographia* (London, 1665) contains many fine plates illustrating vegetable histology, and the first reference in science to the "little boxes or cells, distinct from one another," which the microscope revealed in these structures. This book probably inspired the works of Nehemiah **Grew** (1641–1712) on vegetable histology and physiology (1671, 1682). Grew, whom Haller styled "an industrious observer of nature in every direction," was probably the first to note the existence of sex in plants.

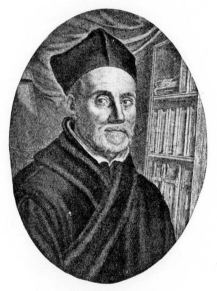

Athanasius Kircher (1602–80).

Jan **Swammerdam** (1637–80), whose interest in natural history was awakened by the fact that his father's apothecary shop contained the finest collection of exotic fauna in Amsterdam, was an expert in microscopic dissecting long before he began to study medicine. Having literally grown up among zoölogic speciments, he never practised, but devoted his short life to arduous and splendid labors in minute anatomy and embryology. His career was that of a scientific enthusiast who lived up to the principle *aliis inserviendo consumor*. His best work is contained in the huge *Bybel der Natuur* or History of Insects (Utrecht, 1669), which was Latinized by Gaub and prefaced by Boerhaave nearly 70 years later (Leyden, 1733). It comprised some 53 plates with

---

[1] Fr. Loeffler: Vorlesungen über die geschichtliche Entwicklung der Lehre von den Bacterien, Leipzig, 1887, pp. 1, 2.

[2] Kircher also treated of the curative powers of magnetism in his *Magnes sive de Arte Magnetica* (1643), which contains a description of "tarantism."

accurate life histories, giving the finer anatomy of the bees, the mayflies, the snail, the clam, the squid, and the frog. The drawings in this collection surpass all other contemporary work in exquisite delicacy and accuracy of detail. Swammerdam was the first to discern and describe the red blood-corpuscles (1658), discovered the valves of the lymphatics (1664), discovered the medico legal fact that the fetal lungs will float after respiration has taken place (1667) and, in 1677, devised the method of injecting blood-vessels with wax, which was afterward claimed by Ruysch. He was also no mean experimental physiologist, studying the movements of the heart, the lungs, and the muscles by plethysmographic methods which are almost modern.[1]

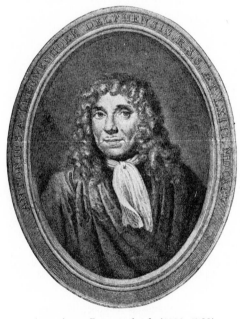

Antonj van Leeuwenhoek (1632–1723).

A very great microscopist was Antonj van **Leeuwenhoek,** of Delft (1632–1723), a draper and city hall janitor, who devoted his private leisure to the study of natural history. He had some 247 microscopes with 419 lenses, most of which were ground by himself, and once sent 26 microscopes to London as a present to the Royal Society, of which he became a Fellow in 1680. The directors of the East India Company sent him specimens, and even Peter the Great visited his collection in 1689. Leeuwenhoek was a strong man of marvelous industry. During his long life he sent as many as 375 scientific papers to the Royal Society and 27 to the French Academy of Sciences. These *Ontledengen en Ontdekkingen* (Leyden, 1696) contain, in addition to a vast amount of work on animalculæ and plant histology, many discoveries of capital importance to medicine. Leeuwenhoek was the first to describe the spermatozoa (originally pointed out to him by the student Hamen in 1674); gave the first complete account of the red blood-corpuscles (1674); discovered the striped character of voluntary muscle, the sarco-

---

[1] See W. Stirling, *Some Apostles of Physiology,* London, 1902, pp. 34, 135, with interesting illustrations. Hermann Klencke's fascinating "culturhistorischer Roman," entitled *Swammerdam oder die Offerbarung der Natur* (3 vols., Leipzig, 1860), is well worth reading for the light it throws upon social life and cultural conditions in the 17th century.

lemma, and the structure of the crystalline lens; was the first to see protozoa under the microscope (1675); found microörganisms in the teeth giving, for the first time, accurate figurations of bacterial chains and clumps as well as of individual spirilla and bacilli (September 17, 1683); and demonstrated the capillary anastomosis between the arteries and veins, which Malpighi had already seen in 1660 without attaching much importance to it. It was Malpighi's discovery and Leeuwenhoek's thorough work on the capillary circulation which finally completed Harvey's demonstration. In the effective study of Paul de Kruif,[1] with its pleasant Batavian flavor, Leeuwenhoek appears as a sturdy, valiant figure, "rich in saving common sense."

The greatest of the microscopists, however, was Marcello **Malpighi** (1628–94), the founder of histology, who was professor of anatomy at Bologna, Pisa, and Messina, and physician to Pope Innocent XII (1691–94). Famed in biology for his works on the anatomy of the silkworm and the morphology of plants, he made an epoch in medicine by his investigations of the embryology of the chick and the histology and physiology of the glands and viscera. The 12 plates accompanying his Royal Society memoirs, *De formatione pulli in ovo* (1673) and *De ovo incubato*, make him the founder of descriptive or iconographic

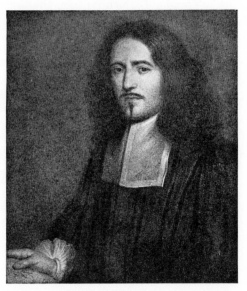

Marcello Malpighi (1628–94). (From the painting by Tabor, Royal Society.)

embryology, surpassing all other contemporary workers on the subject in the accurate notation of such minutiæ as the aortic arches, the head-fold, the neural groove, the cerebral and optic vesicles. Malpighi described the red blood-corpuscles in 1665 (seven years after Swammerdam) as "fat globules looking like a rosary of red coral." He discovered the rete mucosum or Malpighian layer of the skin, and proved that the papillæ of the tongue are organs of taste. Perhaps his greatest work is the *De pulmonibus* (1661), which overthrew the current conceptions of the pulmonary tissues as "parenchymatous," demonstrating their true vesicular nature, the capillary anastomosis between arteries and veins, and how the trachea terminates in bronchial filaments. Of his discov-

---

[1] P. de Kruif: Microbe Hunters, New York, 1926.

ery of the capillaries (1660), Fraser Harris has well said that "Harvey made their existence a logical necessity; Malpighi made it a histological certainty."[1] His work on the structure of the liver, spleen, and kidneys[2] (1666) did much to advance the physiologic knowledge of these viscera, and his name has been eponymically preserved in the Malpighian bodies of the kidney and spleen. This book also contains the first account of those lymphadenomatous formations (general enlargement of lymphatics with nodules in spleen[3]) which were fully described by Hodgkin, in 1832, and which Wilks, in 1856, called Hodgkin's disease, or pseudoleukemia. Malpighi's private life was embittered by the coarse personal attacks of his Pisan colleague Borelli, and by an old-time feud (of which he bore the brunt) between his family and a neighboring clan of the ominous and significant name of Sbaraglia. As in the case of Harvey and John Hunter, some of his best work was lost to posterity by the wanton destruction of valuable manuscripts. In personality, Malpighi was a gentle, fair-minded, sympathetic nature and, among the sick, a patient and devoted Asclepiad. The memory of Malpighi is one of "sweetness and light." Through his capacity for acute observation, he verified the remark of Thoreau that the laws of the universe are "forever on the side of the most sensitive." He is not only one of medicine's greatest names, but one of its most attractive personalities.[4]

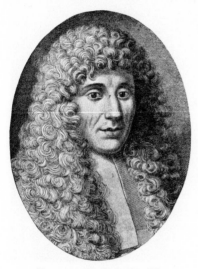

Francesco Redi (1626–97).

The first hard blow to the doctrine of spontaneous generation was dealt by the Italian naturalist, Francesco **Redi** (1626–97), of Arezzo, who confuted the idea, then current, that grubs and maggots develop spontaneously in decaying matter.[5] He exposed meat in jars, some of which were uncovered, the others being covered with parchment and wire gauze. In due course maggots appeared in the first two but, in the latter, developed on top of the gauze. This conclusive object-lesson settled the matter, so far as the spontaneous generation of visible creatures was concerned. Leeuwenhoek's discovery of bacteria and the

[1] Fraser Harris: Nature, Lond., June 29, 1911, 584.

[2] De viscerum structura, Bonn, 1666.

[3] De viscerum structura, Bonn, 1666, 125–126.

[4] A monument to Malpighi was unveiled at Crevalcuore on September 8, 1897.

[5] Experientia circa generationem insectorum, Amsterdam, 1671. Redi is also said to have been one of the first to analyze food.

yeast plant was to raise the question in another form and leave it in dispute until the time of Schwann and Pasteur.

Apart from the productions of the great micrographic or morphologic botanists of the 17th century—Hooke, Grew, Malpighi—some good work was done in systematic or taxonomic botany. The English botanist, John **Ray** (1627–1705), separated flowering from flowerless plants in his *Methodus plantarum* (London, 1682), and further divided the former class into monocotyledonous and dicotyledonous. Ray "stood for the whole plant," as the botanists say, in his classification. Robert Morison (1610–83), the first professor of botany at Oxford, made a systematic arrangement of plants in 18 classes, distinguishing them as woody and herbaceous, flower-bearing and fruit-bearing, after the fashion of Cesalpinus (1672–80).[1] Augustus Quirinus **Rivinus** (1652–1723), of Leipzig, classified the plants by the petals of the flowers (1691–99) and wrote an introduction to botany (1690), illustrating these works at great expense from drawings by capable artists. He wrote a *Censura* of officinal preparations (1701), in which he classifies all useless and undesirable remedies, studied the diseases of Leipzig and Wittenberg, and advanced a *pathologia animata*, ascribing most diseases to mites and minute worms, with a kind of anti-toxic therapy (Neuburger). Toward the end of the century the favorite system of classification of plants was that of Joseph-Pitton de **Tournefort** (1656–1708), the author of *Elemens de botanique* (1694) and *Institutiones rei herbariæ* (1700), in which he described 8000 species, arranged in 21 classes, according to the form of the corolla. This system held the field until the time of Linnæus who, like Tournefort, exaggerated the importance of the flower as a *fundamentum divisionis*.

The zoölogic investigations of Swammerdam, Leeuwenhoek, Redi, and Malpighi were supplemented by the work of Martin Lister (1638–1711), physician to Queen Anne; Oläus Worm (1588–1654), of the Wormian bones; Antonio Vallisnieri, and others who, like the great leaders of the time, devoted their attention mainly to entomology.

Medical theorizing in the 17th century naturally followed the trend of physiologic doctrine and this struck into two different paths, the iatromathematical and iatrochemical. Great advances in chemistry were made by Boyle, Willis, Mayow, and others, and the period was preëminently an age of discoveries in astronomy and mathematical physics.

Following the publication of Copernicus' treatise on the revolution of the planets around the sun (1543), Galileo had invented the telescope (1609), Kepler had stated the laws governing planetary motion (1609–18), and Newton's statement of the law of gravitation (1682) was followed by the publication of his *Principia* (1687). Logarithms were invented by Napier (1614) and Briggs (1617), Descartes founded analytic geometry (1637), Pascal published his contributions to the theory of probabilities (1654), while Newton simultaneously with Leibnitz, created the differential calculus (1665–66), and stated the binomial theorem (1669). Von Guericke, a burgomaster of Magdeburg, invented the air-pump (1641), Torricelli, the barometer (1643), and Hooke, a compound microscope (1665).

Such important discoveries and inventions as these were not without their influence upon medicine. The **Iatromathematical School**, by which all physiologic happenings were treated as rigid consequences of the laws of physics, was represented by Descartes, Borelli, and Sanctorius. The protagonists of the **Iatrochemical School**, which regarded all vital phenomena as chemical in essence, were van Helmont, Sylvius, and Willis.

The *De homine* (1662) of René **Descartes** is usually regarded as the first European text-book on physiology, although it was only a popular

---

[1] Morison: Præludia Botanica, 1672, and Plantarum Historia Universalis, 1680.

17

and theoretic exposition. In this regard, Sir Michael Foster has likened it to Herbert Spencer's *Principles of Biology.* It treats of the human body as a material machine, directed by a rational soul located in the pineal gland. Descartes grasped the dynamic importance of Harvey's discovery, but, like all his contemporaries, was a theoretical Galenist in ascribing the movements of the heart to its internal fire or heat. In his treatise, *Des passions de l'ame* (1649), he gives the first experiment in reflex action—the familiar one of making a person bat his eyes by aiming a mock blow at them—with the correct explanation of the phenomenon.

The mechanical view of the human organism was applied in a striking way by the Neapolitan mathematician, Giovanni Alfonso

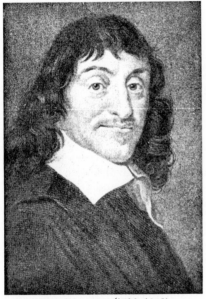

René Descartes (1596–1650).

Borelli (1608–79), whose *De motu animalium* (1680–81) at once suggests a follower of Harvey. A pupil of Galileo, Borelli profited much by a long association with his colleague Malpighi, and his rigorous mathematical reasoning swept away many current superstitions about the true functions of the muscles, the lungs, and the stomach. He treated locomotion, respiration, and digestion (the grinding and crushing action of the stomach) as purely mechanical processes. His ultimate theory of muscular action was dubious, as based upon the erroneous idea that a contracting muscle actually increases in bulk by reason of a fermentation started in its substance from a liquid discharged through the nerves—the *succus nerveus*— which was Borelli's substitute for the Galenic "animal spirits."[1] In this wise, Borelli originated the neurogenic theory of the heart's action, in virtue of which the heart-beat is attributed to the action of extrinsic or intrinsic nerves.

The extreme of iatrophysical doctrine in Italy was reached by Malpighi's pupil, Giorgio **Baglivi** (1668–1706), whom Clement XI appointed to the chair of medical theory in the Collegio della Sapienza. He experimented on muscular physiology and was the first to distinguish between smooth and striped muscle (1700).

---

[1] For the detailed history of this doctrine, see M. del Gaizo: Atti d. r. Accad. med. chir. di Napoli, 1916, lxx, 85–107. Borelli's *succus nerveus* is revived in the experiments of O. Löw: Pflüger's Arch., i, 1921, clxxxix, 239–242.

He pushed the mechanical allegory to the extent of dividing the human machine into innumerable smaller machines: likened the teeth to scissors, the chest to a bellows, the stomach to a flask, the viscera and glands to sieves, the heart and vessels to a waterwork (Neuburger[1]).

But directly he entered the sickroom, Baglivi dropped all these fine theories as the conclusions of immature laboratory logic. He was a highly successful physician, a true follower of Hippocrates at the bedside, and he died of hard work. "To frequent societies," he said, "to visit libraries, to own valuable unread books or shine in all the journals does not in the least contribute to the comfort of the sick."

The men of the Iatromathematical School knew or cared little about the new science of chemistry, and their efforts finally dwindled away into such sterile eccentricities as Archibald Pitcairn's attempt to base the whole of medical practice upon mechanical principles; Edward Barry's attempts to estimate a man's age from the frequency of his pulse, or Clifford Wintringham's efforts to weigh an individual spermatozoön. But the effect of mathematical and experimental physics upon medicine was manifested in more important ways, notably in the first attempt to put pulse counting and clinical thermometry upon a working basis.

In the 15th century Cardinal Cusanus (Nikolaus Krebs of Cues) (1401–64[2]), a Roman Catholic churchman who was a good mathematician, made

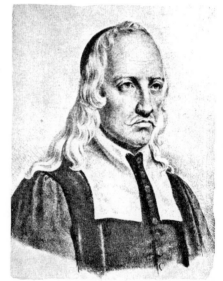

Giovanni Alfonso Borelli (1608–79).

some timely suggestions in his Dialogue on Statics (1450) as to the possible clinical value of weighing the blood and the urine, and of comparing the frequency of the pulse and respiration in disease with that in a normal control, as estimated by the clepsydra or water-clock. These, however, were not put into effect or carried into practice, and remained unnoticed by succeeding generations. Between 1593 and 1597, as Weir Mitchell notes,[3] Galileo had invented a rude thermometer or thermoscope, and as early as 1600, Kepler had used pulse counting to time his astronomic observations. Later, Galileo conceived the idea

---

[1] Neuburger: Puschmann's Handbuch, Jena, 1903, ii, 62.

[2] See C. Binz: Deutsche med. Wochenschr., Leipz. u. Berl., 1898, xxiv, 640; and J. J. Walsh: Old-Time Makers of Medicine, New York, 1912, pp. 336–348.

[3] See S. Weir Mitchell: The Early History of Instrumental Precision in Medicine, New Haven, 1892, p. 10 et seq.

of using his own pulse to test the synchronous character of a pendulum's vibrations, which led him to the converse proposition of measuring the rate and variation of the pulse by a pendulum, much as a metronome is used to check the tempo of music. These ideas were appropriated and utilized in a remarkable way by the celebrated Paduan professor, Santorio Santorio (1561–1636), called Sanctorius. In his commentary on the first book of the Canon of Avicenna (Venice, 1625), Sanctorius describes a clinical thermometer[1] and a pulsilogium, or pulse-clock, of his own devising, inventions which soon passed into the limbo of forgotten things for nearly a hundred years. Sanctorius

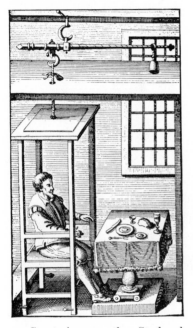

was also the clever inventor of instruments for extracting stones from the bladder and foreign bodies from the ear, as also a trocar, a cannula, and a hygroscope. His medical fame today is best associated with the fact that he founded the physiology of metabolism through his experiments and data upon what he called the "insensible perspiration" of the body. The frontispiece plate in later editions of his Ars de statica medicina (1614), representing the famous Paduan seated in his steelyard chair, in act to weigh himself for a metabolism experiment after a meal, is a familiar human document in the annals of medical illustration.

The physical theory of vision, which might be styled the ground-bass of ophthalmology, owes its development mainly to the work of great astronomers and physicists.

Sanctorius on the Steelyard. (From his Ars de statica medicina, Leyden, 1711.)

The Ad Vitellionem, Paralipomena, of the astronomer Kepler (Frankfort, 1604), contains a treatise on vision and the human eye in which is shown for the first time how the retina is essential to sight, the part the lens plays in refraction, and that the convergence of luminous rays before reaching the retina is the cause of myopia. In the Dioptrica of René Descartes (1637) the eye is compared to a camera obscura, and its accommodation is shown to be due to changes in the form of the lens. It was Edme Mariotte (died 1684) who proved that a luminous eye is due to reflection of light, and discovered the blind spot in the retina (1668). A remarkable pioneer in physiologic optics was the Jesuit astronomer, Christoph Scheiner

---

[1] Drebbel is usually regarded as the inventor of the air thermometer, Galileo, of the alcohol thermometer, and Fahrenheit (1710–14), of the mercurial thermometer.

(died 1650) of Vienna. In 1587, Aranzi had demonstrated the reversal of the image projected on the retina in cattle, and had shown the lateral entry of the optic nerve. In his *Oculus* (Mühldorf, 1619), Scheiner gave an ingenious demonstration of how images fall on the human retina, noticed the changes in curvature of the lens during accommodation, and illustrated accommodation and refraction by the pin-hole test which bears his name.

The founder of the **Iatrochemical School** was the Belgian mystic, Jean Baptiste **van Helmont** (1577–1644) who, before he studied medicine, was some time a Capuchin friar. Like his master Paracelsus, van Helmont believed that each material process of the body is presided over by a special archæus or spirit (which he calls Blas), and that these physiologic processes are in themselves purely chemical, being due in each case to the agency of a special ferment (or Gas). Each Gas is an instrument in the hands of its special Blas, while the latter are presided over by a sensory-motive soul (*anima sensitiva motivaque*), which van Helmont locates in the pit of the stomach, since a blow in that region destroys consciousness. He was the first to recognize the physiologic importance of ferments and gases, particularly of carbonic acid, which he described as *gas sylvestre;* and his knowledge of the bile, the gastric juice, and the acids of the stomach was considerable. He gives a fair account of the nature of wound infection in the jargon of his time, and had some notion of immunity and possible immune sera (Osler).

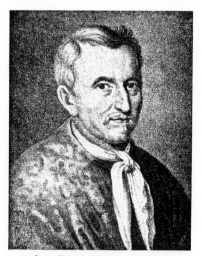

Jean Baptiste van Helmont (1577–1644).

His claims to the discovery of carbon dioxid are somewhat vitiated by the fact that he regarded this "gas sylvestre," formed in vinous fermentation (CO_2) as identical with the gas in the Grotto del Cane in Italy, and with the *dunste*, or deadly vapor of burning charcoal, which is carbon monoxid (CO). Van Helmont introduced the gravimetric idea in the analysis of urine, and actually weighed a number of twenty-four-hour specimens, but drew no deductions of value from his measurements.

Physiological chemistry was divested of many of the fantastic van Helmont trappings by the Leyden professor, Franciscus de le Boë, or **Sylvius** (1614–72), and his pupils: Willis, de Graaf, Stensen, and Swammerdam. Sylvius did for Harvey's ideas what Paré had done for those of Vesalius. He was, as Foster says, an expositor, rather than an investigator, of science; but even as a teacher, and there were none greater in his time, he was wonderfully fertile in original ideas, *e. g.*, as to the function of the ductless glands, acidosis, the thermal and tactile senses, and other things of moment today. He was the first to distinguish between conglomerate and conglobate glands, but his relation to the Sylvian fissure, as described in his *Disputationes medicæ* (1663), is obscure. He regarded digestion as a chemical fermentation, and recognized the importance of the saliva and the pancreatic juice. His best service to medicine was that he took a firm stand upon the ultimate identity of organic and inorganic processes in chemistry, and that, in his little infirmary of twelve beds at Leyden, he was one of the first to introduce ward instruction in medical education.

The Dutch followers of Sylvius (Stephan Blankaart and others) recommended enormous quantities of the newly imported novelties (tea and coffee) as panaceas for acidity and blood-purifiers.

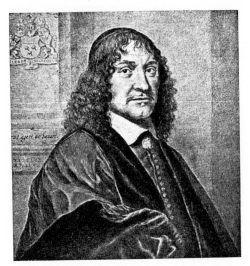

The universities of Jena and Wittenberg espoused his doctrines, and Daniel Sennert, at Wittenberg, was one of his warmest adherents. In Paris, Vieussens, who was the first to make chemical examinations of the blood, was his only follower. The Paris Faculty and Gui Patin condemned his system as the *"nouveauté impertinenté du sècile."*[1]

The leading English exponent of chemiatry was Thomas **Willis** (1621–75), a Wiltshire farmer's son, who graduated from Christ Church College in 1639, was Sedleian Professor of Natural Philosophy at Oxford in 1660 and, moving to London in 1666, acquired the largest

Franciscus Sylvius (1614–72).

fashionable practice of his day. Willis' *Cerebri Anatome* (1664), in the preparation of which he was greatly indebted to Richard Lower and to Sir Christopher Wren (who illustrated it), was the most complete and accurate account of the nervous system which had hitherto appeared. It contains the classification of the cerebral nerves, which held the field up to the time of Soemmerring, the first description of the eleventh cranial (spinal accessory) nerve or "nerve of Willis," and of the hexagonal network of arteries at the base of the brain which is called by his name. Willis accepted the cerebrum as the organ of thought, but argued (from experimental lesions of the cerebellum) that it is the center of vitality, the controller of the involuntary movements of the heart, lungs, stomach, and intestines; and giving free rein to his fancy, he

---

[1] Neuburger: *Op. cit.*, p. 58.

assigned perception to the corpora striata, imagination to the corpus callosum, memory to the cortical gyri, and instinct to the mid-brain. This faulty reasoning, due in part to the clumsiness of Willis' experimental technic and his ignorance of the actual anatomy of his laboratory animals, has led some writers, Sir Michael Foster for instance, to overlook his just merits as a clinician. Willis was, like Sydenham, Heberden, and Bright, a remarkable example of the capacity of the English physicians for close, careful clinical observation. He made the best qualitative examination of the urine which was possible in his time, and was the first to notice the characteristic sweetish taste of diabetic urine, thus

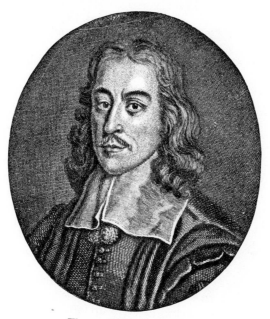

Thomas Willis (1621–75).

establishing the basic principle for the diagnosis between diabetes mellitus and insipidus. In his *London Practice of Physic* (1685, p. 431), he described the Erb-Goldflam symptom-complex (myasthenia gravis). In his *De febribus*, he gave the first account of epidemic typhoid fever as it occurred in the troops of the Parliamentary Wars (1643[1]). He was also the first to describe and name puerperal fever. His works on nervous diseases (1667[2]) and on hysteria (1670[3]) are justly esteemed for their many striking clinical pictures, of which his description of general paralysis (1667) is perhaps the most important. A good example of his talent for locating and isolating important facts is his observation of a

---

[1] De febribus, London, 1659, 171 *et seq.*
[2] Pathologiæ cerebri et nervosi generis specimen, Oxford, 1667.
[3] Adfectionum quæ dicuntur hystericæ, etc., Leyden, 1670.

deaf woman who could hear only when a drum was beating. This phenomenon is known in modern otology as *paracusis* (or *hyperacusis*) *Willisii*, the test for paracutic hearing being made in the clinics by placing a vibrating tuning-fork on the head of a deaf patient or by means of the "noise machine" recently devised by the Viennese otologist, Robert Bárány. Willis' *Pharmaceutice rationalis* (1674) gives a valuable epitome of the materia medica of his time.[1]

Important work in the **physiology of digestion** was done by the Dutchman de Graaf, and the Swiss physiologists, Peyer and Brunner.

Regner **de Graaf** (1641–73), of Schoonhaven, Holland, was the first to study the pancreas and its secretions before the time of Claude Ber-

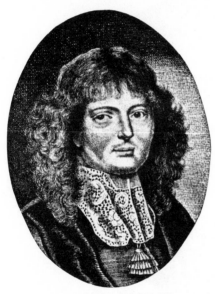

Regner de Graaf (1641–73).

nard. In his disputation on the nature and use of the pancreatic juice (1664[2]) he describes his method of collecting the secretion by means of a temporary pancreatic fistula, noting the small quantity of the juice secreted and its acid character. The monograph is embellished with a picture of the dog employed, showing receptacles depending from a parotid and a pancreatic fistula. De Graaf also employed an artificial biliary fistula to collect the bile, in which he was preceded, however, by Malpighi. In 1668[3] he published a classic account of the testicle, which he described as made up of small tubes folded up into lobules. This work also contains an essay on the use of clysters, which were then coming into fashion. In 1672 appeared his work on the ovary, containing the first account of the structures which Haller called, in honor of his name, the Graafian vesicles (*vesiculæ Graafianæ*).

The name of Johann Conrad **Peyer** (1653–1712), of Schaffhausen, Switzerland, will always be associated with the lesions of Peyer's patches in typhoid fever, although he held that these glands, which he discovered in 1677,[4] were not conglobate or lymphatic, as we now

---

[1] The second part has been praised by Osler (Practice of Medicine, 8th ed., 1912, p. 119) for its description of whooping-cough.

[2] De Graaf: Disp. med. de natura et usu succi pancreatici, Leyden, 1664.

[3] De Graaf: De virorum organis generationi inservientibus, Leyden, 1668.

[4] Peyer: Exercitatio anat. med. de glandulis intestinorum earumque usu et affectionibus, Schaffhausen, 1677.

know them but conglomerate, secreting, as he believed, a digestive juice. He gives an interesting cut of the Peyer glands in the small intestine and of the solitary follicles in the large intestine. He also wrote on the physiology of rumination (*Merycologia*, 1685).

Johann Conrad **Brunner** (1653–1727), of Diessenhofen, Switzerland, discovered Brunner's glands in the duodenum of dogs and man in 1672, publishing his results in 1687.[1] He believed that they secreted a juice similar to that of the pancreas. He also made experimental excisions of the spleen and pancreas in the dog in 1683,[2] keeping the animal alive, with normal digestion, for some time after. In one of these excisions he found that the dog had extreme thirst and polyuria, which would seem to be a pioneer experiment on the internal secretions of the pancreas.

William **Croone** (1633–84), of London, a Cambridge graduate of 1662, succeeded Sir Charles Scarborough as lecturer on the anatomy of the muscles to the Company of Surgeons (1670–84) and is memorable for two monographs on muscular physiology (1667) and embryology of the chick (1671–2), which were far in advance of their time. From the fortune accumulated by his lucrative practice his widow endowed the famous Croonian lectures.

A prominent German physiologist of this period was Johann **Bohn** (1640–1719), of Leipzig, who experimented upon the decapitated frog (1686[3]) in an entirely modern spirit, declaring the reflex phenomena to be entirely material and mechanical, as against the current view of "vital spirits" in the nerve-fluid. The remarkable experiments of Boyle, Redi and Swammerdam on decapitated (decerebrated) snakes, insects, turtles, birds and mammals, led to the same conclusion, and were neatly summarized in Butler's sneer:

> "A convert's but a fly that turns about,
> After his head's pulled off, to find it out."

Bohn showed that the pancreatic juice is not acid and that the nerves do not contain a "nerve-juice." As professor of anatomy (1668) and city physician (1691) at Leipzig, then famous for the medicolegal decisions of its faculty, Bohn made his mark in forensic medicine, particularly by his treatise on lethal wounds (1689).

Niels **Stensen** (1648–86), or Steno, of Copenhagen, was, like Athanasius Kircher, a physician-priest and, also like him, a man of wonderful versatility. He was at once a great anatomist, physiologist, geologist, and theologian, and became Bishop of Titiopolis some time after his conversion from the Lutheran to the Catholic faith in 1667. In anatomy, his name is permanently associated with the excretory duct of the parotid gland (Steno's duct), which he discovered in the sheep

---

[1] Brunner: De glandulis in duodeno intestino detectis, Heidelberg, 1687.

[2] Brunner: Experimenta nova circa pancreas, Amsterdam, 1682.

[3] Bohn: Circulus anatomico-physiologicus, Leipzig, 1686, 460. Cited by Neuburger.

(1661[1]). In the same year he investigated the glands of the eye and, in 1664,[2] came his observations on muscles and glands in which he recognizes the muscular nature of the heart. His Paris discourse on the anatomy of the brain (1669[3]), a violent philippic against the physiological ineptitudes of Willis, argues that it is idle to speculate about cerebral function when so little is known of its actual structure. Stensen's further studies on the physiology of muscles (1667[4]) treat the subject from a purely mechanical and mathematical standpoint. Using the microscope, he saw the muscles as parallelepiped bundles of structural units (fascicles), subdivided into minute fibrils, with the tendon as a tetragonal prism. Explaining contraction *more geometrico*, he reasoned that the total response of a muscle is the summation of the tensile forces developed in each unit (*fibra matrix*), and opposed the view entertained by Borelli that the apparent increase in size of a muscle is due to the influx of hypothetic juices. Animal spirits and nerve-juices he declared to be "mere words, meaning nothing." Stensen was also one of the leading founders of geology. In 1883, a bust over his tomb, in the Basilica San Lorenzo in Florence, was erected and unveiled by geologists of all nations. His treatise, *De solido intra solidum* (1669), contains, after Avicenna and Fracastorius, the most important work on the production of strata, fossils, and other geologic formations. He was led to geology by the dissection of the head of a shark, the teeth of which made it clear to him that the "glossopetræ" found in Tuscany were, in reality, fossil teeth. The story of Stensen's conversion to Catholicism by a sister of the faith, and of his devotion of the better half of his short life to the furthering of its cause alone, is one of the romantic episodes of human history.

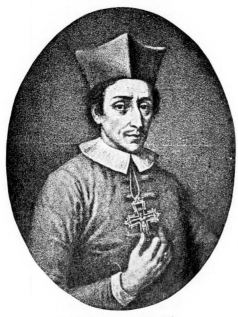

Niels Stensen (1648–86).

[1] Steno: Observationes anatomicæ, Leyden, 1662.

[2] De musculis et glandulis observationum specimen, Copenhagen, 1664.

[3] Discours sur l'anatomie du cerveau, Paris, 1669.

[4] Elementorum myologiæ specimen, seu musculi descriptio geometrica, Florence, 1667.

Francis **Glisson** (1597–1677), of Rampisham, Dorsetshire, was a graduate of Cambridge and Regius Professor of Physic in that University for some forty years. He was also one of the founders of the Royal Society and president of the Royal College of Physicians (1667–69). As anatomist, physiologist, and pathologist, Glisson was highly praised by Haller and Virchow, and his name is famous for four important things: He wrote the original and classic account of infantile rickets, with an early note of Barlow's disease (1650[1]); he gave the first accurate description of the capsule of the liver investing the portal vein (Glisson's capsule) and its blood-supply (1654[2]); and employed suspension in spinal deformities (1660). Before Haller, he introduced the concept of "irritability" as a specific property of all human tissues (1677[3]). Glisson's view of this property was, however, purely metaphysical, bound up with the current notions about "vital spirits" and, in consequence, it had no effect upon the physiology of his time.

The most brilliant outcome of Harvey's experimental method was in the clearing up of the obscure matter of the **physiology of respiration,** which up to the time of Lavoisier was entirely the work of English scientists. Before Harvey's day, men still believed, with Galen, that the object of respiration was to cool the fiery heart; the purpose of the chest movements being to introduce air for generating vital spirits by the pulmonary vein, and to get rid of the heart's smoky vapors by the same channel. This Galenic notion was not a mere piece of symbolism, as in Richard Crashaw's poem on St. Teresa (The Flaming Heart), but was part and parcel of actual belief about the physics of the circulation. "Before Harvey's time," says Allbutt, "respiration was regarded not as a means of combustion but of refrigeration. How man became such a fiery dragon was the puzzle." Harvey's demonstration showed that the blood is changed from venous to arterial in the lungs, but beyond that point, as even Pepys has recorded in his Diary, no one could tell how or why we breathe.[4] The successive steps in what Sir Clifford Allbutt calls "the pathetic quest for oxygen," were as follows: First, the distinguished chemist Robert **Boyle** (1627–91) made experiments with flames and animals *in vacuo* (1660), demonstrating that air is necessary for life as well as for combustion.[5] Next, Robert **Hooke** (1635–1703), in 1667,[6] showed, by attaching a bellows

---

[1] Glisson: De rachitide sive morbo puerili qui vulgo the rickets dicitur, tractatus, London, 1650. The earlier tract of Daniel Whistler: De morbo puerili Anglorum (1645) is without originality and was probably based upon information gained from Glisson (Norman Moore). [2] Glisson: Anatomia hepatis, London, 1654.

[3] Glisson: De ventriculo et intestinis, London, 1677.

[4] "But what among other fine discourse pleased me most was Sir G. Ent about Respiration; that it is not to this day known or concluded among physicians, nor to be done either, how the action is managed by nature, or for what use it is," Pepys' Diary, Mynors Bright's ed., London, 1900, v, 191.

[5] R. Boyle: Nova experimenta physico-mechanica de vi aëris elastica, Rotterdam, 1669.

[6] R. Hooke: "A supply of fresh air necessary for life," Phil. Tr., 1667, Lond., 1700, iii, 66.

to the *arteria aspera* (trachea) of a dog with opened thorax, that artificial respiration can keep the animal alive without any movement of either chest or lungs. This experiment, which had also been performed by Vesalius, proved that the essential feature of respiration is not in its intrinsic movements, but in certain blood changes in the lungs. The next step was made by Richard **Lower,** of Cornwall (1631–91), an able physiologist and successful practitioner, who was the first to perform direct transfusion of blood from one animal to another (February, 1665[1]), and who, with Schneider, overthrew the old Galenic idea (even

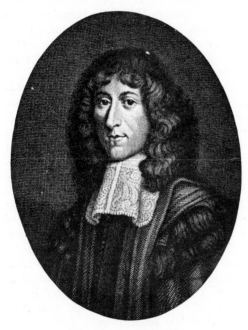

John Mayow (1643–79).

upheld by Vesalius) that the nasal secretions originate in the pituitary body (1672[2]). About 1669,[3] Lower injected dark venous blood into the insufflated lungs, and concluded that its consequent bright color was due to the fact that it had absorbed some of the air passing through the lungs. Finally John **Mayow** (1643–79), another Cornishman, demonstrated, in a series of convincing experiments, that the dark venous blood is changed to bright red by taking up a certain ingredient in this air which, as being a constituent of niter (KNO_3), he termed the igneo-aërial particles or nitro-aërial spirit of air. Mayow was thus, in a sense, very close to the actual discovery of oxygen, and he fully grasped the idea that the object of breathing is simply to cause an interchange of gases between the air and the blood, the former giving up its nitro-aërial spirit (oxygen) and taking away vapors engendered by the blood. He saw that the maternal blood sup-

[1] R. Lower: "A method of transfusing blood," Phil. Tr., 1666, Lond., 1700, iii, 226–232. Denys of Paris was the first to transfuse in man (June 15, 1667), after which Lower performed the operation on Arthur Coga, before the Royal Society (November 23, 1667). The case of Innocent VIII (1492) is probably apocryphal. (See Jour. Am. Med. Assoc., Chicago, 1914, lxii, 553, 633.)

[2] C. V. Schneider: De catarrhis, Wittenberg, 1660–62. R. Lower: "Dissertatio de origine catarrhi in qua ostenditur illum non provenire a cerebro," in his Tractatus de corde, London edition of 1680, 163–175. This discovery localized catarrh in the air-passages and did away with the endless recipes for "purging the brain" (Neuburger).

[3] R. Lower: Tractatus de corde, London, 1669.

plies the fetus not only with food, but with oxygen (*nitro-aër*), and was the first to locate the seat of animal heat in the muscles, an idea which fell into abeyance until Helmholtz demonstrated it anew in 1845. He also discovered the double articulation of the ribs with the spine, and discussed the function of the intercostal muscles in an entirely modern spirit. Mayow was a chemist and physiologist of true genius. His *Tractatus Quinque* (1674) deservedly ranks today with the very best of the English medical classics. Gotch has shown how his ideas were disregarded and discredited through the errors in a garbled English abstract of his Latin text, which some literary hack had made for the Royal Society.[1]

In the latter half of the 17th century, **internal medicine** took an entirely new turn in the work of one of its greatest figures, Thomas Sydenham (1624–89), of Winford Eagle, the reviver of the Hippocratic methods of observation and experience, who ennobled the practice of physic through those qualities of piety, good humor, and good sense, which Edmund Burke declared to be the genius of the English race. Educated at Oxford and Montpellier, but afterward a Puritan captain of horse in the civil wars, a "trooper turned physician," as he was called, Sydenham's relation to medicine was that of a man of action. A typical Saxon, by no means devoid of *nil admirari*, yet rich in the Saxon's special gift of manly independence and "saving common sense," he stood

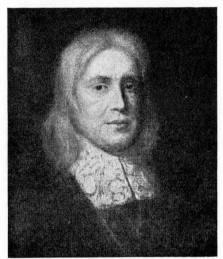

Thomas Sydenham (1624–89). (From a painting by Mary Beale.)

apart from all the medical theorizing and scientific experimentation of his time, disregarded all his predecessors save Hippocrates, and knew nothing whatever of Vesalius, Harvey, Malpighi, or Mayow. His four favorite books were Hippocrates, Cicero, Bacon, and Don Quixote, and his personal attitude toward his contemporaries was indifferent or scornful. This narrowness and aloofness cost him dear, for he complained bitterly of the neglect and opposition of his own profession, yet it was the very secret of his success as an internist. His theory of medicine was simple. The human mind is limited and fallible, and to it final causes must remain inscrutable. Scientific theories are, therefore, of little value to the practitioner since,

---

[1] Sir Francis Gotch: Two Oxford Physiologists, Oxford, 1908, pp. 35–38. See, also, the brilliant chapters on the physiology of respiration in Sir Michael Foster's "Lectures on the History of Physiology," Cambridge, 1901, 174–199; 224–254.

at the bedside, he must rely upon his powers of observation and his fund of experience. Sydenham regarded disease as a developmental process, running a regular course, with a natural history of its own. Each disease belonged to a certain definite species, which could be described and classified as a botanist does plants.[1] Pathology for him was summed up in the Hippocratic theory of concoction of the humors of the body and the subsequent discharge of the *materies morbi*. Hippocrates was his pattern, and more than any other medical man he resembles the Father of Medicine in his mode of portraying disease and his dignified ethical regard for his patients, holding himself "answerable to God" for their care and, himself a martyr to stone and gout, a fellow-sufferer along with them. This power of imaginative sympathy, a trait not usually found in the self-centered Saxon, is prominent in Sydenham's portrait as painted by Mary Beale, representing a Puritan in bearing, like Cromwell or Milton, yet a beautiful face withal, the fine brow, melancholy eye, and sensitive mouth revealing a nature stoical rather than harsh, sad rather than sour, as of a Puritan under protest.

Sydenham's theory of "epidemic constitutions," or *genius epidemicus*, maintains that contagious diseases are influenced by cosmic or atmospheric influences which may change their type—that they may spring from miasms from the bowels of the earth, that they may have long periods of evolution and seasonal variations, and that some diseases may be mere variants or subvarieties of others.[2] Some features were revived in von Pettenkofer's theory of the "soil" (*Boden*) and "soil-water," but the best part of its survives in Pasteur's theory of the origin of epidemics from strengthening or weakening of viruses by environmental conditions. Sydenham's studies in the geography and meteorology of epidemic diseases and the rhythmic periodicity of their recurrence[3] make him, with Hippocrates and Baillou, one of the main founders of epidemiology. Studies of the relation of disease to the weather, a matter of comment even in the diaries of Pepys, Evelyn and Swift, continued to be made even up to the time of Bright. The clinical reputation of Sydenham rests today upon his first-hand accounts of diseases, such as the malarial fevers of his time, gout, scarlatina, measles, bronchopneumonia (*peripneumonia vera*), and pleuropneumonitis (*peripneumonia notha*), dysentery, chorea, and hysteria. His treatise on gout (1683[4]) is esteemed his masterwork. In 1672 he

---

[1] "Primo expedit ut morbi omnes ad definitas ac certas species revocentur, eadem prorsus diligentia ac ἀκριβεία qua id factum videmus a botanicis scriptoribus in suis phytologiis." Cited by Neuburger.

[2] See M. Greenwood: Proc. Roy. Soc. Med. (Sect. Epidem.), 1919, xii, 55–76; F. G. Crookshank: *Ibid.*, 1920, xiii, 159–184; and Sir. H. Rolleston: Jour. Am. Med. Assoc., Chicago, 1920, lxxiv, 1495–1497.

[3] For the mathematical theory of periodicity see Sir Ronald Ross, Proc. Roy. Soc., Lond., 1916, ser. A, xcii, 204–230, and the curves in A. Magelssen's article, "Genius epidemicus," Janus, Amst., 1906, xi, 561–575.

[4] Tractatus de podagra et hydrope, London, 1683.

described the articular and muscular pains of dysentery and, in 1676, its seasonal aspects during 1669–72. In 1675 he gave a full account of scarlatina as it prevailed in London (1661–75), separating the disease from measles and identifying it by its present name. The *Dissertatio Epistolaris* (1682) contains his classic account of hysteria; and his differentiation of chorea minor is to be found in his *Schedula Monitoria* (1686). In therapeutics, Sydenham popularized the use of Peruvian bark and was the innovator of fresh air in sickrooms, horseback riding for consumptives, cooling draughts in small-pox, steel tonics in chlorosis, and the liquid opiate which bears his name. His prescriptions consisted largely of vegetable simples, and he avoided the filthy ingredients recommended, even in the London Pharmacopœia of his time. He was an extensive but not an intensive blood-letter, applying venesection in almost every disease known to him—but with discretion. His *Processus integri* (1692), containing his therapeutic scheme, was the *vade mecum* of the English practitioner for more than a century. An Oxford enthusiast is said to have committed it to memory. The influence of Sydenham lasted unto the advent of the Vienna School and beyond it.

A famous follower and protégé of Sydenham was Walter **Harris** (1647–1732), of Gloucester, physician-in-ordinary to Charles II and William III. His treatise on acute diseases in infants (1689), remarkable for some prevision of the doctrine of acidosis, was reprinted and translated many times and held the field until the days of Underwood (1784).

A group of important monographs which deserve mention in connection with Sydenham's work comprises Tobias Cober's *Observationes castrenses* (1606), noting the relation between typhus fever (*morbus Hungaricus*) and pediculosis; the *De mirabili strumas sanandi* (1609) of André du Laurens, an early historic record of the King's Evil, in which the contagiousness of scrofula is maintained (*struma contagiosus morbus est*); Roger Coke's autopsy of typhoid fever (Record Office, London, 1612); Spieghel's extensive account of malarial fever (*De semitertiana*, 1624); Daniel Sennert's treatises on scurvy (1624), dysentery (1626), and fevers (1627[1]); Diemerbroek on the plague (1646[2]); Glisson's original account of rickets (1650[3]); Thuillier's experimental investigation of ergotism (1657[4]); Höfer on cretinism (1657[5]); Wepfer on the hemorrhagic nature of apoplexy (1658[6]); Solleysel's account of the transmission of glanders from horse to horse (1664[7]); Gideon Harvey on scurvy (1675); Morton's *Phthisiologia*, summing up the knowledge of his time (1689), and Stahl on diseases of the portal system (1698[8]). According to Garrod, black urine (alcaptonuria) was observed by G. A. Scribonius (1609) and Zacutus Lusitanus (1649). Frederik Dekkers, of Leyden, first detected albumen in the urine (1694) by boiling in the presence of acetic acid (Ebstein). In 1614, Felix **Platter** (1536–1614) reported the first known case of death from hypertrophy of the thymus gland in an infant. In 1616, François Citois described "Poitou colic," which long afterward

[1] Sennert: De febribus, Leyden, 1627.

[2] Diemerbroek: De peste, Arnheim, 1646.

[3] Glisson: De rachitide, London, 1650.

[4] Thuillier: J. d. sçavans, Paris, 1676, iv, 79.

[5] Höfer: Hercules medicus, Vienna, 1657, p. 43.

[6] Wepfer: Observationes anatomicæ ex cadaveribus eorum quos sustulit apoplexia, Schauffhausen, 1658.

[7] de Solleysel: Le parfait mareschal, Paris, 1664.

[8] Stahl: De vena portæ, porta malorum, 1698.

was found to be lead colic. Epidemic gangrenous rectitis (*mal de bicho*) was described by Aleixo d'Abreu (1623). Beriberi was first described, from East Indian cases, by the Dutch physicians, Jacob Bontius (1642[1]) and Nicholas Tulp (1652[2]). Bontius also described tropical dysentery in Java. Yaws (*bubas*) was described by Willem Piso, in his *De medicina Brasiliensi* (1648[3]) and yellow fever by Ferreira da Rosa (1694). Sir John Floyer's *Treatise on Asthma* (1698) gives a postmortem of pulmonary emphysema, and assigns as the cause of spasmodic asthma "a contracture of the muscular fibers of the bronchi." The Memoirs of the Earl of Clarendon (1632) contain a case of angina pectoris. In this group we may also include Felix Platter's *Praxis medicæ* (1602–8), containing the first attempt at a systematic classification of diseases, the gynecologic treatise of Rodericus à Castro (1603), the *Sepulchretum* of Théophile Bonet (1679), a collection of all the postmortems made during the 16th–17th centuries; Walter Harris's book on diseases of children (1689[4]), the pediatric treatise (1697) of John Pechey (1655–1716[5]), and the treatises on **medical jurisprudence** by Fortunato **Fedeli** (1602[6]), Rodericus à Castro (1614[7]), and Paolo Zacchias (1621–35[8]). Fedeli's little book has an interesting copper-plate frontispiece, in which the attestation of virginity and time of delivery, the jurisprudence of poisoning, lethal wounds, hereditary disease, torture, monsters, and the formation of the fetus are amusingly "featured," showing the interest which these subjects had acquired. Paolo **Zacchias** (1584–1659), who was protomedicus of Rome, physician to Popes Innocent X and Alexander VII, is replete with medicolegal information, particularly on wounds of the eye and the jurisprudence of insanity, of which he gives an excellent classification. In the *Historiettes* (1657–8) of Tallemant des Réaux (1619–92) there are many amusing details about the delusions, obsessions, phobias, fetichisms, and introversions of the nobles, with genealogic tables, signalizing morbid heredity. An important work on the medicolegal relations of surgery was published in 1684[9] by Nicolas de Blegny (1652–1722), who also founded the first medical journal (1679[10]) and made the first city directory (1684). Medical jurisprudence was not studied in a critical spirit before the 17th century, and up to this time medical ethics and jurisprudence were simply regarded as phases of state medicine. Germany made many contributions to forensic medicine and medical ethics in this period, such as Ludwig Hoernigk's *Politia medica* (1638[11]), Paul Ammann, on lethal wounds (1690[12]), Gottfried Welsch, on lethal wounds (1660) and plural births (1667[13]), Melchior Sebiz, on the signs of virginity (1630[14]), and Johann Bohn on lethal wounds (1689[15]). The most important medicolegal contribution of the century was undoubtedly Swammerdam's discovery that the fetal lungs will float on water after respiration (1667[16]), which was first put to a practical proof by Johann Schreyer in the case of a fifteen-year-old peasant girl accused of infanticide (1681[17]), the sinking of the infant's lungs securing acquittal. The

[1] Bontius: De medicina Indorum, Leyden, 1642, 115–120.

[2] Tulp: Observationes medicæ, Amsterdam, 1652, 300–305.

[3] See E. W. Gudger: Science, N. Y., 1911, n. s., xxxiii, 428.

[4] Harris: De morbis acutis infantum, London, 1689.

[5] Pechey: General Treatise of the Disease of Infants [etc.], London, 1697.

[6] Fedeli: De relationibus medicorum, Palermo, 1602.

[7] à Castro: Medicus politicus, Hamburg, 1614.

[8] Zacchias: Quaesationes medico-legales, Rome, 1621–35.

[9] de Blegny: La doctrine des rapports de chirurgie, Lyons, 1684.

[10] Nouvelles découvertes sur toutes les parties de la médecine, Paris, 1679–81.

[11] von Hoernigk: Politia medica, Frankfurt, 1638.

[12] Ammann: Praxis vulnerum lethalium, Frankfurt, 1690.

[13] Welsch: Vulnerum lethalium judicium, 1660; and De gemellis et partu numeriori, 1667.

[14] Sebiz: De notis virginitatis, 1630.

[15] Bohn: De renuntiatione vulnerum, Leipzig, 1689.

[16] Swammerdam: Tractatus phys.-anat.-med. de respiratione usque pulmonum, Leyden, 1667.

[17] Schreyer: Erörterung und Erläuterung der Frage: Ob es ein gewiss Zeichen (etc.), Zeitz, 1690.

Medicus Peccans of Ahasver Fritsch (Nuremberg, 1684) is an early contribution to **medical ethics.** The *Metoposcopia et Ophthalmoscopia* (1615) of Samuel Fuchs (1588–1630) is an illustrated treatise on physiognomy and the estimation of character by the eyes, not unlike Cardan's or Lavater's. The first English book on dentistry, by Charles Allen, was printed in 1686.[1]

Intravenous injection of drugs (1656) and **transfusion of alien blood** (1665–67) had their scientific origins in the 17th century.

Sir Christopher Wren (1632–1723), assisted by Boyle and Wilkins, first injected opium and crocus metallorum into the veins of dogs in 1656, which experiment was repeated by Carlo Fracassato in 1658. J. D. Major (1662), Caspar Scotus (1664), Elsholtz (*Clysmata nova*, 1665) made the first successful intravenous injections in man. Major published his *Chirurgia infusoria* at Kiel in 1667. Priority in transfusion has been claimed for Francesco Folli (1654), but the first authenticated records are those of R. Lower (1665–67) and A. Coga (1667). Transfusion is mentioned in Pepys' Diary (November 14, 1666[2]).

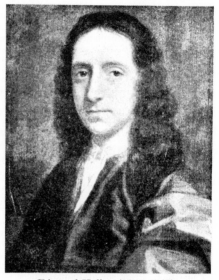

Edmund Halley (1656–1742).

To English medicine belongs the first book on **vital statistics,** the *Natural and Political Observations upon the Bills of Mortality* (London, 1662) of John **Graunt.** The Hebrews and the Romans had, no doubt, taken the census and counted troops, but Graunt was the first to note, from the bills of mortality (1532), that more boys are born than girls, and that the population can be estimated from an accurate death-rate, thus making the first step in the application of mathematical methods to the interpretation of statistics. He describes how the parish clerk delegated women as "searchers" to find out who was dead or about to die (1581). In the absence of compulsory notification of births and deaths these faulty bills of mortality were necessarily valueless. Graunt's book was followed, in 1687, by the *Essays on Political Arithmetic* of Sir William **Petty** (1623–87), who took the first census of Ireland. The English astronomer Edmund **Halley** (1656–1742) compiled the Breslau Table of births and funerals (1693), "to show the proportion of men able to bear arms in any multitude," to estimate mortality-rates, "to ascertain the price of annuities upon lives," and was thus the virtual founder of vital statistics.

---

[1] Printed anonymously as *The Operator for the Teeth* (Dublin, 1686); reprinted under Allen's name as "Curious Observations," [etc.], Dublin, 1687 (Weinberger).

[2] J. M. Fortescue-Brickdale (Oxford thesis): Guy's Hosp. Gaz., Lond., 1904, lvii, 15–80. D. I. Macht: Jour. Am. Med. Assoc., Chicago, 1916, lxvi, 856–860. *Ibid.*, 1914, lxii, 147; 222.

18

In 1672 the Welsh physician, Charles Clermont, published a work with the Hippocratic title, *On the Airs, Waters, and Places of England*, in which he plotted out the medical topography of the country as Daniel Drake did long after for the Mississippi Valley. The mineral waters of England were studied by a goodly number of 17th century physicians, notably Edmond Deane (1626), Edward Jorden (1631), Thomas Guidott (1681), Martin Lister (1682), Sir Patrick Dun (1683), Sir John Floyer (*An Inquiry into the Right Use of the Hot, Cold, and Temperature Baths in England*, 1697), and in Nehemiah Grew's study of Epsom Wells (1698[1]).

The first London *Pharmacopœia* was published in 1618, having been preceded by those of Valerius Cordus (1540), Brice Bauderon (1588), Libavius (1606), Jean de Renou (1615), and other city pharmacopeias of the 16th century.[2] It passed through many editions, all of which were disfigured by the retention of the usual vile and unsavory ingredients, which were not thrown out until William Heberden made an onslaught upon these superstitions in 1745. The *Pharmacopœia Londinensis* was translated into English in 1649 by the famous herbalist and quacksalver, Nicholas Culpeper. Other English Pharmacopeias of the time were Philemon Holland's Latin translation from the French of Bauderon (1639), Salmon's *New London Dispensatory* (1678), and Skipton's *Pharmacopœia Bateana* (1688), compiled from prescriptions of William Bate, physician-in-ordinary to Charles I, Cromwell, and Charles II.[3] Of continental pharmacopeias,[4] we may mention those of Minderer (1621), Poterie (1622), Schröder (1641), Ruland (1644), Zwelfer of Augsburg (1652), Jüngken (1677), Nicolas Lémery (1697), Hadrian à Mynsicht (1697), and C. F. Paulini's *Heilsame Dreckapotheke* (1696), the title of which amply symbolizes the tendency of many 17th century prescriptions.

The most important contribution of the 17th century to **veterinary medicine** was Jacques de Solleysel's demonstration of the transmission of glanders from horse to horse (1664). Andrew Snape's *The Anatomy of an Horse*, was published in London in 1686, and various French works on farriery appeared, in particular, Francini's translation of Carlo Ruini (1607), Beaugrand (1619, 1646), and de Bouvray (1660). The first German works on veterinary medicine were Martin Böhme's Ro s-Artzeney (1618), which held the field for nearly a century, and the *Bellerophon* of Winter von Adlersflügel (1668[5]).

In comparison with the extensive development of anatomy in the 17th century, its literature of **surgery** seems meager.

Among the Italians we find no surgeons commensurate in rank with those of the three centuries preceding. The only names deserving of mention are those of Cesare **Magati** (1579–1647), who followed Paré in holding that gunshot wounds are not poisonous, and taught, in theory at least, the simple expectant treatment of wounds by means of bandages moistened with plain water; and Pietro **de Marchetti** (1589–1673), Professor at Padua, whose *Observationum medico-chirurgicarum sylloge* (Padua, 1664) resembles the *Consilia* and the collections of Benivieni, Amatus Lusitanus, and Peter Forest, containing many strange case-histories and valuable surgical observations. Giuseppe **Zambeccari**, a pupil of Redi, was a pioneer in experimental surgery. He made successful experimental excisions of the spleen, kidneys, gall-bladder, pancreas, and of bits of the liver and intestines. On one dog he performed four successful experimental operations in succession (Neuburger[6]). The gigantic surgical anthology (*Thesaurus Chirurgiæ*) of Peter Uffenbach (1610) deserves mention, although the authors contained in it are all of the 16th century.

In France, owing to disputes of the Paris Faculty with St. Côme, and the decree uniting the surgeons and barbers into one guild, there was little surgical writing of note. The French treatises of the period are forgotten. Jacques de Beaulieu or **Frère Jacques** (1651–1719), a strolling incisor, introduced the lateral

---

[1] These data about mineral baths are given by Handerson in his translation of Baas's History of Medicine, New York, 1889, p. 546.

[2] All mentioned by Baas, *op. cit.*, pp. 436, 437, 546, 547.

[3] Baas: *Op. cit.*, footnote to p. 547.

[4] Baas: *Op. cit.*, p. 547. Scherer: Literatura pharmacopœarum, Leipzig, 1822, and Tschirch: Pharmakognosie, Leipzig, 1910, i, 2. Abt.

[5] Baas, p. 543.

[6] Neuburger: Med.-chir. Centralbl., Vienna, 1896, xxxi, 368.

operation for stone (1697), which was much improved by Rau in Holland. Nicolas de Blegny (1652–1722) invented the elastic truss, described in his treatise on hernia (1676), and wrote on surgical jurisprudence (1684). The surgical treatise of Vauguion (1696) mentions the tourniquet, which was introduced by Morel (1674) and was successfully applied in ligating the femoral artery at the Hôtel Dieu, in 1688. A quiz-compend by Gabriel Le Clerc (*La chirurgie complete*, 1692), which passed through 18 editions, mentions the vitriol buttons used at the Hôtel Dieu for checking hemorrhage, and the mode of manual compression (twenty-four hours at a stretch).

The leading German surgeons of the period were Fabry of Hilden, Scultetus, and the famous army surgeon Purmann.

Wilhelm **Fabry**,[1] of Hilden (1560–1624), called Fabricius Hildanus, whose statue was unveiled at Hilden near Düsseldorf is usually regarded as the "Father of German Surgery." Having a good classic education, he was strongly conservative in theory, supporting the views of the ancients, but in practice a bold and skilful operator and inventor of many new instruments. In his monograph on gangrene (Cologne, 1593[2]) Fabry was the first to recommend amputation above the diseased part, and is said to have been the first to amputate the thigh. In shutting off the circulation before amputation, he improvised a kind of tourniquet by means of a ligature tightened by a stick of wood. He also wrote a treatise on lithotomy (Basel, 1626), but his most important work is his "Century of Surgical Cases" (1606–46), the best collection of case-records of the time. He showed that head

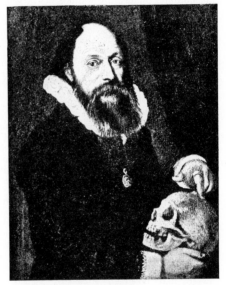

Wilhelm Fabry, of Hilden (1560–1624).

injuries may cause insanity, extracted an iron splinter from the eye with a magnet, explored the auditory canal with a speculum of his invention, and described the first field-chest of drugs for army use, based upon that introduced by Moritz of Nassau in 1612. In 1657, the Brandenburg army surgeon, Janus Abraham a Gehema (1645–1700), author of a little manual for medical officers in the field (1689[3]) recommended that these chests be supplied, as a matter of course, by the government instead of at the expense of the officers, as formerly. Fabry of Hilden was

---

[1] The name is sometimes given in German as "Fabriz," but Sudhoff regards "Fabry" as the genitive of Faber, or Schmidt (Schmitz), a common family name in the Rhineland (München. med. Wochenschr., 1910, lvii, 1401).

[2] Fabricius Hildanus: De gangræno et sphacelo, Cologne, 1593.

[3] Gehema: Der wohlversuchte Feld-Medicus, Rostock, 1689.

a reactionary in his use of the cautery and, like most surgeons of the day, he was a believer in the weapon-salve, which was applied to the weapon instead of the wound.

His contemporary, Johann Schultes (1595–1645), called **Scultetus,** is famous, like Albucasis and Paré before him, as one of the great illustrators of surgery and surgical instruments. His *Armamentarium chirurgicum* (Ulm, 1653) gives us a good side-light on the operations of the time through its interesting plates, representing such procedures as amputation of the breast, reduction of dislocations, passage of sounds, forceps-delivery, etc.

Matthæus Gottfried **Purmann** (1649–1711) was a surgeon in the Brandenburg army in 1675, and acquired great skill and courage through his pillar-to-post operating in the field. With Fabry of Hilden, he is held in the highest esteem by the German historians of today, because he regarded anatomy as the true basis of the surgeon's knowledge. He seems to have performed most of the operations known or proposed in his time, from trephining (40 cases), transfusion, aneurysm, and bronchotomy, to suturing wounds of the intestines. He left many different works, one of the most interesting of which is "Fifty Strange and Wonderful Cures of Gun-shot Wounds" (1693[1]). Needless to say, he was a believer in the weapon-salve and the sympathetic powder for healing wounds at a distance. Another important relic of the Thirty Years' War is the *Medicina Militaris* of Raimund Minderer (Augsburg, 1620). No less than 28 books on contagious diseases in armies were published in this period (Heizmann). Among pioneer operations of the German surgeons in the 17th century may be mentioned the gastrotomies of Florian Matthis (1602) and Daniel Schwabe (1635), Isaac Minnius' open section of the sternomastoid for torticollis (1641), the partial resection of the jaw by Acoluthus of Breslau in 1693, and Schonkoff's "ovariotomy" in 1685. At this time we may judge laparotomy to have been common enough, since plates in Roonhuyze (1663) and Völter's Midwifery (1679) give very plausible representations of the procedure.

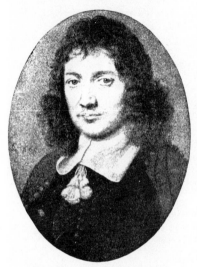

Richard Wiseman (1622–76).

The *Several Chirurgicall Treatises* (1672) of the Royalist surgeon, Richard **Wiseman** (1622–76), is the leading work of a man who played the same part in the English surgery of his day that Sydenham did in the practice of medicine. Wiseman was a skilful operator, amputated above the diseased part, employed primary amputation in gunshot wounds of joints, and was the first to describe tuberculosis of the joints as "tumor albus." He also gave the authentic account of "King's Evil." In his treatise on gonorrhea he mentions the first case of external urethrotomy for stricture, which he performed with Edward Molins in 1652. The first case of amputation by means of a flap is recorded in the *Triumphal Chariot of Turpentine* (1679), by James Yonge (1646–1721). Stephen Bradwell's *Helps in suddain accidents* (1633) is the first book on **first aid.**

---

[1] Purmann: Fünfzig sonder- und wunderbare Schusswundkuren, Frankfurt, 1693.

Seventeenth century **obstetrics** finds expression in the works of Mauriceau, de la Motte, Portal, van Deventer, Roonhuyze; and the midwives: Louise Bourgeois, who attended Marie de Medici through her six labors; Justine Siegemundin, "Court Midwife to the Electorate of Brandenburg," whose treatise of 1690 met with great opposition because it was written in the German language; and the perhaps mythical Jane Sharp, whose *Compleat Midwife's Companion* was first published in London in 1671. Of these writers, François **Mauriceau** (1637–1709), of Paris, is in some respects the leading representative of the obstetric knowledge of his time. His work on the diseases of pregnant and puerperal women (1668[1]), illustrated with exquisite copper plates, was a sort of canon of the art in its time, giving a good account of the conduct of normal labor, the employment of version, and the management of placenta prævia.

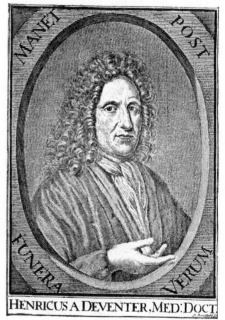

Hendrik van Deventer (1651–1724).

He was the first to correct the ancient view that the pelvic bones are separated in normal labor, and that the amniotic discharge is an accumulation of menstrual blood or milk; he was also the first to refer to tubal pregnancy, difficult labor from involvement of the umbilical cord, and epidemic puerperal fever. His book also gives an account of the author's adventure with the celebrated Hugh Chamberlen, of the Huguenot clan who succeeded in keeping their invention of an obstetric forceps a family secret for nearly two hundred years.[2]

Paul **Portal**[3] (died 1703), of Montpellier, wrote an obstetric treatise in 1685, in which he taught that version can be done by one foot and that face presentations usually run a normal course.

A far more important work is the *Novum Lumen* of Hendrik **van Deventer** (1651–1724), which, although printed in 1701, properly belongs to the 17th century. Van Deventer, a native of Holland, was at first a goldsmith, but turned to medicine at seventeen, and after studying at Groningen, practised obstetrics and orthopedics in his native city, The Hague, until his death. He has been rightly called "the father of

---

[1] Mauriceau: Traité des maladies des femmes grosses (etc.), Paris, 1668.

[2] The forceps was invented by Peter Chamberlen, sr., before 1634 (Doran); with it, Hugh Chamberlen failed to deliver a rachitic dwarf confided to him by Mauriceau.

[3] Portal: La pratique des accouchemens, Paris, 1685.

modern midwifery," for his book, with its interesting plates, gives the
first accurate description of the pelvis and its deformities, and the
effect of the latter in complicating labor. At the same time it is a
pioneer work in the delineation of deformities of the spine. There
was nothing quite like it until *Das enge Becken* of Michaëlis was published one hundred and fifty years later.

Hendrik van **Roonhuyze** (1625?–   ) was a champion of Cesarean
section, which he seems to have performed several times with success.
His *Heelkonstige Aanmerkkingen* (1663) has been described as the
first work on operative gynecology in the modern sense. It is illustrated
with unique copper plates, showing his mode of incision in Cesarean
section, and contains case reports of extra-uterine pregnancy and rupture of the uterus. Roonhuyze was otherwise a skilful operator, excising tumors, treating wounds of the head without trephining, and performing operations for wry-neck and harelip. Stromeyer says he was
the first to practise orthopedic surgery. As Howard Kelly points out,
he first proposed a scientific operation for vesicovaginal fistula, the
features of which were exposure of the fistula by a retracting speculum
with the patient in the lithotomy position; marginal denudation exclusive of the bladder-wall, and approximation of the denuded edges of
the fistula by means of quills fastened by silk threads.[1] He is not to
be confused with his son, Rogier van Roonhuyze, to whom the elder
Hugh Chamberlen is said to have sold the secret of his obstetric forceps
about 1693.[2]

Roonhuyze and Deventer did much to improve the status and
education of midwives in Holland, in which they were followed by
the former's successors in Amsterdam, Frederik Ruysch, and by Cornelis Solingen (1641–87).

A work which compares with Uffenbach's *Thesaurus Chirurgiæ* in size and
shape is the huge *Hebammenbuch* of Gottfried Welsch (1652), consisting of nearly
2000 pages of translations with commentaries, of the works of Mercurio, Pinæus,
and Louise Bourgeois. A gynecologic treatise of the period was *L'hydre féminine*
by Augustin Corrade (Nevers, 1634). The *Callipædia* of the Abbé Claude Quillet
(1656) denounced conventional marriages and was, in some sort, a pioneer work in
eugenics.

The methods of **deaf-mute instruction** practised by the Benedictine monk
Pedro Ponce de Leon (1520–84) were preserved in the treatise of Juan Pablo Bonet
(1620[3]), who had successfully taught the deaf brother of his patron, the constable
of Castile. Sir Kenelm Digby met Bonet at Madrid and bore witness to the success
of his methods. After this, the subject became popular in England and Italy.
Giovanni Bonifacio had published his Art of Signs (*L'Arte de cenni*) at Vicenza in
1616. English treatises on deaf-mute instruction were published by John Bulwer
(1644–8[4]); by John Wallis (1616–1703), Savilian professor of mathematics at Oxford

---

[1] H. A. Kelly: Tr. Am. Gynæc. Soc., Phila., 1912, xxxvii, pp. 8–10.

[2] Fassbender: Geschichte der Geburtshülfe, Jena, 1906, 224. A. Geijl (Janus,
Amst., 1906, xi, 253, 292) is of opinion that the Roonhuyzens and Ruysch knew of
the forceps in 1670.

[3] Bonet: Reduccion de las letras y artes para enseñar á hablar á los mutos,
Madrid, 1620.

[4] J. Bulwer: Chirologia, London, 1644; Philocophus, London, 1648.

(1652[1]); William Holder (1669[2]), and George Dalgarno, of Aberdeen (1661–80[3]). In 1692 Johann Conrad Ammann (1669–1724) published his ingenious method, "*Surdus Loquens*," which was reprinted in 1700.

Daniel **Leclerc** (1652–1728), of Geneva, wrote the first large history of medicine (1696), a work which was translated into English and is still appreciated. Many **medical dictionaries** were published in this period.

The most remarkable were the posthumous glossary of Hippocratic terms by Guillaume Baillou (*Definitionum medicinalium liber*, 1639); the *Quæstiones iatrophilologicæ* of Gabriel Naudé (1647), the Latin-German pharmaceutical lexicon of Friedrich Müller (1661); the etymological lexica of François Thevenin (1669) and J. B. Callard de la Ducquerie (1673); the *Prodromus* of J. L. Hannemann (1672); and the Greek and Latin lexica of Bartolommeo Castelli (1607) and Stephan Blankaart (1679) which passed through many editions. The English version of Blankaart (*Physical Dictionary*, London, 1684) was the first medical dictionary to appear in Great Britain.

There was no printing press in the North American colonies before the year 1639, when one was set up at Cambridge, Massachusetts; its first publication being the Bay State Psalm-Book of 1640. The only medical publication of the New England colonists in the 17th century was the *Brief Rule to Guide the Common People of New England how to Order themselves and theirs in the Small Pocks or Measles* (Boston, 1677[4]) by Dr. Thomas **Thacher**

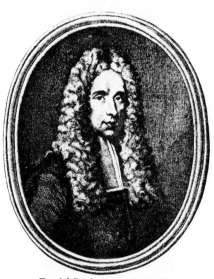

Daniel Leclerc (1652–1728).

(1620–78), an Englishman who settled in New England in 1635, and in 1669 became pastor of the Old South Church, at the same time practising medicine with success. He was a good Hebrew and Arabic scholar, and wrote a Hebrew lexicon and a catechism, which are like the "Brief Rule" in that each of them occupies, as Handerson slyly observes, "only a single sheet of paper."

CULTURAL AND SOCIAL ASPECTS OF 17TH CENTURY MEDICINE

The age of the rise of England and Holland was a time of spiritual and intellectual uplift, and the effect of the continued battle for freedom

---

[1] J. Wallis: De loquela, London, 1652.

[2] W. Holder: Elements of Speech, London, 1669.

[3] G. Dalgarno: Ars signorum, London, 1661; Didascalacophus, Oxford, 1690. For an account of early writings on deaf-mutism, see F. De Land: Volta Rev., Wash., 1920, xxii, 391–421.

[4] Reprinted by H. E. Handerson in Janus, Amst., 1899, iv, 540–547.

of thought was to make it a period of individual scientific endeavor rather than of concerted advancement of science. The stirring events of this age—the burning of Bruno (1600), the Thirty Years' War, the Fronde, the English Revolution, the embarkation of the Pilgrims, the anathemas hurled at Spinoza, the suicide of Uriel Acosta—all go to show that the superior men of the time felt themselves "in the presence of high causes." Although the wars of the Fronde riveted the bonds of monarchy and ecclesiasticism upon France, and although Germany was ruined by the Thirty Years' War, yet England and Holland were free, and the barbarities of feudalism became tempered down into real governmental activities, largely from the growing interest in the study and application of the law. From the time of the perhaps legendary discovery of Justinian's Pandects at Ravenna, about 1135, there had been a gradual attempt to regulate national and civil government as well as the intercourse of nations by the Roman law, and this was brought to a focus through the labors of the two greatest jurists of the period—Hugo Grotius (1583–1645), of Delft (Holland), and Samuel von Pufendorf (1632–94), of Chemnitz, Saxony. With better legal regulations and restrictions, the social status of the physician was correspondingly improved, although the surgeon was still under the ban, unless needed in wartime. In Germany, the physician proper was styled *medicus purus*, and often held definite official positions, such as physician-in-ordinary to a potentate (*medicus ordinarius*), state or city physician (*physicus*), or plague doctor (*medicus pestilentiarius*), all at high salaries; while army surgeons were called *Feldscheerer* because they had to shave the officers. The general run of surgeons were still roughly classed with the horde of barbers, bath-keepers, executioners, and vagrant mountebanks.

The condition of medicine was further improved by the ambitions of princes to found new universities, and by the introduction of two new factors of great moment, viz., the scientific society and periodic literature.

The 17th century marks the rise of many famous Dutch and Germanic **universities**, notably Harderwijk (1600), Giessen (1607), Groningen (1614), Rinteln (1621), Dorpat (1632), Utrecht (1636), Åbo (1640), Bamberg (1648), Herborn (1654), Duisburg (1655), Kiel (1665), Lund (1666), Innsbruck (1673), and Halle (1694). But for centuries the universities had been like Joubert's typical *bourgeois*, the peaceful, idle, and self-satisfied possessors of what they had, transmitters of lifeless tradition. and strongholds of conservatism. The best thinkers and scientists had long since been penetrated with the conviction that the work done in universities was valueless and had as little to do with them as possible. Hence arose the necessity for some organized plan for fostering experimental research, bringing scientific men together and keeping them in touch with one another by means of publications. This haven of research and experiment, dreamed of by Bacon in his *House of Solomon*, was found in the scientific society.[1] The idea of **scientific societies** originated in Italy. Porta's Secret Academy at Naples (1560) was followed by the Academy of the Lynxes (*Accademia dei Lincei*), which was founded at Rome, August 17, 1603, by Marquis Federigo Cesi, its device being a lynx rending

[1] For the best account of this matter in English, see "The Rôle of the Scientific Societies in the seventeenth Century," by Martha Orenstein (-Bronfenbrenner), New York, 1913.

a Cerberus with its claws. At first it consisted of a closed corporation of four members, who met to discuss new experiments, mathematical problems, and "the ornaments of elegant literature and philology, which, like a graceful garment, adorned the whole body of science." Although it encountered much opposition from the Church, it lived to include Galileo as one of its members, and still survives, publishing handsome transactions in quarto. In 1657 a similar society, called the Accademia del Cimento (Academy of Experiment), was established at Florence. In 1645 an "Invisible College," similar to Porta's Secret Academy, was founded in London by Haak, Hartlieb, Boyle, Wren, Goddard, and others and, after combining with an Oxford "Philosophical Society," opened its first journal book on November 28, 1660, and on July 15, 1662, was chartered by Charles II as the Royal Society of London. It began to publish its world-renowned *Philosophical Transactions* in 1664–5. These soon reached such a high level of merit as to include many important works of Leeuwenhoek, Malpighi, and other great names. On March 10, 1681, the first medical congress was opened at Rome, lasting until June 8, 1682, with three to four meetings monthly and a total attendance of 46 physicians (Cumston). The Dublin Philosophical Society was established in 1684, with Sir William Petty as first president and, after some vicissitudes, was reorganized as Trinity College in 1693. Richelieu, in France, founded the famous Académie Française at Paris in 1635, with the object of improving the French language and literature; and in 1665 Colbert founded the Académie des Sciences, which began to publish its transactions (*Histoire* and *Memoires*) in 1699. In Germany the Society of Scientific Physicians (*Gesellschaft naturforschender Aerzte*), or *Academia naturæ curiosorum*, founded at Schweinfurt, January 1, 1652, by Johann Lorenz Bausch and others, became in 1677 the Imperial Leopoldine Academy of Scientists (*Kaiserliche leopoldinische Akademie der Naturforscher*), or *Academia Cæsarea-Leopoldina*, which had begun to publish its "Miscellanea" or Ephemerides in 1670. These were followed by the *Acta medica Hafniensia*, edited by Thomas Bartholinus (Copenhagen, 1671–79), and the *Acta eruditorum* (Leipzig, 1682–1745). Detached **periodical literature** had, meanwhile, taken an independent course. The Acta Diurna of the ancient Romans (brief bulletins of battles, elections, games, and other happenings) and the Chinese *Peking Gazette* founded in the 7th century A. D. and still current, preceded everything else of this kind. The 17th century newspaper derived from the fugitive "news-letters," originally written out in long hand for wealthy patrons, and the consequent formation of "intelligence offices," with hired staffs of clerks, as described in Ben Jonson's comedy, "The Staple of News" (1625). Following the Venetian *gazzette, coranti* or *foglietti* (1531), the *Nieuwe Tijdinghen*, a city newspaper published by Abraham Verhoeven, was licensed to appear at Antwerp in 1605 (no copy extant before 1616), to be followed in turn by the first German newspapers, the *Frankfurter Journal*, founded by Egenolph Emmel in 1615, and the *Frankfurter Oberpostamtszeitung* (1615–66), the London *Weekely News*, first issued on May 23, 1622, and followed by Marchamont Nedham's *Mercurius Britannicus* (August 16, 1643); the *Gazette de France*, issued at Paris by the physician Théophraste Renaudot on May 30, 1631 and, in America, the solitary number one of the *Publick Occurrences*, edited by Benjamin Harris, and published at Boston September 25, 1690. Entirely distinct from newspapers or periodicals proper were such political bulletins as the Scotch *Diurnal of Occurents* (1513–75), Janson's *Mercurius Gallo-belgicus* (1587–94), the *Diurnals* of the English Parliament (1641–2) or Marchamont Nedham's *Mercurius Britannicus* (1643–6). The pedigree of the scientific periodical is out of the scientific society by the newspaper. The new tendency was represented in science by the *Journal des Sçavans* (January 5, 1665) and, in medicine, by the *Nouvelles Découvertes sur Toutes les Parties de la Médecine* of Nicolas de Blegny (Paris, 1679–81), usually regarded as the **first medical periodical** in the vernacular. Its popularity is evidenced by its translation into German as *Monatliche neueröffnete Anmerckungen* (Hamburg, 1680). It was translated into Latin, and continued by Théophile Bonet as the *Zodiacus medico-gallicus* (Geneva, 1680–85). The abortive *Journal de Médecine* (1681–85) of the abbé J. P. de la Roque was continued (1686) by Claude Brunet, who also edited a monthly *Progrès de la Médecine* (1695–1709[1]). The first English medical journal was the *Medicina curiosa* (June 17–October 23, 1684).

De Blegny was also the author of a series of satirical sketches of his contemporaries which, published as the *Mercure savant* (1684), became the original of sub-

---

[1] Sudhoff: München. med. Wochenschr., 1903, 1, 455.

sequent "city directories."[1] Théophraste Renaudot was the originator of pawn-shops and intelligence offices. When we reflect that a postal service did not exist on the continent of Europe before the year 1516,[2] the value of these scientific societies, periodicals, and directories for the more rapid dissemination of knowledge will at once become apparent.

The great centers of **medical education** in the 17th century were Leyden, Paris, and Montpellier. At Leyden were Sylvius, Ruysch, Nuck, and Bidloo; van Deventer and Cornelis Solingen were at The Hague; Roonhuyze and Swammerdam at Amsterdam; Duverney, Vieussens, Pierre Dionis, Mauriceau, Jules Clément, and Paul Portal at Paris; Giorgio Baglivi at Padua; and no less than Sydenham was a pupil of Charles Barbeirac at Montpellier. In Germany, however, medicine had little chance until after the Peace of Westphalia (1648), and even in that period many original scientific investigations all over Europe were made by practising physicians detached from universities. It is not without significance that the huge output of brilliant work in anatomy and physiology followed directly upon the close of the Thirty Years' War.

In 1633, as Baas records, Ingolstadt had only 3 students; in 1647, 2; but 16 in 1648; while Strassburg had but 13 students during the entire period 1612–31, 4 in 1632–48, and 6 in 1649–99. German medical instruction in this period was, moreover, along the old medieval, scholastic lines, a mere blind following of Galen and the Arabians, in opposition to the folk-medicine of Paracelsus. A lively teapot-tempest was stirred up by Thomasius in 1688, when he attempted to emulate the example of Paracelsus by lecturing in the German language, and the same prejudice was even encountered by Schönlein in 1840. Sydenham, Glisson, and Theodore Turquet de Mayerne, the Swiss physician, were the leading exponents of the bed-side study of disease in England. On the continent, the true clinical method, recommended at Leyden (1591) by Jan van Heurne and carried into effect by his son, Otto Heurne, and Ewald Scrivelius (1636[3]) was taught later by Sylvius and perhaps by Barbeirac at Montpellier. The usual method of teaching internal medi-cine was to read off a perfunctory lecture in Latin, followed by a number of pre-scriptions which were variously Galenical, Spagyrical, Iatromathematical, Iatro-chemical or Hermetic, and which the students copied.

Botanic gardens were established at Heidelberg before 1600, Giessen (1605), Strassburg (1620), Oxford (1621), Jena (1629), Upsala (1657), Chelsea (1673), Berlin (1679), Edinburgh (1670), and Amsterdam (1682).

Dissecting as a means of teaching anatomy was more frequent in Italy, Holland, and France than in Germany or England. In England the material was usually obtained by grave-robbing. In Germany dissections, *longo intervallo*, were in the nature of civic events attended by festivities. When Rolfink began to have two annual dissections upon executed criminals at Jena in 1629, the practice was held in holy horror

---

[1] The first being the "Almanac des addresses de Paris," 1691.

[2] Marco Polo describes an extensive courier service among the Chinese of his time, and Louis XI, in 1464, established an official service of mounted messengers (*chevaucheurs en poste*) in France, but the first mounted postal service for purely public use was established between Vienna and Brussels in 1516 by Franz von Thurn und Taxis.

[3] The immediate incentive was an inaugural oration by the Utrecht professor, Willem van der Straten, on March 17, 1636. On August 25, 1637, Heurne and Scrivelius were salaried as bedside professors at 200 guilders each *per annum*. E. C. van Leersum: Janus, Amst., 1926, xxx, 133–155.

by the peasantry who watched newly made graves lest they be "Rolfinked." A skeleton for teaching purposes was a rarity, and although there were anatomic theaters in most of the continental cities in course of time, there was none in Edinburgh until 1697, after which the Scotch capital gained ascendancy under the Monro dynasty. In France Vieussens is said to have made as many as 500 dissections alone. The popularity and frequency of dissecting in Holland are sufficiently evidenced in the canvases of the great Dutch artists of the century. The earliest known of these is the "Anatomie" of Dr. Sebastian Egberts by Arend Pietersz (1603), in the Amsterdam Gallery, representing 28 physicians, with high ruffed collars and Vandyke beards, gathered around the demonstrator, who is about to insert the scalpel in the cadaver before him. Another "Anatomie" by Thomas de Keyser (1619), also in the Amsterdam collection, represents the same physician quizzically tickling the ribs of a hilarious skeleton, to the amusement of five of his friends. A superb document is the canvas of van Mierevelt in the Delft Hospital (1617), representing a body with exposed viscera surrounded by Dr. van der Neer and 17 other figures, with all the accessories of dissecting. Rembrandt's famous Anatomy of Dr. Tulp (1632) at The Hague is sufficiently well known, and the same great master of realistic painting has, in the Amsterdam Gallery, a remarkable unfinished study of a foreshortened cadaver (1656), resembling Mantegna's picture of the Dead Christ, and styled the *Anatomie* of Dr. Johan Deyman. The finest of all these "Anatomies" are Adriaen Backer's, in the Amsterdam Gallery (1670), representing a dissection by Frederik Ruysch, and Johan van Neck's picture of the same master demonstrating the viscera of an infant to five physicians, whilst a child toys with an infantile skeleton in the corner. As we survey the strong, valid faces of these Dutch physicians, richly clad in silk or velvet gowns, or jerkins with high ruffed collars,[1] we get no bad idea of the dignity of the profession in the 17th century. In the Rembrandt pictures, in two Anatomies of Frederik Ruysch, and in Nicholaes Maes' painting of the chiefs of the Surgeons' Guild (Amsterdam, 1680), the ruffed collars have already become Geneva bands. In Rembrandt's Doctor Tulp, as in Greenbury's "Anatomy" of Sir Charles Scarborough (1649) in the Barbers' Hall, London, the short, lace-edged collar, which was evidently a token of wealth or worldly place, is in evidence.[2] An etching representing the Anatomical Theater at Leyden, of date 1610, shows a circular inclosure affording mere fence-rail accommodations for seats; the separate tiers are interspersed with stuffed birds, skeletons of animals, and human skeletons (one on horseback) bearing placards adorned with appropriate mortuary inscriptions. These skeletons and inscriptions were also a feature of Ruysch's famous anatomic museum

---

[1] These ruffed collars are also worn by the lady-patronesses of the Leper Hospital, in Werner van Valckert's painting of 1620 (Holländer, p. 89).

[2] For reproductions and full descriptions of all these pictures see Eugen Holländer, Die Medizin in der klassischen Malerei, Stuttgart, 1903, pp. 34–60.

at Leyden, which was purchased by Peter the Great in 1717 for 30,000 florins (about $75,000), and is still in a fair state of preservation in the Anatomical Museum of the Imperial Academy of Sciences (Leningrad). A second collection which Ruysch afterward made was, on the authority of Hyrtl, scattered and destroyed after his death.

As the great Renaissance physicians had commonly followed botany or zoölogy as special lines of investigation, so we find the physician of the 17th century distinguishing himself as a mathematician and astronomer, a physicist, a microscopist, or a chemist. In university teaching, the most extraordinary versatility was sometimes displayed. Meibom, for instance, presided over philosophy, philology, archeology, and geometry, as well as medicine (Baas). The polyhistorian Hermann Conring taught in all the four faculties. In physics, the work of Des-

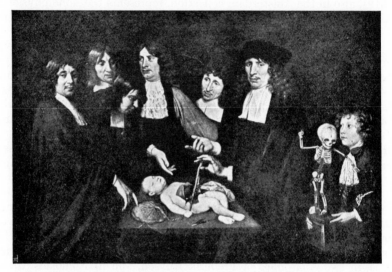

Anatomy of Dr. Frederik Ruysch by Johan van Neck (1683) (Amsterdam Museum),
Hanfstaengl, Munich.

cartes, Kepler, Sanctorius, Hooke, Borelli, and Scheiner has been mentioned; and of physician-chemists we need refer only to van Helmont, who first used the term "gas," and knew the properties of hydrogen, carbon dioxide, and sulphur dioxide; Leeuwenhoek and Redi, who were the first food chemists; Boyle, who first defined chemical "elements," founded analytic chemistry, and discovered that the pressure of a gas is proportional to its density (Boyle's law); John Mayow, who all but discovered oxygen; Minderer, who discovered ammonium acetate (*spiritus Mindereri*); Nicolas Lémery (1645–1715), who discovered iron in the blood; and Thomas Willis, who discovered the sweetish taste of diabetic urine. Johann Rudolph **Glauber** (1604–88), of Carlstadt, whose bust was used as a chemist's sign for nearly 200 years, discovered sodium sulphate (Glauber's salt), made sulphate of copper, arsenic chlorid, and zinc chlorid, distilled ammonia from bones, and obtained hydrochloric acid by distilling sulphuric acid with sea-salt, investigated pyroligneous acid (*acetum lignorum*), did much for the chemistry of wines and spirits, and published a valuable encyclopedia of chemical procedures. He often sold "secrets" to manufacturers, was accused of selling the same secret several times, or of selling secrets which would not work, and his great secret which he expressly declined to sell or publish was the Alkahest, or Universal Solvent. Oliver Cromwell said "This Glauber is an arrant knave"; but Glauber was easily the greatest analytic chemist of his time, and those of his calling who have had their discoveries stolen by their assistants have learned to appreciate his canny sense in keeping his business to himself. The secretive Glauber is particularly interesting because he stands between the scientific chemists, like Boyle or Mayow, and those who deliberately followed **alchemy.** Although the pretended making of gold and silver and other magic practices were opposed by the Church in the famous bulls, *"Spondent pariter"* (1317) and *"Super illius specula"* (1326) of John XXII,[1] alchemy became an intensive cult of extraordinary magnitude in the 16th and 17th centuries, since it appealed particularly to the lust of money, the love of life and the corresponding fear of death. For the philosopher's stone, otherwise known as "the quintessence" or "grand magistery," was not only supposed to transmute the baser metals into gold, make precious stones and a universal solvent, but also conferred perfect health and length of days. It was described by all who claimed to have seen it as of a reddish luster. Raymond Lully called it a carbuncle; Paracelsus likened it to a ruby; Berigard de Pisa, to a wild poppy with the smell of heated sea-salt; van Helmont, to saffron with the luster of glass (Thorpe[2]). The choral symphony in praise of its capacity for maintaining health resembled the testimonials of "Vin Mariani" and other nostrums of our time.

From the universal solvent it was but a step to a universal remedy, like that of Butler's French quack, who

> "Set up physic
> And called his receipt a general specific."

The effect of alchemy upon the medicine of the 16th and 17th centuries had been to create a number of offshoots of the Paracelsian or Spagyric School, which were variously termed Hermetic, Cabalistic, Zoroastrian or Rosicrucian, according to the individual penchant for the doctrines of Hermes Trismegistus (the Egyptian Thoth), the Hebraic "oral

[1] For the Latin text of these bulls, see: Walsh: The Popes and Science, New York, 1908, 414–416.

[2] The Alkahest, the name of Paracelsus' Universal Solvent, which could be prepared by the stone, was supposed to be derived from the Latin *alkali est*, from the German *all Geist* (all gas) or *Alles ist* (it is all), but the chemist Johann Kunkel (1630–1704), who pointed out these derivations, said its true name was *Alles Lugen ist* (It's all a lie); for "if it dissolved everything, no vessel could contain it." Sir E. Thorpe, History of Chemistry, London & New York, 1909, i, 46–56, 81.

tradition" or Cabala, the traditional "living word" (Zendavesta) of the Persian Zoroaster (Nietzsche's Zarathustra), or the Rosicrucian cult. The doctrine of the **Rosicrucians** emanated from three books of mystic and alchemistic jargon, which were published during the years 1614–16 and called the Fama Fraternitatis, the Confessio Fraternitatis, and the Chymical Marriage of Christian Rosencreutz. The supposititious author traveled in the East (as usual), where he learned necromancy, alchemy, and philosophy. Upon his return, he imparted the new knowledge to seven associates, forming the Brethren of the Rosy Cross, who were to follow science and to communicate their results to one another, to render free assistance to the sick poor, and to have no distinctive tokens of their cult except the letters "C. R." It goes without saying that they could manufacture gold, if so inclined, but, like the Spiritualists and Theosophists of our own time, disdained to make any practical use of their superior knowledge which, they admitted, was obtained by direct illumination from God. It was subsequently discovered that the three basic texts of the Rosicrucian cult were written, not by Rosencreutz, but by the Württemberg pastor Johann Valentin Andreas (1586–1654), who perpetrated this solemn piece of mystification in the same spirit in which Meinhold wrote *Sidonia the Sorceress*. All the "six follies of science," viz., circle squaring, multiplication of the cube (fourth dimensional space or spiritism), perpetual motion (Cornelius Drebbel), judicial astrology, alchemy, and magic were rampant in 17th century medicine, and most of them were subjected to keenest ridicule by Butler, the arch satirist of his age. Prominent figures in Butler's *Hudibras* were Ralph, the Judicial Astrologer, who presumably purged and let blood by the signs of the zodiac, and was otherwise

> "For profound
> And solid lying much renowned."

And Sidrophel, the Rosicrucian and veterinarian

> "To whom all people, far and near,
> On deep importances repair
> When brass or pewter hap to stray,
> And linen slinks out of the way:
>
> . . . .
>
> When cattle feel indisposition
> And need the opinion of physician."

The dupes of astrologic physicians of this type were ridiculed in Congreve's *Love for Love* (1695), in the character of "Foresight, an illiterate old fellow, peevish and passive, superstitious, and pretending to understand Astrology, Palmistry, Physiognomy, Omens, Dreams, &c."; and Dr. Johnson, in his criticism of this play, assures us that "the character of Foresight was then common. Dryden calculated nativities; both Cromwell and King William had their lucky days; and Shaftesbury himself, though he had no religion, was said to regard predictions."[1] But the tendency was by no means confined to the learned laity. Kepler is said to have cast a horoscope for Wallenstein. Minderer (of *spiritus Mindereri*) advised the plague doctors to repeat Psalm XXII every time they approached a patient, just as the old Saxon Leechdoms urged the application of holy water and the intoning of Psalms LI, LXVII and the Athanasian Creed over cattle afflicted with pleuropneumonia.[2] That able clinician, Daniel Sennert, believed in witchcraft and pacts with the devil. The affair of the Lancashire Witches, which was dramatized by Thomas Heywood, goes to show that long after Weyer's time people were still credulous about the stigmata of incubi and succubi (hysteric ecchymoses), witches' marks (anesthetic patches), demoniac possession, and other pantomimic phases of hystero-epilepsy (Ormerod[3]). Sebastian Wirdig favored divining-rods and magic. Goclenius and Fabricius Hildanus were patrons of the weapon-salve; and, in 1658, the University of Montpellier heard Sir Kenelm Digby's celebrated discourse on the sympathetic powder, which Madame de Sévigné pronounced "a perfectly divine remedy" (January 28, 1685). **Digby,** an *Uebermensch* in his way, first leaped into prominence as a corsair in the Levantine sea-fight commemorated in Ben Jonson's droll couplet:

> "Witness his action done at Scanderoon
> Upon his birthday, the eleventh of June."

Wealthy and courted, in spite of his father's imprisonment for treason, he dabbled in politics, religion, and science; got a hearing although, according to Lady Fanshawe, "he enlarged somewhat more in extraordinary stories than might be averred," and wrote a unique autobiography. The sympathetic powder, his special hobby, consisted, it is said, of nothing more than green vitriol, first dissolved in water and afterward recrystallized or calcined in the sun. The Duke of Buckingham testified that Sir Kenelm had healed his secretary of a gangrenous wound by simply soaking the bloody bandage in a solution of the powder. Digby claimed to have got the secret remedy from a Carmelite monk in Florence, and attributed its potency to the fact that the sun's rays extracted the spirits of the blood and the vitriol, while, at the same time, the heat of the wound caused the healing principle thus produced to be attracted to it by means of a current of air—a sort of wireless therapy. Quite as amusing are the superstitions of the sympathetic or magnetic cure of wounds and the healing of disease by "stroking." The former originated with Paracelsus, and was exploited in 1608 by Rudolph Goclenius, one of his followers, in the tract, *De magnetica curatione vulneris*. Sympathetic medicine was the subject of a treatise by Sylvester Rattray (1658) and of a collective *Theatrum sympatheticum* (1662). The treatment consisted in anointing the weapon

---

[1] Johnson: Lives of the Poets, *sub voce* Congreve.

[2] Cockayne: Saxon Leechdoms, i, 389.

[3] J. A. Ormerod: St. Barth. Hosp. Jour., Lond., 1913, xx, 91–97.

which had inflicted the wound with the *unguentum armarium*, of the patient's blood and human fat, the wound itself being wrapped in wet lint. This doctrine was supported by Fabry of Hilden, Robert Fludd the Rosicrucian, and van Helmont who attributed the cure to animal magnetism. The clergy held that the weapon cure was wrought by magic and the devil, and their view was set forth by William Foster in *Hoplocrisma Spongus, or a Sponge to Wipe away the Weapon-Salve* (1631). Robert Fludd (1619), van Helmont (1621), Kircher, in *Magnes* (1643), and William Maxwell (1679) were the early theorists about animal magnetism, which was carried into practice by Valentine Greatrakes (Greatorex) (1628–66), one of Cromwell's soldiers in Ireland, who achieved an enormous reputation in his "cures" of disease by laying on of hands (stroking) and the cure of scrofula with carrot poultices. The treatment of scrofula was, however, the special prerogative of royalty. The King's Evil, or *morbus regius*, has latterly been made the subject of an exhaustive and scholarly monograph by Raymond Crawfurd (1911), and the results of his original investigations of the medieval sources are briefly as follows:

> The personal power of healing, in the first instance, always an attribute of the gods, became, by natural association of ideas, a divine right of kings, and many instances of it are recorded by the Roman chroniclers and the fathers of the Church. Thus Helgald, a monk of the 11th century, records that Robert the Pious (996–1031 A. D.) wrought cures by touch, and Guibert, Abbé de Nogent, bears witness that touching for scrofula (*scrophas circa jugulum*) was done by Philip I (1061–1108) of France, and his son Louis VI (1108–37). Shortly before his death, in 1066, Edward the Confessor touched for scrofula in England, on the authority of William of Malmesbury and a monkish chronicler of Westminster. From Clovis on, touching was a power ascribed to the French monarchs, even up to the time of Louis XVI, and was actually revived at the coronation of Charles X in 1824, no less than Dupuytren and Alibert presenting the 121 patients. In England, the Royal Touch fell into disuse among the Norman Kings after the Confessor, but was revived by Henry II, Henry III, and the three Edwards. Items in the wardrobe accounts of the latter show the payment of alms to the scrofulous poor. After Richard II's time, there is complete silence in the chronicles until 1462, when Henry VII revived the royal prerogative with an elaborate ritual and, in 1465, the minting of a special coin, the gold Angel, as a touchpiece. The ceremonial with the use of touchpieces, and of medals as tickets of admission,[1] were features of all subsequent reigns to the time of William of Orange, who treated the practice cavalierly; but Queen Anne revived it, even touching Dr. Johnson (without success). The exiled Stuarts "over the water" also upheld it, but it was practically discarded by George I. It was in the 17th century that the practice of the Royal Touch reached its height. Richard Wiseman, one of the ablest surgeons of the time, wrote the classic account of the King's Evil, in which he bears ample witness to the healing power of Charles II. Shakespeare, in the time of James I (1607), describes (Macbeth, Act IV, sc. 3) how—

> > "strangely-visited people,
> > All swoln and ulcerous, pitiful to the eye,
> > The mere despair of surgery, he cures;
> > Hanging a golden stamp about their necks,
> > Put on with holy prayers."

The Royal Touch was not even subjected to ridicule in the *Pseudodoxia Epidemica; or Enquiries into Vulgar and Common Errors* (1646) of **Sir Thomas Browne** (1605–82), the old Norwich physician

---

[1] For this phase of the subject, see the learned and illuminating monograph of Helen Farquhar on *Royal Charities*, London, 1919 (Brit. Numismat. Jour., xii–xiii).

whose delightful writings, notably *Religio Medici* (1643) and *Urn Burial* (1658), belong to literature proper, in the most exquisite sense. The *Religio Medici*, with its quaint and original modes of expression, is an attempt to reconcile scientific skepticism with faith. The *Vulgar Errors*, while nominally a critical onslaught upon superstition, displays the same delightful whimsicality through its author's credulous attitude toward many of the things he set out to ridicule. Thus while the medical science of the 17th century was making rapid strides forward, its popular medicine was already in process of retrogression to the excesses of the Byzantine Period, which bears out our main thesis, that the folk-ways of medicine are inevitably the same and independent of time and place and circumstance. This can be easily verified by a glance at the **materia medica** of the period.

The first edition of the *London Pharmacopœia*, published in 1618, contains some 1960 remedies, of which 1028 were simples, 91 animal, 271 vegetable. Among these were worms, lozenges of dried vipers, foxes' lungs (for asthma), powders of precious stones, oil of bricks, oil of ants, oil of wolves, and butter made in May (for ointments). Among the 932 compounds, many of which had the names of their Greek and Arabian originators attached, were vegetable syrups, compound senna powder, Neapolitan (blue) ointment, Vigo's plaster (compounded of vipers' flesh, with live frogs and worms), and the celebrated antidote of Mattioli, made up of about 230 ingredients, including the multifarious mithridate (*confectio Damocratis*) and the *theriaca Andromachi*. The Pharmacopœia of 1650 contains cochineal, antimonial wine, the red and white mercurial precipitates, moss from the skull of a victim of violent death, and Gascoyne's powder, compounded of bezoar, amber, pearls, crabs' eyes, coral, and black tops of crabs' claws. In the Pharmacopœia of 1677, the names of the Greeks and Arabians disappear, showing that their influence had also waned, while jalap, cinchona bark, burnt alum, digitalis, benzoin, balsams of copaiba and tolu, steel tonics, and Irish whisky (*aqua vitæ Hibernorum sive usquebaugh*) make their appearance for the first time, as also human urine so highly recommended by Madame de Sévigné (June 13, 1685[1]). Among the queer remedies contained in the three London Pharmacopœias of the period were the blood, fat, bile, viscera, bones, bone-marrow, claws, teeth, hoofs, horns, sexual organs, eggs, and excreta of animals of all sorts; bee-glue, cock's-comb, cuttlefish, fur, feathers, hair, isinglass, human perspiration, saliva of a fasting man, human placenta, raw silk, spider-webs, sponge, sea-shell, cast-off snake's skin, scorpions, swallow's nests, wood-lice, and the triangular Wormian bone from the juncture of the sagittal and lambdoid sutures of the skull of an executed criminal (*ossiculum antiepilepticum Paracelsi*[2]). The Chinese materia medica itself could go no further than this toward demonstrating that the folk-mind is stationary or discontinuous. Yet Minderer prescribed oil of spiders and earthworms for plague, Robert Boyle recommended *album Græcum* as a homely but experienced remedy for dysentery, Nicolas Lémery, cat-ointment and oil of puppies boiled with earthworms, Mattioli, oil of scorpions, and Paracelsus, human ordure (*Zebethum occidentale*). Glauber alone, in an important treatise on salts (1658[3]), urged the employment of chemical preparations in lieu of animal excreta. Old Nicholas Culpeper, the arch herbalist and quacksalver of the time, indulged in a vast amount of scurrilous raillery at the expense of the London Pharmacopœias of 1618 and 1650, but, except for his herb-lore, he was himself only the credulous astrologer described by Nedham, as "a frowsy-headed coxcomb" who had "gallimawfried the Apothecaries' Book into nonsense" in his aim to "monopolize to himself all the knavery and cozenage that ever an apothecary's shop was capable of."

---

[1] She was also a warm advocate of viper meat, to "temper, purify, and refresh the blood." Gossip claimed that Sir Kenelm Digby poisoned his wife with too frequent doses of viper's wine, given in aid of preserving her good looks.

[2] A. C. Wootton: Chronicles of Pharmacy, London, 1910, vol. ii, 2–31.

[3] Glauber: Tractatus de natura salium, 1658.

19

In Germany, Rivinus published a *Censura* of officinal remedies (1701), rejecting as worthless the poisons, parts of animals, perishable and inert substances, adulterated, substituted, faultily prepared or imaginary remedies and incongruous or incompatible mixtures.

Another curious feature of 17th century therapy was the large number of private or **proprietary preparations.** Prominent among these nostrums were the Scot's Pills (Grana Angelica), compounded by Patrick Anderson (1635) of aloes, jalap, gamboge, and anise (the modern pilulæ aloes et myrrhæ), which were, according to Wootton, successfully patented down to 1876, and are still asked for in the shops. John Pechey's cathartic pills were advertised at 1s. 6d. the box in his Sydenham (1695). The *Baume Tranquille*, compounded of herbs, by one of the Capuchins of the Louvre, was highly recommended by Madame de Sévigné (December 15, 1684). The *Baume Fioravanti*, another herbal tincture of the time, is still featured in the French Codex. Daffy's Elixir is still made. Dutch Drops, or Haarlem Oil, a mixture of oil of turpentine with other ingredients, has been used since 1672 as a "medicamentum" or routine preventive of disease. Charles II gave anywhere from £5000 to £15,000 for the formula of "Goddard's Drops," recommended by Sydenham, and said to have been made of raw silk. Carmelite water (*eau de Melisse des Carmes*), an aromatic cordial, made at the pharmacy of the Bare-footed Carmelites near the Luxembourg in 1611, was patented up to 1791, and sold up to 1840. Seignette's salts (*sal polychrestum*), devised about 1672 and a secret up to 1731, were Rochelle salts. The formula of the so-called Frankfurt pills, a popular laxative of aloes and rheum, also called Beyer's pills or *pilulæ angelicæ*, was transmitted by the inventor, Johann Hartmann Beyer (1563–1625), of Frankfurt, to Jacob Flösser, apothecary at the White Swan, in 1528, and handed down, in succession, to other apothecaries until late in the 18th century.[1] The pills of a figurative Dr. Immanuel ("God with us") of Nuremberg, were in use about 1638 as a cure-all, especially when the plague was prevalent.[2] Singleton's Golden Eye Ointment is described in Wootton's Chronicles as the oldest private remedy sold in England, and is still proprietary. Some time before 1630, the Countess of Chinchon, vicereine of Peru, was cured of malarial fever at Lima, by administration of **cinchona bark,** which had long been known to the Peruvian Indians, and was brought to Europe by the Jesuits' in 1632, and later by Juan de Vigo. No other event, says Neuburger, did so much to upset the current school systems of medicine as the discovery of Jesuits' bark. Ramazzini said that cinchona did for medicine what gunpowder had done for war. The fact that it rapidly cured a protracted intermittent fever, for which the older remedies had been employed for months at a time to void the "corrupted humors," was the end of Galenism in medical practice. It was introduced into English practice by Sydenham and Morton, and its use enabled them to differentiate malarial fever from other febrile infections and Torti to isolate the pernicious forms which do not yield to it. **Ipecac** was first mentioned as *igpecaya* by a Portuguese friar in Purchas' *Pilgrimes* (1625), and brought to Paris in 1672. About 1680, it began to be extensively prescribed as a secret remedy for dysentery by Helvetius and, at the instance of Louis XIV, the secret was tried out and purchased by the French government for 20,000 francs (1688). The drug has since had its ups and downs prior to the introduction of emetin (1910). **Antimony** had an extraordinary vogue in the 17th century through the fact that tartar emetic cured Louis XIV of a dangerous illness in 1657. Tartar emetic was first described by Adrian Mynsicht in 1631, and may have been identical with the Earl of Warwick's Powder (1620). Kermes mineral, devised by Glauber in 1651, was a secret for which Louis XIV paid a high figure in 1720, under the guise of *poudre des Chartres.* Antimony cups (*pocula emetica*) were in common use in Germany, but disappeared toward the end of the century.[3] In 1646, Athanasius Kircher described another kind of wooden cup, sent him by the Jesuits in Mexico, which would color water poured into it a deep blue, capable of chameleon-like fluorescence. This was the celebrated *lignum nephriticum*, first noted by Nicolas Monardes (1565) and Francisco Hernandes (1577) as a remarkable diuretic for renal and dropsical troubles. Caspar Bauhin described a similar cup in 1650 and,

---

[1] W. Stricker: Janus, Breslau, 1847, ii, 397–399.

[2] H. Schöppler: Arch. f. Gesch. d. Med., Leipz., 1911–12, v, 446–449; 1912–13, vi, 232.

[3] These remedies are all described at length in Wootton's "Chronicles of Pharmacy," London, 1910, *passim*.

in 1663, Robert Boyle made a careful investigation of the color phenomena. In 1915, W. E. Safford showed that *lignum nephriticum* is obtained from two species, viz., *Eysenhardtia polystacha*, the *palo dulce* of Mexico, which Boyle examined, and *Pterocarpus indica*, a large Philippine tree, from which Kircher's and Bauhin's cups were probably made. In the 17th century these cups were esteemed as gifts fit for royalty.[1] The **moxa,** which Sydenham thought identical with the ὠμόλινον of Hippocrates, was introduced into European practice as a remedy for the gout by Hermann Buschoff, a Batavian clergyman, in 1674, and recommended as a cure-all by Gehema (1682[2]).

Professional poisoning, as bad as that described in Livy and Cicero, was particularly rampant in Italy and France. Much of 16th and 17th century poisoning was, no doubt, intestinal obstruction, extra-uterine pregnancy, appendicitis, or what not. But the objects in the Musée de Cluny[3] and other data indicate that it was an ambition of the time

> To carry pure death in an earring, a casket,
> A signet, a fan-mount, a filigree basket,

and the scene in Swinburne's "Queen Mother," in which Catherine de Medici poisons her clown with a pair of gloves, is probably not exaggerated. Such an Italian poisoner was Exili, who left Rome for Paris, with a record of 150 cases against him, and came in contact with Sainte Croix, the paramour of the depraved Marquise de Brinvilliers. From Exili, Sainte Croix is said to have learned of the subtle compound with which his mistress disposed of her father, two brothers, and many unfortunate patients in hospital. She was caught up with by a love-making detective, tried, and hung in 1676. The white powder she employed defied all analysis. The affair led to a fashionable epidemic of secret poisoning, against which Louis XIV instituted the celebrated "Chambre Ardente." This was a kind of "third-degree" tribunal and, through its official grillings, the female fortune-tellers La Voisin and ·La Vigoureux, with their *poudre de succession*, were exposed and brought to justice. Arsenic was probably the toxic principle of the Aqua Tofana or Aquetta di Napoli of Teofania de Adamo, a diabolic female who, in 1709, owned to having poisoned over 600 persons with it, and was subsequently imprisoned or strangled.

Apothecaries' bills were exceptionally high in the 17th century, and the cost of medicines was often exploited by physicians and surgeons as an excuse for running up their charges. In Germany, the city *Apotheken* were of imposing architecture, the *facade* being sometimes ornamented with stone figures of great physicians of the past, as in those found at Hannover by Hermann Peters and at Lemgo by Arnold Klebs.[4] The Engel apotheke at Darmstadt (1654) became Merck's Fabrik in 1668. In London, Bucklersbury was not only the great drug mart, but had become a fashionable highway of intrigue—a sort of 17th century Bond Street. The grocers were the original drug merchants, even after the apothecaries were duly incorporated by James I (1606); but, in 1617, the druggists succeeded in shedding the grocers by

---

[1] Safford: Ann. Rep. Smithson. Inst., 1915, Wash., 1916, 272–298, 7 pl.

[2] For the history of the moxa, see Reichert: Deutsches Arch. f. Gesch. d. Med., Leipz., 1879, ii, 45; 145.

[3] For a description of these see L. Courtadon: Æsculape, Paris, 1912, ii, 188–192.

[4] H. Peters: Die Heilkunst in der Stadt Hannover, Hannover, 1901. A. C. Klebs: Arch. f. Gesch. d. Naturw., Leipz., 1914–15, v, 102–107, 2 pl.

means of a new charter, after which time they had the physicians against them.   The reason of this was that the apothecaries themselves set up as practitioners, not only selling drugs but prescribing them.   The long wrangle between physicians and apothecaries which came to a head in Garth's *Dispensary* began about the time of the Great Plague in London (1665), when the apothecaries made good in public estimation by staying at their posts, while the physicians (even Sydenham) fled for their lives.   Extortion was the great failing of the apothecaries.   In two drug bills of 1633 and 1635, cited by Handerson, 4s. are charged for a glass of chalybeate wine; "a purge for your worship" is listed at 3s. 6d.; "a purge for your son" at 3s.; and a powder to fume the bedclothes at 4s.   High as these charges were for the time, they are as nothing to the mulcting practised in 1633 by George Buller, who charged 30s. apiece for pills and £37 10s. the boxful.   In the reign of James I, the College of Physicians prosecuted Dr. Tenant for charging £6 each for a pill and an apozeme (decoction); and Pitt, in 1703, stated that apothecaries had been known to make between £150 and £320 out of a single case, and that their prescription charges were at least 90 per cent. more than the shop prices.   At this time, the average London physician's fee was about half a sovereign, while the apothecaries in ordinary to Charles I and Charles II got £40 and £72 per annum respectively. In 1687, the College of Physicians bound their fellows and licentiates to treat the sick poor of London and its suburbs free of charge, which strained the situation still further and, in 1696, 53 influential physicians subscribed £10 each to establish dispensaries for supplying drugs to the poor at cost price.   War was now joined not only between physicians and apothecaries, but an internecine wrangle broke out among the dispensarians and anti-dispensarians, the latter being, of course, favored by the apothecaries.   A lively bout of scurrilous pamphleteering ensued, and in 1699 Garth published *The Dispensary*, a satirical poem in the meter of Pope, urging the injustice of the dilemma forced upon the physicians "to cheat as tradesmen or to fail as fools."   It was described by Dr. Johnson as "on the side of charity against the intrigues of interest, and of regular learning against licentious usurpation of medical authority."   Pope also had a slap at

> Modern pothecaries, taught the art
> By doctor's bills to play the doctor's part,
> Bold in the practice of mistaken rules.

But, in spite of the support of the men of letters, the physicians were in the end beaten by the apothecaries, for a test case against an apothecary who had exceeded his license, which was brought to trial in 1703, and at first decided in the physicians' favor, was subsequently reversed in a higher court.   After this time, the English apothecaries became practitioners to all intents and purposes, and then began to make war upon those of their number who did not come up to certain standards of their own devising.   They were upheld in this, as we shall see, in 1815 and until 1886.

In the 17th century, the control of the **trade routes and the drug marts** passed into the hands of the Dutch and the English.

In the 16th century, Holland had already acquired complete control of the carrying trade between northern and southern Europe, as also of the supply of timber, tar, and wheat; but the secret of the sea route to the East Indies had been jealously guarded by the Portuguese.   In 1595–6, Jan van Linschoten, who had served in the Portuguese Indian fleet, published an account of his travels in the Far East, which gave much of the desired information.   Many brisk sea-fights ensued, until even the Moluccas fell into the hands of Holland.   Torrents of blood were shed for the "apparently inoffensive clove," which today is mainly of value in seasoning pickles and preserves or to conceal the odor of a drunkard's breath.   As Motley said, "The world's destiny seemed to have almost become dependent upon the growth of a particular gillyflower."   To get complete control of the clove, the Dutch extirpated it from the Moluccas and introduced the tree into Amboyna (Flückiger and Hanbury). To monopolize *Myristica fragrans*, the source of nutmegs and mace, they immersed the kernels in milk of lime for three months to prevent propagation outside the Banda Islands, and kept the entire nutmeg crop in stock at Amsterdam for sixteen years (Linton).   Tavernier tells how they monopolized the cinnamon of Ceylon. The English did not succeed in gaining a foothold in the drug marts until late, and for a long time their supplies were obtained by the capture of Portuguese and

Dutch vessels. The capture of Ormuz (1622) and the massacre of the British at Amboyna (1623), the subject of Dryden's play, are features of their clash with the Dutch. Their surest hold was destined to be in the peninsula of Hindustan. The British East India Company was chartered on December 31, 1600, and a permanent station was established on the Malabar coast in 1612.[1]

The extent to which exotic Eastern and American drugs were introduced is evidenced in the remarkable series of pharmacologic tracts published in London during 1672–95 and attributed in part to John Pechey of Gloucestershire. Molucca nuts, ginseng, Angola seed, ipecacuanha, casmunar root, Malabar nuts, Barbado seeds, Bermuda berries, Vanilla beans, salep, Colombo wood, Maldive nuts, *lignum nephriticum, Blatta bizantina*, Bengala beans, Perigua, Mexico seeds, Cylonian plant and cassiny are among these simples.[2] The supposititious author is not to be confused with John Pechey (1665–1716) of London, the translator of Sydenham (1696).

The purchasing power of money in the 17th century is said to have been some seven or eight times what it is now and, with this ratio in mind, we may gain some idea of the **compensation and income** of the physician and surgeon of the time.

The salary of a physician-in-ordinary was £100 annually, but Turquet de Mayerne got £400, with an annuity of £200 settled upon his wife. While the average fee of the English physician was, as stated, about 10s. (worth about $35 today), we find Richard Mead (1673–1754) charging a guinea a little later and a half a guinea for coffee-house practice. Harvey, who was not a successful practitioner, left an estate of £20,000. The annual salary of the Professor of Physic in the University of Cambridge in 1626 was £40. An old bill of 1665 gives 12s. as the fee for a twenty-mile visit; another, £1 and, for an outside visit of two days' duration, £1 10 s. Bleeding a lady in bed cost 10s., as against 2. 6d. for a man. A postmortem cost 3s. 4d.[3]

Thomas Arthur, a physician of Limerick, Ireland, although prevented by religious prejudice from practising among the wealthy, made an average income of about £250, or the equivalent of about $7000 today (Walsh). His fee for the management of a case of gonorrhea (1619) was £2 in advance and, for a putrid sore throat, 8s. The Professor of Physic in the University of Cambridge got £40 per annum in 1626. In Germany, the tariff was fixed by the ordinances of Hesse (1616), Frankfort on the Main (1668), and Prussia (1685). According to the Frankfort ordinance, an office visit was worth 40 pfennige (about 75 cents today), a house visit 1.35 marks, a night visit 1.70 marks, and a consultation one gold gulden (about $12.50). Foreigners were charged half as much again, and the wealthy paid what they liked. The family physician (*Hausarzt*) received a lump sum annually, as high as 100 marks in one case for attendance on a Bavarian countess (Baas). A city physician got over 500 marks if he inspected the city pharmacies; a court physician, 850 marks; and a physician-in-ordinary, 900 marks. The pest-doctor of Prague received 2000 marks a month. In France, Seguin purchased the post of physician-in-ordinary from Guillemeau for 50,000 livres and sold it for 22,000 crowns (about 200,000 francs in present money), while Valot, in 1652, paid Cardinal Mazarin 30,000 crowns for the vacant post of royal physician. Buckle states that the average French doctor's fee was as low as that of an English farrier. According to the *Levamen Infirmi* (1700), cited by Handerson, an English surgeon's fee was 12 pence a mile, 10 groats for bone-setting, a shilling for blood-letting, and £5 for amputation; a licensed physician got a noble or angel (6s. 8d.), although he might demand 10; a graduate in physic 10s., though they commonly demanded 20. Richard Wiseman got £150 as surgeon-in-ordinary in 1661, and de Choqueux £80 in 1665. The medieval custom of paying a life annuity for a successful operation was still in vogue. Wiseman records an annuity of £30 per annum from one patient (Power). According to the Frankfort tariff of 1668, a German barber-surgeon got 10½ marks, for setting a broken arm (20½ marks, if two bones were broken), 30.85 marks for a dislocation of

---

[1] See Tschirch: Pharmakognosie, Leipz., 1910, ii; and Linton: Jour. Am Pharm. Assoc., 1916, v, 473, 574.

[2] See Index Catalogue, S. G. O., 1. s., x, 594–595 *sub voce* Pechey.

[3] See Brit. Med. Jour., London, 1870, ii, 169.

the elbow- or knee-joint, or half as much if the result was poor. A surgeon charged 31 marks for amputating an arm, 41 marks for a leg, 51 marks for a lithotomy, or half price if the patient died. Herniotomy was rated at 51 marks, and a cataract operation 17 marks for one eye, or 25 marks for both. According to Baas' tabulation of the pay of army surgeons in Mark Brandenburg, a company surgeon got about 11 to 15 marks monthly in the infantry, and in the cavalry 11.40 marks in 1639, and 27 in 1655. A regimental surgeon got 30 marks in 1638, 15 marks in 1639, 27 marks in 1655, and 52.80 marks in 1685. During 1635–85 the surgeon of the exiled French mousquetaires got 90 marks monthly. The pay of a Saxon Feldscheerer in 1613 was 33 marks a month. It is interesting to note that, during the Thirty Years' War, and after, the Feldscheerer was at once regimental surgeon, barber, and standard-bearer (*Fähnrich*[1]). In England, under the Commonwealth in 1650, army surgeons at the northern posts got 6s. 8d. *per diem* and £15 for horses and medicine chests, if mounted. An English naval surgeon got £8 1s. for 175 days' services in 1653 and £16 14s. for 51 days' services in 1654.

The administration of **military medicine** during the 17th century was a continuation of the methods established at the siege of Metz (1552). Field medical officers (*medici puri*) were scarce. The armies of Gustavus Adolphus had apparently no regular regimental or company surgeons, but he prohibited pillage, devoting looted goods to "the next hospital," and the enemy's wounded were collected and sent to city hospitals. In the French and English armies, regimental hospitals and company infirmaries were the vogue. Richelieu established the first stationary (base) hospital under a *chirurgien-major* at Pignerol (70 miles from the front) in 1630. In 1666, the engineer Vauban designated places for hospitals in all the captured towns fortified by him. A retreat for superannuated soldiers was established at Hereford by Sir Thomas Coningsby in 1614, and the *Invalides* (Paris) was finally opened in 1676. Permanent general hospitals for soldiers were opened at Chelsea (England), in 1682, at Kilmainham (Ireland) in 1693, and the sailor's hospital at Greenwich in 1695. The medical personnel of the period was of a higher order, including such men as Harvey, Wiseman, Gehema, Purmann and Minderer. In the armies of the Elector of Brandenburg, each regiment had a staff physician and a field barber; and in 1683, the Saxon army acquired a chief surgeon on the staff of the general, with field barber and field apothecary, all with the rank of ensign. At the siege of Rochelle (1627), Richelieu assigned a personnel of civilian assistants (usually Jesuits and cooks) to the field hospitals, and provided for a crude ambulance personnel in an ordinance of 1638. In 1667, Louis XIV held a conference with the surgeons Turbière, Bienaise, and Gayant on increasing the medical personnel, with the result that at the battle of Seneffe (1674), 230 army surgeons were available, with nursing personnel and abundant material for the care of the wounded.[2] The long, tight-waisted *justaucorps* coats, the first distinctive uniform of the army surgeon, appear in this era, and are figured in Purmann and Heister.

The old-time strife and rivalry which, as we have seen, had always existed between the **physicians, surgeons, and barbers,** continued with unabated fervor in the 17th century. After the incorporation of the English barbers and surgeons into one company (1540), the barbers continued to be a nuisance to the surgeons, and the surgeons did not succeed in getting rid of them until 1745. Meanwhile, this united Company of Barber-Surgeons was permitted to have public dissections in its own hall, but nowhere else, and the cause of their education was further advanced by the Arris (1643) and Gale (1698) foundations for public dissections and lectures. In France, the medical profession had consisted for centuries of a *grande bourgeoisie* of physicians, a *petite bourgeoisie* of clerical barber-surgeons, and a proletariate of laic barbers or outcast surgeons (*barbitonsores*), all hating and despising one another and adhering to rigid caste distinctions. When, after the foundation

---

[1] See A. Köhler: Arch. f. klin. Chir., Berl., 1914, cv, 780–783.

[2] C. L. Heizmann: Ann. Med. History, N. Y., 1917–18, i, 287–294

of the College de St. Côme, the surgeon was, in a manner, assimilated to the status of the physician, he began to put on airs like the latter, wearing the square cap and long robe, substituting the device of three boxes of ointment upon his guild banner for the traditional three basins, arrogating to himself the right to examine the barbers, and insisting that his apprentices be "grammarian-clerks." By the 17th century, the physician had become a sterile pedant and coxcomb, red-heeled, long-robed, big-wigged, square-bonneted, pompous and disdainful in manner, making a vain parade of his Latin and, instead of studying and caring for his patients, tried to overawe them by long tirades of technical drivel, which only concealed his ignorance of what he supposed to be their diseases. Among themselves, the physicians were narrowly jealous of their rights and privileges, regarding their fraternity as a closed corporation, yet eternally wrangling about fantastic theories of disease and current modes of treatment. The lay barber, although an outcast and an outlaw, was, in some respects, the most worthy of all three since he was driven to study nature at first hand. He showed little submission or respect toward his rivals, and out of his clan had come Franco and Paré. Thus, while the barbers were crowding the surgeons who in servile imitation of the physicians had formed a syndicate against them, the physicians themselves maintained a supercilious, Malvolio-like attitude toward both. Physicians, as Forgue says,[1] would sometimes join with the barbers in an aristocrat-socialist combine against the surgeons, although sometimes favoring the surgeons' vows of precedence over the barbers, while barbers and surgeons would again solidify as a unit against the doctors. The result of all this intrigue and turmoil was that the barbers finally came into their own through the royal decree of 1660, which unified barbers and surgeons in one guild, but otherwise reduced them to the humblest status and drew down upon them the centupled wrath of the physicians. The curious isolation, the sterile inefficiency of the French internists of the 17th century are strikingly revealed in the letters of **Guy Patin** (1601–72), Dean of the Paris Faculty, who regarded the surgeons as mere "booted lackeys . . . a race of evil, extravagant coxcombs who wear mustaches and flourish razors." In 1686, however, an event occurred which Michelet has deemed "more important than the work of Paré." Louis XIV suffered, it seems, from a fistula in ano which, after remaining obdurate to the exhibition of all manner of ointments and embrocations, was successfully healed by operation at the hands of the royal surgeon, Félix. The latter received for his trouble a farm, 300,000 livres, three times more than the honorarium of the royal physician, and was ennobled, becoming the Seigneur de Stains. Félix was succeeded by Mareschal, and to Mareschal is due the elevation of the French surgeon's social condition in the 18th century. Louis XIV influenced French medicine in three curious ways: His attack of typhoid

---

[1] E. Forgue: Montpellier méd., 1911, xxxii, 601; xxxiii, 8.

fever (1657) gave an immense vogue to the use of antimony; his anal
fistula (1686) brought about the rehabilitation of French surgery; and
the fact that his mistress was attended by Clément, the royal accoucheur,
in 1663, did much to further the cause of male midwifery.[1]

The best sidelight on the pedantic formalism and complacent
ineptitude of the French internist of the period is afforded in the pensive
mockery of **Moliére** (1622–73). The great dramatist had no use whatever for the medical profession, whose ridiculous side early excited his
derision and against whom he seems to have cherished a lasting grudge,
partly because of their inability to do anything for his own malady
(consumption), and partly because he believed that they had killed his
only son and one of his bosom friends with their eternal antimony.
No less than five of his comedies abound in pungent raillery and light-
barbed sarcasm, directed with unerring skill against the tribe of doctors.

The tendency is exhibited in his very earliest farces, such as *Le Docteur
Amoureux, Les Trois Docteurs Rivaux, La Jalousie de Barbouille, Le Médecin Volant.*
In *Le Médecin Volant*, Sganarelle, the valet, cleverly mimics the pedantries of the
Paris Faculty. In *L'Amour Medecin*, we have an inimitable burlesque of professional consultations and discussions among five physicians of different types, one
of the points brought out being the relative merits of the old-fashioned Episcopal
mule and the new-fangled horse as a means of transportation. In the second act,
a strolling drug-vendor chants the virtues of the popular opiate, *orviétan.* In *Le
Médecin Malgré Lui*, Sganarelle is again impressed, by dint of drubbing, into playing
the part of doctor and, having a glib tongue, acquits himself exceeding well. In
Monsieur de Porceaugnac, two physicians, who have been bribed to pronounce M.
Porceaugnac insane, hold a solemn consultation *de lunatico inquirendo* over the pursy
provincial, and their long scholastic tirades seem exactly in the spirit of the times.
But the height of medical satire in Molière is achieved in his last great work, *Le
Malade Imaginaire*, of which the central figure, Argan—the hypochondriac, forever
drugging his imaginary ailments—is of the type portrayed by Butler in The Medicine
Taker. The first act discloses Argan grumbling over his apothecary's accounts,
the principal sources of medical revenue in those days. In order to have a physician
at beck and call about his household, he is desirous of marrying his daughter
Angélique to Thomas Diafoirus, a dense young medical graduate who is a good
match, as matches go, but by no means the young lady's choice. To outwit this
design, Toinette, the maid, disguises as a doctor, and through a clever stratagem
succeeds in making Argan relent his purpose, as well as in restoring him to health
and sanity. In the meantime, however, he is fairly bullied off the stage by M.
Purgon, an irate member of the Faculty who terrorizes him with the prospect of
bradypepsia, dyspepsia, apepsia, lientery, dysentery, dropsy, and general decline.
The doctors defeated, the intrigue is resolved by persuading Argan to become a
physician himself. Then follows what is perhaps the choicest bit of medical satire
ever penned, the intermezzo-ballet, a joyous burlesque of those ceremonies of medical graduation which John Locke described in his French diary. The French routine
of medical examination and graduation in this period was portentous in length and
pomp, and our data are taken from the admirable study of Maurice Raynaud.[2]
The unfortunate candidate, drilled almost to extinction in the scholastic régime of
the "naturals," anatomy and physiology, the "non-naturals," hygiene and dietetics,
and the "contra-naturals," pathology and therapeutics, without any bedside teaching

---

[1] His ordinary physicians were d'Aquin, a creature of Mme. de Montespan's,
and Fagon, who displaced the latter at the instance of Mme. de Maintenon. See,
P. Eloy: Fagon, Archiâtre du Grand Roi, Paris diss., 1918, No. 72.

[2] M. Raynaud: La médecine au temps de Molière, Paris, 1862. Even in the
15th century, it was customary for the regents of the Paris Faculty to have the
recreation of a midwinter visit to the public baths, followed by a supper, all at the
expense of the bachelors. (E. Wickersheimer: Gazette des eaux, Paris, 1914, lvii,
751.)

whatever, was put through his paces every two years by a long string of examinations and argumentation of theses, which lasted a week. The discussion of theses usually began at 5 or 6 A. M., lasting until mid-day, and woe to the luckless candidate who could not cope with the fire of absurd questions which were rained upon him. If he came through successfully and his name was one of those drawn by lot from the fateful urn, he became a licentiate for graduation. Hereupon, the licentiates and bachelors proceeded in solemn array to request the presence of all prominent and influential personages at the graduation ceremonies, the special feature of which was the Dean, the paranymph of the old Greek marriage ritual, who inducted the newly fledged licentiate into a sort of mystic union with the Faculty. At 5 in the morning of the momentous day, a preparatory session was held to determine questions of precedence, which were again decided by the urn. At 10, the hall was opened to visitors, the lists were proclaimed, and the successful candidates fell upon their knees to receive the apostolic benediction. The chancellor then proposed a question of religious or literary character to the candidate, who tackled it at once. This completed, the assembly proceeded in a body to the cathedral to thank the Holy Virgin for her good offices. Then followed, after an interval of six weeks or longer, the doctorate, the object of which was to induct the candidate into the sanctuary of the Faculty, as the licentiate had introduced him to the public. After a close inquiry into his moral character the candidate was first admitted to the *Vesperie*, which consisted in a solemn, intimate presidential discourse on the dignity and importance of the medical profession, followed by the discussion of another thesis, with speeches. Academic full-dress visits to the regents of the Faculty occupied the next few days. On the final day the candidate was sworn to the three articles of medical faith, viz., to obey all laws and observe all prescribed customs of the Faculty, to attend the mass for deceased physicians following St. Luke's Day, and to be unsparing in warfare against all illicit practitioners. The candidate having taken oath to this in the single word, *Juro*, the President (Praeses), making the sign of the cross with the baretta, placed this square bonnet upon his head and, with the administration of a slight tap or *accolade*, the doctor-in-embryo was born into the world. He immediately entered into his rights and privileges by proposing a thesis to be discussed by one of the physicians present, after which he delivered a florid, perfunctory discourse of thanks and praise. On the St. Martin's day following, he presided at the *acte pastillaire*, a general discussion of a thesis of his own choosing, and on the following day his name was inscribed on the registers as a junior for the next ten years.[1] This lengthy ceremony, which was set off everywhere by innumerable dinners, suppers, and banquets of old-time dimensions, forms the substance of Molière's immortal ballet. At the start, the Praeses burlesques, in mock Latin, the solemn discourse of the *Vesperie*. The first doctor then propounds the nice question: Why does opium produce sleep? To which the candidate replies

> Quia est in eo
> Virtus dormitiva,

to be greeted by the obligato chorus:

> Bene, bene, bene, bene respondere,
> Dignus, dignus est intrare
> In nostro docto corpore.

The candidate is then plied with questions as to his probable line of treatment in a string of diseases, for each of which he advances the incontestable merits of the clyster, the lancet, and the purge—

> Clysterium donare,
> Postea seignare
> Ensuita purgare,

followed by the constantly reiterated "Bene, bene." The famous Juro is then administered, and after the Praeses has conferred the bonnet, the candidate delivers a flowery discourse, full of servile praises of his benefactors. The ballet closes with festal dances and cheers, the physicians, surgeons, and apothecaries filing out solemnly at the end.

The good-humored character of Molière's satire, and the apparent indifference with which it was received by the medical profession of

---

[1] M. Raynaud: *La médecine au temps de Molière*, Paris, 1862.

his time and country, suggest that there was plenty of human nature in the French physician of the 17th century, in spite of his innocuous pedantry and sterile fanaticism. Across the Pyrenees, we find the same conditions, if we may trust the Spanish romances of the *picaresco* type, and the medical scenes in Le Sage's Gil Blas which, although published in 1715, is pure 17th century in its characters and local color. The droll consultation in the third chapter of its fourth book, in which Doctors Andros and Oquetos agree that the trouble in Don Vincent's case is "a mutiny of the humors," is fairly typical, the patient losing his life through the consequences of their dispute whether the Hippocratic expression ὀργασμός meant a fermentation or a concoction of said humors. Then there is the slap at the "fellows in this town calling themselves physicians, who drag their degraded persons at the Currus Triumphalis Antimonii, or . . . Cart's Tail of Antimony, apostates from the faith of Paracelsus, idolaters of filthy kermes"; and the sidelight on the use of the seton afforded in the case of Dame Jacinta: "Though a little stricken in years," she cherished her bloom by depletions and "doses of all powerful jelly, . . ." but "what perhaps contributed most to the freshness of this everlasting flower was an issue in each leg, of which I should never have known but for that blab Inesilla." But the medical interest of Gil Blas centers in the figure of Dr. Sangrado, "the tall, withered, wan executioner of the sisters three," whose name has, in fact, become a symbol for the kind of pitiless blood-letting which was rife in the 17th century. Sangrado's procedure of reducing the old canon to death's door in less than two days by drawing off 18 good porringers of blood, with abundant drenches of warm water, may be paralleled by the actual experiences cited by Guy Patin, who bled his wife 12 times for a fluxion in the chest, his son 20 times for a continued fever, himself 7 times for a cold in the head, while his friends, M. Mantel and M. Cousinot, bled 36 and 64 times in a fever and a rheumatism respectively. It is now known that the rationale of this extraordinary therapy (in able bodied people) lay in the copious drafts of water which were given with it, acting as a kind of blood washing in the evacuation of peccant humors. In Italy, where the functions of the physician and surgeon had never been entirely separated, intensive blood-letting had continued in vogue since the days of Botallo. The technic of the practice had become highly specialized, as may be seen in the handsome copper-plates of such books as Malfi's *Il Barbiere* (1626). Costly bleeding-glasses of Venetian type were handed down in families as heirlooms. In Germany, perhaps for some temperamental reason, the degree of blood-letting seems to have been less intense,[1] although the practice was otherwise frequent enough, being a common detail in the numerous pictures of bathing scenes. At these bathing resorts, it was required to spend 124 hours in the water as a cure, with frequent cupping and venesection, set off by the con-

---

[1] On this point, see France méd., Paris, 1912, lix, 365.

sumption of enormous quantities of food. Immorality was frequent, and the bath-keeper, plying his trade as a minor surgeon, is an index of the low status of the art in the Germanic countries, where Fabry of Hilden was almost the only educated surgeon. The German barbers were permitted to let blood, set broken bones, treat wounds and syphilis, but were not allowed to purge. Some of them went on voyages to the East Indies, or on whaling expeditions to Greenland to learn what they could. During the Thirty Years' War and after, many doctors and drug-sellers in the Germanic countries were vagrants.[1] Toward the end of the century, we find another queer substitute for

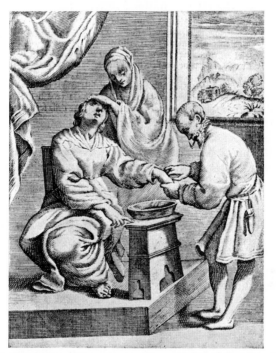

Blood-letting in the 17th century. (From Malfi's Il Barbiere, 1626.)

the surgeon proper, namely, the headsman or executioner. That the ceremonies of medical graduation in 17th-century Germany were as long and as expensive as those ridiculed by Molière is evidenced by an edict of the Elector of Brandenburg (1683), in which, to save the students' purses, banqueting was cut down to a single supper, limited to ten courses. "Ladies" and confectionery were excluded. In the case of needy students, the sumptuary features could be limited to the simple announcement of the candidate's graduation in the auditorium (at half price), the distribution of gloves and the convivium being omitted, unless the student saw fit to invite a few professors to a modest repast,

---

[1] See C. Stichler: Arch. f. Gesch. d. Med., Leipz., 1908–9, ii, 285–300.

at discretion (Baas). Although medical students have always borne a hard reputation for pranks and horse-play, the social customs of the German students, their hazing and "pennalism," were coarse and barbaric beyond belief. As in France, the junior student was a mere *bec jaune*, that is, a novice or aspirant, and treated as such. The lower strata of the profession were made up of all sorts of strolling quacks— tooth-drawers, uroscopists, magicians, rope-dancers, chiropodists, crystal gazers—who were also common in the Low Countries, and a favorite theme of the Dutch and Flemish artists. Of the many pictures of vagabond dentists, the best are the spirited canvases of the Flemish artist Theodore Rombouts in the Prado (Madrid) and, among the Dutchmen, those of Gerard Honthorst (Dresden Gallery), Gerard Dou (Louvre, Dresden, and Schwerin Galleries), Adriaen Brouwer (Cassel Museum; Lichtenstein Gallery, Vienna), and the younger Teniers (Cassel; Dresden). All these tooth-drawers have costumes evidently designed to make the bravest showing consistent with their means, some of them highly fantastic, with fur-trimmed robes and Oriental turbans. The current methods of venesection are well represented by the younger Teniers (Musée du Draguignan), Frans van Mieris (Vienna), in the fainting woman by Eylon van der Neer, and in the Death of Seneca by Rubens, both in the Old Pinakothek at Munich. The pedicurists, or corn-cutters, were a favorite subject of such men as David Teniers, Jr. (Cassel, Budapest, Madrid), and Adriaen Brouwer (Pinakothek; Prado; Schönborn Gallery, Vienna). Venesection in the forehead and the fastening of a seton in the arm or the back are favorite subjects of Adriaen Brouwer. The strangest of the Low Country itinerants were the quacks who pretended to cut stones from the head for the relief of insanity, idiocy, or other mental disorders. In the 16th and 17th centuries, it was a common byword to describe a person mentally unbalanced as having "a stone in his head." The therapeutic imposture consisted in making a superficial incision in the scalp, and palming a stone or stones, which were cast into a convenient basket at stated intervals during the patient's struggles. The trick seems to have been a very old one, and some of its representations in art such as those of van Bosch in Amsterdam, Jan Sanders in the Prado, or the etching of Pieter Breughel, Sr., in the Amsterdam Cabinet, go back to the 15th and 16th centuries. The most comic specimens of 17th century work in this field are the stone-drawers of Frans Hals, Jr., and Jan Steen in the Musée Boijmans (Rotterdam). Steen represents a quack incising the occipital region of a screaming fool, who is tied in a chair, while an old woman holds the pail, into which a giggling lad in the rear tosses the supposititious stones, one by one. A red chalk drawing of the younger Teniers shows a quack, with feathered turban and sword, opening the head of a stoical patient, who sits with folded arms and compressed lips. Physicians of a higher grade are to be seen in the many Dutch pictures of water-casting. Uroscopy is a feature of nearly all the Dutch pictures of the doctor's visit, and was sometimes employed even in the diagnosis of chastity. A solemn consideration of the appearance of the patient's urine seems to have been the favorite procedure in cases of the so-called *minne pyn* or *mal d'amour*, that is, the chlorosis of love-sick young women. To this theme Jan Steen devoted no less than nine canvases; Frans van Mieris, four; and Gabriel Metsu, two. In these pictures, the fur-trimmed jackets and rich gowns of the women indicate the wealthier class, the attending physicians being correspondingly dressed in black velvet robes or doublet and hose, with flat bonnets or bell-crowned hats, according to their social or religious affiliations.

The representation of the pallor and feverish discontent of the greensick, lovelorn maidens is very lifelike, particularly in the fine canvas of Gabriel Metsu (Preyer Collection, Vienna). The *clou* of this group of paintings is undoubtedly the *Mal d'Amour* of Gerard Dou (Buckingham Palace), a charming picture, representing a handsome young doctor, in his fur-trimmed pelisse and fur cap, earnestly scanning a urine flask, while he feels the pulse of a pretty *meisje*, whose upturned face reveals the all-important fact that her interest in his personality is in excess of her confidence in his professional skill.[1]

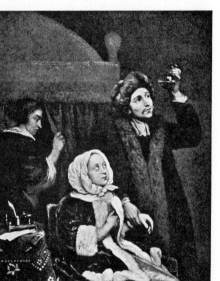

Mal d'Amour, by Gerard Dou. (Buckingham Palace.) Hanfstaengl, Munich.

The 17th century marks the rude beginnings of two new phases of national medicine—the Russian and the American.

In the 15th century, Ivan III (1468–1505), the first Russian ruler to bear the title of Czar, invited foreign physicians to settle in Moscow, with the not very alluring prospect of having their throats cut if they failed to cure. Under the reign of Ivan IV (1533–84), called the Terrible, many English physicians came to Moscow by invitation[2] and

---

[1] For a fuller account of all these pictures, with reproductions, see Eugen Holländer, "Die Medizin in der klassischen Malerei," Stuttgart, 1903.

[2] Among the foreign physicians who visited Russia was John Tradescant, a Fleming, who journeyed to Archangel with Sir Dudley Digges in 1618, and made a unique collection of natural history specimens, coins, medals, and other objects of *virtu*, which became in time the present Ashmolean Museum at Oxford.

some of these also functioned as ambassadors or diplomatists. One of them founded an Apteka, or drug-store, in 1581. Under the Romanoff dynasty (1613–45) and well into the 18th century, there was a great influx of adventurous foreigners who, through the encouragement of Peter the Great and Catherine, undoubtedly did a great deal to stimulate an interest in medicine. Like the Greeks in Rome, they were eyed with suspicion by the natives, who were always ready to sack their houses in popular uprisings. Upon arrival the foreign physicians took an oath of office pledging themselves not to use poisonous drugs. After an audience with the Czar, they were loaded with rich presents, money, provender, horses, and sometimes even acquired an estate of from 30 to 40 "souls." The first native Russian physician was Peter V. Postnikoff, who was sent to Italy to study medicine by Czar Peter and graduated at Padua in 1694.[1] The Russian therapeutic superstitions of the time were similar to those we have found in other countries. There was the same elaborated polypharmacy, including extracts made from insects and parts of animals, and not even the critique of Ambroïse Paré had dispelled the belief in the efficacy of the unicorn's horn, for three specimens of which 100,000 roubles ($30,000) were offered in 1655. Drugs were, however, imported from Germany and Holland, botanic gardens were started and, in 1671, a brief account of native Russian simples was drawn up, "a sort of miniature Siberian pharmacopœia," based upon information gathered from the peasantry by the Siberian *voyevods* (military governors). Under the Romanoffs a Ministry of Medical Affairs was founded, also a central store (Apteka) for the distribution of drugs to the followers of the Moscow court. A later Apteka, of larger scope, which dispensed drugs to soldiers and civilians and looked after the prevention of infectious diseases, was the nucleus of the above mentioned Aptekarski Prikaz (Ministry of Medical Affairs), the starting point of the patriarchal public health service of Russia.[2]

The new-world settlements of Jamestown, Virginia (1607), Plymouth Colony (1620), and the New Netherlands (1623), naturally drew to them a number of European physicians who, as in Russia, were active agents in advancing the interests of legitimate medicine in the colonies.

Prominent among these were Dr. Lawrence Bohun, who became Physician General of Virginia in 1611; Dr. John Pot, the first physician to reside permanently in Virginia, and elected temporary governor of the state in 1628; Herman Van den Boogaerdt, the first physician of New Amsterdam; Dr. Johannes La Montagne, a Huguenot, who was councillor of Wilhelm Kieft, Director General of the New Netherlands; Dr. Samuel Fuller, who came over in the Mayflower and practised in New England until his death in 1633; and Dr. John Winthrop, Jr., who was the first governor of Connecticut (Henderson). One of these emigrant physicians, Thomas Thacher, was, as we have seen, the author of the first and only medical publication printed in the North American colonies in the 17th century (1677).

[1] L. Stieda: Janus, Amst., 1903, viii, 178–189.

[2] For further details, see the article on Russian medicine in Lancet, Lond., 1897, ii, 354–361.

Meanwhile, higher education had a definite start with the foundation and endowment of Harvard College (1636–38), and of the College of William and Mary (Williamsburg, Virginia) in 1693; but native-born students and practitioners soon acquired the habit of going to Leyden, Oxford, or Paris to complete their medical courses. The practice of physic was often combined with the preaching of the gospel. One of these clerical physicians was Giles Firmin who, prior to 1647, delivered the first course in anatomy in New England and whose probable scheme of treatment and instruction has been outlined in the witty imaginative sketch of Oliver Wendell Holmes.[1] His anatomy he got from Vesalius, Paré, Fallopius, and Spigelius; his internal medicine was a mixture of the Greeks, Fernelius, van Helmont, and Sir Kenelm Digby; his pathology was mythology.

"His pharmacopœia consisted mainly of simples, such as the venerable 'Herball' of Gerard describes and figures in abounding affluence. St. John's wort and Clown's All-heal, with Spurge and Fennel, Saffron and Parsley, Elder and Snake-root, with opium in some form, and roasted rhubarb and the Four Great Cold Seeds, and the two Resins, of which it used to be said that whatever the Tacamahaca has not cured, the Caranna will, with the more familiar Scammony and Jalap and Black Hellebore, made up a good part of his probable list of remedies. He would have ordered Iron now and then, and possibly an occasional dose of Antimony. He would perhaps have had a rheumatic patient wrapped in the skin of a wolf or wild cat, and in case of a malignant fever with 'purples' or petechiæ or of an obstinate king's evil, he might have prescribed a certain black powder, which had been made by calcining toads in an earthen pot. . . . Barbeyrac and his scholar Sydenham had not yet cleansed the Pharmacopœia of its perilous stuff, but there is no doubt that the more sensible physicians of that day knew well enough that a good honest herb-tea which amused the patient and his nurses was all that was required to carry him through all common disorders."

Two features of American medicine in the colonial period are especially worthy of note. In the first place, the half-fledged youth, who studied with some physician under indentures of apprenticeship, received actual bedside instruction from the start and, although serving as sweep and stable-boy to his master, was still learning how to bleed and cup, to prepare drugs and apply them. Second, under primitive, frontier conditions, the medieval antagonism between physician and surgeon soon disappeared, for the necessary and sufficient reason that, while midwifery was in the hands of women, the open-country or back-woods doctor was liable to be called upon in any emergency. Thrown upon his own resources, he soon learned to enlarge such native skill as he had in bone-setting, treatment of arrow and gunshot wounds or reducing hernias and so became a bit of a surgeon. Before 1769, the term "Doctor" was not even employed in the colonies (Toner). As Handerson says, "Many of these apprentices doubtless proved as successful physicians (and success is the usual test of merit) as some of their more fortunate colleagues who boasted an M.D. of Leyden, Aberdeen, or Cambridge and slew their patients *secundum artem*."[2]

---

[1] O. W. Holmes: Medical Essays, Boston, 1883, 278–283.

[2] Baas: History of Medicine, New York, 1889, 582.

We may agree with the same authority that, from this period on, American medicine acquired that eminently practical tendency which has been its chief merit and of which we have no reason whatever to feel ashamed. That the profession soon developed a certain *esprit de corps* (backed up by strong public sentiment) is evident in that we find no records of strolling lithotomists, cataract-couchers, or other quacks in this period; that the names of no New England physicians are connected with the scandal of Salem Witchcraft (1692); and that we find records of the latter giving service to the sick poor for a remittance of taxes. Such medical legislation as the colonies had in this period was, as in the Code Hammurabi, mainly concerned with the momentous question of **fees.**

As early as 1636, the Assembly of Virginia passed an act providing that those who had served apprenticeships as surgeons and apothecaries should receive five shillings a visit and university graduates ten. Doctors' bills were usually paid, however, with such articles of barter as corn (in New England), tobacco (in the South), or wampum (among the Indians); and they soon became so exorbitant that, in 1638 and 1639, the Assemblies of Maryland and Virginia passed laws to moderate them. In 1649 the Massachusetts colony passed a law restricting the practice of medicine, surgery, and midwifery to such persons as might be judged competent by "some of the wisest and gravest," or most skilful in the same art, with the additional consent of the patient. A similar law was passed in New York in 1665, and in 1699 an act to prevent the spread of infectious diseases became a law in Massachusetts.

The first hospital in the New World was erected by Cortez in the city of Mexico in 1524. In 1639 an Hôtel Dieu was established in Canada by the Duchesse d'Aguilon, and ultimately located in Quebec. The Montreal Hôtel Dieu was established in 1644, and the General Hospital of Quebec in 1693. The first hospital in what is now the United States was established on Manhattan Island in 1663.

In spite of the serenity of Shakespeare and Spinoza, the light raillery of Molière and Butler, the clear vision of Bacon or La Rochefoucauld, the lusty *joie de vivre* of Rubens and Frans Hals, the spirit of the 17th century was sombre and mortuary, and something of the old medieval feeling about Death, as the King of Terrors, survives in the gloomy forebodings of Pascal or the lines of the Jacobian dramatist, Shirley,

> "Devouring Famine, Plague, and War,
> Each able to undo mankind,
> Death's servile emissaries are."

The actual mortality from wars and **epidemic diseases** was as great as in the Middle Ages.

The **bubonic plague,** if it did not sweep all Europe as formerly, struck with terrific force in some places. The Great Plague of London (1665) carried away 69,000; the Vienna visitation of 1679, 70,000; that of Prague (1681), 83,000; while the Italian epidemic of 1630 numbered 80,000 victims in Milan and over 500,000 in the Venetian Republic. In the opinion of Haeser, these losses, together with the Candian war, contributed materially to the downfall of Venice, whose great fleets once held "the gorgeous East in fee." The earliest visitations were those in Russia (1601–03), in which Moscow lost 127,000 souls from pest and famine. Through the century, England (1603–65), France (1608–68), The Netherlands

(1625–80), Italy (1630–91), Denmark (1654), Germany (1656–82), Sweden (1657), Switzerland (1667–68), and Spain (1677–81) were all severely ravaged. As in the 16th century, the local epidemics were commemorated in coins and medals, some of which were used as amulets, while others, highly ornate, betokened the freeing of a city from the pest. Of these, we may mention the Thuringian silver pennies of 1600, 1602, and 1611; the pest-dollars (of Wittenberg type) of 1619; the coins and medals struck off in memory of the epidemics incident to the Thirty Years' War at Urbino (1631), Venice (1631), Breslau (1631), Ingolstadt (1634), Frankfort on the Main (1635), Munich (1637), and the relics of the later visitations at Vienna (1679), Leipzig (1680), Würzburg (1681), Erfurt (1683), and Magdeburg (1683). All have been described in detail by Pfeiffer and Ruland (*Pestilentia in nummis*, 1882). Famine, always in the train of war and plague, was commemorated in the Annona medals, in praise of the Papal regulation of the price of corn, which were struck off in honor of Popes Clement X (1671–73) and Alexander VIII (1690); and in the medals relating to inundation in Hamburg (1685), to the plague of grasshoppers in Silesia and Thuringia (1693), hard times in the German Empire (1694), and hunger and cold in Holland (1698). The intense popular animosity against the corn pedlars and factors, whose thrifty extortions were not unnaturally confused with the unthrift of bad harvesting as a cause of human misery, is strikingly shown in the curious *Kornjudenmedaillen*.[1] Silesian medals of this type were struck off in 1694–95 and again copied in the 18th century. Besides grasshoppers and pedlars, comets were still regarded with superstitious awe as "God's postillions" (*Gottespostillione*), harbingers of war, pestilence and famine, although Shakespeare had said

"When beggars die there are no comets seen,"

and the astronomer von Littrow has latterly shown that there is no probable connection between the hundreds of comets known and the slightest possible variation in the atmosphere. There were comet medals for the years 1618, 1677, 1680, and 1686, but the appearance of Halley's comet in 1682 was distinguished by the great English astronomer's calculation that it would reappear in 1758. With the verification of this prediction, it was perceived that comets are, after all, like any other periodic phenomenon in nature. The comet theory of disease disappears from medical history after 1758.[2]

State and city ordinances against the plague were many and, while providing for special hospitals, attendance, and sanitary inspection, were sometimes extremely narrow and severe. On August 25, 1683, Colbert, minister to Louis XIV, issued sanitary regulations for the whole of France, giving absolute power to the Board of Health and quarantine station at Marseilles. Not only were plague-stricken houses burned to the ground after the Mosaic method, but persons suspected of spreading the plague by smearing its virus about were put to torture and death. A striking instance is afforded in an episode of the great plague of Milan in 1630, as described by the novelist Alessandro Manzoni,[3] and latterly in the valuable paper of Fletcher.[4] On the morning of June 1, 1630, Guglielmo Piazza, a commissioner of health of Milan, was seen going down the street, writing from an ink-horn at his belt, and wiping his probably ink-stained fingers against the walls of houses. Being accused, by the ignorant women of the neighborhood, of smearing the houses with deadly ointments, he was upon motion of the council haled to torture. The latter barbarity, a survival of the ordeal of feudal times, had an elaborate ceremonial, prescribed by legal code, in which the accused was stripped, shaved to the scalp, and purged before going through his misery; if he survived the atrocities inflicted upon his body three times, God was supposed to have intervened in a miracle. The unhappy Piazza stood for two applications of this hideous rite, but yielding to the "third-degree" suggestions of his tormentors, finally stated that he had obtained a

---

[1] The obverse of these famine medals commonly displayed a sorry looking pedlar, weighted down by a sack of corn which is punctured by a devil. The other side bore a bushel measure, on the inner surface of which was inscribed (in German) the verse of Proverbs (XI, 26): "He that withholdeth corn, the people shall curse him," the outer surface reading: "But blessing shall be upon the head of him that selleth it."

[2] Pfeiffer and Ruland: Pestilentia in nummis, Tübingen, 1882, p. 19.

[3] Manzoni: Storia della colonna infame, 1840.

[4] R. Fletcher: Johns Hopkins Hosp. Bull., Balt., 1898, ix, 175–180.

20

poisonous ointment from a barber named Mora. Following arrest, Mora himself yielded to the first application of torture, and though both unfortunates recanted more than once, the clamors of the superstitious populace against them were such that, upon sentence, they were torn with red-hot pincers, had their right hands cut off, their bones broken, were stretched on the wheel and, after six hours, burned. Their ashes were then thrown into the river, their possessions sold, the house of the crime razed to the ground, and its site converted into a sort of Aceldama by the erection of a "column of infamy" (*colonna d'infamia*). This was less than three centuries ago.

The physicians delegated to treat the plague wore a strange prophylactic garb, consisting of a long red or black gown of smooth material (often Morocco or Cordovan leather) with leather gauntlets, leather masks having glass-covered openings for the eyes, and a long beak or snout, filled with antiseptics or fumigants, for the nose. In his hand the pest-doctor carried a wand to feel the pulse. In spite of this comic opera make-up, he was a highly esteemed functionary, often drawing a large salary.

In the Italian cities, immense pits for burying the dead had sometimes to be dug, the *apparitori* or summoners going before, ringing a bell notifying the people to bring out their dead, the *monatti* attending to the matter, and the *commissari* reporting upon the cases and supervising the whole. Sometimes the rude common graves became filled to overflowing, and the dead lay putrefying in the streets. This is shown in Micco Spadara's picture of the Pest in Naples (1656), in which the Piazza del Mercato is seen swarming with dead and dying bodies which the *monatti* are struggling to remove, under direction of sundry physicians on horseback, while in the heavens God with a drawns word appears, apparently yielding to the entreaties of the Virgin. In "The Plague of the Philistines" by Nicolas Poussin (1593–1665) (Louvre), rats are represented in the background.[1] Nathaniel Hodges, in his *Loimologia* (London, 1672), describes how, during the Great Plague of 1665, rodents and reptiles were seen to come out of their holes to die in the open . Daniel Defoe, in his fictitious "Journal of the Plague Year" (1722), asserts that a purposeful war on rats and mice, as spreaders of pest, was made during the same epidemic (Sticker[2]).

Leprosy had so completely died out by the end of the 16th century that, in 1656 and 1662, Louis XIV was able to abolish the lazar-houses and devote their endowments to charity and general hospital construction. Relics of the disease in art are preserved in Rubens' painting of St. Martin (Windsor Castle) and Murillo's St. Elizabeth in the Prado (Madrid). **Syphilis** had also ceased to be epidemic, and was treated by mercurial fumigation and inunction at the hands of the barber-surgeons. It broke out in Boston, Massachusetts, in 1646, sixteen years after the foundation of the city.[3] Beyond the illustrated books, such as those of Stephen Blankaart, and the views of Sydenham, who regarded it as a modified West-African yaws, the 17th century literature of lues is not important. Next to the plague, **typhus** and **typhoid fevers**, which were often vaguely described as "pest," had the highest mortality, especially in connection with the miseries engendered by the Thirty Years' War. Dysentery and scurvy also added their quota, and so great was the mortality occasioned that, according to the Excidium Germaniæ (cited by Haeser), "one could wander for ten miles without seeing a soul, scarce a cow, only an occasional old man or child, or a pair of old women. In every village, there are houses filled with dead bodies and carrion; men, women, children, servants, horses, swine, cows, and oxen lying pell-mell together, throttled by plague and hunger, devoured by wolves, dogs, crows, and ravens, for want of decent burial." Add to this the sexual atrocities of soldiery, as depicted in Grimmelshausen.[4] In the cities,

---

[1] G. Sticker: Janus, Amst., 1898, iii, 138.

[2] Sticker: Die Pest, Giessen, 1908, i, 178.

[3] Packard: History of Medicine in the United States, Phila., 1901, 39.

[4] H. J. C. von Grimmelshausen: Der abentäuerliche Simplicius Simplicissimus, 1668.

typhus fever was carefully studied by such observers as Stahl and Friedrich Hoffmann in Halle, or Schröckh in Augsburg. Boghurst differentiated the symptoms of the Great Plague from spotted (typhus) fever in an unprinted MS. of 1666. Pepys noted the prevalence of spotted fever among the aristocracy. Willis described typhus among the Parliamentary troops at the siege of Reading (1643) and typhoid at Oxford (1661). Typhoid pneumonia was prevalent in Italy (1602–12, 1633, 1696), as described by Codronchi and others. Hochstätter described an Augsburg epidemic of 1624, and Switzerland was visited in 1652, 1685 (Lake Geneva), and 1694–95. Sir Norman Moore (1882) has described the typhoid of Henry Prince of Wales (1612), from the original autopsy by Roger Coke (Record Office). Malarial fever was pandemic in the years 1657–69 and 1677–95 (Haeser). The English epidemics were well described by Willis, Morton, Sydenham, Morley and Lucas Schacht, the Italian by Cavallari (1602) and Borelli (1661); the Dutch by Fanois (1669) and Sylvius (1677); the French by Chirac (1694). The severe Italian epidemic of 1690–95 was described by Ramazzini and Lancisi. **Dysentery** was epidemic throughout the countries ravaged by the Thirty Years' War, notably Germany, Holland, and France (1623–25). It reinvaded Germany in 1666 and the North in 1676–79. The English epidemics of 1668–72 were described by Willis and Sydenham. During the period 1583–1610, **diphtheria** was confined to Spain. In 1610, it broke out in Italy, where it was again epidemic in 1618–30 and 1650, while Spain was revisited in 1630, 1650, and 1666. Cases occurred at Roxbury, Massachusetts, in 1659 (Jacobi). An epidemic of anthrax (1617) is described by Athanasius Kircher in his *Scrutinium pestis* (i, 9). There were many epidemics of **ergotism** in the Sologne (1630–94), in various parts of Germany (1648–93), and in Switzerland (1650, 1674). **Scurvy** occurred at the siege of Breda (1625), at Nuremberg (1631), and at Augsburg (1632). **Influenza** was common throughout the century, both in the Old World and the New. Crookshank holds that the lethargic encephalitis at Copenhagen, described by Bartholin (1657), the English febrile epidemic of 1661 described by Willis as affecting "brains and nervous stock," the "comatose fever" of Sydenham (1673–5), and a case of encephalitis lethargica noted by J. P. Albrecht of Hildesheim (1695), were all manifestations of influenza. Whitmore describes the anomalous ague (*febris anomala*) of 1658–9 as "so prodigious in its alterations that it seems to outvie even Proteus himself" (Creighton). It was first reported in America in 1647.[1] Yellow fever appeared at New York in 1668, in Boston (1691–93) and Charleston, South Carolina, in 1699, but did not reach the Old World until the following century. Of the exanthemata, **smallpox** was pandemic in Europe in 1614, epidemic in England during 1666–75, while in New England, scattered outbreaks occurred all through the century, the disease reaching Pennsylvania in 1661, and Charleston, S. C., in 1699. The most important accounts are those of Sydenham. The first accounts of unmistakable **scarlatina** are due to Michael Doering (1625–8) and Daniel Sennert (1628), but the disorder became generally known through the descriptions of Sydenham (1676) and Morton (1692[2]). Sydenham first clearly differentiated it from the "morbilli," in which it had been classed. Measles, rubella, and "the purples" (miliary fever) were usually grouped together and not differentiated. **Puerperal septicemia** was first defined and differentiated by Willis in 1660.[3] Infantile conjunctivitis was first reported in America in 1658 (Jacobi[4]). **Infantile mortality** in this period was high. In Restoration England, sometimes half the births were obliterated by disease and two-fifths of the total deaths were of infants under two years. In the hot summers of 1669–71, 2000 babies died of diarrhea in eight or ten weeks. The dense London population had swarmed to the waterside and the alleys of Wapping, Lambeth, Whitechapel, and Spitalfields, living in filthy, overcrowded tenements.[5] The unfortunate newborn child was salted, after the old Galenic teaching, encased in tight swaddling clothes, and allowed no exercise beyond a few minutes dandling in the open air. Later, it learned to walk by means of a walking-chair or leading-strings. Eczema and discharges from unwashed ears were looked upon as part of the scheme of

---

[1] A. Jacobi: Jahrb. f. Kinderh., Stuttgart, 1913 (Baginsky Festschrift), 414.

[2] See Paul Richter's history of scarlatina (Arch. f. Gesch. d. Med., Leipz., 1907–8, i, 161–204), which corrects the errors made by Haeser.

[3] De febribus, 1660, ch. xvi.

[4] *Op. cit.*, 413.

[5] Traill and Mann: Social England, London, 1903, iv, 647. Cited by Forsyth.

nature (Walter Harris, 1689), and artificial feeding, in lieu of wet-nursing, was not known. Pechey (1697) recommended weaning at the appearance of the milk teeth and on the increase of the spring or autumn moon. To overcome the child's dislike for new foods, the mother's nipples were smeared with aloes or wormwood.[1] In France, through the humanitarian efforts of St. Vincent de Paul (died 1660), small asylums for helpless infants were started leading to the establishment of the *Hopital des enfans trouvés* at Paris (1641) by Louis XIII.

As we have seen, the 17th century was the age *par excellence* of medical delineations in oil paintings. Velasquez, the greatest portrait painter of all time, devoted some twelve canvases to the representation of cretinoid or hydrocephalic dwarfs, four to court fools, and three to idiots. Of these, the Prado contains ten, including the hydrocephalic Don Sebastian de Morra, El Primo, the achondroplasic and rachitic specimens in Las Meñinas, the buffoons of "silly Billy" type, and those wonderful figurations of idiocy, El Niño de Vallecas and the strabismic El Bobo de Coria. Ribera has a remarkable picture of unilateral paral- ysis in a boy (Vienna Gallery), showing the characteristic deformity in arm and leg. A hand-bill carried by the lad, bearing the inscription *Da mihi elimosinam propter amorem Dei*, indicates that the speech center is also affected. The lame, the halt, the blind, and various phases of malingering (*les gueux contrefaits*) are well represented in the etchings and engravings of Jacques Callot (1592–1635). Pieter Breughel, the elder, represented the dancing mania, parades of cripples (paralytic gaits), blind men, and other grotesques in his etchings and paintings. The paintings of Breughel and of Heronymus Bosch depict in particular the gaits and deformities of the amputated and the paralytic. Endo- crine (pituitary) obesity may be inferred in the obese, quasi-myxede- matous girl of Juan Careño de Miranda in the Prado. Rubens depicted a microcephalic dwarf in his painting of Count Thomas Arundel and wife (Old Pinakothek, Munich). His colossal paintings of Loyola heal- ing the possessed (Vienna, Genoa) are the great authentic documents of the period for the passional attitudes of the hysterical, and inspired his friend, Arthur Quellinus to carve the remarkable sculpture repre- senting insanity in the City Museum at Amsterdam. His "Death of Seneca" and his crayon studies of muscular anatomy have already been mentioned. Van Dyck depicted leprosy in "St. Martin dividing his cloak" (Windsor Castle). With the exception of his "Tobias healing his father" of cataract, an etching of a leper, and a portrait of a man in the Koppel collection (Berlin), which Holländer regards as syphilitic, Rembrandt adhered rigidly to the normal, even in his etch- ings, in which he depicted every physiologic action of the human body.[2] We have mentioned the success of the Dutch painters in representing chlorosis (*febris amatoria*), and in the same class belong Gabriel Metsu's Feverish Child (Steengracht Gallery, The Hague), Gerard Dou's Dropsi- cal Woman (Louvre), and Frans van Mieris' Physician with a Melan-

[1] Forsyth: Proc. Roy. Soc. Med., Lond., 1910–11, iv, pt. 1, Sect. Dis. Child., 116–120.

[2] Rovinsky Collection, Petrograd, 1890.

cholic Patient (Vienna Gallery). A remarkable painting by Simon
Vouet, in the possession of Professor W. A. Freund, of Berlin, represents a case of suppurative osteomyelitis in a woman whose handsome
appearance is in sharp contrast with her repulsive looking limb. The
Dutch paintings of scenes of medical consultation and urine inspection
are, for costumes and accessories, the finest in existence, in particular
those of Gerard Dou in the Hermitage (Petrograd) and Vienna Gallery,
Adriaen van Ostade and Gerard Terborch in the Old Museum (Berlin),
the elder Teniers in the Uffizi (Florence), Gabriel Metsu in the Hermitage, Frans van Mieris in the old Pinakothek (Munich), and Teniers'
village physicians in the Brussels and Carlsruhe Galleries.[1] Returning

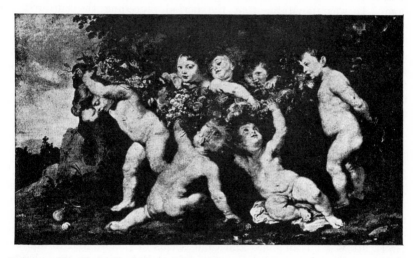

Rubens: The Garland of Fruit (Düsseldorf Gallery). (Eugenic ideal of the late
Renaissance Period.)

to the normal, it is worthy of remark that Rubens excelled all other
artists in conveying the full-bodied maternal type of the later Renaissance ("the justified mother of men") and the charm of healthy infants
and children. His "Garland of Fruit" symbolizes the eugenic ideal of
the period. His handling of this theme in oil reminds us of what Swinburne says of Andrea del Sarto's "round-limbed babies in red-chalk
outline, with full-blown laughter in their mouths and eyes; such flowers
of flesh and live fruits of man as only a great love and liking for newborn children could have helped him to render."[2]

---

[1] For reproductions of these pictures, see Eugen Holländer, Die Medizin in der
klassischen Malerei, Stuttgart, 1903.

[2] A. C. Swinburne: Essays and Studies, London, 1875, p. 356.

THE EIGHTEENTH CENTURY: THE AGE OF THEORIES AND SYSTEMS

The best work of the 17th century, whether of Shakespeare or Molière, Rembrandt or Velasquez, Spinoza or Newton, Harvey or Leeuwenhoek, was either conceived from some deep source of original inspiration or else sprang from a fresh, naïve wonderment over the newly revealed marvels of nature, as when old Pepys declared himself "with child" to see any new or strange thing.[1] The noble sacrifices of the heroes and martyrs of the preceding century engendered rich fruit in science as well as a great gain for spiritual and intellectual freedom. It was inevitable that the period preceding the outburst of political revolution should be as a lull before an approaching tempest, and, indeed, things veered far to the opposite extreme of exaggerated sobriety and apparent content with the old order of things. Tedious and platitudinous philosophizing (upon à priori grounds) was the fashion, even as a device to justify the immoralities of the age.[2] In the literature of France there is sometimes an undertone which seems to tell of coming change—

> The day that dawns in fire will end in storms,
> Even though the noon be calm—

but, in the end, everything tended toward formalism, and every theory, however idealistic, soon hardened into a rational, methodistic "system." In this regard, the most characteristic figures of the century—Kant and Rousseau, Voltaire and Hume, Swedenborg and Wesley, Linnæus and Buffon, Racine and Pope—speak for themselves. Even the music of Mozart, Haydn, and Gluck, although in sheer beauty like something Greek strayed out of place and time, seems of precise and formal cut if compared with the sublime polyphony of Palestrina or the splendor in infinite detail of that contrapuntal giant Bach; while Händel is absolutely square-toed, silver-buckled, and periwigged in manner. The best scientific work done of the period was in the fields of chemistry, mathematical physics, and invention, as witness the names of Lagrange and Laplace, Cavendish and Priestley, Scheele and Lavoisier, Galvani and Volta, Franklin and Count Rumford, Fahrenheit, Celsius, and Réaumur, Watt, Fulton, and Stephenson. For medicine, aside from the work of a few original spirits like Morgagni, Hales, the Hunters, Wolff, and Jenner, the age was essentially one of theorists and system-makers. Linnæus established the vogue of classification in medicine

---

[1] The *Orbis pictus* of Amos Comenius (1657), which so delighted the childhood of Goethe, was a characteristic production of the 17th century, designed to make Latin easy for schoolboys through the illustrations.

[2] The boresome *longueurs* of Rousseau and Crebillon *fils* derive from the illimitable novels of Mlle. de Scudéry, whose "map of affectivity" (*carte du tendre*) affords an amusing purview of 17th century psychology (Psychiat.-Neurol. Wochenschr., 1927, xxix, 369).

as well as in botany and seems to have set the pace everywhere. In this respect, the medicine of the 18th century is as dull and sober-sided as that of the Arabic period. We see the great theorists of the time, as Emerson has described the gods, each sitting apart in his own sphere, "beckoning up to their thrones," yet, as we pass from peak to peak, Hippocrates or Sydenham, Vesalius or Harvey, Celsus or Paré seem somehow nearer and more accessible to moderns than Stahl or Barthez, Bordeu or Boerhaave, Brown or Reil.

The great Swedish botanist, Carl von Linné (1707–78), or **Linnæus,** was himself a physician. He studied medicine in order to win the hand of a wealthy practitioner's daughter, for the father declined to consent to the match unless his prospective son-in-law became a doctor. Linnæus gave the most concise descriptions of plants and animals in all natural history. He originated the binomial nomenclature in science, calling each definite natural object by a generic or family name and a specific or given name, and classifying man himself as *Homo sapiens* in the order of primates. Linnæus believed, however, in the fixity of species (*nulla species nova*) and maintained that "there are just as many species as issued in pairs from the Creator's hands" and no more.

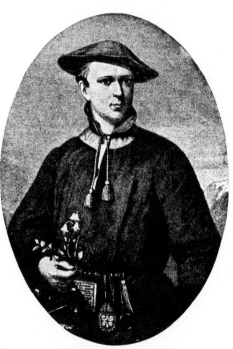

Carl von Linné (Linnæus) (1707–78).

His first work, the *Systema Naturæ* (1735), consists of twelve folio pages containing his classification of plants, animals, and minerals. It became so popular that it passed through twelve editions in his life-time. Specific names were first employed by Linnæus in (1753) his *Species Plantarum* (for plants), and in the tenth edition of the *Systema Naturæ* (1758), for animals. The latter is, in consequence, the most highly prized of all the editions of his great work. The medical writings of Linnæus include his materia medica (1749–52) and his scheme of nosology (*Genera morborum,* 1763). He had some notion of water-borne malarial fever and of the parasitic origin of disease. Hektoen says he gave good descriptions of embolism, hemicrania, and aphasia (1742).

Linnæus based his classification of plants upon characters derived from the stamens and pistils (the sexual organs of the flower). This so-called "Sexual System," which exaggerated the importance of the flower at the expense of the whole plant, and which Linnæus himself admitted to be a faulty but convenient mode of indexing things, dominated European botany for more than a century.

It was further expanded by Michael Adanson (1727–1806), a physician of Aix in Provence, whose *Familles des plantes* (Paris, 1763) comprised an arrangement of genera in 58 families; and by Antoine Laurent de Jussieu (1748–1836) of Lyons. Jussieu was the nephew of Bernard de Jussieu, a botanist who had applied the Linnæan system in arranging the plants in the Royal Garden of the Trianon. When young Jussieu became demonstrator at the Jardin des Plantes, he was called upon to arrange the flora in this garden. He adopted a natural system of one hundred orders arranged in fifteen classes, harking back to the basic principles suggested by Ray—Acotyledones, Monocotyledones, Dicotyledones—and further subdividing these according to the petals. His principal work is his *Genera Plantarum* (Paris, 1789), which was the source of authority until the Geneva botanist de Candolle introduced a morphologic system,[1] based upon the form and development of the organs of plants as opposed to their physiologic functions.

All these systems exerted a profound influence upon medical men in their attempts to classify disease. The system of de Candolle, as we shall see, was the basis of the curious arrangements of pathologic phenomena which were made by Schönlein, Canstatt, Fuchs, Rokitansky, and other members of the German "Natural History School" in the early part of the 19th century.

The ludicrous aspect of this "last century" mania for sterile, dry-as-dust classification was keenly felt by Goethe, the ablest plant morphologist of his time. His sentiments are voiced in the expressive lines in Faust:

> Grau, teurer Freund, ist alle Theorie,
> Und grün des Lebens goldener Baum.

We may dispose of the medical votaries of "gray theory" at once. First of all, Georg Ernst **Stahl** (1660–1734), of Ansbach, Bavaria, in opposition to the mechanistic physiology of Descartes, revamped van Helmont's idea of a "sensitive soul" as the source of all vital phenomena. The Stahlian "animism" (1737) is the ancient doctrine of the identity of soul and life-force (φύσις), the modern "vital principle," the Bergsonian *élan vital* ("*Veteres etiam naturam vocaverunt*"). The body is a passive machine, permeated and guided by an immortal soul. The Stahlian soul acted directly, without the intervention of archæi or ferments, and the criterion of vital processes is that the living body is not subject to putrefaction. Disease to Stahl was a disturbance of vital functions caused by misdirected activities of the soul. Altered tonus and plethora (vascular atony) make up the rest of his pathology. He even doubted the efficacy of drugs like opium or quinin, and was so far behind his time that he still recommended castration in hernia. Plethora he relieved by copious blood-letting and balsamic pills. He was fond of the suggestive effect of "secret" remedies. His conception of "life" was apparently identical with Imlac's definition of immortality in *Rasselas*—"a natural power of perpetual duration as a con-

---

[1] A.-P. de Candolle: Regni vegetabilis systema naturale, Paris, 1818–21. Also his "Prodromus," Paris, 1824–73; and his "Organographie végétale," Paris, 1827.

sequence of exemption from putrefaction." Like Newton, he ended his days in abject melancholia. Apart from his treatise on plethora as a cause of disease (1698[1]), which has won even the commendation of Virchow, and his original account of lacrimal fistula (1702[2]), he left little of value, but he exerted a profound influence upon Whytt, and traces of his influence are discernible in Bichat and even in Driesch. The tendency to confuse what the poet calls "the sublime and irrefutable passion of belief" with the purposes of scientific investigation is, indeed, one of the saddest things in the history of medicine. And Stahl was a well-meaning reactionary in still another direction—in his false theory of combustion which threw back the progress of chemistry for a century. He assumed that when a body burns it is "dephlogisticated," that is, gives off a hypothetic substance (phlogiston), although Mayow before him (as Black and Lavoisier after him) had shown experimentally that a burning substance gains rather than loses in weight.

As a reaction against the empty formalism of the 18th century, the animism of Stahl is of considerable importance to the anthropologist and the psychiatrist. In 1871, E. B. Tylor deliberately employed the Stahlian concept to explain the psychology of primitive man. As an advocate of psychotherapy, Stahl is a connecting link between the present and the past. He observed some of the remarkable effects of the mind upon the body, and his theory of the distraught psyche as a *causa causans* of disease contains the germ of Freudian doctrine.

The principal follower of Stahl was François Boissier de la Croix de Sauvages (1706–67), who considered the soul the activator of the mechanism of the body, but is better remembered by his *Nosologia methodica* (1768), which illustrates the taxonomic mania in a most ludicrous way. Sauvages endeavored to classify diseases as if they were specimens in natural history, subdividing them into 10 classes, with as many as 295 genera and 2400 species.[3]

The "animism" of Stahl became finally merged into the vitalism of the "four B's," Bordeu, Barthez, Bichat, and Bouchut—to find a more recent avatar in the tedious "entelechies" of Driesch. Eighteenth century vitalism assumed a specifically modern form in the *Bildungstrieb* of Johann Friedrich **Blumenbach** (1752–1840), which argues an innate impulse in living creatures toward self-development and reproduction. A great deal of theorizing in the 18th century was part and parcel of the Glisson-Haller doctrine of irritability as a specific property of all living tissues. William **Cullen** (1710–90), a lucid spirit of attractive character, sought to remove some of the difficulties encountered in the theory by regarding muscle as a continuation of nerve, and life itself as a function of nervous energy. In this way, our modern phrase, "nerve force," became a substitute for the old Galenic "animal

---

[1] Stahl: De venæ portæ porta malorum, Halle, 1698.

[2] Stahl: De fistula lachrymali, Halle, 1702.

[3] The other botanic classifiers of disease in the 18th century were Rudolph August Vogel, Sagar, Cullen, MacBride, Daniel, and Plouquet (Wunderlich).

spirits." Even today, when a doctor refers to some indeterminate pathologic condition as "probably nervous," he is unconsciously harking back to Cullen. Upon this sort of reasoning, still another theoretic element was superimposed—the ancient Methodistic doctrine of the *strictum et laxum* of Asclepiades. Friedrich **Hoffmann** (1660–1742), of Halle, assumed a mysterious, ether-like fluid acting through the nervous system upon the muscles, keeping them in a state of partial tonic contraction; and also keeping the humors of the body in the motion necessary for life. Acute diseases should, therefore, be due to a spasmodic condition, chronic diseases to atony. Apart from spasm and atony, Hoffmann admitted humoral changes and faulty excretions as causes of disease. The four conditions were to be relieved by sedatives, tonics, alteratives, and evacuants respectively. In Allbutt's view, Hoffmann was the greatest of the iatromechanists and the first to perceive that "pathology is an aspect of physiology."[1]

As a writer on medicine, Hoffmann was of extraordinary versatility. He revived the use of mineral baths (1696–1731), was one of the first to describe convulsive asthma with dropsy (1707), appendicitis (1716), chlorosis (1730), and rubella (1740), was a careful observer of local epidemics and meterology, wrote notable treatises on personal hygiene (9 vols., 1715–28), physiology (1718), pathology (1719), medical ethics (*Medicus Politicus*, 1738) and pediatrics (1741), sets of *Consilia* (1721–39) and Consultations (1734). Assembled, his many tracts on diseases of the digestive system from apepsia (1695) to esophageal spasm (1733) would make an efficient text-book of the time. His astonishing range of observation is indicated in such themes as convulsive fright from spectres (1682), diseases from metals (1695), *Pumpernickel* (1695), snuffs (1700), traveling for health (1701), oatmeal cure (1714), transmutation of disease (1716), monoxid poisoning at Jena (1716), multiplex causation of death (1717), terminal infections (*quod nemo ægrotorum moriatur ex morbo*, 1717), preparation for reading old authors (1719), sickness from cold drinks (1721), medicated baths (1722), painful heart (1730), metastases (*morbus mutatus*, 1731), and senility as a disease (1731). A great, original physician, whose writings await intensive study.

The Asclepiadean Methodism was pushed to an absurd and yet most logical limit by the celebrated John **Brown** (1735–88[2]). "The disputatious and disreputable Brown," as Allbutt styles him, was a coarse man of low habits, whom Cullen had taken up and launched, but who, like Colombo, Borelli, and other ingrates of medicine, turned against his quiet teacher with the plebeian's usual tactics of reviling his intellectual betters in order to exalt himself. Yet the Brunonian theory, as it was called, actually held the attention of Europe for a quarter-century and, as late as 1802, a *rixa* or students' brawl between Brunonians and non-Brunonians at the University of Göttingen lasted two whole days and had finally to be put down by a troop of Hanoverian horse. As far as it went, the theory was absolutely consistent and complete in all its parts. Brown regarded living tissues as "excitable" in lieu of the Hallerian "irritability," and life itself as non-existent, except as a resultant of the action of external stimuli upon an organized

---

[1] Allbutt: Brit. Med. Jour., Lond., 1900, ii, 1850.

[2] Brown: Elementa medicinæ, 1780.

body. Diseases are then "sthenic" or "asthenic," according as the vital condition or "excitement" is increased or diminished. The essentials of diagnosis are simply whether a disease is constitutional or local, sthenic or asthenic, and in what degree, and the treatment consists in either stimulating or depressing the given condition. To this end opium and, of course, alcohol were Brown's favorite agents. Hippocrates said that no knowledge of the brain can tell us how wine will act upon any particular individual, and Brown proceeded to apply this experimental idea *in propria persona* to elucidate his theory, using successive doses of five glasses at a time. Abuse of opium and alcohol eventually killed him. His method gained little support in France and England, but Rush took it up in America, Rasori, Moscati, Brera and others in Italy, and in Germany, after Christoph Girtanner's plagiarisms of 1790 had been exposed and the "Elementa medicinæ," translated by M. A. Weikard, Brown came into his own. The book hypnotized even Peter Frank and Röschlaub and was greeted by a flood of pamphlets and salvos of praise. Although his errors were pointed out by Humboldt and Hufeland, Brown had the unique distinction of polarizing the German profession. His therapeutic ideas, Baas asserts, destroyed more people than the French Revolution and the Napoleonic wars combined, nor will we dispute the same historian's pronouncement that he was "morally deserving of the severest condemnation."

Another ludicrous phase of theoretic medicine in the 18th century was the so-called "doctrine of the infarctus" of Johann Kämpf, the supposititious *causa causans* of most human ills being simply fecal impaction. This fine theory, of course, fell in with the vogue of clysters and mineral wells, then fashionable, the memory of which is preserved in Molière, in Anstey's *New Bath Guide* (1766), and in the indescribable fantasies of the artists of the period. The *reductio ad absurdum* of the cult is conveyed in a satiric verse:

"And fell all prostrate at Cloaca's shrine."

The leading physician of the age was the founder of the "Eclectic School," Hermann **Boerhaave** (1668–1738), who added to the luster of Leyden as a medical center, and is especially memorable through his pupils, Haller, Gaub, Cullen, Pringle, and the leaders of the "Old Vienna School," van Swieten and de Haen. Boerhaave was educated along the broadest lines, was unquestionably the greatest consultant of his time, but is now principally remembered as a great teacher and especially as an experimental chemist. He taught chemistry, physics, and botany, as well as bedside medicine, and was the first to give a special course of lectures on ophthalmology (1708). His *Elementa chemiæ* (Leyden, 1732), his greatest work, was easily the best book on the subject all through the 18th century. In medicine, Allbutt says, he made no experiments, and "seems to have contented himself with hashing up the partial truths and the entire errors of his time."[1] His *Aphorismi* (Leyden, 1709) suggests his reputation as the "Batavian Hippocrates" (the sedulous de Haen apeing Galen as commentator of the great man), and if this reputation has now evaporated it is due to the simple fact that, in relation to the medicine of his time and country, Boerhaave was a Triton among the minnows. In relation to modern (non-Batavian) medicine his influence is *nil*. Baas (a good critic) says that many of his Delphic utterances seem today "ambiguous rather than profound," while his maxim, *simplex sigillum veri*, "was never manifested in his treatment," and "his prescriptions were less effective than his personal appearance." This is perhaps an extreme view, for

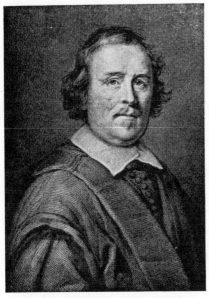

Hermann Boerhaave (1668–1738).

Boerhaave's reputation as a great physician extended even to China. He was consulted by emperors, and left an estate worth two million florins. His writings were enormously influential in their day—his *Institutiones* (1708) and his *Aphorisms* (1709) were translated even into Arabic.[2] He himself knew all the European languages (into which his principal works were translated), as well as Hebrew and Chaldean. He edited Vesalius (1725), Luisinus (1728), Lorenzo Bellini (1730), Aretæus (1731), Prospero Alpino (1733), and Swammerdam (1737) in sumptuous format. In person Boerhaave was tall, robust, ruddy, keen-eyed, of pleasant voice and mien, dignified, simple, and unassuming. He was perhaps the earliest of the great physicians who have loved music and frequently assembled performers at his country home (Oud-Poelgeest) near Leyden. Osler visited this fine mansion with Dock in 1901 and found it deserted, closed, and "somber as the house of Usher." But Boerhaave came into his own again in the Leyden Congress of 1927, at which Welch paid an appreciative tribute.

---

[1] Allbutt: *Op. cit.*, p. 1850. The only physiologic experiment credited to Boerhaave is his attempt to ascertain the effect of extreme heat upon animals. He had his pupils, Prevoost and Fahrenheit, put a dog and a cat in an oven heated up to 73° C.; it was found that they died in twenty-eight minutes, while a sparrow, under the same conditions, lasted seven minutes.

[2] See C. E. Daniëls: Janus, Leyden, 1912, xvii, 295–312, 2 pl. For van Swieten's shorthand notes on Boerhaave's lectures, which give some idea of his mode of speaking in Latin, see E. C. van Leersum, Janus, 1912, xvii, 145–152.

As a clinician Boerhaave stands out, like Sydenham, as a reviver of the Hippocratic method of envisaging clinical problems, which he taught at the bedside. He was the first to describe rupture of the esophagus (case of Baron de Wassenaer, 1724) and the aura-like pain which precedes hydrophobia. In 1728, he described a prodigious dilatation of the heart with suffocation from a fatty tumor of the chest (case of Marquis de Saint Alban), which was not unlike his own sad end, ten years later. It is said that he was the first to establish the site of pleurisy exclusively in the pleura, and to prove that smallpox is spread exclusively by contagion. He used the Fahrenheit thermometer in his clinic and the practice was kept up by his pupils, van Swieten and de Haen. Boerhaave also introduced the idea of "affinity" between chemical substances, together with an improved method of making vinegar (1732).

The theories just reviewed, with the single exception of Hoffmann's perhaps, are not entitled to the respect which we accord to the ideas of an Asclepiades, a van Helmont, or a Sydenham, for it is just these 18th century men who have given currency to the notion, so active in the lay mind, that the progress of medicine itself is only a "succession of forgotten theories." Far abler work was done by a very different group, the systematists, and we may now approach, with all due reverence, the greatest systematist after Galen, and one of the most imposing figures in all medical history, Albrecht von Haller (1708–77), the master physiologist of his time. Haller came out of the old bourgeois aristocracy of Bern (Switzerland), and was an infant prodigy, writing Latin verses

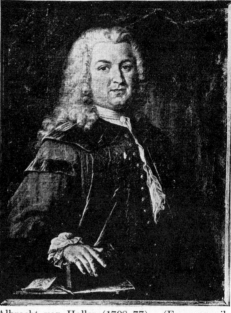

Albrecht von Haller (1708–77). (From an oil-painting by Studer.)

and a Chaldee grammar at ten, and at sixteen, worsting his senior, Professor Coschwitz, in the latter's contention that the lingual vein was a salivary duct (1725[1]). After graduating at Leyden, having for his teachers men like Boerhaave, Albinus, Winslow, and (in mathematics) John Bernouilli, his fame as a poet and botanist soon drew him away from his native city to the newly established university at Göttingen, where he remained for seventeen years, teaching all branches of medicine, establishing botanic gardens and churches, writing some 13,000 scientific papers, and incidentally achieving his best

[1] A. von Haller: Experimenta et dubia circa ductum salivalem novum Coschwizianum, Leyden, 1727.

experimental work. In 1753, at the age of forty-five, he was seized with an attack of *Heimweh*, and retired to Bern for the rest of his days, leading a life of most varied activity as public health officer and savant, with a touch of "Lord High Everything Else." He was equally eminent as anatomist, physiologist, and botanist, wrote poems and historic novels, carried on perhaps the most gigantic correspondence in the history of science, and was the principal founder of medical and scientific bibliography. His patient, arduous labors in this field (1771–78) were marvels of their kind.[1] In anatomic illustration, he did much for the establishment of the norm of the blood-vessels and the viscera. His *Icones anatomicæ* (1743–56) is authoritative for accurate study of these and other structures (Choulant). The Hallerianum at Bern is a symbol of his chief title to fame as the founder of recent physiology, the forerunner of Johannes Müller, Claude Bernard, and Carl Ludwig. His greatest single contribution to the subject is his laboratory demonstration of Glisson's hypothesis that irritability (contractility), *e. g.*, in an excised muscle, is the specific immanent property of all muscular tissues and sensibility an exclusive property of nervous tissue or of tissues supplied with nerve. Haller thus distinguished between nerve impulse (sensibility) and muscular contraction (irritability). This classic research, based upon 567 experiments, of which he himself performed 190, was made at Göttingen in 1757,[2] where he also laid the foundation for his *Elementa physiologiæ corporis humani* (Lausanne, 1759–66). Of this great work, Sir Michael Foster says that to open it is to pass into modern times. To read Professor Kronecker's *Haller redivivus*[3] is to see how many apparently "new" discoveries of modern observers had already been accounted for by this great master and are now forgotten, doubtless because humanity does not take kindly to the theorist on his pedestal. They include a reassertion of the myogenic theory (muscular autonomy) of the heart's action (1736), a recognition of the use of bile in the digestion of fats (1736), and the first experimental injections of putrid matter into the living body (1760). In his concern about sensibility and irritability, Haller saw the parts of the nervous system as tissues, and thus failed to get at some of their functions as organs. He denied irritability to the dura mater and motility to the brain, maintaining a functional equivalence of all its parts and (with Highmore) that one part can function vicariously for another; but *en revanche*, he did oppose Whytt's view that the soul is located or distributed in the central nervous system, since mechanical lesions produce no psychic effects. Akin to the French Encyclopedists in his grasp of detail Haller was the best historian of medicine[4] after Guy de Chauliac. His

[1] Bibliotheca botanica, Zürich, 1771–72; Bibliotheca anatomica, Zürich, 1774–77; Bibliotheca chirurgica, Bern, 1774–77; Bibliotheca medicinæ practicæ, Basel, 1776–78.

[2] "De partibus corporis humani sensibilibus et irritabilibus," in Comment. Soc. reg. Gottingæ (1752), 1753, ii, 114–214.

[3] Mitth. d. naturf. Gesellsch. in Bern (1902), 1903, Nos. 1519–1550, 203–226.

[4] Haller: Methodus studii medici, Amsterdam, 1751.

literary judgments are veritable *lumina sententiarum*. In embryology he was something of a reactionary, and successfully wet-blanketed the correct ideas of Wolff, as will appear. He lectured and wrote on surgery, and made a superb bibliography of the subject,[1] but never performed an operation in his life. In private life, Haller was modest, sensible, kindly, and charitable, and (rare trait) not afraid to affirm his ignorance when he could not explain a phenomenon. But he was complacent as to his infallibility about what he professed to know, did not like to have it questioned, and so left no school of followers behind him. To his contemporaries he seemed a *vir gloriosus*, living apart on a high eminence; but he was probably not the "pursy, play'd-out Philistine" of some of his portraits. As a youth, he was singularly fine-looking. In the history of German literature, Haller has a substantial, honorable place. His *Versuch schweizerischer Gedichte* (1732) was the cause of the famous literary quarrel between Bodmer and Gottsched as to the relative merits of the natural and the artificial in poetry. His poem, *Die Alpen* (1729), first drew attention to the glorious beauties of Swiss mountain scenery, and its influence may be seen in Klopstock, in Schiller, and even in Coleridge. By some irony

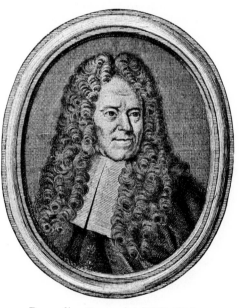

Bernardino Ramazzini (1633–1714).

of fate Haller, the poet, is now chiefly remembered for the following commonplace expression of bourgeois sentiment:

> Ins Innre der Natur dringt kein erschaffener Geist,
> Zu glücklich, wann sie noch die äussre Schale weist.
>
> Of Nature's inmost heart no human mind can tell,
> Happy, indeed, is he who knows its outer shell—

which so excited the derision of Goethe.[2]

With Haller, the systematist, we may class the works of a group of very original men, beginning with the *De morbis artificium diatriba* (Modena, 1700) of Bernardino **Ramazzini** (1633–1714), which opened

---

[1] Bibliotheca chirurgica, Bern, 1774–75.

[2] The lines occur in Haller's apostrophe to Newton, which, of course, stirred the ill-will of Goethe, on account of his own opposition to Newton's theory of colors.

up an entirely new department of modern medicine, viz., trade diseases and industrial hygiene. Ramazzini was the first after Paracelsus to call attention to such conditions as stone-mason's and miner's phthisis (pneumonokoniosis), the vertigo and sciatica of potters, the eye-troubles of gilders, printers, and other occupations. He was a good epidemiologist, and described the outbreak of lathyrism at Modena in 1690, the malarial epidemics of the region, and the Paduan cattle-plague of 1712. Like most clinicians of his time, he made observations of the weather (*Ephemerides barometricæ*, 1710). Italy has done eponymic honor to his memory in the medical periodical which bears his name.

"The Divine Order" (1742[1]) of Friedrich's army chaplain, Johann Peter **Süssmilch** (1707–77), is an epoch-making work in the develop-

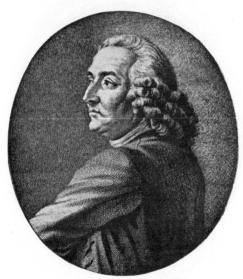

ment of vital and medical statistics. It brings together many data of capital importance in public hygiene, life insurance, and national polity. Although the old theologian's view is entirely teleologic, basing everything upon a divine order in nature, and although the English statist, John Graunt, had long before noticed (1662) that the population can be estimated from an accurate death-rate, yet the importance of Süssmilch to medical men is of a higher order than the mere casting up of figures. He it was who insisted upon the moral and political

Pieter Camper (1722–89).

significance of statistics and affirmed that the true wealth of any nation consists in an industrious, healthy, native population, and not merely in material and financial resources. The intelligent application of this humane, broad-minded principle was the secret of the industrial and military power of the mighty German Empire.

Here, three other famous systematists may be mentioned, viz., Johann Friedrich **Blumenbach** (1752–1840) of Göttingen, Pieter Camper, the founders of anthropology and craniology, and Johann Peter Frank, the founder of public hygiene. Although Blumenbach's thesis, "On the Native Varieties of the Human Race" (1776[2]), was preceded by the essays of Bernier (1684) and Linnæus (1735), yet it

---

[1] J. P. Süssmilch: Die göttliche Ordnung in denen Veränderungen des menschlichen Geschlechts, Berlin, 1742.

[2] Blumenbach: De generis humani varietate nativa, Göttingen, 1776.

may fairly be considered the starting-point of modern ethnology, since he bases his classification upon the shape of the skull and facial configuration, as well as the color of the skin. In describing his large collection of crania, in an atlas of 70 plates (1790–1820[1]), he used the vertical aspect from above downward as a norm in classification, but because a female Georgian skull was the most symmetric, he introduced the unfortunate term, "Caucasian," to represent the Aryan race. He is also remembered by the *clivus Blumenbachii* (occiput). Blumenbach was followed by the learned Pieter **Camper** (1722–89), an artist in training, who illustrated his own works and introduced the "facial angle" as a criterion of race (1760). Camper was Albinus' great rival in anatomic illustration. He painted in oil, aquatint, and pastel, made drawings in chalk and India ink, practised etching and mezzotint, and even made marble busts.

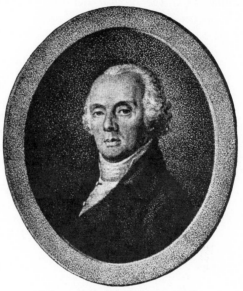

He discovered the processus vaginalis of the peritoneum, the fibrous structure of the lens, and made capital topographic studies of the arm, the pelvis, and the inguinal canal. His comparative researches on the Cetacea, his studies of facial expression of the passions, and his *Icones herniarum* (1779), published by Soemmerring in 1801, are all works of great value. His treatise on the best form of shoes (1781), an important contribution to the physiology of locomotion, was reissued in English translation as late as 1871. Camper, one of the most versatile of men, also introduced a pessary and a correct mode of using the vectis.

Johann Peter Frank (1745–1821).

He practised symphysiotomy on animals, was a promoter of inoculation, lectured to crowded audiences on legal medicine, and was the first to open a surgical polyclinic (Groningen, 1764).

A rare and happy mixture of German thoroughness with French intelligence was Johann Peter **Frank** (1745–1821), of Rotalben (Palatinate), the four volumes of whose "Complete System of Medical Polity" (*System einer vollständigen medicinischen Polizey*), published at Mannheim in 1777–88 by Schwann the printer of Schiller's "Robbers," are the very foundation of modern public hygiene, and a noble monument of a life-long devotion to humanity. The author, a poor waif almost cast adrift at a street door, made himself one of the greatest teachers and practitioners of his time by his own industry. He was the first

---

[1] Another valuable atlas of skulls is to be found in Eduard Sandifort's description of the Leyden Museum of Anatomy (1793–1835).

21

physician to signalize the importance of diseases of the spinal cord (1792[1]), defined diabetes insipidus (1794), and wrote an important treatise on therapeutics (1792–1821[2]). His great work on public hygiene, as covering the whole subject of man's life "from the womb to the tomb"—sewerage, water-supply, even school-hygiene, sexual hygiene, taxation of bachelors, and suitable benches and meals for the children, as well as the ideal of a scientific "medical police"—really left little for Pettenkofer and the moderns. In the preventive medicine of the future, the name of Frank will loom larger with meanings, for he was himself a true modern.

After Haller, the principal landmark of 18th century **physiology** is undoubtedly the *Statical Essays* (1731–33) of Stephen **Hales** (1677–

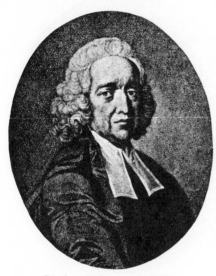

Stephen Hales (1677–1761).

1761), an English clergyman of inventive genius, who enriched practical science in many ways, particularly as the originator of artificial ventilation (1743). In the first part of these essays, Hales investigates the movement of sap in plants. The second part, entitled *Hæmadynamics* (1733), contains his most important work, on the mechanical relations of blood-pressure, marking the first real advance in the physiology of the circulation between Harvey and Poiseuille. By fastening a long glass tube inside a horse's artery, Hales devised the first manometer or tonometer, with the aid of which he made quantitative estimates of the blood-pressure, the capacity of the heart, and the velocity of the blood-current, which in tendency are essentially modern.

The **physiology of digestion** was materially advanced by the experiments of René-A.-F. **de Réaumur**[3] (1683–1757) upon a pet kite, in which he succeeded in isolating the gastric juice and demonstrating its solvent effect upon foods (1752[4]). These results were very ably confirmed and extended by the work of the Abbate Lazaro **Spallanzani** (1729–99), of Scandiano, Italy, an investigator of singular power. Spallanzani dis-

---

[1] Frank: "De vertebralis columnæ in morbis dignitate," in his Delect. opusc. med., Ticini, 1792, xi, 1–50.

[2] "De curandis hominum morbis epitome," Vienna, 1792–1821.

[3] The inventor of the 80 degrees thermometer.

[4] Réaumur: "Sur la digestion des oiseaux," Mém. Acad. roy. d. sc., 1752, Paris, 1756, 266–307.

covered the digestive power of saliva, and reaffirmed the solvent property of the gastric juice,[1] showing that it will act outside the body, and that it can not only prevent putrefaction but will inhibit it when once begun. He failed, however, to recognize the acid character of the gastric juice, a point which was to be brought out by the American physiologist Young (1803).

In 1768[2] Spallanzani founded the doctrine of the regeneration of the spinal cord through his discovery of its new growth during regeneration of the tail in the lizard. He also showed that the sexual posture in the frog is maintained as a spinal reflex after decapitation or after section of the two brachial nerves, fore and aft (1768[3]). He made important investigations of the respiratory exchanges in warm- and cold-blooded animals,[4] showing that hibernating animals can live comfortably for a time in carbon dioxid gas, where ordinary warm-blooded creatures die at once; that cold-blooded animals can live in hydrogen and continue to give off CO_2; and, most important of all, that living tissues, excised from a freshly killed animal, take up oxygen and even give off CO_2 in an atmosphere of air or hydrogen or nitrogen. His experiments on the bat proved that it is very slightly dependent on vision, so that its known deficiency in visual purple (Kühne) may be due to disuse. A most important investigation of Spallanzani's bore upon the doctrine of spontaneous generation. In 1748, John Turberville Needham (1713–81), an English Catholic priest in residence on the continent, published certain experiments on boiled meat-juices, inclosed in vials and sealed with mastic, the subsequent presence of micro-organisms in these liquids leading him to the conclusion that they were produced by spontaneous generation. Spallanzani refuted all this by using glass flasks with slender necks, which could be hermetically sealed in flame, immersing them in boiling water prior to the test. He also overthrew Needham's subsequent objection to the boiling feature by showing that exposure of the sealed fluids to the air again would renew the presumable germinative or "vegetative force" in the liquids, which Needham maintained had been destroyed by the flame. Finally, Spallanzani was, with Réaumur, Trembley, and Bonnet, one of the pioneers of experimental morphology in the strictly modern sense. Réaumur, in 1712, produced regenerations of the claws and scales of lobsters and crabs.[5] In 1740–44,[6] Abraham Trembley cut hydras into several pieces, producing new individuals, and got a third generation by cutting up the latter. In this he was emulated by Bonnet,[7] who experimented on fresh-water worms (1741–45), by Henry Baker, who supplemented Trembley's work on polyps (1743[8]), and by Spallanzani, who produced regenerations of the heads, tails, limbs, and tentacles of earthworms, tad-poles, salamanders, and snails (1768[9]). These experiments were not taken up again until the end of the 19th century, but they contain all the essentials of the modern work of Roux, Driesch, Morgan, Loeb, and others.

An English physiologist, whose work was long forgotten but has come to the front latterly on account of its essential importance, is William Hewson (1739–74), of Hexham, Northumberland, who was a

---

[1] Spallanzani: Della digestione degli animali, in his: Fisica animale, Venice, 1782, vol. i, 1–312, ii, 1–83.

[2] Prodromi sulla riproduzione animale: Riproduzione della coda del girino, Modena, 1768.

[3] Ibid.

[4] See the memoirs on respiration in his collected works.

[5] Réaumur: Mém. de l'Acad. de sc., Paris, 1712, 223–242, 1 pl.

[6] Trembley: Mémoires pour servir à l'histoire d'un genre de polypes d'eau douce, Leyden, 1744.

[7] Bonnet: Traité d'insectologie, pt. 2, Paris, 1745.

[8] Baker: An Attempt towards a Natural History of the Polype, London, 1743.

[9] Spallanzani: Prodromo di un'opera sopra le riproduzioni animali, Milan, 1829.

pupil of the Hunters. John Hunter, in fact, left him in charge of his dissecting-room when he went abroad with the army. Hewson afterward went into partnership with William Hunter in anatomic teaching, shared his profits, and later assisted him at the school in Great Windmill Street from 1769 on. When his pupil married, William Hunter, who seems to have had a natural aversion to Benedicts, abruptly broke off the partnership, much to Hewson's pecuniary disadvantage. He soon retrieved himself, however, having made his reputation through his Royal Society memoir on the lymphatics, which got him the Copley medal in 1769 and the honor of F.R.S. in 1770. Hewson's discovery of the existence of lacteal and lymphatic vessels in birds, reptiles, and

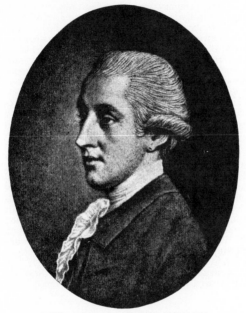

William Hewson, F.R.S. (1739–74).

fishes was esteemed of capital importance in its day, because the two Hunters maintained that absorption is an exclusive function of the lymphatics, against which it was objected that there are animals which have neither lacteals nor lymphatics. Magendie's demonstration that the blood-vessels have an absorbent function of course threw this phase of Hewson's work into the background, and present interest is centered on his *Experimental Inquiry into the Properties of the Blood* (1771). This work, a fine example of the experimental method taught by the Hunters, establishes the essential features of the coagulation of the blood in an entirely modern spirit. Hewson, a man of genius, died of a dissection wound in 1774.

Before Hewson's time, coagulation was ascribed to the supposed cooling off of the blood, to the fact that it had ceased to move, or to the idea that its corpuscles had solidified into rouleaux. Hewson showed that when the **coagulation of the blood** is delayed, as by cold, neutral salts, or otherwise, a coagulable plasma can be separated from the corpuscles and skimmed off the surface, and that this plasma contains an insoluble substance which can be precipitated and removed at a temperature a little over 50° C. Coagulation, in Hewson's view, was due to the formation in the plasma of this insoluble substance, which he called "coagulable lymph," and which we now know to be fibrinogen. Hewson's experiments were soon forgotten, even after Andrew Buchanan had shown (1845) that a substance can be extracted from the buffy coat of the blood, the lymphatic glands, and other tissues, which will coagulate not only blood, but serous fluids not in themselves coagulable. The modern discovery that fibrinogen is a nucleoproteid, and that in coagulation it is converted into fibrin, threw the work of Hewson into stronger relief. He also made the important observation that air is contained in the pleura in pneumothorax (1767), and was one of the first to perform the operation of paracentesis, although in this he was preceded by Monro *secundus*.

William Cumberland **Cruikshank** (1745–1800), of Edinburgh, who succeeded Hewson as William Hunter's assistant, gave the latter such satisfaction that he was made a partner in the Great Windmill Street School which, after Hunter's death, he took over, in conjunction with Matthew Baillie. Cruikshank investigated the reunion and regeneration of divided nerves (1776[1]), the passage of the impregnated ovum through the Fallopian tube (1778[2]), the physiology of absorption (1778–86), and in his *Experiments Upon the Insensible Perspiration of the Human Body* (1778) he demonstrated that the skin, like the lungs, gives off CO_2. His *Anatomy of the Absorbing Vessels of the Human Body* (1786) embodies the re-

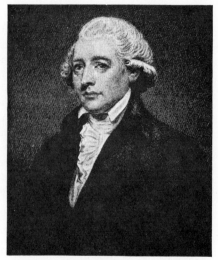

William C. Cruikshank (1745–1800).

sults of his labors with William Hunter.[3] In 1797 Cruikshank demonstrated albuminuria in dropsical fevers. He had a large practice, turning his private office into a public dispensary for the poor on occasion, which won him the lasting regard of his friend, Dr. Johnson, whom he treated in his last illness and who described him, in the Scottish phrase, as "a sweet-blooded man."

While 18th-century physiology was dominated by the Glisson-Haller doctrine of irritability (muscle) and sensibility (nerve), the dominant principle of the psychology and psychiatry of the period was the animism of Stahl (1737), the old van Helmont view of the soul as the motor-power of the human machine, now operating directly without the intervention of gaseous spirits or ferments and allocated vaguely to the total nervous system or some part of it (*sensorium commune*). These views crop out variously in the theoretical systems of Friedrich Hoffmann (spasm and atony), Cullen (life a function of nervous energy), John Brown (life as stimulation), Reil (soul as life-force), Rasori (stimulus and contrastimulus), and even Broussais (irritation)

Robert **Whytt** (1714–66), of Edinburgh, a pupil of Monro *primus*, Cheselden, Winslow, Boerhaave, and Albinus, is memorable as perhaps

---

[1] Phil. Tr., Lond., 1795, lxxxv, 177–189, 1 pl.

[2] *Ibid.*, 1797, lxxxvii, 197–214, 1 pl.

[3] Hunter was accustomed to say that the anatomy of the lymphatic system was developed by himself, his brother John, Hewson, and Cruikshank.

the foremost neurologist of his time. In an age in which disease was an entity (not a reaction) and reaction to stimulus a species of magic, he was remarkably clear-headed. In his memoir *On the Vital and Other Involuntary Motions of Animals* (Edinburgh, 1751), he demonstrated, for the first time, that the integrity of the spinal cord as a whole is not essential for reflex action, but that only a small segment is necessary and sufficient for a reflex arc. He also discovered that destruction of one of the anterior corpora quadrigemina will abolish reflex contraction of the pupils to light (Whytt's reflex, 1768), and was one of the first to notice the phenomena of inhibition and of spinal shock. All these observations would seem to confute the current doctrine of Stahl, that a "rational soul" is the cause of involuntary movements, yet Whytt was, in theory, a pronounced Stahlian animist, and reasoned, from

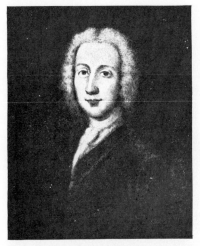

decapitated animals, that the soul is equally distributed throughout the nervous system, that it originates muscular movements, and that it intervenes between sensory stimulus and muscular response in reflex phenomena. In his *Observations on the Dropsy in the Brain* (1768) Whytt first described tuberculous meningitis in children. His book, *On Nervous, Hypochondriacal, or Hysterical Diseases* (1764), was the first important English treatise on neurology after Willis.

Robert Whytt (1714–66). (Courtesy of Dr. John Ruhräh, Baltimore.)

Whytt's doctrine of the immanence of the soul in all parts of the nervous system was opposed by Haller but upheld by the Moravian Georg **Prochaska** (1749–1820), professor at Prague (1785) and Vienna (1791), who surmised that reflexes operate directly through the ganglia and anastomosing nerve filaments by means of physical and psychic stimulation of "ascending nerves," to be reflected (*reflectendæ*) from the *sensorium commune* (Neuburger). He discovered the olivary bodies (1791) and had some inklings of localization of cerebral functions, of Johannes Müller's law of specific nerve energies, and of Bell's law of the spinal nerve-roots. He left a remarkable cabinet of pathologic preparations at Prague.

The intervention of the soul in reflex actions was denied by Johann August **Unzer** (1727–99) of Halle, who first differentiated between voluntary (conscious) and involuntary movements (1746–71), experimented on the possibility of sensation in beheaded people (1746), and described some conditional (Pavloff) reflexes without understanding their real nature.

The doctrine of the life-force as the chemical expression of physiologic function was advanced by Johann Christian **Reil** (1759–1813), of Eastern Frisia, professor of medicine at Halle (1787) and Berlin (1810), and the original editor of the *Archiv für die Physiologie* (Halle, 1795–1815), the first periodical to be devoted to the science. It eventually passed into the elder Meckel's hands, and became in the course of time the epoch-making *Müller's Archiv* (1834–58).

Reil is memorable for his work on the histology of the crystalline lens (1794), in which he employed chemical reagents for his investigation of the structure of nerve-fibers (1796), his figuration of the macula lutea and its postmortem appearance (1797), his description of the "island of Reil" in the brain (1809[1]), and for his "Rhapsodies" on the psychic (humane) treatment of the insane (1803[2]). He founded the first journal of psychiatry (*Magazin für psychische Heilkunde*, 1805–6), which was succeeded by his *Beyträge* (1808–12) and was followed by the *Zeitschrift für psychische Aerzte* (1818–22) of his pupil, C. F. Nasse. Reil's theory of nervous action is summed up in his essay on the life-force (1795[3]), in which the autonomy of cerebral function is established, and vital force, the subjective expression of the chemical interaction of body substances, is defined as the specific function of organic matter, while irritability is not only recognized as a specific property of tissues (Haller), but is regarded, in Glisson's original sense, as the principal manifestation of life as matter in motion. Reil had some notion of metabolism and even of internal secretions (Neuburger). In his clinic, he practised surgery, obstetrics, and ophthalmology, as well as internal medicine. Toward the end of his life, he lost himself in the vagaries of the Nature Philosophy School. A statue was erected to his memory in 1915.

In France, the interest of the Academy of Medicine in head injuries brought the technic of cerebral surgery up to effective standards of laboratory experimentation, which became the key to topical diagnosis. There arose a remarkable school of physiologic (**neurologic**) **surgeons**, of whom François Pourpoir du Petit (1664–1771), an army surgeon up to 1713, contested the alleged cerebral origin of the "intercostal nerve" (sympathetic-autonomic chain), showed the effects of the cervical sympathetic on the eye (1723), and in his letters on the brain (1710), revived by Antoine Louis in 1788, opened out the theory of contralateral innervation by showing that the contralateral paralysis of Hippocrates is complete only when the corpus striatum on either side is injured. He made cortical phenomena basic for diagnosis in brain surgery. Antoine Charles **Lorry** (1725–83), of Paris, by a series of suboccipital and spinal punctures in dogs and cats, concluded that the medulla is the seat of vital functions and even anticipated Flourens in localizing the medulla as the center of respiration.

Nicolas **Saucerotte** (1741–1814), one of the most original of neurologic surgeons, established the theory of contralateral innervation by 28 experiments on dogs (1769) but, through his ignorance of the canine brain, allocated brachial palsies to the hind-brain and *vice versa*. He described the neighborhood symptoms in cerebral compression by blood-clots, the periodic coma and gigantism in acromegaly (1772) and noted the opisthotonos, hyperesthesia, and nystagmus in cerebellar lesions, to which Mehée de la Touche added strabismus in 1773. Saucerotte also noted that cerebral wounds are most dangerous at the base and least so in the fore-brain, He was a skilled lithotomist and one of the most efficient of army surgeons.

The memoirs of the French Academy on contrecoup (began 1760), and the subsequent work of Sabourant, La Peyronie, Chopart, and others added much to the semeiology of head injuries and consequently to cerebral physiology.

Electrophysiology had its origin in the epoch-making experiments on muscle-nerve preparations, summarized in 1792[4] by Luigi **Galvani** (1737–98) of Bologna. John Hunter had studied animal electricity in the torpedo (1773), which had been used in therapy by the Romans; Caldani had already experimented on electrical stimulation of the cerebral cortex (1784), but Galvani's discovery of the electric properties of excised tissues is the starting-point of modern work. On September 20, 1786, he noticed muscular spasms in frogs' legs suspended by copper hooks from an iron balustrade. The difference in potential resulting from accidental contact of the muscle with the iron structure was subsequently superinduced by temporary junction of the nerve in a muscle-nerve preparation with an injured point of the

---

[1] Reil: Arch. f. Physiol., Halle a. S., 1809, ix, 136; 195.

[2] Reil: Rhapsodieen (etc.), Halle, 1803.

[3] Reil: Von der Lebenskraft, Arch. f. d. Physiol., Halle, 1795, i, 8–162.

[4] Galvani: De viribus electricitatis in motu musculari, Modena, 1792.

muscle. It was followed up, with rare skill and insight, by Alessandro
Volta (1745–1827), professor at Pavia (1778–1819[1]), in his "Letters on
Animal Electricity" (1792). Volta divided conductors of electricity
into metallic and liquid (electrolysis), devised the famous Voltaic pile
(1799), and showed that a muscle can be thrown into continuous (tetanic)
contraction by successive electric stimulations. Galvani started the
science of animal electricity; Volta, the electric battery and its manifold applications.

Meanwhile Benjamin Franklin, Kratzenstein (1745), Schaeffer (1752), G. F. Rössle[r]
(electric bath, 1768), Manduyt (1777), William Henly (1779), and many others were
already utilizing electricity in the treatment of disease. Static machines were
installed in the Middlesex Hospital in 1767, in St. Bartholomew's in 1777, and in
St. Thomas's about 1799. An old print, of date 1799, showing the administration
of static electricity to a patient, hangs
on the walls of the Electrical Department of St. Bartholomew's.

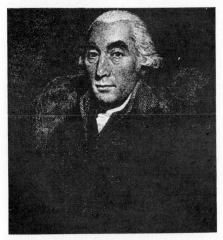

Joseph Black (1728–99).

The Abbate Felice **Fontana**
(1730–1803), author of a treatise
on the venom of the viper
(1767[2]), which was the starting-
point of the modern investigation of **serpent venoms,** experimented on stimulation of the
cerebral cortex with electricity
(1757) and of the central nervous system with viper venom
(1767), but, apart from electrotherapy, the galvanic method
had no immediate effect upon
neurological research. It was
principally employed upon the
cortex of decapitated criminals,
but with such fantastic and frightening effects that experimentation upon
the beheaded came to be interdicted by Prussian law in 1804. The
most telling effect of Galvani's work was to obliterate the outworn
hypotheses of activation of the nervous system by the soul, by animal
spirits, or by nerve-fluid. As Neuburger points out, the physiology of
nerve-currents came to be seen in the light of the electric telegraph
(Soemmerring, 1809), just as the laws of muscular action could be derived from the lever or the rationale of the circulating blood from the
principles of hydrodynamics.

But perhaps the best piece of physiologic work in the 18th century
was the completion of the modern **theory of respiration,** which turned
upon the discovery of the different gases in the atmosphere, viz., carbon
dioxid by Black (1757), hydrogen by Cavendish (1766), nitrogen by
Rutherford (1772), oxygen by Priestley and Scheele (1771), and Lavoisier

[1] A statue of Volta was erected in the Athenæum of the University of Pavia
in 1878.   [2] Fontana: Ricerche fisiche sopra il veleno della vipera, Lucca, 1767.

(1775). The great Scottish chemist, Joseph **Black** (1728–99), is known to physicists for his original definitions of "specific heat" and "capacity for heat" and for his subtle criterion of "latent heat"—that the temperature of a body and the amount of heat it possesses are two entirely different things. In his *Dissertatio de humore acido a cibo orto* (1754) he made a distinction equally important for chemistry and physiology. Chemists of Black's day, following Stahl, believed that when lime is heated it gains phlogiston, that when quicklime is slaked it loses phlogiston. Black's experiments exploded the Stahlian theory by showing that, in reality, quickened lime loses something ($CaCO_3 = CaO + CO_2$), and quicklime, when slaked, gains something ($CaO + H_2O = Ca(OH)_2$). He also noted that the gas or "fixed air" given off by quickened lime and alkalis is also present in expired air, and is physiologically irrespirable, although not necessarily toxic. Thus Black had again isolated the carbonic acid gas which van Helmont had, over a hundred years before, noted in fermentation as *gas sylvestre*. A few steps further and he would have arrived at the conclusion of the whole matter. Joseph **Priestley** (1733–1804) had the truth in his grasp when he isolated oxygen (1772[1]) and saw that vegetating plants renew vitiated air, but, being a confirmed Stahlian, he only made matters worse by seeing respiration as "the phlogistication of dephlogisticated air." It was reserved for the genius of Antoine-Laurent **Lavoisier** (1743–94) to discover

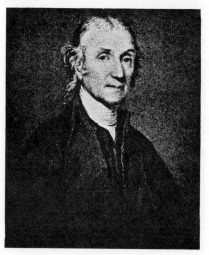

Joseph Priestley (1733–1804).

the true nature of the interchange of gases in the lungs, and to demolish the phlogiston theory by his introduction of quantitative relations in chemistry. As Sir Michael Foster maintains, "he and he alone discovered oxygen" (1775[2]), for Mayow, Priestley, and Scheele had only isolated it. Priestley, deceived by the specious label, "phlogiston," had explained the facts of respiration in an inverted order. But Lavoisier proved that inspired air is converted into Black's "fixed air," the nitrogen or "azote" (which he also discovered) alone remaining unchanged. Further, in conjunction with the astronomer **Laplace** (1780–85[3]), he demonstrated that respiration is in every way the ana-

---

[1] Priestley: Observations on Different Kinds of Air, Phil. Tr., Lond., 1772, lxii, 147–264, 1 pl.

[2] Lavoisier: Hist. Acad. roy. d. sc., 1775, Paris, 1778, pp. 520–526.

[3] *Ibid.*, 1780, Paris, 1784, 355–408.

logue of combustion, the chemical products being carbon dioxid and water. But Lavoisier, whose life was lost to science through the fanaticism of the French Revolutionists, had adopted the erroneous theory that the oxidation of carbon and hydrogen takes place in the tubules of the lungs. This was corrected in 1791 by **Lagrange,** the author of the *Mécanique analytique,* who maintained, through his pupil Hassenfratz,[1] that the dissolved oxygen of the inspired air slowly takes up carbon and hydrogen from the tissues as the blood courses through them. The finishing touch was added when Gustav Magnus, in 1837,[2] showed, with the aid of a Sprengel's air-pump, that venous and arterial blood both contain oxygen as well as CO_2, demonstrating—what Cruikshank toward the end of his life had partly elucidated—that all

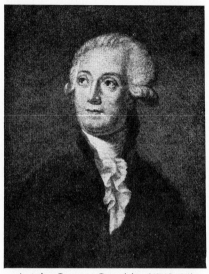

the tissues respire in the sense of assimilating oxygen and giving up CO_2. Thus, the development of the physiology of respiration, from Borelli to Magnus, was almost exclusively the work of three mathematicians, two physicists, and five chemists.

The discovery of oxygen had a singular effect upon medical practice. Louis Jurine, Louis Odier, Pascal Joseph Ferro, G. C. Reich, J. B. T. Baumés, Samuel Latham Mitchill, and other physicians were carried away by their imaginations to the extent of attributing diseases either to lack or excess of oxygen, or to some fine-spun modifications of this theory, too numerous and complex to be mentioned here. Of this group, the most memorable perhaps was **Beddoes** (1760–1808), of Shiffnal, Shropshire, who discovered Humphry Davy. In 1798, he founded the Pneumatic Institute at Clifton for the treatment of disease by **inhalation.**

Antoine-Laurent Lavoisier (1743–94).

The apparatus was constructed by no less than James Watt, who invented the gasometer (1790), while Beddoes' assistant, Davy, discovered the anesthetic properties of nitrous oxid (1799). The essays by Beddoes and Watt *On Factitious Airs* (1794–96) advance the important therapeutic concept of treating certain diseases by placing the patient in a "factitious atmosphere," which has since found some definite vindication in the open-air treatment of phthisis, the modern surgery of the chest, and the treatment of colds by free chlorine. Beddoes' general plan of treating respiratory troubles by inhalations of different gases is now standardized as aërotherapy or pneumotherapy. The plan of Beddoes and Watt was revived by Louis Waldenburg, in his apparatus for differential pneumotherapy (1873). The subject has been further extended by the labors of Demarquay (1866), J. Solis Cohen (1867–76), Paul Bert (1878), M. J. Oertel (1886), P. L. Tissier, and others.[3]

---

[1] Hassenfratz: Ann. d. chim., Paris, 1791, ix, 261–274.

[2] Magnus: Ann. d. Phys. u. Chem., Leipz., 1837, xli, 583–606.

[3] See Neuburger: Einleitung, 108, and Syst. Physiol. Therap. (ed. S. Solis Cohen), 1903, x, *passim.*

The great center of **anatomic teaching** in the 17th century was Leyden; at the beginning of the 18th century, Paris. The rise of Edinburgh as a center of medical teaching was due to the following train of circumstances: In 1700, John **Monro,** a Scotch army surgeon of good family, settled in Edinburgh and, knowing of the superiority of continental training in medicine, conceived the idea of starting a medical school in the northern capital, mainly out of regard for his only son, Alexander, whom he desired to leave well established in this world. In accordance with this plan, young Alexander Monro received a careful medical education at London, Paris, and Leyden, becoming a warm friend of Cheselden and Boerhaave and, on returning to Edinburgh in 1719, was duly examined and qualified by the Surgeon's Guild. In 1720, on recommendation of the Town Council, he was elected professor of anatomy in the newly established university, at the age of twenty-two. Being a teacher of marked ability, his courses were soon followed

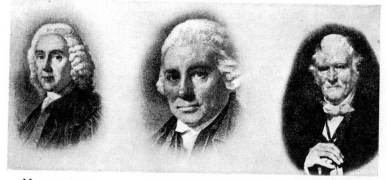

Monro *primus*
(1697–1767).

Monro *secundus*
(1737–1817).

Monro *tertius*
(1773–1859).

The three Monros (1720–1846).

by enthusiastic students in large numbers, the roster climbing from 57 (in 1720) to 182 (in 1749). This steady arithmetic progression was interrupted only by the Rebellion of '45. Alexander Monro followed his father's plan for his own son, who extended the same policy to the grandson. Both were also named Alexander. Thus, the three Monros, *primus, secundus,* and *tertius,* as they were called, held the chair of anatomy at Edinburgh in uninterrupted succession, like some entailed estate, for a period of 126 years (1720–1846). The men of the Monro dynasty were, all of them, original characters of unusual attainments, authors of many remarkable works, morbid on the subject of controversy, it is true, but in every way worthy of the confidence placed in them by their fellow-townsmen. During the period 1720–90 some 12,800 students were taught by Monro *primus* and *secundus* alone. It was largely due to them that Edinburgh became the great center of medical teaching in the "last century."

Anatomic research in this period did not attain the brilliancy it had in the 17th century, nearly every year of which was distinguished by some new discovery. Many of the best anatomists of the 18th century, such as Cheselden, Pott, the Monros, the Hunters, Desault, Scarpa, were so-called **surgeon-anatomists.** The studies of the time were mainly topographic and iconographic. Surgical anatomy, in fact, begins properly with the writings of Joseph **Lieutaud** (1703–80) and, after this time (1724), a great number of fine atlases were published, such as Cheselden on the bones (1733[1]), Albinus on the bones and muscles (1747–53[2]), Eisenmann on the uterus (1752[3]), Zinn on the eye (1755[4]), Scarpa on the ear (1772–99[5]), Soemmerring on the cranial nerves (1778[6]), Eduard Sandifort on the duodenum (1780[7]), or Paolo Mascagni on the lymphatics (1787[8]). These and many others were all gathered together in the great collections of Just Christian von Loder (1794–1803) and L. M. A. Caldani (*Icones Anatomicæ*, Venice, 1801–13). The splendid post-humous MS. illustrations, which Paolo **Mascagni** (1752–1815) had designed for a great anatomic atlas, were entrusted to his prosector, Francesco Antommarchi (Napoleon's physician at St. Helena), for publication, and were issued by him in sumptuous style in 1819, in 1821, and again in 1823–32 by others whom the Mascagni family, disgusted with Antommarchi's dubious methods, had selected as editors. Antommarchi subsequently plagiarized a number of Mascagni's plates in a work purporting to be his own. The surgeons Pierre Dionis and William Cheselden wrote anatomic text-books which were both of them popular in their day, but probably the best all-round treatise on the subject between Vesalius and Bichat was the *Exposition anatomique* (1732) of the Danish teacher, Jakob Benignus **Winslow** (1669–1760), a pupil of Duverney. Winslow did much to condense and systematize what was known, especially in regard to such matters as the origin, insertion, and nomenclature of the different muscles. His work was the authoritative text-book for nearly a century. There was a fair showing of those specialized investigations of physiologic import which added so much luster to 17th century anatomy. Duverney's work on the ear (1683) was very ably supplemented by the investigations of Valsalva (1704) and Cotugno (1774), and with these may be mentioned the monographs of Cowper on the urethral glands (1702[9]), of Abraham Vater on the ampulla of the bile-duct (1720[10]), of Lieberkühn on the intestinal glands (1745[11]), of James Douglas on the peritoneum (1730[12]), of the elder Meckel on the vagus nerve (1748[13]), of Zinn on the ciliary ligaments (1753[14]), the discovery of the Gasserian ganglion (1765) and of the nerve of Wrisberg (1777[15]), Ehrenritter's discovery of the jugular ganglion of the glossopharyngeal and tympanic nerves (1790), Prochaska's discovery of the olivary bodies (1791), Schmidt's account of the spinal nerves (1794), and the varied researches of Santorini (1724[16]). The

---

[1] Cheselden: Osteographia, London, 1733.

[2] B. S. Albinus: Tabulæ sceleti et musculorum corporis humani, Leyden, 1747.

[3] G. H. Eisenmann: Tabulæ anatomicæ quatuor uteri (etc.), Strassburg, 1752.

[4] J. G. Zinn: Descriptio anatomica oculi humani, Göttingen, 1755.

[5] A. Scarpa: De structura fenestræ rotundæ auris et de tympano, Modena, 1772. De auditu et olfactu, Pavia, 1789. De penitiorum ossium structura, Leipzig, 1799.

[6] Soemmerring: De basi encephali et originibus nervorum cranio egredientium, Göttingen, 1778.   [7] E. Sandifort: Tabulæ intestini duodeni, Leyden, 1780.

[8] P. Mascagni: Vasorum lymphaticorum corporis humana historia et iconographia, Siena, 1787.

[9] W. Cowper: Glandularum quarundam, nuper detectarum . . . descriptio, London, 1702.

[10] A. Vater: Dissertatio anatomica qua novum bilis diverticulum circa orificium ductus choledochi (etc.), Wittenberg, 1720.

[11] J. N. Lieberkühn: De fabrica et actione villorum intestinorum tenuium hominis, Leyden, 1745.

[12] J. Douglas: A description of the peritonæum, London, 1730.

[13] J. F. Meckel: De quinto pare nervorum cerebri, Göttingen, 1748.

[14] J. G. Zinn: De ligamentis ciliaribus, Göttingen, 1753.

[15] H. A. Wrisberg: Observationes anatomicæ de quinto pare nervorum encephali, Göttingen, 1777.

[16] G. D. Santorini: Observationes anatomicæ, Venice, 1724.

ganglia were described by Winslow (1723) as "subordinated secondary brainlets (*cerebra secundaria subordinata sive parva*) and by Jacob Johnstone (1771) as "analogous to the brain in their office, subordinate springs and reservoirs of nervous power" (Neuburger). The cerebrospinal fluid was discovered in 1774 by Domenico Cotugno (1736–1822), who also demonstrated albumin in the urine by boiling (1764), seventy years after Frederik Dekker (1694), and described sciatica (1770).

Toward the end of the century, Samuel Thomas **von Soemmerring** (1755–1830), a native of Thorn, Western Prussia, wrote a monumental treatise on anatomy (1791–96[1]), which was reissued nearly half a century later by Rudolf Wagner, Henle, and others (1839–45).

Soemmerring made most important researches on the brain (1799), the eye (macula lutea, 1791), the ear (1806), throat (1806), nose (1809), hernia, the anthropology of the negro (1785[2]), and the injurious effects of corsets (1793[3]), but is now

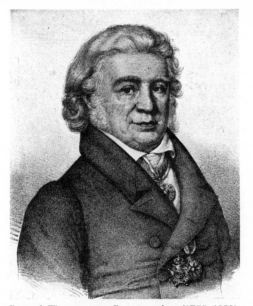

Samuel Thomas von Soemmerring (1755–1830).

best remembered for his remarkable accuracy in anatomic illustration and by his classification of the cranial nerves (1778[4]), which superseded that of Willis. Soemmerring was himself a good artist and trained Christian Koeck to make anatomic drawings under his direction (Choulant). He followed Albinus in fidelity to nature and the quest of the "anatomic norm." His devotion to the "Attic perfection" of his master is seen in his plates of the brain and cranial nerves (1791–99), the embryo (1799), the eye (1801), the ear (1808), the tongue (1808), the nose (1809), and particularly in the exquisitely executed skeleton of a girl of Mainz (1797), which was designed to be a companion-piece to the male skeleton of Albinus (1747). Soemmerring was also one of the inventors of the electric telegraph (1809).

---

[1] S. T. von Soemmerring: Vom Baue des menschlichen Körpers, Frankfort on the Main, 1791–96.

[2] Ueber die körperliche Verschiedenheit des Negers vom Europäer, Cassel, 1784.

[3] Ueber die Wirkung der Schnürbrüste (with copper-plate), Berlin, 1793.

[4] De basi encephali et originibus nervorum cranio egredientium libri quinque, Göttingen, 1778.

A remarkable family of Prussian anatomists were the Meckels, father, son, and two grandsons.

Johann Friedrich **Meckel,** the elder (1724–74), of Wetzlar, graduated at Göttingen in 1748, with a noteworthy inaugural dissertation on the fifth nerve (Meckel's ganglion), became professor of anatomy, botany, and obstetrics at Berlin in 1751, and was the first teacher of midwifery at the Charité. He was the first to describe the submaxillary ganglion (1748), and made important investigations of the nerve-supply of the face (1751) and the terminal visceral filaments of the veins and lymphatics (1772). His son, Philipp Friedrich Theodor Meckel (1756–1803), of Berlin, graduated at Strassburg in 1777 with an important dissertation on the internal ear, was professor of anatomy and surgery at Halle in 1779, and editor of the *Neues Archiv der praktischen Arzneykunst* (Leipzig, 1789–95). He was a favorite and highly honored obstetrician at the Russian court. His son, Johann Friedrich Meckel (1781–1833), of Halle, called the younger Meckel, was an eminent pathologist, and the greatest comparative anatomist in Germany before Johannes Müller. He has been called the German Cuvier. His most important works are his treatises on pathologic anatomy (1812–18), normal human anatomy (1815), his atlas of 33 plates representing human abnormities (1817–26), and his great system of comparative anatomy (1821–30), in which he sets forth the view that the development of the higher animals is an epitome of the ancestral stages which preceded it. He translated Wolff's monograph on the development of the intestines in 1812, and is memorable as the discoverer of the Meckel diverticulum of the intestines. His younger brother, August Albrecht Meckel (1790–1829), of Halle, became professor of anatomy and forensic medicine at Bern in 1821, and was a specialist in the latter branch.

The starting-point of modern **embryology** was the *Theoria Generationis* (1759) of Casper Friedrich **Wolff** (1733–94), of Berlin, one of the most original spirits of his time, who is eponymically remembered by his discovery of the Wolffian bodies. Wolff revived Harvey's doctrine of epigenesis (gradual building up of parts), and took a firm stand against the current theory that the embryo is already preformed and encased in the ovary (*emboitement*); but his negation of germinal continuity, and the opposition of Haller, prevented his evolutionary ideas from gaining any ground until 1812, when the younger Meckel translated his great monograph on the development of the intestines in the chick (1768–69[1]), one of the acknowledged classics of embryology. While the plates and the argument of the *Theoria Generationis* (1759) are far inferior to Malpighi's work, Wolff surpassed himself in the memoir of 1768, described by von Baer as "the greatest masterpiece of scientific observation that we possess." Wolff's view, that the organs are formed from "leaf-like (blastodermic) layers," comes as near as possible to the germ-layer theory of von Baer himself. In 1767, from investigations of the buds of cabbages, beans, and other plants, Wolff arrived at the conclusion that "all parts of the plant except the stem are modified leaves."

This conclusion was reached independently by Johann Wolfgang von **Goethe** (1749–1832), in his essay on plant metamorphosis (1790[2]), in which he argued deductively the fundamental unity of leaf, flower, and fruit, and the descent of all plants from an archetypal form (*Urpflanze*). Like more recent botanists, he was

---

[1] C. F. Wolff: Ueber die Bildung des Darmkanals im bebrüteten Hühnchen, Halle, 1812.

[2] Goethe: Versuch die Metamorphose der Pflanzen zu erklären, Gotha, 1790.

unable to decide whether the direction of evolution was from foliage-leaf to reproductive leaf, or *vice versa*, and he was painfully surprised when Schiller observed,
"This is not an observation, it is an idea." Goethe was, nevertheless, one of the
pioneers of evolution, the first to use the term "morphology," and the discoverer
of the intermaxillary bone (1786[1]). Independently of Oken (1790), he stated that
the skull is made up of modified vertebræ and, before Savigny, he saw that the jaws
of insects are modified limbs. In connection with Goethe's botanic work, a passing
mention should be made of Christian Konrad Sprengel (1750–1816), the old Prussian
pastor who was thrown out of his rectorate at Spandau because he neglected his
congregation for botany, and whose "Newly Discovered Secret of Nature" (1793)
was brought to the front by Darwin. Sprengel pointed out that the colored markings, shapes, nectar, etc., of plants are adaptations to secure cross-fertilizations by
insects, which process is the rule, not the exception. The teleologic significance
of cross-fertilization was afterward proved by Herbert, Gärtner, and others, and
utilized by Darwin. Other forerunners of Darwin were the naturalist Buffon
(1707–88), whose *Histoire naturelle* (1749–1804), although a popular descriptive work,
contained many casual denials of the fixity of species and a veiled suggestion of a
possible common ancestor for horse and ass, ape and man; and Erasmus Darwin
(1731–1802), whose *Loves of the Plants* (1789) and *Zoönomia* (1794) emphasized the
gradual evolution of complex organisms from simple primordial forms, the struggle
for existence in animals and plants, sexual selection, protective mimicry, and the
indirect influence of environment in producing transformations which may modify
species.

Perhaps the greatest comparative anatomist of the 18th century was Felix
Vicq d'Azyr (1748–94), permanent secretary of the Paris Academy of Medicine,
whose studies of the flexor and extensor muscles of man and animals, and the morphology of the brain, the vocal cords, and the structure of birds and quadrupeds, were
the best of the period.

The best specimens of **anatomic illustration** in the 18th century
show the gradual passage from the copper-plate, through the *taille-
douce*, to the steel-plate period, as seen in such splendid folios as Cheselden's *Osteographia* (1733), Haller's *Icones anatomicæ* (1743–56), William
Hunter's *Anatomia uteri humani gravidi* (1774), and the masterpieces
of Haller, Santorini, Albinus, Soemmerring, and Scarpa.

The six beautiful plates of pregnancy and parturition made by Riemsdijk for
Charles Nicholas **Jenty** (1758), of London, are rare examples of **mezzotint,** which
was seldom used in medical illustration.[2] **Colored copper-plates** were introduced
in the 18th century by Jacques-Christophe Le Blon (1667–1741), who left only one
anatomic specimen of his handiwork, a little plate of the genital organs made for
the 1719 edition of Cockburn's treatise on gonorrhea, and now exceedingly rare.
It was followed by the six beautiful anatomic plates which Le Blon's pupil, Jan
Ladmiral (1698–1773), made for Albinus, Ruysch, and others (1736–41); by the
copper-plates in red and black of his pupil Robert (1750), and by the many picturesque atlases of his assistant Jacob-Fabian **Gautier d'Agoty** (1717–86), a layman
whose colored mezzotints are often of striking artistic power, but too grandiose and
showy in their tendency for the ultimate purposes of anatomic illustration. The
flamboyant technique, as Choulant points out, is not suitable for fidelity and delicacy
of detail. Gautier delighted particularly in rendering the graceful physical habitus
of the Parisienne of the 18th century, familiar in the many engravings of the French
artists of the period. These pictures, originally executed life-size in oil, are, in
effect, the last survivors of the skeletons, musclemen, reclining gravid women, and
other stock figures of the old medieval MS. illustrations. Viewed simply as oil-
paintings, the life-sized Gautier panels, sold in Paris in the fall of 1914 and now in
the Wellcome Museum (London[3]), are perhaps the most remarkable examples of
anatomic illustration in this medium. Anatomic copper-plates in two colors (black

---

[1] Goethe: Ueber den Zwischenkiefer des Menschen und der Thiere. Nova
Acta Acad. Leopold-Carol., Halle, 1831, xv, 1–48.

[2] See J. G. de Lint, Janus, Amst., 1916, xxi, 129–135, 4 pl.

[3] For cuts of which, see Lancet, Lond., 1914, i, 557.

and red) were made by Cornelis Ploos van Amstel (for Lavater, 1790) in Giuseppe del Medico's *Anatomia* (1811) and in Jean-Galbert Salvage's *Anatomie du gladiateur combattant* (1812).

One of the greatest anatomic illustrators of his time was Bernhard Siegfried **Albinus** (1697–1770), of Frankfort on the Oder, who had studied under Bidloo, Boerhaave, and Duverney, and held the chairs of anatomy and surgery (1718) and medicine (1745) at the University of Leyden.

Albinus edited the works of Harvey, Vesalius, Fabricius, and Eustachius. His atlases of the bones (1726, 1753), the muscles (1734), the veins and arteries

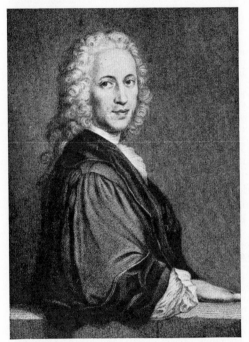

of the intestines (1736), the fetal bones (1737), the skeleton and skeletal muscles (1747, 1762), and the gravid uterus (1749), are all justly renowned for their beauty and accuracy of illustration, and for the elegant style of the accompanying text.

Under Albinus' direction, the artist Jan Wandelaer established a new anatomic norm in illustration, founded upon the closest scientific observation. In this regard, both the scientific and artistic anatomy of the period became, as Choulant says, truly Albinian, as seen in the statuette écorchés of Fischer (1784). Albinus was also held to be an incomparable lecturer, and was a master of the art of anatomic injection. In opposition to Albinus, Pieter **Camper** (1722–89), who made his own drawings, maintained that anatomic subjects should not be represented in perspective, as had been the custom from Vesalius to Haller, but architecturally, *i. e.*, not as if seen from a particular angle, but as if the axes of vision struck each part of the object from the same distance. This mode of ortho-

Bernhard Siegfried Albinus (1697–1770).

graphic projection had been used by Leonardo in some of his drawings. It occasioned bitter controversy between Camper and Albinus.

Of all medical men who have illustrated their own books, probably none have ever exhibited such striking artistic talent as that brilliant Venetian—Antonio **Scarpa** (1747–1832). In appearance like the youthful Napoleon, Scarpa was a virtuoso in the most varied sense, a great anatomist and surgeon, equally skilled as orthopedist and ophthalmologist, an irreproachable Latinist, a master of sarcasm, yet a most attractive teacher, and a draftsman of the first order. He himself trained Faustino Anderloni to execute the copper-engravings from his own drawings (Choulant). Scarpa's greatest work is undoubtedly the magnificent *Tabulæ Nevrologicæ* (Pavia, 1794), which gives the first proper delineation of the nerves of the heart. Executed with the force of genius, and irreproachable in accuracy of detail, Scarpa's illustrations are the crown and flower of achievement in anatomic pen-drawing, while Anderloni's wonderful copper-plates of the same are comparable in *brio* with the work of Sharp, the Drevets, and other masters of the best period of line-engraving.

In anatomy, Scarpa is memorable for his discovery of the membranous labyrinth, the nasopalatine nerve, and the triangle in the thigh which bears his name; he was the first to regard arteriosclerosis as a lesion of the inner coats of the arteries and, in 1832, described cubitodigital neuralgia (Weir Mitchell's causalgia); he wrote important treatises on hernia and eye diseases, and originated the procedure of iridodialysis; he made a shoe for club-foot which is still the model for orthopedists.

In Great Britain, anatomic study received a mighty impulse from the teaching of the brothers Hunter, and the name of William Hunter is inseparably connected with the advancement of **obstetrics.** During the 18th century, the care of labor cases began to pass from the midwife proper to the trained male obstetrician. Peter Chamberlen attended Queen Henrietta Maria in a miscarriage in 1628. In Paris, the pace already had been set during the preceding century, through the cir-

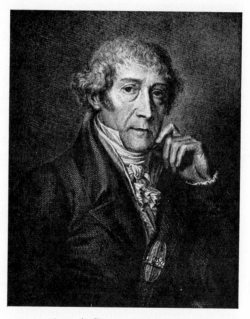

Antonio Scarpa (1747–1832).

cumstance that le sieur Boucher was called upon to attend La Vallière, mistress of the "Grand Monarque," in her first confinement in 1663. In 1670, Julien Clément attended Mme. de Montespan at the birth of the Duc de Maine, afterward delivering the Dauphine (1682). Clément received the title of *"accoucheur"* for his trouble[1]; whereupon, in due course, male midwifery became the fashion among the great ladies of the court. In 1692, Hugh Chamberlen delivered the future Queen Anne. Progress in this matter was of course slow, indeed, when a certain obstetrician told Joseph II that the Viennese women were too modest to have men as midwives, that moral monarch replied, with

---

[1] See Alban Doran: Jour. Obst. and Gynæc. Brit. Emp., Lond., 1915, xxvii, 158–159.

fitting irony: *Utinam non essent adeo pudicae*.[1] At first, as in some court circles today, the obstetrician simply supervised or "assisted at" the conduct of labor among those who could afford his services; but as soon as women began to permit physicians to examine the parts as well as deliver them, the growth of inductive knowledge of the complex details of midwifery was a foregone conclusion. In Great Britain this was principally due to the teaching and influence of two Lanarkshire men (William Smellie and his pupil William Hunter) to Sir Fielding Ould (Dublin) and to Charles White (Manchester). On the continent, the cause of male midwifery was upheld by Röderer in Göttingen,

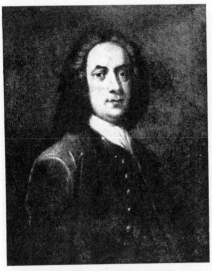

William Smellie (1697–1763).

Camper in Amsterdam, Baudelocque and Levret in Paris, Boër in Vienna, and Saxtorph in Copenhagen.

William **Smellie** (1697–1763), the friend and teacher of Smollett, learned his obstetrics in Paris and, settling in London in 1739, conceived the idea of teaching the subject at his own house, using a leather-covered manikin supported by actual bones, and charging three guineas for the course. In spite of his uncultivated bearing and the bitter opposition of Mrs. Nihell, the Haymarket midwife, who called him "a great horse godmother of a he-midwife," Smellie acquired a large practice, and to him William Hunter came as resident pupil in 1741. Smellie introduced the steel-lock forceps in 1744, and the curved and double-curved forceps during 1751–53. Smellie's *Midwifery* (1752) was the first book to lay down safe rules for using the forceps, and for differentiating contracted from normal pelves by actual measurement. It was deemed worthy of the honor of a special reprint by the Sydenham Society in 1876–78. Smellie's "Set of Anatomical Tables" (1754) is entirely obstetric.

In 1767 John **Harvie**, who married Smellie's niece and succeeded to his lecture room in 1759, published a pamphlet in which the advantages of external manual expression of the placenta over traction or internal manipulation are clearly stated, nearly ninety years before Credé (1854[2]). The same idea was gradually conveyed by the Dublin obstetricians Edward Foster (1781), William Dease (1783), Joseph Clarke (1817), Robert Collins (1835), A. H. McClintock and S. L. Hardy (1848),

---

[1] "Would they were not modest to that extent." (Cited by Moll.) Perhaps the Emperor was thinking of the advice which van Swieten gave to his father.

[2] J. Harvie: Practical Directions, shewing a method of preserving the Perinæum in birth and delivering the Placenta without violence, London, 1767, pp. 45–48.

and, although not known outside of Ireland, became an established mode of procedure there—the "Dublin method."[1]

William Hunter (1718–83) had five years' training at Glasgow University, and three as a pupil of Cullen's. Following the example of his London teachers, Smellie and Douglass, he started, in 1746, a course of private lectures on dissecting, operative surgery, and bandaging. He soon advanced in practice and public esteem, through his refined, courtly ways and his sagacious disposition, and eventually became the leading obstetrician and consultant of London. In 1768, he built the famous anatomic theater and museum in Great Windmill Street, where the best British anatomists and surgeons of the period, including his

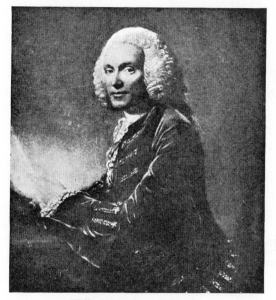

William Hunter (1718–83).

brother John, were trained. Here he labored with ardor to the end of his days, and few men have shown such austere devotion to science. We may contrast his noble gift of a museum worth £100,000 to the city of Glasgow with the Scotch tenacity of purpose and the self-denying stoicism of his private life, as summed up in the terse phrases of Stephen Paget: "He never married; he had no country house; he looks, in his portraits, a fastidious, fine gentleman; but he worked till he dropped and he lectured when he was dying." In relation to his colleagues, William Hunter was a jealous, sensitive, thin-blooded, high-strung man, who embittered his own life by needless controversy with con-

---

[1] See H. Jellett: Tr. Roy. Acad. Med. Ireland, Dublin, 1899–1900, xviii, 305–316; and T. P. C. Kirkpatrick: Jour. Obst. and Gynæc. Brit. Empire, London, 1915, xxvii, 1–7.

temporaries whom he easily overshadowed. His greatest work is his atlas of the pregnant uterus (London, 1774), the only medical publication of the celebrated Baskerville Press, illustrated by Riemsdijk at an enormous expense to the author, and representing the labor of thirty years. His special discovery of the "decidua reflexa" and the separate maternal and fetal circulation, in which his brother had a part, is the foundation of modern knowledge of placental anatomy.

William Hunter also wrote papers of permanent value on old dislocations of the shoulders (1762[1]), symphysiotomy (1778[2]), the jurisprudence of infanticide (1783[3]), and the history of anatomy (1784[4]). He was the first to describe arteriovenous aneurysm (1761[5]) and retroversion of the uterus (1770[6]), and one of the first to recommend the tapping of ovarian cysts (1757[7]); but, unlike Smellie, he opposed the use of the forceps, and sometimes exhibited his own instrument, covered with rust, in evidence of the fact that he never used it.

The obstetric treatise of the Manchester surgeon Charles **White** (London, 1773), stands out in its time as a pioneer work in **aseptic midwifery,** an early brief for surgical cleanliness in obstetrics.

The **mechanism of labor** was first considered by Deventer (1701), by Sir Fielding Ould (1710–89), of Dublin, in his "Treatise on Midwifery" of 1742, and later by Smellie, André Levret, J. J. Fried, J. G. Roederer, Pieter Camper, C. J. Berger, Mathias Saxtorph and Jens Bang.[8]

Prominent continental obstetricians of special note were Jean Palfyn (1649–1730), who reinvented or reintroduced the forceps (*mains de fer*) in 1720[9]; Guillaume Mauquest de La Motte (1665–1737), who extended the use of podalic version to head presentations (1721); Pieter Camper (1722–89), who first proposed symphysiotomy, and Jean Réné Sigault, who first performed it successfully upon Mme. Souchot in 1777; Jean Louis Baudelocque, Sr. (1746–1810), who invented a pelvimeter and advanced the knowledge of the mechanism of labor, but overspecialized in his enumeration of possible positions of the fetus (1781); André Levret (1703–80), who improved the forceps and extended its use (1747); Carl Caspar Siebold (1736–1807), who performed the first symphysiotomy in Germany (1778); and Lucas Johann Boër (1751–1835), who was the ablest German obstetrician of his time and the pioneer of "natural obstetrics" (1791–1806). Before the time of Boër, pregnancy had been regarded as a sort of nine months' disease. He was the first to treat the condition as a physiologic process, and was a forerunner of Ramsbotham in tilting against "meddlesome midwifery." To Mauriceau, Portal, and Mau-

---

[1] W. Hunter: Med. Obs. & Inquiries, Lond., 1762, ii, 373–381.

[2] "Reflections on dividing the Symphysis of the Ossa Pubis." Published as a supplement to the second edition of J. Vaughan's "Cases and Observations on the Hydrophobia," London, 1778.

[3] "On the uncertainty of the signs of murder in the case of bastard children," in Med. Obs. & Inquiries, 1778–83, Lond., 1784, vi, 266–290.

[4] Two Introductory Lectures, London, 1784.

[5] Med. Obs. & Inquiries, Lond., 1753–57, i, 340; 1762, ii, 390.

[6] Med. Obs. & Inquiries, Lond., 1771, iv, 409; 1776, v, 388.

[7] Med. Obs. & Inquiries (1757–61), Lond., 1762, ii, 44–45.

[8] See E. Ingerslev: Arch. f. Gesch. d. Med., Leipz., 1908–9, ii, 141–188.

[9] The instrument was figured by Heister in 1724. Dusée's double-jointed forceps was exhibited in Edinburgh in 1733. Curved forceps was introduced by Pugh (1740), Levret (1747), Smellie (1751–53). Many others followed. For further details about the history of the forceps in the 18th century, see Alban Doran's papers in Jour. Obst. and Gynæc. Brit. Empire, Lond., 1912, xxii, 119, 203; 1913, xxiii, 3, 65; xxiv, 1, 197; 1915, xxvii, 154. The latter entry (1915) gives a good chronology of the history of the forceps.

quest de La Motte is due the improvement of obstetric diagnosis by digital exploration, the standardization of version and its indications, the substitution of a rational
expectant procedure for bungling instrumentation, and the study of contracted
pelves.[1] Duverney was the first to notice simultaneous extra- and intra-uterine
pregnancy (1708[2]).

Operative **gynecology,** as an independent specialty, had no real existence before
the first half of the 19th century. Of stray contributions in the 18th century, we
may mention Robert Houstoun's treatment of an ovarian dropsy (1701), by tapping
the cyst (etymologically an "ovariotomy," but in no sense an excision of the ovary);
William Hunter's proposal of excision for ovarian cyst in 1757, and his description of
retroversion of the uterus (1770); Sigault's symphysiotomy (1777); Matthew Baillie's
description of dermoid cysts of the ovary (1789), and Soemmerring's essay on the
injurious effects of corsets (1793). Georg Ernst Stahl (1660–1734) wrote a lengthy
monograph on the diseases of spinsters in 1724, and Jean Astruc (1684–1766) achieved
a six-volume treatise on diseases of women in 1761–65.

Up to the time of John Hunter, **surgery** was entirely in French
hands, and Paris was the only place where the subject could be properly
studied. In Germany, in consequence of the great setback of the
Thirty Years' War, general surgery was practised mainly by the executioner and the barber (*Chirurgus*), or else by the wandering incisors,
couchers, and bone-setters, while the army surgeon was called a *Feld-
scherer*, because it was his duty to shave the officers. Even with such
talented obstetricians as Heister, von Siebold, and Richter, the art
had no real status before the time of Frederick the Great. In England,
Cheselden and Pott were the only two clinical surgeons of first rank
before John Hunter's time. The whole period before Hunter was one
of enterprise in respect of new amputations, excisions, or other improvements in operative technique, most of which are associated with
French names.

As early as 1673, Pierre **Dionis** (died 1718) was giving courses on
operative surgery on the cadaver. His treatises on anatomy (1690)
and surgery (1707) were, both of them, standard works for half a century, and translated even into Chinese. Dionis' *Cours d'opérations* is
now valued for its anecdotes and pictures of the surgery of the day, in
particular the story of the wandering lithotomist, Frère Jacques, who
began as a bungling experimenter and became a master through his
attention to anatomy.

Jean-Louis **Petit** (1674–1750), of Paris, the leading French surgeon
of the early 18th century, was the inventor of the screw-tourniquet,
gave the first account of softening of the bones and of the formation of
clots in wounded arteries, and made improvements in amputations and
herniotomy. He was the first to open the mastoid process, an operation
which he describes in his posthumous surgical treatise (1774[3]). Petit's
pupil, Dominique **Anel** (1628–1725), of Toulouse, is remembered by his
operation for lacrimal fistula (1712), and by the fact that, like Guillemeau in the 16th century, he treated a traumatic aneurysm by single

---

[1] For details and references, see H. Fassbender: Geschichte der Geburtshülfe,
Jena, 1906, *passim*.

[2] Duverney: Œuvres, Paris, 1708, ii, 355.

[3] J. L. Petit: Traité de mal. chir., Paris, 1774, pp. 153, 160.

ligature (1710) before John Hunter's time. Pierre **Brasdor** (1721–97) is also remembered for his suggestion that aneurysms be treated by distal ligation, which was made accomplished fact by Wardrop in 1828.

Pierre-Joseph **Desault** (1744–95), the teacher of Bichat, was the founder of an important surgical periodical, the *Journal de Chirurgie* (1791–92), did much to improve the treatment of fractures, and developed the technic of ligating blood-vessels for aneurysms.[1] Nicolas **André** (1658–1742) coined the term "orthopedics" in his treatise of 1741, and was the first to describe infra-orbital neuralgia (1756). The real originator of surgical orthopedics was, however, Jean-André **Venel** (1740–91), of Geneva, Switzerland, who in 1780 founded the first orthopedic institute at Orbe, Canton de Vaud, where he achieved many successful results. He was the author of monographs on the treatment of foreign bodies lodged in the esophagus (1769), and on the correction of lateral curvatures and torsion of the spine by mechanical devices (1788). Spinal braces were introduced by Heister (1700), Levascher (1764–68), Portal (1767), Schmidt (1794), and Kohler (1795). Jean-Pierre **David** (1737–84), a Rouen surgeon, in his essay on the effects of movement and rest in surgical diseases (1779) gave a capital description of spinal deformity from caries, with autopsies, contemporaneously with Pott and wrote on necrosis of bone (1782). The name of François **Chopart** (1743–95), of Paris, is associated with his method of amputating the foot (1792), and that of P. F. **Moreau** with the earliest excisions of the elbow (1786–94[2]).

The leading German surgeons of the century were Lorenz **Heister** (1683–1758), who made the first postmortem section of appendicitis (1711), introduced the term "tracheotomy" (1718[3]), and whose *Chirurgie* (Nuremberg, 1718), is of unusual historic interest on account of its instructive illustrations; and August Gottlieb **Richter** (1742–1812), who wrote a good history of surgery (1782–1804), which he left uncompleted, edited an important surgical journal (*Chirurgische Bibliothek*, 1771–96), and wrote a treatise on hernia (1777–79[4]), which is still an acknowledged classic. With Richter's book on hernia may be grouped the important works on the same subject by Percival Pott (1756), Antonio de Gimbernat (1793), Pieter Camper (1801), and Antonio Scarpa (1809).

Johann Ulric **Bilguer** (1720–96), one of Frederick the Great's surgeons general, was the author of a monograph *De amputatione membrorum rarissime administranda aut quasi abroganda* (1761), which was translated into French by Tissot in 1764, and is indeed the most important plea for conservative surgery of the joints before the time of Fergusson, Brodie, and Syme.

Of English surgeons before the time of Hunter, we may consider

---

[1] P. J. Desault: Œuvres chirurgicales, Paris, 1801, 553–580.

[2] P. F. Moreau: Observations pratiques relatives a la résection des articulations affectées de carie, Paris thesis, an. xi (1803).

[3] E. Ebstein: Virchow's Arch., Berl., 1920, ccxxvi, 96–99.

[4] Richter: Abhandlung von den Brüchen, Göttingen, 1777–79

Cheselden and his pupil Sharp, Charles White of Manchester, and Percival Pott.

William **Cheselden** (1688–1752), of Somerby, Leicestershire, a pupil of Cowper's, became surgeon to St. Thomas' Hospital in 1718. On publishing his "Treatise on a High Operation for Stone" in 1723, he was assailed with violent abuse by John Douglass, on the score of alleged plagiarism from the latter's *Lithotomia Douglassiana* (1720). Cheselden accordingly dropped the procedure he had described, and went on to modify the method of Frère Jacques into a "lateral operation for stone," which he performed March 27, 1727, and which has hardly been improved upon since. In 1728, he introduced a new operation for artificial pupil, consisting of a simple iridotomy with a needle.[1] His anatomy (1713) was popular in its day, and his atlas of osteology (1733), illustrated by Van der Gucht, is a work of permanent value. Cheselden was a genial, kind-hearted, versatile man, not unlike Hogarth in appearance. He was a patron of boxing, and a good draftsman; prepared the plans for Old Putney Bridge and the Surgeon's Hall in the Old Bailey, and assisted Van der Gucht in sketching bones for his *Osteographia* under the camera obscura. He was perhaps the most rapid of all the preanesthetic operators, per-

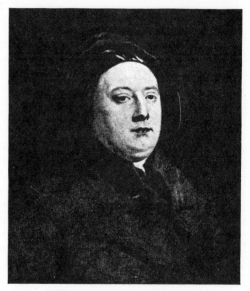

William Cheselden (1688–1752).

forming a lithotomy in fifty-four seconds, which equals or outpaces the time record of even a Langenbeck or a Pirogoff. His social and professional status is embalmed in Pope's couplet:

> "I'll do what Mead and Cheselden advise,
> To keep these limbs and to preserve those eyes."

Charles **White** (1728–1813), of Manchester, one of the pioneers of aseptic midwifery (1773), first excised the head of the humerus in 1768,[2] gave the first account of "white swelling" or phlegmasia alba dolens (1784[3]), and introduced the method of reducing dislocations of

---

[1] W. Cheselden: Phil. Tr., Lond., 1728, xxxvi, 447.

[2] C. White: Phil. Tr., Lond., 1769, lix, 39–46, 1 pl.

[3] White: An inquiry (etc.), Warrington, 1784; also London M. J., 1785, v, 50–57.

the shoulder by means of the heel in the axilla. De Quincey called him "the most eminent surgeon by much in the North of England."

Percival **Pott** (1714–88), of London, was surgeon at St. Bartholomew's Hospital from 1744–87, having, in his own words, served it "man and boy for half a century." Through a fall in the street, he sustained the particular fracture of the fibula which bears his name, and, taking up authorship while confined to his bed, he began to produce in rapid succession such masterpieces as his treatises on hernia (1756), head injuries (1760), hydrocele (1762), fistula in ano (1765), fractures and dislocations (1768), the account of chimney-sweep's cancer (1775) and, above all, the epoch-making pamphlet on palsy

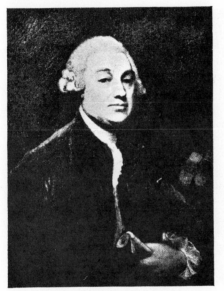

Percival Pott (1714–88).

from spinal deformity (caries) (1779), which was contemporaneous with the more complete account contained in the prize essay of Jean-Pierre David (1779[1]). Toward the end of the century Pott had the largest surgical practice in London. Like Cheselden, he was a man of kindly, charitable nature, and his lectures drew many foreign pupils to St. Bartholomew's.

All the operators before Hunter's time were clinical surgeons, of the stamp of Paré or Richard Wiseman, and knew nothing of pathology. Even long after the publication of Morgagni's great work (1761), surgical pathology had no real existence. For example, the first operation for localized appendicitis was reported by **Mestivier** in 1759,[2] while the pathologic appearances, clearly described in the autopsy, had already been noted by Heister (1711), yet these landmarks left no impression upon practice whatever.

With the advent of **John Hunter** (1728–93), surgery ceased to be regarded as a mere technical mode of treatment, and began to take its place as a branch of scientific medicine, firmly grounded in physiology

---

[1] David: Dissertation sur les effets du mouvement et du repos dans les maladies chirurgicales, 1779. Although spinal caries is now termed "Pott's disease," Pott did not describe the disease or its tuberculous nature, but only the deformity and its sequelæ. The tuberculous nature of gibbous spine, found in Egyptian mummies by Elliot Smith, had been surmised by Hippocrates (Dislocations, §41), confirmed by Galen, revived by J. Z. Platner (1744), and was finally established by Delpech (1816),

[2] H. A. Kelly: Presse méd., Paris, 1903, 437–441.

and pathology. Hunter came up to London in 1748, a raw, uncouth Scotch lad, fonder of taverns and theater galleries than of book-learning. He was taken in hand by his brother, the refined and accomplished

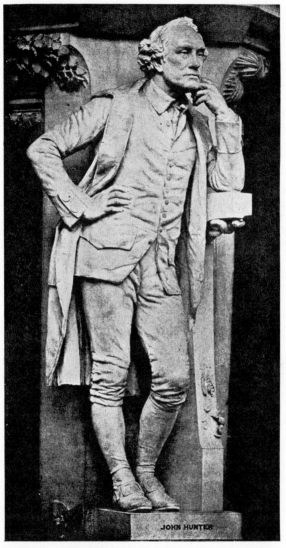

Statue of John Hunter (The Museums, Oxford). (Courtesy of Professor William Stirling, Manchester, England.)

William, and put at dissecting. Here he soon found himself and, at a year's end, was teaching anatomy on his own account and following surgery under Cheselden and Pott. After some experience as staff surgeon with the expedition to Belleisle (1761), where he gained his unique knowledge of gunshot wounds, he settled down in London to a life of ardent original investigation, diversified by extensive surgical practice and a commanding influence as a teacher. In personality, Hunter was very like Ruskin's description of Carlyle—a Northern god struck by lightning—in other words, a Norse or Saxon Scot crossed by Celtic emotionalism and whimsicality. His nature was kindly and generous, though outwardly rude and repelling and, if crossed or thwarted, he was apt to paw the air like a restless, high-spirited horse. Late in life, for some private or personal reason, he picked a public quarrel with the brother who had formed him and made a man of him, basing the dissension upon a quibble about priority entirely unworthy of so great an investigator. Yet three years later, he lived to mourn this brother's death in tears. Of a piece with this was the pathos of John Hunter's own end. Being a victim of angina pectoris, he had said: "My life is in the hands of any rascal who chooses to annoy and tease me," and so it fell out. He was something of a scornful Ishmaelite among his professional colleagues and, being contradicted by one of these in a public discussion, was overtaken by the fatal malady and led out of the room. In a few minutes, the strong, imperious man had passed away. Many years after his death, his brother-in-law, Sir Everard Home, consigned himself to oblivion by burning Hunter's manuscripts after using them as the groundwork for sundry Croonian lectures and other alleged scientific contributions of his own devising. As Hunter was a composite character, so his work was many-sided, and we sense its magnitude not merely in his writings, many of which were destroyed, but in the great museum of over 13,000 specimens which he collected; and by the influence of such pupils as Jenner, Astley Cooper, Abernethy, Cline, Clift, Parkinson, Blizard, Home, Alanson, Wright Post, and Physick. He described the ramifications of the olfactory nerve in the nose, the arterial supply of the gravid uterus, and discovered the lacrimal ducts in man and many features of the lymphatic system. His permanent position in science is based upon the fact that he was the founder of experimental and surgical pathology as well as a pioneer in comparative physiology and experimental morphology. As the phlogiston-chemistry of his day was sadly muddled, he was fortunate in knowing nothing about it. He got up no elaborate experiments, and his mode of questioning nature has been justly praised for its simplicity. Thus he demonstrated the arrest of digestion in hibernation by passing bits of meat down the throats of lizards kept in cool winter quarters. His observations of the collateral capillary circulation in the antlers of deer in Richmond Park led to his method of treating aneurysms. His studies on the repair of tendons began with an accident he sustained while dancing. He accidentally inoculated himself with lues, and purposely delayed treatment in order to study the disease in his own person. As a surgical pathologist, he described shock, phlebitis, pyemia, and intussusception, and made epoch-making studies of inflammation, gunshot wounds, and the surgical diseases of the vascular system. He differentiated clearly between hard (Hunterian) chancre and the chancroid ulcer, but his auto-inoculation seems to have confused gonorrhea[1] with syphilis, a confusion which obtained until the time of Ricord. He introduced artificial feeding by means of a flexible tube passed into the stomach (1790[2]) and invented an apparatus for forced respiration (1793). His greatest innovation in surgery was the establishment of the principle that aneurysms due to arterial disease should be tied high up in the healthy tissues by a single ligature (1786[3]), which displaced the old Antyllus method of securing the aneurysm between two ligatures and evacuating its contents. The novel feature was not the single ligature, which had already been employed by Guillemeau (1594) and Anel (1710), but the sound pathologic reasoning upon which its use was based. Not credited in Hunter's day, it has since saved "thousands of limbs and lives." As a biologist, Hunter dissected and described over 500 different species of animals, but, unlike many modern systematists, declined to publish any monographs on a single animal, aiming to connect morphology with physiology by studying the relation between structure and function. He held that the blood is alive, that structure is the ultimate expression of function (Galen), that abnormities are an expression of "arrested development," and that the embryo, in each successive stage of its existence, resembles the completed form of some order lower than itself, leading to the basic principle of comparative physiology, that the functional activities of the lower forms of life are, as it were, simplifications of those in the higher. In all this, Hunter was sound and modern. His defective education crops out in his various references to the fluid parts of the body as sentient beings, endowed with consciousness, and in such expressions as "the irritation of imperfection," "the stimulus of death," "the blood's consciousness of its being a useful part of the body." Phrases like these not only outvitalize the vitalists, but indicate Hunter's complete ignorance or wilful disregard of the work of his predecessors. In his dispute with the Abbate Spallanzani about digestion, he was hopelessly at fault. His reasoning about phlebitis and pyemia was wrong, since he regarded phlebitis as the cause of thrombosis, a theory which was demolished by Virchow in 1856. But, when all is said, Hunter remains one of the great all-round biologists like Haller and Johannes Müller, and, with Paré and Lister, one of the three greatest surgeons of all time. It is no exaggeration to repeat that Hunter found surgery a mechanical art and left it an experimental science. What he did for the social status of the surgeon is indicated by the remark of one of his colleagues: "He alone made us gentlemen." Here, he is like Beethoven, whose rugged independence

---

[1] See J. Le Petit: Historique du chancre mou. Paris diss. No. 94, 1913.
[2] Tr. Soc. Improvement Med. & Chir. Knowledge, Lond., 1793, i, 182–188.
[3] *Ibid.*, i, 138–181; 1800, ii, 235–256.

made the composer and the musician the reverse of "despised and rejected." Only passing reference can be made to his observations on vital heat in animals and vegetables, fetal smallpox, free-martins, superfetation, electric fishes, postmortem digestion of the stomach, or his experiments on pathologic inoculations and on regeneration and transplantation of tissues, in which he is, in some sort, a forerunner of the experimental morphologists and extra-vital tissue-growers of our own time. His four masterpieces are the *Natural History of the Human Teeth* (1771); the treatise *On Venereal Disease* (1786); the *Observations on Certain Parts of the Animal Œconomy* (1786); and the *Treatise on the Blood, Inflammation and Gunshot Wounds* (1794). Hunter was the first to study the teeth in a scientific manner, and the first to recommend complete removal of the pulp in filling them. He introduced the classes cuspids, bicuspids, molars and incisors, enlarged upon dental malocclusion, and devised appliances for correcting the condition.

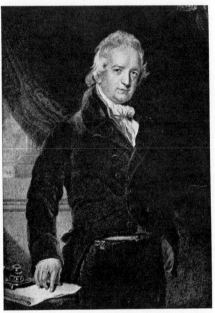

John Abernethy (1764–1831).

His work in dentistry was preceded by a French and a German classic, Pierre **Fauchard**'s *Le Chirurgien Dentiste* (1728), and Philipp **Pfaff**'s *Abhandlung von den Zähnen* (1756). These three books are the most important in the history of dentistry. The second edition of Fauchard's work (1746) contains (pp. 275–277) the first account of pyorrhœa alveolaris, familiarly called Riggs' disease after the American dentist John M. Riggs who, in 1876,[1] introduced the modern heroic treatment of the condition by scraping the teeth to the roots. Fauchard was also the first to employ orthodontal procedure in the treatment of malocclusion.

Hunter's immediate successor in London was his devoted pupil, John **Abernethy** (1764–1831), who constituted himself a sort of champion of his master's physiologic theories, which he dramatized in the lecture room with a poetic imagination and a vigorous style of delivery. Abernethy was the first to ligate the external iliac artery for aneurysm (1796), an operation which he performed four times, twice with success.[2] He ligated the common carotid for hemorrhage in 1798, and improved the treatment of lumbar abscesses by incision, admitting as little air as possible He also described an anomaly of the viscera

---

[1] J. M. Riggs: Penn. J. Dent. Sc., Phila., 1876, iii, 99–104.
[2] J. Abernethy: Surgical Observations, London, 1809, 234–292.

which is not unlike the Eck fistula (1793[1]). He believed that local diseases are either of constitutional origin or due to digestive disturbances and, in practice, treated nearly everything by calomel and blue-mass. Although kind-hearted and generous at bottom, he affected a brusque, downright manner with his patients on the ground that masterful rudeness wins confidence, where amiability might suggest weakness and so diminish respect.

Of **pioneer operations by American surgeons** in the 18th century, a passing notice may be taken of an amputation of the shoulder-joint by John Warren, of Boston, in 1781, three cases of laparotomy for extra-uterine pregnancy by John Bard, of New Jersey, in 1759,[2] and by William Baynham, of Virginia, in 1791 and 1799[3]; and Wright Post's operation for femoral aneurysm by the Hunterian method in 1796.[4]

The **surgery of the eye** owes one of its most telling advancements to Jacques **Daviel** (1696–1762), the originator of the modern treatment of cataract by extraction of the lens (1752). In the early part of the century Brisseau (1706) and Maître-Jan (1707) had brought out the important fact that true cataract is, in effect, a clouding and hardening of the lens. In a postmortem of 1692, Maître-Jan had indeed proved that the opaque lens is cataract, but before 1706–7 it had been regarded as a sort of skin or pellicle immediately inside the capsule. Daviel was a Norman by birth. After studying surgery with an uncle at Rouen, and revealing his courage and humanity in fighting the plague at Toulon and Marseilles, he settled in Paris in 1746, where he soon succeeded in surgical practice. He was appointed eye surgeon to Louis XV in 1749. In 1752, he sent to the Royal Academy of Surgery his only literary production, the memoir on the cure of cataract by extraction of the crystalline lens,[5] with statistics of 100 successful operations out of 115. By 1756, he had a record of 434 extractions, with only 50 failures. From that time on his method became a permanent part of ophthalmic procedure, the principal modification being the addition of iridectomy by von Graefe.[6]

Other ophthalmic contributions of note were Sylvester O'Halloran's treatise on glaucoma (1750), Georg Ernst Stahl's original description of lacrimal fistula (1702[7]), Heberden's account of nyctalopia or night-blindness (1767[8]), John Dalton's account of color-blindness (1794[9]), and Joseph Beer's innovation of iridectomy (1798).

---

[1] J. Abernethy: Phil. Tr., Lond., 1793, 59–68, 2 pl.

[2] Bard: Med. Obs. & Inq., 1757–61, Lond., 1762, ii, 369–372.

[3] Baynham: New York Med. & Phil. Rev., 1809, i, 160–172.

[4] Post: Am. Med. & Phil. Reg., N. Y., 1814, iv, 452.

[5] J. Daviel: "Sur une nouvelle methode de guérir la cataracte par l'extraction du cristallin" in: Mém. Acad. roy. de chir., Paris, 1753, ii, 337–354.

[6] Even in the employment of iridectomy, Daviel was a pioneer, as is shown in his letter to Haller (J. de méd., chir., pharm. [etc.], Paris, 1762, xvi, 245–251).

[7] Stahl: De fistula lachrymali, Halle, 1702.

[8] Heberden: Med. Tr. Coll. Phys., Lond., 3. ed., 1785, i, 60; 1806–13, iv, 56.

[9] Dalton: Mem. Lit. & Phil. Soc., Manchester, 1798, v, pt. 1, 28–45.

An outstanding figure in the history of ophthalmology was Thomas Young (1773–1829), of Milverton, England, a Quaker physician and one of the greatest men of science of all time. Learning Latin and many Oriental languages at an early age, he began to study medicine in 1792 under John Hunter, Matthew Baillie, and William Cruikshank, graduated at Göttingen in 1796, took his M.B. and M.D. at Cambridge in 1803 and 1808, and practised in London from 1799 to 1814. Young was thus the most highly educated physician of his time, and held many scientific positions of honor. Tscherning calls him "the father of physiologic optics," and Helmholtz, "one of the most clear-sighted men who ever lived."

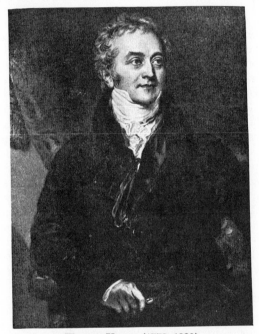

Thomas Young (1773–1829).

In 1792, he read to the Royal Society his paper showing that visual accommodation of the eye at different distances is due to change of curvature in the crystalline lens,[1] which he erroneously attributed to some muscular structure in the latter. In his memoir *On the Mechanism of the Eye* (1801[2]), he gave the first description of astigmatism, with measurements and optical constants. He also stated the present Young-Helmholtz theory that color vision is due to retinal structures corresponding with red, green, and violet, color-blindness being deficient response of these to normal stimuli. In his Croonian lecture of 1808, Young clearly stated the laws governing the flow of blood in the heart and arteries. His *Introduction to Medical Literature* (1813) contains his classification of diseases. His essay on consumption (1815) summarizes the knowledge of his time. In physics, Young is most famous as the author of the wave theory of light (1801–03), that it

[1] Young: Phil. Tr., Lond., 1793, 169–181, 1 pl.
[2] Young: *Ibid.*, 1801, xci, 23–88, 5 pl.

is due to undulations of the ether. In 1809, he showed its application to crystalline refraction and dispersion phenomena, which led to the Fresnel theory of double refraction (1821) and the Helmholtz theory of dispersion for absorbent media. He introduced the modern physical concepts of "energy" and "work done," showing that they are proportional to each other; and in 1804, he stated the theory of capillary attraction, founded upon the doctrine of energy, which was independently advanced by Laplace (1805). He also defined the "modulus of elasticity" (Young's modulus) and regarded heat as the "mechanical vibrations of particles larger and stronger than those of light." His theory of tides (1813) is said to have explained more tidal phenomena than any other hypothesis before the time of Airy. Young was also an accomplished Egyptologist, one of the earliest decipherers of hieroglyphics (Rosetta Stone). He discovered that the demotic characters are not alphabetic, but symbols derived from phonetic signs (hieroglyphs), which view was soon adopted by Champollion. Young's extraordinary versatility is further evidenced in his reports on ship-building, gas-lighting, standardization of the seconds pendulum and the imperial gallon, longitude, and life insurance.

Young was fond of dancing and good society, but was not regarded as a successful practitioner because he studied symptoms too closely, although his treatment was admitted to be effective. In person, he was probably the handsomest of all the great physicians. His fine open countenance was of classic contour, expressing great kindliness and good will, and with that sign of the mathematic mind which the old French poet has also esteemed a criterion of beauty—

"Eyes wide apart and keen of sight."[1]

In 1749 the philosopher Denis Diderot (1713–84) published his *Lettres sur les aveugles*, showing how the blind survive in the struggle for life by supreme adaptability of their four remaining senses, and suggesting the possibility of teaching them to read and write by the sense of touch. For this he was thrown into the Bastile for three months. Rousseau visited him in prison and is said to have suggested a system of embossed printing for the blind. In the 18th century, blind beggars were so numerous that they often fought and jostled for standing room in places where they were likely to receive alms. At the annual fairs, it was customary to utilize the blind, decked out with asses' ears, peacocks' tails, and pasteboard spectacles, as objects of amusement. In 1771, Valentin Hauy (1745–1822), younger brother of the celebrated mineralogist, saw a burlesque concert of this kind, greeted day after day by the coarse guffaws of the vulgar. Deeply affected by the pitiful spectacle, he resolved in his heart to teach the blind to read, write, and play music. In 1785, he founded the *Institut nationale des jeunes aveugles* and began the first printing for the blind in raised characters. By 1786, he was able to make a good exhibition of the success of his pupils before Louis XVI and his court. He then published his *Essai sur l'éducation des aveugles* (1786). This was the origin of modern methods of teaching and caring for the blind.

Otology was very materially advanced in the 18th century.

Among the contributions of capital importance were the studies of the structure and physiology of the ear by Valsalva (1717[2]), Scarpa (1772–89[3]), and Cotugno (1774[4]), and the morphologic essays of Geoffroy (1778[5]) and Comparetti (1789[6]).

---

[1] François Villon, Swinburne's translation.

[2] Valsalva: De aure humana tractatus, Utrecht, 1717.

[3] Scarpa: De structura fenestræ rotundæ auris, Mutinæ, 1772; and his: Anatomicæ disquisitiones de auditu et olfactu, Ticini, 1789.

[4] Cotugno: De aquæductibus auris humanæ internæ, Vienna, 1774.

[5] Geoffroy: Dissertations sur l'organe de l'ouie, Amsterdam, 1778.

[6] Comparetti: Observationes anatomicæ de aure interna comparata, Padua, 1789.

The existence of an elastic fluid in the labyrinth and its rôle in the transmission of sound was noted, even before Cotugno, by Theodor Pyl in 1742 (Neuburger[1]). Catheterization of the Eustachian tube was first attempted by the French post-master Guyot in 1724[2] and subsequently performed by Archibald Cleland in 1741.[3] Eli, a strolling quack, is credited with the first perforation of the tympanic mem-brane for deafness (1760[4]). In 1755, Jonathan Wathen had treated catarrhal deaf-ness by means of injections into the Eustachian tube through a catheter inserted in the nose.[5]

More important still, the mastoid process was opened for the first time in the history of surgery by Jean-Louis Petit in 1736[6] with subsequent successful cases, by the Prussian army surgeon Jasser in 1776,[7] by J. G. H. Fielitz,[8] A. F. Löffler,[9] and the Danish surgeon Alexander Kölpin in 1796.[10]

Inspired by the successes of Rodriguez Pereira, the pioneer of **deaf-mute instruc-tion** in France, the Abbé Charles-Michel de l'Épée (1712–89), founded the first school for deaf-mutes in Paris (1755), maintained at his own expense, and pub-lished many writings on the subject, the most important being his treatise of 1784.[11] He got much from Bonet (1620) and Amman (1692), and may have acquired some of his manual alphabet from Pereira, but the main feature of his hitherto unparalleled success was his intense and lifelong devotion to his pupils, living among them, identifying himself with them, and sparing himself no trouble and expense for their maintenance. In 1838 a monument was erected over his grave in the church of St. Roch. His unfinished dictionary of deaf and dumb signs is said to have been completed by his successor, the Abbé Cucurron Sicard (1742–1822), who succeeded far better in training the minds of deaf-mutes. The earliest advocate of education of the deaf in America was Francis **Green** (1742–1809), of Boston, Massachusetts, who published the treatise *Vox oculis subjecta* (London, 1783), and translated the Abbé de l'Épée's letters.

The salient features of **clinical medicine** in the 18th century were the introduction of postmortem sections, of new methods of precision in diagnosis, and of preventive inoculation, none of which, however, were much appreciated until the following century. In the year 1761, there were published two works which have exerted a profound influ-ence upon the medicine of our own period, viz., the *Inventum Novum* of Auenbrugger and the *De Sedibus et Causis Morborum* of Morgagni.

Leopold **Auenbrugger** (1722–1809), a Styrian by birth, became physician-in-chief to the Hospital of the Holy Trinity at Vienna in 1751, and there he tested and tried out the value of the discovery which afterward made him famous. His little book is the first record of the use of immediate percussion of the chest in diagnosis, based upon observation verified by postmortem experiences and experiment.

---

[1] Pyl: Dissertatio medica de auditu, Greifswald, 1742. (See M. Neuburger, Janus, Amst., 1896–7, i, 380.)

[2] Guyot: Hist. Acad. roy. d. sc., 1724, Paris, 1726, 37.

[3] Cleland: Phil. Tr., 1732–41, London, 1747, ix, 124, 1 pl.

[4] A. Politzer: Gesch. der Ohrenheilk., Stuttgart, 1907, i, 336.

[5] Wathen: Phil. Tr., 1755, Lond., 1756, xlix, 213–222, 1 pl.

[6] Petit: Traité d. mal. chir., Paris, 1774, 153, 160.

[7] Jasser: In Schmucker's Vermischte chirurgische Schriften, Berlin, 1782, iii, pp. 113–125.

[8] Chir. Biblioth. (Richter), Göttingen, 1785, viii, 524; 1788, ix, 553.

[9] *Ibid.*, 1790, x, 613.

[10] See Schmiegelow: Ztschr. f. Ohrenheilk., Wiesb., 1913, lxviii, 55–59.

[11] C.-M. de l'Épée: La véritable manière d'instruire les sourds et muets, Paris, 1784.

Our author's first proposition is that the chest of a healthy subject sounds, when struck, like a cloth-covered drum. He then proceeds to outline his special method of eliciting information by striking the chest gently with the points of the fingers brought together (stretched out straight and afterward flexed), the patient holding his breath; a muffled sound or one of higher pitch than usual indicates the presumable site of a diseased condition. He ascertained the sounds produced by tapping over fluids injected into the chest of a cadaver, localized pectoral fremitus, and carried his findings over into bedside practice, including treatment by thoracentesis. This great discovery was slighted and even snubbed by de Haen, Sprengel, Vogel, Baldinger, and other contemporary writers. Peter Frank gave it but frosty commendation, and only Haller, Stoll, and Ludwig were friendly in Auenbrugger's lifetime. The work remained unnoticed until Corvisart took it up in 1808, one year before its author's death. Although Corvisart might easily have revamped the idea of percussion as his own discovery, he says with fine feeling that he would not sacrifice the name of Auenbrugger to personal vanity: "It is he and the beautiful invention which of right belongs to him that I wish to recall to life." Auenbrugger himself was too well poised and

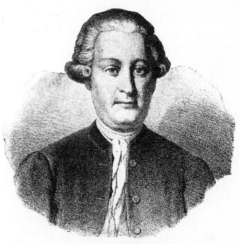

Leopold Auenbrugger, Edler von Auenbrugg (1722–1809).

serene by nature to worry about his posthumous reputation. Grave, genial, inflexibly honest, unassuming and charitable, loving science for its own sake, writing the libretto of a little opera[1] for the delectation of Maria Theresa, and modestly waiving her request that he repeat the experiment on the ground that "one was enough," caring more for the society of his beautiful wife, good music, and *Gemüthlichkeit* generally than for any notoriety, he is, indeed, a noble example of the substantial worth and charm of old-fashioned German character at its very best.[2]

Giovanni Battista **Morgagni** (1682–1771), of Forli, a pupil of Valsalva and later a professor at Padua (1715–71), published the results of his life-work in his seventy-ninth year. It consists of 5 books of letters,

---

[1] It was called "The Chimney Sweep" (Der Rauchfangkehrer). (Composed by Salieri.)

[2] For Dr. Weir Mitchell's beautiful tribute to Auenbrugger, see Tr. Cong. Am. Phys., 1891, New Haven, 1892, ii, 180, 181.

23

70 in number, written in an engagingly communicative manner, and
constituting the true foundation of modern pathologic anatomy, in
that, for the first time, the records of postmortem findings are brought
into correlation with clinical records on a grand scale. As Virchow[1]
said, he introduced the "anatomical idea" into medical practice. In
his preface, Morgagni modestly disavows any special claim to originality,
and gives due credit to the works of his predecessors, such as the
Sepulchretum of Bonet, which contains all the known postmortems up
to 1679. But while others, like Benivieni, Vesalius, or Bonetus, may
have looked at diseased viscera in the dead body with some intelligence,
it was by the vast scope of his work and his many descriptions of new
forms of disease that Mor-
gagni made pathology a
genuine branch of modern
science, even if the seed
sown fell, as Sir Clifford
Allbutt contends, "upon
hard and sterile ground."

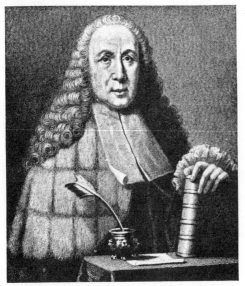

Giovanni Battista Morgagni (1682–1771).

Morgagni gave the first description of cerebral gummata
and diseases of the cardiac valves;
early accounts of syphilitic aneurysm, acute yellow atrophy of
the liver, and tuberculosis of the
kidney, and the first recorded
case of heart-block (Stokes-
Adams disease[2]); identified the
clinical features of pneumonia
with solidification of the lungs,
emphasized the extreme importance of visceral syphilis, and
was the first to show that intracranial suppuration is really
a sequel of discharge from the
ear, a phenomenon which even
Valsalva had conceived the other
way around. Morgagni also de-
scribed what is now known as "Morgagnian cataract." He proved, in many
autopsies, the Valsalva dictum that the cerebral lesion in apoplexy is on the opposite
side from the resulting paralysis.[3] The *De sedibus* abolished humoral concepts
in pathology for a long period of time.

A worthy follower of Morgagni was Matthew **Baillie** (1761–1823),
who, like Smellie, Cullen, and the Hunters, was a native of Lanarkshire,
Scotland. He received a good classic education at Balliol College, was
advised by his uncle, William Hunter, to study medicine, and, in due
course, became a pupil and house-intimate at Windmill Street. He
was physician to George III, and is said to have ruined his health by
devoting sixteen hours a day to his extensive practice. Baillie's *Morbid*

[1] Virchow: Morgagni und der anatomische Gedanke, 1894.

[2] De Sedibus, Venice, 1761, i, 70. Cited by Sir William Osler.

[3] E. Ebstein: Deutsche Ztschr. f. Nervenheilk., Leipz., 1914, liii, 130–136.

Anatomy (London, 1793), illustrated with beautiful copper-plates by William Clift, John Hunter's famulus, differs from Morgagni's work in that it is the first attempt to treat pathology as a subject in and for itself, describing the morbid appearances of each organ in systematic succession, as in a modern text-book, In each instance, the autopsy is correlated with a full case-history, and the author seems to have grasped the idea that postmortem appearances are only end-results, although such results "may then become again the cause of many symptoms." He wisely limited his descriptions, as a rule, to such naked-eye appearances as he actually understood—those in the brain and the viscera—and did not attempt to deal with the nerves or the spinal cord.

Baillie described transposition of the viscera,[1] hydrosalpinx, and dermoid cysts of the ovary[2]; gave the first accurate definitions of cirrhosis of the liver and of "hepatization" of the lungs in pneumonia; distinguished renal cysts from renal hydatids; described endocarditis, gastric ulcer, and the ulceration of Peyer's patches in typhoid fever (without understanding their significance). He showed that death from "polypus of the heart" is really due to a clot of fibrin, and that pulsation of the abdominal aorta is not necessarily a sign of internal disease. In his second edition (1797), he mentions rheumatism of the heart, to which Pitcairn first called attention in his lectures of 1788.

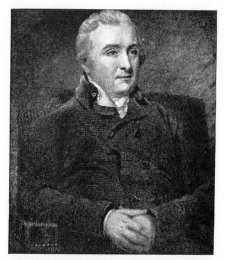

Matthew Baillie (1761–1823). (From the painting by John Hoppner.)

In consultation, Baillie had the same gift of clear, concise expression which distinguished his writings. He was the last inheritor of the "Gold-headed Cane," and his bust is in Westminster Abbey.

The Hallerian doctrine of irritability was carried over into pathology by Hieronymus David **Gaub** (1705–80), of Heidelberg, one of Boerhaave's pupils, who became lector (1731), and professor of chemistry at Leyden (1734). His Institutes of Medical Pathology (1758[3]), was a favorite text-book on the continent for a long time. Gaub envisaged irritability as a pathologic increase of vital power and applied this concept to disease. This did great harm, as his book, which passed through many editions and translations, was in the hands of all students, to most of whom Morgagni and Matthew Baillie were unknown. Gaub was more of a chemist than a medical man. His best work is his treatise on prescriptions (1739[4]).

During the 18th century there were some noteworthy attempts to employ instruments of precision in **diagnosis**. In 1707, Sir John **Floyer**

---

[1] Baillie: Phil. Tr., Lond., 1788, lxxvii, 350–363.

[2] London Med. Jour., 1789, x, 322–332.

[3] Gaub: Institutiones pathologiæ medicinalis, Leyden, 1758.

[4] Gaub: Libellus de methodo concinnandi formulas medicamentorum, Leyden, 1739.

(1649–1734), of Staffordshire, published his *Physician's Pulse Watch*, which records the first effort in a century to revive the forgotten lore of Galileo, Kepler, and Sanctorius. Floyer, in Haller's phrase, "broke the ice," in that he tried to get the pulse-rate by timing its beats with a watch, which ran for exactly one minute. He tabulated his results, but his work was neglected or its intention even vitiated by a revival of the old Galenic doctrine of specific pulses, *i. e.*, a special pulse for every disease. Of the pulse-lore of the 18th century, Dr. Weir Mitchell, the historian of instrumental precision in medicine, says: "It is observation going minutely mad; a whole Lilliput of symptoms; an exasperating waste of human intelligence," and he adds that "it was not until a later day, and under the influence of the great Dublin school,

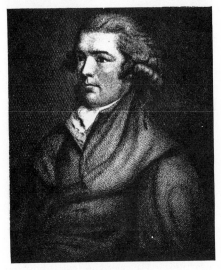

James Currie (1756–1805).

that the familiar figure of the doctor, watch in hand, came to be commonplace."

The clinical thermometry dreamed of by Sanctorius, and couquetted with by Boerhaave, Haller, and de Haen, was revived in the classic *Essays and Observations* (1740) of George **Martine** (1702–41), of Scotland, which is the only scientific treatment of the subject before the time of Wunderlich. Martine's ideas were carried into practice in the *Medical Reports* (1798) of James **Currie** (1756–1805), another Scot, the editor and biographer of Robert Burns, who, after an adventurous experience in America, attained eminence as a practitioner in Liverpool. Long before Brand of Stettin, Currie used cold baths in typhoid fever and checked up his results with the clinical thermometer. He used sea-water, as a rule, pouring it over the patient's body and making the douches colder and more frequent, the higher the temperature, as measured by the thermometer. Dr. S. Weir Mitchell saw "absolute genius" in Currie's book which, like those of Floyer and Martine, was neglected, if not soon forgotten.

In Germany, the use of the cold pack in exanthematous fevers was revived by the Silesian, Sigmund Hahn (1662–1742), and his sons, particularly in the *Psychroluposia* (1738) of Johann Sigmund Hahn (1696–1773), which, as late as 1898, was reissued in a sixth edition by Wilhelm Winternitz (1835–1917).

One of the ablest clinicians of his time was William **Withering** (1741–99), of Shropshire, England, memorable as the pioneer in the correct use of digitalis. An Edinburgh graduate of 1766, afterward enjoying a large and lucrative practice at Birmingham, Withering was not only an admirable observer of the English school, but a man of unusual versatility. He described the epidemics of scarlatina and scarlatinal sore throat of 1771 and 1778 and, in 1793, recommended an admirable modern treatment for phthisis. He was one of the greatest of medical botanists, wittily called "the flower of physicians." His *Botanical Arrangement of all the Vegetables* (1776) is esteemed his masterpiece. He also made analyses of minerals and mineral waters, was an opponent of phlogiston, a member of the famous "Lunar Society," a climatologist, a breeder of dogs and cattle, and solaced his leisure hours with the flute and harpsichord. In 1776, Withering learned from an old grandame in Shropshire that foxglove is good for dropsy. He immediately set about trying it in heart diseases, afterward recommending its use where he could and, by 1783, it was introduced into the Edinburgh Pharmacopœia. His views were supported by Cullen and fiercely opposed by Lettsom.[1] His *Account of the Fox-glove* (1785), a pharmacological classic, was incidentally a protest against the abuses of digitalis, which were already creeping in. In Withering's time, dropsy was regarded as a primary disease, and he himself did not know of the distinction between cardiac and renal dropsy, which was afterward made by Bright. He was disappointed to find that "cerebral dropsy" (hydro-

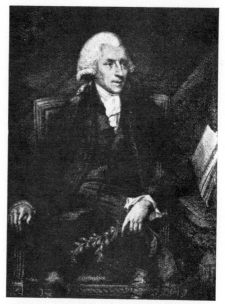

William Withering (1741–99). (From a painting by C. F. Breda.)

cephalus) and ovarian (cystic) dropsy did not yield to the drug. Withering was buried in the old church at Edgbaston, and the foxglove adorns the monument over his grave.

Among the English clinical teachers of the 18th century there is no name more justly and highly esteemed than that of William **Cullen** (1712–90). A pupil of Monro *primus*, he was instrumental in founding the medical school of Glasgow (1744), and, during his long life, held the chairs of medicine and chemistry at both Glasgow and Edinburgh. He was one of the first to give clinical or infirmary lectures in Great Britain, and these lectures were the first ever given in the vernacular

---

[1] G. Foy: Med. Press & Circ., Lond., 1915, cli, 39.

instead of Latin (1757). Having a mind of philosophic bent, Cullen was probably greater as an inspiring teacher than as a clinician, and was particularly noted for his kindness in assisting needy students. Although he introduced some new remedies into practice, Sir William Hamilton was perilously near the truth when he said that "Cullen did not add a single new fact to medical science." His best innovation was hydrotherapy with quick changes of temperature, which Despine, of Aix les Bains, called the "Scotch douche" (1760). The basis of Cullen's teaching was to the effect that life is a function of nervous energy, muscle a continuation of nerve, disease mainly nervous disorder, and fever an effect of diminished cerebral power from local (external) lesions. The *Synopsis nosologiæ methodicæ* (1769), which divides

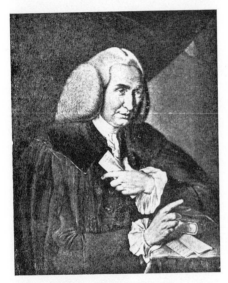

diseases into fevers, neuroses, cachexias, and local disorders, even including gout among the neuroses, and differentiating 34 varieties of chronic rheumatism, is now forgotten, although it made Cullen's reputation; but his "First Lines of the Practice of Physic" (1776–94) was for years authoritative on medical practice, even among the pioneers and "forty-niners" in the Far West.

A typical practitioner of the period, whose life-time covered nearly the whole century, was the distinguished William **Heberden** (1710–1801), of London, Soemmerring's *medicus vere Hippocraticus*, whom Dr. Johnson called *"ultimus Romanorum,* the last of our great physicians."

William Cullen (1712–90).

A Cambridge graduate of superior attainments, Heberden was esteemed as one of the finest Greek and Hebrew scholars of his time, and he resembles the classic writers in his careful portrayals of disease. His *Commentaries* (1802), written in Latin, are the result of a lifetime of conscientious note-taking. They contain his original pictures of varicella (1767[1]), angina pectoris, synthetized from 20 cases (1768[2]), and his notation of the nodules in the fingers which occur in arthritis deformans (1802), a disease which was clearly differentiated by Haygarth

---

[1] Heberden: "On the Chickenpox," Med. Tr. Coll. Phys. Lond., 1767, 3. ed., 1785, i, 427–436.

[2] *Ibid.,* 1768–70, ii, 59–67. Hans Kohn shows that Rougnon's case (Lettre à Lorry, Paris, 1768) was not angina pectoris, but pulmonary emphysema, with dyspnea and cardiac dilatation.

in 1805.[1] Heberden also described "night-blindness, or nyctalopia" (1767[2]). As Sir Dyce Duckworth points out,[3] Heberden's *Commentaries* are rich in the subtle notation of such clinical minutiæ as the diminished liability to diphtheria after adolescence, the lightning flashes before the eyes in hemicrania, or the tendency of phthisis to rebate in pregnancy, but not after it. An actual case of angina pectoris was described in the memoirs of the Earl of Clarendon (1632) in the person of his own father, but it was Heberden's classic account that put the disease upon a scientific basis, and his work was soon confirmed by the observations of Parry (1799) and Edward Jenner. In his *Essay on Mithridatium and Theriaca* (1745), Heberden did a most important service to therapeutics by dispelling current superstitions about these curious concoctions, and banishing them forever from the pharmacopeia. This little book is one of the shining monuments of medical scholarship.

William Heberden, Jr. (1767–1854), son of the above, was also an able classical scholar, and author of a Latin *Epitome* of pediatrics (1804, Englished 1805), which is of such superlative excellence and brevity that it might well be attributed to the father.

A group of men who resembled Heberden in character, if not in learning, were Fothergill, Lettsom, and Parry.

John **Fothergill** (1712–80), of Carr End, Yorkshire, a Quaker pupil of Monro *primus*, became a very successful and wealthy

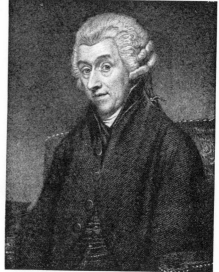

William Heberden (1710–1801).

London practitioner, was noted for his generous philanthropies, his magnificent botanic garden, his splendid collections of shells, insects, and drawings, which after his death fell into the hands of his friend, William Hunter. He stands out as a true follower of Sydenham, in his *Observations on the Weather and Diseases of London* (1751–54), and his original descriptions of diphtheritic sore throat (1748) and facial neuralgia (1773). Fothergill was a warm friend of the American colonies. He advocated the repeal of the Stamp Act in 1765, collaborated with Franklin in a plan for reconciliation with the mother-country in 1774,

---

[1] Heberden: Commentarii, London, 1802, Cap. 28, p. 130. Haygarth: A clinical history of acute rheumatism, London, 1805, 158 (Arnold Klebs).

[2] Med. Tr. Coll. Phys. Lond., 3d ed., 1785, i, 60; 1806–13, iv, 56.

[3] St. Bartholomew's Hosp. Rep., 1910, Lond., 1911, xlvi, 1–12.

and played an important part in the founding of the Pennsylvania Hospital (1751).

John Coakley **Lettsom** (1744–1815), of Little Vandyke (Virgin Islands), also a Quaker and, like Fothergill, lavish in expenditure and munificent in philanthropy, was one of the original founders of the Medical Society of London (1773), which commemorates his name, with Fothergill's, in the Lettsomian and Fothergillian lecture foundations.

Lettsom was a prolific writer on such subjects as effects of stuffy air (1772), substitutes for wheaten bread (1774), tea, chlorosis in boarding-schools (1795), effects of hard drinking (1791), and the like, but his only contribution of value to modern medicine is his original account of alcoholism, which is incidentally the first paper on the drug habit (1789[1]). He wrote an admirable *History of the Origin of Medicine* (1778), with interesting illustrations.

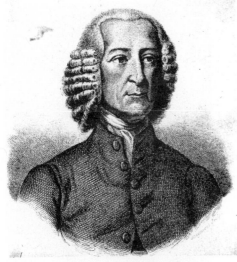

John Fothergill (1712–80).

Caleb Hillier **Parry** (1755–1822), a highly esteemed practitioner of Bath, who, like Heberden, acquired a lifelong habit of taking notes, described the first recorded cases of facial hemiatrophy (1814[2]), and of congenital idiopathic dilatation of the colon (1825), and, in 1786, left an account of exophthalmic goiter[3] so complete and original that it more justly entitles him to the honor of its discovery than either Flajani (1800), Graves (1835), or Basedow (1840).

The work of these men illustrates the eminently practical tendencies of English physicians since the time of Sydenham and, as careful, common-sense observers, studying their patients' symptoms rather than books, they were true followers of the master. The same thing may be said of two physicians of a more provincial stamp, Huxham and Baker. John **Huxham** (1692–1768), of Totnes, Devon, one of Boerhaave's pupils who had studied Hippocrates in the original, made meteorologic observations like Fothergill's, won the Copley medal for his essay on antimony (1755), and in his *Essay on Fevers* (1755) gave careful and original observations of many infectious diseases, differentiating, in particular, between the "putrid malignant" and the "slow

[1] Lettsom: Mem. Med. Soc. Lond., 1779–87, i, 128–165.

[2] Parry: Collected Works, London, 1825, i, 478–480.

[3] Parry: *Ibid.*, iii, 111–128.

nervous" fevers, that is, between typhus and typhoid. Huxham devised the familiar tincture of cinchona bark with which his name is associated, and in 1747 recommended that 1200 sailors of Admiral Martin's fleet, who had been disabled by scurvy, be put upon a vegetable diet.[1] In his essay on malignant sore throat (1757), he was the first to observe the paralysis of the soft palate which attends diphtheria, and which he confused with scarlatina. In 1739, he described Devonshire colic[2] (from cider-drinking) without, however, ascertaining its true cause. This was discovered in 1767[3] by Sir George **Baker** (1722–1809), another Devonshire man, who noticed that the cider-time colic, endemic in Devon, was somehow correlated with large pieces of lead used in the vats and cider presses, which were not so employed in other counties of England. He completed his chain of induction by extracting lead from the Devonshire cider, and proving that none could be found in the cider of Herefordshire. Although he was denounced from the pulpit as a "faithless son of Devon" for his pains, yet, in course of time, the colic disappeared from the county and Baker extended his investigations of lead-poisoning to iron pipes, glazed earthenware, and the linings of iron vessels. Public service of the same high character was rendered by Sir John **Pringle** (1707–82), the founder of modern military medicine and the originator of the Red Cross idea. Pringle, a Scotch pupil of Boerhaave and Albinus, and a friend of van Swieten's, was a surgeon on the continent in the mid-century wars, and surgeon general of the English army from 1742 to 1758. In his *Observations on the Diseases of the Army* (London, 1752), he lays down the true principles of military sanitation, especially with regard to the ventilation of hospital wards. Both Pringle and Stephen Hales were instrumental in securing better ventilation for those confined in ships, jails, barracks, and mines. Pringle was also a pioneer of the antiseptic idea; left a

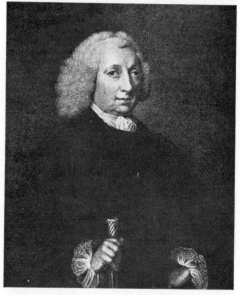

John Huxham (1692–1768).

---

[1] Huxham: "De scorbuto," Venice, 1766.

[2] De morbo colico Damnoniensi, London, 1739.

[3] Baker: An essay concerning the cause of the endemial colic of Devonshire, London, 1767.

good description of typhus fever; showed that jail fever and hospital fever are one and the same; correlated the different forms of dysentery, and named influenza. As he relates, it was about the time of the battle of Dettingen (1743) that the Earl of Stair made the historic suggestion that the military hospitals of both the French and the English sides should be regarded as neutral and immune from attack.

"But the Earl of Stair, my late illustrious patron, being sensible of this hardship, when the army was encamped at Aschaffenburg, proposed to the Duke of Noailles, of whose humanity he was well assured, that the hospitals on both sides should be considered as sanctuaries for the sick, and mutually protected. This was readily agreed to by the French General, who took the first opportunity to show a particular regard for his engagement. . . . This agreement was strictly observed on both sides all that campaign; and though it has been since neglected, yet we may hope that on future occasions the contending parties will make it a precedent."[1]

This rule remained loosely in force until it was put upon an absolute basis through the efforts of Henri Dunant (Geneva Convention, 1864).

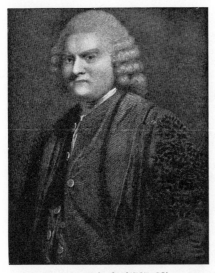

Sir John Pringle (1707–82).

In connection with Pringle's work in military medicine, mention may be made of van Swieten's monograph on camp diseases (1758[2]), the sterling *Œconomical and medical observations on military hospitals and camp diseases* (1764) of Richard Brocklesby (1722–97), Hugues Ravaton's *Chirurgie d'armée* (1768), de Meyserey's *La médecine d'armée* (1754), Jean Colombier's *Code de médecine militaire* (1772), Jourdain le Comte's *La santé de Mars* (1790), Thomas Dickson Reide's *View of Diseases of the Army* (1793), and Robert Jackson's *Scheme of Medical Arrangement for Armies* (1798). Prominent contributions to naval medicine were James Lind's essay on the hygiene of sailors (1757), and Thomas Trotter's *Medicina nautica* (1797–1803).

James **Lind** (1716–94), a native of Scotland, who was surgeon in the Royal Navy (1739–48) and became physician to the Royal Naval Hospital at Haslar (1758–83), four years after its foundation (1754), was the founder of **naval hygiene** in England. His fame rests upon three epoch-making treatises, those on scurvy (1754), naval hygiene (1757), and tropical medicine (1768).

Scurvy became an all-important subject at this time through its ravages among the sailors of Lord Anson's expedition of 1740 (75 per cent. of the total complement of men). The Channel Fleet had 2400 cases after a ten-weeks' cruise in 1779, and

---

[1] Pringle: Observations on the Diseases of the Army, London, 1752, preface, pp. viii–ix.

[2] van Swieten: Kurze Beschreibung und Heilungsart der Krankheiten welche am öftesten im Feldlager beobachtet werden, Vienna, 1758.

Lind had met with 350 cases in a ten-weeks' voyage. He points out that orange and lemon juice had been employed by the Dutch (Ronssius, 1564), in the voyages of Sir Richard Hawkins (1593) and by Commodore James Lancaster (1600), after which it had been recommended in John Woodall's *Surgeon's Mate* (1636, p. 165). Huxham, as we have seen, recommended a vegetable diet (1747). Lind, in his treatise of 1754, even urged the use of preserved orange and lemon juice. Through his influence, Admiral Watson employed lemon juice in 1757, and Sir Gilbert Blane (1749–1834) cured an outbreak in 28 ships of the line in 1782 by means of fresh lemons, limes, and oranges, also recommending lime juice in his *Observations on the Diseases of Seamen* (1785). Through the powerful influence of Blane, an Admiralty order enjoining the use of lemon juice was at length issued in 1795, after which scurvy disappeared from the Navy as if by magic. Earl Spencer could not find a single case at Haslar in 1797 (Rolleston). In his study of jail (typhus) fever, Lind recommended all the essentials of delousing, viz., bathing, clean apparel, and baking of lice-ridden clothing in ovens. He introduced regular uniforms, powdered foods, and portable soups into the Navy; recommended that the sick in tropical ports should be kept on "hospital ships," and devised a method of distilling sea water for drinking purposes (1761–62). Trotter, who also wrote on scurvy (1786), says that "Lind stands alone in the Navy" as "the father of nautical medicine."[1]

Perhaps the most important English statist of the period was John **Heysham** (1753–1834), of Lancaster, who commenced practice at Carlisle in 1778, where he founded its first poor-law dispensary, described jail-fever there in 1781 and, in 1779–88, made those statistical observations of births, marriages, diseases, and deaths which became the basis of the celebrated "Carlisle Tables" of the actuary, Joshua Milne (1816).

The epoch-making reforms of John **Howard** (1726–90) in relation to the management of the prisons, hospitals, and lazarettos of Europe (1777–89[2]) had much to do with the suppression of that vermin-carried disease, typhus fever.

Howard found the jails endemic nests of fever, which was spread thence to armies, ships, and fleets. He established a relation between the death-rate in prisons and floor-space per capita, showed the social injustice of debtor rates as enhancing property values above public health, recommended smooth floors for easy flushing, pumps, daily baths, ovens for baking clothes (virtual delousing plants), attachment of physicians and apothecaries to jails, location of suspects, and separation of the infected from susceptibles—altogether a modern program.

The work of Johann Conrad Amman (1669–1724), on the education of **deaf-mutes** (1692–1700[3]), the efforts of the Abbé de l'Épée (1712–90) to get an alphabet of communication for the deaf and dumb (1771[4]), the work of Valentin Hauy (1745–1822) in educating the blind (1785), and Pestalozzi's work in the cause of popular education (1781–1803), are remarkable features of social medicine in this period. In 1787, C. G. Gruner showed the possibility of venereal infection from a common drinking-cup.[5]

There was little of value in the **clinical medicine** of France in the 18th century. Its principal representative, Théophile **de Bordeu** (1722–76), the founder of the Vitalistic School of Montpellier, is now remembered as a theorist pure and simple. He graduated at Montpellier in

---

[1] H. D. Rolleston: Jour. Roy. Naval Med. Serv., Lond., 1915, i, 181–190.

[2] Howard: The State of the Prisons in England and Wales, Warrington, 1777; and his "An Account of the Principal Lazarettos in Europe," Warrington, 1789. See, also, W. A. Guy: John Howard's Winter's Journey, London, 1882.

[3] Amman: Surdus loquens, Amsterdam, 1692; reprinted, 1700.

[4] De l'Épée: Institution des sourds et muets par la voie des signes méthodiques, Paris, 1776.

[5] C. G. Gruner: Der gemeinschaftliche Kelch, Jena, 1785; Die venerische Ansteckung durch gemeinschaftliche Trinkgeschirre, Jena, 1787.

1794, was director of the baths in the Pyrenees, but spent the greater part of his life in Paris, where he held a high reputation in spite of his wrangles with the Faculty. Like most medical leaders of his time, Bordeu maintained a rigid, dogmatic "system," not unlike that of van Helmont.

He held that the organs of the body, with their several functions, are federated with and dependent upon one another, but presided over and regulated by the stomach, the heart, and the brain, which he called the "Tripod of Life." Next in importance were the nerves and the glands, the former centralizing the different functions of the body, and consequently governing the secretions of the latter. Each separate part of the body had a *vita propria*, and the brain as many areas as there were organs governed by it—a foreshadowing of localization. Bordeu first stated the doctrine that not only each gland, but each organ of the body, is the workshop of a specific substance or secretion, which passes into the blood, and that upon these the integration of the body as a whole depends. Thus Bordeu, as Neuburger has shown,[1] was very close upon the modern theory of the internal secretions and "hormonic equilibrium," but, as he made no experiments, his ideas can be regarded as sheer theory only. Disease he regarded as passing through the stages of irritation, coction, and crisis, dependent upon the glandular and other secretions of the blood. In consequence, he classified diseases, not according to their clinical or pathologic manifestations, but arbitrarily as *cachexias*. Of these, he unrolled an extraordinary list, corresponding to the different organs and secretions, as bilious, mucous, albuminous, fatty, splenic, seminal, urinary, stercoral, perspiratory, and so on, with an equally complex classification of the pulse as critical, non-critical, simple critical, compound critical, nasal, tracheal, gastric, renal, uterine, seminal, etc. The most interesting part of his theory is his observation of the effects of the testicular and ovarian secretions upon the organism. He regarded the *aura seminalis* of the sexual secretions as giving

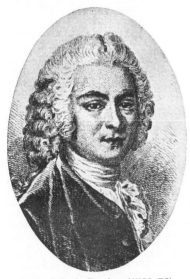

Théophile de Bordeu (1722–76).

a "male (or female) tonality" to the organism, "setting the seal upon the animalism of the individual," and, in effect, "the particular stimulus of the machine (*novum quoddam impetum faciens*)." In this connection, he made clever studies of the obesity, retiring disposition, and other characteristics of eunuchs, capons, and spayed animals, suggesting some phases of the modern pituitary and gonadal syndromes.

Bordeu's successor, Paul-Joseph Barthez (1734–1806), of Montpellier, who was successively a theologian, physician, soldier, editor, lawyer (even a counselor of justice), philosopher, and again a physician, is memorable for his introduction of the term "vital principle" (*vitalis agens*) to denote the cause of the phenomena in the living body. The vitalism of Bordeu and Barthez underwent a third transformation in the nineteenth century as the " semi vitalism" of Bouchut.

---

[1] M. Neuburger in Janus, Amst., 1903, viii, 26–32; and Wien. klin. Wochenschr.' 1911, xxiv, 1367. Neuburger cites the following from Bordeu's "Analyse médicinale du sang" (1774): "J'en conclus que le sang roule toujours dans son sein des extraits de toutes les parties organiques . . . chacun (des organes) aussi sert de foyer et de laboratoire à une humeur particulière qu'il renvoie dans le sang après l'avoir préparée sans son sein, après lui avoir donné son caractère radical," pp. 943, 948.

The rise of the **Old Vienna School,** under Gerhard **van Swieten** (1700–72), of Leyden, was a feature of the ascendancy of Austria under Maria Theresa and Joseph II. Van Swieten, who was in special favor with the Empress, did much to advance Austrian medicine, and created the world-famed Vienna clinic after the Leyden pattern. As prefect of the Imperial Library at Vienna, which he raised to the first rank, he had great influence upon the advancement of higher and medical education by his reorganization of the University. He took the censorship of prohibited books away from the Jesuits, and his stenographic notes, with the characteristic *"damnatur"* and *"Nil mali inveni"* have been preserved.[1] He was a great friend of the poor, but a poor friend to Mozart. As army surgeon, he wrote an important work upon the hygiene of troops in camp (1758). As clinician, he noted such things as the aura in hydrophobia, the occurrence of symmetric gangrene in spinal affections, used the Fahrenheit thermometer, was instrumental in bringing about the internal use of corrosive sublimate (*liquor Swietenii*) in syphilis, and left a commentary upon the aphorisms of Boerhaave (1741–76), which occupied him for over thirty years.

Besides van Swieten, the Vienna group included such prominent figures as the quarrelsome, pragmatic Anton **de Haen** (1704–76), of The Hague, the rabid defender of belief in witchcraft, who wrote a treatise on hospital therapeutics in 15 volumes (1758–69), maintained the supremacy of clinical experience over physiologic experimentation, used the thermometer at the bedside, first noted that there is an elevation of temperature in the algid stage of ague, and employed electrotherapy; the bureaucratic Anton **Stoerck** (1731–1803), of Swabia, who was the great champion of emetics and did some careful work in pharmacology and toxicology, notably his investigations of hemlock (1760–61), stramonium, hyoscyamus, and aconite (1762), colchicum (1763), and pulsatilla (1777); the epidemiologist Maximilian **Stoll** (1742–87), of Swabia, who followed Sydenham in meteorologic studies of the *genius epidemicus,* influenced even Bretonneau in therapeutics, wrote well upon medical ethics, and brought the Old Vienna School to its high-water mark; Marcus Anton **von Plenciz, Sr.** (1705–86), who, in his tract on scarlatina (1762[2]), advanced the idea of a *contagium animatum,* with a special *seminium verminosum* for each disease in man, animals, and plants; the dermatologist Joseph Jacob **von Plenck** (1732–1807), who followed the method of Linnæus in classifying diseases of the skin (1776[3]); Johann Valentin von Hildenbrand (1763–1818), who had some inklings of the difference between typhus and typhoid fevers (1810[4]); and, above all, the sterling figures of Auenbrugger and Frank.

The leading practitioners in Germany were Stahl, Hoffmann, Kämpf, Werlhof, Zimmermann, Wichmann, Senckenberg, Reil, and Heim. Of these, Paul Gottlieb **Werlhof** (1699–1767), of Helmstädt, court physician at Hannover, was a great friend of Haller and, like him, wrote poems in the German language and medical works in Latin.

---

[1] See Sitzungsb. d. k. Akad. d. Wissensch. in Wien, Phil.-hist. Cl., 1877, lxxxiv, 387 *et seq.;* and Janus, Amst., 1906, xi, 381. 446, 501, 588 (E. C. van Leersum). Haller is said to have disliked van Swieten because he suspected him of tabooing his poems in Austria.

[2] Plenciz: Tractatus III de scarlatina.

[3] Plenck: Doctrina de morbis cutaneis, Vienna, 1776.

[4] Hildenbrand: Ueber den ansteckenden Typhus, Vienna, 1810.

He is now remembered by his original description of purpura hæmorrhagica, or morbus maculosus Werlhofii (1735[1]).

The snobbish Johann Georg **Zimmermann** (1728–95), of Brugg, Switzerland, a practitioner of great repute, who succeeded Werlhof as ordinarius at Hannover, was the author of an important monograph on "Epidemic Dysentery in the Year 1765,"[2] and of the famous *Treatise on Solitude*, which so tickled the sentimental palates of our grandfathers.

Johann Ernst **Wichmann** (1740–1802), a contemporary of Werlhof's at Hannover, is notable for his monograph on scabies (1786[3]); and Johann Christian Senckenberg (1702–72), for his public-spirited endowment of the Senckenberg Foundation at Frankfort on the Main (1768). Ernst Ludwig **Heim** (1747–1834), a wealthy, witty, very honest, and very independent practitioner of Berlin, is said to have introduced Jennerian vaccination into that city in 1798, and as *"der alte Heim,"* is remembered for his many sharp sayings.

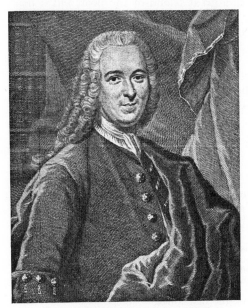

Paul Gottlieb Werlhof (1699–1767).

Christian Wilhelm **Hufeland** (1762–1836), of Langensalza, professor at Jena (1793) and Berlin (1800), was one of the great philanthropic physicians who are true friends of the human race. At Weimar (1783–93), he was the friend and physician of Goethe, Schiller, and Herder, and did much to correct popular misconceptions about Mesmerism, Brunonianism, phrenology, and other current fancies. He was one of the first to espouse the cause of Jenner and took the keenest interest in combating smallpox and cholera.

He described the typhoid and typhus epidemics of 1806–7 and 1813 respectively, and wrote much on popular medicine, in particular his treatise on long life (*Makrobiotik*, 1796) and his *Encheiridion medicum* (1836). He is now best remembered as one of the great pioneers of medical journalism in the 18th century. He edited four different periodicals, the most important of which was "Hufeland's Journal" in 82 volumes (*Journal der praktischen Arzneikunde*, 1795–1836).

---

[1] Werlhof: Opera omnia, Hannover, 1775, ii, 615–636. (Dissertation published at Brunswick, 1735.)

[2] J. G. Zimmermann: Von der Ruhr unter dem Volke im Jahr 1765, Zürich, 1767.

[3] Wichmann: Aetiologie der Krätze, Hannover, 1786.

Simon-André **Tissot** (1728–97), the famous practitioner of Lausanne, was one of the leading propagandists of variolation (1754), wrote considerable treatises on epilepsy (1770) and nervous diseases (1782), and became widely known through his popular writings on onanism (1760), the hygiene of literary men (1766), and the diseases of men of the world (1770). His best known achievement in this kind was the *Avis au peuple sur la santé* (1760), a tract on popular medicine which ran through ten editions in less than six years, and was translated into every European language.

Théodore **Tronchin** (1709–81), of Geneva, Boerhaave's favorite pupil, Voltaire's favorite physician, and one of the wealthiest and most fashionable practitioners of his time, is notable for his compilation *De colica Pictonum* (1757), in which he showed that "Poitou colic" was caused by water poisoned from passing through the gutters of lead roofs. He introduced inoculation into Holland (1748), Switzerland (1749), and France (1756), with 20,000 successful cases to his credit; and was a pioneer of the open-air cult, of psychothérapy, and of suspension in spinal curvature (1756).

The greatest Italian clinician of the period was Giovanni Maria **Lancisi** (1655–1720), of Rome, who was physician to several popes, one of whom (Clement XI) placed in his hands the forgotten 47 copper plates of Eustachius, executed in 1552, which Lancisi edited with marginal notes and published, with a title-page vignette by Pier Leone Ghezzi, in 1714.

Lancisi was a great epidemiologist. He described the epidemics of influenza in 1709–10, of cattle-plague in 1713, and of malarial fever in 1715. His great treatise on swamp fevers (1717[1]), while stating the doctrine of miasms, shows a clear insight into the theory of contagion and the possibility of transmission by mosquitoes (*Culices*), of which he gives a naturalist's account. He was the author of two works of capital importance on sudden death (1707[2]) and on aneurysm (1728[3]). In the former, he notes hypertrophy and dilatation of the heart as causes of sudden death, first describes valvular vegetations and gives a classification of cardiac diseases. In the latter, he notes the frequency of cardiac aneurysm, distinguishes between aneurysmal cavities with thin and thick walls, and signalizes heredity, syphilis, asthma, palpitation, violent emotions, and excesses as prominent causes. He was the first to describe cardiac syphilis.

Francesco **Torti** (1658–1741), professor at Modena, and a good pharmacologist, wrote an important treatise on the pernicious malarial fevers (1712[4]), which brought about the employment of cinchona bark into Italian practice and introduced the term *mal aria*.

Pellagra was originally described by Gaspar Casal (1691–1759), a Spanish physician, in a book written by him in 1735, but not published until 1762.[5] At court, Casal met François Thiéry who, from what he had seen or heard of Casal's

---

[1] Lancisi: De noxiis palundum effluviis, Rome, 1717.

[2] Lancisi: De subitaneis mortis, Rome, 1707. Written on account of the fright of the Roman population at the number of sudden deaths in 1706.

[3] Lancisi: De motu cordis et aneurysmatibus, Naples, 1728.

[4] Torti: Therapeutice specialis ad febres quasdam perniciosas, Modena, 1712.

[5] Casal: Historia natural y medica de el principado de Asturias, Madrid, 1762.

description, published an account of the disease in 1755,[1] antedating him in priority of publication, but not of first-hand description. Both Casal and Thiéry called the new disease "rose sickness" (*mal de la rosa*). In 1771[2] Francesco Frapolli, an Italian physician, published a careful account of pellagra, in which he gave the malady its present name.

Connected with the history of internal medicine on the continent is the revival of Athanasius Kircher's hypnotic idea, under the guise of "animal magnetism," by Franz Anton **Mesmer** (1734–1815), of Itznang, Switzerland. Mesmer's graduating dissertation dealt with the subject of planetary influence on man (1771) and, in experimenting with the magnet, he got the idea that a similar power is possessed by

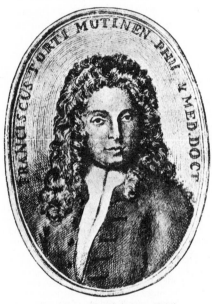

Francesco Torti (1658–1741).

the human hand. Attempting to practise mesmerism in Vienna, his private séances were investigated by one of Maria Theresa's "commissions," and he was compelled to leave the city inside of twenty-four hours. Arriving in Paris in 1778, after some failures at Spa, he at length gained a foothold, and in a very short time, was making a great deal of money by his hypnotic séances. In these, he appeared clad in a lilac suit, playing upon a harmonica, touching his patients with a wand, staring into their eyes, and attending them in a private chamber in case of a "crisis." A prominent feature of the mesmeric treatment was a number of so-called magnetic tubs, or *baquets*, containing a *mixtum composition* of hydrogen

sulphide and other ingredients, and provided with iron conductors from which depended a ring for contact with the patients, who stood around the tubs, joining hands. Being investigated by another committee, Mesmer was again driven from the field, and, after the Revolution, dropped out of sight. His book, containing his ideas on mesmerism, was published in 1779.[3] Although the subject did not gain a scientific foothold until the time of Braid, mesmerism, like Lavater's ideas on physiognomy (1772[4]), attracted a great deal of public and private notice and was exploited in various mystic

---

[1] Thiéry: Jour. de méd., chir. et pharm., Paris, 1755, ii, 337–346.

[2] Frapolli: Animadversiones in morbum, vulgo pelagram, Milan, 1771.

[3] Mesmer: Mémoire sur la découverte du magnétisme animal, Geneva and Paris, 1779.

[4] Joh. Caspar Lavater: Von der Physiognomik, Leipzig, 1772.

forms by Charles d'Eslon, a pupil of Mesmer's, the brothers Puységur, Lavater, the novelist Justinus Kerner, and by Baron Karl von Reichenbach, whose concept of "odic force" still survives in the ouija-boards and odic telephones of the present time. Somnambulism (witness Bellini's opera) and ventriloquism (witness Brockden Brown's *Wieland*) began to have their vogue also, and in the "wonder-cures" of the exorcist Joseph Gassner and the necromancer Schröpfer, the magic medicine of primitive man began to loom large again. In London, Mesmer's charlatanry cropped out in the notorious "Temple of Health" (1780) of the quack James Graham, in the ministrations of which, Emma Lyon, the future Lady Hamilton, played a prominent choreographic part.

With all its lack of instrumental precision, the internal medicine of the 18th century, as a whole, was far superior to its surgery, in that the systematic tendencies of the age led to the composition of specialized text-books, the introduction of new drugs, and the accurate description of many new forms of disease. Among these isolated clinical discoveries we may mention Friedrich Hoffmann's descriptions of chlorosis (1730[1]) and rubella (1740[2]); Freke's case of myositis ossificans progressiva (1736[3]); Fothergill's accounts of diphtheria (1748[4]); facial neuralgia (1773[5]), and sick headache (1784[6]); J. Z. Platner on the tuberculous nature of gibbous spine[7]; Nicolas André on infra-orbital neuralgia (1756[8]); the description of pellagra by François Thiéry (1755[9]), William Hunter on arteriovenous aneurysm (1757[10]); Tronchin on lead colic (1757[11]); Mestivier's operated case of appendicitis (1759[12]); Robert Hamilton on orchitis in mumps (1761[13]); Heberden on varicella (1767[14]) and angina pectoris (1768[15]); Robert Whytt's clinical picture of tuberculous meningitis (1768[16]); Rutty's account of relapsing fever (1770[17]); Cotugno on sciatica (1770[18]); van Swieten on the paralytic type of rabies (1771); Rouelle's discovery of urea (1773); J. W. Tichy's Observations of sediments in febrile urine (1774); Werlhof on purpura hæmorrhagica (1775[19]); Matthew Dobson's proof that the sweetness of the urine and blood-serum in diabetes is due to sugar (1776[20]); Bylon and Benjamin Rush on dengue (1779–80); Pott on pressure paralysis from spinal caries (1779[21]);

[1] F. Hoffmann: De genuina chlorosis indole, 1730.

[2] Opera omnia, Geneva, 1748, ii, 63.

[3] J. Freke: Phil. Tr., 1732–44, Lond., 1747, ix, 252.

[4] J. Fothergill: An account of the sore throat, London, 1748.

[5] Med. Obs. Soc. Phys., Lond., 1771–76, v, 129–142.

[6] Med. Obs. & Inquiries, Lond., 1784, vi, 103–137.

[7] J. Z. Platner: De iis, qui ex tuberculis gibberosi fiunt, Leipzig, 1744, with plate by Schönemann.

[8] N. André: Observations pratiques sur les maladies de l'urétre, Paris, 1756.

[9] F. Thiéry: J. de méd., chir. et pharm., Paris, 1755, ii, 336–346.

[10] W. Hunter: Med. Obs. & Inquiries, Lond., 1757, i, 340.

[11] T. Tronchin: De colica Pictonum, Geneva, 1757.

[12] Mestivier: J. de méd., chir. et pharm., 1759, x, 441.

[13] Hamilton: Tr. Roy. Soc. Edinb. (1773), 1790, ii, pt. 2, 59–72.

[14] Heberden: Med. Tr. Coll. Phys., Lond., 3. ed., 1785, i, 427–436.

[15] Heberden: Med. Tr. Coll. Phys., Lond., 1768–70, ii, 58–67.

[16] Whytt: Observations on the Dropsy in the Brain, Edinburgh, 1768.

[17] Rutty: A chronological history (etc.), London, 1770.

[18] Cotugno: De ischiade nervosa, Vienna, 1770.

[19] Werlhof: Opera omnia, Hannover, 1775, ii, 615–636.

[20] Dobson: Med. Obs. & Inq., Lond., 1776, v, 298–316.

[21] Pott: Remarks on that kind of palsy (etc.), London, 1779.

24

the yeast test for sugar in diabetic urine by Francis Home (1780[1]) and Johann Peter
Frank (1791); Lettsom on the drug habit and alcoholism (1786[2]); Parry on exophthalmic goiter (1786[3]); George Armstrong (1771[4]) and Hezekiah Beardsley (1788[5])
on congenital hypertrophic stenosis of the pylorus; Soemmerring's case of achondroplasia (1791[6]); Charles Stewart's description of paroxysmal hematuria (1794[7]);
Wollaston's discovery of urates in gouty joints (1797[8]); Nikolaus Friedreich's description of peripheral facial paralysis (1797[9]); and John Haslam's description of general paralysis (1798[10]). Besides this brilliant array of original work, which would
honor any century, there were many admirable treatises or text-books on special
branches of internal medicine, such as Astruc (1736), Girtanner (1788–89), and
Benjamin Bell (1793) on venereal diseases; Senac on diseases of the heart (1749),
Plenciz on scarlatina (1762), Zimmermann on dysentery (1767), Lind on tropical
diseases (1768), Millar on asthma and whooping-cough (1769), Walter on peritonitis
(1785), Chabert on anthrax (1780), Malacarne (1788) and Fodéré (1792) on cretinism and goiter, and John Rollo on the success of meat diet in diabetes (1797),
Benjamin Martin in *A New Theory of Consumptions* (London, 1720) discusses parasitic microörganisms as the cause of phthisis.[11] The transmission of yaws by flies
was noted by Edward Bancroft (1769[12]). There was a great increase in the literature
bearing on the diseases of children, as evidenced in the pediatric treatises of William
Cadogan (1748), Nils Rosén von Rosenstein (1752), George Armstrong (1767),
Mellin (1783) and Michael Underwood (1784), which contains the first account of
infantile poliomyelitis. Sir John Floyer wrote the first treatise on diseases of old age
(*Medicina gerocomica*, 1724). Gout and scurvy were favorite subjects of the English
practitioners of the period, notably George Cheyne (1720) and Cadogan (1764) on
the former; Lind (1753) and Thomas Trotter (1785) on the latter. Of all these
special monographs, the best was unquestionably the treatise of Robert Willan
(1757–1812) on diseases of the skin (1796–1808), which marks an epoch in the history
of dermatology, but belongs essentially to the modern period. The outstanding
books and classifications of skin diseases in the 18th century were those of Plenck
(1776) and Lorry (1777). Of original contributions to descriptive dermatology, we
may mention John Machin's observation of ichthyosis hystrix in the Lambert
family (1733[13]), which was followed through successive generations by Henry Baker
(1755[14]), and Tilesius (1802[15]); the observation of scleroderma in Curzio's clinic at
Naples by William and Robert Watson (1754[16]); Wichmann on the parasitic origin
of scabies (1786[17]), and Sir Everard Home's description of cutaneous horns (hyperkeratosis) in 1791.[18]

Medical jurisprudence, which had hitherto been a part of state
medicine and public health, was carefully systematized in the 18th

---

[1] F. Home: Clinical Experiments, Edinburgh, 1780.

[2] Lettsom: Mem. Med. Soc. Lond., 1779–87, i, 128–165.

[3] Parry's works, London, 1825, ii, 111.

[4] G. Armstrong: Essay, London, 1771. An account, [etc.], Lond., 1777, 49
(J. A. Foote).

[5] Beardsley: Cases & Obs. Med. Soc., New Haven County, 1788, 81–84.

[6] Soemmerring: Abbildungen . . . einiger Missgeburten, Mainz, 1791, 30, pl. xi.

[7] Stewart: Med. Comment., Edinb., 1794, Dec. II, ix, 332.

[8] Wollaston: Phil. Tr., Lond., 1797, lxxxvii, 386–400.

[9] Friedreich: Med. chir. Ztg., Salzburg, 1798, i, 415.

[10] Haslam: Observations on insanity, London, 1798.

[11] See C. Singer: Janus, Amst., 1911, xvi, 81–98.

[12] Bancroft: Essay on the Natural History of Guiana, London, 1769, 385.
Cited by E. W. Gudger.   [13] Machin: Phil. Tr., Lond., 1733, xxxvii, 299–301, 1 pl.

[14] Baker: Phil. Tr., Lond., 1755, xlix, pt. 1, 21–24.

[15] Tilesius: Ausführliche Beschreibung . . . der beiden sog. Stachel-
schweinmenschen, Altenburg, 1802.

[16] Watson: Phil. Tr., Lond., 1754, xlviii, 579–587.

[17] Wichmann: Aetiologie der Krätze, Hannover, 1786.

[18] Home: Phil. Tr., Lond., 1791, lxxxii, 95–105.

century, and the leaders in this field were the Germans, who were the first to found professorships of forensic medicine and turned out the most important treatises.

The earliest of these was the *Corpus juris medico-legale* of Michael Bernhard Valentini (1657–1729), published in 1722, a huge storehouse of well-arranged facts. It was followed in 1723 by the *Institutiones* of Hermann Friedrich Teichmeyer (1685–1746), which was for a long time the standard authority, and, in 1736–47, by the *System* of Michael Alberti (1682–1757) of Halle, a six-volume work, not unlike Valentini's in scope and thoroughness. In France, Antoine Louis (1723–92) was the pioneer in applying medical knowledge to court-room practice. He wrote an important memoir on the differential signs of murder and suicide in cases of hanging (1763). In his discussion of the celebrated Villebranche case (1764), he ridiculed the possibility of extremely protracted pregnancy, and tried to set the time-limits of normal gestation, which, under the Code Napoleon, were finally fixed at three hundred days, as in the Roman laws of the Twelve Tables. Fodéré's great treatise on legal medicine (1798) really belongs to the modern period. The first English work was the *Elements* of Samuel Farr (1788), but William Hunter's essay on the signs of murder in bastard children (1783) is probably the most important English contribution.

Medical ethics was treated in Friedrich Hoffmann's *Medicus politicus* (1738), in Johann Wilhelm Baumer's *Fundamenta politica medica* (1777), and by Stoll.

Medical history was systematically treated in the works of Freind (1725–27), J. H. Schulze (1728), J. C. Lettsom (1778), Blumenbach (1786), J. C. G. Ackermann (1792), and Kurt Sprengel (1792–1803).

Of these, John Freind (1675–1728), of Croton, Northamptonshire, who was highly educated at Oxford in the humanities and in medicine, and delivered the Ashmolean lectures on chemistry in 1704, was an intellectual light of considerable prominence in his day. He accompanied the Earl of Peterborough on his Spanish campaign (1705), as physician to the English forces and, subsequently mixing in politics as a partisan, was committed to the Tower on the charge of high treason in March, 1922–23; but was soon released through the good offices of Mead, and became physician to Queen Caroline in 1727. During his short imprisonment, Freind planned his *History of Physick from the Time of Galen to the Beginning of the Sixteenth Century* (London, 1725–26), dedicated to Mead, and intended as a continuation of Leclerc. This is usually regarded as the best English survey of the period of which it treats although, as Sir Clifford Allbutt says, the author "spread his net too widely" and produced a general history "from the time of Galen," where he might have done better by confining himself to English medicine in detail.

The greatest medical historian of the 18th century was the eminent Pomeranian botanist Kurt Polykarp **Sprengel** (1766–1833), whose work,[1] also translated into French and Italian, has been the great source-book for facts and footnotes for all subsequent investigators.

Although Sprengel's uncompromising vitalism makes him an unfair critic of the 17th century scientists, his history is still a marvel of solid learning and contains a valuable chronology. He also wrote a series of medico-historical essays (*Beytrage*, 1794–96), and a history of surgical operations (1805–19). Hardly inferior to Sprengel as original investigators were such men as Johann Karl Wilhelm **Möhsen** (1722–95), of Berlin, who investigated the medical MS. in the Royal Library there (1746–47); also the medical portraits (1771), medical medals (1772–73), the earliest important contribution to medical numismatics, and wrote a learned history of science in Mark Brandenburg (1781); Christian Gottfried **Gruner** (1744–1815), a prolific writer on the history of diseases (*Morborum antiquitates*, 1774), in particular syphilis (1793) and sweating sickness (1847); the army surgeon Ernst Gottfried **Baldinger** (1738–

[1] Sprengel: Versuch einer pragmatischen Geschichte der Medicin, Halle, 1792–1803.

1804), biographer of his contemporaries (1768), of Haller (1778), and Tode (1778), a sturdy organizer, who poured many learned essays into his *Magazin für Aerzte* (1795–99); Johann Heinrich Eder (1687–1744), author of the earliest German history of medicine (1728) and the first to attempt photography; Philipp Gabriel Hensler (1733–1805), historian of syphilis (1783–89) and leprosy (1790); Christoph Girtanner (1760–1800), another syphilographer (1783–89); August Friedrich Hecker (1763–1811), editor of many periodicals, and Antoine Portal (1742–1832), author of a seven-volume history of anatomy and surgery (1770–73). Haller's 1751 edition of the *Methodus studii medici* of Boerhaave is an introduction to medical literature similar to that compiled by Thomas Young (1813), and is remarkable for those sententious critical *aperçus* for which Haller is so justly famous. The earliest periodicals devoted to the history of medicine were F. Aglietti's *Giornale per servire alla storia ragionata della medicina di questa secolo* (Venice, 1783–95), and P. L. Wittwer's *Archiv für die Geschichte der Arzyneykunde* (Nuremberg, 1790).

In an age in which medico-historical studies were so assiduously cultivated, **medical lexicography** became effectively specialized.

The exegesis of Greek medical terms by J. G. Hebenstreit (1751), the glossary of Erotian, Galen and Herodotus of J. G. Franz (1780), the lexica of Latin-French terms by Elie Col de Villars (1741) and of Latin-German by G. Mathæus (1748) and C. E. H. Knackstedt (1784–5) follow the old Renaissance lines. Dictionaries of special terms abounded, notably those of anatomy by Peras (1753), P. Tarin (1753), J. F. Dufieu (1766) and F. Vicq d'Azyr (1786), of surgery by A. F. T. Levacher de la Feutrie (1767), Antoine Louis (1772), and P. François (1773), of drugs by Nicolas Lemery (1714), and Julliot (1758), of prognosis (1770) and semeiology (1777) by Michel du Tennetar. The principal medical dictionaries in English are those of John Quincy (1719), Robert James (1743), and Robert Hooper (1798). An important three-volume treatise on **medical geography** was published by Leonhard Ludwig Finke (1747–1828) in 1792–95.[1] The *Observations on Epidemical Diseases in Minorca* (1751) of George Cleghorn (1716–89), still useful to practitioners in the island, contains many postmortems, and clarifies obscurities in the Hippocratic books, particularly as to the modification of acute and chronic diseases by concurrent malarial fever. The *Observations* of William Hillary (died 1763) on the epidemic diseases of Barbadoes (1759) contains a valuable account of sprue.

Toward the end of the century came one of the greatest triumphs in the history of medicine—the successful introduction of **preventive inoculation** by Edward **Jenner** (1749–1823), son of a Gloucestershire clergyman, who, in 1770, became a friend and pupil of John Hunter's, and helped him not a little in his experiments. It had long been a countryside tradition in Gloucestershire that dairy-maids who had contracted cow-pox through milking did not take smallpox, and similar observations had been noted in Germany and France. On learning of this fact from a milkmaid, Jenner early conceived the idea of applying it on a grand scale in the prevention of the disease. When he communicated his project to Hunter, the latter gave him the characteristic advice: "Don't think, try; be patient, be accurate." On returning to his home at Berkeley, Jenner began to collect his observations in 1778 and, on May 14, 1796, performed his first vaccination upon a country boy, James Phipps, using matter from the arm of the milkmaid, Sarah Nelmes, who had contracted cow-pox in the usual way. The experiment was then put to the test, by inoculating Phipps with smallpox virus on July 1st, and the immunization proved successful. By 1798,

[1] L. L. Finke: Versuch einer allgemeinen medicinisch-praktischen Geographie, Leipzig, 1792–95.

Jenner had 23 cases, which he embodied in his work, *An Inquiry into the Causes and Effects of the Variolæ Vaccinæ*, a thin quarto with four colored plates, printed in 1798, and dedicated to Parry of Bath. This book establishes Jenner's main thesis that a vaccination with cow-pox matter protects from smallpox, and was followed, during the years 1799–1806, by five successive pamphlets, recording his subsequent experiments and improvements in technic up to the stage of recommending ivory points as the best vectors in inoculation. The idea was rapidly taken up on the continent and in America; good statistics began to pour in in less than a year's time and, by 1800, as many as 6000 people had been vaccinated. In 1802 and 1807, Parliament voted grants amounting to £20,000 to Jenner in aid of prosecuting his experiments. At the same time he met with bitter opposition from jealous contemporaries, such as Ingen-Housz, Woodville, and Pearson, who either claimed priority or acted upon the parliamentary principle that the duty of the opposition is to oppose.

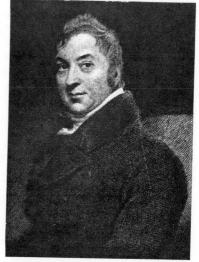

Edward Jenner (1749–1823). (From the painting by Sir Thomas Lawrence.)

The mere idea of inoculation is apparently as old as the hills. Human inoculation of variolous virus is said to be mentioned in the Atharva Veda (Baas), certainly in the *Flos* of the School of Salerno, and was known to most Oriental peoples. The idea was introduced into England by Timoni's and Pilarini's communications to the Royal Society in 1713–16, and was afterward taken up by Sir Hans Sloane (1717). On March 18, 1718, Lady Mary Wortley Montagu had her three-year-old son inoculated in Turkey, and her five-year-old daughter was inoculated in England, in April, 1721. During the sixth epidemic of smallpox in Boston, Massachusetts, Zabdiel Boylston (1679–1766) courageously inoculated his son and two negro slaves on June 26, 1721, and had inoculated 244 persons before its close, exciting great opposition and even threats of hanging. In the Boston epidemic of 1752, 2109 were inoculated, and nearly 20,000 in England, under Daniel Sutton in 1764–65.[1] Apart from the huge 18th century literature on inoculation, one of the most important items of which is the proposal of preventive inoculations against the plague (1755) by the Hungarian physician, Stephan Weszprémi (1723–99), there had been successful cow-pox vaccinations by the Dorset farmer Benjamin Jesty, in 1774–89, and by Plett of Holstein in 1791. All these efforts were, however, "as an arrow shot in the air or a sword-stroke in the water."

The merit of Jenner's work rests upon the fact that, like Harvey, he started out with the hope of making his thesis a permanent working principle in science, based upon experimental demonstration, and he

[1] See Reginald H. Fitz, on Zabdiel Boylston in Bull. Johns Hopkins Hospital, Balt., 1911, xxii, 315–327, and A. C. Klebs: *Ibid.*, 1913, xxiv, 69–83, *passim*. Inoculation was a common preventive measure in America during the War of the Revolution.

succeeded to the extent of carrying his inoculations successfully through several generations in the body and, above all, in overcoming the popular aversion to vaccination. In short, Jenner transformed a local country tradition into a viable prophylactic principle, and, although he was preceded by really scientific experts in human inoculation (variolation), his reputation in his own field is fairly safe from the priority-mongers. Faults of diffuseness and lack of skill in marshaling facts have been imputed against the *Inquiry*, but, on the whole, it remains an unimpeachable record of careful scientific work, the effect of which is seen today in the rapid advance of serotherapy and immunology, and in the results of compulsory vaccination in Prussia and Holland, where the mortality curve of smallpox approaches zero as its limit. Striking, indeed, was the relative immunity of the German Army of the Franco-Prussian War in 1870–71, in which the unvaccinated French prisoners lost 1963 out of 14,178 cases of smallpox, while the Germans, who had been revaccinated within two years, had 4835 cases and 278 deaths (Myrdacz). Kitasato's statistics of vaccination in the Russo-Japanese War (1911[1]) show that, with smallpox endemic in Japan, there were only 362 cases and 35 deaths in an army of over a million soldiers. It has been well said that the scar on the arm of the chorus girl is a measure of the success of Jenner's experiment; it is better to escape smallpox itself than to incur the risk of death or pitting by smallpox. Propagandists like the late Charles Creighton, who spoiled a brilliant career by his opposition to vaccination, or Bernard Shaw, who regards it as a semi-savage rite, have been prone to forget the bevies of great ladies in the past, whose pock-marked cuticles would cut but a sorry figure in these days of frank physical exposure.

Jenner's monograph of 1798 contains an early reference and a clear explanation of **anaphylaxis** or allergy. In case 4 he notes that inoculations of variolous matter in a woman who had had cow-pox thirty-one years before produced a palish red efflorescence of the skin, which he regards as almost a criterion of whether the infection will be received or not, attributing the phenomenon to the dynamic effect of a permanent change in the blood during life.[2]

In 1814, Jenner made his last visit to London, of which capital he had been made an honorary citizen. He died at Berkeley of apoplexy in 1823. A monument was erected to his memory in Trafalgar Square in 1858. In personality, Jenner was the typical English country gentleman, blond, blue-eyed, of handsome figure. A well-known account describes him ready for a mount, in blue coat, nankeen riding-breeches, and top-boots, with whip and silver spurs. He was a bird-fancier, played the flute and violin, botanized, and wrote clever verses, of which the "Address to a Robin" and the "Signs of Rain," rodolent of the English countryside, deserve a place in any anthology of minor

---

[1] Cited by Osler in his Principles and Practice of Medicine, eighth edition, New York, 1912, p. 330.

[2] Jenner: Inquiry, 1798, footnote to p. 13, cited by L. Hektoen in Jour. Am. Med. Assoc., Chicago, 1912, lviii, footnote to p. 1087.

poets. Jenner's kidness of heart is seen in his regard for his first vaccination patient, James Phipps, for whom he built a cottage, planting the roses in the garden with his own hands. Like Newton, Harvey, Sydenham, Darwin, and Lister, he is one of the great men of purely Saxon genius, a happy combination of rare common sense with extreme simplicity of mind and character.

In Germany, Jenner's work was immediately taken up about 1798–99 by Hugo von Wreden, G. F. Ballhorn, and C. F. Stromeyer in Hannover (1799), by Heim and Brenner in Berlin (1800), by A. H. MacDonald in Altona (1800), by Hirt in Saxony. The Berlin Vaccine Institution was founded on December 5, 1802. Vaccination was introduced into Vienna by Jean de Carro and Pascal Ferro (1799). De Carro was also the first to introduce Jennerian vaccination into Asia. Pinel and Thouret in France, Vrancken in Holland, Demanet in Belgium, Luigi Sacco in Italy (1799), Heinrich Callisen in Denmark, Amar and others in Spain, were among the earliest promoters of the practice, which reached India and Mexico in 1802. In the United States, the Harvard professor of medicine, Benjamin Waterhouse (1754–1846) made the first vaccinations upon his four children in July, 1800,[1] procuring his virus from Dr. Haygarth of Bath, England. He was speedily followed by Crawford and Smith in Baltimore, James Jackson in Boston, David Hosack in New York, and John Redman Coxe in Philadelphia. The first Vaccine Institute was organized in Baltimore by James Smith in 1802 and a national Vaccine Agency was established by Congress under his direction in 1813. Waterhouse said that, before the introduction of vaccination, the fear of smallpox compelled the New Englanders, "the most democratical people on the face of the earth," to endure "restrictions of liberty such as no absolute monarch could have enforced."[2] The early American tracts of the colonial pamphleteers on inoculation, such as Benjamin Colman (1721–22), Isaac Greenwood (1721), Increase Mather (1721), William Cooper (1721–30), William Douglass (1722–30), Zabdiel Boylston (1726), Adam Thomson (1750), Nathanael Williams (1752), Lauchlin MacLeane (1756), Benjamin Franklin (1759), John Morgan (1776), and Benjamin Rush (1781), with the Waterhouse pamphlets on vaccination (1800–02), are now among the rarest and most highly prized of medical curiosities.

There was no **American medical literature** to speak of until long after the American Revolution. The first medical book to be published on the North American continent was printed by the Spaniards in the city of Mexico in 1570, and the first medical school was founded by them in 1578. Thacher's *Brief Rule* (Boston, 1677), a mere tract, was the only medical publication of the American colonists in the 17th century. The first medical book of the Colonies appears to have been a duodecimo (1708) reprint of Nicholas Culpeper's *English Physician* (Ballard).

"At the commencement of the Revolutionary War," says Billings, "we had one medical book by an American author, three reprints, and about twenty pamphlets"; and of the book in question, John Jones's *Plain, Concise, Practical Remarks on the Treatment of Wounds and Fractures* (New York, 1775), he goes on to say that "it is simply a compilation from Ranby, Pott, and others, and contains but one original observation."[3] This book contains, however, an appendix on camp and military hospitals, and was of great use to the young military and naval surgeons of the Revolution, for whom it was primarily designed, being, in fact, the first American

---

[1] In the "Columbian Sentinel" of March 12, 1799, Waterhouse refers to vaccination in down-East phrase, as "Something curious in the medical line."

[2] Cited by Dock.

[3] J. S. Billings in "A Century of American Medicine," Philadelphia, 1876, p. 293.

book on military medicine. Jones was a skilful lithotomist and was remembered by Benjamin Franklin in his will for a successful performance of the operation. Of pamphlet literature, there were some now curious colonial productions on the various anginas and eruptive fevers of the time by John Walton (1732) Cadwallader Colden (1735), William Douglass (*Angina ulcusculosa*, 1736), praised by Hirsch and Creighton as an exquisite account of scarlatina, Jabez Fitch (1736) and the tracts on inoculation, already mentioned. The early inaugural dissertations of the students Elmer, Potts, and Tilton at the University of Pennsylvania (1771), the latter a product of the celebrated Bradford Press, are now only collectors' curiosities, and the same thing applies to the oration *Antiqua novum orbem decet medicophilosophica*, delivered at Williamsburg, Virginia, June 12, 1782, by Jean-Francois Coste (1741–1819), medical director of the French forces in America, published at Leyden in 1783 and dedicated to Washington. Better than those are the essays on yellow fever by John Bard, Colden (1743), Mitchell (1741), John Lining (1753), and William Currie (1793); and, more important still, the clinical studies of Thomas Cadwalader (1708–79) on the West-Indian dry-gripes (lead-poisoning), which was printed by Benjamin Franklin (Philadelphia, 1745); John Tennent on pleurisy (1736), John Bard on malignant pleurisy (1749), and the essay of Samuel Bard (1742–1821) on diphtheria or "angina suffocativa" (1771), which was translated by Bretonneau and signalized by Osler as "an American classic of the first rank." The *Cases and Observations of the Medical Society of New Haven County* (founded 1784), contains the first American case of congenital hypertrophic stenosis of the pylorus (1788[1]) by Hezekiah Beardsley (1748–90), of Southington, Connecticut, which Osler rescued (in Lessing's sense of the term) by reprinting it in 1903.[2] It was preceded by the description of George Armstrong (1771). The history and geography of yellow fever in the United States were treated of by William Currie (1793) and Noah Webster (1796–99). The work of Matthew Carey (1760–1839) on the Philadelphia epidemic of yellow fever (1793) stands with that of Benjamin Rush (1794) as the most graphic, realistic, and complete account of the disease which had yet appeared.[3]

Some good botanic works were printed abroad, notably a first account of senega (1736) by John Tennent, of Virginia (1742), John Clayton's *Flora Virginica* (Leyden, 1739), probably the first work on American botany; *An Experimental Inquiry into the Properties of Opium*, by John Leigh of Virginia (Edinburgh, 1786), which gained the Harveian prize in 1785; and the still more interesting *Materia medica Americana* (Erlangen, 1787) of the old Anspach-Bayreuth surgeon, Johann David Schoepf (1752–1800), who came out to America with the Hessian troops in 1777, remained over after the war, and recorded his experiences in his *Travels in the Confederation* (1788), later translated and published in Philadelphia (1911). The first pharmacopœia to be printed in America, a pamphlet of 32 pages, was prepared by Dr. William Brown, of Virginia, who succeeded Rush as Physician General of the Middle Department. It was designed for use in the Continental army and was issued anonymously from the military hospital at Lititz, Pa., in 1778 (Handerson[4]). Daniel Turner published the first American books on dermatology (1714) and venereal diseases (1727). The first American contributions on medical education, medical ethics, and medical history were written by John Morgan (1765), Samuel Bard (1769), and Peter Middleton (1769) respectively. The *Syllabus* (1732) of Abraham Chovet (1704–99) is a relic of early anatomical teaching in Philadelphia (W. S. Miller).

The War of the Revolution was the making of medicine in this country, and it was in the nature of things that it should bring to the front the three leading American physicians of the time, Morgan, Shippen, and Rush. The war found us in a state of "unpreparedness," with noth-

---

[1] Beardsley: *Loc. cit.*, pp. 81–84.

[2] Arch. Pediat., N. Y., 1903, xx, 355–357.

[3] Charles Brockden Brown's novel of *Arthur Mervyn* (1799) contains another interesting account of this epidemic.

[4] Pharmacopœia simpliciorum et efficiarum in usum Nosocomi militaris ad Exercitum Federatum Americæ Civitatum, Philadelphia, Styner & Cyst (1778). A copy is in the Surgeon-General's Library. For a facsimile of the title-page of the second edition (1781), see Handerson's translation of Baas, p. 820. Brown's booklet was followed by the *Compendium* of J. F. Coste (Newport, 1780).

ing of military, still less of medical organization. Every one was on the fighting line, and there was little time for building hospitals, making instruments, or obtaining drugs. After drafting the Declaration, the ablest members of the Continental Congress were called, like every one else, to immediate and pressing duties in their several states; and Congress itself became, by all accounts, a feeble, bungling, almost impotent thing, accomplishing little in aid of the medical administration of the war, in some respects the most important feature of all. As Mumford says, there was but one man who was found "steadfast, patient, imperturbable," and that was Washington.[1] All honor to his two Surgeons General, Morgan and Shippen, who did so much for the organization of American medical education. Only brief mention can here be made of other physicians, many of whom played a noble and self-sacrificing part, such as John and Joseph Warren of Massachusetts, the latter serving in the ranks and losing his life at Bunker Hill; Benjamin Church, the first Surgeon General of the American Army; Hugh Mercer, of Virginia, who was killed at Princeton in 1777; James Thacher, the first American medical biographer, whose *Military Journal* (Boston, 1827) gives a picturesque account of the struggle and perhaps the best word-picture of the personality of Washington; and James Tilton, whose *Observations on Military Hospitals* (Wilmington, 1813) is a contribution of permanent value to his subject.

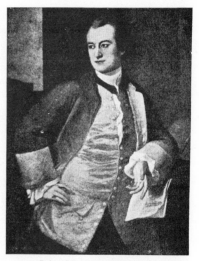

John Morgan (1735–89).

John **Morgan** (1735–89), a native of Philadelphia, was a student of John Redman's, served as surgeon in the French wars, and graduated at Edinburgh in 1762, where he was trained by such masters as William Hunter, the Monros, Cullen, and Whytt. Returning to his native city in 1765, he published, in the same year, his *Discourse upon the Institution of Medical Schools in America*, which files the first brief for adequate medical education in this country and commemorates the organization, at the College of Philadelphia (founded 1740), of the Medical Department of the University of Pennsylvania (1765), of which Morgan was, with Shippen, the principal founder and in which he held the first chair of practice of medicine. In 1775, Congress appointed Morgan "Director General and Physician in Chief" of the American Army, to

---

[1] Mumford: Narrative of Medicine in America, Philadelphia, 1903, 122.

succeed Church. He entered upon his duties with vigor, insisting upon rigorous examinations for medical officers and subordinating the regimental surgeons to the hospital chiefs, but the enmity of his subalterns and the shiftiness of politicians led to his unjust dismissal by Congress in 1777, and Shippen was appointed in his place. Morgan thereupon published his spirited *Vindication* (1777), in which he ably defends himself, with all loyalty to the cause and his great chief, demanding at the same time a court of inquiry. After two years' deliberation, the latter met and honorably acquitted him of all the charges in 1779. Broken in spirit, poor, and injured in health, Morgan retired to private practice and died twelve years later.

William **Shippen**, Jr. (1736–1808), of Philadelphia, who succeeded Morgan as Surgeon General in 1777, was also an Edinburgh graduate

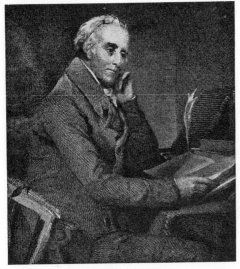

Eenjamin Rush (1745–1813).

(1761), coming under the Hunters, Cullen and Monro *secundus*. Returning to America in 1762, he began to give private and public instruction in anatomy and obstetrics, and was, indeed, the first public teacher of obstetrics in this country, and a prime mover of the cause of male midwifery. In 1765, he collaborated with Morgan in organizing the Medical Department of the University of Pennsylvania, in which he was, at the same time, appointed professor of anatomy and surgery. Upon his accession to the surgeon-generalcy in 1777, Shippen, who was more practical, less sensitive, better off in worldy wisdom than Morgan, was none the less court-martialed on grave charges in 1780, but secured acquittal. He resigned in 1781, to devote his entire attention to medical teaching, which he had kept up intermittently during his period of military service. By this he is best remembered, for he left no literary contributions of moment,[1] but he was the second in seven generations of American physicians bearing his name.

Benjamin **Rush** (1745–1813), of Pennsylvania, was of English Quaker stock and a graduate of Princeton (1760) and Edinburgh (1768), his graduating thesis dealing with "coction of food in the stomach." In 1769, he was elected professor of chemistry in the Col-

---

[1] Shippen's Edinburgh dissertation, *De placentæ cum utero nexa* (1761), is now only of bibliographic interest.

lege of Philadelphia, and succeeded Morgan as professor of practice in the same institution in 1789, attaining the chair of institutes of medicine, when the latter was merged into the University of Pennsylvania in 1791. He was also physician to the Pennsylvania Hospital (1783–1813), where he introduced clinical instruction; chief founder of the Philadelphia Dispensary (the first in this country) in 1786, and Treasurer of the United States Mint (1799–1813). Rush was a man of highly original mind, well read, well trained in his profession, an attractive, straightforward teacher, of wide human interests, sometimes wrong-headed as well as strong-headed. A signer of the Declaration and sometime Surgeon General for the Middle Department under Shippen (1776–78), he deserted Washington at Valley Forge to join the infamous "Conway Cabal" against the latter's "Fabian policy." As a medical theorist, he opposed Cullen's elaborate classification of diseases by a modified Brunonianism. His own therapeutic scheme was upon the most arbitrary basis. He looked upon inflammation as the effect rather than the cause of disease, and in regard to his statement that "Medicine is my wife and science my mistress," Dr. Holmes has added the caustic comment: "I do not think that the breach of the seventh commandment can be shown to have been of advantage to the ligitimate owner of his affections." A typical 18th century theorist, and a man whose social propagandism against war, slavery, alcoholism, and the death penalty was perhaps not entirely dissociated from a personal interest in increasing his practice, Rush was easily the ablest American clinician of his time, and his writings and reputation won him golden opinions abroad. Lettsom called him the American Sydenham, where effusive but more uncritical compatriots had dubbed him the Hippocrates of Pennsylvania, and he was the recipient of a diamond and various medals from royalty. He belongs to the school of Sydenham in his adherence to blood-letting and in his careful accounts of the diseases under his observation. He described cholera infantum in 1773; he was the first, after Bylon of Java (1779), to describe dengue (1780[1]), and one of the first to note the thermal fever occasioned by drinking cold water when overheated. His monograph on insanity (1812) was pronounced by Mills[2] to be, with that of Isaac Ray, the only systematic American treatise on the subject before the year 1883. His account of the Philadelphia epidemic of yellow fever (1793) is only approached by that of Matthew Carey for its realism. In fighting this epidemic, Rush played a commendable part, breaking down his health by treating 100–150 patients a day. He incurred civic and professional hatred by insisting that the disease was not imported from without but arose *de novo* in the city. His scheme of treatment was the exhibition of large doses of calomel and jalap, copious blood-letting, low diet, low temperature in the sick-room, and abundant hydrotherapy, within and without. As a

---

[1] Rush: Medical Observations and Inquiries, Phila., 1789, v, 104–121.

[2] C. K. Mills: Benjamin Rush and American Psychiatry, 1886. Cited by Mumford.

blood-letter, Rush has been likened to Sangrado, but he saved many patients and, when down, as he thought, with yellow fever, consistently submitted to his own line of treatment. Apart from his clinical memoirs, Rush wrote a valuable pamphlet on the hygiene of troops (1777). His papers on the diseases of North American Indians (1774) and their vices (1798), with his account of the German inhabitants of Pennsylvania (1798), are perhaps the earliest American contributions to anthropology. The original bent of his mind is shown in his inquiries into the effects of ardent spirits on the mind, the cure of diseases by the extraction of decayed teeth, and the effect of arsenic on cancer. Like Shippen and Physick, Rush was a well-featured man of aquiline profile, suggesting native shrewdness and penetration.

The name of **Benjamin Franklin** (1706–90), of Boston, is intimately connected with American medicine through his invention of bifocal lenses (1784[1]), a flexible catheter and a stove, his letters on the treatment of paralysis by electricity (Franklinism, 1757), and on lead-poisoning (1786), his observations on gout, the heat of the blood, sleep, deafness, nyctalopia, the infective nature of colds, infection from dead bodies, death-rate in infants, and medical education. He was the principal founder and the first president of the Pennsylvania Hospital (1751), of which he wrote a history, by request, printed at his own press in 1754. Of special bibliographic interest are his *Dialogue with the Gout* and his pamphlet on inoculation in smallpox (London, 1759), which was accompanied by William Heberden's directions for performing the operation.

Thomas **Cadwalader** (1708–79), of Philadelphia, a pupil of Cheselden, was a pioneer of inoculation (1730), a founder of the Philadelphia Library (1731) and its director (1731–39), and the first to teach anatomy by dissections in the city (1730–31).

His *Essay on the West-India Dry-Gripes*, printed by Benjamin Franklin in 1745, and sometimes wrongly catalogued as an "Essay on the Iliac Passion,"[2] is an account of lead colic and lead palsy from the habitual use of Jamaica rum distilled, as Franklin showed in 1786, through leaden pipes. It contains Cadwalader's autopsy of a case of mollities ossium (1742).

Apart from the work of Morgan, Rush, and Shippen, the writings of the colonal pamphleteers on inoculation, the clinical observations of Cadwalader, Samuel Bard, Beardsley, Rush, and Carey, and the pioneer exploits in pelvic and vascular surgery by John Bard, William Baynham, and Wright Post, most of the productions of American medicine in this period, although of a respectable character, are aside from the main current of scientific progress. As Sainte Beuve said to Matthew Arnold about Lamartine's poems, they are "important to *us*," in the sense of having a definite local historic interest.

---

[1] In his letter to George Wheately of London, May 2, 1785.

[2] See C. W. Dulles: Med. Library & Histor. Jour., Brooklyn, 1903, i, 181–184.

CULTURAL AND SOCIAL ASPECTS OF EIGHTEENTH CENTURY MEDICINE

The rise of Prussia and Russia and the American and French revolutions are perhaps the only historic events which exerted much influence upon the condition of medicine in the 18th century, and then only in relation to the development of surgery. The tendencies of the age were artificial and theoretic rather than sincere or realistic. This periwigged period is conceded to have been the "Golden Age," alike of the successful practitioner and the successful quack. The reason is to be sought in the stationary condition of society prior to the French Revolution, which kept all occupations in a definite groove; so that the internist or physician proper was in every sense of the word a family doctor (*Hausartz*), who was given a voluntary annual honorarium for his continuous services during the year, thus relieving him of the necessity of competing with his fellow practitioners or of struggling for his existence beyond a certain point. Nearly every one of the great physicians of the time stood upon a pedestal all his own, and many of these, as Welch has said, "let it be known" that they were in possession of private or secret remedies which were superior to all others. Practice was inherited from father to son, or passed on to favorite pupils. In this way, a certain elegant leisure was acquired by the well-to-do members of the profession, giving them exceptional opportunities for the acquisition of culture. Haller, William Hunter, Scarpa, Heberden, and Thomas Young yield to none in scholarship and variety of attainments. Arbuthnot, Garth, and other physicians of Queen Anne's reign were coffee-house intimates of the wits and poets of the period.[1] Lessing had studied medicine. Goldsmith and Schiller were medical graduates; and such men of letters as Garth, Arbuthnot, Blackmore, Akenside, Haller, Zimmermann, and Werlhof were practitioners. There is plenty of evidence that the social status of the 18th century physician was, if anything, better than it is today. In some countries, he wore a sword, his color was the "austere scarlet," and people commonly took off their hats to him, even when he bore a muff, to preserve his delicacy of touch in diagnosis. In England, the fashionable physician wore a powdered wig, a handsome coat of red satin or brocade, short breeches, stockings and buckled shoes, a three-corned hat, and bore a goldheaded cane. Werlhof, at Hannover, on the occasion of his second marriage, wore a violet velvet coat. Toward the end of the 17th century, ruffled collars gave place to Geneva bands, an appropriate symbol of the clerical origin of the medical profession. The summit of its grandeur, in cos-

---

[1] Every reader of Pope will recall his grateful tribute to Arbuthnot:
"Friend to my life; (which did you not prolong,
The world had wanted many an idle song),

. . . .

The muse but serv'd to ease some friend, not wife,
To help me through this long disease, my life,
To second, Arbuthnot! thy art and care,
And teach the being you preserved to bear."

tume at least, is to be seen in the portrait of the elder Baron, the pleasant-faced dean of the Paris Faculty (1730–34), which is reproduced in the beautiful album of its artistic collections published in 1911.[1] The handsome dean wears a long, carefully curled wig, an ermine cape, a delicate, transparent *rabat* in place of the stiff Geneva band, a red ecclesiastic cope or "regal dalmatic," with lace-ruffled sleeves and, over his breast, a decoration suspended by a long black ribbon. Solemn elegance could go no further. Careless elegance, as well as political sympathies, were sometimes evinced in the loosely knotted "Steenkirk tie."[2]

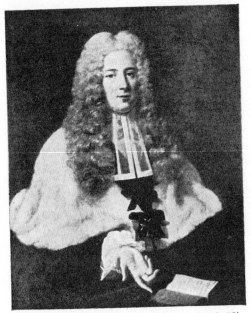

Hyacinthe-Théodore Baron père (1710–58), Dean of the Paris Medical Faculty, 1730–34. (Courtesy of M. Noé Legrand, Paris, from his "Les Collections Artistiques de la Faculté de Médecine de Paris," 1911.)

Except in caricature, the art of the 18th century throws but little light upon the status of the medical profession. Reynolds and Gainsborough, Fragonard and Watteau are unusually reticent about medicine in their canvases, although a few portraits of physicians were, of course, painted by Raeburn and others, with Sir Joshua's great portrait of John Hunter at the head of the list. The status of Bichat by David d'Angers belongs in the Napoleonic (transition) period.

Hogarth's "Company of Undertakers" (1736), with the legend, *Et plurima mortis imago*, portrays twelve hard-featured individuals, all bewigged and armed with gold-headed canes, who are supposed to represent Spot Ward, the Chevalier Taylor, Madame Mapp (in a zany's coat of many colors), and other quacks of the period. Hogarth also made two pictures of Maria Toft's miraculous birth of rabbits, a celebrated imposture of the 18th century, and has various broad or slanting allusions to prostitution, pregnancy, alcoholism, and insanity in his copper-plates, including the quack with the syphilitic girl in *Mariage à la Mode* (Plate III). His "Pool of Bethesda" (St. Bartholomew's Hospital) has representations of lameness, rickets, consumption, psoriasis, and other diseases (Norman Moore). Greuze's paralytic grandfather has the 18th century tendency toward artificial sermonizing which so irritated Carlyle. Gillray and Rowlandson, those masters of the coarse and grotesque, in-

[1] Les Collections Artistiques de la Faculté de Médecine de Paris. Inventaire raisonné par Noé Legrand et L. Landouzy, Paris, 1911.

[2] So called from the disordered condition of rich cravats at the battle of Steinkirk (1692). After this event, the studiously disarranged tie became fashionable in France and, if we may trust the Restoration dramatists, even in England. See Vanbrugh's Relapse, act 1, sc. 3, and Scott's Rob Roy, ch. xxxi.

dulged their animal spirits abundantly at the expense of medicine, but their plates belong mainly to the Georgian period. Those on The Dying Patient, or the Doctor's Last Fee (Rowlandson, 1786), Transplantation of Teeth (Rowlandson, 1787), The Gout (Gillray, 1799), The Midwife (Rowlandson, 1800), and Metallic Tractors (Gillray, 1801) are all true 18th century in implication. Animal magnetism, vaccination, clysters, Macassar oil, men-midwives, metallic tractors, phrenology, and other foibles of the period were all abundantly caricatured in the fugitive anonymous plates of the time. That prolific Danzig artist, Daniel Chodowiecki, the illustrator of the Zopfzeit, has some clever etchings of German interiors, representing inoculation, animal magnetism, dissecting, fashionable physicians (Modedoctoren), miraculous healers (Wunderdoctoren), Frederick the Great having a vein opened, a sick person receiving extreme unction, an absurd proposal of marriage by a corpulent physician to an equally stout patient, and a plate showing Prussian police in the act of ordering patients to the Charité. Leonard Mark has noted that the various etchings and mezzotints of one Richard Dickinson, a shoe-cleaner and gingerbread-seller of Scarborough Spa, afford striking representations of the acromegalic facies, made over 200 years ago (1725–26[1]). Boucher's cartoon of the orviétanvendor (1736) was reproduced in Gobelin tapestry. The excellence of Tiepolo's dwarfs has been emphasized by Charcot. A clever painting by Pietro Longhi represents an Italian apothecary shop of the period.

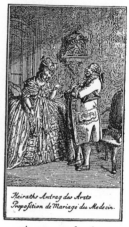

Heiraths Antrag des Arzts
Proposition de Mariage du Medecin.

A proposal of marriage. Etching by Daniel Chodowiecki (1726–1801).

In the secular literature of the 18th century the physician was especially satirized by Smollett (Count Fathom), Sterne (Dr. Slop), and Le Sage (Gil Blas). In Smollett's Count Fathom the adventurous knave takes it into his head to enroll himself among "the sons of Pæan." His experiences give an amusing purview of the "solemnities of dress and address," the trade tricks (being called out of church or riding aimlessly about in a chariot) which were resorted to even by practitioners of better repute. The capable Huxham, a butcher's son, who first practised among non-conformists and afterward went over to the Established Church, often had himself summoned out of conventicle at stated intervals, whereupon he would gallop through the town to create the impression of an extensive practice. He usually stalked about in a scarlet coat, flourishing a gold-headed cane, a footman bearing his gloves at a respectful distance. Le Sage throws much light upon medicine in Spain, where blood-letting and cathartics were almost the only known remedies, where cleaning the streets of offal was opposed for a fantastic reason, where there was not a single apothecary for over half a century, and where, as late as 1795, permission to practise outside of Madrid cost only $45 (Baas). The ignominious position of the army surgeon in Germany after the time of Frederick the Great is alluded to in the early writings and poems of Schiller.[2] In Roderick Random, Smollett describes the exceedingly low status of the medical

---

[1] L. Mark: Lancet, Lond., 1914, ii, 1412 (with cuts).

[2] For Schiller's medical career, see Neuburger, Wien. klin. Wochenschr., 1905, xviii, 488–497.

profession on board ship, and the humbuggery and corruption which attended the competitive examinations for the position of surgeon's mate. His picture of M. Lallemant, the shabby, nimble-shilling apothecary, is equally significant. In an age in which caste distinctions were on an ironclad basis (witness the French Revolution), it is obvious that the imposing dress and manners of the upper-class physicians should lend themselves readily to imitation at the hands of unscrupulous impostors. The 18th century was the age *par excellence* of successful

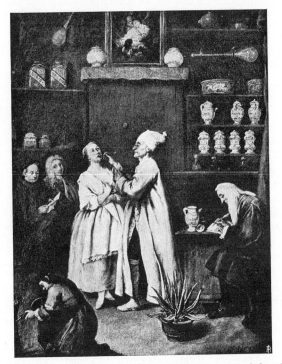

The Apothecary, by Pietro Longhi (1702–85). (Italian interior of the 18th century.)

quacks, and it yields only to the 19th century in respect of those patented or secret preparations of which the poet Crabbe, the satirist of quacks, laments:

"From the poor man's pay
The nostrum takes no trifling part away."

Quackery, if not universal, was at least, in Thoreau's phrase, "universally successful." Rolling stones, like Cagliostro and Mesmer, managed to ply their trade for a long while without interruption. Casanova paid a decorous visit to Haller at Bern, and his stay with the great man was supposed to be not so much "the homage which vice pays to virtue" as a manifestation of genuine esteem, for Casanova not only affected to enjoy the commerce of the learned, but had written

Latin dissertations or had some one write them for him. In England, there was a long line of successful medical charlatans of both sexes. The earliest of these was Sir William Read, who started out as a tailor, but in 1694 set up in the Strand as an oculist, having hired some one to write a book on eye diseases under his name and a Grub Street poet to praise him in verse. His success in this specialty attracted the attention of Queen Anne, whose bad eyesight made her an easy victim of such impostors. Gaining her good graces, he was actually knighted, subsequently becoming oculist to George I. Read frequented the society of Swift and the other coffee-house wits, who made fun of him while accepting his lavish hospitality, and he is even mentioned in the Spectator (September 1, November 27, 1712). Other quack oculists of importance in their day were Dr. Grant (who was also patronized by Queen Anne), Thomas Woolhouse (oculist to James II and William III) who is said to have proposed iridectomy in 1711 (before Cheselden), and the Chevalier Taylor. The latter, the son of a female apothecary of Norwich, had actually worked with Cheselden at St. Thomas's and had invented a cataract needle and other instruments but, failing of success in London, decided for the adventurous career of a roving oculist. It has been remarked that even Daviel, in the early part of his career, did practically the same thing, trumpeting his praises abroad after the fashion of the wandering eye-couchers of the Middle Ages, but with this difference that Daviel was really a great ophthalmic surgeon in the making, where Taylor was only a clever buffoon.[1] Clad in black, with a long flowing wig, possessed of a good address and undoubtedly of some skill in eye surgery, Taylor went about, lecturing like a mountebank at a fair, expressing himself in queer sentences with inverted syntax, in imitation of Latin, which style he called "true Ciceronian." He numbered even Gibbon and Händel among his patients, but did not impose upon Horace Walpole or Dr. Johnson. The latter says of him (Boswell, 1779): "Taylor was the most ignorant man I ever knew, but sprightly: Ward, the dullest. Taylor challenged me once to talk Latin with him [laughing]. I quoted some of Horace, which he took to be a part of my own speech. He said a few words well enough." The Ward to whom Dr. Johnson refers was Joshua Ward, another famous quack, also known as "Spot" Ward, on account of a claret mark on one side of his face. Ward was originally a drysalter who had tried politics without success, but soon made his fortune by the sale of antimonial pills and drops, a "liquid sweat," a "dropsy purging powder," and other nostrums. General Churchill constituted himself press-agent for Ward's pills. Ward's "essence for headache" and "Ward's paste" (for fistula and piles) afterward appeared in the pharmacopeia as compound camphor liniment and confection of pepper. He won the absolute confidence of George II by reducing a dis-

---

[1] Taylor's writings, translated into many languages, contain matters in advance of his time, e. g., the first delineation of conical cornea after that of Duddell (in 1736). G. Coats: Roy. Lond. Ophth. Hosp. Rep., 1915, xx, 1–92.

located thumb with a sharp wrench, after which he was given a room in Whitehall and liberally patronized by the great, numbering Chesterfield, Walpole, and Gibbon among his patients. He was specially exempted from the penalties of the Parliamentary Act of 1748, restricting the practice of medicine and, in his will, had the impudence to request burial in Westminster Abbey. Pope has embalmed him in a couplet:

> "Of late, without the least pretence to skill,
> Ward's grown a famed physician by a pill."

Notable female impostors of the period were Mrs. Mapp, a bonesetter, who was so successful that she could drive in from Epsom in a chariot and four, with gorgeously liveried servants; and Joanna Stevens, a widow, who, in 1739, actually succeeded in having her remedy for stone purchased *pro bono publico* by Act of Parliament. Her philanthropy went to the extent of agreeing to part with this valued recipe for £5000, but even a titled subscription list could not raise this sum in the first instance, and powerful influence was brought to bear upon Parliament, even Cheselden, Sharp, and Cæsar Hawkins vouching for her merits. The recipe was published in the London Gazette of June 19, 1739, and turned out to be a set of mixtures of egg-shells, garden-snails, swines' cresses, soap, and such vegetable ingredients as burdock seeds, hips, and haws. In each one of her certified "cures," the stone was found in the bladder after death.

Of secret or **proprietary medicines** patented in England, Timothy Byfield's *sal oleosum volatile* (1711) was the first to take advantage of the old Statute of Monopolies of 1624. It was followed by Stoughton's Great Cordial Elixir (1712), Betton's British Oils (1742), John Hooper's Female Pills (1743), and a long list of other nostrums, down to Ching's Worm Lozenges (1792) and Della Lena's Powder of Mars (1799). The Duke of Portland's Powder is mentioned in Fielding's Voyage to Lisbon (1755). The most famous of these were the antimonial fever powder (1747) and analeptic pills (1794) of Dr. Robert James, a physician of solid ability, who wrote a bulky Dictionary of Medicine and a Pharmacopœia Universalis, and was an esteemed friend of Dr. Johnson. The original James's powder was, in the opinion of Christison, more effective than its antimonial substitute in the Pharmacopœia. The *eau medicinale de Husson*, a secret remedy for gout, probably contained colchicum (introduced by Stoerck in 1763). "Tuscora Rice," for consumption, was the first American patent medicine (1711).

Among the therapeutic fads of the time were quassia-cups, saffron drops, purging sugar-plums, anodyne necklaces for pregnant women and teething children, Macassar oil (for the hair), and the metallic or magnetic tractors patented by Elisha Perkins of Connecticut in 1798. These were compass-like contrivances, with one blunt-pointed and one sharp-pointed arm, made of combinations of copper, zinc, and gold, or iron, silver, and platinum. Cures were effected by stroking, and their principle of action was supposed to be analogous to that of galvanism or animal magnetism. Perkin's tractors had a remarkable vogue in England, were abundantly satirized in such colored prints and pamphlets as "A Terrible Tractoration," until John Haygarth, a Bath physician, showed that similar cures could be effected with wooden tractors, whence it was perceived that it was all imposture. Electricity and animal magnetism were exploited as a special mode of appealing to the baser passions by James Graham of Edinburgh, who was the coryphæus of "celestial beds" for rejuvenating senility. Graham was a man of handsome physique, aquiline features, and pontifical manner, who had half studied medicine and picked up some knowledge of electricity from hearing about Franklin's experiments in America. His "Temple of Health," opened in London in 1780, consisted of a sumptuously appointed apartment, with all the implications and accessories of a strictly Oriental interior, including mysterious perfumes, soft music, and bacchantic poses. The entrance fee was six guineas and, in a plain-spoken lecture which "tickled the ears of the groundlings," immediate conception was guaranteed to the childless for a £50 bank note. The fraud did not last long and, when the crash came in 1782, Graham was driven to preach mud-baths (fangotherapy), evincing his sincerity by remaining in them for hours at a time each day. "Half knave, half enthusiast," as Robert Southey called him, he did not profit by his hygienic theories, and died at an early age. More respectable, and hardly to be classed among out-and-out quacks, were the "Whitworth doctors," otherwise the Taylor brothers, two village farriers who took up human ailments, buying Glauber's salts by the ton, and dispensing it in proportion, bleeding the poor free of charge on Sunday mornings, setting broken bones and treating cancers, apparently with some show of success. Although the elder Taylor cared more for horse-doctoring than for human patients, Whitworth was crowded with the visiting sick, who were treated strictly as they came, without preference or deference for rank. Even royalty had to taste the same rustic independence. The "Whitworth Red Bottle" and "Whitworth Drops" were famous a century ago. When John Hunter asked Taylor the composition of one of his ointments, he replied, "No, Jack, that's not a fair question. I'll send you as much of it as you like, but I won't tell you what it's made of."[1]

Toward the close of the century, a Mr. and Mrs. Loutherbourg acquired an enormous following by reviving Valentine Greatrakes' old method of curing disease by touch ("stroking"), a variant of faith cure. They were besieged by great crowds of patients whom they professed to treat gratis, declining to take any fee whatever, but it was discovered that they were in collusion with certain agents who sold their "free" tickets for whatever they could get. Dr. Katterfelto, another sharp practitioner, traveled about the north of England in a van drawn by six horses, containing a number of black cats and attended by many outriders in gay liveries. Dr. Myersbach, in spite of Lettsom's opposition, continued to make a large income out of fashionable people. On the continent, Villars had

---

[1] For further information, see Brit. Med. Jour., 1911, i, 1264–1274; Wootton's Chronicles of Pharmacy, Lond., 1910, ii, 203–219, and the separate biographic notices in Leslie Stephen.

enormous success with a five-franc nostrum of niter and water, and
Ailhaud, whose powders are said to have destroyed as many people
as Napoleon's campaigns, though he was put out of business by Tissot
in his *Avis au peuple* (1803), had already attained to three baronies
and was known as the Baron de Castelet.[1] Johann Andreas Eisenbart
(1661–1771), of Magdeburg, the hero of the student's song,

> "Kann machen dass die Blinden gehn,
> und dass die Lahmen wieder sehn,"

was a very real impostor of the *Zopfzeit*, who held forth with drum as a
"barker" (*Marktschreier*) at fairs. Johann Christoph Ludemann (1685–
1757), of Harburg, practised astrology and uroscopy in Amsterdam up
to the end of his life. His success was largely due to a female companion who, like the Wise Woman of Hogsdon, in Heywood's comedy,
played the part of informant and procuress.[2]

In Farquhar's *Recruiting Officer* (act iv, sc. 3) there is a scene in
which Sergeant Kite whiles away his time by passing himself off as a
conjurer. Assuming the power of prediction, he tells a butcher that,
from his skill in swinging the cleaver, he will some day become surgeon
general of the army. This was at the beginning of the century, and,
only a little while before, the witty and dissolute Earl of Rochester is
said to have diverted himself by hiring a stall on Tower Hill, where he
practised as a quack doctor, delivering himself of truly Paracelsian
tirades,[3] and selling cosmetics and remedies for female complaints. It
is obvious that the great army of adventurers, card-sharpers, quacks,
and other financial crooks who flourished in the 18th century succeeded,
then as now, by the kind of bullying assurance which the Germans
call *imponiren*. They dared to be themselves with a vast amount of
swagger and with the trait of clever brutality which is always an asset
among rogues. Yet the same aplomb was noticeable in more honorable
branches of activity, and, as Jeaffreson says, "the physician, the divine, the lawyer, the parliament-man, the country gentleman, the
author by profession—all had peculiarities of style, costume, speech, or
intonation, by which they were well pleased that they should be recognized. . . . The barrister's smirk, the physician's unctuous smiles,
the pedagogue's frown, did not originate in a mean desire to be taken
for something of higher mark and esteem than they really were."[4]
Indeed, Thomas Sergeant Perry maintains that the uneasy sense of
inferiority and concern about the opinion of others, which is snobbery,
first made its appearance in literature in the episode of Mrs. Tibbs in
Goldsmith's "Citizen of the World" (1762[5]). The professional jealousy
and rancor which obtained among some members of the profession can

---

[1] J. C. Jeaffreson: A Book about Doctors, New York, 1861, 101–114.

[2] J. G. de Lint: Janus, Leyden, 1913, xviii, 165–196.

[3] For an amusing speech by Rochester, see Wootton's Chronicles of Pharmacy,
London, 1910, ii, 204–205.

[4] J. C. Jeaffreson: *Op. cit.*, 83.

[5] T. S. Perry: The Evolution of the Snob, Boston, 1887, 57–60.

be sensed in the virulent character of their medical controversies, which form such a large segment of 18th century pamphleteering. On the evening of June 10, 1719, in the quadrangle of Gresham College, Richard Mead and John Woodward began a duel with swords about their views on the treatment of smallpox, which was stopped by by-standers when Woodward lost his footing, and terminated in a war of words. On December 28, 1750, Drs. John Williams and Parker Bennet, of Jamaica, being involved in a wrangle about their respective views on bilious fever, came to blows and, the next day, proceeded to a desperate hand-to-hand combat with swords and pistols, which ended fatally for both.[1] It is said that Johann Peter Frank was so disgusted with the behavior of doctors in consultation that he advised the calling in of the police on all such occasions (Jacobi). In 1799, the Medical and Chirurgical Faculty of Maryland imposed a fine of 10 dollars upon any member guilty of disorderly conduct in its meetings, with orders to eject him, if necessary (Cordell[2]). But these cases are hardly typical. The general tendency of the age was toward sobriety, urbanity, extremely artificial manners, and the control of the body by the mind. The 18th century physician of better type was in position to make large sums of money without using his profession as a trade and enjoyed social and cultural advantages far above the average. Let us glance for a moment at some of the fashionable London practitioners of the period. In England, Garth was the idol of the Whigs, Arbuthnot of the Tories. Sir Samuel **Garth** (1661–1719) was the only physician who belonged to the famous Kit-Kat Club and, while making a name for himself in literature and taking an occasional hand in politics, had no mean success as a practitioner. John **Arbuthnot** (*Martinus Scriblerus*) (1667–1735), the author of "The History of John Bull," was the friend and familiar of Pope and Swift and eventually became physician to Queen Anne. Sir Richard **Blackmore** (died 1729), although a total failure as a poet, was accounted one of the most successful men in the medical profession, the oracle of the wealthy, whom he emulated in "style." Sir Hans **Sloane** (1660–1753), the first physician to be made a baronet, enjoyed the highest scientific and professional reputation, was a founder and later the secretary and president of the Royal Society. His museum and library, after his death, became the nucleus of the present British Museum collections. John **Radcliffe** (1650–1714), although of humble origin, was appointed physician to Princess Anne of Denmark, which position he lost through his arrogant demeanor. He had financial luck from the start, commencing practice about the time that Richard Lower was losing ground, and was making more than 20 guineas a day at the end of his first year. He was a Jacobite, and, says Jeaffreson, "contrived by his shrewd humor, arrogant simplicity, and immeasurable insolence to hold both Whigs and Tories in his

---

[1] J. Williams and P. Bennet: Essays on Bilious Fever, London, 1752.

[2] Cited by Cook: New York Med. Jour., 1915, ci, 140; 205.

grasp. The two factions of the aristocracy bowed before him." His disposition was somewhat soured by the fact that he had been once jilted and once rejected in a proposal of marriage, yet, though he pretended to be miserly, he was frequently generous with his money. After liberally providing for his relatives in his will, he left funds to Oxford for the present foundations known as the Radcliffe Library, the Radcliffe Infirmary, the Radcliffe Observatory, and the Radcliffe Travelling Fellowship. Toward the close of his life, he took a fancy to young Richard **Mead** (1673–1754), who flattered his vanity and so inherited his practice. "Mead, I love you," said Radcliffe, "and I'll tell you a sure secret to make you a fortune—use all mankind ill." Mead was a complete contrast to his predecessor—a scholar where Radcliffe was ignorant of books, courtly and polished where Radcliffe was crude and overbearing. "Dr. Mead," said Dr. Johnson, "lived more in the broad sunshine of life than almost any man." Through Radcliffe's influence, Mead was summoned to the death bed of Queen Anne, and became the most prosperous practitioner of his time, making in one year as much as £7000. Upon moving into Radcliffe's house in Bloomsbury Square, he inherited the latter's famous gold-headed cane, which passed successively through the hands of Askew, Pitcairn, and Baillie, and is now in the Library of the Royal College of Physicians. Mead afterward moved into a handsome establishment in Ormond Street and lived to be eighty-one. After him came such men as Heberden, Lettsom, Fothergill, Parry, and the Hunters.

On the continent we find Werlhof, court physician at Hannover and, after the battle of Dettingen (June 27, 1743), physician-in-ordinary to George II. He was succeeded by Zimmermann and Wichmann, who, says Baas, flourished a barber's bowl before he entered the gymnasium. In Leyden, Boerhaave was preëminent; in Halle, Stahl and Hoffmann, and later Reil; in Berlin, Heim; in Jena, Hufeland; in Vienna, van Swieten and de Haën; in Paris, Théophile de Bordeu; in Modena, Torti; at Pavia, Borsieri de Kanilfeld and Peter Frank; in Geneva, Tronchin; and at Lausanne, Tissot.

All these physicians were fortunate above the average, and one characteristic seems common to most of them. As they were not specially exposed to commercial competition and the petty human traits it brings forth, they could afford to be charitable in the best sense. No other single group of physicians was probably so generous to the poor. Take, for example, this little note which Garth scribbled to Sir Hans Sloane:

"Dear Sir Hans:
"If you can recommend this miserable slut to be fluxed, you'll do an act of charity for, dear sir,
"Your obedt sert
"Sl Garth."

or this of John Hunter to his brother William:

"Dear Brother:
"The bearer is very desirous of having your opinion. I do not know his case. He has no money, and you don't want any, so that you are well met.
"Ever yours,
"John Hunter."

Rough kindness this, yet it shows a degree of fraternal confidence between physicians which seldom exists today, and toward the humble poor the sentiment of Empedocles:

> "Thou art my friend, to thee
> All knowledge that I have,
> All skill I wield are free."

That this sentiment was reciprocated by the mass of mankind, we need no better evidence than the experience of Jenner, or the extraordinary popularity of such books as Tissot's *Avis au Peuple* or Hufeland's *Makrobiotik*. The Chimney Sweeper's Act of 1788 was motivated by Pott's account of chimney sweep's (scrotal) cancer (1775), which set forth the misery and virtual slavery of the poor "climbing boys," and was followed by Jonas Hanway's *Sentimental History of Chimney Sweepers* (1785). Yet, in spite of Lord Ashley's Acts of 1834 and 1840, a child of seven and a half years was lifted into a chimney in 1873, and the mortality from cancer was still high in 1902 (Legge).

One of the kindest and most liberal of the 18th century physicians was Richard **Brocklesby** who, in 1788, gave Edmund Burke £1000 with an offer to repeat the gift "every year until your merit is rewarded as it ought to be at court"; who encouraged Young and who offered to settle £100 a year upon Dr. Johnson for life. Boswell records that "a grateful tear" gathered in Johnson's eye, "as he spoke of this in a faltering tone." In 1792, Benjamin Thomson, **Count Rumford** (1753–1814), of Woburn, Mass., established the People's Soup Kitchens at Munich, with provision for warm **meals for school children,** the first venture of this kind.

Another side-light on the social status of 18th century physicians is afforded by the incomes they made, and the **fees** some of them received. The guinea came into currency in Restoration England (1660), and afforded an opportunity to raise the doctor's fee from a noble or angel to this sum, a fee which has persisted even to our day, although the guinea ceased to be coined in 1813 (Power). Mead commonly charged a guinea as an office fee, two guineas or more for a visit to patients in good standing and, like Radcliffe, he wrote half-guinea prescriptions for the apothecaries while sitting in his coffee-house, without seeing the patient. His average income was between £5000 and £6000 per annum, which had a purchasing power of over three times its equivalent in modern money. Mead attended to Freind's practice when the latter went into politics, and handed him 11,400 guineas as the amount collected. Radcliffe's consultation fee at Bow was 5 guineas. Later on, we find Fothergill making £5000 a year, and Lettsom £12,000. Baas considers 3000 to 4000 marks ($2250 to $3000 in present value) as a mediocre 18th-century income in a city of size, and he states that, in 1782, Heim in Berlin got 4200 marks from 784 patients, 6600 marks from 383 patients in 1784, 26,400 marks from 1000 patients in 1790; by 1805, his annual income had gone up to 36,000 marks. Orräus, in Moscow, was making 90,000 marks in a short time.[1] The phenomenal fee of the period was that acquired by Thomas Dimsdale for inoculating Catherine of Russia and her son, viz., $50,000, with $10,000 additional for traveling expenses, a pension of $2500 for life, and the rank of baron of the empire. Quarin got a pension of $10,000 per annum and was made a baron for his consultation with Joseph II. University professors were also well paid. Baas assumes an average salary of 3000–7500 marks for the North German universities, but points out that the cost of comfortable living was about 6000

---

[1] Baas: *Op. cit.*, pp. 745; 751; 763.

marks annually in Hannover and 7500 in Berlin. De Haën got 10,000 and Johann Peter Frank 9000 marks in Vienna, Morgagni about $4500 in Padua. Frank got 342 marks as court physician at Baden, 1370 marks and many perquisites as physician-in-ordinary to the Bishop of Speyer, and 9600 marks as imperial physician in Russia.

Three new editions of the London Pharmacopœia were issued during the 18th century, each of them characterized by changes which show the status of **therapeutics** and the gradual advance of pharmacology.[1] The fourth Pharmacopœia (1721), edited by Sir Hans Sloane, drops many of the old syrups and waters, but retains theriac, extracts of excreta and other animal products, and introduces stramonium, gamboge, Secale cornutum, hepar, ipecac, tartar emetic, lunar caustic, lime-water, Ethiops mineral, spirit of sal volatile, iron sulphate, tincture of perchlorid of iron, and other inorganic preparations. The fifth London Pharmacopœia (1746), revised by Mead, Heberden, Freind, and others, professes to condemn the old astrologic and folk remedies, and while it drops human fat, spider-webs, moss from human skulls, unicorn's horn, virgin's milk, bones from the stag's heart, and the like, still retains mithridate, theriac, crabs' eyes, wood-lice, pearls, bezoars, vipers, coral, etc. Syrups and medicated waters diminish in number, but there are many new tinctures, including those of valerian and cardamoms. Glauber's salts, sweet spirits of niter, syrup of squills, liquor potassæ, and potassium acetate are added. One year before this pharmacopeia was printed, William Heberden published his famous essay, *Antitheriaka* (1745), in which he showed that the belief in the efficacy of theriac and mithridate was based upon a tissue of absurdities, since the actual formula for theriac found in the cabinet of Mithridates after his death called for 20 leaves of rue, 1 grain of salt, 2 nuts, and 2 dried figs, in striking contrast with the long-winded recipes for its composition which had been imagined by later authorities.[2] Heberden successfully ridiculed these nostrums out of existence, but it was too late to make any changes in the Pharmacopœia of 1746. The effect of his destructive criticism appears to advantage in the sixth Pharmacopœia (1788), in which practically all the animal materia medica has disappeared, along with theriac and mithridate; while among the new drugs and compounds added are aconite, arnica, castor oil, colombo, cascarilla, kino, quassia, magnesia, senega, simaruba, ether, tartrate of iron, oxide of zinc, Dover's powder, Hoffmann's anodyne, Huxham's tincture, James' powder, spiritus Mindereri, sarsaparilla decoctions, compound tincture of benzoin, extract of chamomile, tincture of opium, and tinctura opii camphorata (paregoric). Of these, kino and catechu were introduced by Fothergill, colombo by Gaub, quassia by Daniel Rolander, senega by John Tennent of Virginia. Dover's powder was introduced by the famous buccaneer physician, Thomas Dover (1660–1742), who was once in residence with Sydenham and, in 1709, rescued Alexander Selkirk (Robinson Crusoe) from the island of Juan Fernandes. Dover's formula for his "diaphoretic powder" is given in his "Ancient Physician's Legacy to His Country" (1732). Digitalis was introduced by William Withering in 1785, but did not appear in the London Pharmacopœia until 1809. Stoerck of Vienna made careful studies of conium, stramonium, hyoscyamus, colchicum, pulsatilla, clematis, and recommended their use (1760–71). Thomas Fowler introduced his solution of arsenic in 1786. Compound licorice powder was the invention of E. G. Kurella of Berlin, and first appeared in the Prussian pharmacopeia of 1799. In 1724, Friedrich Hoffmann discovered a mineral spring at Seidlitz, Bohemia, which owed its medicinal properties to a combination of magnesium and sodium sulphates; but of "Seidlitz powders" only the name remains attached to the present formula, which was patented by the Bond Street chemist Savory in 1815. Many physicians of the 18th century, including Hoffmann, Stahl, Sloane, and Mead, made money by selling preparations with secret formulas, and a token of the popular faith in drugs was the large-sized medicine spoon which often formed part of a bride's dowry. In this period, both physicians and surgeons compounded and dispensed their own remedies, and, as the practitioners themselves were usually "family doctors," their incidental charges were made for their prescriptions and not for their visits. This largely accounts for the terribly long-winded prescriptions which abound in the 18th century and, as Billings remarks, the sur-

---

[1] Wootton: *Op. cit.*, ii. pp. 65–67.

[2] Most remarkable of these was the complex *thériaque céleste* of Strassburg, the formula of which, as given by Marc Mapp (1695), was repeated in the Strassburg pharmacopeias of 1725 and 1757 and charmingly represented, as a lay-out in colors, in an advertisement of the Strassburg druggist Stroehlin (1744). See E. Wickersheimer: La thériaque céleste, Paris, 1920.

geons "kept on prescribing and using their oils, ointments, plasters, vulnerary drinks, etc.," for the same reason.[1] That English clergymen dabbled in therapeutics is plain from the lucubrations of Bishop Berkeley on the virtues of tar-water (1720–48) and John Wesley's *Primitive Physick* (1747).

Except in France, the status of **surgery** was exceedingly low during the greater part of the 18th century. The French surgeon owed the improvement in his social condition to the fistula of Louis XIV and its successful treatment by Félix, which made the latter and his successor, Mareschal, royal surgeons. In 1724, Mareschal obtained from Louis XV the creation of five chairs of surgical instruction at St. Côme. The Paris Faculty immediately went into revolt and, in spite of the king's order, made a public demonstration against the surgeons.[2] Decked out in their scholastic robes, the physicians, headed by the dean of the Faculty, preceded by a beadle and an usher, marched to St. Côme in solemn array, in spite of the bitter cold weather, the snow and sharp sleet, which made their red robes almost unrecognizable. Cheering one another on with cries and oaths and followed by a great crowd of people, they at length ranged themselves in a long line against the wall, while the dean presented himself at the door of the College accompanied by the only anatomist of the Faculty, who stood behind him holding a skeleton. Cries and imprecations, knocks, and threats to break down the door, were only greeted by the jeers of the students from within, and when an usher tried to make himself heard as to what the surgeons owed to the physicians, the people suddenly turned against these formalities, which they had once respected like a religion, and drove the doctors away without regard for their furs and costly raiment. Two steps more put the surgeons on a social and scientific level with the doctors, viz., the foundation of the Academy of Surgery, the first session of which was held on December 18, 1731; and the ordinance of Louis XV (1743), delivering the surgeons from further association with barbers and wig-makers, who were forbidden to practise, while no one could be a master in surgery thereafter without being a master of the arts. This was the French surgeon's declaration of independence. Henceforth, he was a lettered man, prepared for his life-work by a special scientific education. The King was inspired to make this wise move by François **de la Peyronie** (1678–1747) the eminent Montpellier surgeon who, with Georges Mareschal (1658–1736) had founded the Academy of Surgery and, in fact, devoted his entire fortune to the advancement of his beloved art.

In addition to Mareschal's five surgical professorships of 1724, La Peyronie founded a sixth at his own expense, with an assistant to each professor, and also obtained four chairs of surgery for Montpellier, laying upon each incumbent the obligation of lecturing on obstetrics to both surgeons and midwives. In his will, he left a legacy of annual prizes in surgery, his two houses in the Grande Rue, and 100,000 francs to build the amphitheater of St. Côme, now the Bourse and the Chamber of Commerce. It was due to La Peyronie that Paris became the surgical center of the world in the 18th century.

[1] J. S. Billings: History of Surgery (Dennis's "System"), New York, 1895, i, 70.

[2] E. Forgue: Montpellier méd., 1911, xxxiii, 10, 11.

During the French Revolution, the 18 medical faculties and 15 medical colleges of France were abolished by vote in 1792, and along with them the *Société royale de médicine* (founded 1776) and the *Académie de chirurgie* (1731). This was modified in 1794, by the creation of *Écoles de santé*, the title of "health officer" (*officier de santé*) being substituted for that of "doctor." All distinction between physicians and surgeons as separate guilds or cliques was broken down, and practice was thrown open to anyone who could pay for a license.[1] Hospital internes, externes, physicians, and "ordinary professors" were appointed by competitive trials (*concours*), and medical societies became *Sociétés libres de médicine*. The *Écoles de santé* were created to supply the urgent need for military surgeons for the armies of the Republic, so that the schools at Paris, Montpellier, and Strassburg were, in reality, schools of military medicine. It was soon found that this chaotic device of mob-rule was fatal to further progress, and under the Consulate, the medical and surgical faculties were restored (1803–04), with the revival of examinations and diplomas. The *concours* were finally abolished by the Bourbons after 1821.[2]

In 18th century England, there were no surgeons of first rank before the time of Pott and Cheselden, Hunter and Abernethy.

On June 24, 1745, through the good offices of Mr. Ranby, serjeant surgeon to the king, the surgeons were formally separated from the barbers as the "Masters, Governors, and Commonalty of the Art and the Science of Surgeons of London," and it was declared to be a penal offense for any one to practise surgery in London or within a radius of seven miles from it, without being duly examined and licensed by ten of their number. In getting rid of the barbers, the surgeons left them the hall, library, and plate, only appropriating to themselves the Arris and Gale endowments. By 1790, the company of surgeons had a local habitation. but Mr. Gunning, the master, reminded them that "Your theater is without lectures, your library room, without books, is converted into an office for your clerk, and your committee room is become his parlor."[3] In 1800, the Corporation of Surgeons was rechartered by George III as the Royal College of Surgeons of London and, in 1843, this body became the present Royal College of Surgeons of England. Cheselden began to lecture at St. Thomas's Hospital about 1720, Pott at St. Bartholomew's in 1763, and there had been some haphazard lecturing on anatomy in the latter institution from the year 1734 on. The London Hospital began to take in students in 1742, and was fully organized by 1785. When Guy's Hospital was opened to students in 1769, it was agreed that all surgeons of the hospital should lecture on their subject now and then. In those days, "students went for their anatomy to Windmill Street, for their midwifery to Queen Street, and for their 'Chymistry, Materia Medica and Practice of Physic' to that new home of other delights—Leicester Square." The fees were £50 for one year's dressing under a surgeon and £25 for "walking the hospital" (Charles[4]), Surgical teaching in Edinburgh began vaguely with the Monro dynasty, whose whole concern was anatomy. The only Edinburgh surgeons of prominence were Benjamin Bell and John Bell whose unfortunate passion for controversy kept him out of the Royal Infirmary and thus deprived students of the only surgeon who could have taught them properly. In Ireland, the guild of barbers chartered by Henry VI in 1446, was combined with the surgeons by the charters of Elizabeth (1572) and James II (1687); but they began to break asunder in 1745, and in 1784, the surgeons

---

[1] For a specimen "examination" of 1803, with the illiterate answers given, see E. Wickersheimer: Paris méd., 1912–13, suppl., 749–751.

[2] Baas: *Op. cit.*, pp. 749, 760, 774.

[3] Cited by Billings, *op. cit.*, p. 83.

[4] Charles: Univ. Durham Coll. Med. Gaz., Newcastle, 1916, xvi, 59.

were given their own autonomy through the creation of the Royal College of Surgeons in Ireland. Through a bequest of Sir Patrick Dun (1704), president of the College of Physicians in Ireland, medical and surgical teaching began at Dublin in 1714.

In Germany, there was little advancement of the surgeons' status before the time of Frederick the Great. Heister's illustrated treatise, printed in the vernacular (1743), was, it is true, the most popular surgical work in the 18th century[1]; but Haller lectured and wrote on the subject without having performed an operation in his life, and there was no adequate teaching, until Richter began to lecture at Göttingen (in 1766) and von Siebold at Würzburg (in 1769). Surgical practice was mainly in the hands of the barber, the executioner, and the strolling bone-setters, cataract-couchers, herniotomists and lithotomists, of whom the famous Dr. Eisenbart was the type. In Goethe's Autobiography, the barber who shaved his father is styled *der gute Chirurgus*. Even Theden, Surgeon General of the Prussian Army, was once a barber. The barber's apprentice was usually an illiterate lad, practically a servant in the household, advertised for as a bond slave if he ran away. Superstitious belief in charms and magic prevailed, and the executioner was believed to have a compact with the devil, power to deal with diseases caused by witchcraft and, from his occasional duty of breaking bones upon the wheel, he was credited with a special talent for setting fractures and dislocations. Judicial torture was, in fact, still very common in the 18th century, and approved of, for instance, by Maria Theresa.[2] Even Frederick the Great, in 1744, allowed the Prussian executioners to treat wounds, ulcers, and fractures on the ground that, if competent, they were better for the uncared masses than bungling surgeons or no surgeons at all.[3] Indeed, owing to the great need for competent surgeons in the Prussian Army, the *Theatrum Anatomicum* at Berlin (founded in 1713) was expanded in 1724 to include a *Collegium Medico-Chirurgicum*, and the Charité Hospital at Berlin was founded, in 1727, by Friedrich Wilhelm I to furnish clinical instruction to the students at the Collegium. But Frederick the Great, in his Silesian campaigns, still found his army sadly deficient in surgeons, and not only sent medical cadets to Paris and Strassburg to complete their surgical education but, in 1743, engaged 12 French surgeons, with assistants, to look after his troops. The Prussian Army surgeon of the day was ranked above a drummer and beneath a chaplain. Being a barber's

---

[1] For the library of a German surgeon in 1712 (110 volumes), see W. von Brunn: Arch. f. Gesch. d. med., Leipz., 1924–5, xvii, 199–201.

[2] Her codification of laws, the *Constitutio criminalis Theresiana* (1768), was as iron-clad in this respect as the earlier code of torture of Guazzini (1612), and while the practice was abolished by Frederick in Prussia in 1740–54, and in Saxony in 1770, it was not until 1776 that Maria Theresa consented to do away with it. Austria owes this advance to the humanitarian writings and efforts of Ferdinand von Leber and Joseph von Sonnenfels. See Max Neuburger: Wien. klin. Wochenschr., 1909, xxii, 1075–1078, and H. Schneickert: Arch. f. Krim.-Anthrop., Leipz., 1907, xxvii, 341–345.

[3] For the surgical status of the executioner in the 18th century, see K. Caröe, Janus, Amst., 1897–8, ii, 309–312.

apprentice, he had to shave the officers, and if he proved delinquent in line of duty, he could be beaten with sticks at their instance. The general ignorance and incompetence of these army surgeons gave so much dissatisfaction that, in 1785, under Surgeon General Görcke, the *Collegium Medico-Chirurgicum* was converted into a Medico-Chirurgical *Pepinière*, devoted exclusively to the education of army surgeons and retaining its connection with the Charité. This institution was also known as the *Friedrich-Wilhelms Institut* and, since 1895, has been called the *Kaiser-Wilhelms Akademie.*

The leading Prussian Army surgeons of this period were Holtzendorf, the first surgeon general (1716); Schmucker, who left some valuable collections of surgical cases (1774–82); Bilguer, who filed the first brief for a conservative attitude toward amputation (1761); Theden who was an early advocate of methodical bandaging, and Görcke, who reorganized the Prussian Army medical department. In October, 1810, the University of Berlin was opened, with such men as Hufeland, Riel, Ernst Horn, Rudolphi, and the elder Graefe in the medical faculty, and here many of the young army surgeons of the *Pepinière*, including Helmholtz, were educated. In 1748, a similar *Collegium Medico-Chirurgicum* was established at Dresden, and in 1785, under Joseph II, the Medico-Chirurgical Academy or *Josephinum* was founded at Vienna, in charge of Brambilla, for instruction in military medicine, with permanent military hospitals at Prague, Budapest, Brünn, and other cities. The pupils at the Josephinum, like those in Berlin, were usually barbers or sons of poor officials, but these institutions undoubtedly did much to elevate the status of surgery in Prussia, Saxony, and Austria. The Vienna school of ophthalmology was established, under royal patronage, by Michel Barth, in 1773.

In Russia, Peter the Great, who visited Boerhaave and Ruysch, tried to nationalize medicine, and to this end built the first hospital and medical school in Russia (copied from the Greenwich Hospital) in 1707. Being of wood, this structure was often burned down and as often rebuilt, in spite of the grumbling of the ecclesiastics, who "had to find the funds." There were 50 pupils in 1712, but the constant disputes between Synod and Senate about finances led to the neglect of the hospital, and it gradually fell into ruins. In 1754, under Elizabeth, it passed into the hands of the Military Collegium, the War Department of the period. The students were clad in a caftan or long cloak, a camisole, and breeches. There was much brawling and drunkenness among them, they were often subjected to imprisonment or beating with the knout, and from various side-lights upon this period in literature and painting, some of them may have answered to the thumb-nail sketch of the Russian poet:

> "Buried in his cravat, his coat reaching down to his heels,
> Heavily mustached, with a dull look and a falsetto voice."

Peter the Great opened the St. Petersburg Admiralty Hospital in 1716 and, in 1717, the Dry Land Hospital, which was rebuilt in 1733. In 1799, the Russian Army Medical Academy was founded, and the ancient hospital and medical school became the purely military institution which it is to-day. In 1763, the 17th century *Apteka* became a *Collegium medicum* under an "Archiater," the first of these being a Scotchman, Robert Erskine, who was also "*Leib-medik*" of Peter the Great.

A prominent feature of the bureaucratic machinery founded by Czar Peter was the institution of the "tchins" in 1722, consisting of a series of grades of nobility conferred upon the *tchinovniks*, or public servants, a very complicated scheme of degrees of gentility and precedence. Under this system it was possible for medical men to rise to almost any rank.[1]

The administration of **military medicine** became, in the 18th century, a function of government.

Limited periods of enlistment, strongly advocated by the Maréchal de Saxe in 1732, were carried out in England (three-year periods) in 1755, and permanently adopted by Venice (1766) and in the British Army in 1775. Medical examination of recruits was carried out in France during 1726–75, adopted by Prussia in 1788 and by England in 1790. Regular government barracks for troops were substituted for billeting and their hygienic requirements were discussed by all writers on the art of war and military medicine, as were also the clothing, rationing and food-supplies of troops. The common daily ration was 2 lbs. bread, 1 lb. meat, 1 pint wine, or 2 pints beer. In 1799, this issue was made at the expense of the French government and not out of the soldier's pay. Army hospitals were put under military regulation by the French in 1718 and by the English in 1762. Schools of military medicine, such as the Prussian Pepinière (1785) or the Austrian Josephinum (1785), were established, and the first journal of military medicine appeared in France in 1766. Red Cross agreements were effective at the battle of Dettingen (1743) and the Bridge of Lodi (1796). At the Berlin exposition of military medicine in 1914, five precursors of the Geneva Convention, between 1743 and 1864, were placarded. In 1748, the British Army had flying, fixed, and convalescent hospitals. Disposition of the wounded, even in Marlborough's time, being like that at the siege of Metz (1552), attempts were made to devise plans for evacuation which would not interfere with military movements. These came to a remarkable focus at the battle of Fontenoy (May 11, 1745), where, as Heizmann says, the wounded were treated on the front line by regimental surgeons, then collected at ambulance stations, where capital operations were performed and to which the walking wounded came, and finally transferred to general hospitals in near cities, or to cities further back, when these became overcrowded.[2] Yet during the Seven Years' War (1756–63), due to Frederick's methods of flank and frontal attack in close order, and of volley firing at close range, rescue of the wounded during a battle was impossible.

Many new scientific and medical societies were founded in the 18th century.

The more important were: The Royal Academies at Berlin (1700), Göttingen (1751), and Munich (1759); the Paris Académie de chirurgie (1731), and the medical societies of Edinburgh (1737), London (1773), Paris (1776), the Physical Society of Guy's Hospital (1771); the Society for Improvement of Medical Knowledge (1782), the Society for Improvement of Medical and Surgical Knowledge (1783), both of which published transactions; the Lyceum Medicum Londinense (1785), the Abernethian Society (London, 1795), and the Royal College of Surgeons at London (1800). An exclusive "Medical Society" of seven members (1752), dominated by William Hunter, published six volumes of valuable "Medical Observations and Enquiries." Of **medical libraries,** Lancisi founded the Biblioteca Lancisiana at Rome (1711) and, in 1733, the Faculty of Medicine of Paris, which possessed only 32 books, acquired from François Picoté de Bélestre some 2273 volumes, the nucleus of its present splendid collection, the largest in the modern world.[3] Similar collections by Sir Hans Sloane and John Radcliffe were the origins of the Library of the British Museum and of the Radcliffe Camera at Oxford. The earliest **medical periodicals** of the 18th century were the *Weekelijk Discours over de Pest* (Amsterdam, 1721–22), *Esculapius* (Amsterdam, 1723), *Der patriotische Medicus* (Hamburg, 1724–26), which were followed by over 100 others, of which 55 were German, 3 French, 4 English, and 1 American. It is in the files of these forgotten periodicals, Sudhoff thinks, that the unwritten cultural history of 18th century medicine is to be found.[4]

---

[1] Lancet, Lond., 1897, ii, 354–361.

[2] C. L. Heizmann: Ann. Med. History, N. Y., 1917–18, i, 294–300.

[3] For its history, see A. Chéreau: Notice sur l'origine de la Bibliothèque de la Faculté de médecine de Paris, Paris, 1878.

[4] For further details, see the histories of medical libraries and medical journalism by the present writer in Stedman's Ref. Handb. Med. Sc., N. Y., 1915, v, 706; 901.

Advancement of **medical education** in the 18th century was mainly effected in anatomy and clinical medicine.

Before the advent of John Hunter, surgery was well taught at Paris only; prior to the Monro dynasty, anatomy flourished principally on the continent. Berlin and Strassburg seem to have had the best opportunities for obtaining material for dissection. A Theatrum anatomicum founded at Berlin in 1713, was especially favored by medical legislation and, by 1876, was supplied with some 200 dead bodies of suicides and workhouse paupers. It was much frequented by foreigners. In Strassburg, under Salzmann, there were daily dissections and thrice weekly demonstrations, as early as 1708. He is said to have had 30 cadavers in 1725, and 60 in 1760, affording opportunities even for surgical work on the cadaver. At Tübingen, however, Haller, the student, did most of his dissecting on dogs and, in Paris, he had to flee for his life for body-snatching. At Leyden, Albinus got only one cadaver a year, and Friedrich Hoffmann, at Halle, only 20 bodies in twenty-four years. In Prague, there were only three dissections during the period 1692–1712. In Vienna, there was hardly a dissection as late as 1741, although an anatomic theater had been opened in 1718. In Great Britain, chairs of anatomy were established at Edinburgh (1705), Cambridge (1707), Glasgow (1718), Oxford ("lecturer on anatomy," 1762), Dublin (1785), while the four cadavers allotted to the Company of Surgeons (1540) and the College of Physicians (1565) had been increased by Charles II to six. The first professor of the subject was Robert Elliot, who assumed his Edinburgh chair in 1705, at an annual salary of £15, and resigned in favor of Monro *primus* in 1720. The matriculation tickets and certificates of attendance at Edinburgh in these early days were written or printed upon the backs of ordinary playing cards. The ticket of Ralph Asheton, of Philadelphia, to the second course of anatomy in 1758, is made out upon the back of a deuce of spades (Packard[1]). Even under the Monro dynasty, instruction was very rudimentary, the whole demonstration being done upon a single cadaver, while the vessels and nerves were studied in a fetus and surgical operations taught upon a dog. The dissecting rooms of the time, as depicted in old engravings, were unwholesome places. Jesse Foot recalled five lecturers on anatomy who had died of "putrid myasma" from foul cadavers furnished by the resurrection men. John Bell,[2] in his reply to Gregory's diatribes, gives some grim details of bungling, incompetent surgery as a result of anatomic ignorance. In one operation for stone (1808), the patient was kept in intense suffering for over thirty minutes and, even then, the stone could not be extracted, although the normal time limit for a lithotomy in those pre-anesthetic days was about five minutes, and Cheselden usually did it in three. In Italy, before the time of Scarpa, Felice Fontana's wax preparations[3] were used in lieu of cadavers for teaching purposes. In Spain, until the middle of the century, there was no anatomic teaching at all.

With such a great leader as Linnæus, it was natural that botany should have been extensively cultivated in this period. In England, Fothergill, Cruikshank, and others had private botanic gardens of their own. Kew Gardens was established as a royal preserve about 1730, and a Physic Garden was added to it in 1759, with William Aiton, and later Sir Joseph Banks, as managers. Other gardens were established at St. Petersburg (1713), Vienna (1754), Cambridge (1762), Madrid (1763), St. Vincent (1764), Coimbra (1773), Calcutta (1786), Sydney (1788); and the garden of the Royal Dublin Society at Glasnevin was opened about 1796. It is said that there were about 1600 botanic gardens in Europe at the end of the 18th century. The interest in botany in the New World is sufficiently evidenced by the generic names Claytonia, Coldenia, Kuhnia, Gardenia, Mitchella, Bigelowia, Marshallia, Bartonia, etc., which were bestowed upon colonial plants by Linnæus and others in honor of American botanists (H. A. Kelly[4]).

---

[1] Packard: History of Medicine in the United States, Philadelphia, 1901, plate opposite p. 158.

[2] John Bell: Letters on Professional Character and Manners, Edinburgh, 1810, pp. 590–592.

[3] The Museum of the Abbate Felice Fontana (1730–1803) was the most famous anatomic collection of its kind in the 18th century, containing over 1500 preparations in wax, many of them made after Mascagni's dissections. These still exist, "beautiful to look at, but inaccurate and of little scientific value" (J. S. Billings).

[4] H. A. Kelly: Jour. Am. Med. Ass., Chicago, 1911, lviii, 437–441.

Except at Leyden, there was no **clinical instruction** on the continent until 1745, when an ambulatory clinic was established at Prague, which lasted about one year. In 1745, van Swieten organized a clinic at Vienna, consisting of 12 beds at the Bürgerspital, in charge of de Haën, who published clinical reports of the work. The example was followed by Borsieri de Kanilfeld at Pavia (1770), at Prague under von Plenciz (1781), at Göttingen under Frank (1784), at Jena under Hufeland about 1793. Bedside instruction was reintroduced into France by Desbois de Rochefort in 1780. In England, chairs of clinical medicine were established at Edinburgh in 1741 and Oxford in 1780. About 1757, Cullen began to lecture on medicine in English instead of Latin. English physicians, no doubt, got a great deal of their early clinical knowledge from association with a patron or preceptor, as we have seen in the case of Mead, who inherited his practice from Radcliffe. The special feature of modern English clinical instruction, the **hospital medical school,** had its beginnings in such institutions as Guy's Hospital (1723), the Edinburgh Hospital (1736), or the Meath Hospital (Dublin, 1756), and attained a definite status at the London Hospital Medical School (1785), and at St. Bartholomew's under Abernethy (1790). Private instruction, such as that of Smellie in obstetrics, Cullen in internal medicine, Black in chemistry, or the Hunters in anatomy, surgery, and obstetrics, was the feature of the period. The private medical school of Sir William Blizard and Maclaurin became, in 1785, the London Hospital Medical School. On June 14, 1710, the School of Physic in Trinity College, Dublin, was founded by a grant for a chemical laboratory and anatomic theater, and on February 22, 1711, Thomas Molyneux was chosen professor of physic. The scope of this school was further enlarged by the acts of 1785 and 1800, and, in 1825 it acquired a new set of buildings, which made the reforms of Graves and Stokes possible. Private instruction in midwifery was first given by Grégoire, sr., in Paris in 1720, but by 1797 there was a school for midwives at the Maternité under Baudelocque. Obstetric instruction was first given at Strassburg (1728), followed by a school for midwives (1737), and at Vienna (1748). The first German institution for the instruction of male obstetricians was founded under Röderer at Göttingen (1751), to be followed by schools for midwives and obstetricians at Berlin (1751), at Tübingen (1759), at Berne, under Venel (1782), at Cassel about 1760, at Jena (1788), at Marburg (1790), and at Würzburg under von Siebold (1778–99). In Edinburgh, instruction for midwives was given by Joseph Gibson (1726), in England by John Maubray (1724) and Richard Manningham (1736), in Dublin by Bartholomew Mosse (1746) and his successor Sir Fielding Ould (1759). Mosse's private lying-in hospital at Dublin (opened March 15, 1745) was the first institution of the kind in the United Kingdom. In 1751, Mosse, a surgeon and obstetrician of philanthropic turn, began the construction of the Rotunda Hospital, Dublin (opened December 8, 1757). Chairs of midwifery were established at Edinburgh (1739), at Dublin (1743), and at Glasgow (1815). The British Lying-in Hospital was founded in 1749, the City of London Lying-in Hospital in 1750, the Queen Charlotte Hospital in 1752, and an obstetric polyclinic was opened at Meath Hospital (Dublin) by Fleury in 1763. In Italy, schools for midwives were opened at Piedmont (1728), Padua (1769), and Rome (1786). Bedside instruction in pediatrics was introduced by Rosenstein (Stockholm) in 1760 (Jacobi). In 1795, Trommsdorff established a Chemico-Pharmaceutical Institute at Erfurt, which raised pharmacy to the dignity of a science. **Medical history** was taught at the Paris Faculty by Goulin (1795–99) and Cabanis (1799–1808), but the chair was abolished up to 1818, when it was again occupied by Moreau de la Sarthe (1818–22[1]).

Many new **hospitals** were built in the 18th century, but, in respect of cleanliness and administration, these institutions sank to the lowest level known in the history of medicine. The principal London hospitals were the Westminster (1719), Guy's (1725), St. George's (1733), the London (1740), the Middlesex (1745), and the Small-pox Hospital (1746), and there were provincial hospitals at York (1710), Salisbury (1716), Cambridge (1719), Bristol (1735), Windsor (1736), Northampton (1743), Exeter (1745), Worcester (1745), Newcastle (1751), Manchester (1753), Chester (1755), Leeds (1767), Stafford (1769), Oxford (1770), Leicester (1771), Norwich (1771), Birmingham (1778), Nottingham (1782), Canterbury (1793), and Stafford (1797). In Scotland, hospitals were founded at Edinburgh (Royal Infirmary, 1729, 1736), Aberdeen (1739), Dumfries (1775), Montrose (1780), Glasgow (1794), and Dundee (1795); in Ireland, at Cork (1720–22), Limerick (1759), and Belfast (1797), while the earliest of the Dublin hospitals were the Jervis Street (1726), Steevens's (1733),

---

[1] L. Hahn: Janus, Amst., 1899, iv, 26.

Mercer's (1734) and the Meath Hospital (1756). The Royal Sea-Bathing Infirmary for Scrofula, a new departure in the treatment of surgical tuberculosis, was opened at Margate in 1791. Children's hospitals were founded at London by George Armstrong (1769), at Vienna by J. J. Mastalier and L. A. Gölis (1787). The Charité at Berlin (1710), the Albergo dei poveri at Naples (1751), the Allgemeines Krankenhaus at Vienna (1784), the Necker (1779), Cochin (1780), Beaujon (1785), and St. Antoine (1795) at Paris were among the larger hospitals founded on the continent. To Catherine II, Moscow owed the Catherine, Pavlovski, and Golitzin Hospitals, an insane asylum and a foundling asylum (1764); St. Petersburg the Obukhovski Hospital (1784), a Foundling Hospital (1770), and a "Secret Hospital" for venereal diseases (1763), the linen of which was marked "Discretion."

In 1788, Jacobus-René **Tenon** published a series of memoirs on the **hospitals** of Paris,[1] containing his famous description of the old Hôtel Dieu, which was at that time a veritable hotbed of disease. There were some 1220 beds, most of which contained from four to six patients, and also about 486 beds for single patients. The larger halls contained over 800 patients crowded on pallets or often lying about miserably on heaps of straw, which was in vile condition. Acute contagious diseases were often in close relation to mild cases, vermin and filth abounded, and the ventilation was often so abominable that the attendants and inspectors would not enter in the morning without a sponge dipped in vinegar held to their faces. Septic fevers and other infections were the rule. The average mortality was about 20 per cent., and recovery from surgical operations was, in the nature of things, a rarity. The same thing was true of the *Allgemeines Krankenhaus* of Vienna, the Moscow Hospital, and many other institutions of size, and it was not until John Howard had made his exhaustive studies of the condition of European hospitals, prisons, and lazarettos (1777–89), and after Tenon had published his report (1788), that any attempts at reforms were made. Baas says that, in Frankfurt am Main and other cities, "even physicians declined hospital service as equivalent to a sentence of death." Under Louis XVI and Joseph II, reforms were finally made in Paris and Vienna, with a very creditable and significant reduction of mortality. One result of Tenon's report was the foundation of the present *Hôpital des enfants malades* (1802), at the time the largest children's hospital in Europe. When the Czar Paul came to the throne, he was so horrified with the condition of the Moscow Hospital that he ordered its reconstruction in 1797, with the result that the new Moscow Hospital, with accommodations for 1280 patients, was completed in 1802. But hospitals remained notorious for uncleanliness and general danger to life well into the 19th century, indeed, there are persons alive today who recall the horror in which they were held. The real angel of purity and cleanliness was Florence Nightingale, and there was no such thing as surgical cleanliness before the time of Lister.

Bad as was the management of hospitals, the **treatment of the insane** was even worse. They were either chained or caged when housed, or, if harmless, were allowed to run at large, the Tom o' Bedlams

---

[1] J.-R. Tenon: Mémoires sur les hôpitaux de Paris, Paris, 1788.

of England or the wizards and warlocks of Scotland (Lochiel in Campbell's poem). The earliest insane asylums in the northern countries were Bedlam (1547), the Juliusspital at Wurtzburg (1567), St. Luke's in London (1751), the Quaker or County Asylum near York (1792, and the *Narrenthurm*, or "Lunatics' Tower" (1784), one of the showplaces of old Vienna, where, as in ancient Bedlam, the public were allowed to view the insane, like animals in a menagerie, on payment of a small fee. The latter institution was described by Richard Bright in 1815 as a fanciful, four-story edifice having the external appearance of a large round tower, but consisting on the inside of a hollow circle, in the center of which a quadrangular building arose, joined to the circle by each of its corners. The inclosed structure afforded residence for the keepers and surgeons. The circular part contained 300 patients, "whose condition," says Bright, "is far from being as comfortable as in many of the establishments for the insane which I have visited."[1] It was not closed until 1853. Until well into the 19th century, insanity was regarded not only as incurable, but as a disgrace rather than a misfortune. Heinroth (1818) even regarded it as a divine punishment for personal guilt of some kind, just as the recent tendency is to attribute all kinds of personal guilt to insanity. In such later asylums as those erected at Munich (1801), Sonnenstein (1811), Siegburg (1815) and Sachsenburg (1830), the sad lot of the insane was that of Hogarth's engraving and Kaulbach's celebrated drawing. Mönkemöller's researches on German psychiatry in the 18th century, based on the records of Hanoverian asylums at Celle and elsewhere,[2] confirm what Reil wrote of German asylums in his "Rhapsodies" of 1803, and go to show that the theoretic part of the science in this period was nebulous philosophic speculation. Insanity was still attributed to yellow and black bile or to heat in the dog days, and symptoms, such as exaggerated self-esteem, jealousy, envy, sloth, self-abuse, etc., were regarded as causes. Kant, in his *Anthropologie* (1798) actually improvised a semeiology of insanity and maintained that, in criminal causes, it was the province, not of the medical, but of the philosophical faculty. The cases treated were all of the dangerous, unmanageable, or suicidal type, and no hope of recovery was held out. There was an extensive exhibition of drugs and unconditional belief in their efficacy. A case that did not react to drugs was regarded as hopeless. Melancholia was treated by opium pills, excited states by camphor, pruritus by diaphoresis, and a mysterious power was ascribed to belladonna: if it failed, everything failed. Other remedies were a mixture of honey and vinegar, a decoction of *Quadenwurzel*, large doses of lukewarm water, or, if this failed, "that panacea of psychiatry, tartarus tartarisatus." The costly aqua benedicta Rolandi, with three stout ruffians to admin-

---

[1] Bright: Travels . . . through Lower Hungary, Edinburgh, 1818, 87, 88.
[2] Mönkemöller: Zur Geschichte der Psychiatrie in Hannover, Halle, 1903. Also: Allg. Ztschr. f. Psychiat., Berl., 1902, lix, 193–210. Also: Psychiat.-neurol. Wochenschr., Halle, 1911–12, xiii, 211, 220, 232.

ister it, a mustard plaster on the head, venesection at the forehead and both thumbs, clysters, and plasters of Spanish fly, were other resources. Barbarities were kept in the background, but the harsh methods of medieval times were none the less prevalent. A melancholic woman was treated with a volley of oaths and a douche of cold water as she lay in bed. If purgatives and emetics failed with violent patients, they came in for many hard knocks, with a régime of bolts and chains to inspire fear. A sensitive, self-conscious patient was confined in a cold, damp, gloomy, mephitic cell, fed on perpetual hard bread, and otherwise treated as a criminal. The diet—soup, warm beer, a few vegetables and salad—was of the cheapest. There were some attempts at open-door treatment, such as putting the patients to mind geese, sending them to the mineral baths at Doberan, Töplitz, Pyrmont, Vichy, Bath or Tunbridge Wells, or sending them as harvest hands to Holland (*Hollandgeherei*). Marriage was also recommended as a cure.

The Quaker retreat, founded by William Tuke in 1794 at York, England, was the first attempt at humane treatment of the insane before the advent of Philippe **Pinel** (1745–1826), who, on May 24, 1798, with the consent of the National Assembly, struck off the chains from 49 insane patients at Bicêtre, as depicted in the painting of Tony-Robert Fleury.

In *Emile* (1762), Jean-Jacques **Rousseau** made his famous protest against the disinclination of French mothers to nurse their own children, as a source of weakness to the nation. At this time, the rate of **infantile mortality** was appalling. Of 31,951 children admitted to the Paris Foundling Hospital during 1771–77, 25,476 (80 per cent.) died before completing the first year, as against 7601 out of 15,104 during 1820–22. At the Dublin Foundling Asylum, during 1775–96, only 45 survived out of 10,272 (99.6 per cent. mortality). Sir Hans Sloane stated that the ratio of mortality of dry-nursed to breast-fed infants was as three to one. In the early 19th century, Marshall Hall said that 7 in 10 dry-nursed children died. At the British Lying-in Hospital, compulsory feeding at the mother's breast lowered the mortality 60 per cent. The hired wet-nurse had her palmiest period at the end of the 18th century, usually getting 25 guineas a year or 10 a quarter. In order to make money in this way, young unmarried women deliberately had illegitimate children, who were destined to die through baby-farming or in the foundling hospitals. In England, the wet-nurse became a tyrant in the household until she was put out of business by the nursing bottle. In France, the evil grew apace and added to the depopulation caused by the Revolution and the Napoleonic wars. The earliest substitute for mother's milk was water-pap, made of boiled bread or baked flour moistened. To this panada, Lisbon sugar was sometimes added. Then followed French bread, Uxbridge rolls, turtle-doves, and small beer. With clear insight, Michael Underwood (1784) recommended boiled cow's milk diluted with barley-water, and added rice, tapioca, and semolina to the semi-solid foods. He curtailed the period of suckling to a twelvemonth, introduced Mrs. Relf's nipple-shield, and suggested a special diet for infants in sickness and fever. Thus **artificial infant feeding** had its origin in the 18th century. In the early 19th century, the term of weaning was less than a year, but the attempt to regulate it was given up in favor of subsequent mixed feeding. Oatmeal, cowslip tea, boiled barley, star-of-anise in milk and German beer-soup came into vogue, to be followed by sago-milk, arrowroot, "tops and bottoms" (tiny baked and browned bits of dough), isinglass and jellies. "Liebig's food" (malted milk) and flour came in in 1867. The original sucking-bottle was a cow's horn, already known in 1783, and highly recommended by Heberden. This was followed by the glass bottle, the pap-boat, and the pap-spoon. The nipple was made successively of parchment and leather, sponge, heifer's teats kept in spirit, wood and india-rubber. M. Darbo's *biberon* came in with the Paris Exposition (1867), and, in

1869, C. H. F. Routh introduced a simpler form, which underwent the usual improvements.[1]

Outbreaks of epidemic diseases were more scattered and isolated than in former centuries. Malarial fever, influenza, and scarlatina were often pandemic; smallpox, diphtheria, and whooping-cough were widely diffused, but plague, syphilis, ergotism were far less malignant and, with the return of Halley's comet in 1758, people began to get rid of various superstitious theories in regard to the origin of epidemic diseases. During 1702–05, southern Italy was visited by a series of earthquakes (described by Baglivi) which destroyed some 20,000 lives, and the winter of the year 1708–09 was beset with such intense cold that even Venice was icebound. Lancisi said that this winter was as fatal to life as the pest, and the general destruction of vegetation and consequent shortening of the food-supply brought on famine, diseases of cattle, and ergotism. Inundations and fluctuations of heat and cold were followed by epidemics of malarial and typhus fevers in the first quarter of the century, and during 1720–50 these gave place to diphtheria and the exanthemata. At the beginning of the century, the principal focus of the plague was in Turkey and the Danube region; by 1703, it was devastating the Ukraine, whence, through the war of Charles XII with Russia, it gradually spread to the Baltic Sea and the Scandinavian countries. Danzig sustained a mortality of 32,599 (January 5 to December 7, 1709) and Prussia and Lithuania lost 283,733 during 1709–10. The epidemic suddenly disappeared after a hurricane which swept over all Europe on February 27, 1714; but it was again introduced, this time in the south of France, devastating Provence during 1720–22. It was again prevalent along the Danube and in the Ukraine (1734) and, in 1743, cost Messina (Sicily) 30,000 lives. The most severe epidemic was that at Moscow in 1770–71, in which the total mortality was 52,000 out of a population of 230,000. This epidemic was checked through the prophylactic measures of Orräus, but matters were further complicated by the outbreak of a revolution. In England, Richard Mead's Discourse on the plague (1720) effected the humane sanitary reform of isolating plague patients outside the city limits, instead of incarcerating them in their own houses. Typhus or camp fever was, of course, especially prevalent during all the wars of the century, in particular the long contest between Frederick the Great and Maria Theresa (1740–48), the Seven Years' War (1756–63), and the French Revolution (1789–99), with the events preceding it. One Prussian outbreak of typhus (1757) was described by the statician Süssmilch, one of Frederick's army chaplains. Typhus was particularly fatal at Prague (1742), around Mainz (1760), and, as "famine fever," in Ireland (1740), where a failure of the potato crop cost 80,000 lives, in Saxony (1778), and Italy (1783). Jail fever was again rife at the Black Assize at the Old Bailey (London) in 1750, carrying off the Lord Mayor, 3 judges, 8 of the Middlesex jury and over 40 others, all on the left side of the court-room. At the instance of Stephen Hales and Pringle, the Corporation of London tried to ventilate Newgate Prison and to remove the distemper, but without avail. Lind, from experiences on board ship, stated that ventilation would not stop jail fever, which he regarded as "the most fatal and general cause of sickness in the Royal Navy." He recommended such modern delousing procedures as stripping, bathing, and baking infestated clothing in ovens, yet, because sulphur does not destroy lice, concluded that "contagion is not propagated by animalcules."[2] At this time, the clinical minutiæ were well known and preventive measures at hand, yet disregarded, as plainly sensed in Burns' lines *To a Louse*. In 1774, on recommendation of John Howard, Alexander Popham (1729–1810), M. P. for Taunton, introduced his celebrated bill for the prevention of the gaol distemper, an admirable bit of sanitary legislation, the provisions of which were, however, largely evaded. The old window-tax of March 25, 1696 (7. and 8. William and Mary, Cap, 18) was pushed to an exorbitant extreme in 1746–7 (20.–21. George II) and, says Creighton,[3] "was enforced by a galling and corrupt machinery of commissioners, receivers-general and collectors paid by results," with consequent circumvention by the rich and self-stifling by the poor, until abated by the law of 1803, which went back to the original plan of rating houses and their windows as a whole. This tyrannous tax on light and air (abolished 1851) was an activator of infection, in dark houses throughout the entire 18th century. In France, the window-tax and the salt-tax

---

[1] Forsyth: Proc. Roy. Soc. Med., Lond., 1910–11, iv, Sect. Dis. Child., 121–141. H. Brüning: Arch. f. Gesch. d. Med., Leipz., 1907–8, i, 326–328.

[2] MacArthur: Tr. Roy. Soc. Trop. Med., Lond., 1927, xx, 494–502.

[3] Creighton: History of Epidemics in Britain, Cambridge, 1894, ii, 88–90.

(*gabelle*) were among the many sources of discontent which led to the Revolution. Infection with typhus was a commonplace in darkened, vermin-infested houses. In keeping track of the course of communicable diseases by the bills of mortality, remarkable work was done by such pioneer epidemiologists as Haygarth at Chester (1772–81), Percival (1772–6) and Ferriar (1790–1804) at Manchester, Lettsom in London (1773–1808), Aikin and Price at Warrington (1773–81), John Clark at New Castle (1777–89), Heysham at Carlisle (1779–1814) and Currie at Liverpool (1791–8), almost the only physicians of the time who followed these diseases among the poor.[1] Typhus and typhoid fevers were, of course, confused, and were variously termed "putrid," "gastric," or "nervous." Baglivi described typhoid as "mesenteric fever"; Huxham, during the Plymouth epidemic of 1737, clearly distinguished between "putrid" (*febris putrida*) or typhus, and "slow nervous fever" (*febris nervosa lenta*) or typhoid fever. During the heavy typhoid epidemic at Göttingen (1757–63), a careful account of the disease was published, in 1762, by Johann Georg Roederer, professor at the Göttingen clinic, and his assistant Wagler, who made autopsies of the cases.[2] The intestinal lesions were carefully noted, but the authors regarded the disease as identical with intermittent fever and dysentery. Perhaps for this very reason the unique monograph was soon forgotten, although Cotugno is said to have made similar postmortem observations in Italy. The old theory of epidemic constitutions was still in the ascendant, and Stoll of Vienna thought that the diseases of "bilious type," which had been prevalent since 1760, began to take on a "putrid" character about 1779–82, a view which won much consideration in Germany and Italy. Stoll regarded nearly all fevers and inflammatory diseases as "gastro-bilious," with emetics as the standard remedy. Malarial fever and dysentery played havoc in camps and were clearly defined and distinguished in the careful observations of Pringle. **Malarial fever** was spread by inundations, pollution of streams, and the unsanitary condition of streets and sewers. The Italian epidemic of 1715 was described by Lancisi and Baglivi. **Dysentery** was widely prevalent on the continent throughout the century. The term **"puerperal fever"** was introduced by Edward Strother (*Criticon febrium*, 1716). Its contagious (epidemic) character was noted at the Hôtel Dieu by Malouin (1746), at the British Lying-in Hospital (London) by Leake (1760), at the Dublin Lying-in Hospital (1767–88) by Joseph Clarke, at Aberdeen (1760–92) by Alexander Gordon (1795). A classic description of the Swiss epidemic in the cantons of Bern and Thurgau was published by Zimmermann in 1762. **Scarlatina** was common, and, from 1776 on, spread over both hemispheres. The monograph of Plenciz (1762) describes the disease to a *contagium animatum*. It was still confused with measles, which also caused a high mortality in the French and German cities and in Brazil (1749). Experimental inoculations of measles were made by Francis Home in 1759. There were several pandemics of **influenza** in both the old world and the new. Lancisi described the influenza epidemic of 1709–10. In 1712, epidemics occurred at Tübingen (*Schlafkrankeit*) and at Turin, which, as described by Camerarius (1712) and Guidetti (1725), were probably identical with the encephalitis lethargica (Economo 1917). A similar outbreak occurred at Tübingen in 1729. The term "influenza" was first employed in English by Huxham (1767) in his account of the vernal catarrh of 1743, which was first called *grippe* by the flippant Parisians. A Swedish epidemic of 1757–8, with the same symptoms, was attributed by Rothmann (1763), a pupil of Linnæus, to radish seeds in threshed grain, and called Raphania. The first case of botulism was described in Germany in 1755. In describing the Upsala epidemic of 1756–8, Boström (1760) was the first after Fernel (1544) to note the protean nervous manifestations. In Saillant's *Tableau historique* (1780), which became a source of authority down to the time of Leichtenstern, the semeiology was limited to the banal febrile catarrh of the air-passages. This narrow view was maintained later by Andral, ridiculed by Broussais and perpetuated by Hirsch (1860), even beyond the period of Creighton's exegesis (1891–5[3]). Infantile poliomyelitis, a possible nervous sequel, afflicted Sir Walter Scott (1773) and was first described by Underwood (1784). Diphtheria, yellow fever, whooping-cough, and epidemic pneumonia were wide-spread; croup and erysipelas were occasionally epidemic. The term "yellow fever" was first employed by Griffith Hughes in his "Natural History of Barbadoes" (1750). Puerperal fever was often confused with "miliary" or sweating fever (*Schweissfriesel*). **Smallpox** was so common everywhere that it was taken for

---

[1] Creighton, ii, 134 and *passim*.   [2] These findings were challenged by Murchison.

[3] F. G. Crookshank: Influenza, Lond., 1922, 42–80, *passim*.

granted and only the heavier epidemics were recorded, *e. g.*, in Paris (1719), Sweden 1749–65), Vienna (1763, 1767), Tuscany (1764), and London (1766, 1770). It was particularly destructive in the East Indies (1770–71), and among the Indians of the new world (Haeser). The great success of Jennerian vaccination has obscured the early history of the other preventive measure which it eventually displaced, viz., inoculation of human virus or **variolation.** Arnold Klebs, in his interesting study of variolation,[1] divides its history into an introductory period (1713–21), a period of stagnation (1727–46), a second revival (1746–64), and a scientific and experimental period (1764–98). The practice was introduced into Europe by Emanuel Timoni and Pilarini, who published accounts of it in 1713 and 1716, respectively. Timoni's daughter was inoculated in 1717, and the inoculation of the children of Lady Wortley Montagu followed (1718–21). In 1721, Boylston began to inoculate in Boston, Massachusetts, and, by 1752, had 2124 inoculations, with 30 deaths, while in Charleston (South Carolina), Kirkpatrick had inoculated between 800 and 1000 in 1743, with only 8 deaths. Attenuation of the virus was attempted by passing it through several human subjects (Kirkpatrick's arm-to-arm method), by dilution with water, or by choosing the virus at the crude or unripe stage. By 1728, there had been 897 inoculations in England and Scotland, with 17 deaths. In 1760, Robert and Daniel Sutton introduced inoculation by puncture, with dietetic preparation, and had some 30,000 cases, with about 4 per cent. mortality. In Paris, Angelo Gatti, of Pisa, was given permission to inoculate by the scientific method of preparatory treatment and puncture inoculations in 1769. Gatti maintained that smallpox is caused by the introduction of a living specific virus, capable of reproducing itself. Prior to Sutton, the great danger of inoculation had been the large amount of virus used and the extensive sores, which tended to make the subject a veritable smallpox carrier. The success of the Suttons and Gatti was such that in 1768, at the instance of Voltaire, Catherine of Russia permitted herself and the Grand Duke Paul to be inoculated by Dimsdale, and, in the same year, Ingen Housz inoculated three of the imperial family in Austria after preliminary experiments upon 200 children of the Viennese suburbs. In 1770, George Motherby was inoculating at Königsberg. By 1774, Benjamin Jesty had performed his first vaccination. The subsequent success of Jenner's experiments soon swept variolation from the field, although it had well-nigh attained the status of a modern preventive inoculation. The success of vaccination was due to its relative harmlessness, there being little mortality and no possibility of convection of the disease by the vaccinated person. In England, variolation was declared a felony by Act of Parliament in 1840.

Until after the Revolution, there was little advancement in the status of **American medicine.**

Before 1800, there were five good **medical schools** established, viz., those of the University of Pennsylvania (1765), King's College, New York (1767), which became the Medical Faculty of Columbia College (1792), Harvard University (1782), the College of Philadelphia (1790), and the Medical School of Dartmouth College (1798). In 1720, Yale College conferred an honorary medical degree upon Daniel Turner, who published the first American treatises on dermatology (1714) and venereal diseases (1727). The first American to graduate abroad (Edinburgh) was John Moultrie, of South Carolina (1749). The first medical diploma to be awarded after a course of study in America was that given to John Archer at the University of Pennsylvania in 1768. It is now in the Library of the Medical and Chirurgical Faculty of Maryland. There were 63 American medical graduates at Edinburgh during 1758–88 (Packard[2]). **Medical societies** were organized in Boston (1735–41), New York City (1749), Philadelphia (1765–81), again in New York City (about 1769), Philadelphia (American Medical Society, 1773), Boston (1780), New Haven County (1784), and state medical societies in New Jersey (1766), Massachusetts (1781), South Carolina (1789), Delaware (1789), New Hampshire (1791), Connecticut (1792), and Maryland (1798). Of these, the Massachusetts Medical Society (1781), the College of Physicians of Philadelphia (1787), and the Medical and Chirurgical Faculty of Maryland (1789,

---

[1] A. C. Klebs: Die Variolation im achtzehnten Jahrhundert, Giessen, 1914.

[2] Packard: History of Medicine in the United States, Philadelphia, 1901, 156, 160. The most important were Moultrie (1749), Thomas Clayton (1758), Shippen (1761), Morgan (1763), Samuel Bard (1765), Adam Kuhn (1767), Rush (1768), William Brown (1770), Caspar Wistar (1768), Samuel L. Mitchill (1786), Physick (1792), William Gibson (1809) and S. G. Morton (1823).

incorporated 1799) are remarkable for solid performance as well as for ancient lineage and continuous descent. The societies of New Jersey (1766[1]), Massachusetts (1790), and the College of Physicians of Philadelphia (1703) issued transactions and, in 1788, the Medical Society of New Haven County, Connecticut (instituted 1784), published a thin little volume of *Cases and Observations.* The first medical periodicals of the period were the *Medical Repository* of New York (1797–1824), edited by Samuel L. Mitchill, Elihu H. Smith, and Edward Miller, a single number of a translation of the *Journal de médecine militaire* of Paris (1790), and John Redman Coxe's *Philadelphia Medical Museum* (1804). These had all been preceded by the *Mercurio volante* (October 17, 1772), the earliest Mexican medical periodical, edited by Josef Ignacio Bartolochi. The memoirs of the American Academy of Arts and Sciences were begun in Boston in 1785. The hospitals of the early period were the Pennsylvania Hospital of Philadelphia, organized in 1751, and opened in a permanent building in December, 1756, the Philadelphia Dispensary (1786), the New York Dispensary (organized 1791, incorporated 1795), and the New York Hospital, which was begun in 1773, destroyed by fire in 1775, and not rebuilt until 1791. The original of Bellevue Hospital[2] was a large room for patients in the Public Workhouse of New York City (erected in 1736). Dr. John Van Buren was the first medical officer, at £100 a year. A new building was put up on the present site of Bellevue in 1796, and here a new almshouse and hospital was opened on April 28, 1816. A fever hospital was added in 1825, a new wing in 1855, and the first ambulance service in the world was established here in 1869. The first lying-in hospital was Shippen's private institution of 1762. The first insane hospital was the Eastern Lunatic Asylum at Williamsburgh, Virginia, chartered 1772, opened 1773. The first American botanic garden was established by John Bartram at Philadelphia in 1728, and the first museum of natural history at Charleston, S. C., in 1773. Medical libraries were founded in the Pennsylvania Hospital (1762), the New York Hospital (1776), and the College of Physicians of Philadelphia (1788), the latter being now one of the finest in the country. The favorite text-books of the period were Albinus, Cowper, Cheselden, Monro, and Winslow in anatomy, Haller's First Lines of Physiology, Boerhaave and van Swieten on internal medicine, Heister's surgery, Smellie's midwifery, and, of course, Sydenham, Huxham, Pott, and other well-known authors. There was strong prejudice against dissecting, and material was usually obtained by body-snatching. There was little study of physiology or pathology, but surgery was ably taught by such men as John Jones, William Shippen, Jr., Thomas Bond, John Warren, Richard Bayley, and Wright Post. Obstetric cases were usually handled by midwives. The first male obstetricians were pupils of Smellie and William Hunter. William Shippen, jr., first lectured on the subject in Philadelphia in 1762. There were a few strolling dentists and oculists here and there but, with the exception of Perkin's tractors, we hear little of quackery in the colonial period, for the simple reason that no very rich harvest was held out to its practitioners. Witch-doctoring, in the sense of averting malign influence, was, however, still common among the Germans of southeastern Pennsylvania. It is said that the expense account of General Washington for October, 1797, shows that he paid his employee, Christopher, $25 for a visit to a German hex- and herb-doctor at Lebanon, Pa., to secure treatment for hydrophobia, which probably consisted of an infusion of red chickweed or pimpernel.[3] The *Long Hidden Friend* of George Hohman (1819), a German redemptioner who came over in 1799, is the authoritative compilation of the folklore of hex-doctoring. It is made up of herbal remedies, acrostic charms, and pious invocations, like those in Aetius and Alexander Trallianus. Acts to regulate the practice of medicine and surgery were passed in New York City (1760) and New Jersey (1772), a special ordinance for midwives in New York City (1716), quarantine acts in Pennsylvania (1700), Massachusetts (1701), Virginia (1722), New York (1758), and other states. The establishment of the Marine Hospital Service by Act of Congress (July 16, 1798) was followed by a general quarantine (National) act (February 23, 1799). The earliest Canadian medical laws were the "Quebec Ordinance" of 1788, "To Prevent Persons practising Physic and Surgery" in Lower Canada; and the Newark (Upper Canada) "Act to Regulate the Practice of Physic and Surgery" (1795), which was variously modified as time went on.

---

[1] The transactions of the Medical Society of New Jersey for 1766–1859 remained in MS. until 1875, when they were printed in one volume.

[2] "Bellevue: A Short History of Bellevue Hospital," New York, 1915.

[3] Burdick: Dietet. & Hyg. Gaz., N. Y., 1912, xxviii, 423–426. See, also, J. N. Bertloet: Phila. Month. Med. Jour., 1899, i, 730–732.

THE NINETEENTH CENTURY: THE BEGINNINGS OF ORGANIZED ADVANCEMENT OF SCIENCE

In the evolution of modern medicine, as in the development of pure science of which it was a part, three factors seem of especial moment. First of all, the great industrial or social-democratic movement of civilized mankind, which, following close upon the political revolutions in America and France, intensified the feeling for intellectual and moral liberty and upheld the new idea of the dignity and importance of all kinds of human labor, as exemplified in Napoleon's famous device: "The tools to those who can handle them" (*La carriére ouverte aux talens*). Some immediate corollaries of this proposition were the removal of the civil disabilities oppressing the Jews, and the opening out to talented womankind of occupations and modes of thought which had hitherto been closed to them. Second, the publication of such works as Helmholtz's *Conservation of Energy* (1847) and Darwin's *Origin of Species* (1859) did away forever with many of the silly antropomorphisms and appeals to human conceit which have always hampered the true advancement of medicine in the past. Third, as an inevitable consequence, physics, chemistry, and biology came to be studied as objective laboratory sciences, dissociated from the usual subjective human prepossessions. Hardly any one today doubts the theorem sustained by Emile Littré that the real advancement of biological and medical science has nothing to do with theological dogma or metaphysical speculation, but simply depends upon collateral improvements in physical and chemical procedure. Medicine owes much to the great mathematicians and physicists of the 17th and 18th centuries, who developed the theory of vision and almost the whole physiology of respiration. In the 19th century, the extension of the three fundamental branches of pure science has not been surpassed in variety by the work of any preceding age.

Of modern mathematicians, we need only mention the names of Euler, Gauss, Riemann, Jacobi, Abel, Weierstrass, Cayley, Sylvester; of physicists, Young, Carnot, Fourier, Kirchoff, Clausius, Helmholtz, Ohm, Maxwell, Lord Kelvin, Boltzmann, Gibbs, J. J. Thomson, Edison, Tesla, Arrhenius; of chemists, Dalton, Dumas, Chevreul, Berzelius, Liebig, Wöhler, Berthollet, Mendelejeff, Ostwald, van't Hoff, Ramsay, Rutherford, and the Curies.

The physical principle of Conservation of Energy was demonstrated by Robert Mayer (a physician of Heilbronn) and James Prescot Joule in 1842, and applied to the whole field of chemistry and physics by Helmholtz in 1847. The principle of Dissipation of Energy was first stated by Sadi Carnot (1824), developed by Clausius (1850) and Lord Kelvin (1852), and applied to all physical and chemical phenomena by the Yale professor, Willard Gibbs (1872-78). The generalization of Gibbs was so complete and far-reaching that it made engineering, geology, biology, medicine, and every other phase of science that deals with states of substance a branch of chemistry. An immediate consequence of Gibbs' work was the development of the new science of physical chemistry by Ostwald, Le Chatellier, van't Hoff, Roozeboom, and the chemists of the Dutch school. In physical or thermodynamic chemistry all changes of substance are treated as rigid consequences of the laws of dynamics.

In 1859, Kirchhoff and Bunsen devised spectrum analysis. Faraday (1821–54) and Maxwell (1865) worked out the whole theory of electricity and electromagnetism, upon which followed such practical consequences as electric lighting, heating, and motor power, telephonic communication, and the realization of wireless telegraphy (radio) by Hertz (1887) and Marconi (1895). The Roentgen rays were discovered in 1895. The Curies isolated radium chloride in 1898. Among physicians, Thomas Young described astigmatism (1801), stated the wave theory of light (1802), and the surface tension theory of capillarity (1805); John Dalton stated the chemical law of multiple proportions (1802) and the atomic theory (1803); William Hyde Wollaston investigated the pathological chemistry of calculi (1797–1809), suggested stereochemistry (1808), showed that gas explosions will not pass through a small tube (1814), which led to Sir Humphry Davy's safety lamp (1815); and invented the camera lucida (1807); Helmholtz invented the ophthalmoscope and the ophthalmometer (1850), the teleostereoscope (1857), and elaborated the theories of vision (1853–67) and of tonal perception (1856–63). Another physician, William Charles Wells (1757–1817), a native of Charleston, S. C., developed the theory of dew and dewpoint (1814). Photography was developed by Niepce (1814), Daguerre (1839), Draper (1840), and Fox Talbot (1840). Following Amici (1812) and Chevalier (1820), Joseph Jackson Lister (1830) devised the improved achromatic lenses of the compound microscope to which Amici gave the idea of water-immersion, Chevalier the compound objective, Purkinje stereopticon effects and reagents, and E. Abbé the modern illuminating apparatus, apochromatic objective, oil immersion, and compensating ocular (1886).

It will be seen, from the dates of these discoveries, that the modern scientific movement did not attain its full stride until well after the middle of the century. The medicine of the early half was, with a few noble exceptions, only part and parcel of the stationary theorizing of the preceding age. Up to the year 1850 and well beyond it, most of the advancements in medicine were made by the French. After the publication of Virchow's "Cellular Pathology" (1858), German medicine began to gain its ascendancy. The descriptions of new forms of disease, and the discoveries of anesthesia (1847) and antiseptic surgery (1867), were the special achievements of the Anglo-Saxon race.

On the continent of Europe, Immanuel Kant, who pointed out the limitations of thought and the subjective character of human observation, had little effect upon medical theories, but the so-called "Nature Philosophy" of Schelling, which aimed to establish the subjective and objective identity of all things, and the system of Hegel, which, like evolution today, regarded everything as in a state of becoming something else (Werden), exerted a very baneful effect upon German medicine by diverting mental activity away from the investigation of concrete facts into the realm of fanciful speculation. The "therapeutic nihilism" formulated by Skoda put a decided limitation upon Austrian medicine and, in France and Italy, a vast deal of energy, and even of human life, was wasted over the doctrines of Broussais and Rasori. It took a long time to demonstrate that the advancement of internal medicine as a science can never be accomplished by hugging some pet theory out of a regard for its author's personality, but only through the performance of a vast amount of chemical, physical, and biological research by thousands of willing workers. The first step in this direction was taken by Broussais, who did away with metaphysical conceptions of disease only to substitute something worse.

François-Joseph-Victor **Broussais** (1772–1838), the son of a Breton physician, had sworn at troops as a sergeant in the Republican Army in 1792, and swung a cutlass as a privateersman in 1798. After graduating in medicine (1803), he served for three years as an army surgeon in Napoleon's campaigns. He carried his rough schooling into his medical teaching, in which his methods were Napoleonic and his therapeutics sanguinary. Broussais modified the Brunonian theory by saying that life depends upon irritation, but, in particular, upon heat, which excites the chemical processes in the body. Disease, however, depends upon localized irritation of some viscus or organ, *e. g.*, the heart, or, above all, the stomach and in-testines. Specific morbid poisons, such as the syphil-itic virus, were to Broussais non-existent. The only mer-it in his reasoning was that he substituted the diseased organ for the hazy concept "fever" as the all-important factor, the *foyer de maladie.* To describe a mere group of symptoms as a "clinical entity" and label it with a name was to Broussais a fictive process (ontology). Gastro-enteritis he thought the "basis of all pathology,"[1] as Cullen regarded nearly everything as a neurosis or Cruveilhier as a phlebitis. Nature had no healing power and it was necessary to abort disease by active measures. To this end, he

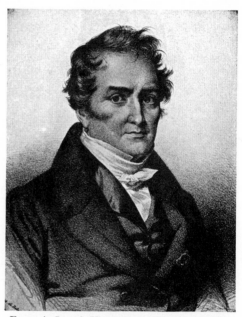

François-Joseph-Victor Broussais (1772–1838).

adopted a powerful antiphlogistic or weakening régime, the main features of which were to deprive the patient of his proper food and to leech him all over his body. As many as 10 to 50 leeches were applied at once; as many as 5 to 8 were prescribed in cases of extreme debility. Of the scarcity of leeches in Broussais' time, Baas records that "in the year 1833 alone 41,500,000 leeches were imported into France, and only nine or ten million exported. Yet in 1824–25, two or three million were sufficient to supply all demands." As he ap-proached his dotage, which O. W. Holmes has so humorously described, Broussais scolded, bullied, and wrangled with the vigor of the proverbial

---

[1] Max Neuburger says that the supposed gastric origin of most diseases (gas-tricism) had been long before advanced by Tissot, Grant, Finke, and Stoll. (Pusch-mann Handbuch, Jena, 1903, ii, 96.)

vieux militaire, and although his follower, Bouillaud, was moved to let even greater torrents of blood, students had already begun to edge away from the elder vampire, whose extravagances were finally exploded by the good sense and temperate judgment of the clinician Chomel, the statistical inductions of his pupil Louis and the sarcasms of Laennec, who slyly likened Broussais to Paracelsus. Broussais' doctrine of irritation was taken up in Germany by Roeschlaub, and occasioned a pale temporary reflex in the writings of Benjamin Travers, Pridgin Teale, and other English physicians of the period, who ascribed various diseases to "spinal irritation."

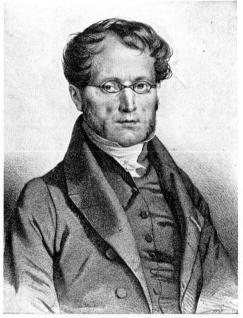

At Milan, about 1807, Giovanni Rasori began to revamp the Asclepiadean theory of constricted and relaxed conditions (which Brown had called sthenic and asthenic and Hoffman tonic and atonic) by considering diseases as states of stimulus or contrastimulus. Diagnosis of these conditions was effected by means of venesections, which were supposed to turn out beneficially in overstimulated conditions or *vice versa*. Overstimulus was opposed by sedatives, opium, and copious blood-letting; contrastimulus by huge doses of gamboge, aconite, ipecac, nux vomica, and the like. This

Pierre-Charles-Alexandre Louis (1787–1872).

method, which did as much harm as that of Broussais, had to run its course and, like the latter, eventually died out.

The arbitrary doctrines of Broussais were finally overthrown by Pierre-Charles-Alexandre **Louis** (1787–1872), the founder of medical, as distinguished from vital, statistics. After passing six years in Russia, where his despair over the impotence of medicine in a diphtheria epidemic convinced him of the necessity of deeper study, he returned to Paris to complete his medical education and, entering Chomel's clinic, devoted the rest of his life to teaching, combined with incessant dissecting and hospital practice. His principal works are his researches on phthisis (1825[1]), based upon 358 dissections and 1960 clinical cases, which point to the frequency of tubercle in the apex of the lung; his

[1] Louis: Recherches anatomico-physiologiques sur la phthisie, Paris, 1825.

work on typhoid fever (1829[1]), which gave the disease its present name (*fièvre typhoïde*), and his polemics against Broussais (1835[2]), which finally demolished the latter's "system," and, by a statistical proof that blood-letting is of little value in pneumonia, did away with its abuse in that disease. Louis thought that the fallacies of an *a priori* theory, like that of Broussais, can easily be brought out and thrown into relief by good statistics[3] and that statistics can sometimes be used as an instrument of precision in cases where proper experimental methods are wanting. Although Gavarret wrote a treatise on statistics in which therapeutic problems were especially considered (1840[4]), the idea met with no special support in Louis' lifetime, indeed, some of his own findings turned out to be jejune and without true correlation; but it has since proved its own worth in testing etiologic and hereditary data or the value of different therapeutic methods, especially through the great increase in medical periodicals, with corresponding improvements in bibliography and census-taking, which, of course, furnish the materials for good statistics. Its value was shown by Fournier and Erb in demonstrating the causal nexus between tabes, paresis, and syphilis; and by others, in testing the value of hydrotherapy in typhoid, of antitoxin in diphtheria, of operative intervention in appendicitis and other surgical conditions, or in trying out new drugs, such as "606." Louis was the first, after Floyer, to use the watch in timing the pulse, in which he was followed by the clinicians of the Irish, English, and American schools. Through his American pupils, Holmes, Gerhard, the Jacksons, the Shattucks and others, he exerted a powerful influence upon the advancement of medical science in the Eastern United States. The strong stand which Louis took in favor of facts and figures, as against the sterile theorizing of the past, appealed especially to the keen, practical common sense of these northern physicians.

The most distinguished and important internist of the early French school was Réné-Théophile-Hyacinthe **Laennec** (1781–1826), a native of Quimper (Brittany), who, like Bichat, was a regimental surgeon in the Revolution, and was also, like him, an early victim of phthisis. He was physician to the Hôpital Beaujon in 1806 and to the Hôpital Neckar in 1816. Laennec made his name immortal by his invention of the stethoscope in 1819 (at first only a cylinder of paper in his hands), and by the publication of the two successive editions of his *Traité de l'auscultation médiate* in 1819 and 1826. This work placed its author among the greatest clinicians of all ages, and had better luck than Auenbrugger's, for it was immediately taken up and translated every-

---

[1] Recherches . . . sur la maladie connue sous les noms de gastro-entérite (etc.), Paris, 1829.

[2] Recherches sur les effets de la saignée (etc.), Paris, 1835.

[3] The use of statistics in medical investigations was first suggested by the astronomer Laplace. To establish his own results, Louis made over 5000 postmortems (Neuburger, *op. cit.*, p. 139).

[4] Gavarret: Principes généraux de statistique, Paris, 1840.

where. It is the foundation stone of modern knowledge of diseases of the chest and of their diagnosis by mediate auscultation. In the first edition (1819), Laennec pursues the analytic method, giving the different signs elicited by percussion and auscultation, with the corresponding anatomic lesions (he was an expert pathologist). In the second edition (1826), the process is turned about and the method is synthetic, each disease being described in detail in respect of diagnosis, pathology, and (most intelligent) treatment, so that this edition is, in effect, the most important treatise on diseases of the thoracic organs ever written.[1] Laennec not only put the diagnostic sounds of cardiac[2] and pulmonary

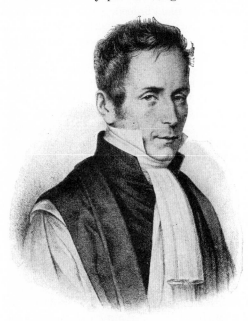

disease upon a reliable basis, but was the first to describe and differentiate bronchiectasis (first noted by his assistant Cayol in 1808), pneumothorax, hemorrhagic pleurisy, pulmonary gangrene, infarct and emphysema, esophagitis, subdeltoid bursa, and that form of cirrhosis of the liver which is now termed "chronic diffuse interstitial hepatitis." He left masterly descriptions of bronchitis, peritonitis, and pneumonia, with a full account of the pathologic appearances, and his accounts of pulmonary gangrene and emphysema needed only the retouching of Rokitansky's microscope to make the pictures classic.

Réné-Théophile-Hyacinthe Laennec (1781–1826).

He established the etiologic unity of tubercle and has been defined as "the greatest of teachers on pulmonary tuberculosis" (Heise). Laennec was also the first to discover and describe the "anatomic tubercle" or postmortem wart,[3] which McCall Anderson, in 1879, showed to be identical with lupus verrucosus; and he was the originator of such terms as "egophony," "pectoriloquy," the sonorous and sibilant "râles," and other

---

[1] Laennec's book passed through 5 French editions, viz., 1819, 1826, 1831, 1837, and 1879 (issued by the Paris Medical Faculty); two Belgian (1828, 1834); seven English (London) translations (1821, 1827, 1829, 1834, 1838, 1846, 1923) and four American (1823, 1830, 1835, 1838); three German versions (1822, 1832, 1839) and an Italian (Leghorn) translation in four volumes (1833–36). (Lawrason Brown.)

[2] For the history of our knowledge of the heart sounds before and after Laennec, see G. Joseph, Janus, Gotha, 1853, ii, 1, 345, 565.

[3] Also noted by Sir Samuel Wilks as "verruca necrogenica," in 1862.

well-recognized signs of moment in the exploration of the chest. Personally, he was a slight, nervous, aquiline figure, of generous, tolerant, unaffected nature and refined feelings. Like Auenbrugger, he was modest about his work and cared more for his proficiency in horseback riding than for fame. A statue, erected to his memory in 1868, stands in the Place Saint-Corentin, Quimper.

Of French internists contemporaneous with Louis and Laennec, Gaspard-Laurent **Bayle** (1774–1816), of Vernet (Provence), a Paris graduate of 1801, made his mark in pathology by his original description of the coarse characters of tubercle, and its identity with the pulmonary, granular and other varieties of tuberculosis (1803), which he expanded in his *Recherches sur la phthisie pulmonaire* (1810), the basis of Laennec's and of subsequent work.

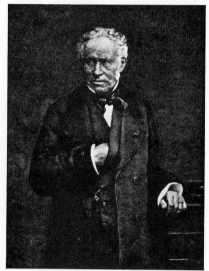

Pierre **Bretonneau** (1771–1862), of Tours, wrote important monographs on the contagion of "dothienenteritis" or typhoid fever (1819–29[1]), on diphtheria (1826[2]), giving the disease its present name; and, on July 1, 1825, performed the first successful tracheotomy in croup.[3] He located and understood the typhoid lesions in Peyer's patches as early as 1820, predicted that typhoid would some day be differentiated from typhus (1828), and, in 1855, clearly stated the doctrine of specificity (germ-theory) in disease.[4] His correspondence with his pupils, Velpeau and Trousseau, is the most interesting collection of medical letters since Guy Patin.

Pierre Bretonneau (1771–1862). (From the painting by Moreau of Tours.)

Jean-Baptiste **Bouillaud** (1796–1881), of Angoulême, although a furious blood-letter, was one of the ablest diagnosticians of his time. He was the first to point out that aphasia is correlated with a lesion in the anterior lobes of the brain (1825[5]) and he established a "law of coincidence" between the occurrence of heart disease and acute articular rheumatism (1836[6]). These researches were further extended in his

---

[1] Bretonneau: Arch. gén. de méd., Paris, 1829, xxi, 57–78.

[2] Des inflammations spéciales du tissu muqueux et en particulier de la diphthérite, Paris, 1826.

[3] Bretonneau: Des inflammations spéciales (etc.), Paris, 1826, 300–338.

[4] For these references see Paul Triaire: Bretonneau et ses correspondants, Paris, 1892, i, 303; ii, 593.

[5] Bouillaud: Arch. gén. de méd., Paris, 1825, viii, 25–45.

[6] Bouillaud: Nouvelles recherches sur le rhumatisme articulaire (etc.), Paris, 1836.

important clinical treatise on articular rheumatism of 1840.[1] Regarding fever as the effect of endocarditis or of inflammation of the intima of the blood-vessels, he favored pitilessly rapid bleeding, *"coup sur coup."*

Jean-Nicolas **Corvisart** (1755–1821), Napoleon's favorite physician, and the teacher of Bayle, Bretonneau, Dupuytren, Laennec, and Cuvier, is now remembered chiefly through his revival of Auenbrugger's work on percussion (1808), a previous translation of which had already been made by Rosière de la Chassagne (1770), but forgotten. Corvisart's *Essay on the Diseases and Organic Lesions of the Heart and the Great Vessels* (1806), the most important French treatise on cardiac disease after Senac's, was reprinted in 1818, with some simplifications and improvements of Auenbrugger's method.

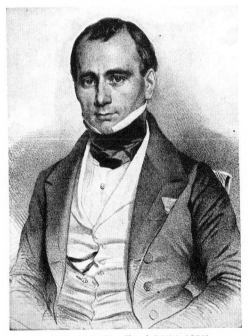

Jean-Baptiste Bouillaud (1796–1881).

The noble-minded Philippe **Pinel** (1745–1826), of Saint-Paul (Tarn), stands high in medical history as the first to treat the insane in a humane manner. On May 24, 1798, at the risk of his own life and liberty, he struck off their chains at Bicêtre, placing them in hospitals under lenient physicians, and doing away with the abuses of drugging and blood-letting to which they were subjected. In this regard he is the real founder of the modern "open-door" school of psychiatry, although his classifications of insanity and disease are now forgotten. His *Traité médico-philosophique sur l'alienation mentale* (1801) is one of the most important of medical classics. It was followed by such psychiatric milestones as Reil's Rhapsodies on the Psychic Treatment of Insanity (1803), Heinroth's books on insanity (1818), the jurisprudence of insanity (1825), and the psychology of lying (1834[2]); Calmeil on general paralysis of the insane (1826[3]); Prichard's *Treatise on Insanity*, containing the first description of moral insanity (1835); Esquirol's great work (1838[4]), Falret's original description of circular

---

[1] Traité clinique du rhumatisme articulaire, Paris, 1840.

[2] J. C. A. Heinroth: Die Lüge, Leipzig, 1834.

[3] L.-F. Calmeil: De la paralysie générale (etc.), Paris, 1826.

[4] J.-E. D. Esquirol: Des maladies mentales, 2 vols. and atlas, Paris, 1838.

insanity (1853[1]), and John Conolly on *The Treatment of the Insane without Mechanical Restraints* (1856).

Gabriel **Andral** (1797–1876), of Paris, was a clear, methodic, analytic spirit who opposed all scholastic eccentricity and fanaticism, edited the works of Laennec, joined hands with Louis in his propaganda against blood-letting, favored cold baths in typhoid and other fevers, and is to be especially remembered as the first to urge a chemical examination of the blood in morbid conditions (1843[2]).

His *Clinique medicale* (1829–33) was the first work of the kind made famous by Trousseau, Dieulafoy, and others, in which a series of medical cases is employed as a means of establishing the data of internal medicine. In Andral's series, the clinical pictures of the development of morbid processes were masterly. His chemical studies of the blood (with Gavarret), the only thing of the kind after Hunter and Hewson, led him to the conclusion that there are primary blood diseases, a phase of humoral pathology which was again to be revived by Ehrlich.

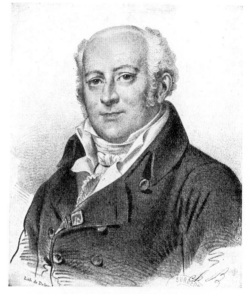

Jean-Nicolas Corvisart (1755–1821).

Pierre-Adolphe **Piorry** (1794–1879), of Poitiers, was the inventor of the pleximeter (1826) and the pioneer of mediate percussion (1828[3]).

He wrote much, including a treatise on pleximetry (1866), and, although a "poet," affected an exaggerated and pedantic nomenclature, employing such high-sounding terms as "cardiodysneuria," "hypersplenotrophy," and so forth.

Pierre-François-Olive **Rayer** (1793–1867), of Calvados, was the author of a number of works of capital importance. His treatise on skin diseases, with atlas (1826–27), succeeded Biett. His classification of skin diseases (1831) antedated Hebra in stressing pathology. He first described adenoma sebaceum. His monograph on glanders and farcy in man (1837[4]) is a classic. His three-volume treatise on diseases of the kidney, with atlas (1837–41), marks an epoch in the development of the subject. His memoir on endemic hematuria (1839) is another milestone.

Philippe **Ricord** (1799–1889), born of French parents in Baltimore,

---

[1] J.-P. Falret: Bull. Acad. de méd., Paris, 1853–4, xix, 382–400.

[2] Andral: Essai d'hématologie pathologique, Paris, 1843.

[3] Piorry: De la percussion médiate, Paris, 1828.

[4] Rayer: De la morve et du farcin chez l'homme, Paris, 1837.

Md., and a graduate of the Paris Faculty, was the greatest authority on venereal diseases after John Hunter. His treatise on the subject (1838[1]) is memorable in the history of medicine for overthrowing Hunter's erroneous ideas as to the identity of gonorrhea and syphilis (2500 inoculations), establishing the autonomy of these diseases (1831–37).

He divided lues into its primary, secondary, and tertiary stages, described vaginal, uterine, and urethral chancres, and noted the rarity of reinfection, and wrote on such subjects as the use of the speculum (1833), gonorrhea in women (1834), epididymitis (1839), gonorrheal conjunctivitis (1842).

Ricord is credited with a vast number of risky *bons mots* and anecdotes (Ricordiana) relating to his specialty. Dr. Oliver Wendell Holmes styled him "the Voltaire of pelvic literature—a skeptic as to the morality of the race in general, who would have submitted Diana to treatment with his mineral specifics, and ordered a course of blue pills for the vestal virgins."

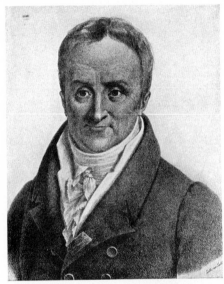

Philippe Pinel (1745–1826).

Modern **dermatology** derives from the work of Willan, and his pupil Bateman, as continued and carried forward by the French and the New Vienna schools. Robert **Willan** (1757–1812), a Yorkshire Quaker who had studied the pathologic work of Matthew Baillie to advantage, did much to clear up the nature of eczema and lupus, and divided cutaneous diseases, according to their objective appearances, into eight classes: the papular, squamous, exanthematous, bullous, vesicular, pustular, tubercular, and macular. By collating all the Greek, Latin, and Arabic terms, he established a definite classic nomenclature. His classification, which was awarded the Fothergillian gold medal in 1790, was the starting-point of modern dermatology, and is still more or less in use. Among his pupils were Bright and Addison. Willan's great work *On Cutaneous Diseases* (1796–1808), published in parts, was left unfinished at his death, and was completed by Bateman. It contains original descriptions and figurations of prurigo, pityriasis, and ichthyosis, while psoriasis (the Biblical "leprosy" of Gehazi and Naaman), sycosis, tinea versicolor, lupus, and impetigo are more clearly defined and differentiated. Osler says that the first case of Henoch's

---

[1] Ricord: Traité pratique des maladies vénériennes, Paris, 1838.

purpura (with visceral symptoms) is here described. Willan also defined erythema iris as a species of his original genus "iris" (herpes iris), and separated out the forms of eczema due to external irritation (eczema solare, impetiginodes, rubrum, mercuriale). He gave a clearer description of the "urticaria tuberosa" described by Frank in 1792. This part of his work is included in the *Delineations of Cutaneous Diseases*, an atlas of 72 colored plates published in 1817 by Thomas **Bateman** (1778–1821), of Whitby, Yorkshire. Bateman was the first to describe lichen urticatus, molluscum contagiosum, and ecthyma, which Willan had depicted as "phlyzacia."

Ecthyma terebrans or "pemphigus gangrenosa" was first described by Whitley Stokes of Dublin (1807[1]), and xanthoma by Addison and Gull (1851[2]).

The founder of the modern French school of dermatology was Jean-Louis **Alibert** (1768–1837), of Villefranche de l'Aveyron, Dr. Holmes' "jolly old Baron Alibert, whom I remember so well in his broad-brimmed hat, worn a little jauntily on one side, calling out to the students in the courtyard of the Hôpital St. Louis, *Enfans de la méthode naturelle, êtes-vous tous ici?*" This "natural method" of classifying diseases was, indeed, the passion of Alibert's life. A picture of his

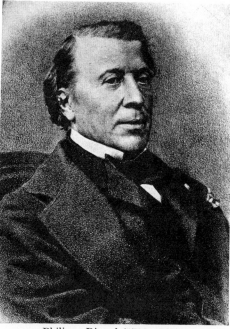

Philippe Ricord (1799–1889).

"family tree" of dermatoses, standing grim, gaunt, and solitary in the foreground of a barren, uninviting landscape, forms the initial plate of his principal work.[3] Alibert was the first to describe mycosis fungoides (*pian fungoïde*) in 1806 and keloid (*cancroïde*) in 1810 (later as *keloide* or kelis, 1835). He also described, as *pustule d'Alep* (1829[4]), the endemic ulcer now correlated with the Leishman-Donovan bodies, and introduced many new terms, such as "syphilides," "dermatoses," "dermatolysis," etc. *Un visuel et un artiste*, as Sabouraud styled him, Alibert prided himself upon the fact that he was the first to employ

[1] W. Stokes: Dublin Med. and Phys. Essays, 1807–8, i, 146–153.
[2] Guy's Hosp. Rep., Lond., 1851, 2. s., vii, 265.
[3] Alibert: Monographie des dermatoses, Paris, 1842, vol. i, plate opposite p. 1.
[4] *Ibid.*: Rev. méd. franç. et étrang., Paris, 1829, iii, 62–71.

27

the painter's palette and the burin in the delineation of skin diseases. In his clinical lectures, he was at pains to visualize everything to his pupils by long, personal, circumstantial case-histories, like those of John Bell. In his efforts to make these picturesque, he sometimes pushed the devices of rhetoric to a ludicrous and pompous extreme. Alibert's family tree was discarded for the system of Willan by his pupil Biett, who described lupus erythematosus. The ideas of Biett were further extended by Rayer (1826) and Cazenave and Schedel (1828), who made the first classifications of skin diseases upon an anatomic basis, *e. g.*, inflammations, hypertrophies, disorders of secretion and sensation, hemorrhagic manifestations, etc. This classification was the forerunner of the second phase of modern dermatology, the

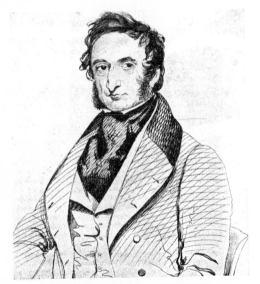

Robert James Graves (1796–1853).

pathologic or histologic period inaugurated by von Hebra and his followers, of the New Vienna School.

Laennec's teaching had an immediate outcome in Great Britain in the brilliant clinical work of two physicians of the **Irish school.** The founders of the Dublin school were John Cheyne (1777–1836), who described acute hydrocephalus (1808[1]) and Cheyne-Stokes respiration (1818[2]); Abraham Colles (1773–1843), who stated "Colles' law"; and Robert Adams (1791–1875), who left classic accounts of essential heart-block (1826[3]) and rheumatic gout (1857[4]). Other important

---

[1] Cheyne: An essay on hydrocephalus acutus, Edinburgh, 1808.

[2] Cheyne: Dublin Hosp. Rep., 1818, ii, 216. See, also, "The case of the Honourable Colonel Townshend" in George Cheyne's "English Malady" (London, 1733, 209–212).   [3] Adams: Dublin Hosp. Rep., 1827, iv, 396.

[4] Adams: Treatise on rheumatic gout, London, 1857.

members of this school were Corrigan (of "Corrigan's pulse"), William Wallace (1791–1837), who introduced the use of potassium iodide in syphilis (1836), and Francis Rynd (1801–61), who first employed hypodermic injections by a gravity device (of his invention) for the relief of pain (1845–61[1]). The true leaders of the Dublin school, however, were Graves and Stokes.

Robert James **Graves** (1796–1853), the son of a Dublin clergyman, took his medical degree in 1818, and, while making the usual continental tour, had such adventurous experiences as being arrested as a German spy in Austria on account of his fluency as a linguist, and of successfully quelling a mutiny on board ship during a storm in the Mediterranean, afterward assuming command and saving the vessel through his pluck. Returning to Dublin in 1821, he became chief physician to the Meath Hospital and one of the founders of the Park Street School of Medicine. Here he immediately went in for the widest reforms, introducing the continental methods of clinical teaching, such as making his advanced students handle and report on clinical cases, and suppressing the maltreatment and abuse which hospital patients had to endure from the rough-spoken Irish M.D.'s of the day. Tall, dark, and *distingué*, Graves had a warm heart in spite of his sarcastic speech, and once even did a stint of literary work for a poor student. His

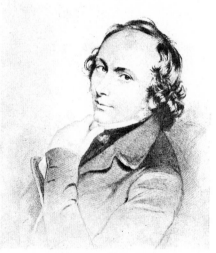

William Stokes (1804–78).

Clinical Lectures (1848), which Trousseau read and re-read with highest admiration, introduced many novelties, such as the "pin-hole pupil," timing the pulse by the watch, and discarding the old lowering or antiphlogistic treatment of fevers. He requested that the phrase "He fed fevers" should be his epithaph. Graves also left early accounts of angioneurotic edema, scleroderma and erythromelalgia (1843–8). In 1835, he published a description of exophthalmic goiter so admirable that the disease still goes by his name.[2]

William **Stokes** (1804–78), Graves' colleague at Meath Hospital, was the son of Whitley Stokes, Regius Professor of Medicine at Dublin, and succeeded his father in this position in 1845. As early as 1825, he

---

[1] Rynd: Dublin M. Press, 1845, xiii, 165; and description of instrument in Dublin Quart. Jour. Med. Sc., 1861, xxxii, 13. For a full account of Rynd's invention, see C. A. Pfender, Wash. Med. Ann., 1912, x, 346–359.

[2] Graves: London Med. & Surg. Jour., 1835, vii, pt. 2, pp. 516, 517.

put himself on record as a disciple of Laennec by the publication of his "Introduction to the Use of the Stethoscope." During the Dublin epidemic of typhus fever in 1826, he worked hard for the poor, and had an attack of the disease himself in 1827. He reported the first case of cholera in the Dublin epidemic of 1832, and, in 1846, published his celebrated accounts of Cheyne-Stokes breathing and the Stokes-Adams disease.[1] His treatises on diseases of the chest (1837) and diseases of the heart and aorta (1854) won him lasting fame. He was one of the few physicians who ever received the Prussian order *"pour le mérite."*

Sir Dominic John **Corrigan** (1802–80), who described the "famine fever" of 1847, also wrote upon diseases of the heart, and, in 1832, published an original description of insufficiency of the aortic valve (with

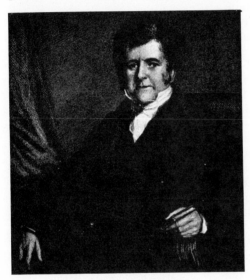

a superb plate) which is accepted as the classic account of the disease,[2] although it had been earlier noted by Cowper (1705), Vieussens (1715), and Hodgkin (1829).

Corrigan was the first to throw into relief the characteristic receding or "waterhammer" pulse in aortic regurgitation (Corrigan's pulse), and suggested that a flagging heart may be stimulated by tapping the precordial region with a hot spoon (Corrigan's hammer). He also noted the "cerebral breathing" of typhus and the expansile pulsation of aneurysm (Corrigan's sign), and described cirrhosis of the lungs or fibroid phthisis, which, like aortic incompetency, sometimes goes by his name.

Richard Bright (1789–1858).

The **English clinicians** of the early 19th century assimilated the ideas of Laennec and Bichat in their practice, and, like Heberden, Parry, Fothergill, and Huxham, showed themselves true followers of Sydenham in their descriptions of disease. Of special importance is the clinical and pathologic work which was done by the long line of brilliant workers at Guy's Hospital—the "great men of Guy's." Of these, Richard **Bright** (1789–1858), of Bristol, had studied under Astley Cooper and James Currie, and for twenty-three years (1820–43) was physician at Guy's where he worked for six hours a day in the wards and postmortem room, besides lecturing on materia medica and clinical medicine. His experience was further widened by extensive continental travel, in the course of which he came to know and admire Johann

---

[1] Stokes: Dublin Quart. Jour. Med. Sc., 1846, ii, 73–85.

[2] Corrigan: Edinb. Med. & Surg. Jour., 1832, xxxvii, 225–245, 1 pl. (Hodgkin: London Med. Gaz., 1828–29, iii, 433–443).

Peter Frank. Bright was the leading consultant of London in his day. His *Reports of Medical Cases* (1827), containing his original description of essential nephritis, with its epoch-making distinction between cardiac and renal dropsy, at once established his reputation all over Europe. White clouds in the urine had been noticed even by Hippocrates[1]; Saliceto, the Italian surgeon, had pointed out the association of dropsy, scanty urine, and hardened kidneys (*durities in renibus*) in 1476[2]; and the correlation between dropsy and albuminous urine had been established by William Charles Wells (1811[3]) and John Blackall (1813[4]); but Bright was the first to correlate these symptoms with the glomerular nephritis[5] which he found in so many postmortems, and his epoch-making synthesis soon made its way everywhere, on account of its immense importance in medical practice.[6] In work of this kind, he is one of the greatest of modern pathologists. In the spring of 1842, as Thayer records, he had two clinical wards at Guy's set apart for a semester of study of renal disease, a complete clinical unit, with consulting room and clinical laboratory between. This was the first coöperative investigation of disease ever undertaken. The results were published by Barlow and Rees in the Hospital Reports (1843) after Bright's retirement. As an original delineator of disease, he ranks next to Laennec. "Bright could not theorize," says his biographer, Wilks, "but he could see, and we are struck with astonishment at his powers of observation, as he photographed pictures of disease for the study of posterity." He advanced no special views of pathology and affixed no particular labels to his many descriptions of morbid states, but he collected an extraordinary number of facts and knew how to use them. Thus, he left original accounts of pancreatic diabetes and pancreatic steatorrhea (1832[7]), acute yellow atrophy of the liver (1836[8]), unilateral convulsions or Jacksonian epilepsy (1836[9]), and "status lymphaticus" (1838[10]), which, had they been tagged with appropriate names, would

---

[1] For instance, in the case of Thasus, wife of Philinus, in Epidemic Diseases, Book I, §13, Case iv.

[2] "Signa duritiei in renibus sunt, quid minoratur quantitas urinæ, et quod est gravitas renum et spinæ cum aliquo dolore; et incipit venter inflari post tempus et fit hydropicus secundum dies. Et ut plurimum fit talis durities post apostema calidum in renibus et post febrem ejus." Saliceto: Liber in scientia medicinali, 1476, ch. 140.

[3] Wells: Tr. Soc. Improve. Med. & Chir. Knowledge, 1804–12, Lond., 1812, iii 194–240.

[4] Blackall: Observations on the nature and cure of dropsies, London, 1813.

[5] Aschoff points out that while Bright included all nephritides in his clinical category, the essential Brightic nephritis is glomerular, with secondary contraction of the kidney, toxic and inflammatory albuminuria and renal dropsy without hypertension. The arteriosclerotic contracted kidney with cardiac edema does not belong in this category. Lancet, Lond., 1927, ii, 133.

[6] For the history of Bright's disease (1827–47), see C. P. Falck, Janus, Breslau, 1848, iii, 133, 456.

[7] Bright: Med. Chir. Tr., Lond., 1832–33, xviii, 1–56.

[8] Guy's Hosp. Rep., Lond., 1836, i, 36–40.

[9] *Ibid.*, 604–637.   [10] *Ibid.*, 1838, iii, 437.

have been better known before our day. His Medical Reports contain
accurate notations of such novelties as scarlatinal otitis, otitic abscess
of the brain, laryngeal phthisis, pressure paralyses, the cerebral hemi-
phlegias, the hysteric equivalents of disease, and striking plates of the
pathologic appearances in typhoid fever, nephritis, acute yellow atrophy
of the liver, and cerebral disease. Sir Samuel Wilks further records
that he was one of the first, if not the first, to describe pigmentation
of the brain in melanemia, condensation of the lung in whooping-
cough, small echinococci in the interior of hydatid cysts, and the bruit
of the heart in chorea. Bright was a capable and accomplished artist, a
collector and connoisseur of engravings, and his early volume of Hun-

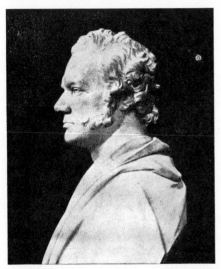

Thomas Addison (1793–1860). (Courtesy of Dr. Herbert L. Eason, Guy's Hospital, London.)

garian travels (1818) is illustrated with charming pictures
drawn by himself. This great
physician was also an able
botanist and geologist, and personally a simple, unprejudiced,
truth-loving man.

Thomas **Addison** (1793–
1860), of Longbenton, North
Cumberland, Bright's colleague
at Guy's, was more the brilliant
pathologic lecturer and diagnostician than the successful
practitioner. On account of
a haughty, repellent manner
which, on his own showing,
concealed excessive shyness and
sensibility, he never had a large
practice and lived almost entirely for his pupils and hospital work. He attached so
little importance to drugging

that (it is said) he sometimes forgot to prescribe; yet "Addison's
pill," of calomel, digitalis. and squills, for hepatic dropsy in syphilis,
is still used. He was also the first to employ static electricity in
the treatment of spasmodic and convulsive diseases (1837), and,
in collaboration with John Morgan, wrote the first book in English
on the action of poisons on the living body (1829). In 1839,
he published a good account of appendicitis. In 1849, Addison read
a paper before the South London Medical Society,[1] in which he
described pernicious anemia (twenty years before Biermer) and disease
of the suprarenal capsules (*melasma suprarenale*). These clinical notations were afterward expanded at full length in his great monograph
On the Constitutional and Local Effects of Disease of the Suprarenal

---

[1] Addison: London M. Gaz., 1849, xliii, 517.

Capsules (London, 1855). This book was regarded merely as a scientific curiosity in Addison's time, but it is now recognized as of epoch-making importance, since, in connection with the physiologic work of Claude Bernard, it inaugurated the study of the diseases of the ductless glands and of those disturbances of chemical equilibrium known as "pluri-glandular syndromes." It was Trousseau who first proposed to call the suprarenal syndrome "Addison's disease." In 1851, Addison and Sir William Gull described the skin disease "vitiligoidea," now known as xanthoma. "Addison's keloid" is a circumscribed form of scleroderma.

The pathologist, Thomas **Hodgkin** (1798–1866), of Tottenham, England, a member of the Society of Friends, always wearing their characteristic dress, was a philanthropist and reformer by nature and was driven away from Guy's, says Wilks, by his eccentric independence of spirit. His reputation rests upon his original description of that simultaneous enlargement of the spleen and lymphatic glands or lymphadenoma (1832[1]), which, as he himself records, was vaguely outlined by Malpighi in 1665, and which Wilks, in 1865, called "Hodgkin's disease." He also wrote an account of insufficiency of the aortic valve (1829[2]),

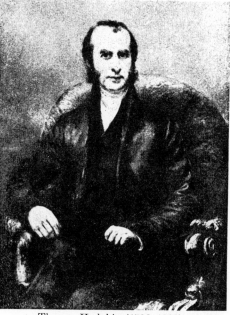

Thomas Hodgkin (1798–1866).

which antedated Corrigan's classic paper by three years. His essay on medical education (1823) is an interesting contribution, and his *Lectures on the Morbid Anatomy of the Serous and Mucous Membranes* (1836–40) is one of the earliest English treatises on pathology. Being generous to his patients and careless about collecting fees, Hodgkin gradually fell out of practice and devoted the rest of his life to various philanthropies. He died at Joppa, while traveling in the East with Sir Moses Montefiore, who erected the monument over his grave.

Probably the greatest of all illustrators of gross pathology was Sir Robert **Carswell** (1793–1857), of Paisley, Scotland, an Aberdeen gradu-

---

[1] Hodgkin: Med. Chir. Tr., Lond., 1832, xvii, 68–114.
[2] Hodgkin: London M. Gaz., 1828–29, iii, 433–443.

ate of 1826, who became professor of pathology at University College, London (1828). From a wonderful series of 2000 water-color drawings of diseased structures (1828–31) came his *Illustrations of the Elementary Forms of Disease* (1837), a folio of colored plates, drawn and set upon the stone by himself, which has never been surpassed.

Other eminent English clinicians of the early period were Parkinson, Wells, Hodgson, and Hope.

James **Parkinson** (1755–1824), of London, one of John Hunter's pupils, is remembered today by his unique and classic description of paralysis agitans or "Parkinson's disease" (1817[1]), and by the fact that he reported the first case of appendicitis in English (1812[2]), this case being also the first in which perforation was recognized as the cause of death (H. A. Kelly). Parkinson was a radical, a reformer and political agitator, sometime in hot water with the government, and what little is known of his life is almost entirely due to the recent interesting researches of L. G. Rowntree (1912[3]). He wrote political and controversial pamphlets, a number of small treatises on domestic medicine, and a good book on medical education (*The Hospital Pupil*, 1800); but his most important contributions outside of medicine are his works on fossil remains (1804–22). An able geologist and palæontologist, he is memorable, with Avicenna, Fracastorius, Stensen, Hutton, Wollaston, Owen, and Huxley as one of the many medical men who have contributed something of permanent value to these sciences.

William Charles **Wells** (1757–1817) was born in South Carolina, but his people being Tories in the Revolutionary period, he must be accounted, by his own choice, a British subject. Wells was a highly original observer, both in medicine and in physics, to which he contributed the now classical *Essay on Dew* (1814). He described the albuminous urine of dropsy in 1811,[4] and published perhaps the earliest clinical report on the cardiac complications of rheumatism (1810[5]). His essays on vision (1793–1814) contain observations of the highest originality.

Joseph **Hodgson** (1788–1869), of Birmingham, a successful lithotomist, wrote an important *Treatise on Diseases of the Arteries and Veins* (1815), in which he gave the first description of aneurysmal dilatation of the aortic arch, which the French call *maladie d' Hodgson*. This book is a wonderful storehouse of knowledge on the subject of vascular disease, and contains many valuable historic data about aneurysms and the early ligations of important arteries. Of the same period is Allan Burns' "Observations" on Heart Disease (1809), the second edition of which contains the first observation of chloroma (1811).

---

[1] Parkinson: An Essay on the Shaking Palsy, London, 1817.

[2] Parkinson: Med. Chir. Tr., London, 1812, iii, 57.

[3] Rowntree: Bull. Johns Hopkins Hosp., Balt., 1912, xxiii, 33–45.

[4] Wells: Tr. Soc. Improve. Med. and Chir. Knowledge, 1804–12, Lond., 1812, iii, 194–240.

[5] *Ibid.*, 372–412.

James **Hope** (1801–41), of Stockfort (Cheshire), an Edinburgh graduate (1825) afterward associated with St. George's Hospital, did much for our knowledge of heart-murmurs, aneurysm and valvular disease, as summarized in his treatise on *Diseases of the Heart and Great Vessels* (1831). In 1833–4, he produced an atlas of plates of anatomy, drawn by himself, which was, however, surpassed by that of Carswell (1837).

The most important English treatise on the practice of medicine in the first half of the 19th century was the "Lectures on the Principles and Practice of Physic," published in 1843 by **Sir Thomas Watson** (1792–1882). For more than a quarter century, this work continued to pass through many editions and enjoyed a well-deserved popularity on account of its author's attractive and elegant style and his clear presentation of his subject.

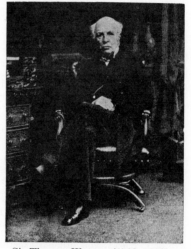

Sir Thomas Watson (1792–1882).

The treatise on practice by Bright and Addison, of which only the first volume was ever published (1800), is a strictly scientific production, in which the phenomena of disease are treated in rigid categories, as in a work on mathematical physics. It is remarkable for its frankly agnostic spirit in regard to obscure phenomena, such as the nature of fever. Most of the text is said to have been written by Addison.

Other clinical treatises of the period, now almost forgotten, were Scudamore on gout (1816), Thackrah on the blood (1819), Sir Charles Hastings on inflammation of the lungs (1820), Sir James Clark on phthisis (1835), Francis Sibson on position of the internal organs (1844), Golding Bird on urinary deposits (1845), and the works on James Hope (1832), Peter Mere Latham (1845), Alison (1845), and Chevers (1851) on heart disease.

A prominent feature of English medicine in this period was the publication of admirable systems and encyclopedias of medicine, such as those of Forbes (1833–35), Todd (1835–59), Tweedie (1840), South (1847), and Reynolds (1866–79). These, with Panckoucke's sixty-volume *Dictionnaire des sciences médicales* (1812–22) and the 100-volume *Encyclopedie* of Dechambre (1834–89[1]), were the forerunners of such later works as Quain's Dictionary of Medicine and the systems of Ziemssen, Eulenburg, Allbutt, and Osler. A remarkable compiler of the day was James Copland (1791–1870), of the Orkney Islands, a "polyhistorian" of the type ridiculed in Germany, who made his living by hack work, and whose "Dictionary of Practical Medicine" (1834–59) consists of 3509 double column pages, all written by himself. Norman Moore likens it to the *Continens* of Rhazes, adding that our own generation leaves it, "as undisturbed on the shelves as the Continent itself." As president of the Pathological Society of London, Copland excited many a chuckle of derision when he claimed various modern discoveries as his own.

---

[1] The 17th century encyclopedias of medicine were really anthologies. The modern idea of dictionary compilations originated in such works as the Konversations-Lexika of Hübner (1704) and Brockhaus (1796–1808), the encyclopedias of Ephraim Chambers (1728), Diderot (1751–72), and Voltaire (*Dictionnaire philosophique*, 1764), and the Encyclopædia Britannica (1768–71). For a good list of early medical encyclopedias, see Brit. Med. Jour., London, 1913, i, 725.

A most important feature of British medicine in the 19th century was the work of the Anglo-Indian surgeons. The East India Company was chartered by Queen Elizabeth in 1600 and established its first trading station in 1612. Even in the early days, two surgeons, Gabriel Boughton, who, in 1645, was sent from Surat to the court of Shah Jahan at Agra, and William Hamilton, who accompanied the mission to Delhi in 1714–17, were both of them instrumental in securing trading concessions and charters for the company, leading up to the establishment of the three great centers at Bombay, Calcutta, and Madras; but it was not until well after Clive's victory at Plassey in 1757 that we see the Indian Medical Service playing much of a part in colonial and tropical medicine., It was formally constituted as such on January 1, 1764. The earliest treatise on tropical medicine was, in fact, published in 1768 by James Lind (1716–94), whose important work was followed in due course by an imposing array of books on the Indian climate and diseases, notably those of John Peter Wade (1791–93), William Hunter (1804), Sir James Annesley (1825), William Twining (1832), Sir James Ranald Martin (1841), Allan Webb (1848), Charles Morehead (1856) and Goodeve's perennial little treatise on tropical pediatrics (1844). Aside from the development of tropical medicine, the organization of hospitals, of medical education, of public hygiene, and other administrative duties connected with the building up of the Indian Empire. the most important achievements of these army surgeons[1] were their remarkable first-hand accounts of heat stroke (those of Green, Barclay, Longmore et al., being among the closest to fact that we have), the descriptions of various forms of snake-bite, of native modes of poisoning, and of the properties of far eastern drugs, their many contributions to Indian botany, zoölogy, geology, and ethnography, the original accounts of cholera, beri-beri, scurvy, dysentery, leprosy, and filarial elephantiasis, and the introduction of such novelities as mesmeric anesthesia, the British Army bamboo splint, the Hindu method of teaching surgical incision upon plants, and the reintroduction of the use of ipecac in dysentery by Surgeon-Major E. S. Docker (1858).

The literary organ of the Indian Medical Service at this time was the *India Journal of Medical Science* (1834–45), which up to 1842 was edited by Frederick Corbyn. The earlier volumes contain interesting engravings of some of the medical nabobs of the period.

Two of the Anglo-Indian surgeons will always hold a high place in the history of serpent venoms, viz., Patrick **Russell** (1727–1805), of Braidshaw, Scotland, whose *Account of Indian Serpents* (4 volumes, 1796–1809) was the earliest venture in the field, containing the original description of the celebrated Russell's viper (*Daboia Russellii*); and **Sir Joseph Fayrer** (1824–1907), who played a spirited part in the Mutiny, and whose *Thanatophidia of India* (1872) is one of the great classics of zoölogy, describing all the venomous snakes of the Indian Peninsula, with magnificent life-size plates from drawings by Hindu pupils in the Government School of Art in Calcutta; and original experiments on the venoms, which were, however, preceded by the early work of the Abbate Fontana (1767) and Weir Mitchell (1870). The greatest of the Anglo-Indian zoölogists was Thomas Caverhill Jerdon, whose accounts of the birds (1844–64) and mammals (1854) are famous. Among the many botanic works were William Roxburgh's *Plants of the Coromandel Coast* (1795–1819) and *Flora Indica* (1820–24), Nathaniel Wallich's *Tentamen Floræ Nepalensis* (1824–26) and *Plantæ Asiaticæ Rariores* (1830–32), Robert Wight's *Icones Plantarium Indiæ Orientalis*, 6 volumes with over 2000 plates (1838–53), William Griffith's *Icones Plantarum Asiaticarum* (1847–51), and Thomson and Hooker's *Flora Indica* (1855). Important original monographs on tropical diseases were John Peter Wade on fever and dysentery (1791–93), John MacPherson's *Annals of Cholera* (1839), Edward Hare on the treatment of remittent fever and dysentery (1847), N. C. MacNamara's *History of Asiatic Cholera* (1876), and the original investigations of Henry Vandyke Carter, (1831–97) on mycetoma (1874), leprosy, and elephantiasis (1874) and spirillosis (1882), and of Leonard Rogers on Indian fevers (1897–1908), and dysenteries (1913). Beri-beri had already been described in the 17th century by Bontius (1642) and Tulp (1652), but the treatise of John Grant Malcolmson (1835) will always be accounted a classic source of recent knowledge of the disease. The treatises on tropical pediatrics by Frederick Corbyn (1828) and Henry Hurry Goodeve (1844) were new departures. The latter enjoyed a popularity of nearly fifty years standing. Some of the Indian surgeons, who left the service early, attained

---

[1] D. G. Crawford: History of the Indian Medical Service (1600–1913), 2 v., London, 1914.

distinction in other fields of activity, notably Murchison, Esdaile, Playfair, whose midwifery passed through nine editions (1876–98), Ireland, memorable for his writings on insanity, and Edward John Waring (1819–91) who compiled the first official Indian pharmacopœia (1868), a bilingual work on *Bazar Medicines* (1860), also a Haller-like *Bibliotheca Therapeutica* (1878), and afterward did good service in public hygiene.

Charles **Murchison** (1830–79), born in Jamaica of Scotch parentage, entered the Bengal army in 1853, and published a treatise on the climate and diseases of Burmah in 1855. Returning to England, he became a prominent physician at the London Fever Hospital (1856–70) and St. Thomas' Hospital (1871–79), in connection with his wonderful special knowledge of fevers. In 1873, he was presented with a testimonial by the residents of West London for tracing an epidemic of typhoid to a polluted milk supply. He was noted for his solid accuracy, promptitude, and decision in diagnosis, and although he opposed the bacterial theory of infection, his *Treatise on the Continued Fevers of Great Britain* (1862) is as important a work for England as Drake's *Diseases of the Mississippi Valley* is for the United States. Murchison translated Frerichs' book on diseases of the liver in 1861 and wrote a number of important monographs on the same subject himself. Like his famous brother, he was an able geologist.

The name of Esdaile, of the Indian Medical Service, is prominently associated with the history of **hypnotism,** particularly of hypnotic anesthesia in surgical operations. After the time of Mesmer, hypnotism was only a peg for arrant charlatanry. The pioneer of scientific hypnosis before Charcot was James **Braid** (1795–1861), a surgeon of Fifeshire, Scotland, who settled in Manchester and became attracted to the subject of animal magnetism about 1841. Braid at first believed that the phenomena produced by professional mesmerists were due to "collusion and illusion"; but he soon became convinced, upon experimentation, that there can be a genuine self-induced sleep brought about by a fixed stare at a bright inanimate object (Braidism). The importance of Braid's work is that he proved that the mesmeric influence is entirely subjective or personal, and that no fluid or other influence passes from the operator to the patient. This subjective trance he called neurohypnotism or hypnosis (1842). His treatise on the subject was entitled *Neurypnology, or the Rationale of Nervous Sleep* (1843). Braid's views met with violent opposition, especially from the professional mesmerists, who wished to keep their exhibits upon a miraculous basis, but his ideas were taken up by Azam, Broca, Charcot, Liébeault, Bernheim, and became the true starting-point of the French school.[1] Hypnotism was first used in surgical operations by John **Elliotson** (1791–1868[2]), a professor of practice in the University of London and president of the Royal Medical and Chirurgical Society, who, in 1843, published a pamphlet describing *Numerous Cases of Surgical Operations without Pain in the Mesmeric State.* Dispute about this led to his resignation

---

[1] Wilhelm Preyer translated Braid's complete works into German in 1882.
[2] To whom Thackeray dedicated his "Pendennis."

from his various offices. A far more impressive record was made by James **Esdaile** (1808–59), of Montrose, Scotland, who, in 1845, began to try hypnotism in operating on Hindu convicts. He performed over 100 such operations with success, having been put to a severe test by the Deputy Governor of Bengal, and eventually had a record of 261 painless operations with a mortality of 5.5 per cent., as described in his book, *Mesmerism in India* (1846). On returning to Scotland, Esdaile found that, except in disease, the self-contained Europeans differed from the impressionable, neurotic Hindus in not being specially susceptible to the hypnotic trance.

German medicine, in the first half of the 19th century, labored under the disadvantage of being split up into schools. Exhausted by the Napoleonic wars, and existing mainly as a set of petty principalities, with only a vague racial and political solidarity, the German people had to endure a long period of brutal military régime, as a natural sequel of the previous struggle against foreign invasion. In consequence, the best minds of the time were driven into various idealistic modes of thought, a fermentation which came to a head in the Revolution of 1848. Brunonianism, Mesmerism, and the various phases of "magical medicine" which followed in its train, had prepared the ground for the wildest kind of speculation. During this period of idealism, the favorite philosophers were Schelling, Fichte, and Hegel. Clinical medicine was dominated by the fanciful reveries of the **Nature-Philosophy School** of which Schelling himself was, indeed, the founder. Its principal spirit was the Bavarian naturalist, Lorenz **Oken** (1779–1851), editor of the journal *Isis* and a founder of the first German Congress of Naturalists and Physicians (1822). Oken combined great originality of thought with much ineptitude. He accepted and expanded Goethe's vertebrate theory of the skull (1806), regarded the flesh as a conglomeration of infusoria (cells), and glorified the male element in nature to the extent of declaring that "Ideally every child should be a boy." Other members of the school, such as Döllinger, Görres, Treviranus, and Steffens, drifted into a maze of incomprehensible jargon and fanciful distinctions as to the real and the ideal, identity, imponderables, polarities, irritability, metamorphosis, and the like. Hard upon the Nature-Philosophy School followed the Natural History School, which aimed to name and classify diseases after a rigid system, as in botany or zoölogy. It was succeeded by the Rational or Physiologic School of Roser and Wunderlich, Henle and Pfeufer, the forerunners of the scientific movement of German medicine, which was headed by the pupils of its prime mover, Johannes Müller. Apart from these, many strayed into such devious by-paths as Phrenology, Homœopathy, Rademacherism, Baunscheidtism, Hydropathy, Odic Force, Animal Magnetism, and other narrow and exclusive ways of conceiving the facts of medicine. The tendency of all these hole-and-corner schools was toward wholesale contempt for the scientific achievements of men like Bichat and Magendie, Laennec and Louis, or the practical sense of such clinical workers as Bright, Stokes, or Graves. This tendency reached the limit of exaggeration in the doctrines of the New Vienna School, as stated by Skoda, Hammernijk, and Dietl. Skoda said that while we can diagnose and describe disease, we dare not expect by any manner of means to cure it: *Nichts tun ist das beste der inneren Medizin.* Dietl, in an oft-quoted utterance of 1851, announced that a physician must be judged, not by the success of his treatment but by the extent of his knowledge: "As long as medicine is art, it will not be science. As long as there are successful physicians there will be no scientific physicians." These ingenious paradoxes, which amounted virtually to a plea of impotence, made up the "therapeutic nihilism" of the New Vienna School. The Revolution of 1848 dissipated the silly doctrines of the Nature-Philosophy School into space, but the New Vienna School died hard, and Rokitansky had to be overthrown by Virchow, and Semmelweis had to sacrifice

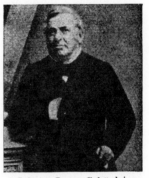

his life in proving his thesis before German medicine could finally emerge from the Happy Valley of speculation to gain the tableland of reality.[1]

The first to break away from the jargon of the Nature-Philosophy School was Johann Lucas **Schönlein** (1793–1864), of Bamberg, the founder of the so-called **Natural History School,** the ambition of which was, as we have said, to study medicine as descriptive botany and zoölogy are studied. Schönlein, his pupil, Carl Canstatt, and Conrad Heinrich Fuchs, all of them inspired by de Candolle's classification of

Johann Lucas Schönlein (1793–1864).

plants, proceeded to make arbitrary classifications of disease, based, in each case, upon a very hazy *fundamentum divisionis*, not unlike those of Boissier de Sauvages in the 18th century. Schönlein, in particular, indulged in such whimsies as forcing gangrene of the uterus into the class "neurophlogoses" and cholera into the catarrhs. In his progress from Würzburg to Zürich and Berlin, he passed through all three of the developmental phases of the Natural History School, the parasitic, the nosologic, and the scientific.[2] The real merits of Schönlein, however, are of a different order. In his clinic at the Charité, in Berlin, he was the first to lecture on medicine in German instead of Latin (1840), and was the founder of modern clinical teaching in Germany, introducing examinations of the blood and urine, chemical analysis, auscultation, percussion and microscopic investigations. He wrote little,[3] his only

---

[1] For the intellectual follies of the period, see Jacobi: New York Med. Jour., 1901, lxxiii, 617–623.

[2] Neuburger. (Puschmann Handbuch, ii, 145.)

[3] As to certain submerged writings of Schönlein, see E. Ebstein: Arch. f. Gesch. d. Med., Leipz., 1911–12, v, 449–452.

contributions of importance being his observation of triple phosphates in the excreta of typhoid fever (1836), his description of peliosis rheumatica (Schönlein's disease) in 1837,[1] his discovery of the parasitic cause of favus (achorion Schönleinii) in 1839,[2] and his proposal of the terms "typhus abdominalis" and "typhus exanthematicus" to differentiate these diseases (1839), and of the term "hemophilia" for the hemorrhagic diathesis. Schönlein was a man of peculiar character. During his later years in Berlin he often affected the eccentricities of a recluse, denying himself to patients when it suited his whim, and otherwise treating them with the "godlike coarseness" of demeanor (göttliche Grobheit[3]) which was then the vogue. His scientific abilities have been ably set forth in the well-known eulogy of Virchow (1865[4]), but he seemed, alike to the delicate perception of Fanny Hensel and the plain common sense of Augustin Prichard, something of a boor.

Schönlein's pupil, Carl Friedrich **Canstatt** (1870–50), of Ratisbon, wrote a sterling text-book on practice, absolutely free from metaphysical dogma, which, says Jacobi,[5] was the "Bible of German medicine" until it was superseded by Niemeyer, as the latter was, in due course, supplanted by Strümpell.

The scientific movement in modern. German medicine was started and kept in pace mainly through the medium of four important periodicals which stood out for exact investigation and exerted great influence upon the younger spirits in the speculative period, viz., Müller's Archiv für Anatomie, Physiologie und wissenschaftliche Medicin (1834), Henle and Pfeufer's Zeitschrift für rationelle Medicin (1841–69), Roser and Wunderlich's Archiv für physiologische Heilkunde (1842–59), and Virchow's Archiv für pathologische Anatomie (1847–1913). Of these able editors, Müller, Henle, and Virchow were the leaders in Germany of comparative, histologic, and pathologic anatomy respectively, and Müller, in particular, was the greatest German physiologist of his time. Wunderlich was perhaps the most original clinician.

Carl Reinhold August **Wunderlich** (1815–77), of Württemberg, graduated at Tübingen in 1837 and taught medicine there until 1850, when he succeeded to Oppolzer's chair at Leipzig (1850–77). He described renal apoplexy (1856), wrote a good treatise on practice (1858) and an excellent history of medicine (1859), but his masterpiece is undoubtedly his treatise on the relations of animal heat in disease (1868[6]), which is the very foundation of our present clinical thermometry.

[1] Schönlein: Allg. u. spec. Path. u. Therap., Herisau, 1837, ii, 1848.

[2] Müller's Arch., Berlin, 1839, 82, 1 pl. (A contribution of only 20 lines.)

[3] The Homeric phrase occurs for the first time in Friedrich Schlegel's celebrated romance of "Lucinde." Virchow gives one (perhaps apocryphal) instance of Schönlein's rudeness. The latter was once consulted by an elderly physician, who, disconcerted by his brusque manner, pointed to his gray hair. Schönlein retorted: Auch die Esel sind grau!

[4] Virchow: Gedächtnissrede auf Lucas Schönlein, Berlin, 1865.

[5] Jacobi: Op. cit., p. 622.

[6] Wunderlich: Das Verhalten der Eigenwärme in Krankheiten, Leipzig, 1868.

Before Wunderlich's time, Reil and others had written five-volume treatises on fever as a disease. About 1850, Clausius, Helmholtz, and Sir William Thomson had worked out the mathematical relations of the laws governing heat-transformations, and, in 1849, Thomson (Lord Kelvin) had established his "absolute scale of temperature," without which no thermometers could be reliable. Upon this hint, Wunderlich made many careful observations of temperature in disease, tabulating his results, and, after the true significance of the thermal changes in the body were better understood, thermometry became a recognized feature in clinical diagnosis, and new studies were made of fever and other pathologic problems in which the idea of temperature is involved. Before the time of Clausius, heat (caloric) was still

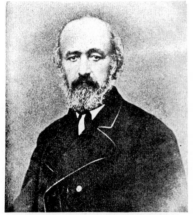

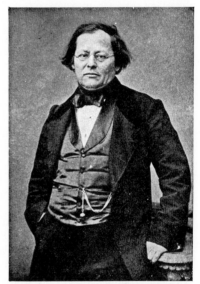

Carl R. A. Wunderlich (1815-77). (By kind permission of Frau Geheimrat Franz Hofmann-Wunderlich, Leipzig.)

Josef Skoda (1805-81). (Collection of A. C. Klebs.)

regarded by many as a material substance, an ideal which threw back the progress of medicine as much as did its parent and forerunner, the phlogiston theory of Stahl.[1] By utilizing the advanced thermodynamic knowledge of his time, Wunderlich made his book a permanent scientific classic. He found fever a disease and left it a symptom.

Josef **Skoda** (1805–81), of Pilsen, Bohemia, was the leading clinician of the **New Vienna School** and the exponent of its therapeutic nihilism. He was the first medical teacher in Vienna to lecture in German (1847), and taught nearly all his life in the Allegemeines Krankenhaus. His

---

[1] It is now charitably supposed that when Stahl and his followers maintained that if a body undergoes combustion, it gives off something (becomes "dephlogisticated"), they were clumsily groping in the direction of Carnot's principle that "Heat cannot flow from a colder to a warmer body." Even as late as 1865, we find an able engineer like the hard-headed Rankine still confident that heat is an indestructible substance.

principal contribution to medicine is his treatise on percussion and auscultation (1839[1]), in which he attempts to classify the different sounds in the chest by categories, ranged according to musical pitch and tonality, and alternating from full to hollow, clear to dull, tympanitic to muffled, high to deep. Skoda's resonance, the drum-like sound heard in pneumonia and pericardial effusion, is a permanent aid in modern diagnosis. Although little was known of the physics of sound in Skoda's day, his acoustic refinements were, in some respects, an improvement upon the loose descriptive terms used by the French clinicians of the period, as wittily exemplified in the "Stethoscope Song" of Dr. Holmes:

> "The *bruit de râpe* and the *bruit de scie*
> And the *bruit du diable* are all combined;
> How happy Bouillaud would be,
> If he a case like this could find."

None the less, so effective an expression as Laennec's "egophony" still means a great deal to the ear of the modern practitioner. In recent times, Skoda's work has found further elaboration in the complicated instruments with Helmholtz resonators which some clinicians use to analyze the sounds of the chest for teaching purposes. Skoda was a whimsical, top-heavy old bachelor, who, as Baas relates, put up with queer clothes all his life for fear of offending his tailor (a personal friend), yet once sued a clergyman to obtain payment of a fee.[2] He looked upon his patients as objects of investigation merely, and, when it came to treatment, said, with a shrug: *Ach, das ist ja alles eins!* This set a bad example. The humane or psychic side of medical treatment was entirely ignored, and a diagnosis confirmed by a postmortem came to be a sort of shibboleth in Vienna, where snap-diagnoses (*Schnell-Diagnosen*) were the fashion, even among practitioners who could not have differentiated the pitch and tonality of a heart-sound from a band of music.

Carl **Rokitansky** (1804–78), Skoda's colleague and also a Bohemian, was a man of different type, genial and unassuming, where Skoda was pragmatic and pedantic; a graceful and witty writer, where Skoda was dry and dull. His Viennese *bonhomie* is sensed in his jest about his four sons, two of whom were physicians, the other two singers: *Die Einen heilen, die Anderen heulen.* Rokitansky did an enormous amount of pathologic work, and, it is said, had the disposal of between 1500 and 1800 cadavers annually. He made over 30,000 postmortems in his life. He was the first to detect bacteria in the lesions of malignant endocarditis, and to differentiate between lobar and lobular pneumonia, as also between Bright's disease and *Speckniere* (Virchow's amyloid degeneration of the kidney). He first described acute dilatation of the stomach (1842), left a classic account of the pathologic appearances in

---

[1] Skoda: Abhandlung über Perkussion und Auskultation, Vienna, 1839.
[2] Baas: *Op. cit.*, footnote to p. 954.

acute yellow atrophy of the liver, giving the disease its present name
(1843); described and defined the bronchitic and pulmonary complications of typhoid as bronchotyphus and pneumotyphus; and completed
Laennec's picture of emphysema of the lungs by describing the microscopic appearances. In obstetrics and orthopedics, he is memorable as
the first to describe the spondylolisthetic deformities (1839[1]). The
value of the first edition of Rokitansky's treatise on pathologic anatomy
(1842-46[2]) was seriously impaired by his doctrine of "crases" and
"stases," in which chemical states of substance were actually conceived
of as being susceptible to "disease," and which was mercilessly chaffed
out of existence by Virchow (1846[3]). The latter intimated that Rokitansky was in reality an adherent of the
Natural History School, since he
employed a bizarre terminology to
describe things of which he had
no ken, his chemical hypotheses of
tissue changes being susceptible of
a simpler and more purely mechanical explanation, while his attempt
to revamp the ancient drivel about
solidism and humoralism was a mon-
strous anachronism (*ein ungeheurer
Anachronismus*). Virchow knew
more chemistry than Rokitansky,
but he cordially admitted that, in
picturing what was actually before
him on the postmortem table, his
jolly Viennese rival was the ablest
descriptive pathologist of his time.
It is said that when Rokitansky
read Virchow's criticism, he could
never bring himself to look at
his unfortunate first edition again.

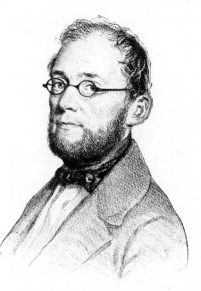

Carl Rokitansky (1804-78).

Rokitansky's finest productions are unquestionably his monograph on
diseases of the arteries (1852[4]), illustrated with 23 folio plates; and his
great memoir on defects in the septum of the heart (1875[5]), the result
of fourteen years' labor, giving his transposition theory of the deviation
of the aortic septum. These works have been the subject of deep study
by modern pathologists, in connection with the English classic (1866)
of Thomas Bevill Peacock (1812-82) on malformations of the human
heart (1866), and the later memoir of Maude Abbott (1908).

[1] Rokitansky: Med. Jahrb. des österreichischen Staates, Vienna, 1839, xix, 41,
195.   [2] Rokitansky: Handbuch der pathologischen Anatomie, Vienna, 1842-46.

[3] Virchow: Med.-Ztg. (Verein f. Heilk. in Preussen), Berl., 1846, xv, Lit. Bei-
lage, Nos. 49, 50, pp. 237, 243.

[4] Rokitansky: Ueber einige der wichtigsten Krankheiten der Arterien, Denkschr. d. k. Akad. d. Wissensch., Vienna, 1852, iv, 1-72.

[5] Rokitansky: Die Defekte der Scheidewände des Herzens, Vienna, 1875.

Johannes **von Oppolzer** (1808–71), also a Bohemian, was a clear-headed, extremely competent practitioner who steered clear of all haphazard theorizing, and, as professor at Leipzig, did much to popularize the Viennese innovations in Germany. He was noted for his quickness in offhand diagnosis. Hamernijk of Prague and Dietl of Cracow were the extremists in therapeutic nihilism, the latter is now remembered only by the painful symptoms in floating kidney (Dietl's crises), attributable to a kink in the ureters or renal vessels, which he described in 1864.

Perhaps the most brilliant name of the New Vienna School, after Skoda's and Rokitansky's, was that of **Ferdinand von Hebra** (1816–80),

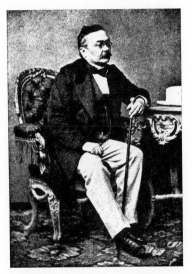

Ferdinand von Hebra (1816–80).
(Boston Medical Library.)

of Brünn (Moravia), a pupil of both these masters, and the founder of the histologic school of **dermatology,** the second phase in its modern development. Prior to this period, French dermatology had been dominated by such humoral (diathetic) concepts as dartrous, psoric or herpetic dyscrasias, a viewpoint which even influenced Allbutt. Hebra's classification of skin diseases (1845[1]) was based upon their pathologic anatomy. While complicated, erroneous, artificial, and lacking the simplicity of Willan's, it opened out new lines of investigation, in which Hebra's pupils, Kaposi, Neumann and Pick, played a prominent part. Hebra regarded most cutaneous disorders as purely local, and, from this viewpoint, devised mainly local (external) remedies. Yet, as a champion of nihilistic therapy, he is said to have followed Skoda in feigning treatment in some cases in order to demonstrate to his own satisfaction that they could get well of themselves.

Hebra's clinic was one of the most popular in Vienna, on account of his genial, offhand style of lecturing, and his keen, often sarcastic, humor. Among his pupils were Neumann, Auspitz, Pick, Wertheim, and Carl Heitzmann. Hebra revived the use of mercurials in syphilis and left the classic accounts of lichen ruber (1857[2]) and eczema marginatum (1860[3]) accepted Bateman's view that molluscum contagiosum is non-contagious (1817) until Vidal proved the contrary (1877). He tried to clear up obscure points in classification and nomenclature, segregated erythema multi-

[1] F. von Hebra: Versuch einer auf pathologischer Anatomie gegründeten Eintheilung der Hautkrankheiten, Ztschr. d. k. k. Gesellsch. d. Aerzte zu Wien., 1845, i, 34, 142, 211.

[2] Allg. Wien. med. Ztg., 1857, ii, 95.

[3] Handb. d. spec. Path. u. Therap. (Virchow), 1860, iii, 1. Abth., pp. 316–363.

forme, pityriasis rubra lichen scrofulosorum, rhinoscleroma, and was the first to describe impetigo herpetiformis (1872[1]), the definitive account of which was completed (1887[2]) by his son-in-law, Moritz Kaposi (1807–1902).

The greatest single achievement of the New Vienna School was the determination of the true cause and prophylaxis of **puerperal fever**. That the disease is fatal and contagious ("few escape it") had been noted in the Hippocratic treatise on female maladies, by Malouin, at the Hôtel Dieu (1746), by Gordon in Aberdeen (1795). In the 18th century, Charles White, in Manchester, England, had enlarged upon the advantages of scrupulous cleanliness in these cases. On February 13, 1843, **Oliver Wendell Holmes** (1809–94) read to the Boston Society for Medical Improvement his paper *On the Contagiousness of Puerperal Fever*,[3] in which he affirmed that women in childbed should never be attended by physicians who have been conducting postmortem sections or cases of puerperal fever; that the disease may be conveyed in this manner from patient to patient, even from a case of erysipelas; and that washing the hands in calcium chloride and changing the clothes after leaving a puerperal fever case was likely to be a preventive measure. Holmes' essay stirred up violent opposition on the part of the Philadelphia obstetricians, Hodge and Meigs, and, in 1855, he returned to the charge in his monograph on *Puerperal Fever as a Private Pestilence*, in which he reiterated his views and stated that one "Senderein" had lessened the mortality of puerperal fever by disinfecting the hands with chloride of lime and the nailbrush. This Senderein was Ignaz Philipp **Semmelweis** (1818–65), a Hungarian pupil of Skoda's and Rokitansky's who, in 1846, had become an assistant in the first obstetric ward of the Allgemeines Krankenhaus in Vienna. This ward had acquired such a high mortality in puerperal cases that women begged in tears not to be taken into it. Semmelweis had noticed that the first ward differed from the second (which had a lower mortality-rate) in that students came into it directly from the dissecting-room for

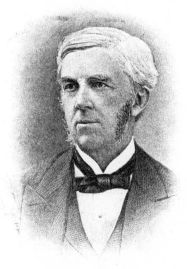

Oliver Wendell Holmes (1809–94).

---

[1] Wien. med. Wochenschr., 1872, xxii, 1197–2101.

[2] Kaposi: Vrtljschr. f. Dermat., Vienna, 1887, xiv, 273–296, 5 pl.

[3] Holmes: N. Engl. Quart. Jour. Med., Bost., 1842–43, i, 503–530.

instruction, often making vaginal examinations with unclean hands, while in the second ward, devoted to the instruction of midwives, much greater attention was paid to personal cleanliness. With this idea in mind, he also made a careful study of the autopsies in the fatal puerperal cases. In 1847, Kolletschka, Rokitansky's assistant, died of a dissection-wound, and Semmelweis was present at the postmortem. As he stood beside the body of his former instructor, he noticed that the pathological appearances were the same as in the unfortunate puerperæ of the first ward, and he now had his chain of evidence complete. He immediately instituted such precautions in the handling of labor cases that the mortality curve sank from 9.92 to 3.8 per cent. In the following year,

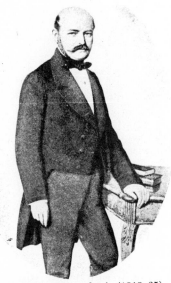

Ignaz Philipp Semmelweis (1818–65).

he had a mortality as low as 1.27 per cent., and all through the simple expedient of washing the hands in a calcium chloride solution in connection with pregnancy and the conduct of labor. Semmelweis is thus the true pioneer of antisepsis in obstetrics, and while Holmes antedated him in some details by five years, the superiority of his work over that of his predecessor lies not only in the stiff fight he put up for his ideas, but in the all-important fact that he recognized puerperal fever as a blood-poisoning or septicemia (1847–49[1]). Like Holmes, he met with fierce opposition, and while Rokitansky, Hebra, Michaelis, and, to his lasting honor, Skoda stood by him, he was persecuted by Scanzoni, Carl Braun, and the orthodox obstetricians of the day. Disgusted, he suddenly left Vienna for Budapest, where he became in due course professor of obstetrics at the University (1855) and published his immortal treatise on "The Cause, Concept, and Prophylaxis of Puerperal Fever" (1861[2]), as well as his scathing "Open Letters to Sundry Professors of Obstetrics" (1861). But his sensitive nature was not equal to the strain of violent controversy, and brooding over his wrongs brought on insanity and death. He is one of medicine's martyrs and,

---

[1] The original communication is "Höchst wichtige Erfahrungen über die Aetiologie der in Gebäranstalten epidemischen Puerperalfieber," Ztschr. d. k. k. Gesellsch. d. Aerzte in Wien, 1847–48, iv, pt. 2, 242; 1849, v, 64.

[2] Semmelweis: Die Aetiologie, der Begriff und die Prophylaxis des Kindbettfiebers, Budapest and Vienna, 1861.

in the future, will be one of its far-shining names, for every child-bearing woman owes something to him.

Medicine is also indebted to the New Vienna School for the introduction of **laryngoscopy** and **rhinoscopy**.

The dentist's mouth mirror appears to have been long known and is mentioned by Celsus (lib. vii, cap. xii, 1) as *"specillum."* Various oral specula had also been employed, the most important being that described by the osbtetrician André Levret in 1743,[1] and the "light conductor" of Philipp Bozzini (1773–1809) of Mainz, in which the idea of illumination and reflection by mirrors was utilized (1807[2]). On March 18, 1829,[3] a rude "glottiscope" was exhibited to the Hunterian Society of London by Benjamin Babington (1794–1866), of Guy's Hospital, and, in 1837, the Scotch surgeon, Robert Liston, described his mode of exploring the larynx.[4] These efforts passed unnoticed, however, so that the modern laryngoscope came to be invented by Manuel **Garcia** (1805–1906), a Spanish singing teacher in London, who sent an account of his instrument to the Royal Society in 1855.[5] Three years later, his method of examining the throat was made a permanent part of laryngology by Johann Nepomuk **Czermak** (1828–73), of Bohemia, and his colleague, the Viennese neurologist, Ludwig **Türck** (1810–68), both publishing their initial communications in the same year (Czermak, March 27, Türck, June 26, 1858[6]). Separate treatises on laryngoscopy by the same writers appeared in 1860, and, about the same time, Czermak devised a method of exploring the nose and nasopharynx by means of small mirrors (1859–60[7]). Türck wrote an important treatise on diseases of the larynx, with atlas (1866[8]), and was an able neurologist. His studies on the sensible cutaneous areas of the separate spinal nerves (1856–68) are classic. He was also the first to note the correlation of retinal hemorrhage with tumors of the brain (1853[9]).

Other prominent members of the New Vienna School were Josef Hyrtl, the great anatomist, the physiologist Ernst von Brücke, the ophthalmologists Beer, Arlt, Stellwag von Carion, and Jaeger von Jaxtthal, Adam Politzer the otologist, the clinicians Bamberger, Winternitz, and Nothnagel, and the neurologists Meynert, Benedikt, and Ritter von Rittershain. Virchow was almost the only German spirit of his time who appreciated Bichat and Magendie, Bright and Addison, and it was largely due to the eminently practical tendency of these physicians of the New Vienna School—most of them Slavs—that German medicine finally crossed the Rubicon.

One other prominent feature of German medicine in the early part of the 19th century was the rise of **homeopathy,** which, in point of time, is really one of the many isolated theoretic systems of the preceding century. Its founder, Samuel Christian Friedrich **Hahnemann** (1755–1843), of Meissen, took his degree at Erlangen in 1779, and toward the

[1] Levret: Mercure de France, Paris, 1743, p. 2434.
[2] Bozzini: Der Lichtleiter, Weimar, 1807.
[3] Babington: London Med. Gaz., 1829, iii, 555.
[4] Liston: Practical Surgery, London, 1837, p. 350.
[5] Garcia: Proc. Roy. Soc., Lond., 1854–55, vii, 399–410.
[6] Czermak: Wien. med. Wochenschr., 1858, viii, 196. Türck: Ztschr. d. k. k. Gesellsch. d. Aerzte zu Wien, 1858, xiv, 401; 1859, xv, 817. Czermak: Sitzungsb. d. k. Akad. d. Wissensch. Math.-naturw. Cl., Vienna, 1858, xxix, 557–584. See also, Louis Elsberg: Phila. Med. Times, 1873–4, iv, 129–134.
[7] Czermak: Wien. med. Wochenschr., 1859, ix, 518; 1860, x, 257.
[8] Türck: Klinik der Krankheiten des Kehlkopfes, Vienna, 1866.
[9] Türck: Ztschr. d. k. k. Gesellsch. d. Aerzte zu Wien, 1853, ix, pt. 1, 214–218.

end of the century, as the result of certain experiments, some of them made upon his own person, began to formulate the theories which characterize his system. These are, first, a revival of the old Paracelsian doctrine of signatures, namely, that diseases or symptoms of diseases are curable by those particular drugs which produce similar pathologic effects upon the body (*similia similibus curantur*); second, that the dynamic effect of drugs is heightened by giving them in infinitesimally small doses, which are to be obtained by carrying dilution or trituration to an extreme limit; third, the notion that most chronic diseases are only a manifestation of suppressed itch or "Psora." These doctrines were embodied in Hahnemann's *Organon der rationellen Heilkunde* (1810), and found wide acceptance, especially in the New World.

The difference between Hahnemann and Paracelsus was, as Neuburger says, that Hahnemann directed his arcana, not against the causes of disease, but against symptoms or groups of symptoms. Hence his therapeutic method is not a true iso-therapy, nor were the isopathic systems which followed it quite the same thing as treatment by sera, vaccines, bacterins, hormones, and animal extracts.[1] Among the later offshoots of homeopathy was the system of Johann Gottfried Rademacher (1772–1850), in which pathologic processes and findings were ignored, diseases being diagnosed and classified as "universal" or "organic," from the effect of remedies upon them. The natural child of this system was the school of "specificists," which re-jected the fantastic "universal remedies" of Rademacher for the doctrine of the spe-cific relation of certain remedies to definite parts of the body. This system, which is strongly suggestive of Ehrlich, was favorably regarded by Virchow. It was but natural that this aimless theorizing should finally dwindle and fade into a colorless, footless "eclecticism." The impotence of eclecticism was sufficiently manifested in the floods of turgid verbosity and fustian inspired by the cholera epidemic of 1831–37.[2] Neuburger says that the masterpieces of Skoda and Rokitansky were greeted with frigid silence, "a silence that speaks volumes."

The extreme popularity of Hahnemann's doctrines is probably due to the fact that they lessened the scale of dosage of drugs in practice. He was, in fact, the introducer of the small dose. Otherwise his system is but an offshoot of 18th century theorizing. He died a millionaire in Paris in 1843.

Of the earlier **American clinicians,** those who did the most original work were Otto, the Jacksons, North, Ware, the elder Mitchell, Gerhard, and Drake.

John Conrad **Otto** (1774–1844), born at Woodbridge, New Jersey, of German-American stock, took his medical degree at the University of Pennsylvania in 1796, succeeded Benjamin Rush at the Philadelphia Dispensary in 1813, and taught clinical medicine at the Pennsylvania Hospital for twenty-one years. He played an active part in the cholera epidemic of 1833, and is especially remembered by his paper on hemophilia (1803[3]), an investigation of a family of "bleeders," which apart from the Talmudic reference, and notations by Albucasis, Hochstetter (1635), Banyer (1743), and Fordyce was the first clear account of the condition in literature.

James Jackson (1777–1868), of Boston, a pupil-apprentice of Edward Augustus Holyoke (1797–8) and later a dresser at St. Thomas's Hospital and a student of Astley Cooper's, was the first physician to the Massachusetts General Hospital

---

[1] The isopathy (*aequalia aequalibus*) of G. F. Müller, proposed the treatment of scabies by psorin, tænia by tæniin, dental caries by odontonekrosin, phthisis by phthisin (*i. e.,* phthisical sputa, as originally proposed by Robert Fludd), liver diseases by hepatin, etc.

[2] Neuburger: Puschmann-Handbuch, Jena, 1903, ii, 125–129.

[3] J. C. Otto: Med. Repository, New York, 1803, vi, 1–4.

(1810), wrote an early text-book on practice (1825), and was widely read in his attractive *Letters to a Young Physician* (1855). He left one of the earliest accounts of alcoholic neuritis, which he described as "arthrodynia a potu" (1822[1]), outlining the mental symptoms, and his report on typhoid fever (1828[2]) played a great part in getting the disease upon a definite basis in this country.

Jackson's son, James Jackson, Jr. (1810–34), whose early death robbed American medicine of one of Louis' most promising pupils, left a valuable memoir on the cholera epidemic of 1832 and first described the prolonged expiratory sound as an important diagnostic sign of incipient phthisis (1833[3]).

Elisha North (1771–1843), of Goshen, Connecticut, was a pioneer in Jennerian vaccination (1800), established the first eye infirmary in the United States at New London (1817), and, in 1811, published the first book on cerebrospinal meningitis ("spotted fever"), in which he recommends the use of the clinical thermometer. North's book was preceded by the graduating dissertation of Nathan Strong, Jr. (Hartford, 1810).

John Ware (1795–1864), of Hingham, Massachusetts, a Harvard graduate, who was professor of practice at Harvard from 1832 to 1858, wrote an important monograph on croup (1842[4]), and his exhaustive study of delirium tremens (1832[5]) is, in connection with the earlier paper of Thomas Sutton (1813), the classic account of this neurosis.

John Kearsley Mitchell (1798–1858), of Virginia, was educated in Scotland, graduated from the University of Pennsylvania in 1819, and after making three sea voyages as a ship's surgeon, commenced practice in Philadelphia, where he became eminent as an internist, neurologist, and teacher. The volume of monographs collected after his death by his distinguished son (1859[6]) reveals an originality of mind far above the average.

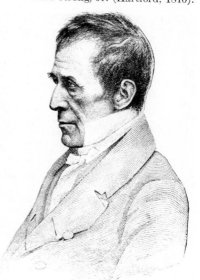

James Jackson (1777–1868). (Boston Medical Library.)

He wrote ably and suggestively on mesmerism, osmosis, liquefaction, and solidification of carbonic acid gas and ligature of limbs in spastic conditions, and he was the first to describe the neurotic spinal arthropathies (1831[7]), which have since been developed by Charcot, Bechtereff, Strümpell and Marie. His essay *On the Cryptogamous Origin of Malarious and Epidemic Fevers* (1849) files the first brief for the parasitic etiology of disease on *a priori* grounds—a rigorous, logical argument which, as pure theory goes, ranks with Henle's essay on miasms and contagia (1840).

Jacob **Bigelow** (1787–1879), of Massachusetts, was one of the greatest of American botanists. His "American Medical Botany"

---

[1] J. Jackson: New Engl. Jour. Med. and Surg., Bost., 1822, ii, 351.

[2] J. Jackson: Report founded on the cases of typhoid fever, Boston, 1838.

[3] Communicated to the Société médicale d'observation de Paris in 1833.

[4] Ware: "Contributions to the History and Diagnosis of Croup," Boston, 1842.

[5] Ware: Med. Communicat. Mass. Med. Soc., Bost., 1830–36, v, 136–194.

[6] J. K. Mitchell: Five Essays, edited by S. Weir Mitchell, Philadelphia, 1859.

[7] Am. Jour. Med. Sc., Phila., 1831, viii, 55–64.

(3 vols., 1817–20), illustrated with 60 plates and 6000 colored engravings, technically devised by himself, was a work of international reputation, approached only in America by the writings of Barton, Raffinesque, Porcher, and Asa Gray. Bigelow was visiting physician to the Massachusetts General Hospital, professor of materia medica at Harvard, and a great medical reformer. During the cholera epidemic of 1832, his wise sanitary rulings limited the mortality in Boston to 100, as against 3000 in New York City. His discourse *On Self-limited Diseases* (1835) exerted a powerful influence upon medical practice in the United States, and, in the words of Holmes, did "more than any

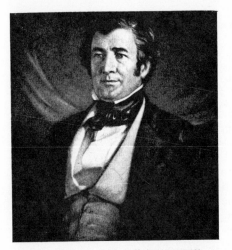

John Kearsley Mitchell (1798–1858).

other work or essay in our own language to rescue the practice of medicine from the slavery to the drugging system which was a part of the inheritance of the profession." In 1855, Bigelow published an anonymous volume of clever poetic travesties entitled "Eolopoesis."

William Wood **Gerhard** (1809–72), born in Philadelphia, of German extraction, perhaps the most brilliant American pupil of Louis, is memorable for the first definite separation of typhus and typhoid fevers (1837). He was resident physician to the Pennsylvania Hospital (1834–68), taught the institutes of medicine at the University of Pennsylvania (1838–72), and was much beloved in his native city for his geniality and kindliness.

He investigated the endermic application of medicines (1830), described (with Pennock) the cholera epidemic at Paris in 1832, and wrote interesting papers on smallpox (1832[1]) and pneumonia (1834[2]) in children. His treatise on diseases of the chest (1842) was the most authoritative American work on the subject before the time of Flint. He left two contributions of enduring value, his monograph on tuberculous meningitis in children (1833–4[3]), the first accurate clinical study of the disease, and his paper on differential diagnosis of typhus and typhoid fevers (1837[4]), which, in the United States at least, definitely settled the clinical and pathologic status of the two affections. Isolated observers, like Willis (1643[5]), Huxham (1737[6]), or Hildenbrand (1810[7]), had no doubt distinguished between the two diseases to their own satisfaction; but they were not differentiated in general practice before the time of

---

[1] Gerhard: Am. Jour. Med. Sc., Phila., 1832, xi, 368–408.

[2] *Ibid.*, 1834, xiv, 328; 1834–35, xv, 87.

[3] *Ibid.*, 1833–4, xiii, 313; 1834, xiv, 99.

[4] *Ibid.*, 1837, xx, 289–322.

[5] Willis: De febribus, 1659, ch. xiv, xvii.

[6] Huxham: Essay on Fevers, 1755.

[7] J. V. von Hildenbrand: Ueber den ansteckenden Typhus, Vienna, 1810.

Gerhard. Even Louis' masterpiece of 1829 took no cognizance of typhus fever, and British practitioners, with the possible exception of A. P. Stewart (1840[1]) or Perry of Glasgow, did not clearly separate typhus from typhoid until Sir William Jenner pointed the way in 1849.[2]

The greatest physician of the West, and one of the most picturesque figures in American medicine, was **Daniel Drake** (1785–1852), who was the first after Hippocrates and Sydenham to do much for medical geography, and has a unique position of his own in relation to the topography of disease. He was born in New Jersey in abject poverty and was reared in a log-cabin among the Kentucky pioneers. The story of his struggles to gain an education, self-aided and single-handed, his rise to the height of his profession in the face of almost every obstacle, is typical of the hardships endured by Western physicians in this early period. As a pupil of William Goforth, the pioneer of Jennerian vaccination in the West, Drake's diploma, made out in Goforth's handwriting, was the first to be issued west of the Alleghanies. Although he practised, Drake did not complete his medical education until 1815, when he received an academic degree at the University of Pennsylvania. He was one of Osler's "peripatetic physicians," constantly moving from place to place in aid of the cause of medical educa-

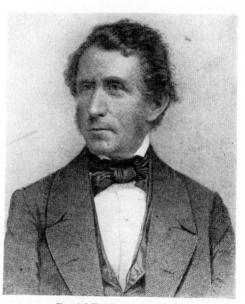

Daniel Drake (1785–1852).

tion, "ever at war with man" (for his nature was combative), and apparently dissatisfied with every condition he met. He changed his locality as a teacher no less than seven times during his life, and two important medical faculties, the Medical College of Ohio (1821) and the Medical Department of Cincinnati College (1835), were founded by him. In the latter venture, he had as associates some of the best American teachers of his day, including Samuel D. Gross and Willard Parker. Drake was also founder of the *Western Journal of the Medical and Physical Sciences* (1827–38), the most important medical periodical of the West in its time. It contains his celebrated essays on Medical Education, which were reprinted in 1832, and are, far and away, the

[1] Stewart: Edinb. Med. & Surg. Jour., 1840, liv, 289–369.
[2] Sir W. Jenner: Med.-Chir. Tr., Lond., 1849–50, xxxiii, 23–42.

most important contributions ever made to the subject in this country. They are written in a style which, for clarity and beauty is, even to-day, a perfect model of what such writing should be. In 1841, Drake published one of the first accounts in literature on the local disorder known as "the trembles," or milk sickness.[1] He also described epidemic cholera as it appeared in Cincinnati in 1832, and wrote a number of papers on the evils of city life (1831), mesmerism (1844), moral defects in medical students (1847), and an entertaining posthumous work on *Pioneer Life in Kentucky* (1870); but his crowning achievement was the great work on the *Diseases of the Interior Valley of North America* (1850–54), the result of thirty years' labor, based largely upon personal observation made during extensive travel. The first volume is a wonderful encyclopedia of the topography, hydrography, climate, and meteorology, plants and animals, population (including diet, habitat, and occupations), of the Mississippi Valley. The second volume, not published until after his death, treats of the autumnal malarial and other fevers, yellow fever, typhus fever, the exanthemata, and the unclassified "phlogistic fevers," in relation to topographic, meteorologic, and sociologic features. There was nothing like this book in literature, unless it might be Hippocrates on Airs, Waters, and Places, and even Hippocrates made no attempt to map out or triangulate the geographic locale of disease. In its practical intention, Drakes' book belongs in the class described by Billings as distinctively and peculiarly American, "in subject, mode of treatment, and style of composition."[2] When Alfred Stillé reported upon it to the American Medical Association in 1850, Drake was greeted with prolonged and thunderous demonstrations of enthusiasm and applause, such as had seldom been accorded to any physician before. "He covered his face with his hands and wept like a child." Two of his earlier pamphlets are among the rarest of medical Americana. The first, a pamphlet on the Climate and Diseases of Cincinnati (1810), was the germ of the greater work; the second, his *Narrative of the Rise and Fall of the Medical College of Ohio* (1822), is one of the choicest bits of medical humor in existence. Drake, as described by Gross, was a tall, commanding figure, simple and dignified in manner. "He was always well dressed, and around his neck he had a long gold watch-chain, which rested loosely upon his vest." As a lecturer he had a splendid voice, and was possessed of fiery eloquence, causing him at times to sway to and fro like a tree in a storm. He was gentle, fond of children, hating coarseness, and had a genuine poetic

---

[1] Early accounts were those of Thomas Barbee, in "Notices Concerning Cincinnati" (1809), and by Alexander Telford and Arthur Stewart in Med. Repository, N. Y., 1812, xv, 92–94.

[2] J. S. Billings, in "A Century of American Medicine," Philadelphia, 1876, p. 314. Billings was the first to emphasize the importance of Drake in American medicine. The elaborate and excellent biography by the late Otto Juettner, of Cincinnati (Daniel Drake and his Followers, Cincinnati, Harvey Publ. Co., 1909), gives a detailed account of Western medicine in the early days, and should be read by all who wish to understand the conditions of the time.

side, writing very creditable verses. Yet, although he practically created decent medical teaching in Cincinnati, he was subjected to many snubs and insults by snobs who affected to look down upon his origin and early chances. He assigned as a reason for not going to Europe that he did not wish to meet physicians who might plume themselves upon possessing greater advantages than himself, and said, with pathetic feeling, "I think too much of my country to place myself in so awkward a position."

Other prominent American physicians of the early period were George Bacon Wood (1797–1879) and Franklin Bache (1792–1864), of Philadelphia, who collaborated in the huge "Dispensatory of the United States" (1833), which ran through 17 editions; Alonzo Clark (1807–87), of New York; who introduced the opium treatment of peritonitis (1855[1]); Elisha Bartlett (1804–55), of Rhode Island, John Y. Bassett (1805–81), Osler's "Alabama student," and Samuel Henry Dickson (1798–1872), of South Carolina, a trio of elegant and attractive medical litterateurs; that belligerent Celt, Charles Caldwell (1772–1853), of North Carolina, who founded two medical schools in the West, and whose *Autobiography* (1855) is a remarkable repository of medical scandal; Robley Dunglison (1798–1869), of Keswick, England, who compiled an excellent medical dictionary (1833) and wrote an amazing array of text-books on nearly every subject except surgery; David Hosack (1769–1835), in his day the best known practitioner in New York City, and editor of the *American Medical and Philosophical Register* (1810–14), in which work he was assisted by John Wakefield Francis (1789–1861), a German-American physician who came to enjoy something of Hosack's popularity in New York, was an attractive teacher and writer and something of a medical Mæcenas in the city; Nathaniel Chapman (1780–1853), of Virginia, a prominent teacher of clinical medicine at the University of Pennsylvania, who, with Matthew Carey, founded the *Philadelphia Journal of the Medical and Physical Sciences* (1820), which, in 1827, under the guidance of Isaac Hays (1796–1879), became the *American Journal of the Medical Sciences* (Hays' Journal); Theodoric Romeyn Beck (1791–1855), of New York, whose *Elements of Medical Jurisprudence* (1823) was easily the best American work on the subject in its day, running through 10 editions and many translations; and Isaac Ray (1807–81), of Beverly, Massachusetts, who wrote the first treatise on the medical jurisprudence of insanity (1838), a solid, well-written book which is still of value.

Of isolated discoveries in internal medicine in the first half of the 19th century, we may mention the original description of "kondee," or sleeping sickness, in the African travels of Thomas Winterbottom (1803[2]); the first accounts of cerebrospinal meningitis by Gaspard Vieusseux (1746–1814) at Geneva (1805[3]), and by L. Danielsson and E. Mann at Medfield, Massachusetts (1806[4]); Charles Badham's little monograph on bronchitis, to which he gave the name (1808[5]); Allan Burns on endocarditis (1809[6]); William Charles Wells on rheumatism of the heart (1812[7]); Romberg's thesis on achondroplasia (1817[8]); John Clarke's account of laryngismus stridulus and tetany in children (1815[9]); John Bostock on hay-fever (1819[10]); Louyer-Villermay's

---

[1] Clark: On the treatment of puerperal peritonitis by large doses of opium, New York, 1855.

[2] Winterbottom: An Account of the Native Africans, London, 1803, ii, pp. 29–31.

[3] Vieusseux: Jour. de méd., chir., pharm., etc., Paris, 1805, xi, 163–182.

[4] Danielsson and Mann: Med. & Agric. Register, Boston, 1806–7, i, 65–69.

[5] Badham: Observations on the Inflammatory Affections of the Mucous Membrane of the Bronchiæ, London, 1808.

[6] Burns: Observations on Some of the Most Frequent and Important Diseases of the Heart, Edinburgh, 1809.

[7] Wells: Tr. Soc., Improve. Med. & Chir. Knowledge, 1804–10, Lond., 1812, iii, 373–412.

[8] M. H. Romberg: De rachitide congenita, Berlin, 1817.

[9] J. Clarke: Commentaries on some of the most important diseases of children, Lond., 1815, pp. 86–97.   [10] Bostock: Med.-Chir. Tr., Lond., 1819, x, 161–165.

classic paper on appendicitis (1824[1]); Kopp's description of "asthma thymicum" and "thymus-death" (1830[2]); Lobstein's account of fragility of the bones, or osteopsathyrosis (1833[3]), John Badham's clinical description of infantile paralysis (1835[4]); Carl Adolph Basedow's important paper on exophthalmic goiter, giving the three basic symptoms or "Merseburg triad" (1840[5]); Mohr's case of tumor of the pituitary body with obesity (1840[6]); Jakob Heine's monograph on infantile poliomyelitis (1840[7]); Henry Burton's notation of the blue line along the gums in lead poisoning ing (1840[8]); Perrin on intermittent hydrarthrosis (1845[9]); the independent accounts of leukemia by Virchow and John Hughes Bennett (1845[10]); the allocation of the symptoms myosis, ptosis, and enophthalmus (Horner's triad) as an expression of cervical sympathetic nerve lesion (1869) by Johann Friedrich Horner (1831–86); and Curling's note of the connection of absence of the thyroid with "symmetric swellings of fat tissue at the sides of the neck connected with defective cerebral development" or myxedema (1850[11]).

The earliest 19th century exponent of **anatomy** and of scientific medicine in France was Marie-François-Xavier **Bichat** (1771–1802), the

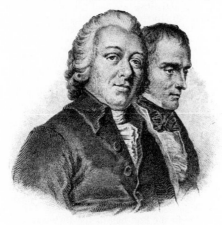

Desault (1744–95) and Bichat (1771–1802).

creator of descriptive anatomy. The son of a physician, the favorite pupil, assistant, and household intimate of the surgeon Desault, and some time an army surgeon in the French Revolution, Bichat soon developed from a light-hearted, rollicking, happy-go-lucky student into a successful surgeon and a master-worker in the science which sustained one of its gravest losses by his early death. His *Traité des membranes* (1799–1800), his five-volume *Anatomie descriptive* (1801–3), and his work on general anatomy applied to physiology and medicine (1802) opened out an entirely new field for anatomists, that of a detailed description of the parts and tissues of the body in health and disease. Before Bichat's time, such text-books as those of the Monros

---

[1] Louyer-Villermay: Arch. gén. de méd., Paris, 1824, v, 246–250.

[2] J. Kopp: Denkwürdigkeiten in der ärztlichen Praxis, Frankfurt a. M., 1830, i, 1, 368.

[3] Lobstein: Traité de l'anat. path., Paris, 1833, ii, 204–212.

[4] Badham: London Med. Gaz., 1835–36, xvii, 215. First described by Michael Underwood (1784).

[5] Basedow: Wchnschr. f. d. ges. Heilk., Berl., 1840, vi, 197, 220.

[6] Mohr: Wchnschr. f. d. ges. Heilk., Berl., 1840, vi, 565–571.

[7] Heine: Beobachtungen über Lähmungszustände der untern Extremitäten und deren Behandlung, Stuttgart, 1840.

[8] Burton: Med.-Chir. Tr., Lond., 1840, xxiii, 63–79.

[9] Perrin: Jour. de méd., Paris, 1845, ii, 82. Union méd., Paris, 1878, 3, s. xxv, 821.

[10] Virchow: "Weisses Blut," in Neue Notizen a. d. Geb. d. Nat. u. Heilk., Weimar, 1845, xxv, 151–155. Bennett: Edinb. Med. & Surg. Jour., 1845, lxiv, 413–423.   [11] Curling: Med.-Chir. Tr., Lond., 1850, xxxiii, 303.

were woefully rudimentary in spots and said next to nothing about the detailed anatomy of the nerves and viscera; while teaching by dissection, as Robert Knox has recorded, was on the most rough-and-ready basis. Bichat was a forerunner of Henle and the histologists, dividing the tissues into 21 (non-microscopic) varieties, which he treated as indivisible parts, like the elements in chemistry, each tissue having its own particular kind of sensibility and contractility (*propriétés vitales*). He was profoundly influenced by Bordeu, and, like Hunter, he regarded disease as an alteration of vital properties or principles. His error was to assign a specific vital property, a different mode of vitalism, to each tissue. This physiologic doctrine, now obsolete, is summed up in his famous and fallacious definition of life as "the sum of the forces that resist death,"[1] which, as has been often observed,[2] is only a question-begging truism in the form of a reversible equation, in fact, a simple case of arguing in a circle.

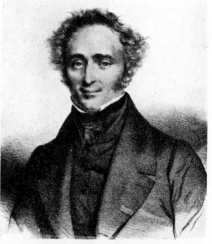

Jean Cruveilhier (1791–1873).

In connection with Bichat's work may be mentioned the splendid atlas, *Anatomie de l'homme* (Paris, 1821–31), by Jules-Germain Cloquet (1790–1883), consisting of five volumes illustrated with 300 folio plates; and the discovery of the third corpuscles or blood-platelets by Alexandre Donné (1801–78) in 1842.[3]

Bichat's ideas were carried over into pathology by Jean **Cruveilhier** (1791–1873), of Limoges, a pupil of Dupuytren's, who held the first chair of pathology in the Paris Faculty (1836), gave the first description (with plates) of disseminated sclerosis[4] and left an early description of progressive muscular atrophy of the Aran-Duchenne type (Cruveilhier's palsy). Like John Hunter, Cruveilhier reasoned from the false assumption that pyemia is the result of phlebitis, and even went to the extent of asserting that "Phlebitis dominates all pathology." His atlases of pathology (1842) are among the most

---

[1] Bichat: Recherches sur la vie et la mort, Paris, an viii (1800), p. 1.

[2] For example, in the inaugural dissertation of Dr. Abraham Jacobi (Congitationes de vita rerum naturalium, Cologne, 1851, p. 24): "Prioribus iam temporibus Bichat alio modo vitam definire conatus est. Vitam igitur qualitatum et actionum materiæ *morte resistentium*, complexum nominat. Sed hæc num definitio est? num aliud est, quam circulus? Statim interrogandum erit, *quidnam sit mors*, et quod solum respondere poteristis, id erit, mortem absentiam esse vitæ. Mors, constituta notione vitæ, vitæ negatione definienda est, non vice versa."

[3] Donné: Compt. rend. Acad. d. sc., Paris, 1842, xiv, 366–368.

[4] Cruveilhier: Anatomie pathologique, Paris, 1835–42, ii, livraison xxxviii, pl. 5.

splendidly illustrated books on the subject. He did not use the microscope, and his errors were afterward corrected, as we shall see, by
Virchow.

Sir Charles Bell (1774–1842), the leading British anatomist of the
period, is now more celebrated as a physiologist and neurologist. He
was the son of a Scotch Episcopal clergyman, and a brother of John
Bell, the well-known surgeon, who opened a private school of anatomy
at Edinburgh in 1790. Both the Bells had an uncommon artistic gift,
and Charles, in particular, illustrated his *System of Dissections* (1798),
his *Engravings of the Brain and Nervous System* (1802), and his Bridgewater treatise on the hand (1833) with exquisite sketches. Coming

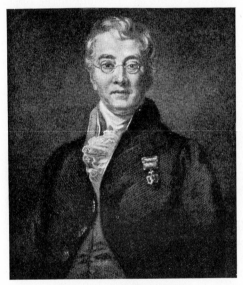

Sir Charles Bell (1774–1842).

up to London in 1804, he
began teaching anatomy in
his own house and later at
Great Windmill Street. He
also lectured to artists, his
"Anatomy of Expression"
(1806) being a sequel of
these studies. Through his
ardent devotion to private
investigation, he never acquired the practice he had
hoped for in London, and
eventually accepted the
chair of surgery at Edin-
burgh in 1836. In 1811,
Bell published *A New Idea
of the Anatomy of the Brain
and Nervous System*, which
contains the following sentence: "On laying bare the
roots of the spinal nerves,
I found that I could cut
across the posterior fasciculus of nerves which took its origin
from the posterior portion of the spinal marrow without convulsing
the muscles of the back, but that, on touching the anterior fasciculus with the point of the knife, the muscles of the back were
immediately convulsed." This is the first experimental reference to
the functions of the spinal nerve-roots in literature, but Bell vitiated
the effects of his discovery, to some extent, by holding fast to the old
theory that all nerves are sensory, classifying them as "sensible and
insensible," and, in reality, he demonstrated clearly the functions of
the anterior roots only. An anatomist by training, his subsequent discoveries were all, in his own phrase, "deductions from anatomy,"
largely, no doubt, on account of his dislike of vivisection, and he failed
to understand the true bearings of the experiment he had made or to
interpret it correctly. The conclusive experimental proof that the

anterior roots are motor, the posterior sensory, was made by Magendie upon a litter of eight puppies (1822[1]), and confirmed by Johannes Müller in the frog (1831[2]). In 1826, Bell himself (in a letter of January 9th) had acquired a clear idea of the difference between sensory and motor nerves. In 1829, he demonstrated that the fifth cranial nerve is sensory-motor; discovered "Bell's nerve"; also the motor nerve of the face (portio dura of the seventh nerve), lesion of which causes facial paralysis (Bell's palsy). These discoveries are incorporated in his book on the nervous system (1830), which also contains early cases of pseudohypertrophic paralysis and "Thomsen's disease." Bell was a genial, unaffected, kind-hearted man, with a captivating twinkle behind his eye-glasses, a bit of a dandy in attire. He was much lionized during his London life, and in 1829 was knighted for his physiologic discoveries by the enthusiastic Lord Brougham. He was an able surgeon, and attended the wounded after Corunna and Waterloo, making interesting sketches of what he saw.

The main supporter of Bichat's ideas in Great Britain was the Scotch anatomist, Robert **Knox** (1791–1862), who was the first to teach general anatomy from the descriptive, histologic, and comparative angles, and attracted Edinburgh students in great numbers by his dramatic style of delivery and his showy appearance in the lecture-room. At this time, there were no public regulations to supply dissecting material for teaching purposes, and the needs of the large anatomy classes were met by surreptitious methods. Body-snatching and even murder were rife. On November 29, 1827, the dead body of an old man who owed £4 to his landlord, William Hare, was sold by Hare to Knox for £7 10s., to recoup the debt, and this stroke of business led Hare and his associate Burke to the idea of smothering their lodgers, or any other unfortunates who fell into their hands, as a money-making scheme. The victim was first intoxicated, and then suffocated by closing the hands tightly over the nose and mouth ("Burking"). Sixteen dead bodies were thus secured and sold before the crime was detected, and the last body was found in Knox's rooms. All Edinburgh went wild on the instant. Knox himself was mobbed by the horrified populace, vituperated by press and pulpit, and threatened with hang-ing. The fact that "Daft Jamie," a harmless imbecile of the "Old Town," and the voluptuous body of "a beautiful Lais" had been among those victimized and dissected, added greater fuel to the flames. Knox, a man of powerful physique and self-possessed character, braved the clamor, made bold to outface his opponents, and eventually defended himself in writing, but he was never popular afterward. His only adherents were his faithful pupils, he eventually lost his hold and dropped out of professional activity, leading a wandering existence until his

---

[1] Magendie: Jour. de physiol. expér., Paris, 1822, ii, 276–279.

[2] Müller: Froriep's Notiz. a. d. Geb. d. Nat. u. Heilk., Weimar, 1831, xxx, 113, 129. The experiment was further confirmed in fish by Wagner (1846) and Stannius (1849), and in birds by Panizza (1834) and Schiff (1858).

death.[1] This sensational and entirely discreditable episode led at least
to one good reform, Lord Warburton's Anatomy Act of 1832 (2d and
3d William IV, cap. 75), which provided that all unclaimed bodies
should, under proper conditions, go to the medical schools. Knox was
an able and interesting writer on artistic anatomy and natural history.
His fragment on *The Races of Man* (1850), although full of eccentric
views, is one of the most original and readable contributions ever made
to anthropology. It was highly praised by Emerson.

An interesting work on artistic anatomy, which may be mentioned in connection
with Knox, is the "Anatomical Studies of the Bones and Muscles for the Use of
Artists" (London, 1883), which were engraved from the posthumous drawings of
John **Flaxman** (1755–1836) by Henry Landseer.

The leading **comparative anatomists** of the early 19th century were Lamarck,
Cuvier, Owen, and Agassiz. Of these, Jean-Baptiste **Lamarck** (1744–1829), who
gave up soldiering for medicine, medicine for botany, and botany for zoölogy, once
famous for his Natural History of Invertebrates (1815–22), is now best remembered
by his *Philosophie Zoölogique* (1809). In this he appears as a great pioneer of evolution, in his theory that variations are produced by the effects of use and disuse
upon organs, by response to external stimuli, and by the direct inheritance of these
acquired characters. Like Galen and Hunter, Lamarck believed that structure follows function (*La fonction fait l'organe*). His doctrine of the heredity of acquired
characters has been hotly contested in consequence of Weismann's glittering gener-
alities, but, while not true in all its parts, has latterly found some confirmation.
Lamarck is now regarded as one of the greatest of philosophic biologists.

Georges **Cuvier** (1769–1832), whom Lamarck·helped and who afterward turned
against him, had, as Flourens said, "*l'esprit vaste.*" His great works on comparative anatomy (1801–05), on the fossil bones of Paris (1812), on the structure of
fishes (1828), and on the animal kingdom (1836–49) are on the most extended scale.
He was the founder of vertebrate paleontology, first stated the theory of morphologic types (vertebrate, molluscan, articulate, radiate), the doctrine of the structural correlation of parts of an organism, and the catastrophe theory of geologic
formations. But he believed in spontaneous generation, the fixity of species, and the
preformation of the embryo.

Sir Richard **Owen** (1804–92), of Lancaster, England, a pupil of Abernethy's,
and the associate and son-in-law of John Hunter's secretary, William Clift, edited
Hunter's posthumous works, and began his studies in morphology with his great
Catalogue of the Physiological Series of Comparative Anatomy (1833–40) in Hunter's
collection. His *Anatomy and Physiology of the Vertebrates* (1866–68) was pronounced
by Flower to rank next to Cuvier's Comparative Anatomy in scope. In 1840–45,
he published his *Odontography*, a monumental treatise on the morphology of the
teeth of living animals, illustrated with 150 plates. In paleontology, his monographs
on British fossil mammals, birds, and reptiles (1846–84), extinct mammals of Australia (1877), and extinct wingless birds of New Zealand (1879), are of the highest
importance. He described the Archæopteryx, the oldest known bird, the Apteryx,
Notornis, and Dinornis, the latter class including the dodo and the giant moa. He

---

[1] Of the odium which Knox incurred from the Burking incident, it may be said
that, while he was technically guiltless, the aversion of his fellow-townsmen was
not entirely without foundation, since they knew that the bodies of poor people
were liable to be spirited away by "sham mourners" at funerals and other devices
of the "Resurrectionists," while the showy, sensational methods of the lecturer
himself were not strictly in accord with the best modern taste as to the dignity of
medical teaching. Dissection and vivisection, to be respectable and scientific,
should always be private and under proper legal restrictions. Even the public dissections depicted on the title-pages of Vesalius and Columbus reek a little too much
of the Barnum's show-bill for modern taste, and a blood-pressure experiment demonstrated on a vivisected animal to a public audience, hardly any of whom understand its bearings, can best be judged in the light of the "Law" of Hippocrates:
"Those things which are sacred are to be imparted only to sacred persons; and it is
not lawful to impart them to the profane until they have been initiated into the
mysteries of the science."

was also the first to describe the Trichina spiralis (1835[1]), but he classified the spermatozoa as internal parasites under "Entozoa." Owen was one of the early workers with the microscope in England, a founder and charter member of the Royal Microscopic Society, and an accomplished violoncellist and chess-player. He was Hunterian professor at the Royal College of Surgeons (1836–56), and superintendent of the Natural History Department of the British Museum (1856–83). In 1843 he introduced the well-known distinction between serial homologies (organs of similar structure and development) and morphologic analogies (different organs of similar function). He followed Goethe and Oken in upholding the vertebrate theory of the skull,[2] and while admitting variation of species through an innate tendency to deviate from an ancestral archetype, was an opponent of Darwinism, but being worsted by Huxley in two important controversies, he eventually went over to it. After Owen's death, Huxley wrote an appreciative study of his work.

Louis **Agassiz** (1807–73), of Mottier, Switzerland, settled in Cambridge, Mass., in 1846, and his *Contributions to the Natural History of the United States* (1857–62) is of especial interest to Americans.
His Lowell Institute lectures on comparative embryology (1846) followed by those of Jeffries Wyman on comparative physiology (1849), introduced new ideas into American teaching. His Fossil Fishes (1833–44), describing over 1000 species, is his masterpiece, although his empirical classification by scales is now discarded. He was an opponent of Darwinism, and upheld the old Linnæan idea of the fixity of species; also the Recapitulation Theory, that "the history of the individual is but the epitomized history of the race."

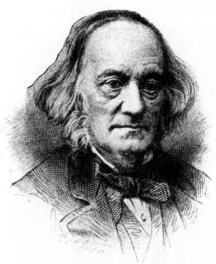

Sir Richard Owen (1804–92).

The pioneers of American anatomy in the first half of the century were Wistar, Horner, Godman, and Morton.

Casper **Wistar** (1760–1818), born in Philadelphia of German extraction, taught anatomy at the University of Pennsylvania from 1791–1818, and his "System of Anatomy" (1811–14), now forgotten, was the earliest treatise on the subject published in this country. His description of the ethmoid bone was praised by Soemmerring, and his memory survives in the wistaria vine, which was named after him; in the still popular "Wistar parties" of old time, weekly literary gatherings at which he was a cultured and amiable host, and in the present Wistar Institute of Anatomy and Biology in Philadelphia (1892).

William Edmonds **Horner** (1793–1853), of Warrenton, Virginia, studied medicine at Edinburgh and Philadelphia, and after serving as army surgeon in the war of 1812, settled in the latter city, where he became prosector to Wistar, Dorsey, and Physick, eventually suc-

---

[1] Owen: Tr. Zoöl. Soc., Lond., 1835, i, 315–324. See, also, Hilton: London Med. Gaz., 1833, xi, 605.

[2] Owen: On the Archetype and Homologies of the Vertebrate Skeleton, London, 1848.

29

ceeding the latter as professor of anatomy in the University of Pennsylvania (1831), his successor being Joseph Leidy.

Horner discovered the tensor tarsi muscle (Horner's muscle) supplying the lacrimal apparatus (1824[1]), and investigated the odoriferous axillary glands in the negro, the muscular tube of the rectum, and the membranes of the larynx. He performed and described important surgical operations, particularly on the eye, and published treatises on anatomy (1826) and pathology (1829). In 1834,[2] he showed that the rice-water discharges in Asiatic cholera consist of epithelium stripped from the small intestine.

John D. **Godman** (1794–1830), of Annapolis, Maryland, an anatomist of great talent, could not realize what was in himself, because, as Gross puts it, "poverty literally pursued him from the cradle to the grave." Orphaned in infancy, friendless, cheated out of his inherit-

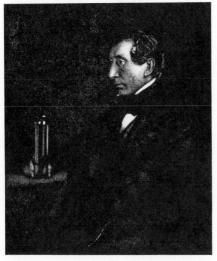

William Edmonds Horner (1793–1853).

ance through fraud, by turns a printer's apprentice and a sailor, he succeeded in gaining his medical education through a noble perseverance, attracted the kindly notice of Daniel Drake, who gave him a chair in surgery, and became editor of the short-lived *Western Quarterly Reporter of Medical, Surgical, and Natural Science* (1822–23), the first medical journal to be printed west of the Alleghanies. His life was one of grinding toil, his lectures were popular, but never remunerative, and he was an early victim of phthisis; but he produced three works of importance and originality—his treatise on the *Fascia* (1824), his *Contributions to Physiological and Pathological Anatomy* (1825), and his *American Natural History* (1826).

Samuel George **Morton** (1799–1851), of Philadelphia, a graduate of the University of Edinburgh, published an elaborate treatise on general and microscopic anatomy (1849), but he is now best remembered as craniologist, paleontologist, and phthisiographer. His *Crania Americana* (1839) and *Crania Ægyptiaca* (1844) are fine atlases, among the earliest of their kind, of permanent value and reputation. His book on organic remains (1834) is said to be the starting-point of all systematic studies of American fossils. His valuable *Illustrations of Pulmonary Consumption* (1834) sums up the knowledge of his time. He believed that the races of mankind are of diverse origin, and his essay on

---

[1] Horner: Phila. Jour. Med. and Phys. Sc., 1824, viii, 70.

[2] Horner: Am. Jour. Med. Sc., Phila., 1834, xv, 545; 1835, xvi, 58; 277, 2 pl.

hybridity (1847) demonstrated the fertility of hybrids, which views made him a target for controversial abuse and theological hatred.

Among the earlier American works on zoölogy and morphology are Thomas Say's *Crustacea of the United States* (1817–18) and *American Entomology* (1824–28), Richard Harlan's *Fauna Americana* (1825), Godman's work on North American mammals (1826), Audubon's *Birds of America* (1827), Isaac Lea's *Fresh Water Mussels* (1829), Nuttall's *Ornithology of the United States and Canada* (1823–34), Holbrook's *North American Herpetology* (1836–40), De Kay's *Zoölogy of New York* (1846–49), and Audubon and Bachmann's *Quadrupeds of North America* (1846–54).

In Germany, the development of anatomy and physiology went hand in hand, and the ablest of the earlier morphologists and histologists—Müller, Schleiden, Schwann, Henle, Remak— were also, in the best sense of the term, physiologists. The founder of scientific medicine in Germany was, indeed, Johannes **Müller** (1801–58), of Coblenz, who was also the greatest German physiologist of his time, and like Haller and John Hunter, one of the great all-round medical naturalists. He was equally eminent in biology, comparative morphology, physiologic chemistry, psychology, and pathology, and through his best pupils—the histologists Schwann, Henle, Kölliker, and Virchow, the physiologists Du Bois Reymond, Helmholtz and Brücke, most

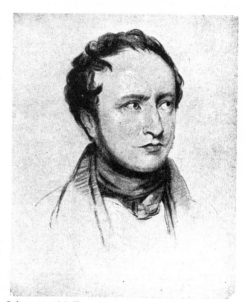

Johannes Müller (1801–58). (From a chalk drawing in the Surgeon General's Library.)

of whom followed the same trend—we may trace the main currents of modern German medicine. Müller's *Handbuch der Physiologie des Menschen* (1834–40) resembles Haller's great treatise as a rich mine of novel facts and original ideas, and introduces two new elements into physiology—the comparative and the psychologic.

His principal contributions to the science were his investigation of specific nerve energies (1826[1]), his explanation of the color sensations ("pressure-phosphenes") produced by pressure on the retina (1826[2]), his experimental proof (in the frog) of the Bell-Magendie law of the spinal nerve-roots (1831[3]), his discovery of the lymph-hearts in the frog (1832[4]), his law of the eccentric projection of sensations from the

---

[1] "Ueber die fantastischen Gesichtserscheinungen," Coblenz, 1826; and Zur vergleichenden Physiologie des Gesichtssinnes, Leipzig, 1826.

[2] Zur vergleichenden Physiologie des Gesichtssinnes, p. 73.

[3] Notizen a. d. Gebiete d. Natur. u. Heilk., Weimar, 1831, xxx, 113, 129.

[4] Phil. Tr. Lond., 1833, pt. 1, 89–94.

peripheral sense organs to other nerve-terminals (1833), his experiments on the vocal cords and the voice (1835–57[1]), his theory of color contrast (1837[2]), his isolation of chondrin and glutin (1837[3]), his demonstration of the function of the bristle cells of the internal ear (1840[4]), and his examination of the slimy secretions of the club-cells of the myxinoid fishes (1845[5]). His broadest generalization, the Law of Specific Nerve-energies,[6] which maintains that each sense organ, when stimulated, gives rise to its own peculiar sensations and no other, has since been extended far beyond its author's original intention, to the idea that each nerve-fiber, as well as each organ or nerve, has its specific sensations, differing in degree if not in kind under stimulation. As a morphologist, Müller made investigations of the first rank on the structural relations of the myxinoid and ganoid fishes (1834–44), the Plagiostoma (with Jacob Henle in 1838–41), and the echinoderms (1846–52). In embryology, his name is associated with the discovery of the Müllerian duct (1825[7]). As a histologist, he worked out the whole finer anatomy of the glandular and cartilaginous tissues (1830[8]), grouped the connective tissues, and thus cleared the ground for the cell theory of his pupil, Schwann. In pathology, as in histology, he was one of the first to use the microscope, particularly in his monumental work on tumors (1838[9]), and he introduced the idea that fever is a nervous reflex (1840). In 1841 he described the parasitic disease now recognized as psorospermosis.[10] In 1834 he founded the journal everywhere known as *Müller's Archiv*, which was continued after his death by His, Reichert and Du Bois Reymond, and later by His and Waldeyer, Engelmann and Rubner. As containing a host of classic contributions, it has exerted a profound influence upon the advancement of scientific medicine.

Like every great investigator who has approached his subject from the broadest angle, Müller made a few mistakes. Following Hewson, Mascagni, and the Hunters, he maintained that absorption is the special and exclusive function of the lymphatics, although Magendie, in 1836, had shown that the blood-vessels also possess this power. As late as 1840, Müller held that respiration in the fetus is effected not (as John Mayow had shown in 1674) by the placenta, but by a special juice or plasma secreted in the maternal blood. In 1840, Müller stated that no one could ever hope to measure the velocity of a nervous impulse. Ten years later his pupil, Helmholtz, had done so. Temperamentally, Müller was a mystic, and, by the same token, a vitalist in theory. Interesting, in this connection, is his correspondence with Goethe on the phenomena now known as eidetics. He believed that there is something in vital processes which does not admit of a mechanical or material explanation, but he also believed that such explanation may be pushed to the limit "so long as we keep to the solid ground of observation and experiment." Strongly built, with broad shoulders and a massive Achillean head—Virchow said it "seemed like that of some warrior of old"—Müller was a striking, magnetic, impressive

---

[1] Handb. d. Physiol., Coblenz, 1840, ii, 184–222.

[2] Handb. d. Physiol., 1840, ii, 372.

[3] Ann. d. Pharm., Heidelb., 1837, xvi, 277–282.

[4] Handb. d. Physiol., 1840, ii.

[5] Untersuchungen über die Eingeweide der Fische, Berlin, 1845, p. 11.

[6] Handb. d. Physiol., 1840, ii, 258.

[7] Nova acta Acad. Nat. Curios., Bonn, 1825, pt. ii, 565–672, 6 pl.

[8] De glandularum secernentium structura penitiori, Leipzig, 1830.

[9] Ueber den feinern Bau und die Formen der krankhaften Geschwülste, Berlin, 1838.

[10] Müller's Arch., Berl., 1841, 477–496, 1 pl.

teacher, of rare personal charm, who influenced and inspired his pupils for good as only a great man can.

After Müller's time, the main trend of German anatomy was along histologic and functional lines, and this new departure turned upon three important factors—the foundation of modern **embryology** by von Baer (1827–28), the improvement of the achromatic microscope by Joseph Jackson Lister in 1830, and the development of the cell theory by Schleiden and Schwann (1838–39).

Carl Ernst **von Baer** (1792–1876), the father of the new embryology, was a native of Esthland, in the Baltic Sea provinces of Russia, and was successively professor at Dorpat, Königsberg, and St. Petersburg. The special service of von Baer was that, where his predecessors had only studied the chick, he made embryology a comparative science, established the modern theory of the germ-layers, and the beginnings of histogenesis, organogenesis, and morphogenesis.

Caspar Friedrich Wolff, in 1768, had already been close upon the germ-layer concept when he saw that the intestines are produced by the folding in and rolling together of "leaf-like" embryonic layers. In 1817[1] Christian Pander (1793–1865), assisted by von Baer, in his observations upon the chick, extended the number of these layers to three. Von Baer, in his great work on the development of animals (1828–34[2]), showed, from comparative studies of all kinds, that these leaf-like layers are not true tissues of the developing organism, but the germs or germ-layers from which the alimentary canal, the nervous system and its other parts are unfolded, disappearing as the latter are completed.

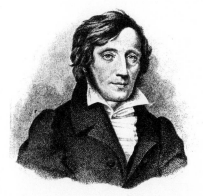

Carl Ernst von Baer (1792–1876). (From an engraving in the Surgeon-General's Library.)

He recognized four layers in all, from the fact that the middle layer is made of two sheets; but this double layer was afterward shown to be a single structure by Robert Remak, who first defined the three categories, ectoderm, endoderm, and mesoderm (1845).

The supreme merit of von Baer's work lies in the wonderful patience shown in working out, as Minot says, "almost as fully as was possible at this time, the genesis of all the principal organs from the germ-layers, instinctively getting at the truth as only a great genius could have done." This was in the trying early days of the modern microscope, and the clear and beautifully accurate results obtained, from sections cut without the aid of a microtome, have set the pace for all subsequent work, down to the recent phase of tracing the embryonic cell-lineage in minutest detail. Von Baer discovered the

---

[1] Pander: Diss. sistens historiam metamorphoseos quam ovum incubatum prioribus quinque diebus subit, Würzburg, 1817.

[2] von Baer: Ueber Entwickelungsgeschichte der Thiere, Königsberg, 1828–34.

mammalian ovum in 1827,[1] and, at the same time, the chorda dorsalis or notochord. From his exhaustive studies in comparative embryology, he was led to classify animals into four groups, viz., Vertebrata, Articulata, Mollusca, and Radiata, which makes him, with Cuvier, the founder of modern morphology (Haeckel). Von Baer went to Russia in 1834, and devoted the rest of his life to investigating the physical geography and antropology of that country. In coöperation with Rudolf Wagner, he was instrumental in calling together the first Congress of Anthropologists in 1861. He was of a deeply religious nature, and his autobiography, privately printed in 1864, gives an interesting account of his experiences.

Contemporaneous with von Baer were Wagner's discovery of the germinal spot (1835), Purkinje's characterization of the formative substance ("protoplasm") of the embryo (1839), Schwann on respiration in the embryonic chick (1834), Reichert on the visceral arches in vertebrata (1837), Bischoff on the development of the rabbit (1848) and the guinea-pig (1852); but the newer embryology of von Kölliker, His, Haeckel, Balfour, Hertwig, and Minot is part and parcel of the doctrine of the nucleated cell.

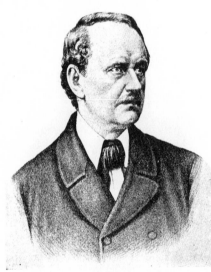

Matthias Jacob Schleiden (1804–81).

The development of the **cell-theory**, one of the fundamental principles of modern science, was almost entirely the work of botanists. In the 17th century, Robert Hooke (1665), Malpighi (1675), and Nehemiah Grew (1682) had noticed the "small boxes or bladders of air" (cellular cavities) in cork and green plants. In 1831, the cell-nucleus was discovered by the botanist Robert Brown (1773–1858), who also discovered the rôle of pollen in the generation of plants. The cell nucleolus was discovered by Gabriel Valentin in 1836. The significance of the nucleus in vegetable histology was first emphasized by the Hamburg botanist, Matthias Jacob **Schleiden** (1804–81), who, after studying law and medicine, became professor of botany at Jena, Dorpat, and Frankfort on the Main. In his important paper on *Phytogenesis* (1838[2]) Schleiden saw and proved that plant tissues are made up of and developed from groups of cells, of which he recognized the nucleus (or "cytoblast") as the important feature; but he held that young cells originate spontaneously from the cytoblast, which he thought to be encased in the solid cell wall. He regarded the young cell as resting upon and expand-

---

[1] von Baer: De ovi mammalium et hominis genesi, Leipzig, 1827.
[2] "Beiträge zur Phytogenese," Müller's Arch., Berl., 1838, 137–176, 2 pl.

ing over the cytoblast like a watch-crystal over a watch, the "watch-glass theory" (*Uhrglastheorie*). Thus, Schleiden regarded cell reproduction as endogenous (free internal formation) instead of by division, and the cell wall as a solid structure instead of a semipermeable membrane. But he was a true physiologic botanist in tendency, with a lively contempt for the mere herbarium collector, and his *Grundzüge* (1842–43)[1] is perhaps the most important landmark in the modern history of the science. He was keen at controversy and, lawyer-like, did not hesitate to indulge in personalities to put his adversaries in a corner. A friendly after-dinner conversation between Schleiden and Schwann, who in the meantime had discovered nucleated cells in the animal tissues, led Schwann to look for cells in all the tissues he knew of and to formulate the most important generalization in the science of morphology, viz., the principle of structural similarity in animal and vegetable tissues: "There is one universal principle of development for the elementary parts of organisms, however different, and that principle is the formation of the cells." To Schleiden's concept of the cytoblast, Schwann added the "cytoblastema" or matrix of cell development, analogous to the mother liquor from which crystals spring. This, as Virchow pointed out, was a tacit acceptance of "spontaneous generation," the very thing which Schwann afterward did so much to overthrow.

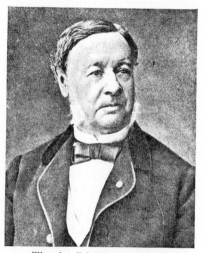

Theodor Schwann (1810–82).

Theodor **Schwann** (1810–82), born at Neuss near Düsseldorf, was a pupil of Müller's at Bonn and his prosector at Berlin. After the publication of his classic on the cell theory in 1839,[2] Schwann was called to the University of Louvain, and, in 1848, became professor of anatomy and physiology at Liège.

A most careful and accurate investigator, he discovered the sheath of the axis-cylinder of nerves, which goes by his name (1838[3]), and the striped muscle in the upper part of the esophagus (1837[4]). His inaugural dissertation (1834[5]) showed that air is necessary for the development of the embryo; and, applying the same idea to

---

[1] Grundzüge der wissenschaftlichen Botanik, Leipzig, 1842–43.

[2] Mikroskopische Untersuchungen über die Uebereinstimmung in der Struktur und dem Wachsthum der Thiere und Pflanzen, Berlin, 1839.

[3] Froriep's Neue Notizen, Weimar, 1838, v, 228, and Schwann's book on the cell-theory.

[4] Joh. Müller: Handbuch d. Physiologie, Coblenz, 1840, ii, 36.

[5] De necessitate aëris atmosphærici ad evolutionem pulli in ovo incubato, Berlin, 1834.

the problem of spontaneous generation, he was able to prove, in 1836,[1] that putrefaction is produced by living bodies, which are themselves destroyed if the surrounding air be heated or vitiated. In 1837,[2] about the same time as Cagniard Latour, he discovered the organic nature of yeast, and showed that the yeast-plant causes fermentation which can be suppressed by heating the culture-medium and sterilizing the surrounding air by heat. As a physiologist, Schwann discovered pepsin in 1835,[3] showing its power to change nondiffusible albumens into peptones; and, in 1841,[4] demonstrated, by means of an artificial biliary fistula in a dog, that bile is absolutely essential to digestion. He was the first to investigate the laws of muscular contraction by physical and mathematical methods, in his classic experiment, demonstrating that the tension of a contracting muscle varies with its length (1837[5]).

In personality, Schwann was an amiable, unpretentious nature, somewhat below the middle height, with an open, pleasant, genial countenance, not unlike that of Claude Bernard. He is said to have visited London twice without making himself known to any one. He was a devout Catholic, submitting the manuscript of his work on the cell theory to the Bishop of Malines for approval before publication, but he did not hesitate to declare the Louise Lateau affair an arrant imposture. During the last forty years of his academic life he seems to have done little scientific work. Professor Ray Lankester records that "to sit with him in front of a café in the pleasant streets of Louvain and hear him discourse on the progress of histology and the germ theory of disease" was "a pleasure no less startling than that which could be conferred by one risen from the dead."

Following the researches of Schleiden and Schwann, cells were discovered which had not a cell wall, but merely what physicists call a "surface of discontinuity" in relation to the surrounding medium; and it was found that the nucleus is contained, not in the cell wall, as Schleiden had supposed, but in the ground substance of the cell itself. From this time on, the nature and significance of this fundamental substance became the main object of investigation.

In 1835, the French zoölogist Felix Dujardin (1801–60) had described and defined it in the protozoa as "sarcode."[6] Schleiden, in his paper of 1838, had noted it in plants and regarded it as a gum. Purkinje was the first to employ the term "protoplasm," applying it to the germinal ground substance of the embryo (1839). In 1846–51, the botanist Hugo von Mohl (1805–72), of Stuttgart, described part of the contents of the vegetable cell (just under the cell-membrane) as "protoplasm,"[7] and the chemical nature of the same was investigated by a Swiss botanist, Carl Nägeli (1817–91), in 1862–63.[8] Ferdinand Cohn (1828–98), of Breslau, eminent for his work in bacteriology, declared, after a study of the protococcus, that animal and vegetable protoplasm are analogous, if not identical, substances (1850–53[9]). Heinrich Anton de Bary (1831–88), a Frankfort botanist, showed this identity further

[1] Ann. d. Physik. u. Chemie, Leipz., 1837, xli, 184–193.

[2] Mitth. a. d. Verhandl. d. Gesellsch. naturf. Freunde zu Berlin, 1837, ii, 9–15.

[3] Müller's Archiv, Berl., 1836, 90–114.   [4] Ibid., 1844, 127–159.

[5] Described in Müller's "Physiologie," 1840, ii, 59–62.

[6] Dujardin: Ann. d. sc. nat. (zoöl.), Paris, 1835, iv, 343–376.

[7] Von Mohl: Botan. Ztg., 1846, iv, 337, 353, 369, 385.

[8] Nägeli: Sitzungsb. d. k. bayer. Akad. d. Wissensch., München, 1862, ii, 280. 1863, i, 161, 483; 1863, ii, 119.

[9] Cohn: Zur Naturgeschichte des Protococcus pluvialis, Breslau, 1850, and Untersuchungen über die Entwicklungsgeschichte der mikroskopischen Algen und Pilzen, Bonn, 1853.

in his work on the myxomycetes (1859[1]). In the meantime (1858), Virchow had already announced the continuity of cell development and its importance in pathology. Finally, Max Schultze, in 1861,[2] showed that the likeness between animal and vegetable protoplasm is not only structural and chemical, but also physiologic.

Thus the cell gradually came to be recognized as the structural and physiological unit in all living organisms, whether animals or plants, simple or complex, embryonic or adult, healthy or diseased, while, in our own time, the cell-nucleus is regarded as the chemical "center of oxidation," the chromosome as the transmitter of inherited characters and the determinant of sex.

It was in this way that anatomic studies came to be more and more histologic or microscopic, and the "seats and causes" of disease itself to be referred to the cellular elements in the body and the unicellular organisms which may attack them.

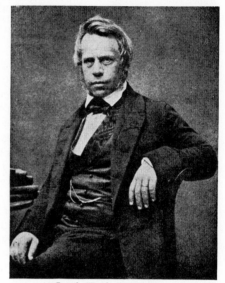

Jacob Henle (1809–85).

The importance of the cell theory is immediately sensed in the work of Jacob **Henle** (1809–85), the greatest German histologist of his time and one of the greatest anatomists of all time. Born of Jewish parents at Fürth, near Nuremberg, Henle was one of Johannes Müller's favorite pupils, one of his prosectors at Berlin, and later professor of anatomy at Zürich (1840), Heidelberg (1844), and Göttingen (1852–85). Henle did many important things for medical science. In his classic researches of 1836–37[3] he was the founder of modern knowledge of the epithelial tissues of the body.

He first described the epithelia of the skin and intestines, defined columnar and ciliated epithelium, and pointed out that this tissue constitutes the true lining membrane of all free surfaces of the body and the inner lining of its tubes and cavities. In 1840,[4] he demonstrated the presence of smooth muscle in the middle (endothelial) coat of the smaller arteries, a discovery which was the starting-point of the present physiological theory of the vasomotor mechanism. He also discovered the external sphincter (striated muscle) of the bladder, the central chylous vessels, the internal root-sheath of the hair, the Henle tubules in the kidney (1862[5]) and gave the first

---

[1] de Bary: Die Mycetozoen, Leipzig, 1859.

[2] Schultze: Müller's Arch., Berl., 1861, 1–27.

[3] Henle: Symbolæ ad anatomiam villorum intestinalium imprimis eorum epithelii et vasorum lacteorum, Berlin, 1837.

[4] In his "Allgemeine Anatomie," Leipzig, 1841, pp. 510, 690.

[5] Contained in his "Handbuch der systematischen Anatomie," 1862, ii, 300–305.

accurate account of the histology of the cornea and of the morphology and development of the larynx. He first pointed out many important structures in the brain, notably the relations of the hippocampus, and the vestigial character of the posterior lobe of the pituitary body.

Altogether, the histological discoveries of Henle[1] take rank with the anatomical discoveries of Vesalius.

As a morphologist, he collaborated with Müller in his monograph on the plagiostomes (1838–41), and described the electric fish Narcine, and the annelid Enchytræus. In pathology he was, with his friend Pfeufer, the founder of the celebrated *Zeitschrift für rationelle Medizin* (1842–69), which exerted a powerful influence upon the advancement of German medicine and contains some of the best monographs of the period. His essay "On Miasms and Contagia" (1840[2]) contains the first clear statement of the idea of a *contagium animatum*. His essay on fevers[3] elaborates Müller's idea that fever is only a symptom, occasioned by disturbances in the central nervous system. In practical medicine, Henle first connected the catarrhs and exanthemata with inflammation (1838), pointed out the preponderance of left-sided varicocele and the relation of left-sided intercostal neuralgias to the hemiazygos vein, and first showed the significance of urinary casts in renal disease (1844).

In his "Handbook of Rational Pathology" (1846–53[4]) he maintains that the physician's duty is to prevent and cure disease; that disease is a deviation from normal physiologic processes; death the cessation of metabolism; and the hypothesis of a vital force, "just as good or as weak as that of electric attraction or gravitation." Of Henle's two books on anatomy, the earlier *Allgemeine Anatomie* (1841) was, in reality, the first treatise upon microscopic histology, and marks a great advance upon Bichat in that the tissues are considered in their developmental and functional, as well as their structural, relations. The classification of the tissues is the simplest and best ever made, and the book contains an admirable history of microscopy and histology, as also some of Henle's most important discoveries. The later" Handbook of Systematic Anatomy" (1866–71[5]) is an exhaustive three-volume treatise of the highest scientific order. It contains the first logical account and nomenclature of the axes and planes of the body, the terminology is greatly simplified and the sections on the ligaments, the muscles, the viscera, and the vascular and nervous systems are of epoch-making importance. The illustrations of this work, made with Henle's own hand, are, as he puts it, architectural rather than diagrammatic, in that only so much of a structure is given in light and shade as is necessary for its comprehension, while the idea of plan and elevation is freely resorted to. As a lecturer, Henle was vivid and inspiring, making his own drawings with his crayon as he went along, and winning love and admiration by his sincerity and charm. He was not only a skilful artist, but something of a poet, and an accomplished musician, beginning with the violin and eventually learning to play both viola and violoncello, so that he might take any part at

---

[1] These discoveries are to be found in Henle's two treatises on anatomy.
[2] In his "Pathologische Untersuchungen," Berlin, 1840, pp. 1–82.
[3] *Ibid.*, 206–274.   [4] Handbuch der rationellen Pathologie, Braunschweig, 1846–53.
[5] Handbuch der systematischen Anatomie des Menschen, Braunschweig, 1866-71.

need in an impromptu string quartet. The experiences of his life, his peripatetic career as student and professor, the romantic circumstances of his first marriage, his friendships with such men as Humboldt, Gustav Magnus, and Felix Mendelssohn, make an interesting narrative.

Robert **Remak** (1815–65), of Posen, also of Jewish descent, was an assistant of Schönlein's at the Charité, and apart from his reputation as a microscopist, did a number of important things in other directions. In histology he is memorable for his discovery of the non-medullated nerve-fibers (fibers of Remak) in 1838,[1] and of the ganglionic cells in the sinus venosus of the frog's heart (1848[2]), now regarded as the autonomous centers causing the heart-beat. He was one of the first to point out that the proliferation of cells to form tissues is accomplished by cell division (1852[3]), and not, as Schleiden and Schwann had supposed, by endogenous formation. As we have seen, he simplified von Baer's classification of the germ-layers (1851[4]). In 1842, in Schönlein's clinic, he produced favus experimentally, *in propria persona*, separating the fungus from the genus Oïdium, and calling it Achorion Schönleini, after the master (1845[5]). He was the first to describe ascending neuritis (1861), and he was, with Addison and Duchenne of Boulogne, one of the pioneers of electrotherapy, substituting the galvanic for the induced current (1856[6]).

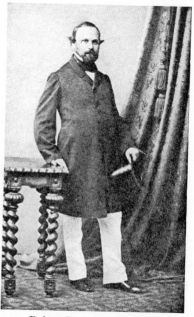

Robert Remak (1815–65).

Another important pioneer in the use of the microscope was Johannes Evangelista **Purkinje** (1787–1869), of Bohemia, who was also a physiologist of genius. He began life as a teacher, having previously taken orders, but graduated in medicine at Prague (1819) with an inaugural dissertation on subjective visual phenomena,[7] which won for him the

---

[1] Remak: Observationes anatomicæ et microscopicæ de systematis nervosi structura, Berlin, 1838.

[2] Remak: Müller's Archiv, Berl., 1848, 139.   [3] *Ibid*, 1852, 47–57.

[4] Remak: Untersuchungen über die Entwickelung des Wirbelthiereies, Berlin, 1851.

[5] Remak: Diagnostische und pathogenetische Untersuchungen, Berlin, 1845, pp. 196, 205, 208.

[6] Remak: Galvanotherapie der Nerven- und Muskelkrankheiten, Berlin, 1858.

[7] Purkinje: Beiträge zur Kenntniss des Sehens in subjectiver Hinsicht, Prague, 1819.

friendship and protection of Goethe. It was perhaps through Goethe's influence that Purkinje was appointed professor of physiology and pathology at the University of Breslau in 1823. At Breslau, he was at first coldly received, on account of the current prejudice against Slavs, which he soon lived down, winning every one over by his superior knowledge and urbane demeanor. Purkinje remained at Breslau until 1850, when he was called to the chair of physiology at Prague. During his Breslau period he did some important work for the development of German science which is frequently overlooked. He was the founder of laboratory training in connection with German university teaching.

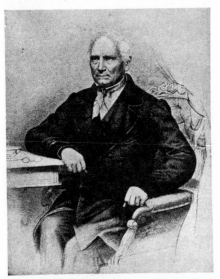

Johannes Evangelista Purkinje (1787–1869).

In 1824, he started a physiologic laboratory in his own house. The work done by the master and his pupils proved to be of such high character that the Prussian government finally erected a Physiological Institute for him at Breslau in 1842. As in the case of Carl Ludwig, many dissertations of Purkinje's pupils represent the ideas of the great physiologist himself.

As a microscopist, Purkinje was the first to use the microtome, Canada balsam, glacial acetic acid, potassium bichromate, and the Drummond lime light (1839). In 1825,[1] he described the germinal vesicle in the embryo, and he was the first histologist to employ the term "protoplasm," which he applied to the embryonic ground substance in 1839.[2] He discovered the sudoriferous glands of the skin with their excretory ducts (1833[3]), the pear-shaped ganglionic (Purkinje) cells in the cerebellum (1837[4]), the lumen of the axis-cylinder of nerves,[5] and the ganglionic bodies in the brain.[6] In 1834–35, he wrote (with Gabriel Valentin[7]) his famous essay on ciliary epithelial motion; described the "Purkinje fibers" of the cardiac muscle (1839[8]) and

---

[1] Symbolæ ad ovi avium historiam ante incubationem, Breslau, 1825.

[2] Uebersicht d. Arb. u. Veränd. d. schles. Gesellsch. f. vaterl. Kultur, 1839, Breslau, 1840, p. 82. Also, De formatione granulosa in nervis aliisque partibus organismi animalis, student's dissertation by Joseph Rosenthal, Breslau, 1839.

[3] In student's dissertation, "De epidermide humana," by Adolph Wendt, Breslau, 1833.

[4] Ber. ü. d. Versamml. deutsch. Naturf. u. Aerzte, 1837, Prague, 1838, xv, 180, plate, Fig. 18.

[5] *Ibid.*, 177.

[6] *Ibid.*, 178–179.

[7] Müller's Arch., Berl., 1834, 391–400. Also "De phænomeno generali et fundamentali motus vibratorii continui in membranis tum externis tum internis animalium plurimorum et superiorum et inferiorum ordinum obvii, Breslau, 1835.

[8] In student's dissertation by Bogislaus Palicki: De musculari cordis structura, Breslau, 1839.

of the uterus (1840[1]). In 1837,[2] two years before Schwann, he pointed out the probable identity of structure in animal and plant cells and he also antedated the latter by two years in his work on artificial digestion (1838[3]). In 1823,[4] long before Francis Galton, he pointed out the importance of finger prints, giving accurate figurations of the same, and he also noted that deaf mutes can hear through the bones of the skull. He was an important pioneer in the description of most of the subjective visual figures (1819–23), notably those obtained by galvanic stimulation, the recurrent images, the entoptic appearances from the shadows of the retinal vessels, the dependence of brightness of color upon intensity of light, the choroidal figure, the rosettes of light produced by the use of digitalis, and the peculiar radiations following the instillation of belladonna. Purkinje was also the first to employ the terms "enchyma" for the basic substance of glands, "cambium" for the same thing in plants, and "protoplasm" for the ground substance of tissues. Altogether a physiologist of extraordinary range and keenness of perception, he was further distinguished as a pharmacologist, his experiments on the action of camphor, belladonna, stramonium, and turpentine having been made upon himself (1829[5]).

In relation to clinical medicine, Purkinje was the first to study the vertigo and rolling of the eyes produced by rotating the erect body in a vertical axis (1820–25[6]), and, although he did not connect the phenomenon with the semicircular canals, his description is the starting-point of modern work on vestibular and cerebellar nystagmus.

After Henle's time, perhaps the most distinguished histologist of the early period was Albert **von Kölliker** (1817–1905), a Swiss who had heard Johannes Müller's lectures at Berlin, graduated at Heidelberg in 1842, and was Henle's prosector at Zürich in 1843. He became professor of anatomy at Zürich in 1846, and, the following year, received a call to Würzburg, where he remained for the rest of his active life. Kölliker was a follower of pure science and was equally remarkable in comparative embryology, histology, and morphology. In his monograph on the development of invertebrates (1843[7]) he was one of the first to apply Schwann's cell-theory to descriptive embryology, treating the ovum as a single cell and its segmentation as normal cell division only.

In 1847, he first demonstrated the true development of the spermatozoa, showing that they are not extraneous bodies, but originate in the testicular cells and fertilize the ovum.[8] He was the author of the first work on comparative embry-

---

[1] In student's dissertation by Wilhelm Kasper: De structura fibrosa uteri nongravidi, Breslau, 1840.

[2] Ber. d. Versamml. deutsch. Naturf. u. Aerzte, Prague, 1837, 175.

[3] Purkinje and Pappenheim: Ueber künstliche Verdauung, Müller's Arch. Berl., 1838, 1–4.

[4] Commentatio de examine physiologico organi visus et systematis cutanei, Breslau, 1823. In this Purkinje describes the three entoptic images of a flame placed in front of the eye in a dark room.

[5] Neue Breslau. Samml. a. d. Geb. d. Heilk., 1829, i, 423–444.

[6] "Beiträge zur Kenntniss des Schwindels aus heautognostischen Daten," Med. Jahrb., Vienna, 1820, vi, 79–125, and Rust's Mag. f. d. ges. Heilk., Berl., 1825, xxiii, 284–310. See, also, the student's dissertation "De cerebri læsi ad motum voluntarium relatione, certanque vertiginis directione ex certis cerebri regionibus læsis pendente," by Heinrich Carl Krause, Breslau, 1824.

[7] Müller's Arch., Berlin, 1843, 68–141.

[8] Kölliker: Neue Denkschr. d. allg. schweiz. Gesellsch. f. d ges. Naturwissensch Zürich, 1847, viii.

ology (1861[1]), which embodies his important study of the relation of the vertebrate notochord to the adult spine and skull. In histology, he was the first to isolate smooth muscle (1846–48[2]), confirming Henle's discovery of the latter in the walls of blood vessels; and he demonstrated the relation of the nerve-cell to medullated nerve-fiber (1889–94). He also confirmed Sharpey's theory of ossification and growth of bone (1860) and Corti's discoveries on the finer anatomy of the ear. Kölliker's "Microscopic Anatomy" (1850–54[3]) and "Handbook of Human Histology" (1852[4]) were the first formal text-books on the subject. The fifth edition of the Handbook was so enlarged by an added wealth of material as to be, in effect, a new book, the second volume literally creating the science of the comparative histology of the central nervous system in vertebrated animals. Minot says that "Kölliker knew more by direct personal observation of the microscopic structure of animals than any one else who has ever lived." In physiology, he applied Matteucci's "rheoscopic frog" effect to the heart (1855) and first investigated "veratrinized muscle" (1856). In zoölogy, Kölliker's name will always be assocated with the Cephalopoda, the Cœl-

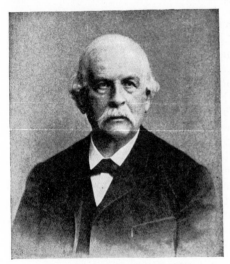

enterata, the Gregarinidæ, Rhodope, Actinophrys, and other animals investigated by him. In 1849 he founded, with von Siebold, the *"Zeitschrift für wissenschaftliche Zoologie,"* the leading German organ of the science, which he edited for half a century. Kölliker was not only unrivaled in his notations of fact, but was also an able theorist and in advance of his time. Although ignorant of Mendel's work, he rejected the theory of natural selection in favor of saltatory or spontaneous variations (mutations); he regarded the cell nucleus as the transmitter of hereditary characters, and his theory of the mechanism of the male generative process (1863[5]) was confirmed by Eckhard. In 1862, he rediscovered the branched muscle plates in the heart, which Leeuwenhoek had seen two hundred years before.[6]

Albert von Kölliker (1817–1905).

Personally, von Kölliker was a strong, grave, handsome, dignified figure, a veteran of pure science, whose prodigious industry was rewarded by a patent of nobility from the Bavarian government and the Prussian order *"pour le mérite."* Like his great predecessor, von Baer, he left an interesting autobiography (1899).

The first and greatest teacher of topographic and regional anatomy in the 19th century was Josef **Hyrtl** (1810–94), of the New Vienna School, who was born at Eisenstadt, in Hungary. His father, a musician in Count Esterhazy's band, had played an oboe under Haydn, and Hyrtl, himself a chorister in his youth, had something the look of

---

[1] Entwicklungsgeschichte des Menschen und der Thiere, Leipzig, 1861.

[2] Mitth. d. naturf. Gesellsch. in Zürich, 1847, i, 18–28, and Ztschr. f. wissensch. Zool., Leipz., 1848, i, 48–87, 4 pl.

[3] Mikroskopische Anatomie, Leipzig, 1850–54.

[4] Handbuch der Gewebelehre des Menschen, Leipzig, 1852.

[5] Würzb. naturw. Ztschr. (Sitzungsb., 1863), 1864, v, p. v.

[6] Proc. Roy. Soc., Lond., 1862–63, xii, 65–84.

Haydn. As a student, he became Czermak's famulus at Vienna, made discoveries for which he was appointed prosector in 1833, and, at the age of twenty-six, became professor of anatomy at Prague. Appointed to the professorship of anatomy at Vienna in 1844, he was for thirty years the most fascinating and popular lecturer on the subject in Europe, his courses being followed by enthusiastic crowds of every race and class, even foreign nobles and consuls. His lectures were clear, concise, eloquent presentations of what he himself knew, interspersed to an extraordinary degree with witty epigrams, classic quotations, anecdotes, and veiled allusions of a questionable character.

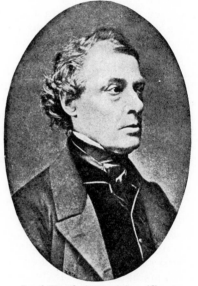

Josef Hyrtl (1810–94). (Courtesy of Captain Henry J. Nichols, U. S. Army.)

Hyrtl did not go in for merging his science into histology, like Henle, but kept up the straight Vesalian tradition of teaching gross or regional anatomy, and, for once, he succeeded, both as writer and lecturer, in making a dry subject piquant as well as interesting. Zuckerkandl said: "He spoke like Cicero and wrote like Heine." He made no great discoveries, and, as an independent investigator, he is not anywhere in Henle's class, but is to be regarded rather as the unapproachable teacher and technician and one of the greatest of medical philologists, a man to whom written and spoken Latin were as his mother tongue. His famous *Lehrbuch* (1846) passed through twenty-two editions, was translated into most languages, and has been pronounced by von Bardeleben to be the least soporific of all scientific treatises. Before reaching its twentieth edition (1889), it had no illustrations, the deficiency being largely supplied by Hyrtl's clear, beautiful, straightforward style, closing immediately with the subject in hand, and his wealth of historic and cultural allusions. Following the example of the French surgeons, Hyrtl published, in 1847,[1] the first topographic anatomy in the German language, which, despite its lack of illustrations, is doubly fascinating by reason of the same extraordinary display of historic and philologic knowledge. Hyrtl's manual of dissecting, published in 1860, is a classic of the same rank with Virchow's book on postmortem sections, and his *Corrosions-Anatomie* (1873) is a permanent memento of his unique skill in making anatomic preparations. These, the wonder and admiration

---

[1] Hyrtl: Handbuch der topographischen Anatomie, Vienna, 1847.

of Europe, included his unrivaled collection of fish skeletons, all prepared by himself; his models of the human and vertebrate ear; his microscopic slides and the corroded preparations (his own invention), consisting of injections of the blood-supplies of the different organs and regions, with the adjacent parts eaten away by acids, to show the finest ramifications. His favorite fields of investigation were, in fact, the vascular and osseous systems. He discovered the portal vein of the suprarenal capsules, the branchial veins of fishes, the origin of the coronary arteries (1854), and made a collection of hearts devoid of blood-supply (*gefässlose Herzen*). Everything he did was stamped with originality and self-will. He once had the Laokoön represented as a life-sized skeletal group in support of his belief that bodily grace and poise depend, in the last analysis, upon bony structure. He opposed Brücke's theory of the autonomy of the heart with such harsh personalities that there came to be a Hyrtl faction and a Brücke faction in Vienna. Hyrtl had known the bitterness of poverty in his youth, but when he came into his own, and he was accounted wealthy as physicians go, his charity and humanity knew no bounds. Generous to a fault with his money, he endowed churches, orphanages, universities, with the same innate kindliness and liberality which prompted him to cheer his students at their work by his engaging presence and witty sallies. Nothing delighted him more than to lavish praise upon the work of a younger man, and in this unique regard he is like Müller and Ludwig, Virchow and Pasteur, those incomparable teachers of youth. Having filled his chair for thirty years, he resigned it voluntarily in 1874, in order to escape the (to him) humiliating experience of being pensioned off at seventy, retiring to a hermit-like existence at his country villa at Perchtoldsdorf. Here, in the society of his gentle, poetic wife, he produced his three masterpieces on Hebraic and Arabic elements in anatomy (1879[1]), on anatomic terminology (1880[2]), and on old German anatomic expressions (1884[3]). Hyrtl ranks with Emile Littré as one of the greatest of modern medical scholars, and these books show him at his best in a field which was his very own. His declining years were clouded by a phase of pessimism that belied his cheerful, kindly nature.[4]

The group of investigators just considered includes a number of men who, under the influence of those great morphologists, John Hunter and Johannes Müller, approached physiologic problems largely from the point of view of structure. Müller and his pupil Schwann employed both physical and chemical procedures in experimentation, but, after Müller's time, physiologic investigation proceeded along two broadly

---

[1] Hyrtl: Das Arabische und Hebräische in der Anatomie, Vienna, 1879.

[2] Onomatologia anatomica, Vienna, 1880.

[3] Die alten deutschen Kunstworte der Anatomie, Vienna, 1884.

[4] See, "Ein Besuch bei Hyrtl," in Wien. med. Wochenschr., 1894, xliv, 1406. Contrast this with the jolly discourse of 1880 (*Las Culebras*) in Allg. Wien. med. Ztg., 1880, xxv, 521.

divergent lines. The physical school, which aimed at purely mechanical modes of experimentation and interpretation, includes such names as Flourens, Poiseuille, Marshall Hall, the brothers Weber, Brücke, Carl Ludwig, du Bois Reymond, and Helmholtz. The chemical school, the followers of Liebig and Wöhler, was represented by Schwann, Beaumont, Tiedemann, Gmelin, Pettenkofer, and attained its highest development in the epoch-making work of Claude Bernard and Pasteur.

The pioneer of **experimental physiology** in France was François **Magendie** (1783–1855), of Bordeaux, who, like Müller, employed both physical and chemical procedure in his investigations, and was incidentally the modern founder of experimental pharmacology. Unlike Bichat, Magendie had not the slightest use for vitalistic or other theories, but regarded medicine as "a science in the making" (*une science à faire*) and sought to explain everything in terms of physics and chemistry. Pathology he was fain to regard as "the physiology of the sick man." Physiology he sought to advance by closer revision of the facts. He compared himself to a rag-picker (*chiffonier*), who wanders through the domain of science collecting whatever he finds. This expressive phrase sums up

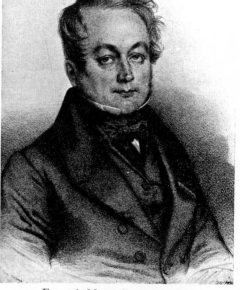

François Magendie (1783–1855).

the hard limitations which Magendie put upon himself or which existed in his own mind. He discovered only isolated facts, did not try to connect them with one another by any special hypotheses, and so arrived at no important generalizations. As the ardent protagonist of experimentation on living animals he is, of course, the particular aversion of the anti-vivisectionists, and there is no doubt that many of his experiments were without aim and needlessly cruel. But, before his time, physiology was made up of what Claude Bernard called *rêveries systématiques*, and it is the special distinction of Magendie to have headed the recent line of illustrious laboratory experimenters from Bernard himself to Pavloff, Loeb, and Ehrlich. Magendie was the founder of the first periodical devoted

30

exclusively to physiology, the *Journal de physiologie expérimentale* (Paris, 1821–31[1]).

His greatest contribution to the science was his experimental proof (on a litter of puppies) of the truth of Bell's law, that the anterior roots of the spinal nerves are motor, the posterior sensory in function (1822[2]). Through his bold vivisecting and lucid seasoning he arrived at a much clearer conception of these functions than Bell; and, in adjusting the two claims, it seems proper to assign to Bell priority of discovery and demonstration in reference to the anterior roots, to Magendie priority of conclusive demonstration and interpretation of the functions of both motor and sensory roots. Magendie also made important investigations of the mechanism of deglutition and vomiting (1813[3]); of the effects of excision or section of the cerebellum (1825[4]), and of the "circus movement" (*mouvement de manège*) obtained by lesion of the optic thalamus. He demonstrated that the pumping power of the heart is the main cause of the blood-flow in the veins, that chemical differences between the blood and the lymph will cause osmosis through the vessel walls, and that the absorption of fluids and semisolids is a function of the blood-vessels as well as of the lymphatics (1821[5]); in other words, that absorption is not a specific vital property of the lymphatics, but only imbibition by vascular tissues. With Poiseuille, he was one of the first to notice that arterial blood-pressure rises with expiration, and his experiments on the circulation demonstrated the absurdity of the ancient idea of "points of election" in blood-letting, since the effects of venesection are the same at any site. Magendie thought deeply on the cerebrospinal fluid, which he regarded as a secretion of the pia mater, but being inept at generalization, could only envisage its movement as a Galenic ebb and flow about the intracranial spaces (Cushing). What might have helped him was the doctrine of Monro Secundus and George Kellie (1822) that the fluid and solid content of the intracranial chamber must always remain constant in bulk, the self-same mathematical postulate which was Harvey's mainstay in demonstrating the circulation of the blood.

Magendie's investigations in pharmacology introduced bromine, iodine compounds, and such alkaloids as strychnine (showing its action on the spinal cord in paralysis), morphine, veratrine, brucine, piperine, and emetine into medical practice (1821[6]). In experimental pathology, he induced Gaspard to repeat Haller's experiment of injecting putrid matter into the veins (1822[7]). His proof that secondary or subsequent injections of egg-albumen cause death in rabbits tolerant to an initial injection was the first experiment in anaphylaxis or supersentization of the tissues (1839[8]), a phenomenon which Edward Jenner had already observed in variolous inoculations in 1798.

The most important French physiologists between Magendie and Claude Bernard are Legallois, Flourens, and Poiseuille.

Julien-Jean-César **Legallois** (1770–1814), a Breton who took part in the French Revolution, was some time in hiding for his political affilia-tions, and, after studying at the École de santé, received his medical degree in 1801. He was one of the earliest of the experimental physiolo-gists, and his procedure was cruder and more brutal than Magendie's.

---

[1] For a study of this periodical, see Robert Grammont: Paris diss. No. 296, 1926.
[2] Magendie: Jour. de physiol. expér., Paris, 1882, ii, 276–279.
[3] Magendie: Mémoire sur le vomissement, Paris, 1813.
[4] Jour. de physiol. expér., Paris, 1825, v, 399.
[5] *Ibid.*, 1821, i, 1–31.
[6] Formulaire (etc.), Paris, 1821.
[7] Jour. de physiol. expér., Paris, 1822, ii, 1–45; 1824, iv, 1–69.
[8] In his "Lectures on the Blood," Phila., 1839, 244–249.

He made such experiments as investigating the effect of submersion upon newly born animals or the temperature relations of brainless animals subjected to artificial respiration. In 1812,[1] he showed that bilateral section of the vagus nerve may produce fatal bronchopneumonia, and he greatly extended the observation of Robert Whytt (1750) that absolute integrity of the spinal cord is not necessary for the maintenance of the reflex functions.[2] His discovery that a lesion of a small circumscribed area of the medulla inhibits breathing (1811[3]) was the first attempt to localize the center of respiration and was afterward completed by the work of Flourens. Legallois is principally remembered today by his *Expériences sur le principe de la vie* (1812), in which he was the first, after Borelli, to revive the neurogenic theory of the heart's action. He maintained that the motor power of the heart is a principle or force contained throughout the spinal cord, and transmitted to the heart by the branches of the sympathetic nerve. This was soon shown to be erroneous, but the neurogenic theory was further fortified by Robert Remak's discovery of intrinsic nerve-ganglia in the heart (1844), and held in its own until the revival of the myogenic theory by Gaskell and Engelmann.

Marie-Jean-Pierre **Flourens** (1794–1867) is memorable as the discoverer of the *nœud vital*, or "vital node," the bilateral center of respiration in the medulla oblongata, a lesion of which causes asphyxia (1837[4]). Although the exact situation and extent of this vital spot have been in dispute down to the present time, the crucial feature of Flourens' experiment has never been set aside.

In 1822–24,[5] he made his classic observations on the effects of removal of the cerebrum and cerebellum in pigeons, showing the absolute maintenance of reflexes with loss of cerebration and volition in the former case and the disturbance of equilibrium in the latter. These important

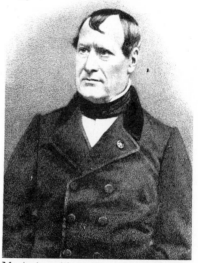

Marie-Jean-Pierre Flourens (1794–1867).

experiments demonstrated that the brain is the organ of thought and of will power, while the cerebellum presides over the coördination of bodily movements. Flourens, however, denied the possibility of any cortical localization of functions. In 1828,[6] he announced that a lesion of the semicircular canals in the internal ear will cause motor incoördination and loss of equilibrium, section of an individual canal producing rotatory motion around an axis at right angles to the plane of cleavage. From the analogy of these phenomena with the effects of a deep lesion in the cerebellum, Flourens inferred that both organs have to do with coördination of movements. Thus, where Purkinje had described only a presumable visual nystagmus, Flourens located the existence of a true cerebellar and labyrinthine vertigo. His results were confirmed physiologically by Vulpian,

---

[1] Legallois: Expériences sur le principe de la vie, Paris, 1812.

[2] Legallois: Œuvres, Paris, 1830, i, p. 135.

[3] *Ibid.*, i, p. 248. Expériences (etc.), Paris, 1812, p. 37.

[4] Flourens: Recherches expérimentales, Paris, 2. éd., 1842, p. 204. Compt.-rend. Acad. d. sc., Paris, 1858, xlvii, 803; 1859, xlviii, 1136.

[5] Flourens: Arch. gén. de méd., Paris, 1823, ii, 344, 351; 1825, viii, 422–426; and Recherches expérimentales, Paris, 1824.

[6] Flourens: Mém. Acad. d. sc., Paris, 1828, ix, 455–477.

Goltz, Cyon, Ferrier; on the clinical side by Ménière; and have been ably elucidated, both surgically and clinically, by Robert Bárány as "vestibular nystagmus."

Jean-Léonard-Marie **Poiseuille** (1799–1869), of Paris, a medical graduate of 1828, was the first experimenter between Stephen Hales and Carl Ludwig to make any real advance in the physiology of the circulation. His name is permanently associated with the study of blood-pressure and the viscosity of the blood.

Starting from Hales' original blood-pressure experiment of 1733, Poiseuille improved upon it by substituting a mercury manometer for the inconvenient long tube, connection with the artery being established by means of a hollow lead tip filled with potassium carbonate to prevent coagulation. This was Poiseuille's hemo-dynamometer (1828[1]), with which he showed that the blood-pressure rises and falls on expiration and inspiration, and measured the degree of arterial dilatation (about $\frac{1}{2\overline{3}}$ of the normal) at each heart-beat. To this instrument Carl Ludwig added a float (1847[2]), and, as Professor Stirling says, "had the genius to cause this float to write on a recording cylinder, and thus at one *coup* gave us the kymograph, or wave-writer, and the application of graphic method to physiology." With these improve-ments, the science of blood-pressure (hemodynamics) became a definite part of recent medicine. Poiseuille's other great contribution to physiology was an investigation in mathematical physics, namely, on the flow and outflow of liquids in capillary tubes (1840[3]). He found that the average velocity of capillary flow varies directly with the sectional area of the tube, the grade of pressure, and the viscosity or stickiness of the moving fluid; also that the quantity of outflow is inversely as the length of the tube and directly proportional to the fourth power of its diameter, the pressure grad-ient, and the viscosity coefficient $\left(Q = \dfrac{D^4PV}{L}\right)$, whence, for unit length, diameter, and pressure, the viscosity coefficient can be computed from the following formula:

$$V = \frac{QL}{D^4P}.$$

This important equation is the mathematical expression of "Poiseuille's law," which, in recent times, has become fundamental in estimating the viscosity of the blood. The instrument used for the purpose (viscosimeter) was also invented by Poiseuille. He now stands, with Harvey, Hales, and Ludwig, as one of the founders of hemo-dynamics.

In applying the methods of laboratory physics to physiologic prob-lems, remarkable work was done by the brothers Weber, of Witten-berg. Of these, **Ernst Heinrich Weber** (1795–1878) was professor of anatomy and physiology at Leipzig (1821–66) up to the time of Carl Ludwig's advent, and afterward held the chair of anatomy there until 1871, when he was succeeded by Wilhelm His. He made an event in medical history by his discovery of the inhibitory power of the vagus nerve (1845[4]) a find which threw much light upon such problems as

---

[1] This instrument is described in Poiseuille's graduating dissertation: "Re-cherches sur la force du cœur aortique," Paris, 1828.

[2] Ludwig: Arch. f. Anat., Physiol. u. wissensch. Med., Berl., 1847, 261.

[3] Poiseuille: Compt. rend. Acad. d. sc., Paris, 1840, xi, 961, 1041; 1841, xii, 12; 1843, xvi, 60.

[4] The discovery was communicated by the Webers to the Congress of Italian Scientists at Naples in 1845 ("Experimenta quibus probata nervos vagos rotatione machinæ galvano-magneticæ irritatos, motum cordis retardare et adeo intercipere," in Omodei's Ann. univ. de med., Milan, 1845, 3 s., xx, 227). It was afterward pub-lished at length in Wagner's Handwörterbuch der Physiologie, 1846, iii, 45–51.

the motion of the heart, the nature of fever, and the like. His original experiment, made with his brother, **Eduard Friedrich Weber** (1806–71), consisted in bringing the heart to a standstill by placing one pole of an electromagnetic apparatus in the nostril of a frog, the other on a cross-section of the cord at the level of the fourth vertebra. The field of inhibition was then localized to a region between the optic lobes and the calamus scriptorius, the vagi were found to be the channels of communication, and the results were extended to warm-blooded animals. Although the Webers at first thought that stimulation of both vagi was necessary for inhibition, and although Ludwig and Schmiedeberg afterward showed that the vagus contains accelerator as well as inhibitory fibers (1870–71), the original proof remains unshaken as one of the great monuments of physiologic discovery. Ernst Heinrich and Eduard Friedrich Weber also collaborated in the famous *Wellenlehre* or Hydrodynamics of Wave-Motion (1825), in which the velocity of the pulse-wave was measured for the first time and it was shown that it is delayed $\frac{1}{6}''$ to $\frac{1}{7}''$ in transmission, thus overthrowing Bichat's theory that the pulse is synchronous in all the arteries. In 1837, these two brothers again did clever work together in measuring and comparing

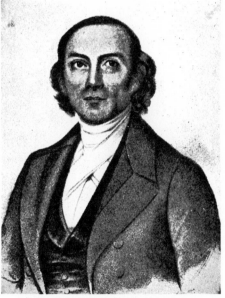

Ernst Heinrich Weber (1795–1878).

the velocity of the blood and lymph corpuscles in the capillaries.[1] Ernst Heinrich Weber is again memorable for his model to illustrate the hydrodynamics of the circulation (1850[2]), but the coping-stone of his single achievement is undoubtedly his great work on touch and temperate sense (*Der Tastsinn und das Gemeingefühl*, 1846), which was the starting-point of the experimental psychophysics of Fechner and Wundt. Johannes Müller, while assigning to each sense organ its proper, particular functions, did not admit the existence of any "common sensation" (such as pain or malaise) apart from the sense of touch. Weber was the first to show that this common sensation can be analyzed into its visceral and muscular components, and that these

---

[1] Weber: Müller's Arch., Berl., 1837, 267–272.

[2] E. H. Weber: Ber. ü. d. Verhandl. d. k. sächs. Gesellsch. d. Wissensch., Leipz., 1850, 186.

can be separated from tactile sensations. He boldly applied the idea of measurement to sensations of pain, heat, pressure, smell; noted that the threshold of painful sensation is also the threshold of nerve-injury, and stated the generalization known as Weber's law, viz., that intensity of sensation is not directly proportional to the degree of stimulus, but depends upon its mode of application. A given stimulus is less perceptible when added to a larger stimulus than to a smaller one; in other words, when the sensation increases in arithmetic progression, the stimulus must vary by geometric progression. Fechner afterward expressed this idea by saying that intensity of sensation varies with the logarithm of the stimulus (Weber-Fechner law), since the curve produced is a logarithmic curve.

A third brother of the Weber family was the celebrated electrician, **Wilhelm Eduard Weber** (1804–91), who was professor of physics at Göttingen all his active life (1831–91), constructed the first electromagnetic telegraph in 1833, made an atlas of the earth's magnetism (1840), and further distinguished himself by his important work in electric measurements. He collaborated with Eduard Friedrich Weber in the well-known classic on the mechanics of the human locomotor system (*Mechanik der menschlichen Gehwerkzeuge*, 1836), the most important study of the time on the physiology of motion and locomotion and the mechanism of the joints.

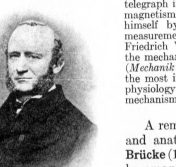

A remarkable all-round physiologist and anatomist was Ernst Wilhelm **von Brücke** (1819–92), of Berlin, who, in 1849, became professor of physiology at Vienna, where he was associated with the New Vienna School for the rest of his life.

Ernst Wilhelm von Brücke (1819–92).

His investigation covered all branches of the subject, including the luminosity of the eye in animals (1845), phonetics (1856–62), the semilunar valves (1855), and artistic anatomy (1892), the latter one of the most attractive books ever written on the subject. He was the first to hold that normal urine may contain sugar (1858), and he introduced the emulsion test for fatty acids (1870).

The leading English exponent of physical experimentation in the early period was **Marshall Hall** (1790–1857), of Nottingham, whose Royal Society memoir on *The Reflex Function of the Medulla Oblongata and Medulla Spinalis* (1833[1]) established the difference between volitional action and unconscious reflexes.

The idea that peripheral impulses can be reflected outwardly from the nerve centers connected with the brain, without relation to consciousness, had originally been suggested by Descartes in 1644 in his discussion of the batting of the eyes upon a threatened blow. Robert Boyle had noted that a viper, three days after decapitation, still wriggles upon being pricked. Johann Bohn had discussed the reflex movements of the decapitated frog as "a material phenomenon" (1686). Stephen Hales had shown that the movements of the decapitated frog are nullified when the spinal

---

[1] Hall: Phil. Tr., Lond., 1833, 635–665.

cord is destroyed. Robert Whytt, of Edinburgh, showed that destruction of the anterior optic lobe abolishes the contraction of the pupil to light (Whytt's reflex), and that a mere fragment of the spinal cord will suffice for the maintenance of reflex movements. But most of these observers believed that reflex phenomena are bound up with sensation and ideation. The Bell-Magendie experiment (1811–22) was a great step forward and the discovery of the respiration center by Legallois (1826) and Flourens (1837) threw further light upon the problem.

Independently of these last, and in apparent ignorance of the work of his predecessors, Marshall Hall showed that strychnine convulsions cease upon destruction of the spinal cord, that reflexes are more readily produced by stimulating the nerve-endings than the nerves themselves, and that there is a reflex contraction of sphincter muscles. He introduced the concept of traumatic "shock" (1850).

It was Hall's work which gave "reflex action" a permanent place in physiology, although he did not realize, as Sherrington and others have pointed out, that volitional and reflex processes can pass from one to the other and that many nervous phenomena lie between the two extremes. He thought that the chief merit of his work lay in the discovery of special reflex paths dissociated from sensation and volition, an idea which was borne out by R. D. Grainger's discovery that the gray matter in the cord and its afferent roots is the true medium of reflex action (1837).

William **Sharpey** (1802–80), of Arbroath, Scotland, who was all his life a prominent teacher of physiology at University College, London (1836–74), is memorable for his papers on cilia and ciliary motion (1830–36[1]), and for his discovery of the "fibers of Sharpey" (1846[2]). Modern English physiology owes its origins to Huxley and to Sharpey, who was the teacher of the Cambridge and Oxford pro-

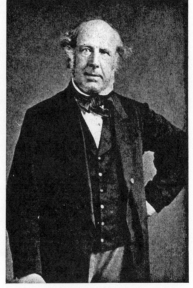

William Sharpey (1802–80). (Boston Medical Library.)

fessors, Michael Foster and Burdon-Sanderson. "Sharpey," says Foster, "was the only pure physiologist in England; . . . the only man of the time who devoted all his life to physiology." In describing Ludwig's work on blood-pressure curves to his students, he would sometimes use his old cylinder hat as a kymographion.

Sir William **Bowman** (1816–92), of Cheshire, England, eminent as physiologist and ophthalmic surgeon, discovered and described striated muscle (1840–41[3]), basement membranes (1842), the ciliary region of

---

[1] Sharpey: Edinb. Med. and Surg. Jour., 1830, xxxiv, 113–122, and Todd's Cyclopedia, London, 1835–36, i.

[2] Sharpey: in Jones Quain's Anatomy, 5. ed., Lond., 1846, ii, pp. cxxxii–clxiii.

[3] Bowman: "On the Minute Structure and Movements of Voluntary Muscle," Phil. Tr., Lond., 1840, 457–501, 4 pl.; 1841, 69–73, the drawings by Bowman himself.

the eyeball (1847). To Bowman is due the scientific treatment of lacrimal disorders. In 1842,[1] he stated his theory of the urinary secretion that the renal tubes and their capillaries are probably the parts concerned in the secretion of the basic principles of the urine, and the Malpighian bodies an apparatus destined to separate the watery portion from the blood.

The chemical tendency in modern experimental physiology, which led up to the magnificent work of Claude Bernard and Pasteur, was initiated by Liebig and Wöhler in Germany, and by Dumas and Chevreul in France.

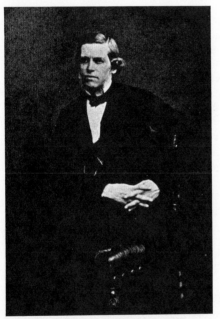

Justus **von Liebig** (1803–73), of Darmstadt, a pupil of Gay-Lussac, was the founder of agricultural chemistry, one of the principal founders of physiological chemistry and the chemistry of the carbon compounds, and the originator of laboratory teaching in chemical science. Liebig's laboratory, established at Giessen in 1826, was the first institution of the kind to be connected with university teaching, and, bare and simple as were its appointments, was soon thronged with enthusiastic, hard-working students. Here Liebig made his famous investigations of cyanides, cyanates, amides, aldehydes, benzoyls, benzoates, organic acids, and chemical fertilizers of soils, and here he founded Liebig's *Annalen* (1832–74), the leading literary organ of chemistry during his lifetime.

Sir William Bowman (1816–92).

Liebig's most important contributions to medicine were his discoveries of hippuric acid (Poggendorff's Ann., 1829), chloral and chloroform (1831[2]), his studies of uric acid compounds, his mode of estimating urea (1853[3]), and his important work on fats, blood, bile, and meat juice (Liebig's extract). His book on "Organic Chemistry in its Applications to Physiology and Pathology" (1842[4]) was the first formal

---

[1] Bowman: Phil. Tr., Lond., 1841–2, 57–80.

[2] Liebig: Ann. d. Pharm., Lemgo and Heidelb., 1832, i, 182–230. Chloroform was discovered independently in the same year by Soubeiran (Ann. de chim., Paris, 1831, xlviii, 113–157), and by Samuel Guthrie, M. D., (1782–1848), of Bloomfield, Mass. (Am. Jour. Arts and Sc., 1831, xxi, 64; xxii, 105), at Jewettsville, near Sackett's Harbor, N. Y., where he hit upon the modern method of making chloroform by distilling alcohol with chlorinated lime.

[3] Liebig: Ann. d. Pharm., Lemgo and Heidelb., 1853, lxxxv, 289–328.

[4] Liebig: Die organische Chemie in ihrer Anwendung auf Physiologie und Pathologie, Braunschweig, 1842. Schwann introduced the phrase "metabolic phenomena" in 1839 (Fraser Harris).

treatise on the subject, introducing the concept of "metabolism" (*Stoffwechsel*). His Familiar Letters on Chemistry (1844) did more than any other work to popularize that science.

Liebig's investigations of fermentation and putrefaction were vitiated by his purely materialistic view of these phenomena, as based upon his theory of catalysis. He defined catalysis as the tuning-fork power of a system of molecules to set up sympathetic vibrations in another system, producing chemical change, and he affected only contempt or disbelief in regard to such vital agencies as bacteria or living ferments. He believed that fermentation and putrefaction are only physical disturbances of equilibrium which can be communicated by contact to other bodies. He refused to believe that yeast is alive and declined to look through a microscope. When, after long and bitter controversy, Liebig saw that his materialism had been refuted by Pasteur, he reluctantly stated that he had only attempted to assign a chemical cause for a chemical phenomenon. Yet Liebig was otherwise an uncompromising vitalist. Lord Kelvin relates that when he once asked the great chemist if he believed that a leaf or a flower could be formed or could be made to grow by chemical forces,

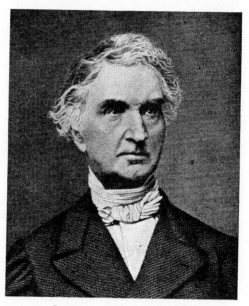

Justus von Liebig (1803–73).

Liebig replied: "I would more readily believe that a book on chemistry or on botany could grow out of dead matter by chemical processes."[1]

Friedrich **Wöhler** (1800–82), of Eschersheim, Hesse-Nassau, was associated with Liebig in his investigations of uric acid, the cyanogen compounds, and the oil of bitter almonds, the artificial synthesis of sugar, morphine and salicin, and himself made many important discoveries, two of which were epoch-making in the history of physiology. In 1828, Wöhler succeeded in effecting an artificial synthesis of urea[2] by heating ammonium cyanate, according to the equation: $NH_4CNO = CO(NH_2)_2$. This was the first time that an organic substance had ever been built up artificially from the constituents of an inorganic

---

[1] Lord Kelvin: Popular Lectures, London, 1894, ii, foot-note to p. 464.

[2] Wöhler: Ueber künstliche Bildung des Harnstoffs, Ann. d. Phys. u. Chem., Leipzig, 1828, xii, 253–256.

substance, without any intervention of vital processes, and it soon
became clear that there is no essential difference between the structural chemistry of life and that of inanimate nature. This discovery
led to a brilliant line of synthetic work, of which the highest point has
so far been attained by Emil Fischer. In 1824, Wöhler made, and in
1842 confirmed, a discovery which became the starting-point of the
modern chemistry of metabolism, viz., that the benzoic acid taken in
with the food appears as hippuric acid in the urine.[1] This at once did
away with the idea, current in Wöhler's time, that while plants can
synthetize their complex materials, animals have to receive their constituent substances already synthetized from plants or other animals.
Other modes of animal synthesis, such as those of uric acid from ammonium carbonate or of glucose from glycogen in the liver, were soon
discovered and the problem of building up artificial foods from elementary materials had its inception here. Liebig and Wöhler were, in
fact, the inaugurators of what von Noorden calls the qualitative period
of metabolism experiments.

Among the earlier chemical investigations of importance to medicine were
Sertürner's isolation of morphine (1806[2]); Wollaston's investigation of cystin calculi (1810[3]); Kirchhoff's conversion of starch into sugar (1811[4]); Blackall and Wells
on albumen in the urine (1812–14); the isolation of strychnine (1818[5]), brucine (1819),
quinine,[6] and veratrine (1820) by Caventou and Pelletier; Alexander Marcet's investigation of black urine (1822[7]); Dutrochet's work on endosmosis and exosmosis
(1827–35[8]); Geiger and Hesse's isolation of atropine (1833[9]); F. Rose's biuret test
for albumen (1833[10]); the investigations of Cagniard Latour[11] and Schwann on yeast
cells and vinous fermentation (1837–38); the proof of Bouchardat and Péligot that
the sugar of diabetic urine is grape-sugar (1838[12]); Trommer's test for grape-sugar
in the urine (Mitscherlich, 1841); Pettenkofer's test for bile (1844[13]); the quantitative
test for sugar in the urine (1848[14]) of Hermann von Fehling (1847–1925); Henry
Bence Jones' discovery of a special proteid (albumose) in the urine of patients with
softening of the bones (myelopathic albumosuria, 1848[15]); Adolf Strecker's investigations of ox bile (1848–49[16]); Millon's discovery of a special reagent for proteids

[1] Wöhler: Ann. d. Phys. u. Chem., Leipz., 1842, lvi, 638–641. One year before
this, Alexander Ure, of Edinburgh, had pointed out that benzoic acid is changed to
hippuric in the body (Provincial Med. and Surg. Jour., London, 1841, ii, 317).
Wöhler's original experiment was given in Tiedemann's Ztschr. f. Physiol., 1824, i,
142, but his views were not definite until after Liebig's discovery of hippuric acid in
1829.   [2] Sertürner: J. d. Pharm., Leipz., 1806, xiv, 47: 1811, xx, 99.

[3] Wollaston: Phil. Tr., Lond., 1810, 223–230.

[4] Kirchhoff: Jour. f. Chem. u. Physik, Nuremb., 1815, xiv, 389–398.

[5] Caventou and Pelletier: J. d. pharm., Paris, 1819, v, 142–177.

[6] Ann. de chim. et phys., Paris, 1820, xv, 289. 337.

[7] Marcet: Med.-Chir. Tr., Lond., 1822–23, xii, 37–45.

[8] Dutrochet: Ann. de chim. et phys., Paris, 1827–35, vols. 35, 37, 49, 52, 60.

[9] Geiger and Hesse: Ann. d. Pharm., Lemgo and Heidelb., 1833, v, 43; vi, 44.

[10] Rose: Poggendorff's Ann., Leipz., 1833, xxviii, 132.

[11] Cagniard Latour: Ann. de chim. et phys., Paris, 1838, lxviii, 206–221.

[12] Péligot: Ann. de chim. et pharm., Paris, 1838, lxvi, 140.

[13] Pettenkofer: Ann. d. Chem. u. Pharm., Heidelb., 1844, lii, 90–96.

[14] Fehling: Arch. f. d. physiol. Heilk., Stuttg., 1848, vii, 64–73.

[15] Bence Jones: Phil. Tr., Lond., 1848, 55–62.

[16] Strecker: Ann. d. Chem. u. Pharm., Heidelb., 1848, lxv, 1; lxvii, 1; 1849, lxx,
149.

(1849[1]). The chemistry of the urine derived a strong impetus from the brilliant work of Johann Florian **Heller** (1813–71), of the New Vienna School, a pupil of Liebig and Wöhler who devised the ring test for albumen (1844[2]), the caustic potash tests for sugar in the urine (1844[3]), was the first to notice the retention of chlorides in pneumonic urine (1847[4]), introduced the caustic potash test for blood in the urine (1858[5]), invented the ureometer for estimating specific gravity (1848), and wrote a famous classic on urinary concretions (1860[6]). Great impetus was given to chemical investigation in France by the work of Jean-Baptiste **Dumas** (1800–84), who isolated methyl alcohol, established the quantitative analysis of air and water, studied the chemical changes in the development of the chick, and (with Coindet) showed the value of iodine treatment in goiter (1820[7]). Michel-Eugène **Chevreul** (1787–1889) investigated the sugar in diabetic urine (1815[8]), and made an important study of animal fats (1823). In England, Thomas **Graham** (1805–69), of Glasgow, did work of capital importance in modern physiology by his discovery of the laws governing diffusion of gases (1829–31[9]), his investigation of osmotic force (1854[10]), and his method of separating animal and other fluids by dialysis, introducing the distinction between colloid and crystalloid substances (1861[11]). Graham's definition of osmosis as "the conversion of chemical affinity into mechanical power" still remains the most scientific ever made, as borne out by recent investigations of semi-permeable membranes.

The most important advance made by chemical investigation in the early period was in the physiology of **digestion**. The first work in this field, in order of time, was the graduating thesis of John R. **Young**, of Maryland, "An Experimental Inquiry into the Principles of Nutrition and the Digestive Process" (Philadelphia, 1803).

The labors of the earlier physiologists on digestion—Van Helmont, Sylvius, Borelli—were to a great extent impaired by their theories of innate heat and vital spirits, and, as William Hunter derisively remarked, they were fain to regard the stomach as a mill, a fermenting vat, or a stewpan.

In the 18th century, Réaumur isolated the gastric juice and demonstrated its solvent effect upon foods (1752). Spallanzani confirmed the fact of its solvent and antiseptic character (1782), and thus did away with the various views of concoction, putrefaction, trituration, and fermentation in favor of a chemical theory of solution; but he failed to recognize that the solvent action of the gastric juice is due to its acidity. Young took up his work at this point and, by experiments made upon bullfrogs, snakes, and even *in propria persona*, showed that the solvent principle of the gastric juice is an acid, turning litmus paper red and softening bones into a pulp, and that this acid does not arise from any vinous or other fermentation in the stomach, but is part of the normal gastric secretion.

Young arrived at the important deduction, demonstrated in our own time by Pavloff, that the flow of gastric juice and of saliva are associ-

---

[1] Millon: Compt.-rend. Acad. d. sc., Paris, 1849, xxviii, 40–42.

[2] Heller's Arch. f. Physiol. u. path. Chem., Vienna, 1844, i, 192–199.

[3] *Ibid.*, 1844, i, 212, 292.

[4] *Ibid.*, 1847, iv, 522–525.

[5] Heller: Ztschr. d. k. k. Gesellsch. d. Aertze zu Wien, 1858, n. F., i, 751. L. Teichmann gave an earlier test for hæmin in Ztschr. f. rat. Med. Heidelb., 1853, iii, 375–388 (Erich Ebstein).

[6] Heller: Die Harnconcretionen, Vienna, 1860.

[7] Coindet: Ann. de chim. et phys., Paris, 1820, xv, 49–59.

[8] Chevreul: Ann. de chimie, Paris, 1815, xcv, 319.

[9] Graham: Quart. Jour. Sc., Lond., 1829, ii, 74–83; Phil. Mag., Lond., 1833, ii, 175–190.

[10] Graham: Phil. Tr., Lond., 1854, cxliv, 177–228.

[11] *Ibid.*, 1861, cli, 183–224.

ated and synchronous, but he wrongly inferred that the acid principle of the stomach is phosphoric acid. In 1824, William **Prout** (1785–1850), an English chemist, was able to prove, by careful titration and distillation, that the acid of the gastric juice is free hydrochloric acid.[1] This result was soon confirmed by other chemists, notably in the classic monograph on "Digestion, Experimentally Considered" (1826–27[2]), by Friedrich **Tiedemann** (1781–1861), of Cassel, and Leopold **Gmelin** (1788–1853), of Göttingen.

In this work Gmelin's nitric acid test for the bile-pigments in chyle, blood-serum, and urine is given (preface, p. 11[3]), the limited quantity of the gastric secretion is pointed out, and it is shown that the saliva contains a sulphocyanate, and the pancreatic secretion a principle which turns red with chlorine water. This principle (tryptophan) was afterward shown by Claude Bernard to be a by-product of pancreatic digestion and not a true constituent of the pancreatic juice.

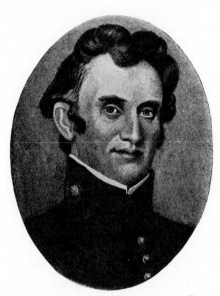

William Beaumont (1785–1853). (Courtesy of Dr. Jesse S. Myer, St. Louis.)

In 1833, William **Beaumont** (1785–1853), of Connecticut, a surgeon in the United States Army, published his famous "Experiments and Observations" on an accidental gastric fistula in the Canadian half-breed, Alexis St. Martin, which threw a new light upon the nature of the gastric juice, the process of digestion in the stomach, and the early stages of gastritis. As far back as 1664, Regner De Graaf had published his account of artificial salivary and pancreatic juice in a dog, giving a picture of the dog; and there were earlier cases of gastric fistulæ; but Beaumont was the first to study digestion and the movements of the stomach *in situ* (1825[4]). He began by carefully reviewing the work of his predecessors in a fair-minded spirit; gave an accurate description of the normal and pathologic appearances of the gastric mucous membrane in life, and of the movements of the stomach up to

---

[1] Prout: Phil. Tr., Lond., 1824, 45–49.

[2] Tiedemann and Gmelin: Die Verdauung nach Versuchen, Heidelberg and Leipzig, 1826–27.

[3] Erich Ebstein (Ztschr. f. Urol., Leipz., 1915, ix, 283) points out that Gmelin's nitric acid test for bile was employed about forty years before (November, 1787) by Francesco Marabelli, a pupil of Johann Peter Frank, and apothecary to the hospital at Pavia (Atti d. Accad. d. sc. di Siena, 1794, vii, 224–232). Marabelli's scattered essays (Leipzig, 1795) also contain analyses of dropsical fluid (1791), diabetic urine (1792), and of maize (1787) and various fruits and drugs.

[4] Beaumont: Med. Recorder, Phila., 1825, viii, 14; 840: 1826, ix, 94.

the completion of digestion; showed that the gastric juice is secreted only when food is present and that mechanical irritation of the mucous membrane produces congestion, but only a limited local secretion of gastric juice, thus foreshadowing the results of Pavloff, and overthrowing the doctrine of Magendie that the gastric secretion is continual. Beaumont's experiments on the effect of gastric juice upon different foods and the relative digestive values of the latter are the foundation of modern dietetic tables and scales. His chemical examination of the gastric juice led him to the conclusion that it contains free hydrochloric acid plus some other active chemical substance, which Theodor Schwann, in 1835, proved to be pepsin. Beaumont's was the most important work on the physiology of gastric digestion before the time of Pavloff, and the difficulties under which the experimenter completed his labors, first begun at an isolated military post in the primeval forests of Michigan, and completed only by dint of following up his patient, and bringing him nearly 2000 miles to Plattsburgh Barracks, N. Y., make his experience one of the romantic episodes in the history of medicine. "Every physician who prescribes for digestive disorders," says Vaughan, "and every patient who is benefited by such a prescription, owes gratitude to the memory of William Beaumont, who, in 1825, on the island of Mackinaw, began his studies of digestion, which he pursued with labor and skill for the benefit of mankind." He was the true leader and pioneer of experimental physiology in our country.

Early 19th century **surgery** was mainly a continuation of the surgery of the 18th century, with this difference, that the center of gravity had shifted from Paris to London, as a result of the mighty influence of Hunter's teaching, and of the evil effects of the fanatical prohibitions of 1792–93, which abolished medical faculties and societies in France. Many bold operative feats were performed in this period, plastic surgery was revived, most of the larger arteries were successfully ligated, American and Russian surgery came into existence, but of general operating within the cranium, joints, abdomen, and female pelvis, or in isolated organs like the eye and ear, there was no sign until well after the year 1867.

The leading surgeons of the pre-Listerian period were the Bells, Cooper, Colles, Brodie, Liston, Syme, and Fergusson in Great Britain; Larrey, Dupuytren, Lisfranc, Delpech, Velpeau, Malgaigne, and Nélaton in France; the elder Langenbeck, Dieffenbach, the elder Graefe, and Stromeyer in Germany; Pirogoff in Russia; Physick, Post, Mott, the Warrens, and McDowell in America.

The brothers John and Charles Bell were leading figures among the London and Edinburgh surgeons of their day, but the fame of Sir Charles Bell now rests largely upon his discoveries in anatomy, physiology, and pathology. **John Bell** (1763–1820), of Edinburgh, belongs, in part, to an earlier period, but his great works upon surgical anatomy exerted a powerful influence upon the men of a later time, and he was, with Desault and John Hunter, a founder of the modern surgery of the vascular system. He himself had tied the common carotid and the posterior branch of the internal iliac successfully, and was the first to ligate the gluteal artery.[1] Like his brother Charles, John Bell was an artist of talent, one of the great medical men who have illustrated their own books. His *Anatomy of the Human Body* (1793–1803) once important, was later reissued with original plates drawn by Sir Charles Bell (1811); and his *Engravings*, illustrating the different parts and organs of the body (1794–1804), the drawings and almost all the etchings and engravings being his own, is one of the milestones in the history of anatomic delineation. The third volume, dealing with the brain, nerves, sense organs, and viscera (1804), is

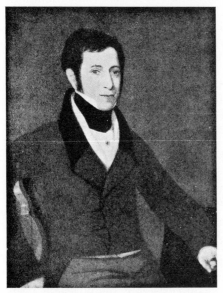

almost entirely the work of Sir Charles. John Bell's most enduring contributions to surgery are his *Discourses on the Nature and Cure of Wounds* (1795), the second of which is a valuable historic discussion of the surgery of the arteries; and his monumental *Principles of Surgery* (1801–1807), embellished with beautiful original engravings and full of unique historical and clinical matter relating to the ligation of the great vessels, fractures, trephining, tumors and lithotomy, of which he gives a detailed history (248 pages). The writings of John Bell are characterized by great sincerity and depth of feeling. He took his profession with a fine ethical seriousness, which, given his combative tempera-

John Bell (1763–1820). (Courtesy of Mr. Henry S. Wellcome.)

ment, often involved him in hot and bitter controversy. He railed at the mistakes of Benjamin Bell and Monro *secundus*, which did not increase his popularity. He was kept out of practice in the Royal Infirmary through the machinations of James Gregory, who assailed him in a bulky volume under the now-forgotten pseudonym of "Jonathan Dawplucker." Toward the end of his life, broken in health by a fall from a horse, John Bell went to Italy to die, leaving an enduring memento of his visit in his posthumous *Observations on Italy* (1825), one of the best books of travel ever written by a physician. This work is again remarkable for beautiful original drawings, some of which exhibit a feeling for the details of Italian architecture akin to that of Piranesi.

---

[1] John Bell: "Principles of Surgery," 1801, vol. i, pp. 421–426.

Sir Astley Paston **Cooper** (1768–1841), of Norfolk, a pupil of John Hunter's, was the most popular surgeon in London during the first quarter of the century. A clergyman's son, he was something like Hunter in his youthful pranks, and became demonstrator of anatomy of St. Thomas's Hospital at the age of twenty-one (1789), and surgeon at Guy's Hospital in 1800. He was one of the pioneers in the surgery of the vascular system, in experimental surgery, and in the surgery of the ear. In 1808, he successfully ligated the common carotid and the external iliac arteries for aneurysms, and made postmortem dissections of his cases in 1821[1] and 1826[2] respectively. In 1817, came his celebrated feat of ligating the abdominal aorta.[3] Valentine Mott has left

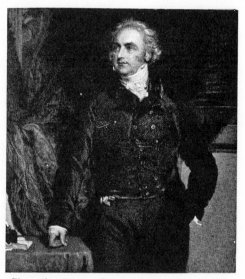

Sir Astley Paston Cooper, Bart. (1768–1841).

an interesting account of Cooper's attempt to tie the subclavian in 1809.[4] Cooper also made experimental ligations of the arteries and nerves in dogs.[5] In 1824, he amputated at the hipjoint. His Royal Society memoir, on perforating the tympanic membrane for deafness resulting from obstruction of the Eustachian tube in 20 cases (1801[6]), gained him the Copley Medal in 1802, and a slight operation performed on George IV (1820) was followed by his baronetcy. Cooper's professional life was thus one long trail of success, which can be sensed in the enormous number of engravings which were made of his likeness. "No surgeon, before or since," says Bettany, "has filled so large a space in the public eye." Although his early income was very small, his wife's fortune made his circumstances easy. Yet few medical men have ever worked so hard and so incessantly. He dissected every day of his life, even when traveling, paying large fees and liberal *douceurs* to the body-snatchers. With these, his experiences were such that he once stated before a House of Commons committee that "there was no person, whatever his worldly place, whom he could not dissect if

---

[1] Bell: Guy's Hosp. Rep., Lond., 1836, i, 53–58, 1 pl.

[2] *Ibid.*, 43–52, 2 pl.

[3] Cooper & Travers' "Surgical Essays," London, 1818, pt. 1, 101–130, 2 pl.

[4] Mott: Med. Repository, N. Y., 1809–10, xiii, 331–334.

[5] Guy's Hosp. Rep., Lond., 1836, i, 457, 654.

[6] Phil. Tr., Lond., 1801, 435–450, 1 pl.

he would." His daily course of life was to rise at six, dissect until eight, breakfast on two hot rolls and tea, see poor patients until nine, attend to his regular consulting practice until one, when he would drive rapidly to Guy's Hospital to visit the wards. At two he lectured on anatomy at St. Thomas's Hospital, after which he went through the dissecting rooms with the students and visited or operated on private patients until seven. He would then bolt his dinner, snatch forty winks of sleep, and start out again for a possible clinical lecture, with another round of visits until midnight. He dictated whatever he wrote while in his carriage. He read little, but managed to absorb the best current knowledge, and his books on *Hernia* (1804–07), *Injuries of the Joints* (1822), *Diseases of the Testis* (1830), and the

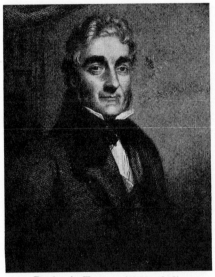

Benjamin Travers (1783–1858).

Anatomy of the Thymus Gland (1832) are still remembered, as also Cooper's fascia, Cooper's hernia, and other eponyms. Cooper was one of the first surgical teachers to substitute practical demonstration upon an actual case for the old didactic theory-mongering of the past; and one of his best achievements was the large number of capable and spirited young surgeons he formed through contact with himself. In personality, he was no pedant or Philistine, but "courteous-eyed, erect and slim," the tall, handsome, engaging figure of Sir Thomas Lawrence's portrait, with a lively, expressive countenance, cheeks aglow with color, a clear voice and chuckling laugh, and, in spite of his quick, imperious temper, idolized by the students, who followed his clinics in enthusiastic throngs. As an operator, he was unaffected, elegant, rapid but unhurried, thorough, masterful, "all ease, all kindness to the patients, and equally solicitous that nothing should be hidden from the observation of the pupils." He attributed his professional success to his uniform and unfailing courtesy to rich and poor alike, as well as to his zeal and industry, "but for this I take no credit, as it was given to me from above." Few men have so fully realized the truth of the poet's device, "We receive but what we give," in the possession of a cheerful, manly, and generous disposition.

Charles **Aston Key** (1793–1849), of Southwark, one of Cooper's juniors at Guy's successfully ligated the external iliac artery for femoral aneurysm in 1822,[1] and the

---

[1] Key: Guy's Hosp. Rep., Lond., 1836, i, 68–70.

subclavian for axillary aneurysm in 1823.[1] He also tied the carotid in 1830 and introduced such improvements as the use of the straight staff in lithotomy (1824) and the principle of dividing the stricture outside the sac in strangulated hernia (1833). Like Cooper, he was a swift, neat operator and a popular teacher, smart in attire, but, unlike his chief, condescending, over-dictatorial, and self-important in manner.

Benjamin **Travers** (1783–1858), of London, another of Cooper's pupils, collaborated with the latter in the valuable *Surgical Essays* (1818–19), to which he contributed a noteworthy paper on wounds of the veins. In 1809 he successfully ligated the common carotid artery in a case of aneurysm by anastomosis in the orbit.[2] He was one of those who followed Broussais in regarding constitutional irritation as a cause of disease, particularly in the nervous system (1824–34). His specialty was ophthalmology, in which field he introduced the use of mercury in non-specific iritis and wrote the best systematic treatise on diseases of the eye of his time (1820).

Abraham **Colles** (1773–1843), of Dublin, professor of surgery in that city for thirty-two years (1804–36), was the leading Irish surgeon of his day. He tied the subclavian artery twice (1811–15[3]), and was the first to tie it within the scaleni (1816). He is said to have been the first man in Europe to tie the innominate successfully.[4] He wrote treatises on surgical anatomy (1811) and on surgery (1844–45), but his most important works are his original description of fracture of the carpal end of the radius or "Colles' fracture" (1814[5]), and his *Practical Observations on the Venereal Disease* (1837), in which he states "Colles' law," relating to the supposed immunity which a healthy mother acquires in bearing a syphilitic child.

Robert **Liston** (1794–1847), of Scotland, was an Edinburgh graduate who became professor of clinical surgery in University College, London, in 1834.

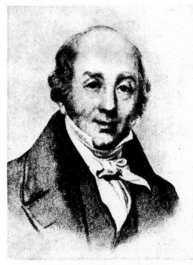

Abraham Colles (1773–1843).

Like the Bells and Astley Cooper, he was a fine anatomist, keeping up his dissections all his life, and this helped to make him one of the most brilliant and skilful operators of his time. He excelled in emergency cases which called for swiftness of decision and originality of procedure, and introduced many novelties, such as his popular mode of flap-amputation, his shoe for club-foot, and his devices for reducing dislocations and crushing and cutting for stone. He was especially successful in plastic operations. In 1836, he successfully excised the

---

[1] Med.-Chir. Tr., Lond., 1823–27, xiii, 1–11.

[2] Travers: Med.-Chir. Tr., London., 1817, ii, 1–16.

[3] Colles: Edinb. Med. and Surg. Jour., 1815, xi, 1–25.

[4] I have been unable to verify this statement, which is made in all biographies of Colles.

[5] Edinb. Med. and Surg. Jour., 1814, x, 182–186.

upper jaw, and, in 1837,[1] he described a method of laryngoscopy, in which he was one of the early pioneers. His most important works were his *Elements of Surgery* (1831) and his *Practical Surgery* (1837), which passed through many editions and still contain things of permanent value. Liston was often rough, abrupt, and contentious in public relations, but kind and charitable to the poor, soft and gentle in the sick-room. He was possessed of such Herculean strength that he could amputate a thigh with the aid of only one assistant, while compressing the artery with his left hand and doing all the sawing and cutting with his right.

James **Syme** (1799–1870), of Edinburgh, was a cousin of Liston's and taught anatomy with the latter in 1822. Having quarreled with

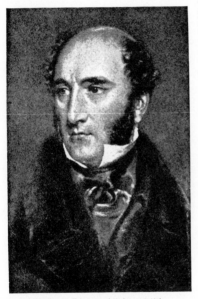

his partner, he could get no appointment in the Royal Infirmary until 1833, but when Liston went down to London in 1834, he succeeded to his very large Scotch practice. The enemies were soon reconciled, and, after Liston's death in 1847, Syme succeeded him in London, but not liking the atmosphere, returned to Edinburgh. Syme's most important contribution to surgery is his work on amputations and excisions. In his *Excision of Diseased Joints* (1831), he was the first to show that excision is usually preferable to amputation, and the adoption of this new principle is due to him, although it was afterward developed *in extenso* by Fergusson.

Robert Liston (1794–1847).

He made his first three successful excisions of the elbow-joint in 1828–29.[2] On September 8, 1842,[3] he performed his first successful amputation at the ankle-joint (Syme's amputation) of which he described eight cases in his *Contributions to the Pathology and Practice of Surgery* (1847). In 1864, he published his work on "Excision of the Scapula" and, in the same year, successfully excised a large part of the tongue. He treated aneurysm by tying the artery above and below and incising the tumor, performing this operation for carotid and iliac aneurysms in 1857. In 1862, he successfully treated an iliac aneurysm by ligation of the common, external, and internal iliac arteries.[4]

Syme was a genial, happy, even-tempered man who "never wasted a word, nor a drop of ink, nor a drop of blood," yet a broad-minded,

---

[1] In his "Practical Surgery," London, 1837, p. 350.

[2] Syme: Edinb. Med. and Surg. Jour., 1829, xxxi, 256–266.

[3] Syme: Lond. and Edinb. Month. Jour. Med. Sc., 1843, iii, 93–96.

[4] Syme: Proc. Roy. Med. and Chir. Soc., Lond., 1862, iv, 114–116.

liberal spirit withal, welcoming all surgical innovations of value. He was, with Pirogoff, perhaps the first European surgeon to adopt ether anesthesia (1847), and, in 1868, he was the first to welcome the antiseptic method of his best and greatest pupil, his son-in-law, Lord Lister.

Sir William **Fergusson** (1808–77), of Prestonpans, Scotland, was the founder of conservative surgery, that is, of the preservation of parts of the body which were needlessly sacrificed by earlier operators. Before Fergusson's time, denuded bones, diseased or painful (even neurotic) joints, were regarded as a sufficient reason for amputation.

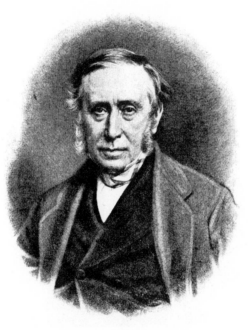

James Syme (1799–1870).

He held it to be "a grand thing when by prescience even the tip of a thumb can be saved." Fergusson was a pupil and prosector of Robert Knox, and soon became surgeon to the Edinburgh Royal Dispensary (1831) and the Royal Infirmary (1839); but Syme's huge practice drove him to London, where, after slow progress, he eventually attained the summit. He was one of the first in Scotland to tie the subclavian artery, and his progress in substituting excisions for amputation was rapid. He excised the head of the femur for incurable hip disease (1845), the scapula, in place of the interscapular-thoracic amputation (1847), and the knee-joint (1850). Between 1828 and 1864 he had operated 400 times for harelip, with only three failures, and 134 times for cleft-palate, with 129 successful cases. In lithotomy, he proceeded with such lightning speed and skill that some one advised a prospective visitor at his clinic to "look out sharp, for if you only wink, you'll miss the operation altogether." Yet he carefully planned every detail in advance, silently working out each step as he went along, even to the bandaging. He wrote a *System of Practical Surgery* (1842), and his *Progress of Anatomy and Surgery During the Present Century* (1867) is a historic work of permanent value. He was an indifferent lecturer and is said to have had a poor bedside manner, but he fascinated his patients and was adored by the children. He was highly accomplished, a good violinist, an inventor of many surgical

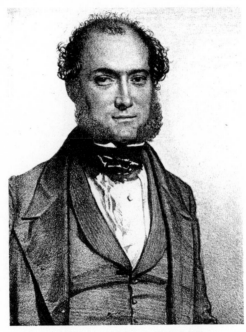

Sir William Fergusson (1808–77).

instruments, so expert in carpentry and metal work that he could devise any necessary apparatus out of hand, an enthusiast at fly-fishing and in dancing Scotch reels. He was noted for his great generosity and hospitality to struggling authors, dramatists, and medical students.

Sir Benjamin Collins **Brodie** (1783–1862) was the son of a Wiltshire clergyman who was descended from a Jacobite exile in England. He was a pupil of Sir Everard Home, lectured at Great Windmill Street (1805–12), and was subsequently assistant surgeon, and later full surgeon, at St. George's Hospital (1808–40). Being profoundly influenced by Bichat, he at first devoted himself to physiologic experimentation.

During 1810–14, he produced four papers, important in their day, on the influence of the brain on the action of the heart (1810[1]), the effects of certain vegetable poisons (1811[2]), the influence of the nervous system on the production of animal heat (1812[3]), and the influence of the pneumogastric on the secretions of the stomach (1814[4]). In these researches, the first two of which gained him the Copley Medal (1811), he used the woorara poison which had just been brought from Guiana.

In 1819 he published his classic treatise *On the Pathology and Surgery of Diseases of the Joints*, his most important work, clearly describing the various articular diseases and differentiating the local lesions from the hysteric and neuralgic forms. He was a pioneer in subcutaneous surgery, performing his first operation in a case of varicose veins in 1814, and made many improvements in surgical instruments and appliances. Brodie was the acknowledged head of the medical profession in London for over thirty years, his income often averaging £10,000 annually, and largely made up of guinea fees at that. He did not regard operative intervention as the highest part of surgery: "his vocation was more to heal limbs than to remove them." Brodie had been all his life assisted by influential friends and family connections, but he held high places, such as the presidency of the Royal College of Surgeons, with dignity, grace, and the kind of tactful self-effacement which aims to stimulate and bring out the ideas of other men. He seems to

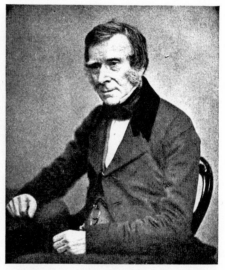

Sir Benjamin Collins Brodie (1783–1862).

have been "servile to none, deferential to none," standing on an equal footing of friendliness and confidence with the poor in hospital or his titled intimates at Holland House or Windsor Castle. "I hear you are ill," he once wrote to an almost unknown student; "no one will take better care of you than I; come to my country house till you are well," making the student remain with him two months.

Here may be mentioned two other surgeons of the Scotch group—Wardrop and Lizars.

James **Wardrop** (1782–1869), of Scotland, an Edinburgh graduate who settled in London in 1809, is now best remembered by his *Essays on the Morbid Anatomy of the Human Eye* (1808) and by his method

---

[1] Brodie: Phil. Tr., 1811, 36–48.

[2] *Ibid.*, 1811, 178–208; 1812, 205–227.

[3] *Ibid.*, 1812, 373–393.   [4] *Ibid.*, 1814, 102–106.

of treating aneurysm by ligating on the distal side of the tumor, which was first suggested by Brasdor in the 18th century. Wardrop performed this operation twice with success on the carotid artery (1809[1]) and once on the subclavian in a case of innominate aneurysm (1827[2]). A curious side of Wardrop is that he stood in the way of his own success and estranged his colleagues through his acrimonious and abusive papers in the Lancet of 1826–27, and through the famous *Intercepted Letters*, in the same journal for 1834, in which he foisted off more personal abuse by using the leading names of the London profession as stalking-horses.

John **Lizars** (1783–1860), of Edinburgh, a pupil of John Bell's, was originally a naval surgeon, but became professor of surgery to the College of Surgeons in his native city in 1831. He was one of the first to remove the lower jaw, but he is now best remembered as the follower of McDowell (his fellow-pupil) in ovariotomy (1825), and by his *System of Anatomical Plates* (1825), a superb series of 110 colored illustrations in folio, made largely from his own dissections.

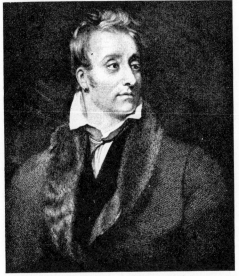

James Wardrop (1782–1869).

Other prominent English surgeons during the pre-antiseptic period were William Hey (1736–1819), of Leeds, who first described infantile hernia (1764), internal derangement of the knee-joint (1782–1803), fungus hæmatodes, and devised a useful saw for operating in fractures of the skull (1803), and whose "Practical Observations on Surgery" (1803) passed through three editions; Edward Alanson (1747–1823), of Newton, Lancashire, a pupil of John Hunter's, who was the first scientific surgeon of Liverpool in his period, published a valuable treatise on amputation (1779), and displayed wonderful insight in his rulings about absolute cleanliness and proper ventilation in hospital wards; Allan Burns (1781–1813), of Glasgow, who wrote an important work on the *Surgical Anatomy of the Head and Neck* (1811), and first described the falciform process of the fascia lata in relation to femoral hernia; Samuel Cooper (1780–1848), whose *Surgical Dictionary* (1809) was the first thoroughgoing work of its kind to be published, passing through eight editions; Joseph Constantine Carpue (1764–1848), who was a pioneer in electrotherapy (1803[3]), revived the Hindu method of rhinoplasty (1816), and wrote a valuable *History of the High Operation for Stone* (1819); John Flint South (1797–1882), the historian of early British surgery, who translated Chelius, and whose posthumous manuscript of a *History of the Craft of Surgery in England* was edited and published by D'Arcy Power in 1886; O'Bryen Bellingham (1805–57), whose book on the treatment of aneurysm by compression (1847) preserves his name and fame in connection with the procedure; Thomas Pridgin Teale (1801–68), of Leeds, memorable for his treatise on abdominal hernia

[1] Wardrop: Med.-Chir. Tr., Lond., 1825, xiii, 217–226.

[2] Wardrop: Lancet, Lond., 1827, xii, 471, 601, 798; 1827–8, i, 408.

[3] J. C. Carpue: An Introduction to Electricity and Galvanism, London, 1803.

(1846), his method of amputation by a long and short rectangular flap (1858), and for his attempt to apply the Broussais doctrine of irritation to the nervous system (1829); Sir William Lawrence (1783–1867) and Sir William Bowman (1816–92) who did much to advance the surgery of the eye; Sir William Wilde (1815–76), of Castlerea, Ireland, one of the pioneers of aural surgery (1843–53) and cerebral surgery (Wilde's incision), who also discovered prehistoric lake dwellings on the Irish crannogs (1839) before Keller; William Henry Porter (1790–1861), who wrote an important work on the surgical pathology of the larynx and trachea (1826); and John Hilton (1804–78), of Guy's Hospital, whose *Rest and Pain* (1863) is one of the permanent classics of surgery. Robert Chessher (1750–1831), an estimable surgeon of Hinckley, Leicestershire, achieved a great reputation through his double inclined-plane to support fractured legs, his apparatus for weak spines and for massage of contractures. He is mentioned in George Eliot's *Middlemarch* ("Mr. Chessher and his irons"). Joseph Fox, in his *Natural History of the Human Teeth* (1803), gave the first explicit directions for correcting dental irregularities, which were in use for nearly half a century (Weinberger).

Of isolated operations and **operative procedures by English surgeons** of the period, we may mention the interscapular-thoracic amputation (excision of arm, scapula and clavicle), which was first performed by Ralph Cuming of the Royal Navy in 1808[1]; Anthony White's excision of the head of the femur for hip disease (1822[2]); the first English cases of gastrostomy (1858–59[3]) by John Cooper Forster (1824–96), of Guy's Hospital; Pridgin Teale's method of amputation by a long and a short rectangular flap (1858); Richard Carden's single flap amputation (1864[4]); and four successful cases of ligation of the external iliac artery by William Goodlad (1811[5]), William Stevens (1812[6]), John Smith Soden (1816[7]), and T. Cole (1817[8]). In Stevens' case, the patient lived ten years, the parts being dissected eight years later (1830[9]) by Sir Richard Owen. The first successful ligation of the common carotid artery was performed by David Fleming, surgeon of H. M. S. Tonnant, in October, 1803.[10]

The leading English military surgeon of the time was George James **Guthrie** (1785–1856), of London, who had served in America and in the Napoleonic wars. At Waterloo, Guthrie successfully amputated the hip-joint[11] and ligated the peroneal artery (1815[12]). His most important work is his *Treatise on Gunshot Wounds of the Extremities requiring Amputation* (1815), which was epoch-making and ran through six editions. Guthrie was also a skilled ophthalmic surgeon and left two important works on artificial pupil (1823) and the surgery of the eye (1812). He was the step-father of Margaret Gordon, of Carlyle's "Reminiscences."[13]

Dominique-Jean **Larrey** (1766–1842), the greatest French military surgeon of his time, also served in the Napoleonic wars. In his will,

---

[1] Cuming: Lond. Med. Gaz., 1829–30, v, 273.

[2] White: Lancet, Lond., 1849, i, 324.

[3] Forster: Guy's Hosp. Rep., Lond., 1858, 3. s., iv, 13; 1859, v, 1.

[4] Carden: Brit. M. J. Lond., 1864, i, 416–421.

[5] Goodlad: Edinb. Med. and Surg. Jour., 1812, viii, 32–39.

[6] Stevens: Med-Chir. Tr., Lond., 1824, v, 422–434.

[7] Soden: *Ibid.*, 1816, vii, 536–540.

[8] Cole: London Med. Repository, 1820, xiii, 369–375.

[9] Owen: Med.-Chir. Tr., London, 1830, xvi, 219–325.

[10] Fleming: Med.-Chir. Jour. and Rev., Lond., 1817, iii, 1–4.

[11] In his Treatise on Gunshot Wounds, second ed., London, 1820, 332–340.

[12] Guthrie: Med.-Chir. Tr., Lond., 1816, vii, 330–337.

[13] For an interesting account of him, see R. C. Archibald: "Carlyle's First Love," London, 1910, 53–61.

Napoleon left 100,000 francs to "Larrey, the most virtuous man I have ever known." Larrey was one of the first to amputate at the hip-joint (1803[1]), performing the operation twice with success. He was surgeon-in-chief to the *Grande Armée*, taking part in 60 battles and 400 engagements. He was three times wounded, performed as many as 200 amputations in 24 hours at Borodino, was the inventor of the celebrated "flying ambulances" (1792), and later professor at the École de médicine militaire at Val-de-Grâce, which was founded in 1796. He was the originator of "first aid to the wounded," in the ultra-modern sense, "taking the hospital to the wounded" with his hundreds of ambulances, directly a battle was joined and not after it.

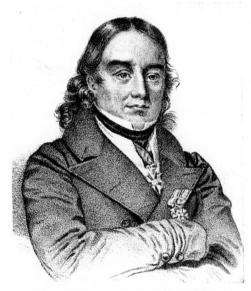

Dominique-Jean Larrey (1766–1842).

Like Ambroïse Paré, he was adored by his comrades in arms for his good nature, courage, and humanity. His most interesting work is contained in the four volumes of his "Mémoires de Médicine Militaire" (1812–17), which contains the first account of "trench foot" (1812, iii, 60). In a memoir published at Cairo in 1802, he was the first to point out the contagious nature of Egyptian ophthalmia or granular conjunctivitis. Wound excision (1812) he got from Desault (1789).

The ablest and best trained French surgeon of his time was Guillaume **Dupuytren** (1777–1835), at once a shrewd diagnostician, an operator of unrivaled aplomb, a wonderful clinical teacher, and a good experimental physiologist and pathologist. Dupuytren rose from poverty and fought his way up. His achievements are sometimes overlooked on account of the peasant-like meanness of his character. In 1808, he became one of the staff at the Hôtel Dieu, and on September 9, 1814, he was appointed surgeon-in-chief. Here his lectures and his extensive practice soon made him the leading surgeon of France, and he died a millionaire and a baron of the Empire. His clinics drew crowds of students from all countries, and he turned out many brillaint pupils. He had an immense practice, about 10,000 patients annually outside his hospital work.

---

[1] Larrey: Mém. de chir. mil., Paris, 1812, ii, 180–195.

He was the first to excise the lower jaw (1812[1]) and to treat aneurysm successfully by compression (1818[2]); the first to treat wry-neck by subcutaneous section of the sternomastoid muscle (1822[3]), and performed many feats in vascular surgery, such as the successful ligation of the external iliac (1815[4]) and two ligations of the subclavian (1819–29[5]). He also substituted ligation for amputation in fractures complicated by aneurysm (1815), devised an original method of treating artificial anus by means of a compressing enterotome of his invention (1828[6]), but his most enduring title to modern fame is in the field of surgical pathology. His original descriptions of fracture of the lower end of the fibula (Dupuytren's fracture, 1819[7]), congenital dislocation of the hip-joint (1826[8]), and retraction of the fingers from affection of the palmar aponeurosis, for which he devised an operation (1832[9]), are his greatest works. He also described fractures on children (1811), vaginitis in maidens (1827), varicose aneurysms (1829), and subluxation of the wrist or radius curvus, afterward known as Madelung's deformity. His memoirs On Injuries and Diseases of the Bones and on other phases of surgical pathology were reprinted in translation by the Sydenham Society in 1847 and 1854. He also left a treatise on wounds in war (1834), and his *Leçons orales* (1839) were often translated. In 1803, he founded the *Société anatomique de Paris* and he also endowed the well-known Musée Dupuytren at Paris, founded by Orfila.

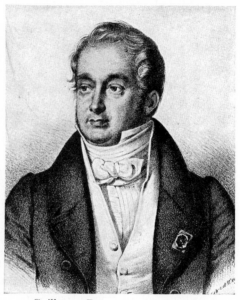

Guillaume Dupuytren (1777–1835).

Dupuytren was the type of man whom grinding poverty in youth, perhaps also some youthful disappointment in love, had made overambitious and overbearing. He had the utmost *sangfroid* and self-control, even when a patient had died on the table before him. His personality was olympian. In Paris, he was regarded as "nobody's friend," since he tolerated no rivals, and persecuted and intrigued against those who, like Duméril or Velpeau, aspired to that eminence, even pursuing them with vindictive hatred. He was cold, hard, con-

[1] Dupuytren: Leçons orales, Paris, 1839, ii, 421–453.

[2] Bull. Fac. de méd. de Paris, 1818, vi, 242.

[3] Described in Dupuytren: Leçons orales, Paris, 1839, iii, 455–461, and in Charles Averill's "Short Treatise on Operative Surgery," London, 1823, 61–64. The operation was repeated by Bouvier (1836) and J. Guérin, (1837).

[4] Repert. gén. d'anat. et de physiol. path., Paris, 1826, ii, 230–250.

[5] Edinb. Med. and Surg. Jour., 1819, xv, 476, and Arch. gén. de méd., Paris, 1829, 7. s., xx, 566–573.

[6] Mém. Acad. de méd., Paris, 1828, i, 259–316, 3 pl.

[7] Annuaire méd.-chir. d. hôp. de Paris, 1819, i, 1–212.

[8] Repert. gén. d'anat. et de physiol. path., Paris, 1826, ii, 82–93.

[9] J. univ. et hebd. de méd. et de chir. prat., Paris, 1832, 2. s., v, 348–365.

temptuous, unscrupulous, and overbearing, and more respected than beloved. Percy called him the first of surgeons and the least of men. Lisfranc dubbed him "the brigand of the Hôtel Dieu." Yet his fame was such that, when he visited Italy, he was treated *en prince.*

Alexis **Boyer** (1757–1833), a pupil of Desault and surgeon at the Charité even after the Revolution, wrote a treatise on diseases of the bones (1803), but was best known by his treatise on surgical diseases (1814–26), a huge compilation in 11 volumes defined by Malgaigne as "a summary of the works and opinions of the French Academy of Surgery." Boyer, like Hippocrates and Delpech, noted that caries of the spine is occasioned by *"le vice scrofuleux."*[1]

Jacques **Lisfranc** (1790–1847), surgeon at La Pitié, devised many new operations, in particular his partial amputation of the foot at the tarsometatarsal articulation (Lisfranc's amputation, 1815[2]), his methods of disarticulating the shoulder-

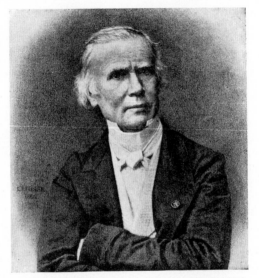

Alfred-Armand-Louis-Marie Velpeau (1795–1867).

joint (1815), of excision of the rectum, of lithotomy in women, and of amputation of the cervix uteri. He was little admired for his many aspersions of his colleagues.

Philibert-Joseph **Roux** (1780–1854), a pupil and friend of Bichat, was surgeon at the Charité in 1810, and succeeded Dupuytren at the Hôtel Dieu in 1835. He was the first French teacher to give a definite course of lectures (1812). He was a pioneer in plastic surgery, performing the first staphylorrhaphy in 1819 (described in detail in his memoir of 1825[3]), and the first suture of the ruptured female perineum (1832[4]).

Jacques-Mathieu **Delpech** (1777–1832), of Toulouse, graduated in Montpellier (1801) and, in 1812, became professor of surgery there. He was the pioneer of orthopedic surgery in France, his principal work

---

[1] Boyer: Traité des maladies chirurgicales, Paris, 1814, ii, 492.

[2] Lisfranc: Nouvelle méthode opératoire (etc.), Paris, 1815.

[3] Roux: Arch. gén. de méd., Paris, 1825, vii, 516–538.

[4] Roux: Gaz. méd. de Paris, 1834, 2. s., ii, 17–22.

being *De l'orthomorphie* (1828). On May 9, 1816, he performed, for the first time, a subcutaneous section of the tendo Achillis for club-foot,[1] the object being to exclude the air and obtain union by first intention. This operation, hitherto done by the open method, was twice repeated by Stromeyer in 1821–22. Delpech was also one of the first after Hippocrates to point out that Pott's disease (spinal caries) is of tubercular nature (1816[2]). He erected a large orthopedic institute at Montpellier, and, one morning, while on the way to it in his car-riage, he and his coachman were shot and killed by a vindictive patient, who thought that an operation for varicocele had rendered him unfit for marriage.

Alfred - Armand - Louis-Marie **Velpeau** (1795–1867), a pupil of Bretonneau's, originally a blacksmith's son who had once been appren-ticed to his father's trade, was surgeon to the Hôpital St. Antoine (1828–30), La Pitié (1830–34), the Charité (1834–67), and professor of clinical surgery at the Paris Faculty (1834–67). He was not a scientific surgeon, but a strong, capable, hard-working teacher and oper-ator, of whom Oliver Wen-dell Holmes said that "a good sound head over a pair of wooden shoes is a good deal better than a wooden head belonging to an owner

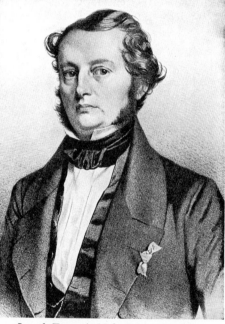

Joseph-François Malgaigne (1806–65).

who cases his feet in calf-skin." His principal works are his Treatise on Surgical Anatomy (1823), the first detailed work of its kind, his three-volume treatise on operative surgery, with atlas (1832), im-portant for its historic data, and once edited in translation by Valentine Mott (1847), and his great treatise on Diseases of the Breast (1854[3]), the most important work on the subject in its time.

Joseph-François **Malgaigne** (1806–65), the son of a French health officer, is described by Billings as "the greatest surgical historian and critic whom the world has yet seen," and he is, with Pétrequin, an

---

[1] In his Clin. chir. de Montpellier, 1823, i, 147–231, pl. x.

[2] Delpech: Précis élémentaire des maladies réputées chirurgicales, Paris, 1816, iii, 629, 638, *et seq.* Also: De l'orthomorphie, Paris, 1828, i, 241–251.

[3] Velpeau: Traité des maladies du sein, Paris, 1854.

authority on the surgery of the Hippocratic period. He served in the Napoleonic wars, wrote important works on operative surgery (1834), experimental surgery (1838), fractures and dislocations (1847–55), and edited the authentic modern edition of Ambroïse Paré, with a fine biography of the latter (1840). Malgaigne's *Manuel de médicine opératoire* (1834) passed through seven editions and five translations, one of them Arabic. In practical surgery his name is associated with the hooks of his invention used in treating fracture of the patella, but he is perhaps best remembered by the clinical and historical discourses which Billings classes "among the most delightful reading in surgical literature."

Auguste **Nélaton** (1807–73), of Paris, who presided with Malgaigne at the Hôpital St. Louis, held the same unapproachable rank as

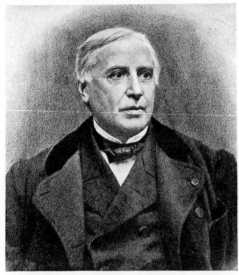

Auguste Nélaton (1807–73).

an operator and teacher which Dupuytren had attained at an earlier period, but in personality he was the logical opposite of his self-seeking predecessor. He was modest, quiet, helpful, and friendly, generous to the unfortunate—in brief, a gentleman. He invented a bullet-probe (first used in Garibaldi's case) and a valuable flexible rubber catheter (1860), and improved the treatment of nasopharyngeal tumors. In gynecology he is memorable as the first to describe pelvic (retro-uterine) hematocele (1851–52), and he did most to establish ovariotomy in France. His principal work is his *Éléments de pathologie chirurgicale* (1844–59).

Paul **Broca** (1824–80), who was, in succession, surgeon at St. Antoine, La Pitié, the Hôpital des Cliniques, and the Hôpital Necker, was the founder of the modern surgery of the brain and also of the modern French school of antropology. In 1861,[1] he discovered that the third left frontal convolution of the brain is the center of articulate speech, a point which is now disputed, but which, in the first instance, undoubtedly led to mapping out the different centers of the brain for surgical operations. Broca was, in fact, the first to trephine for a cerebral abscess diagnosed by his theory of localization of function. In connection with his discovery, he introduced the term *aphemia* or "motor

---

[1] Broca: Bull. Soc. d'anthrop. de Paris, 1861, ii, 235–238, and Bull. Soc. anat. de Paris, 1861, xxxvi, 330, 398.

aphasia" (1861[1]), which has undergone destructive criticism at the hands of Pierre Marie. In anthropology, Broca is, with Topinard and Quatrefages, the greatest name of modern France. He originated the modern methods of determining the ratio of the dimensions of the brain to those of the skull (craniometry), and to this end devised the occipital crochet, a craniograph, a goniometer, and did much to standardize the measurements of bones and the classification of colors of the hair and skin. He opposed the polyphyletic theory that the different races were originally developed from several separate pairs of species of his law of "eugenesis," which maintains that the different varieties of the genus Homo are, and always have been, fertile with each other. This drove the "polygenists" to their last resort, diversity of language. Broca is also credited with the aphorism: "I would rather be a transformed ape than a degenerate son of Adam."

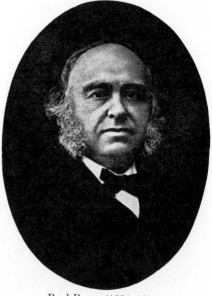

Paul Broca (1824–80).

Among the isolated French contributions of importance are Richerand's resection of the fifth and sixth ribs (1818); the introduction of lithotrity by Leroy d'Étiolles (1822), Civiale (1824), and Heurteloup (1824–31), which occasioned a bitter dispute as to priority. Béclard's excision of the parotid (1823[2]); Gensoul's incision of the upper jaw (1826); Lembert's method of enterorrhaphy (1826[3]); Maisonneuve's hair catheter (1845[4]); Sédillot's introduction of gastrostomy, which he performed for the first time on November 13, 1849[5]; Pravaz's hypodermic syringe (1851[6]); and Lallemant's method of autoplasty (1856).

Plaster-of-Paris bandages were introduced by Anthonius Mathijsen (1805–78), of Brabant, in 1852, and popularized by J. H. P. van de Loo.

Among the prominent German surgeons of the period were Vincenz von Kern (1760–1829), professor at Vienna (1805–24), who simplified wound-dressings by using bandages moistened with plain water (first proposed by Cesare Magati in 1616) as a substitute for the salves and plasters then in vogue; Christian Ludwig Mursinna (1744–1823), who

[1] Broca: Bull. Soc. d'anthrop. de Paris, 1861, ii, 235–236, and Bull. Soc. anat. de Paris, 1861, xxxvi, 332.

[2] Béclard: Arch. gén. de méd., Paris, 1824, iv, 60–66.

[3] Lembert: Repert. gén. d'anat. et physiol. path., Paris, 1826, ii, 100–107, 1 pl.

[4] Maisonneuve: Compt. rend. Acad. d. sc., Paris, 1845, xx, 70–72.

[5] Sédillot: Gaz. méd. de Strasbourg, 1849, ix, 366–377.

[6] Pravaz: Compt. rend. Acad. d. sc., Paris, 1853, xxxvi, 88–90.

was successively weaver, bath-keeper, barber's apprentice, and surgeon general of the Prussian Army (1787–1809); Conrad Johann Martin **Langenbeck** (1776–1851), professor of anatomy and surgery at Göttingen and surgeon general of the Hannoverian Army (1814), who devised the operation of iridocleisis for artificial pupil (1817), and attained such supreme swiftness in operating that he is said to have amputated a shoulder while a colleague present was taking a pinch of snuff; and Max Joseph von Chelius (1794–1876), whose *Handbuch der Chirurgie* (1822–23) was the standard text-book in Germany until the middle of the century, and who, according to Baas, was "the only professor in Heidelberg who kept a carriage." The most important German surgeons before 1850 were Dieffenbach, the elder von Graefe, the younger Stromeyer, Langenbeck, and Gustav Simon.

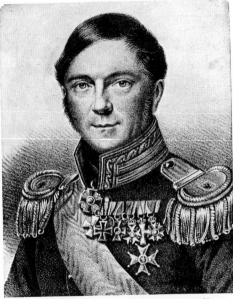

Carl Ferdinand von Graefe (1787–1840).

Carl Ferdinand **von Graefe** (1787–1840), of Warsaw, was one of the surgeons-general in the German struggle for independence (1813–15), and having previously been professor of surgery at the University of Berlin in 1810, resumed this position after the war. He was the founder of modern plastic surgery and devised the operation for congenital cleft-palate in 1816.[1] In 1818, he introduced rhinoplasty (simultaneously with Bünger) and blepharoplasty (simultaneously with Dzondi). In the same year, he improved the technic of Cesarean section and excised the lower jaw for the first time in Germany. He was also the first German surgeon to ligate the innominate artery (1822), his patient living 68 days.[2] His *Rhinoplastik* (1818) was the first handling of the theme of artificial nose-making after Tagliacozzi (1575) and Carpue (1816).

Johann Friedrich **Dieffenbach** (1792–1847), of Königsberg, also fought (as a rifleman) in the German war for independence. His doctor's dissertation at Würzburg (1822), on regeneration and transplantation of tissues,[3] already shows his leaning toward plastic surgery.

[1] von Graefe: Jour. f. Chir. u. Augenheilk., Berlin, 1820, i, 1–54, 2 pl.

[2] London Med. and Phys. Jour., 1823, xlix, 475.

[3] Dieffenbach: Nonnulla de regeneratione et transplantatione, Würzburg, 1822.

He was surgeon at the Charité (Berlin) in 1829, and, in 1840, succeeded von Graefe as professor at the university. In 1829, following Stromeyer's proposal, he first treated strabismus by severing the tendons of the eye muscles (with success[1]).

This success perhaps led him to attempt the erroneous procedure of subcutaneous division of the lingual muscles for stammering (1841[2]), which produced many untoward results in his patients; but he got wonderful results in tenotomy, skin-grafting, and orthopedic surgery, and was a pioneer in the transplantations and experimental surgery on animals, first essayed by John Hunter and Giuseppe Baronio (1804[3]). He wrote on treatment of urethral stricture by incision (1826); transfusion of blood (1828), bandaging (1829), nursing (1832), treatment of preternatural anus (1834), and urethral fistula (1836), and a great treatise on operative surgery (1845–48[4]). He also made a brave attempt to treat vesicovaginal fistula by every known method, and left a classic account of the sufferings entailed by the condition (1845).

Dieffenbach was a genial, humane, attractive man, and an admirable teacher, upholding the highest ideals of his profession. He maintained that the surgeon should be a many-sided Odysseus, full of native invention and resources not to be found in books. All great surgeons, he says, are, or ought to be, clear thinkers, and therefore good writers.

Georg Friedrich Louis **Stromeyer** (1804–76), of Hannover, professor at Erlangen, Munich, Freiburg, and Kiel, and successively

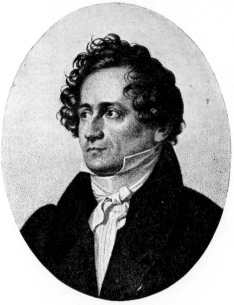

Johann Friedrich Dieffenbach (1792–1847).

surgeon-general of the Schleswig-Holstein and Hannoverian armies, was the father of modern military surgery in Germany. He greatly extended the fields of conservative surgery of the joints and subcutaneous surgery. Stromeyer performed his first subcutaneous section of the tendo achillis in 1831,[5] fifteen years after Delpech (1816), but if Delpech was the discoverer, Stromeyer developed the field. He practically created the modern surgery of the locomotor system by applying subcutaneous tenotomy to all deformities of the body depending upon muscular

---

[1] Dieffenbach: Ueber das Schielen, etc., Berlin, 1842.

[2] Dieffenbach: Die Heilung des Stotterns (etc.), Berlin, 1841.

[3] G. Baronio: Degli innesti animali, Milan, 1804.

[4] Dieffenbach: Die operative Chirurgie, Leipzig, 1845–48.

[5] Stromeyer: Mag. f. d. ges. Heilk., Berl., 1833, xxxix, 195–218.

defects. He is thus one of the founders of orthopedics in recent times. His methods were introduced into England by Little, who established the Royal Orthopedic Hospital in London (1837), and published a standard treatise on deformities (1853). Stromeyer's Maxims of War-Surgery (1855) made an epoch in German military medicine. He was a poet and wrote an attractive autobiography.

Bernhard **von Langenbeck** (1810–87), the nephew of Conrad, succeeded Dieffenbach at Berlin in 1847, and became the greatest clinical surgeon and teacher of his day in Germany, having trained nearly every prominent operator up to the present time. In 1861, he started the *Archiv für klinische Chirurgie* (known as Langenbeck's Archiv), and founded the German Society of Surgery, both of which have exerted a profound influence ever since. He has 21 operations credited to his name, of which the most important are his methods of excising the ankle, knee, hip, wrist, elbow, shoulder, and lower jaw, and of plastic surgery of the lip, palate, and nose.

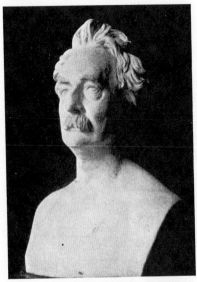

Georg Friedrich Louis Stromeyer (1804–76). (New York Academy of Medicine.)

Gustav **Simon** (1824–76), of Darmstadt, professor at Rostock (1861) and Heidelberg (1867), was a highly original operator and the author of admirable monographs on the treatment of vesicovaginal fistula (1854), the excision of the spleen (1857[1]), on plastic surgery (1868[2]), and the surgery of the kidneys (1871–76[3]). He was the first in Europe to excise the kidney (1869[4]), but killed his second patient by sepsis from a digital exploration on the twenty-first day after the operation. The fatal result in Paul von Bruns' case of 1878 made an end of nephrectomy until antisepsis was firmly established.

Albrecht Theodor **von Middeldorpf** (1824–68), of Breslau, performed the first operations for gastric fistula (1859) and esophageal tumor, was a pioneer in the use of the galvanocautery (1854), and made important contributions on fractures and dislocations.

The greatest of Russian surgeons, and one of the greatest military surgeons of all time, was Nikolai Ivanovich **Pirogoff** (1810–81), who, like Paré and Hunter, had a remarkable career of self-development.

---

[1] Simon: Die Exstirpation der Milz am Menschen, Giessen, 1857.

[2] Simon: Beiträge zur plastischen Chirurgie, Prague, 1868.

[3] Simon: Chirurgie der Nieren, Erlangen, 1871–76.

[4] Simon: Deutsche Klinik, Berl., 1870, xxii, 137.

Graduating in 1832, he studied for two years at Berlin and Göttingen, where he was disgusted with the small attention paid to anatomy. Langenbeck was, in his estimation, the only man who was well informed on the subject. Upon returning to Russia, he taught at Dorpat for five years, and, in 1840, was appointed professor of surgery at the Medico-Chirurgical Academy at St. Petersburg. In his forty-five years of service there he introduced many important reforms, among others the teaching of applied topographic anatomy, for the first time in Russia, to which end he invited Hyrtl's pupil, Gruber, from Vienna. He

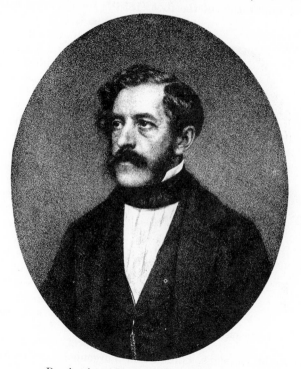

Bernhard von Langenbeck (1810–87).

made 11,000 postmortems, among them 800 of cholera victims in 1848. He saw a great deal of military surgery, serving in the field during the campaigns in the Caucasus (1847) and the Crimea (1854), and also reported upon the Franco-Prussian and Russo-Turkish campaigns. He served fourteen months in and around Sebastopol, and, in trenches and tents, witnessed all the horrors of pyemia, hospital gangrene, erysipelas, and purulent edema. Here he got himself into hot water with the governmental authorities by his sharp criticism of the bad management of the campaign, his attempts at segregation and other improvements, and was forced to resign his professorship. His experiences with sepsis led him to define war as a "traumatic epidemic."

32

Through the aid of the Grand Duchess Helena Pavlovna, he introduced female nursing of the wounded in the Crimea, and, all his life, he was a warm advocate of freedom and higher education for women. In 1847, he was already using ether anesthesia in his surgical practice.[1] He devoted his latter days to advancing the cause of medical education in his native country, in which he was again subjected to bitter enmity and persecution at the hands of the official and military tchinovniks. Pirogoff is, in the esteem of cultivated Russians, the most important figure in their medical history. He is noted for his method of complete osteoplastic amputation of the foot (1854[2]); for his great atlas of 220 plates (1851–54[3]), in which frozen sections were first utilized on a grand scale in anatomic illustration[4]; and for his treatise on military surgery (1864[5]), in which he holds large hospitals responsible for the spread of epidemic diseases and recommends small, barrack-like pavilions, such as were suggested by his Crimean experiences. In speed, dexterity, and strength of hand, Pirogoff, the operator, was like those Slavic virtuosi of music whose execution is the astonishment of our times. The usual portraits of the great surgeon in his old age represent a broad-browed, serious face of venerable aspect, strongly resembling

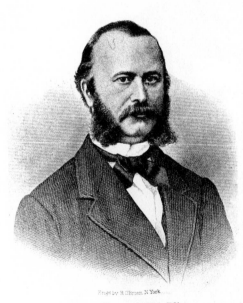

Engr by R.G.Brien N York.

Gustav Simon (1824–76).

two other great Russians, Glinka and Turgenieff. In relation to his country, we may apply to him the exquisite tribute which Henry James paid to the latter: "His large nature was filled with the love of justice but he was also of the stuff of which glories are made."

American surgery in the pre-Listerian period was distinguished principally by a great deal of bold operating on the vascular and osseous

[1] Pirogoff: Recherches pratiques et physiologiques sur l'éthérisation, St. Petersburg, 1847.

[2] Voyenno Med. Jour., St. Petersburg, 1854, lxiii, 2. sect., 83–100.

[3] Anatome topographica sectionibus per corpus humanum congelatum triplice directione ductis illustrata, St. Petersburg, 1851–54.

[4] Frozen sections in anatomy were first used by Pieter de Riemer (1760–1831) in his "Afbeeldingen" (The Hague, 1818) and later by E. Weber (1836) and Huschke (1844).

[5] Pirogoff: Grundzüge der allgemeinen Kriegschirurgie, Leipzig, 1864.

systems, by the foundation of modern operative gynecology at the hands of McDowell and Sims, and by the permanent introduction of surgical anesthesia. Its leading representatives in this period were Physick, the two Warrens, Post, Mott, Gibson, the two Smiths, Willard Parker, McDowell, and Sims.

Philip Syng **Physick** (1768–1837), of Philadelphia, a pupil of John Hunter's, and sometimes called the Father of American Surgery, was an Edinburgh graduate of 1792, surgeon to the Pennsylvania Hospital in 1794, and professor of surgery in the University of Pennsylvania (1805–18). He wrote nothing of consequence and all his teaching is preserved in the treatise on surgery of his nephew, John Syng Dorsey (1813).

Physick is now remembered principally by such procedures as the introduction of absorbable kid and buckskin ligatures (1816[1]), the use of the seton in ununited fracture (1822[2]), an operation for artificial anus (1826[3]), the advocation of rest in hip-joint disease (1830[4]), and the invention of the tonsillotome (1828[5]). His modification of Desault's splint for fracture of the femur is still in use. He seems to have been the first to describe diverticula of the rectum (1836[6]), and he was the first American to wash out the stomach with a syringe and tube in a case of poisoning (1802[7]).

John Warren (1753–1815), of Roxbury, Massachusetts, rendered distinguished army service in the Revolution and was founder and the first professor

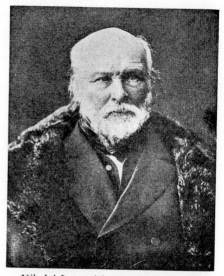

Nikolai Ivanovich Pirogoff (1810–81).

of anatomy and surgery of the Harvard Medical School (1783). He was seventh president of the Massachusetts Medical Society, an office which he held until his death (1804–15). He amputated at the shoulder-joint in 1781,[8] and excised the parotid gland in 1804.[9] His son, **John Collins Warren** (1778–1856), of Boston, was a pupil of Astley Cooper and Dupuytren, and succeeded to his father's

---

[1] Physick: Eclect. Repertory, Phila., 1816, vi, 389.

[2] Phila. Jour. Med. and Phys. Sc., 1822, v, 116–118.

[3] *Ibid.*, 1826, xiii, 199–202.

[4] Am. Jour. Med. Sc., Phila., 1830, vii, 299–308, 1 pl.

[5] *Ibid.*, 1828, ii, 116.

[6] Am. Cycl. Pract. Med. and Surg., Phila., 1836, ii, 123–136.

[7] Eclect. Repertory, Phila., 1812–13, iii, 111, 381. Matthews: Med. Recorder, Phila., 1826, ix, 825–827. Physick acknowledges the priority of Monro *secundus* in the invention of a similar instrument (1767).

[8] Warren: Boston Med. and Surg. Jour., 1839, xx, 210.

[9] In J. C. Warren: Surgical Observations on tumors, Boston, 1837, p. 287.

professorship in 1815. He was a pioneer in the excision of bones and joints, such as the hyoid (1804) and the elbow (1834), introduced the operation of staphylorrhaphy for fissure of the soft palate in 1828,[1] and was the first in this country to operate for strangulated hernia. He was the founder of the Massachusetts General Hospital (1811) and of the Warren Museum, and he practically introduced ether anesthesia in surgery (1847). His principal work is his *Surgical Observations on Tumors* (1837).

Nathan **Smith** (1762–1829), of Rehoboth, Massachusetts, a medical graduate of Harvard (1790), studied also in the Scotch and English schools, commenced practice at Cornish, N. H., and in 1798 became a professor in Dartmouth College, filling, as O. W. Holmes said, not a chair, but "a whole settee of professorships," viz., anatomy, surgery, chemistry, and practice.

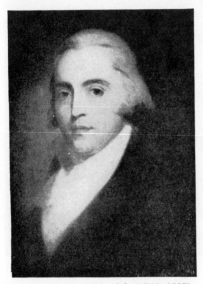

Philip Syng Physick (1768–1837).
From an oil-painting by Thomas Sully.
(Surgeon General's Library.)

For fourteen years Smith labored at building up the Dartmouth school, when, in 1821, he was asked to establish a medical department at Yale, with the same multifarious duties. This accomplished, in the face of many obstacles, he did a similar good turn for Bowdoin College (1820) and later for the University of Vermont. He was more the great organizer and teacher than a writer on medicine, but his essay on typhus fever (1824) and his observations on necrosis (1827) are still memorable. An able and successful operator, particularly in lithotomy, he performed the second ovariotomy in the United States (July 25, 1821), amputated at the knee-joint (1825), and did the first staphylorrhaphy.

The pioneer surgeon of the Middle West was Daniel **Brainerd** (1812–66), of New York, a graduate of Jefferson Medical College (1834), who settled in Chicago in 1835 and secured a charter for Rush Medical College (1837), which, after some Parisian study, he organized in 1843, occupying the chair of surgery until his death. He invented the bone-drill, and made several good contributions to surgery, notably a prize essay of 1854 on a new method of treating fractures and deformities.

Wright **Post** (1766–1822), of Long Island, N. Y., was the first in America to ligate the femoral artery successfully (for popliteal aneurysm) according to John Hunter's method (1796[2]), and the second to ligate the external iliac successfully (1814[3]), having been preceded by

---

[1] Am. Jour. Med. Sc., Phila., 1828, iii, 1–3, 1 pl.

[2] Post: Am. Med. and Phil. Register, N. Y., 1814, iv, 452.

[3] Post: *Ibid.*, 1813–14, iv, 443–453. Also in: Med. Repository, N. Y., 1815, n. s., ii, 196–199.

Dorsey in 1811.[1] Post was also the first surgeon to tie the primitive carotid in its continuity with success (1813[2]), an operation which he successfully repeated in 1816,[3] and the subclavian artery was first successfully ligated outside the scaleni by him in 1817.[4]

Valentine **Mott** (1785–1865), of Long Island, was a pupil of Astley Cooper, and, like him, a great pioneer in vascular surgery. The innominate artery was ligated for the first time in the history of surgery by Mott in 1818,[5] the first successful operation being that of Smyth, of New Orleans, in 1864.

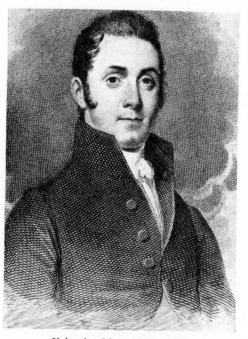

Valentine Mott (1785–1865).

In addition, Mott has to his credit the remarkable record of successfully ligating the common iliac at its origin (1827[6]), the carotid for subclavian aneurysm (1829[7]), the carotid for anastomosing aneurysm in a three-months' infant (1829[8]), the external iliac for femoral aneurysm (1831), the right subclavian within the scaleni (1833[9]), both carotids simultaneously (1833[10]), and the right internal iliac (1837[11]). Besides

---

[1] Dorsey: Elect. Repertory, Phila., 1811, ii, 111–115.

[2] Post: Am. Med. and Phil. Register, N. Y., 1814, iv, 366–377.

[3] Post: Med. Repository, N. Y., 1817, n. s., iii, 412.

[4] Post: Tr. Phys. Med. Soc., N. Y., 1817, i, 387–394.

[5] Mott: Med. and Surg. Register, N. Y., 1818, i, 9–54.

[6] Phila. Jour. Med. and Phys. Sc., 1827, xiv, 176–181.

[7] Am. Jour. Med. Sc., Phila., 1829, v, 297; 1830, vi, 532.

[8] *Ibid.*, 1829, v, 255; 1830, vii, 271.

[9] *Ibid.*, 1831, viii, 393–397. [10] *Ibid.*, 1833, xii, 354. [11] *Ibid.*, 1837, xx, 13–15.

the innominate artery, says Billings, Mott "tied the subclavian 8 times, the primitive carotid 51 times, the carotid twice, the common iliac once, the external iliac 6 times, the internal iliac twice, the femoral 57 times, and the popliteal 10 times"— in all, 138 ligations of the great vessels for aneurysm. Mott was also a bold and successful operator on the bones and joints. He excised the right side of the lower jaw, after tying the carotid artery (1821[1]); successfully amputated at the hip-joint (1824[2]); excised the left clavicle for osteosarcoma (1828[3]), and removed a large fibrous growth from the nostril by dividing the nasal and maxillary bones (1841[4]).

In connection with the work of Post and Mott, it is proper to mention here some other early ligations of arteries by American surgeons in the same field. The primitive carotid artery was successfully ligated for primary hemorrhage by Mason Fitch Cogswell (1761–1830), of Connecticut, in 1803,[5] and, for secondary hemorrhage by Amos Twitchell (1781–1850), of New Hampshire, in 1807,[6] eight months prior to Sir Astley Cooper's case. Both primitive carotids were first successfully tied in continuity, within a month's interval, by James Macgill, of Maryland (1823[7]), to be followed by Reuben D. Mussey (1827) and Mott (1833). The primitive and internal carotids were first simultaneously tied by Gurdon Buck (1807–77), of New York City (1848[8]); and John Murray **Carnochan** (1817–87), of Savannah, Georgia, ligated the carotid on both sides for elephantiasis (1867[9]). Carnochan was also the first to excise the superior maxillary nerve (including Meckel's ganglion) for facial neuralgia (1858[10]). John Kearny Rodgers (1793–1851), of New York City, a pupil of Wright Post, was the first to tie the left subclavian artery within the scaleni for aneurysm (1845[11]), but with fatal result, the first successful case being that of Professor W. S. Halsted, of Johns Hopkins (1892[12]). William Gibson (1788–1868), of Baltimore, Maryland, was the first American surgeon to tie the common iliac artery (1812[13]). In the preceding year, John Syng Dorsey (1783–1818) had successfully tied the external iliac,[14] to be followed by Post (1814), Horatio Gates Jameson (1821[15]), and Edward Peace (1841[16]). The internal iliac was successfully tied by S. Pomeroy White (1827[17]); the femoral, by Henry M. Onderdonk (1813[18]); David L. Rodgers (1824), and Carnochan (1851); the gluteal artery, by John B. Davidge, of Baltimore, and George McClellan, of Philadelphia; the aorta, for the first time after Sir Astley Cooper, by Hunter McGuire (1868[19]). In addition, Gurdon Buck (1807–77), of New York, successfully ligated the femoral, profunda, external and common iliac arteries for femoral aneurysm (1858[20]); Willard Parker (1800–84), of Francistown, N. Y., ligated the left subclavian inside the scalenus, together with the common carotid and vertebral arteries, for subclavian aneurysm (1864[21]) the patient dying on the forty-second day. Andrew Woods Smyth (1833–1916), of New

---

[1] Mott: New York Med. and Phys. Jour., 1822, i, 385.

[2] Phila. Jour. Med. and Phys. Sc., 1827, xiv, 101–104.

[3] Am. Jour. Med. Sc., Phila., 1828, iii, 100–108.

[4] *Ibid.*, 1842, n. s., iii, 257; 1843, v, 87.

[5] Cogswell: New Engl. Jour. Med. and Surg., Bost., 1824, xiii, 357–360.

[6] Twitchell: New Engl. Quart. Jour. Med. and Surg., Bost., 1842–43, i, 188–193.

[7] Macgill: New York Med. and Phys. Jour., 1825, iv, 576.

[8] Buck: New York Med. Times, 1855–56, v, 37–42.

[9] Carnochan: Am. Jour. Med. Sc., Phila., 1867, n. s., liv, 109–115.

[10] Carnochan: *Ibid.*, 1858, n. s., xxxv, 134–143.

[11] Rodgers: *Ibid.*, 1846, n. s., ix, 541.

[12] Halsted: Johns Hopkins Hosp. Bul.., Balt., 1892, iii, 93.

[13] Gibson: Am. Med. Recorder, Phila., 1820, iii, 185–193, 2 pl.

[14] Dorsey: Eclect. Repertory, Phila., 1811, ii, 111–115.

[15] Jameson: Am. Med. Recorder, Phila., 1822, v, 118–124.

[16] Peace: Med. Exam., Phila., 1842, n. s., i, 225–228.

[17] White: Am. Jour. Med. Sc., Phila., 1827, i, 304–306.

[18] Onderdonk: Am. Med. and Phil. Register, N. Y., 1814, iv, 176.

[19] McGuire: Am. Jour. Med. Sc., Phila., 1868, n. s., lvi, 415–419.

[20] Buck: New York Med. Jour., 1858, 3 s., v, 305–311.

[21] Parker: Am. Jour. Med. Sc., Phila., 1864, n. s., xlvii, 562.

Orleans, first successfully ligated the innominate artery, together with the common carotid, and subsequently the right vertebral, for subclavian aneurysm (1864[1]) exhibiting his patient alive in 1869. The specimen is now in the U. S. Army Medical Museum.

Of early American operations upon the bones and joints, we may mention the first amputation at the hip-joint in the United States, by Walter Brashear (1776–1860), of Maryland (1806[2]); the successful excision of part of the lower jaw, by William Henry Deadrick (1773–1858), of Winchester, Va. (1810[3]); the first successful excision of the clavicle, by Charles McCreary (1785–1826), of Kentucky (1813[4]); the excision of the superior maxilla, by Horatio Gates Jameson (1788–1855), of York, Pa. (1820[5]); the successful amputation at the elbow-joint, by James Mann, U. S. Army (1821[6]); an excision of the fifth and sixth ribs, with a portion of gangrenous lung, by Milton Antony (1789–1839), of Georgia (1821[7]); excision of nearly the whole of both upper jaws, by David L. Rogers, of New York (1824[8]); amputation at the knee-joint, by Nathan Smith (1762–1829), of Massachusetts (1824[9]); osteotomy for ankylosis of the hip-joint, by John Rhea Barton (1794–1871), of Lancaster, Pa. (1826[10]); successful wiring of an ununited fracture of the humerus (1827[11]), by J. K. Rodgers (1793–1851), of New York City; excision of the coccyx, by Josiah Clark Nott (1804–73), of Columbia, S. C. (1832[12]); excision of the elbow-joint, by John Collins Warren (1778–1856), of Massachusetts (1834[13]); the interscapular-thoracic amputation, by Dixi Crosby (1801–73), of New Hampshire (1836[14]); and, in two stages, by Reuben Dimond Mussey (1818–82), of New Hampshire, in 1831–37[15]; excision of the olecranon process, by Gurdon Buck (1807–77), of New York City (1842[16]); the Fergusson operation for fissure of the hard and soft palates, by Jonathan Mason Warren (1811–67), of Boston (1842[17]); S. D. Gross's amputation at the ankle-joint in 1851[18]; Bigelow's excision of the hip-joint (1852[19]); exsection of the ulna (1853[20]), the radius (1854[21]), and the os calcis (1857[22]), by John Murray Carnochan (1817–87), of Savannah, Ga., and Sayre's resection of the hip for ankylosis (1855[23]). In 1836 Paul Fitzsimmons Eve (1806–77), of Georgia, removed a large fibrous polyp from the base of the cranium,[24] and, in 1850, William Detmold (1808–

[1] Smyth: Am. Jour. Med. Sc., Phila., 1866, n. s., lii, 280–282. (Exhibition of living patient). New Orleans Jour. Med., 1869, xxii, 464–469. Repeated by J. Lewtas, of Murdan Hospital, Punjab (Brit. Med. Jour., Lond., 1889, ii, 312).

[2] Brashear: Tr. Kentucky Med. Soc., 1852, Frankfort, 1853, ii, 265.

[3] Deadrick: Am. Med. Recorder, Phila., 1823, vi, 516.

[4] McCreary: Tr. Kentucky Med. Soc., 1852, Frankfort, 1853, ii, 276.

[5] Jameson: Am. Med. Recorder, Phila., 1821, iv, 221–230, 1 pl.

[6] Mann: Med. Repository, New York, 1822, n. s., vii, pp. 17–19.

[7] Antony: Phila. Jour. Med. and Phys. Sc., 1823, vi, 108–117, 1 pl.

[8] Rogers: New York Med. and Phys. Jour., 1824, iii, 301–303.

[9] Smith: Am. Med. Rev. and Jour., Phila., 1825, ii, 370.

[10] Barton: North Amer. Med. and Surg. Jour., 1826, iii, 279–292, 400, 1 pl.

[11] Rodgers: New York Med. and Phys. Jour., 1827, vi, 521–523.

[12] Nott: New Orleans Med. Jour., 1844–45, i, 58–60.

[13] J. C. Warren: In Hodge's (J. M.) Excision of Joints, Boston, 1861, p. 69.

[14] Crosby: Med. Record, N. Y., 1875, x, 753–755. (Crosby was preceded by the English naval surgeon, Ralph Cuming, in 1808.)

[15] Mussey: Am. Jour. Med. Sc., Phila., 1837, xxi, 390–394.

[16] Buck: Ibid., 1843, n. s., v, 297–301.

[17] J. M. Warren: New Engl. Quart. Jour. Med. and Surg., Bost., 1842–43, i, 538–547.

[18] Gross: Cited on p. 457 of Am. Jour. Med. Sc., Phila., 1876, n. s., lxxi.

[19] Bigelow: Am. Jour. Med. Sc., Phila., 1852, xxiv, 90.

[20] Carnochan: Am. Med. Monthly, N. Y., 1854, i, 180–188.

[21] Carnochan: Am. Jour. Med. Sc., Phila., 1868, n. s., xxxv, 363–370.

[22] Carnochan: Am. Med. Gaz., N. Y., 1857, viii, 321–323.

[23] Sayre: New York Jour. Med., 1855, n. s., xiv, 70–82.

[24] Eve: South. Med. and Surg. Jour., Augusta, 1836–37, i, 78–80.

94) opened the lateral sinus of the brain for abscess,[1] the report of which operation Virchow treated with scornful skepticism. Carnochan's three cases of excision of the fifth nerve for neuralgia (1858[2]) were followed by the ingenious and successful method of Joseph Pancoast (1805–82), of New Jersey (1872[3]), who was also the first to perform a successful plastic operation for exstrophy of the bladder in February, 1858.[4] This operation was repeated with success upon the female bladder by Daniel Ayres, of Brooklyn, N. Y., in November, 1858.[5] Cystotomy for inflammation and rupture of the bladder was first performed (1846–54[6]) by Willard Parker (1800–84) of Francistown, N. Y., who was also the first, after Hancock, of London (1848), to operate for appendicitis (1864[7]), and tied the subclavian artery five times. In lithotomy, Benjamin Winslow Dudley (1785–1870) was especially successful, having performed this operation 225 times, with scarce a death. Next to Dudley, Physick is said to have cut for stone oftener than any other American surgeon, and his removal of over a thousand calculi from Chief Justice Marshall is a famous early case. The kidney was first excised (before Gustav Simon) by Erastus Bradley Wolcott (1804–80), of Benton, N. Y., in 1861.[8] John Stough Bobbs (1809–70), of Pennsylvania German descent, was the first to perform cholecystotomy for gall-stones (1868[9]), in which he was followed by Marion Sims (1878[10]). Among the special procedures introduced by American surgeons in this period are Nathan Smith's method of treating necrosis of bones with the trephine (1827[11]), Jonathan Knight's successful treatment of aneurysm by digital compression (1847[12]), the method of reducing dislocations by manipulation, without weights or pulleys, introduced by William W. Reid, of Rochester, New York, in his classic papers of 1851–55,[13] based upon dissections and experiments; the treatment of fractures of the femur by Nathan Ryno Smith's anterior splint (1860[14]), and by the weight and pulley apparatus of Gurdon Buck (Buck's extension, 1861[15]).

The Civil War in the United States (1861–65) brought forth the remarkable *Medical and Surgical History of the War of the Rebellion* (1870–88), by Joseph Janvier Woodward, Charles Smart, George A. Otis, and David L. Huntington, a splendid collection of case histories and pathologic reports, embellished with fine plates, and, altogether, a work that is unique in the annals of military medicine. It was the subject of enthusiastic praise by Virchow.[16] Another important surgical work which came out of this war was the study of "Gunshot Wounds and Other Injuries of Nerves" (1864) by S. Weir Mitchell, George R. Morehouse, and William W. Keen, who were then acting as army surgeons at the Turner's Lane Hospital in Philadelphia. This book was the first full-length study of the traumatic neuroses, introducing the use of massage in these cases, and was the starting point of Mitchell's subsequent work on ascending neuritis, traumatic neurasthenia, and the psychic phenomena in those who have undergone amputation.[17]

The only successful amputation at the hip-joint during the Civil War was performed in a case of gunshot injury by Edward Shippen, of Philadelphia.[18]

---

[1] Detmold: Am. Jour. Med. Sc., Phila., 1850, xix, 86–95.

[2] Carnochan: *Ibid.*, 1858, n. s., xxxv, 134–143.

[3] Pancoast: Phila. Med. Times, 1872–72, ii, 285–287.

[4] Pancoast: North Am. Med.-Chir. Rev., Phila., 1859, iii, p. 710 (bracketed case, reported by S. D. Gross).   [5] Ayres: Am. Med. Gaz., N. Y., 1859, x, 81–89, 2 pl.

[6] Parker: New York Jour. Med., 1851, n. s., vii, 83–86. Also, Tr. Med. Soc., N. Y., 1867, 345–349.   [7] Parker: Med. Rec., New York, 1867, ii, 25–27.

[8] Wolcott: Med. and Surg. Reporter, Phila., 1861–62, vii, 126.

[9] Bobbs: Tr. Med. Soc. Indiana, 1868, 68–73.

[10] Sims: Richmond and Louisville Med. Jour., 1878, xxvi, 1–21.

[11] N. Smith: Phila. Month. Jour. Med., 1827, i, 11; 66.

[12] Knight: Boston Med. and Surg. Jour., 1848, xxxviii, 293–296.

[13] Reid: Buffalo Med. Jour., 1851–52, vii, 129–143.

[14] N. R. Smith: Maryland and Virginia Med. and Surg. Jour., 1860, xiv, 1, 177.

[15] Buck: Bull. New York Acad. Med., 1860–62, i, 181–188.

[16] Virchow: Die Fortschritte der Kriegsheilkunde, Berlin, 1874, p. 7.

[17] Mitchell: Injuries to Nerves and their Consequences, Philadelphia, 1872.

[18] Surgeon-General's Office: Circular No. 7, Washington, 1867.

The early history of the introduction of **ether anesthesia** in America has been the subject of rabid controversy, but the principal facts may be briefly stated as follows: The use of the soporific draught of Dioscorides and the soporific sponge of the Salernitans was unknown to Paré and died out in the 17th century, but it was sometimes customary for early 19th century surgeons to intoxicate the patient with alcohol or opium in cases requiring complete muscular relaxation, such as reduction of dislocations, ligations of large arteries, or operation for hernia. Hypnotism was also employed, and even suggestion, as where Dupuytren induced a convenient fainting spell by a brutal remark. In March, 1842, Dr. Crawford Williamson Long (1815–78), of Daniels-ville, Ga., a graduate of the University of Pennsylvania (1839), having previously noted some accidental anesthetic effects of ether, removed a small cystic tumor from the back of the neck of a patient under its influence, and subsequently used it in other cases (1842–43), which have been amply certified and vouched for by resident physicians of his locality.[1] But Long published no reports of his results, and, as Welch has said, "we cannot assign to him any influence upon the historical development of our knowledge of surgical anesthesia or any share in its introduction to the world at large." Long had no one to take up and expand his work, as Lizars did for McDowell's. In 1800, Sir Humphry Davy (1788–1829), of Penzance, England, experimented upon himself with nitrous oxide, and stated that "it may probably be used with advantage in surgical operations in which no great effusion of blood takes place." In 1844, Horace Wells (1815–48), a dentist of Hartford, Connecticut, began to use nitrous oxide in dentistry, communicating his results to his friend and former partner, William Thomas Green Morton (1819–68), of Charlton, Massachusetts; but a fatal case caused Wells to withdraw from practice, and he eventually put an end to his life. Morton had, in the meantime, been studying medicine, having for his preceptor Dr. Charles T. Jackson, a chemist of ability, who pointed out to him the anesthetic effects of chloric ether, which he proceeded to apply in filling a tooth in July, 1844. Becoming interested, Morton pushed his inquiries further and subsequently learned from Jackson that sulphuric ether is also an anesthetic, whereupon he applied it at once in extracting a deeply rooted bicuspid tooth from one of his patients. Morton then visited Dr. John Collins Warren, of the Massachusetts General Hospital, and persuaded him to give the new anesthetic a trial in surgical procedure, without, however, disclosing the name of the drug. The operation took place at the hospital on October 16, 1846, the case being a "congenital but superficial, vascular tumor, just below the jaw, on the left side of the neck." The tumor was dissected out by Warren in five minutes, and, as the patient came back to consciousness, he exclaimed, "Gentlemen, this is no humbug."

---

[1] The original documents in support of Long's claim have been effectively brought together by Dr. H. H. Young in Bull. Johns Hopkins Hosp., Balt., 1896–97, viii, 174–184.

The next day a large fatty tumor of the shoulder was removed by
Hayward, with Morton as anesthetist, and again with success. On
November 18, 1846, the discovery was announced to the world in a
paper by Henry J. Bigelow, published in the Boston Medical and
Surgical Journal.[1] It was largely due to the high character and repute
of such men as Warren and Bigelow that ether anesthesia was taken
up all over the world and became a permanent part of operative surgery, for Morton tried to patent the drug as "letheon" (1846[2]), squab-
bled with Jackson about their respective legal rights, and did not
announce it as sulphuric ether until 1847.[3] In the meanwhile, Robert
Liston had amputated a thigh under ether in December, 1846; Syme
took it up in Edinburgh (1847), and Pirogoff wrote a little manual on
etherization (1847), used later in Crimean experiences. The terms
"anesthesia" and "anesthetic" were proposed by Oliver Wendell
Holmes. On January 19, 1847, Sir James Young Simpson (1811–70),
professor of obstetrics at Edinburgh, used ether in midwifery practice
for the first time in Great Britain, but on November 4, 1847, he was
led to substitute chloroform, the discovery of Liebig, Guthrie, and
Soubeiran, and was so much impressed with its advantages over ether
in obstetric work that he published his results a week later.[4] The
effect of these discoveries upon medicine and surgery was remarkable in
many ways. First of all, the surgeon, who, in pre-anesthetic days, had
to rush through an operation at lightning speed and under great disadvantages occasioned by the struggles and distress of the patient, could
now take his time and therefore perform many new operations impossible
under the old conditions.[5] The days of sleight-of-hand feats were over,
and the prestidigitations of a Cheselden, a Langenbeck, a Fergusson, or
a Pirogoff gave place to careful, deliberate procedure. Again, a few
whiffs of chloroform enabled the lying-in woman to confront the fierce
pangs of labor with greater ease and security, and the obstetrician was
able to work under the same advantages as the surgeon. Both surgeon
and obstetrician specialized at need, as operative gynecologists, while
laboratory workers in physiology and other branches of experimental
medicine could have no further misgivings about the sufferings of
vivisected animals. In these fields anesthesia was, in the memorable
phrase of Weir Mitchell, the "Death of Pain."

---

[1] Bigelow: Boston Med. and Surg. Jour., 1846–47, xxxv, 309, 379.

[2] T. W. Morton: Circular, Morton's letheon, Boston, 1846.

[3] Morton: Remarks on the proper mode of administering sulphuric ether, etc.,
Boston, 1847.   [4] Sir J. Y. Simpson: Account of a new anesthetic agent, Edinb., 1847.

[5] "When I was a boy, surgeons operating upon the quick were pitted one against
the other like runners on time. He was the best surgeon, both for patient and on-
looker, who broke the three-minutes record in an amputation or a lithotomy. What
place could there be in record-breaking operations for the fiddle-faddle of antiseptic
precautions? The obvious boon of immunity from pain, precious as it was, when
we look beyond the individual, was less than the boon of time. With anesthetics
ended slapdash surgery; anesthesia gave time for the theories of Pasteur and Lister
to be adopted in practice." Sir Clifford Allbutt: Johns Hopkins Hosp. Bull., Balt.,
1898, ix, 281.

Operative gynecology, which had no special existence before the beginning of the 19th century, was largely the creation of certain surgeons from the Southern States and had its origin mainly in the attempt to repair the errors and omissions of backwoods obstetrics. In the 18th century, William Baynham (1749–1814), of Virginia, operated twice with success for extra-uterine pregnancy (1790–99[1]) and, in 1816,[2] John King, of Edisto Island, South Carolina, performed a remarkable operation for abdominal pregnancy, saving both mother and child by cutting through the walls of the vagina and applying the forceps, with abdominal pressure exerted upon the fetus from above. He afterward expanded his observations in a thin volume of 176 pages, published at Norwich, England, in 1818, entitled "An Analysis of the Subject of Extra-uterine Fœtation, and of the Retroversion of the Gravid Uterus," the first book on the subject. The founders of operative gynecology were McDowell and Sims.

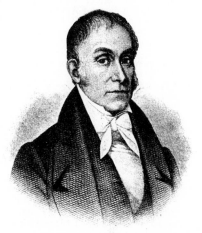

Ephraim McDowell (1771–1830), of Virginia, was a pupil of John Bell, of Edinburgh, in 1793–94, and, through Bell's eloquent teaching, was early impressed with the sad and hopeless fate of women afflicted with ovarian disease. In 1795, he settled in the village of Danville, Kentucky, then one of the outposts of civilization, and soon became known as a skilful and successful surgeon, especially in lithotomy, which he performed 22 times in succession without losing a case. In December, 1809, he performed his first ovariotomy upon Mrs. Crawford, a woman of forty-seven, who thereupon lived to be seventy-eight. McDowell reported this case with two others in April, 1817,[3] following up with a report of two more cases in 1819.[4] He performed the operation 13 times in his life, with a record of 8 recoveries. Although he may have been preceded by Weyer's swineherd of the 16th century, and by the partial operation (tapping of cyst) by Houstoun, of Edinburgh (1701), yet one swallow does not make a summer, and ovariotomy had no existence in surgical practice before McDowell produced his results and put it upon a permanent basis. He had sent a manuscript copy of his first paper to his old preceptor, John Bell, who was then ending his days in Italy and never saw it. It came, however, into the hands

Ephraim McDowell (1771–1830).

[1] Baynham: New York Med. and Phil. Rev., 1809, i, 160–170.
[2] King: Med. Repository, N. Y., 1817, n. s., iii, 388–394.
[3] McDowell: Eclect. Repertory and Analyt. Rev., Phila., 1817, viii, 242–244.
[4] McDowell: *Ibid.*, 1819, ix, 546–553.

of Bell's pupil, John Lizars (1787–1860), of Edinburgh, who took up McDowell's work with interest, publishing his results in his *Observations on Extraction of Diseased Ovaria* (1825), the next important contribution to the subject.

In the meantime, Dr. Nathan Smith had performed an ovariotomy at Norwich, Vermont, in July, 1821,[1] in ignorance of McDowell's work which was destined to receive its greatest impetus at the hands of the brothers, John L. and Washington L. Atlee, of Pennsylvania, the former of whom performed the operation 78 times, with 64 recoveries (1843–83), and the latter 387 times (1844–78). Ovariotomy was firmly established in English surgery through the labors of Charles Clay (1801–93), of Manchester, and Sir Spencer Wells (1818–97), of London. Benedikt Stilling did an ovariotomy by the extraperitoneal route in 1837. The introduction of ovariotomy in France was due to Auguste Nélaton, to Jules Péan (1830–98), who performed the first successful operation in Paris (1864), and to the Alsatian surgeon Eugène Koeberlé (1828–1915), who performed his first ovariotomies on June 2 and September 29, 1862.[2] Before the time of Sims, much important work of a scattered character was done in Europe and America, notably Osiander's 8 cases of excision of the portio for cancer (1801–8[3]), C. J. M. Langenbeck's vaginal hysterectomy for cancer (1813[4]), which was followed by the cases of J. N. Sauter (1822) and J.-C.-A. Récamier (1829); Ritgen's case of gastro-elytrotomy (1821[5]), Roux's operation for ruptured perineum (1834[6]); William Campbell's *Memoir on Extra-uterine Gestation* (1840); Récamier's invention of the *speculum plein et brisé* (1842[7]), the simultaneous invention of special uterine sounds, in 1843, by Huguier, of Paris, Kiwisch, of Prague, and Sir James Young Simpson[8]; Heath's abdominal section for fibroids (1843), Bennett's treatise on *Inflammation of the Uterus* (1845); C. D. Meigs' *Females and their Diseases* (1849); Tilt on *Ovarian Inflammation* (1850); Nélaton's description of pelvic hematocele (1851–52[9]); Emil Noeggerath's operation of epicystotomy (1853[10]), and Daniel Ayre's plastic operation for congenital exstrophy of the female bladder (1859[11]). In 1836, Michaëlis, of Kiel, reported the celebrated case of Frau Adametz, upon whom four Cesarean sections had been successively performed, his own operation being as successful as the rest.[12] In America, John Lambert Richmond performed the first Cesarean section at Newton, Ohio, on April 22, 1827.[13] François Prevost (1764–1842), of Donaldsonville, Louisiana, performed the operation four times prior to 1832,[14] with three successful cases; and William Gibson, of Baltimore, performed the Cesarean operation twice with success upon the same patient (1835–38[15]), who lived for fifty years after her first experience. Myomectomy for fibroid tumors of the uterus was performed twice with success by Washington L. Atlee in 1844,[16] and by

---

[1] Smith: Am. Med. Recorder, Phila., 1822, v, 124–126.

[2] Koeberlé: Mém. Acad. de méd., Paris, 1862–63, xxvi, 371–472, 6 pl.

[3] Osiander: Göttingen gelehrte Anz., 1808, 130; 1816, 16.

[4] Langenbeck: N. Biblioth. f. d. Chir., Hannover, 1817, i, st. 3, 557.

[5] Ritgen: Heidelberg. klin. Ann., 1825, i, 263–277.

[6] Roux: Gaz. méd. de Paris, 1834, 2. s., ii, 17–22.

[7] Récamier: Bull. Acad. de méd., Paris, 1842–43, viii, 661–668.

[8] Simpson: London and Edinb. Monthly Jour. Med. Sc., 1843, iii, 547, 701 1009; 1844, iv, 208.

[9] Nélaton: Gaz. d. hôp., Paris, 1851, 3. s., iii, 573, 581; 1852, iv, 54, 66.

[10] Noeggerath: New York Med. Jour., 1853, 3. s., iv, 9–24.

[11] Ayres: Am. Med. Gaz., N. Y., 1859, x, 81–89, 2 pl.

[12] Michaëlis: Mitth. a. d. Geb. d. Med. (etc.), Altoona, 1836, iv, 7.–8. Hft., p. 60.

[13] Richmond: West. Jour. Med. & Phys. Sc., Cincin., 1830, iii, 485–489.

[14] Prevost: Am. Jour. Med. Sc., Phila., 1835, vi, 347. (See Harris: New Orleans Med. & Surg. Jour., 1878–79, n. s., vi, 935–937.)

[15] Gibson: Am. Jour. Med. Sc., Phila., 1835, xvi, 351; xvii, 264; 1838, xxii, 13; 1885, n. s., xc, 422.

[16] Atlee: The Surgical Treatment of Certain Fibrous Tumors of the Uterus, New York, 1853.

Walter Burnham, of Lowell, Massachusetts, in 1853.[1] In the same year, Gilman Kimball (1804–92), of Lowell, Massachusetts, first performed this operation with deliberate intention (1853[2]). Eugène Koeberlé, the pioneer of hysterectomy and *morcellement* of tumors, excised the uterus for uterine fibroma on March 14 and April 20, 1863, excised the uterus and adnexa for tumor in 1869, and performed his first myomectomy in 1878. He had many disputes with Jules Péan as to priority in the invention and use of the hemostatic forceps. Before the time of Sims and Koeberlé operations upon the uterus had been attempted here and there, but the various procedures had fallen into disrepute through failure (*exitus lethalis*). A system of uterine gymnastics for prolapse and other female complaints was introduced by Thure Brandt (1809–95), a pupil of Ling, about 1864–70.

Prior to the year 1852, the stumbling-block of gynecology was the relief of **vesicovaginal fistula.** Many surgeons, from the time of Paré onward, had attempted to operate for this condition, with no better result than to entail an additional amount of suffering and inconvenience upon their unfortunate patients.

Roonhuyze (1672) and Fatio (1752) left admirable accounts of their operative methods, but no reports of successful cases. Dieffenbach left a classical account of the wretched plight of the women upon whom all his wonderful resources were tried in vain (1845). Jobert de Lamballe had written a whole treatise upon female fistulæ (1852[3]), but his autoplastic operation *par glissement* had only resulted in repeated failures and the death of many of his patients. Six successful operations for the condition had been reported in America by John Peter Mettauer (1787–1875), of Virginia (1838–47[4]), others by George Hayward (1791–1863), of Boston, in 1839[5]; by Joseph Pancoast, of Philadelphia (1847[6]); and, in France, by Maisonneuve (1848[7]).

The whole matter was changed, as Kelly says, "almost with a magic wand" by James Marion **Sims** (1813–83), of South Carolina. A graduate of Jefferson Medical College, Philadelphia (1835), Sims settled in Alabama, where he soon became known as a capable and original surgeon, operating successfully for abscess of the liver in 1835, and removing both the upper and the lower jaw in 1837. In 1845, he was called to see a country woman who had sustained a displacement of the uterus from a fall from a horse. In making a digital examination to correct the displacement, he hit upon the peculiar lateral posture (Sims' position), and was led to the invention of the special curved speculum, which were to be the particular factors of his success in operating for vesicovaginal fistula. To the Sims position and the Sims speculum, which enabled the operator to see the condition "as no man had ever seen it before," he added a special suture of silver wire, to avoid sepsis, and a catheter for emptying the bladder while the fistula was healing. With these four coefficients, Sims perfected his operation for repairing this almost irremediable condition, and

---

[1] Burnham: Nelson's Am. Lancet, Plattsburgh, N. Y., 1853, vii, 147.

[2] Kimball: Boston Med. and Surg. Jour., 1855, lii, 249–255.

[3] A.-J. Jobert de Lamballe: Traité des fistules vésico-utérines, Paris, 1852.

[4] Mettauer: Boston Med. and Surg. Jour., 1840, xxii, 154. Also, Am. Jour. Med. Sc., Phila., 1847, n. s., xiv, 117–121.

[5] Hayward: Am. Jour. Med. Sc., Phila., 1839, xxiv, 283–288.

[6] Pancoast: Med. Examiner, Phila., 1847, n. s., iii, 272; 1851, vii, 650.

[7] Maisonneuve: Clinique chirurgicale, Paris, 1848, vii, 660 et seq.

published his paper in 1852.[1] It created a profound impression, and, in 1854,[2] was followed by a monograph of Gustav Simon, suggesting a method of uniting the edges of the fistula by means of double sutures. Sims removed to New York in 1853, and established the State Hospital for Women (1855), which soon became the center of the best gynecological work of the time. Visiting Europe in 1861, Sims performed his fistula operation with great *éclat* before Nélaton, Velpeau, Larrey, and other surgical leaders, and was soon in request all over Europe as an operator in diseases of women. His *Clinical Notes on Uterine Surgery* (1866) was trans-

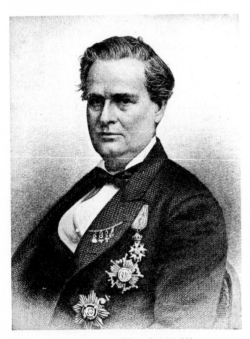

James Marion Sims (1813–83).

lated into German, and Robert Olshausen and August Martin have borne testimony to the high esteem in which Sims was held in that country.[3] Among his other important contributions were his methods of amputating the cervix uteri (1861[4]), his description of the condition "vaginismus" (1861[5]), his operation of cholecystotomy (1878[6]), and his great paper on "The careful aseptic invasion of the peritoneal cavity for the arrest of hemorrhage, the suture of intestinal wounds, and the cleansing of the peritoneal cavity, and for all intraperitoneal conditions" (1881[7]). Sims, a kindhearted but impulsive man, was one of the most original and gifted of American surgeons. A statue, erected to his memory in 1894 by European and American admirers, is in Bryant Park, New York City.

In the Woman's Hospital in New York, Sims was assisted by Thomas Addis **Emmet** (1828–1919), a native of Virginia, who, under his training, became a great master of the plastic surgery of the perineum,

[1] Sims: Am. Jour. Med. Sc., Phila., 1852, n. s., xxiii, 59–82.

[2] Simon: Ueber die Heilung der Blasen-Scheidenfisteln, Giessen, 1854.

[3] Olshausen: Ueber Marion Sims und seine Verdienste um die Chirurgie, Berlin, 1897. Martin: Ztschr. f. Geburtsh. u. Gynäk., Stuttgart, 1913, lxxiii, 946–948.

[4] Sims: Tr. Med. Soc. New York, Albany, 1861, 367–371.

[5] Sims: Tr. Obst. Soc. Lond., 1861, iii, 356–367.

[6] Sims: Richmond and Louisville Med. Jour., 1878, xxvi, 1–21.

[7] Sims: Brit. Med. Jour., Lond., 1881, ii, 925, 971; 1882, i, 184, 222, 260, 302.

the vagina, the cervix uteri, and the bladder. As Kelly says, he "caught Sims' idea at once, acquired his methods, and improved upon them, and did more than any other surgeon to teach the members of the profession in this country how to do these operations."

Emmet's principal contributions were his papers on the treatment of dysmenorrhea and sterility resulting from anteflexion of the uterus (1865[1]); on the surgical treatment of lacerations of the cervix uteri (1869–74[2]), his monograph on vesicovaginal and rectovaginal fistula (1868[3]), and his papers on vaginal cystotomy (1872[4]) and the plastic surgery of the perineum (1882[5]). He also wrote a treatise on gynecology (1879) and an entertaining autobiography (1905).

Sims' work was further extended by Nathan **Bozeman** (1825–1905), of Alabama, who did many successful operations on vesical and fecal fistulæ in women, paying special attention to the complication of pyelitis, which he treated by catheterizing the ureter through a vesicovaginal opening (1887–88[6]).

In the group of Southern gynecologists may be included Prevost, of Donaldsonville, Louisiana, and William Gibson, of Maryland, both pioneers in Cesarean section, and Josiah Clark **Nott** (1804–73), of South Carolina, who, in 1844, described the condition which Sir James Y. Simpson, in 1861, called "coccygodynia."[7] Nott was also one of the first to suggest the "mosquito theory" in reference to the transmission of yellow fever (1848[8]), and wrote a number of works on ethnology.

Theodore Gaillard **Thomas** (1831–1903), of Edisto Island, South Carolina, practised in New York. In 1868, he published a treatise on diseases of women, which was esteemed the best that had yet appeared,[9] and was translated into French, German, Italian, Spanish, and Chinese. In 1870, Thomas revived Ritgen's operation of gastro-elytrotomy as a substitute for Cesarean section,[10] and was the first to perform vaginal ovariotomy (1870[11]).

Robert **Battey** (1828–95), of Augusta, Georgia, a graduate of the Jefferson Medical College of Philadelphia, was the first to suggest the operation of oöphorectomy, or excision of the uterine appendages, for such non-ovarian conditions as painful menstruation and neuroses. This operation was first performed by him on August 17, 1872.[12] "Bat-

---

[1] Emmet: New York Med. Jour., 1865, i, 205–219.

[2] Am. J. Obst., New York, 1868–69, i, 339–362; 1874–75, vii, 442–456.

[3] New York, 1868.

[4] Am. Pract., Louisville, 1872, v, 65–92.

[5] Tr. Am. Gynec. Soc., 1882, N. Y., 1884, viii, 198–216.

[6] Bozeman: Tr. Internat. Med. Cong., Wash., 1887, ii, 514–558; and Am. Jour. Med. Sc., Phila., 1888, n. s., xcv, 225, 368.

[7] Nott: New Orleans Med. Jour., 1844–45, i, 58–60. Simpson: Med. Times and Gaz., Lond., 1861, i, 317.

[8] Nott: New Orleans Med. Jour., 1848, iv, 563, 601.

[9] Thomas: A Practical Treatise on the Diseases of Women, Phila., 1868.

[10] Thomas: Am. Jour. Obst., N. Y., 1870, iii, 125–139.

[11] Thomas: Am. Jour. Med. Sc., Phila., 1870, n. s., lix, 387–390.

[12] Battey: Atlanta Med. and Surg. Jour., 1872–73, x, 321–339.

tey's operation" was afterward applied in the treatment of uterine myomata by E. H. Trenholme (1876[1]), to other pelvic conditions by Alfred Hegar (1830-1914) in Germany, and Lawson Tait in England, and has more recently acquired a special physiological significance in connection with modern work on the chemical correlation of the internal secretions.

The **advancement of scientific medicine in the second half of the 19th century** was characterized by the introduction of a biological or evolutionary view of morphology and physiology, out of which came the sciences of cellular pathology, bacteriology, and parasitology, new modes of seeing disease and its causes, which had in them the germ of

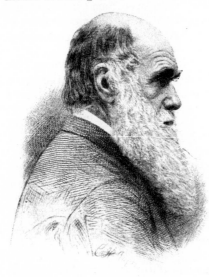

novel methods of treatment by means of sera and vaccines. The discoveries of Pasteur led immediately to Listerian or antiseptic surgery, with its remarkable applications in such regions as the abdomen, the brain, the joints, the thorax, and special sense organs, and its extension to operative gynecology. Great improvements in medical education, public hygiene, and military medicine followed upon these developments in due course, and were further helped out by a marked increase in the number and quality of scientific periodicals and through the growth of rapid means of national and international communication by railway, steamship, telegraph, and cable. At this stage, specialties like ophthalmology, otology, laryngology, orthopedics, dentistry, and veterinary medicine became something more than mere names.

Charles Robert Darwin (1809–82).

The immense growth of general **biology** in our time was principally due to the evolutionary theories of Charles Robert **Darwin** (1809–82), of Shrewsbury, England, a Cambridge graduate, whose bent toward natural history was set by his boyhood interest in botany and his five years' cruise as naturalist on H.M.S. Beagle (1831–36), an experience which rendered him an expert geologist and zoölogist. Although an invalid for the rest of his life, Darwin labored for twenty years before publishing his great work *On the Origin of Species by Means of Natural Selection* (1859), perhaps the most wonderful piece of synthesis in the history of science. This theory was arrived at independently by Alfred

---

[1] Disputed by Lawson Tait, who claimed priority in an alleged case of 1872. See Trenholme: Med. News, Phila., 1886, xlix, 530.

Russel Wallace (1822–1913) in 1858, although Darwin's priority dates back to 1838. Both Darwin and Wallace owed much to the Essay on the Principle of Population of the English clergyman, Thomas Robert Malthus (1798). Darwin's extraordinary marshaling of facts, in evidence of the survival of the fittest by natural selection in the struggle for existence, had the same far-reaching influence upon biological speculation that the discoveries of Copernicus had upon astronomy. It dispensed with the ancient Linnæan concept of the fixity of species, that animals and plants were originally created as we find them today, and the ghostly metaphysical abstractions which were invoked to "explain" why this should be. It created the sciences of comparative physiology and pathology, by pointing to the close structural and functional relationship between human tissues and those of animals and plants. And though the idea of evolution was known to the Greeks and was more or less definitely outlined by Bacon, Buffon, Erasmus Darwin, Goethe, Lamarck, Lyell, and Herbert Spencer, it became the salient fact of modern science through Darwin's work. The application of the idea of continuous development in *The Descent of Man* (1871) made an end of the anthropocentric theory that the universe was created for man. It began to be perceived that there is a rude and noble dignity in the story of man's painful evolution from the lower forms of life, even as Darwin's picture of the struggle for existence illuminated the true causes of human misery as never before. That there are flaws and gaps in Darwin's hypotheses; that he did not take sufficient account of those spontaneous accidental variations or mutations which, as Mendel and De Vries have indicated, may also originate species; that his theory of sexual selection is not borne out by the facts; that many specific characters in animals and plants are not true survival values, is all clear enough now. But it should not be forgotten that Darwin himself regarded natural selection "as the main, but not the exclusive, means of modification," and that a true specific character is a survival value only in regard to its possessor's essential environment, and not in respect of some accidental enemy. Darwin's essay on The Variation of Animals and Plants under Domestication (1868) is now mainly memorable for his attempt to explain the mechanism of inheritance by "pangenesis," or the transportation of gemmules from all parts of the organism to the ovum, to insure their reproduction, which has found an avatar in Starling's theory of the hormones. The great monograph on *The Expression of the Emotions in Man and Animals* (1873) ranks with the contemporaneous work of Duchenne of Boulogne (1862), and the theory of evolution itself is the starting-point of comparative psychology. The investigations in botany and geology, the monographs on *Climbing Plants* (1875), *Cross and Self-Fertilization* (1876), *Power of Movement in Plants* (1880), *Formation of Vegetable Mould* (1881), *Coral Reefs* (1842), and *Volcanic Islands* (1844), can only be mentioned. In Huxley's view, Darwin saw selection and the struggle for existence as morphological relations, but failed, through

33

his ignorance of the meaning of cell division and of the mechanism of reproduction, to grasp the physiological significance of species. Bearing in mind the grave, self-possessed, entirely human figure of Darwin himself, the magnificent sincerity of his work, and its profound effect upon modern biology, his fame can endure unlimited caviling.

Darwin's work was popularized and extended in the "Principles of Biology" (1866–67), "Principles of Psychology" (1871), and "Descriptive Sociology" (1873–81) of Herbert Spencer (1820–1903) in the "Geographical Distribution of Animals" (1876) of Alfred Russel Wallace (1823–1913); and by Huxley and Haeckel.

Thomas Henry **Huxley** (1825–95), of Ealing, England, was a medical graduate of the London University (1845) who became a surgeon in the Royal Navy. As with Darwin, his interest in biology was awakened

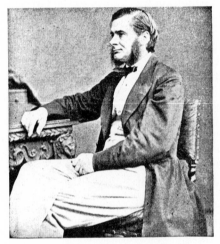

Thomas Henry Huxley (1825–95).

by a sea voyage, a five years' cruise on H. M. S. Rattlesnake (1846–50). Prior to this experience he had already discovered the layer of cells in the root-sheath of hair which goes by his name (1845[1]), and upon his return he made many important contributions to marine zoölogy, in recognition of which he became Fellow and gold-medallist of the Royal Society (1851–52). Resigning from the navy, he became lecturer on natural history at the Royal School of Mines, and introduced the idea of teaching morphology by means of a series of typical animals, as norms of their species, which afterward became the feature of Huxley and Martin's *Elementary Biology* (1875). He applied evolution to paleontology, in his extended studies of fossil fishes, crocodiles, and other vertebrata, and in his work on the ancestry of the horse. His Croonian Lectures on the theory of the vertebrate skull (1858) overthrew Owen's concept of an archetype in favor of a morphologic type, an assemblage of features common to all its class, as in a composite photograph. With this may be bracketed Huxley's important lectures on the craniology of birds (1867). In 1861,[2] he demonstrated the inaccuracy of another contention of Owen's, relating to the supposed backward projection of the cavities of the brain into the posterior horn and the hippocampus minor, as a specific character in man. The essays on the *Comparative*

---

[1] Huxley: Lond. Med. Gaz., 1845, n. s., i, 1340.

[2] Huxley: Nat. Hist. Rev., Lond., 1861, 67–84. Proc. Zoöl. Soc., Lond., 1861, 247–260.

Anatomy of Man and the Higher Apes (1859–62), and *On Evidence as to Man's Place in Nature* (1863), reveal the follower of Darwin, of whose ideas Huxley was indeed the ablest modern interpreter. From first to last, Huxley maintained that the logical foundations of natural selection are insecure, "since selection cannot explain the origin of species unless experimental selective breeding can be made to produce species" (varieties infertile with one another). He boldly told Darwin of his error in believing that *Natura non fecit saltum.* Huxley's own observations on the spontaneous appearance of short-legged Ancon sheep and six-fingered children anticipated Mendelism or what he himself called "the doctrine of transmutation." A master of vigorous English, Huxley wrote several volumes of essays, which are among the most delightful of modern contributions to popular science; and his text-books on physiology (1866), which passed through 30 editions, on vertebrate and invertebrate anatomy (1871–77), and on physiography (1877) are little masterpieces of their kind. Huxley defined himself as one who cared more for freedom of thought than for the mere advancement of science, and this is the interest of his personality. Vigorous and resolute in form and features, a stalwart, masculine-minded man who ruined his health

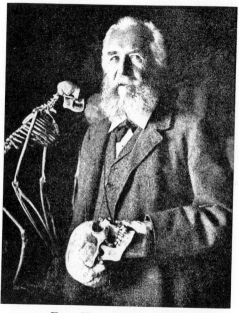

Ernst Haeckel (1834–1919).

by sedentary labors, he was, in the circumstances of his marriage, as in his championship of Darwinism or his Napoleonic warfare on theologians, a romantic, like Vesalius. No man ever fought more bravely and openly for truth and honesty, for the right of people to think and express their own thoughts. No man ever admitted his own errors more readily or was more generous to a fallen adversary. His conviction that "there is no alleviation for the sufferings of mankind except veracity of thought and action and the resolute facing of the world as it is, when the garment of make-believe by which pious hands have hidden its uglier features is stripped off," is the final justification of Darwininism and sounds the keynote of the social medicine of the future.

Ernst **Haeckel** (1834–1919), of Jena, a great morphologist, carried

Darwinism into Germany, where the opposition of Virchow created the necessity for such a champion.[1] Haeckel's greatest work is his *Generelle Morphologie* (1866), in which organisms and the forms of organic structures are considered and classified in relation to serial homology, heredity, and evolution. In 1868 appeared his "Natural History of Creation"; in 1874, the *Anthropogenie*, a great treatise on human embryology; and, in 1884, his monograph on the Gastræa Theory, which regards the two-layered gastrula as the ancestral form of all multicellular animals. These were all contributions of the most effective kind, the result of years of patient investigation. Haeckel's popular writings include his delightful letters of East Indian travel and such uncritical works as The Riddle of the Universe. In the latter, he combines an iron-clad materialism, like that of the French Encyclopedists, with the notion that aggregations of molecules have souls (*Plastidul-Seelen*), which was ridiculed by Virchow. In his lifetime Haeckel, the sage of Jena, was highly revered among scientific men, and looked up to as one of the greatest of fighters for freedom in thought and teaching. His Phyletic Museum at Jena is said to be the most wonderful collection of serial illustrations of evolution and development in the world.

The problem of **heredity** was attacked in four different ways by Mendel, Hering, Galton, and Weismann.

Gregor **Mendel** (1822–84), abbot of the Augustinian monastery at Brünn, Austria, discovered the mathematical law governing the dominant and recessive characters in hybrids (1866–67), the application of which belongs to the 20th century.

Ewald **Hering** (1834–1918), a Saxon professor, advanced the psychophysical theory (1870) that facultative memory, the automatic power of protoplasm to do what it has done before, is the distinctive property of all living matter. The transmission and reproduction of parental characters are supposed to be the result of the organism's unconscious memory of the past, the mechanism being, in Hering's view, the persistence of wave motions of molecules. This idea was also advanced by Haeckel (Perigenesis of Plastidules) and by Samuel Butler (1835–1902), of Langar, England, who translated Hering's essay and applied the doctrine in his polemics against Darwinism.

Sir Francis **Galton** (1822–1911), a cousin of Darwin's, began to investigate heredity experimentally in 1871. His observations upon the inheritance of transfused blood in rabbits, of tricolored spots on the coat of Bassett hounds, of stature and other characters in human families, led him to reject the Lamarckian theory of the inheritance of acquired characters as well as the Darwinian Pangenesis. In his book on *Natural Inheritance* (1889), he proceeds, by statistical induction, to the Law of Filial Regression, which asserts that the offspring of parents unusual in height, talent, etc., regress to the average of the stock; also to the Law of Ancestral Inheritance, in virtue of which each parent contributes one-fourth $[(\frac{1}{2})^2]$ of the total inheritance, each of the four grandparents one-sixteenth $[(\frac{1}{2})^4]$, each of the eight great-grandparents $\frac{1}{128} = (\frac{1}{2})^5$, while, in general, the ancestors in n degrees removed contribute $(\frac{1}{2})^{2n}$ each. The latter theorem has been confirmed, with slight mathematical changes, by the biometric methods of Karl Pearson. Galton's work on finger-prints (1892) is the first contribution of importance after Purkinje. He introduced the doctrine of eugenics (a term of his coinage), founded the Eugenics Laboratory in London (1904), and, with Pearson and Weldon, founded *Biometrika* (1901), a journal for the study of biologic problems by advanced statistical methods.

---

[1] It is said that Fritz Müller was the first German to support the Darwinian theory ("Für Darwin," 1864), Haeckel the second (1866), and Weismann the third (1868).

An important extension of evolutionary theory is the idea of the unbroken continuity or immortality of the germ-plasm, which was elaborated by August **Weismann** (1834–1914), of Frankfort on the Main, between 1893 and 1904. The general idea of continuity of growth and development by direct cell-lineage was already inherent in Virchow's cell-theory. Owen, in his paper on Parthenogenesis (1849), distinguished between cells forming the body and germ-cells. Haeckel emphasized the idea of continuous descent all through his *Generelle Morphologie* (1866). Jaeger coined the phrase "continuity of the germ protoplasma" in 1878, and the capacity of the latter for transmitting hereditary qualities was clearly stated by Nussbaum in 1875. Weismann insisted on the continuity of descent in unicellular organisms, and, in tracing the gradual evolution of multicellular organisms from these, pointed out that the complex organism, made up of body-cells, is only the vehicle of the germ-cells. The germ-plasm, a complex structure contained in the nuclei in these reproductive cells, is the parent of the germ-cells of the succeeding generation, securing a relative immortality for the species, although individuals die out. The union of the two germs or "amphimixis" is the principal agent in evolution. Weismann maintained that variation is produced by sexual selection, and latterly by a nutritional selection among the components of the germ-plasm (germinal selection). He held that the germ-plasm in the sex-cells is to be found in the chromosomes (idants) and predicted the "reduction division" (by one-half) in the maturation of the sex-cells and the "equation divisions" or equal division of the chromosomes. His assumption that the determinants in the chromosomes are arranged in a linear series has been confirmed by T. H. Morgan. Another feature of Weismann's theory is his experimental proof that acquired characters are not directly transmitted. This apparent overthrow of the Lamarckian theory has caused much controversy, but the balance of experimental evidence seems in favor of Weismann. If true, the Weismann theory is of far-reaching social significance, since it seems probable that moral qualities cannot be transmitted to children, but have to be acquired, in each case, by intensive early training.

Another outgrowth of biologic and evolutionary thinking was the 19th century science of **anthropology**. With nothing to start with but the meagre data in Hippocrates, Herodotus, Tacitus (*Germania*) and the early travellers, it was built up by the labors of such men as Darwin, Huxley, Lyell, Spencer, Prichard, and Tylor in England; in France, by Broca, who invented some 27 craniometric and cranioscopic instruments; in Germany, by Virchow, who was an expert in craniology, and took the whole field of anthropology for his province; in Italy, by Cesare Lombroso (1836–1909), who developed the study of the criminal and the morbid side of the man of genius. Following the publication of Darwin's *opus magnum* (1859), anthropological societies were founded in Paris (by Broca) in 1859, in London in 1863, in Madrid in 1865, in Berlin in 1868, in Vienna in 1870, in Italy in 1871, and in Washington, D. C., in 1879. Physical anthropology was developed through the craniological investigations of Broca and Virchow, the treatises of Paul Topinard, Quatrefages' studies of fossil and savage men (1861) and pygmies (1887), Virchow's statistics on the physical anthropology of the Germans (1876), Lombroso's books on genius and insanity (1864), criminal man (*L'uomo delinquente*, 1876) and criminal anthropology (1899), Adolf Bastian's theory of "elemental ideas" (1881), the Ratzel-Smith theory of the geographic diffusion of ethnic culture by convection (1882–1915), Alphonse Bertillon's method of identifying criminals by selected measurements (*Bertillonage*, 1886), and Francis Galton's simpler mode of identification by finger-prints (1892), which superseded Bertillonage in England in 1900. Ethnological societies had been founded in Paris (1839), New York (1842), and London (1844. The principal monuments of the science are the monographs of Prichard (1813), Pickering (1848), Knox (1850), Latham (1850–59), Nott and Gliddon (1857), Waitz (1859–72), Herbert Spencer (1873–81), Friedrich Müller (1873), Peschel (1873), Ratzel (1885–88), Haddon (1894–1909), Achelis (1896), and Ripley (1900). In the field of ethnic craniology, we may mention Morton's albums of American and Egyptian skulls (1839–44), the *Crania ethnica* of de Quatrefages and Hamy (1872–82), Rütimeyer and His on Swiss skulls (1864), the albums of Finnish and Swedish skulls (1878–1900) by Gustaf Magnus Retzius (1842–1919) and Virchow's *Crania ethnica Americana* (1892). The subject was carried into a singular excess of detail in Sergi's polysyllabic subdivisions of racial types of skulls, and in Aurel von Török's *Systematic Craniometry* (1890), with its 5000 proposed measurements of a single skull. Medical anthropology, yet in its infancy, has for its basic data such finds as Dupuytren's radius curvus, Hutchinson's teeth, Manouvrier's sincipital-T, the sabre-shaped tibia, the graphic representation of disease and deformity in art, and such interesting recent developments as the studies of Sir Marc Armand Ruffer (1859–1917) on palæo-pathology (1909–14), the investigation of the clinical significance of the scaphoid scapula by William W. Graves (1910–20), the study of disease in autochthons, of ethnic incidence and racial equation in disease; and the application of the Binet-Simon tests to determine the mental age of children, adults and soldiers (R. M. Yerkes, 1917–18). Military anthropometry on a large scale is exemplified in such measurements as those conducted by J. H. Baxter and Robert Fletcher on U. S. troops in the Civil War (1875), by Rodolfo Livi (1856–1920) on the Italian army (1896) and by Albert G. Love and Charles B. Davenport on our drafted troops in the European War (1919–20). Ethnic psychology was developed by Andrew Lang (1884–1901), Adolf Bastian (1886–90), Alfred Fouillée (1903), Wilhelm Wundt (1904), and in such monographs as those of the Torres Straits Expedition (1898). Other phases of comparative ethnology are the studies of Pitt-Rivers on technology (1860–75), Sir Henry Maine on *Ancient Law* (1861), J. J. Bachofen on the matriarchate (*Das Mutterrecht*, 1861), F. MacLennan on *Primitive Marriage* (1865), Sir Edward Burnett Tylor (1832–1917) on *Primitive Culture* (1871), L. H. Morgan on *Systems of Con-sanguinity* (1871), Herbert Spencer on *Descriptive Sociology* (1873–81), William Black (1883) and Max Bartels (1893) on medical folk-lore, J. G. Frazer on *Totemism* (1887), *Totemism and Exogamy* (1910), and *The Golden Bough* (1890–1913), Westermarck on *Human Marriage* (1891), Alfred C. Haddon on *Evolution in Art* (1895), Edwin Sydney Hartland on *Primitive Paternity* (1910), and W. I. Thomas on *Social Origins* (1909). The excavations of bones and flint implements by M. Boucher de Perthes at Abbeville (1805–47), the later unearthing of similar finds in the Devonshire caves, the exploration of lake-dwelling remains in the Irish crannogs by Sir William Wilde (1839), and of the Swiss *Pfahlbauten* by Ferdinand Keller (1853–54), led to extensive and intensive study of these prehistoric objects all over the world. The results were systematized in Gabriel de Mortillet's classic, *Lé Préhistorique* (1883), and carried forward by Sir John Evans in England, Virchow in Germany, Piette in France, and Holmes in America. The discovery of the prehistoric skull and skeletal remains at Neanderthal in 1856, which Virchow pronounced diseased, Broca normal, and Huxley human but ape-like, led Huxley to his famous assignment of man's place in nature as "more nearly allied to the higher apes than the latter are to the lower" (1860). The subsequent cranial finds only added fuel to the ensuing controversy which is bound up with the question of the monophyletic or diverse origin of man. In general, man is now classed, where Linnæus left him in 1735, with the Hominidæ. The unity of the human species has been maintained by Linnæus, Buffon, Prichard, Sir William Law-rence, Broca, the English anthropologists and the followers of Haeckel, while the multiple or polyphyletic theory has been favored largely by those Germans who have followed the somewhat official leadership of Virchow.

After the labors of such masters as Bichat, Bell, Henle, and Hyrtl, there was little to be added to the subject of descriptive human an-atomy and most investigation in this field became merged into morphol-ogy and histology.

Splendid atlases of gross or macroscopic anatomy were published, such as those of the Bells, Cloquet (1821–31), Werner Spalteholz (1904), Carl Toldt [1864–1920] (1896–1900), Sir William MacEwen's Atlas of Head Sections (1893), and the albums of John C. Dalton (1885), the younger Retzius (1896) and Carl Wernicke (1897–1904) on the brain. Frozen sections, introduced by Pieter de Riemer (1760–1831) in 1818, were utilized in Pirogoff's epoch-making *Anatome topographica* (1852–59) and in the atlases of the pregnant uterus (1872) and of normal topographic anatomy (1872) by Christian Wilhelm Braune (1831–92). Among the many excellent treatises on topographical and surgical anatomy were those of Velpeau (1825–26), Hyrtl (1847), Malgaigne, (1859), J. H Power (Anatomy of the Arteries, 1863), C. Heitzmann (1870), N. Rüdinger (1873–79), Luther Holden 1876), W. Henke (1884), F. S. Merkel (1885–89), A. W. Hughes (1890), G. McClellan (1891–92), Sir F. Treves (1892), and K. von Bardeleben (1894). Artistic anatomy was ably treated by John Flaxman (1833), Robert Knox (1852), Mathias Duval (1881), the physiologists, Paul Richer (1890) and Ernst Wilhelm Brücke (1891); and by direct photography from the nude, in the different works of Carl Heinrich Stratz (1858–1924), the mo-tion pictures of Eadweard Muybridge (1901), and the splendid treatise of 1886 by Julius Kollmann (1834–1918). Treatises on gross anatomy were published by Jones

Quain (1828), Erasmus Wilson (1840), M.-P.-C. Sappey (1850–64), H. Gray (1859), C. Gegenbaur (1883), Léon Testut [1849–1925] (1889–91), K. von Bardeleben (1896), J. Sobotta (1904), A. Van Gehuchten (1906–09), and the coöperative treatises edited by D. J. Cunningham (1902) and the Americans, F. H. Gerrish (1899) and G. A. Piersol (1911). Special treatises of great use and value were the manuals of dissecting of Luther Holden (1850) and Hyrtl (1860), Holden's *Osteology* (1855), D. N. Eisendrath's *Clinical Anatomy* (1903), L. F. Barker's *Laboratory Manual* (1904), the *Applied Anatomy* (1910) of Gwyllym George Davis (1858–1918) and the *Cross-section Anatomy* of A. C. Eycleshymer and D. M. Schoemaker (1911). The history of anatomy was taken up by Hyrtl, Knox, Robert von Töply (1898), the history of anatomic methods by William W. Keen (1852), the history of anatomic illustration by Ludwig Choulant (1852), translated by Mortimer Frank (1920), and the history of plastic anatomy by Mathias Duval and Edouard Cuyer (1898). There were isolated discoveries in plenty, such as the island of Reil (1809), Clarke's columns (1851), Broca's convolution (1861), Auerbach's plexus (1862), Bigelow's demonstration of the Y-ligament (1869), or Waldeyer's ring (1884). Perhaps the most important of these was the description of the parathyroid glands by the Swedish anatomist, Ivar Sandström, in 1879.

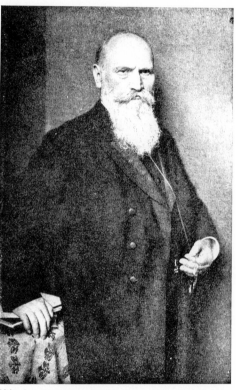

Wilhelm Waldeyer (1837–1921). (Berlin Photographic Company.)

The leading German anatomist of recent times was Wilhelm **Waldeyer** (1837–1921), of Hehlen, Brunswick, a pupil of Henle, professor at Berlin (1883), who made important researches on the development of cancer (1867–72), retroperitoneal hernia (1868), ovary and ovum (1870), the topographical relations of the pregnant uterus (1886), pelvic viscera (1892) and pelvis (1899), and the neuron theory (1891), to which he gave the name. He first described the open ring of lymphoid tissue[1] formed by the faucial, lingual, and pharyngeal tonsils (1884), which is now regarded as a prominent portal of infection. Waldeyer also referred the lymphatic constitution to persistence of the thymus gland.

Karl **von Bardeleben** (1849–1918), of Giessen, a graduate of Berlin (1871), assistant to His at Leipzig (1871–2), prosector to Gustav Schwalbe at Jena (1873–88), and professor extraordinarius at Jena

---

[1] Waldeyer: Deutsche med. Wochenschr., Leipz. and Berl., 1884, x, 313.

(1889–1918), was the author of a topographical atlas (1894), a manual of dissecting (1896), a *Lehrbuch* (1906), edited a great *Handbuch der Anatomie* (1896–1915), and made many special investigations in the skeletal, muscular, and vascular systems. He was for thirty years the general secretary and leading spirit of the *Anatomische Gesellschaft* (founded 1886).

English anatomy sustained a grave loss in the early death of Henry **Gray** (1825–61), who gained the triennial prizes of the Royal College of Surgeons and the Royal Society by his memoirs on the optic nerves

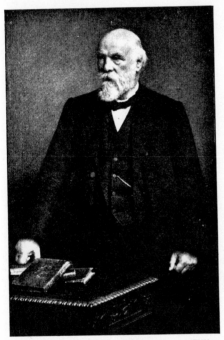

Sir William Turner (1832–1916). (Elliot and Fry, London.)

(1849) and the spleen (1853), and whose anatomic treatise (1858), recently adapted to the B. N. A. terminology by E. A. Spitzka (1913), has been the standard text-book of English-speaking students for over half a century. The superb drawings by H. Vandyke Carter have, most of them, been retained in the latest edition.

John **Goodsir** (1814–67), of Anstruther, Fifeshire, succeeded to the chair of Monro *tertius* at Edinburgh (1845), and did much to lift anatomic teaching from the disrepute into which it had fallen through the latter's incompetence. Goodsir's *Anatomical and Pathological Observations* (1845) contain the germinal idea of the cell-theory of Virchow, who dedicated his Cellular Pathology to him. Goodsir also discovered the Sarcina ventriculi (1865).

Sir William **Turner** (1832–1916), of Lancaster, England, became Goodsir's assistant (1854) and successor (1867) at Edinburgh, where he made its anatomic school the foremost and the largest in Great Britain. Shrewd, broad-minded, and exceeding wise, he became president of the Council (1898–1905) and ultimately principal of the University (1903). As teacher, investigator, and administrator, Turner was a tower of strength, sometimes grim and pawky in his humors, but big, jovial, kind-hearted *au fond*.

He made able contributions on placentation in the Cetacea (1870–89), comparative anatomy of the placenta (1875–6), Indian craniology (1899), Scottish anthropology (1915), craniocerebral topography, and wrote the history of anatomy in the Encyclopædia Britannica (1875), the best monograph on the subject in English.

Sir Arthur **Keith,** Hunterian professor at the Royal College of Surgeons, discovered (with Flack), the sino-auricular node in the heart (1907) and has written with ability on the anthropoid apes (1896), human embryology and morphology (1901), the antiquity of man (1914), and the endocrine aspects of race (1911–25).

Joseph **Leidy** (1823–91), of Philadelphia, who succeeded Horner as professor of anatomy at the University of Pennsylvania, was the leading American anatomist of his time, and a biologist of the type of Hunter and Müller, doing important work in botany, zoölogy, mineralogy, and paleontology, as well as in comparative and human anatomy. He was our greatest descriptive naturalist. His *Fresh Water Rhizopods of North America* (1879) is one of our biological classics. He made valuable researches on the comparative anatomy of the liver (1848), the bones, trichinosis in hogs, etc., and his *Elementary treatise on Human Anatomy* (1861, revised 1889) has a special interest in that it was illustrated by himself.

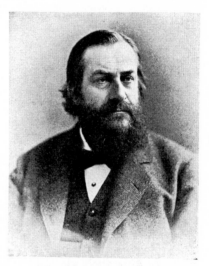

Joseph Leidy (1823–91).

He was the first to find Trichina spiralis in hogs (1846[1]), discovered the bacterial flora of the intestines (1849[2]), made the first experiment in transplanting malignant tumors (1851[3]), and, in 1886, found the hookworm in the cat, and suggested that it might also be found in man as a cause of pernicious anemia.[4] As army surgeon during the Civil War, he performed some 60 autopsies, and, in the hospital wards, he surmised that flies may be transmitters of wound infection.[5] He was the first to separate out the parasitic amebæ (1879). The discoveries in his *Researches in Helminthology and Parasitology,* edited by his nephew, Joseph Leidy, Jr., in 1904, would suffice to make a reputation in themselves. He was the founder of vertebrate paleontology in America, and his great memoirs of 1869[6] and 1873[7] upon extinct fossils have never been surpassed. Like Gebhard and Gross, Leidy was a fine type of the American physician of German origin, as modest and unassuming as he was learned and versatile.

Oliver Wendell **Holmes** (1809–94), of Boston, whose work on puerperal fever has been mentioned, was Parkman professor of anatomy at the Harvard Medical School (1847–82), and resembled Hyrtl in his

[1] Leidy: Proc. Acad. Nat. Sc., Phila., 1846, iii, 107.

[2] *Ibid.,* 1848–49, iv, 225–233.

[3] *Ibid.,* 1851, v, 212.

[4] Tr. Coll. Phys., Phila., 1886, 3. s., viii, 441–443.

[5] Proc. Acad. Nat. Sc., Phila., 1871, xxiii, 297.

[6] Leidy: Jour. Acad. Nat. Sc., Phila., 1869, 2. s., vii, 1–472.

[7] Rep. U. S. Geol. Survery, 1873, i.

skill in making a dry subject interesting through his liveliness and wit. He made no discoveries of importance, but he wrote many clever medical poems, and his "Medical Essays" (1883) was easily the most important American book dealing with medical history in its day.

Prominent among the **comparative anatomists** of the transition period were Gegenbaur and Wiedersheim. Carl **Gegenbaur** (1826–1903), a native of Würzburg and a fellow-student of Haeckel's, established the point that comparative morphology, and not embryology, is the true criterion for determining the relation of homologies or pedigrees of organs (phylogeny), thus bringing the matter of the genealogy of organs back to Owen's original concept. In recent times, a large number of facts in corroboration of Owen's theory were produced, but many others which showed that similar structures may arise in different ways. At present, embryology is studied as a phase of morphology. Gegenbaur also gave the *coup de grâce* to the vertebrate theory of the skull (Goethe-Owen), by showing that, in the embryo, there are a large number of head segments corresponding to the brachial clefts and the cranial nerves; that, in the lowest order of fishes, the head, instead of being composed of vertebræ, is unsegmented, while in the higher, many cranial bones arise from the skin. In 1861, Gegenbaur demonstrated that the ovum of every vertebrate is a single cell. His principal works are his Comparative Anatomy of Vertebrates (1864–72), his Elements of Comparative Anatomy (1870), and his Text-book of Human Anatomy (1883). He was editor of the *Morphologisches Jahrbuch* (1875–1902), and professor of anatomy at Heidelberg, where he had many American pupils.

Robert **Wiedersheim** (1848–   ), professor of anatomy at Freiburg, was the author of important works on the Comparative Anatomy of Vertebrates (1882–3) and The Structure of Man as an Evidence of his Past (1887).

After the time of Schleiden, Schwann, and Henle, the study of the finer or **microscopic anatomy** of the tissues became the word of ambition. Histological investigation was rapidly improved by the introduction of new staining methods, microtomy, and other technical procedures. Purkinje, as we have seen, had a microtome and used Canada balsam, glacial acetic acid, and potassium bichromate, but these things were not generally known, and the common procedure was to examine the tissues in the fresh state, sliced by a razor between layers of vegetable pith. Hardening of the tissues in alcohol came long after. In 1847, Joseph **von Gerlach**, Sr. (1820–96), of Mainz, began to inject capillaries with a transparent mixture of carmine, ammonia, and gelatine; by 1855, he was employing carmine as a nuclear stain for the tissues. Virchow did practically all his work with carmine. Gerlach was also a pioneer in the use of aniline and gold chloride, and, after his time, differential staining became rapidly specialized. The microtome was definitely introduced by Wilhelm His in 1866, but was not perfected until about 1875, after which it became an important labor-saving device.

The master worker in histology was Max **Schultze** (1825–74), of Freiburg, who was professor of anatomy at Halle (1854–9), and, succeeding Helmholtz at Bonn in 1859, became director of the Anatomical Institute there in 1872.

Schultze introduced the dilute chromic acid solution, the osmic acid stain, iodated serum as a preservative, and invented the heatable object-stand. An important contributor to marine zoölogy through his studies on the Turbellaria (1848–

51), the Polythalamia (1854–6), and the embryology of Petromyzon (1856), he made an epoch in histology by his great monographs on the nerve-endings of the sense organs, in particular, in the internal ear (1858[1]), the nose (1863[2]), and the retina (1866[3]). In 1865, he founded the *Archiv für mikroskopische Anatomie*, which he edited until his death. Schultze had a lasting influence upon the cell theory through his essay of 1861,[4] in which, contemporaneously with Brücke, he defined the true cell as a clump of nucleated protoplasm, thus emphasizing the point which Leydig had made in 1856, that the cell membrane, even in the ovum, is a secondary physico-chemical formation, probably due to surface-tension condensation of the cell contents. In his memoir on the protoplasm of rhizopods and plant cells (1863[5]), Schultze definitely introduced the term "protoplasm," and showed that it is practically identical in all living cells. In 1863, he gave the most accurate contemporary account of the furrowing and segmentation of the frog's egg.[6]

Schultze was a striking, keen-eyed investigator, an accomplished draftsman, an amateur of music, devoting his leisure to the violin.

The next most important step in the cell doctrine was taken by Walther **Flemming** (1843–1905), of Schwerin, professor at Prague (1873–6) and Kiel (1876–1905), whose important monograph, *Zellsubstanz, Kern- und Zelltheilung* (1882), gives the classic account of cell division and karyokinesis. Some phases of karyokinesis had been observed by Virchow and Schneider; and Heitzmann had noted (1873) that all protoplasm is a continuous network, the granular appearance of which is only optical. Flemming's memoir put the whole matter in a new light. He worked out the phenomena of nuclear division, as crystallized in his aphorism

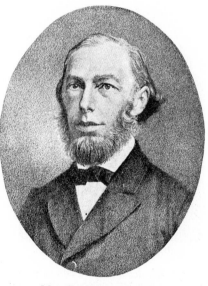

Max Schultze (1825–74).

"*Omnis nucleus e nucleo*"; and showed that protoplasm is a complex structure, made up of an active, contractile, net-like material, and an inert, semifluid, inter-reticular substance, which, from their behavior toward various stains, he called chromatin and achromatin, respectively. Histologists hold this to be the most important work on the cell after Schwann's and Virchow's.

---

[1] Schultze: Müller's Arch., Berl., 1858, 343–381.

[2] Abhandl. d. naturf. Gesellsch. zu Halle, 1863, vii, 1–100.

[3] Zur Anatomie und Physiologie der Retina, Bonn, 1866.

[4] Arch. f. Anat., Physiol. u. wissensch. Med., Leipz., 1861, 1–27.

[5] Das Protoplasma der Rhizopoden und der Pflanzenzellen, Leipzig, 1863.

[6] De ovorum ranarum segmentatione, Bonn, 1863.

Many important discoveries and innovations in **histology** were made in this period, such as the investigation of the mammalian cochlea (rods of Corti, 1851[1]) by Alfonso Corti (1822–88), Virchow's discovery of the neuroglia (1854[2]), Wilhelm His' investigations of the structure of the lymphatic glands (Leipzig, 1861) and lymphatic vessels (1863), Willy Kühne's memoir on the peripheral end-organs of the motor nerves (Leipzig, 1862), Deiters' memoir on the brain and spinal cord in man and mammals (Brunswick, 1865), the islands of Langerhans (1869[3]), F. S. Merkel's description of the tactile corpuscles in the papillæ of the skin (1875), the investigations of the histology of the nervous system (nodes of Ranvier, 1878) by Louis-Antoine Ranvier (1835–1922), Ehrlich's investigations of the leukocytes (1880[4]), and his intravital (methylene-blue) stain for nerve substance (1886[5]), and Camillo Golgi's epoch-making work on the nervous system (1873–86[6]). The third elements of the blood, the so-called blood plaques or platelets, were first noticed by Alexander Donné (1801–78[7]) in 1842, afterward by Max Schultze, and more fully described by Sir William Osler (1873[8]) and Giulio Bizzozero (1883[9]).

One of the most eminent of modern histologists was Magnus Gustav **Retzius** (1842–1919), a graduate of Lund (1871) and professor of histology at the Karolingska

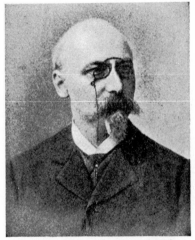

Walther Flemming (1843–1905).

Institut (1877–1900), who investigated the organ of hearing in bony fishes (1872) and vertebrates (1881–4), also the macroscopic anatomy of the human brain (1896), published remarkable albums of Finnish and Swedish skulls (1898–9), and a series of splendid histologic studies in folio (1890–1914).

Toward the close of the 19th century, the storm center of histologic controversy was the **neuron theory,** the doctrine of the physiologic autonomy of the nerve-cell and its branches. The cell theory seemed adequate to account for this as far as the nerve-cell itself was concerned, but the real stumbling-block was the origin and true significance of the far more abundant nerve-fibers, which had always been described as detached formations, separate from the cells. In 1850, Augustus Volney **Waller** (1816–70), of Faversham, England, showed that if the glossopharyngeal and hypoglossal nerves be severed, the outer segment, containing the axis-cylinders cut off from the cells, will undergo degeneration, while the central stump will remain relatively intact for a long period of time.[10] This "law of Wallerian degeneration" indicated that the nerve-fibers are simply prolongations of the cells from which, as Waller maintained, they receive their nourishment. The classical researches of Deiters (1865[11]) showed that each nerve-cell has an axis-cylinder or nerve-fiber process growing from it, and a number of protoplasmic processes or dendrons, which branch into

---

[1] Corti: Ztschr. f. wissensch. Zoöl., Leipz., 1851, iii, 109–169.

[2] Virchow: Arch. f. path. Anat., Berl., 1854, vii, 135–138.

[3] Paul Langerhans: Berlin dissertation, 1869.

[4] Ehrlich: Ztschr. f. klin. Med., Berl., 1879–80, i, 553–560.

[5] Ehrlich: Deutsche med. Wochenschr., Leipz. and Berl., 1886, xii, 49–52.

[6] Golgi: Sulla fina anatomia degli organi centrali del sistema nervoso, Milan, 1886.

[7] Donné: Compt. rend. Acad. d. sc., Paris, 1842, xiv, 366–368.

[8] Osler: Proc. Roy. Soc., Lond., 1873–74, xxii, 391–398.

[9] Bizzozero: Di un nuovo elemento morfologico del sangue, Milano, 1883.

[10] Waller: Phil. Tr., Lond., 1850, 423–430.

[11] Otto F. C. Deiters: Untersuchungen über Gehirn und Rückenmark (etc.), Brunswick, 1865.

dendrites, forming arborizations. The material continuity of the nerve-fibers with the terminal arborizations was demonstrated by Gerlach's gold chloride stain in 1871, and later the use of carmine with Weigert's mordant showed the continuity of the nerve-body with the axis-cylinder. In 1883,[1] Camillo **Golgi** (1843–1926), of Pavia, applied his silver nitrate stain of 1873[2] to the central nervous system, and strikingly demonstrated the existence of multipolar nerve-cells, having long and short axis-cylinder processes (Golgi cells) with the arborizations of dendrites. In 1886,[3] Wilhelm **His** showed how the nerve-cell develops from a columnar epiblastic cell into a neuroblast by thrusting out a pseudopodium, which becomes the axis-cylinder, the polar pseudopodia remaining protoplasmic and becoming the dendrites. Progress was now rapid. Forel, in 1887, confirmed the work of His on the pathologic side by studying experimental degenerations. A host of investigations by von Kölliker (Switzerland), von Lenhossék (Hungary), the younger Retzius (Sweden), A. Van Gehuchten (1861–1914) (Belgium), and the eminent Spanish histologist, Santiago **Ramón y Cajal** (1852–   ) greatly extended the knowledge of those terminal arborizations in the brain and cord, which Obersteiner likened to an espalier growth and Ramón y Cajal to the network of lianas and mosses in a tropical forest. Many new staining methods were introduced, in particular, that of Bethe, who made Ehrlich's intravital (methylene-blue) stain a permanent one by adding ammonium molybdate, and thus clearly demonstrated the continuity of the cell-body and axis-cylinder (1895[4]). The neurofibrillæ, which Max Schultze had seen in the electric lobe of the torpedo in 1872, were beautifully brought out in violet by the gold chloride stain of the Hungarian, S. Apáthy (1987[5]), who thought he saw them extending from one neuron into another. This was, however, confuted by the remarkable staining methods of Ramon y Cajal (1903), Bielschowsky (1903), and Donaggio (1905). Meanwhile the whole doctrine had been brought to a focus in the celebrated essay of Wilhelm **Waldeyer** (1891[6]), which affirmed that the nervous system is made up of epiblastic cells or neurons each consisting of a cell-body with two sets of processes, an axon (axis-cylinder) having efferent (cellulifugal) functions and one or more dendrites with afferent (cellulipetal) functions. Upon these countless neurons the functional activity of the nervous system depends, the nerve-fibers being nowise independent, but axonic and dendritic outgrowths. In America, the whole subject was ably and critically expounded in the treatise of Lewellys F. Barker (1899[7]), who has dealt particularly with the controversies which raged up to this time. Implicit in the neuron doctrine itself is the basic idea of the autonomy of its units, viz., that the branches of the neurons are contiguous, but not continuous, transmitting sensations and impulses by contact alone. But Gerlach believed that the *sensorium commune* is made up of a continuous network *(rete mirabile)*; Apáthy, Held, and Bethe upheld the notion of a continuum of neurofibrillæ, Henson, the concept of a system of intercellular bridges, Franz Nissl (1860–1919), the theory that the gray matter *(nervöse Grau[8])* is the conducting medium, Held and Bethe that nerve-fibers can be formed by a fusion of certain cells (pluricellular doctrine). In battling over these views, many able investigators wandered away from actual facts into journalistic pettifogging. The conclusion of the whole matter was reached in a series of beautiful and convincing experiments by Ross Granville **Harrison** (1870–   ), who eventually demonstrated the ameboid outgrowth of the nerve-fibers from the cell in an extravital culture (1910[9]). Thus, by purely physical and chemical methods, the whole nervous system was finally brought under the cell doctrine of Schwann and Virchow.

---

[1] Golgi: Riv. sper. di freniat., Reggio-Emilia, 1882, viii, 165, 361; 1883, ix, 1, 161, 385; 1885, xi, 72, 193.

[2] Golgi: Gazz. med. ital. lombard., Milano, 1873, 6. s., vi, 244–246, 1 pl.

[3] His: Abhandl. d. math.-phys. Kl. d. k. sächs. Akad. d. Wissensch., Leipz. 1887, xiii, 477–513, 1 pl.

[4] Albrecht Bethe: Arch. f. mikr. Anat., Bonn, 1894–5, xliv, 579–622.

[5] Apáthy: Mitth. a. d. zoöl. Station zu Neapel, 1897, xii, 495–748.

[6] Waldeyer: Deutsche med. Wochenschr., Leipz. and Berl., 1891, xvii, 1244, 1267, 1287, 1331, 1352.

[7] Barker: The Nervous System and its Constituent Neurons, New York, 1899.

[8] Franz Nissl: München. med. Wochenschr., 1909, xlv, 988, 1023, 1060.

[9] Harrison: J. Exper. Zoöl., Phila., 1910, ix, 784–846, 3 pl.

By the close of the 19th century, **embryology** had become a highly complex science, its main developments being along such paths as the investigation of the origin of tissues, the morphology and pathology of the embryo as a whole, the significance of maturation and fertilization of the ovum, the tracing of cell lineage (cytogenesis), the study of embryology in the light of evolution (Recapitulation Theory), the structural relations of the placenta, and the beginnings of experimental embryology.

Highest among contemporary names, perhaps, stands that of Wilhelm **His** (1831–1904), of Basel, Switzerland, who did the best work of his time on the origin of tissues and the serial and morphological study of the embryonic and adult organism. As Bichat dealt with the coarser aspects of tissues, Henle and Kölliker with their

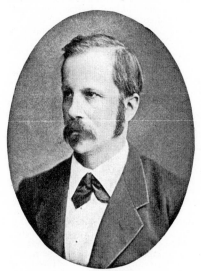

microscopic appearances in health, Virchow with the same in disease, so the name of His will always be associated with the science of their origins (histogenesis). His came of a distinguished Basel family, and apart from the advantages derived from his parentage, his education was of the very best, his teachers being Johannes Müller, Robert Remak, Virchow, and Kölliker. Professor of anatomy at Basel from 1857 to 1872, he was, through the influence of Carl Ludwig, appointed in the latter year to the same chair at Leipzig where he remained for the rest of his life (1872–1904).

Wilhelm His (1831–1904). (Courtesy of Miss Davina Waterson.)

His earlier studies were on such themes as the normal and pathological histology of the cornea (1853–6), the structure of the thymus gland (1859–61), the histology of the lymphatic glands (1861) and the lymphatic vessels (1862–3), the latter illustrated with unrivaled plates. In 1865, he published his great academic program, "On the Tissue-layers and Spaces of the Body,"[1] introducing a new classification of tissues as a guide in embryological research. It contains a sympathetic appreciation of Bichat, a defense of his classification as being related to the germ-layers, and points out that all the serous spaces arise in the mesoderm and are lined with the special membrane which His called endothelial. His monograph on the embryology of the chick appeared in 1868, and during 1880–5 his famous *Anatomie menschlicher Embryonen*, in which, from carefully selected specimens, the human embryo was studied as a whole for the first time. In 1886, His established, by embryological investigation, the fact that the axis-cylinder is a process of the nerve-cell. In 1900, he introduced his concepts of the lecithoblast and angioblast (the *Anlage* of the blood and capillaries).

In the meantime, His had been approaching his subject from a larger angle. A beautiful draftsman and a skilful photographer from

---

[1] His: Die Häute und Höhlen des Körpers, Basel, 1865.

boyhood up, his aim in teaching was to visualize everything to his pupils by means of microphotography, lantern-slides, models, and his own unrivaled drawings, and he was able to utilize the advantages given him at Leipzig in a most remarkable way. In 1866, he invented a microtome which he gradually improved, and, from the serial sections so obtained, he conceived the idea of a graphic reconstruction of the embryo in two and three dimensions (1868), the former process being attained by means of the "embryograph" (his invention), the latter by the models of his assistant, F. J. Steger, and afterward, by the device, invented by Born, of drawing the sections upon wax plates and setting them in juxtaposition. These serial sections, all from the same embryo, soon obviated the errors made by comparing chance sections of embryos of different sizes and ages. The His-Steger models, now seen in all anatomical museums, are permanent memorials of his success in demonstrating morphological relations in three-dimensional space. This is especially true of his *Präparate zum Situs viscerum* (1878), which included models of the female pelvic viscera. In 1874, he published *Unsere Körperform*, which argues that the form of an organism is due to such mechanical effects as the migrations of cells, tissues and organs, although a mechanical causation of cell growth is denied. While not the same thing as developmental mechanics, this idea may be said to have led up to it. His was one of the founders of the Anatomische Gesellschaft, and in 1895 he drew up its report on the revision of anatomical nomenclature (B. N. A.), which, it is said, reduced current anatomical terms by about 80 per cent. This was presented in English dress by Lewellys F. Barker in 1907. In 1876, His founded the *Zeitschrift für Anatomie und Entwicklungsgeschichte*, which, in 1877, became merged into the old Müller-du Bois Reymond *Archiv*, His and Braune editing the *Anatomische Abteilung* (1877–1903). The great Anatomisches Institut at Leipzig was constructed under the direction of His, and opened April 26, 1875. He was also one of the founders of the *Archiv für Anthropologie* (1876), and his interest in the subject is evidenced in the monograph on Swiss crania which he made with Rütimeyer in 1864, his studies of the Rhætian population (1864), of the skeletons belonging to Vesalius and Platter (1879), of the development of human and animal physiognomies (1892), and his identification of the remains of Johann Sebastian Bach (1895) which had been found in a coffin in the yard of the old Johanniskirche. By comparative measurements and averages taken from other cadavers, His enabled the sculptor Seffer to construct a bust in clay which was at once recognizable as a counterfeit presentment of the great composer. Unlike his colleague, Ludwig, His founded no school, believing that it is best for the student to go his own way and follow his own bent. His work on the anatomy of the human embryo has been carried forward to a unique conclusion by his pupils, Franz Keibel and Franklin P. Mall (1910–12[1]).

---

[1] Keibel-Mall: Manual of Human Embryology, 22, Jena, 1910–12.

The problem of the dynamics of the maturation, fertilization, and segmentation of the ovum, which had remained insoluble since Harvey's time, was worked out in the following way: In 1826,[1] Prévost and Dumas first described the segmentation of the frog's egg. The mammalian ovum was discovered by von Baer (1827), and was shown to be unicellular in every vertebrate by Gegenbaur (1861). The spermatozoa, discovered by Hamen in 1677, were shown, in a filtration experiment of Spallanzani's, to be essential to fertilization (1786), and their cellular origin was demonstrated by Kölliker (1841). In 1865, Schweigger-Seidel and La Valette St. George proved that the spermatozoön is a cell possessing a nucleus and cytoplasm.[2] Its union with the ovum was first observed (in the rabbit) by Martin Barry in 1843. Virchow clearly stated that the ovum is derived, in continuous line of descent, from preëxisting fertilized ova (1853). In 1875, Oscar Hertwig (1849–1922) demonstrated that the spermatozoön enters the ovum and that fertilization is accomplished by the union of the male and female pronuclei so formed.[3] Huxley conceived that, "regarded as a mass of molecules, the entire organism may be compared to a web of which the warp is derived from the female and the woof from the male" (1878). The polar bodies, given off by the ripe ovum, were shown to be formed by division of its nucleus by Bütschli (1875) and by Fol (1876). In 1880, the splitting of chromosomes in the cell-nucleus (karyokinesis) was discovered by Flemming; and in 1883, Van Beneden discovered that the associated male and female pronuclei in the fertilized egg each contain half as many chromosomes as the normal body cells in the same species. Weismann believed that the object of this partition was to keep the number of chromosomes constant in the given species. Theodor Boveri (1862–1915) defined the splitting of the chromosomes as a definite act of reproduction (1888), and he showed that there are two varieties of Ascaris megalocephala which differ only in the number of chromosomes. In 1875, Flemming discovered a minute body in the ovum of the Anodon, usually lying outside the nucleus and often paired. This was discovered independently by Édouard Van Beneden (1876), and was termed the "centrosome" by Boveri (1888). The centrosome was soon found to be common to many other cells of the body and to unicellular organisms, and came to be regarded as the special organ of cell division, the "dynamic center" of the cell. Boveri supposed it to be the specific organ of fertilization in the spermatozoön, initiating mitosis by its own division, or, as Wilson once put it, "the web is to be sought in the chromatic substance of the nuclei," while "the centrosome is the weaver at the loom." While the latter point has not been entirely substantiated, the study of the reduction of the chromosomes has led to an exact comprehension of oögenesis and spermatogenesis (Oscar Hertwig, 1890), and latterly to the elucidation of the part they play in heredity and the determination of sex by McClung, Morgan, Wilson, Miss Stevens, and others.

The science of the germ-layers was founded by von Baer (1828–34) and Robert Remak (1845). In 1849, Huxley showed that the embryonic epiblast (ectoderm) and hypoblast (endoderm) can be assimilated to the two layers of cells which make up the body of the adult Hydra. This was regarded as a great advance at the time, but later investigation has shown that the developments from the germ-layers in different animals are by no means constant; that the mesoderm may originate from either ectoderm or endoderm, and that many organs can be traced back to certain predestined cells, rather than to cell-layers. Cell lineage, or cytogenesis, has therefore become a subject of ardent investigation, and, since the initial labors of Blochmann (1882), most of this work has been done in America. In such finely illustrated monographs as those of Charles Otis Whitman on the embryology of Clepsine (1878), Edmund B. Wilson on Nereis (1892), C. A. Kofoid on Limax (1895), Frank R. Lillie on the Unionidæ (1895), H. S. Jennings on Asplanchna (1896), W. E. Castle on Ciona (1896), and E. G. Conklin on Crepidula (1897), the germ layers have been traced out, cell by cell, from the beginning of segmentation, and it has been shown that there is nothing constant about the development of the mesoderm and its derivatives.

The net result of the vast amount of embryological investigation, up to the year 1881, was summed up in the master-work of Francis Maitland **Balfour** (1851–82), of Edinburgh, whose tragic death robbed

---

[1] Prévost and Dumas: Ann. d. sc. nat., Paris, 1827, xii, 415–443.

[2] F. Schweigger-Seidel: Arch. f. mikr. Anat., Bonn., 1865, i, 309–335.

[3] O. Hertwig: Morph. Jahrb., Leipz., 1875–6, i, 347–434, 4 pl.

science of one of its brightest, most attractive and most promising spirits. At Cambridge, Balfour came under the influence of Michael Foster, and from that master he acquired his interest in embryology, collaborating with him in the well-known Elements (1874), which was the standard text-book of its time in English and American schools. In 1873, Balfour went to study under Anton Dohrn at the Naples Zoölogical Station, and here he made an important research upon the embryology of Elasmobranch fishes,[1] which was particularly strong in regard to the early stages of the ovum and embryo, the development of the kidneys, and the origin of the spinal nerves. In the meantime, Balfour had been appointed fellow and lecturer on animal morphology at Cambridge, and was soon attracting large classes of enthusiastic pupils. In 1880–81, appeared his great *Treatise on Comparative Embryology*, which is not only indispensable as a digest of all that was known up to that time, but, as embodying the work of himself and pupils, is the most compact and lucid exposition of the science which has yet appeared. Foster describes it as brushing away many cobwebs and mooted points "with a firm but courteous sweep." In acknowledgment of the value of this work, Balfour was made professor of animal morphology at Cambridge in 1882, but he was not to enjoy the fruits of his labors. Taking up Alpine climbing to improve his health, he attempted, in July, 1882, to make an ascension of a virgin peak and was never seen alive again. His body and that of his guide were found at the bottom of a chasm a day later. Balfour was described by Foster as a keen, quick observer and logician, a high-minded, fascinating, and very able man. Had he lived, he would undoubtedly have been one of the topmost figures of modern science. Locy says that "the speculations contained in the papers of the rank and file of embryological workers for more than two decades, and often fondly believed to be novel, were for the most part anticipated by Balfour, and were also better expressed, with better qualifications."

The close resemblance between the early stages of the embryo in different animals had been noticed by Meckel and Oken. Von Baer is said to have admitted that he could not distinguish between three unlabeled embryos of a bird, a reptile and a mammal before him. Agassiz, in his *Essay on Classification* (1859), stated that the developmental phases of all living animals correspond to the morphological changes in their fossal successors throughout geological time. Fritz Müller, in 1863, showed that the larval stages of crustaceans can be interpreted as a recapitulation of the evolution of the race. Kovalevsky, in 1866, showed that the early stages of Amphioxus (the lowest vertebrate), and of the invertebrate order of Tunicata are identical. He also demonstrated that all animals pass through the so-called gastrula stage, which led Haeckel to his Gastræa Theory (1884), viz., that the two-layered gastrula is the analogue of the hypothetic ancestral form of all multicellular animals (gastræa). Haeckel's biogenetic law asserts that the developmental history of the individual (ontogeny) tends to recapitulate the developmental history of the racial type (phylogeny). The most critical and conservative statements of the **Recapitulation Theory** are those of von Baer and Balfour. Von Baer's "laws" assert that the resemblance of early embryonic stages in different vertebrates is limited to a certain short period at which the embryo in question not only differs, in special class features, from all other embryos, but has already begun to put on generic and specific

[1] Balfour: Jour. Anat. and Physiol., Lond., 1876–8, *passim.*

characters of its own. Balfour pointed out that the recurrence of certain ancestral characters, such as the fish-like branchial clefts and the two-chambered heart in the frog, indicate that these "were functional in the larva of the creature after they ceased to have any importance in the adult." The De Vries theory, that species can originate by sudden jumps or mutations, has created a great spirit of antagonism to the old Darwinian idea of the slow, gradual evolution of species through accidental variations, although it is perfectly possible that both processes may coexist in the scheme of nature. In any case, the Recapitulation Theory is now regarded as a mere literary analogy or formal interpretation, as something read into the facts of comparative embryology by human prepossessions. Concerning the hypothetic family tree of the vertebrata through the Amphioxus, the Annelida, the worms of Sagitta type, the spiders, Limulus and the Echinoderms, Driesch quotes the scathing remark of du Bois Reymond that "phylogeny of this sort is of about as much scientific value as are the pedigrees of the heroes of Homer."

Among the important embryological researches of the century may be mentioned Wilhelm Waldeyer's studies on the ovary and ovum, including his discovery of the germinal epithelium (1870), Édouard Van Beneden (1846–1910) on the early development of the mammalian ovum (1875) and the history of the germinal vesicle and embryonic nucleus (1876), the work of Alexander Agassiz (1835–1910) on the Echinoderms (1872–83) and the Ctenophora; the discovery of the atrio-ventricular bundle of the heart by Wilhelm His, Jr. (1893), Johannes Sobotta on the formation of the corpus luteum (1896), Alfred Schaper on the earliest phases of differentiation in the central nervous system (1897), the work of Florence Sabin on the lymphatics, and the important investigations of George Howard Parker on the evolution of the nervous system.

Of Americans, William Keith **Brooks** (1848–1908), of Cleveland, Ohio, professor at the Johns Hopkins University (1876–1908), is memorable for his monographs on the oyster (1891), the genus Salpa (1893), which corrected the earlier views entertained as to its "alternation of generations," the Stomatopoda of the Challenger expedition, the genera Lucifer and Macrura, and his books on *Pangenesis* (1877), *Heredity* (1883), and *The Foundations of Zoölogy* (1899). He founded the Chesapeake Zoölogical Laboratory (1878), and was a fascinating, inspiring teacher, especially through his unusually beautiful drawings.

Charles Otis **Whitman** (1842–1910), of Woodstock, Maine, professor of zoölogy in the University of Chicago (1892), founded the *Journal of Morphology* (1887) and the *Biological Bulletin* (1899), and is memorable for his papers on the embryology of Clepsine (1878) and the inadequacy of the cell theory of development (1895).

Franklin Paine **Mall** (1862–1917), of Belle Plaine, Iowa, professor of anatomy at the Johns Hopkins University, a pupil of His and Carl Ludwig, did good work on the physiology of the circulation under the latter, and is known for his important investigations on monsters, the pathology of early human embryos (1899–1908), and the structural unit of the liver (1905). He collaborated with Franz Keibel in valuable *Manual of Human Embryology* (1910–12), the best modern work of its kind.

Charles Sedgwick **Minot** (1852–1914), of West Roxbury, Massachusetts, professor of embryology and comparative anatomy at Harvard University, was the author of an important treatise on *Human Embryology* (1892), which introduced many novel theories, also of a Bibliography of Vertebrate Embryology (1893), and a *Laboratory Text-book of Embryology* (1903). He invented two different kinds of automatic microtomes, and is widely known for his original investigations, particularly those on the origin and structure of the placenta (1891). His *Age, Growth, and Death* (1908) states the "law of cytomorphosis," in virtue of which these processes result from the steady change of protoplasm into more highly differentiated forms.

Thomas Hunt **Morgan** (1866–   ), of Lexington, Kentucky, professor of experimental zoölogy at Columbia College (1904), wrote the first treatise on experimental embryology in English (1897), has made many important investigations in embryology and the mechanism of heredity, and is the author of outstanding monographs on *Regeneration* (1901), *Evolution and Adaptation* (1903), *Experimental Zoölogy* (1907), *Heredity and Sex* (1913), *The Mechanism of Mendelian Heredity* (1915), *Experimental Embryology* (1927), and *Theory of the Gene* (1928).

George Howard **Parker** (1864–   ), of Philadelphia, professor of zoölogy at Harvard University (1906), is the author of important researches on the survival of primitive types of neuromuscular mechanism in the higher vertebrates, summarized in his work on *The Elementary Nervous System* (1919). He discovered that differentiation of muscle precedes differentiation of the nervous system in the lower multicellular animals, which accords with Galen's law that structure follows function.

Experimental embryology is a branch of experimental morphology or developmental mechanics (*Entwicklungsmechanik*), a phrase introduced by Wilhelm **Roux** (1850–1924), of Halle, who may be regarded as the founder of the science.

Roux was a pupil of Virchow and Haeckel, and his bent was already shown in his graduating dissertation (Jena, 1878), which dealt with the hydrodynamic conditions governing the formation of the lumina of branching blood-vessels. In 1894, he founded the *Archiv für Entwicklungsmechanik*, the principal organ of his science to date. Most of the early work in experimental embryology was done upon the frog's egg, as being the easiest to obtain. The first step was taken by the physiologist Eduard **Pflüger** (1829–1910), who, in 1822–83, made a number of experiments on cross-fertilization with different species of the frog. In 1883, Pflüger made a series of still more important experiments upon the effect of gravity upon the development of the egg, showing that the initial planes of cleavage will be vertical and the development normal, no matter how the egg is placed. In 1884, Born showed that gravity brings about a slow rearrangement of the contents of a rotated egg, according to their specific gravity. In the same year, Roux demonstrated that eggs whirled in a centrifugal machine do not differ in development from the normal controls. Pflüger, in 1884, showed that compression of the unsegmented egg between two planes of glass modifies the planes of cleavage according to the direction of pressure. Later, in 1892, Hans **Driesch** (1867–   ) showed that continued pressure applied to an Echinus egg can produce a flat plate of 16 or 32 cells, which will proceed to an normal development in three dimensions, directly the pressure is removed. In 1888, Roux published his celebrated experiment of killing one of the two initial blastomeres with a hot needle, producing a typical half-embryo. This led to the Roux-Weismann hypothesis of mosaic or qualitative development, which assumes that the center of formative changes is the complex structure of the nucleus, the sifting of the differential characters in the daughter cells being purely qualitative. Driesch, however, found, in 1891, that if the two blastomeres could be separated and set free by shaking, the segmentation in each would go on unilaterally up to the blastula stage, after which the open side of the latter would close over, resulting in a fully developed but small-sized embryo. Thomas Hunt **Morgan** (1866–   ), by rotating the surviving blastomere in Roux's hot-needle experiment, so that the white pole was turned upward, produced a whole embryo of half size (1894), showing that the completed development was due to a rearrangement of the contents; and Schultze, in 1894, produced double monsters by inverting a fertilized frog's egg between two glass plates, so that the dark pole of the egg came uppermost. In 1895, Driesch and Morgan, by cutting off a piece of the protoplasm of a Ctenophore egg, prior to segmentation, without damaging the nucleus, produced the same half-embryo which ordinarily results from isolating the blastomeres of this egg. In 1889, Boveri had succeeded in fertilizing a non-nucleated piece of sea-urchin egg with the sperm of another species, producing an organism destitute of maternal characteristics. Later, Jacques Loeb produced the fatherless sea-urchin and fatherless frog. All this indicated that the protoplasm, rather than the nucleus, is the principal agent in the production and regulation of form (morphogenesis). Herbst pointed out (1894–1901) that the formative and directive stimuli are usually external in plants and internal in animals. From a number of facts of this order, including the many novel experiments upon regeneration in adult marine hydroids by Loeb, Morgan, Miss Bickford, and others, Driesch was led to formulate his quantitative theory of cell-division, viz., that the "prospective value" of any embryonic cell is simply a function of its location; and that protoplasm is a "polar bilateral structure," capable of regulating its development symmetrically in any of the three dimensions of space, also a "harmonious equipotential system," having the same potency for development in all its parts. From the totipotency of protoplasm, Driesch argued that its functions can never be explained mechanically, since a machine, the smallest part of which is identical in structure and functional capacity with the whole machine itself, is unthinkable. The same sharp distinction which is made in mechanics and patent law between a "tool" and a "machine" is, therefore, to be observed between a machine and a living organism or substance, since the former is always a clumsy imitation of the latter, and never *vice versa*. If this point were constantly observed by biologists, the superfine vitalism of Driesch would soon dwindle into a truism, for the eminent morphologist has latterly invoked, as a substitute for the medieval vital principles, the old

Aristotelian "entelechies," which is, again, only a *petitio principii*. Driesch has given up experimentation to philosophize in the Cloud-Cuckoo-Land of "harmonious equipotential systems," but his quantitative theory of the development of the ovum had the advantage of being identical with the "epigenesis" of Wolff and von Baer, while Roux's "mosaic theory" is only a modified form of the old "preformation" hypothesis of Bonnet and Haller. Roux, having become enmeshed in these difficulties, devoted a great deal of labor to the task of extricating himself by means of "sage provisos, sub-intents and saving clauses." Thus, two of the ablest experimental morphologists of recent times have elapsd into scientific inactivity through the effect of their own theories.

The masters of **physiology** in the second half of the 19th century were Helmholtz, Claude Bernard, and Carl Ludwig. In the second rank come du Bois Reymond, Brücke, Goltz, Pflüger, Brown-Séquard, and, among the physiological chemists, Willy Kühne, Hoppe-Seyler, Salkowski, and Kossel. About the middle of the century, the physical principles of the Conservation, Transformation, and Dissipation of Energy came into prominence, and we may begin with the great mathematician and physician who made these an essential part of the physiological theory.

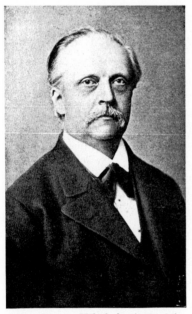

Hermann von Helmholtz (1821–94).

Hermann **von Helmholtz** (1821–94), of Potsdam, was of mingled German, English, and French extraction, and was educated as a surgeon for the Prussian army. At the University of Berlin, he came under Johannes Müller and Gustav Magnus, and met such younger men as Virchow, du Bois Reymond, Brücke, Kirchhoff and Clausius. His inaugural dissertation dealt with the origin of nerve-fibers from cells in the ganglia of leeches and crabs, which he had observed with a rudimentary compound microscope (1842). During his barrack life at Potsdam, he published his essay, *Uebdr die Erhaltung der Kraft* (1847), which established his reputation, although, at first, appreciated only by the mathematician Jacobi. In 1849, Helmholtz was appointed professor of physiology and pathology at Königsberg, subsequently occupying the chairs of anatomy and physiology at Bonn (1855–8), physiology at Heidelberg (1858–71), and physics at Berlin (1871–94).

The essay on the Conservation of Energy established the first law of thermodynamics, viz., that all modes of energy, *e. g.*, heat, light, electricity, and all chemical phenomena, are capable of transformation from one to the other but otherwise indestructible and impossible of creation. This had actually been demonstrated for physiological processes by the Heilbronn physician, Robert Mayer, and, for physical phenomena, by James Prescot Joule, in 1842, but Helmholtz gave it universal application. During the years 1850–2, Clausius and Lord Kelvin established the second law of the thermodynamics, which asserts that energy, in all its modes, is continually flowing or tending to flow from states of concentration to phases of dissipation and never otherwise. This was applied to all physical and chemical phenomena by one of Helmholtz's pupils, the Yale professor, Willard Gibbs (1872–8), of whose work Helmholtz wrote an appreciative study in 1882. That the muscles are the main source of animal heat was demonstrated by Helmholtz in isolated preparations (1848[1]). In 1850–2,[2] he measured the velocity of the nervous impulse with the pendulum-myograph of his invention. His invention of the ophthalmoscope (1851[3]) made ophthalmology an exact science. It was followed by his phakoscope and ophthalmometer (1852). With the latter, he was able to determine the optical constants and explain the mechanism of accommodation (1854), particularly the part played by the lens. His great Handbook of Physiological Optics (1856–67) is a permanent classic, containing his revival of the Young theory of color vision, which he regarded as a special case of Müller's law of specific nerve energies. The *Tonempfindungen* (1863) shows the same wonderful sweep and mastery, revealing, at the same time, the accomplished musician. Never has the subject of acoustics been so exhaustively dealt with, except, perhaps, in Lord Rayleigh's treatise. Helmholtz also made an important study of the mechanism of the tympanum and ossicles of the middle ear (1869), which did much to elucidate the phenomenon of audition. After assuming the chair of physics at Berlin (1871) and the directorship of the Physico-Technical Institute at Charlottenburg (1887), he devoted the rest of his life to the field in which his true genius lay and in which he was only equaled, in modern times, by such men as Clerk Maxwell and Lord Kelvin. In mathematical physics, Helmholtz made contributions of the first rank to the principles of dynamics, hydrodynamics, thermodynamics, and electrodynamics. He investigated the spin or vortex motion of an ideal, frictionless fluid (1858–73); he introduced the idea of the convection of electricity by moving material systems, and, in his Faraday lecture of 1881, stated his belief that the chemical atoms are, in their ultimate nature, electric. Independently of Gibbs, he defined the "free (available) energy" of a chemical system as the difference between its total (intrinsic) energy and its molecular (unavailable) energy. He was the first to introduce the idea that the "hidden motions" of material bodies are those of cyclic systems with reversible circular motions (as in the gyroscope or the governor of a steam-engine), in other words, rotational stresses in the ether or "whirls of energy." The Gibbs-Helmholtz equation, which asserts that the electromotive force of a galvanic cell (the actual work it can do) is equal to its free energy per electro-chemical equivalent of decomposition, is now one of the basic principles of physical and physiological chemistry, containing, as Nernst says, "all that the laws of thermodynamics can teach concerning chemical processes." It was in Helmholtz's laboratory that Rowland investigated the properties of a moving body charged with electricity, so important in colloidal chemistry, and that Hertz discovered the electric (Hertzian) waves, which led to wireless telegraphy.

Yet, although he stood at the summit of the highest department of human thought, Helmholtz never forgot that he was a physician. "Medicine," he said, with pride, "was once the intellectual home in which I grew up; and even the emigrant best understands and is best understood by his native land." He even made a little contribution to medical practice, the application of quinine sulphate to the nasal mucous membrane in hay-fever (1869[4]). As a lecturer on "popular science," Helmholtz was approached only by Huxley, Tyndall, and Ernst Mach. His writings in this field have an elevation and dignity,

---

[1] Helmholtz: Arch. f. Anat., Physiol. u. wissensch. Med., Berl., 1848, 144–164.

[2] *Ibid.*, 1850, 71, 276; 1852, 199. See, also, E. Ebstein: Janus, Amst., 1906, xi, 322.

[3] Beschreibung eines Augen-Spiegels zur Untersuchung der Netzhaut im lebenden Auge, Berlin, 1851.

[4] Ueber das Heufieber, Arch. f. path. Anat., Berl., 1869, xlvi. 100–102.

a genial command of vast resources, which is peculiarly his own. In them one senses the personal nobility of the scientific gentleman. Helmholtz was of middle height, a man of extremely serious, dignified manner, his head of Goethean proportions, with fine, earnest eyes. With the sincere, he was absolutely sincere and helpful. With shallow or trivial persons, he was apt to invest himself with "the subtle ether of potential disapprobation," which, as some have testified, made them feel as if they were dealing with the fourth dimension of space. He had the northern tendency toward the impersonal, and this was manifested even in his attitude toward religion. As to his ultimate views of the

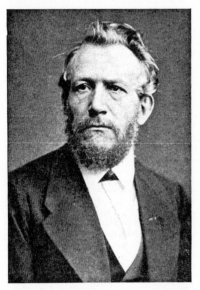

Emil du Bois Reymond (1818–96).

great questions of life, death, and immortality, Helmholtz was inscrutable and gave no sign. And, in this regard, his impersonal contributions to mathematical and physiological science are a true expression of his strong and dignified character.

Emil **du Bois Reymond** (1818–96), of Berlin, the founder of modern **electrophysiology,** was of French extraction, and he wrote in German with the clarity and precision commonly associated with the French language and literature. Like Helmholtz, he was one of Johannes Müller's pupils, and succeeded the latter as professor of physiology at Berlin in 1858, holding the chair for the rest of his life. Here he added new lustre to the Berlin Faculty, turning out many fine pupils, and supervising the construction of the palatial Physiological Institute (opened November 6, 1877), the best equipped laboratory of its kind in the world. The studies of du Bois Reymond relate almost entirely to the physiology of those muscle-nerve preparations which he did so much to introduce into laboratory experimentation. His numerous investigations were twice printed in collective form—in 1848–60 and 1883.

After the discovery of muscular electricity by Galvani, and of physiological teta-nus by Volta, in 1792, there was little done in electrophysiology beyond the intro-duction of the astatic galvanometer by Leopoldo Nobili (1784–1834), of Florence (1825); and the brief investigations of Stefano Marianini (1790–1866), and of Carlo Matteucci (1811–68), who introduced the word "tetanize" (1838), established the difference of potential existing between a nerve and its damaged muscle (1838), and first demonstrated the "rheoscopic frog" effect, viz., that the muscle of a muscle-nerve preparation will contract if its nerve be laid across another contracting muscle (1842[1]). Du Bois Reymond introduced faradic stimulation by means of the interrupted

---

[1] Matteucci: Compt. rend. Acad. d. sc., Paris, 1842, iv, 797.

(make-and-break) current from the special induction coil which is called after him (1849), made a thoroughgoing investigation of physiological tetanus, and was the first to describe and define electrotonus (1843), representing both conditions graphically by means of algebraic curves. In 1843, he noted that difference of potential between the cut end of an excised muscle or nerve and the uninjured end produces a current which can be demonstrated with a galvanometer, by closing the circuit. He wrongly inferred that this difference of potential exists in normal uncut muscle, but Hermann has since shown that it is due to chemical changes in an injured end. Since du Bois Reymond's time, a tetanic condition of injured or uninjured muscle has been regarded as the summation of individual responses evoked by rapidly succeeding stimuli. He discovered and elucidated the "currents of rest" or negative variations in stimulated resting muscle or nerve (1843-8). He showed that tetanized muscle yields an acid, resting muscle a neutral, reaction; that stimulation with a constant current has no effect upon nerve, and stated the "law of stimulation," in virtue of which the excitation of nerve depends, not upon the intensity of the current, but upon the rapidity of its variation or upon maximum variations in unit time. He believed that the "currents of rest", and other electric phenomena which he found in muscle, nerve, and the glands, were due to electromotive molecules of prismatic form, arranged in series end to end, unbroken circuits being maintained by the fact that these tissues are all moist conductors. He applied the same reasoning to the organs of electric fishes, which he was the first to study in detail, and summed up his view by stating that electrophysiological stimulation is merely a phase of electrolysis.

During his long life, du Bois Reymond wrote many fascinating essays and many fine biographical memoirs, in particular, his scientific studies of the French materialists, Voltaire, La Mettrie, Diderot, Maupertuis; and of Johannes Müller and Helmholtz, the latter being the standard sources of information in regard to their achievements. These lectures are written with great verve and *esprit*, displaying wide culture, but are more loaded with erudition than those of Helmholtz. Two have attracted especial attention—those on the Limits of Natural Science (1872) and the "Seven World-Riddles" (1880), in which their author professes a rigid denial of final causes in regard to such problems as the nature of force and matter, the origin of motion, the origin of life, the purposeful character of natural phenomena, the origin of sensation, thought, and speech, and the freedom of the will, summing up his view in the oft quoted phrases, *Ignorabimus, Dubitemus*. In person, du Bois Reymond was a man of middle height, of ruddy countenance and energetic features, strong and athletic, with fiery glance and lively gestures. He left two sons, both of whom became well-known physicians.

The work of Helmholtz and du Bois Reymond proved an efficient stimulus to the study of the **physiology of muscle and nerve,** and to the introduction of new instrumental procedures. Many of these, such as the cosine lever, the myotonograph, and the improved thermopile, were introduced by Adolf **Fick** (1829–1901), of Cassel, a pupil of Ludwig's, who wrote two important works on medical physics (1856[1]) and on mechanical work and heat production during muscular activity (1882[2]). The method of obtaining myograms, introduced by Schwann (1837) and Helmholtz (1850) was vastly improved by Étienne-Jules **Marey** (1830–1904), of Paris, who showed that, in order to avoid the errors from inertia and other causes, it is best to have a very light writing style for the tambour (1860). Investigation was also materially aided by such instruments as Gabriel Lippmann's capillary electrometer (1872), d'Arsonval's mirror galvanometer (1881), Fick's tension writer (1882), the

---

[1] Fick: Die medizinische Physik, Braunschweig, 1856.

[2] Fick: Mechanische Arbeit und Wärmeentwicklung bei der Muskelthätigkeit, Leipzig, 1882.

ingenious improvements of the Scandinavian, Magnus Blix, for synchronous records of isometric and isotonic curves (1892), Bernstein's differential rheotome (1890), Mosso's ergograph (1890[1]), for the study of voluntary muscular contractions in man, and his myotonometer (1896). Photography was effectively employed by Sir John Burdon Sanderson (1828–1905) and by Julius Bernstein (1839–1917) in measuring the time relations of the period of latent stimulation of muscle, which they reduced from the figures Helmholtz gave to about 0.0035 inch.[2] Bernstein, one of du Bois Reymond's best pupils, also did most important work upon the thermodynamics of muscular contractions (1902–8). Injury currents in quiescent muscle, which du Bois Reymond had termed currents of rest, were investigated as "demarcation currents" by Ludimar Hermann (1879), Bernstein (1897), and J. S. Macdonald (1900–1902), the phenomenon being due to concentration of ions at the injured surface of discontinuity. The effect of veratrine upon muscular contraction ("veratrinized muscle") was first investigated by Kölliker (1856[3]) and later by Bezold and Hirt (1867). Willy Kühne proved that muscle plasma is coagulable (1859) and fluid within the living fiber (1863). Ludimar Hermann investigated muscular metabolism (1867), showing that there is increased elimination of CO_2 upon contraction.

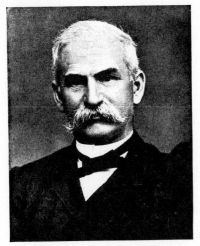

Hugo Kronecker (1839–1914).

Angelo Mosso (1846–1910), of Turin, investigated muscular fatigue with the ergograph (1890–91[4]), and, by injection experiments with the blood of a fatigued animal, indicated that fatigue is due to a toxic product of muscular contraction (1890[5]). Auguste Chauveau (1827–1917) investigated the heat and energy relations of muscular work (1891), and Theodor Wilhelm Engelmann (1843–1909), the mechanics and thermodynamics of muscular contraction, illustrating his theory by an artificial muscle made of a violin-string (1875–95). He believed that evolved heat contracts muscle just as it shortens catgut, but Fick showed that chemical energy in muscle is converted directly into the work of contraction, any heat evolved being negligible and incidental to the work done (1882). Gad found the contraction to be due to lactic acid formation (1893), which Sir Walter Fletcher and Gowland Hopkins found to derive from glycogen in the muscle (1902–7). Some of the best work on muscle was done in Carl Ludwig's laboratory, notably, Bowditch's demonstration of the *Treppe* in smooth (heart) muscle (1871[6]), von Kries upon the effect of tension upon the response of muscle to stimuli (1880), and the work of Kronecker and A. V. Hill.

Hugo Kronecker (1839–1914), of Liegnitz, Silesia, a pupil of Helmholtz, Wundt, Kühne, Traube and Ludwig, and professor of physiology at Berne (1885–1914), distinguished himself particularly by his work on fatigue and recovery of striped muscle (1871[7]), his proof that heart muscle cannot be tetanized (1874[8]), his investigation of the mechanism

[1] Mosso: Arch. ital. de biol., Turin, 1890, xiii, 124–141.

[2] Sanderson: Jour. Physiol., Lond., 1895, xviii, 146. Bernstein: Arch. f. d. ges. Physiol., Bonn., 1897, lxvii, 207.

[3] Kölliker: Virchow's Arch., Berl., 1856, x, 257–272.

[4] Mosso: La fatica, Milan, 1891.

[5] Tr. Internat. Med. Cong., 1890, Berl,. 1891, ii, 2. Abth., 13.

[6] Bowditch: Ber. d. k. sächs. Gesellsch. d. Wissensch., Leipz., 1871, xxiii, 652–689.

[7] Kronecker: Arb. a. d. physiol. Anst. zu Leipz., 1871, 177–266.

[8] Kronecker: Ludwig Festschrift, Leipz., 1874, pt. 1, pp. clxxiii–cciv.

of deglutition (with S. J. Meltzer, 1880–3), his inventions of the phrenograph, the thermo-esthesiometer, the graduated induction coil, the frog-heart manometer, and a perfusion-cannula, his studies of reflex action, animal heat, innervation of respiration, and many other things of importance. The classic experiments of Bowditch and Kronecker on heart muscle established the principle that the heart's motto is "all or none," *i. e.*, no matter what the stimulus, it will either contract to the fullest extent possible or not at all. Kronecker also investigated the importance of inorganic salts for the heart-beat, the rationale of transfusion, and the physiology of mountain sickness. He directed and assisted von Basch in the first sphygmomanometric studies on human beings, and was instrumental in the foundation of Mosso's Monte Rosa Institute in the High Alps, of the Hallerianum at Berne, and of the Institut Marey at Paris. He was the soul of Ludwig's laboratory and a lifelong promoter of cordial relations among scientific men (Meltzer). His American pupils include Meltzer, Stanley Hall, Cushing, Mills, and H. C. Wood, Jr.

The **mechanics of locomotion** was first investigated by the Weber brothers (1836), later by Samuel Haughton (1873), and along rigid mathematical lines by Christian Wilhelm Braune and Otto Fischer (1891–95). The idea of investigating locomotion by serial (cinematographic) pictures was first suggested by the astronomer Janssen, who observed the transit of Venus in this way (1878). The method was perfected and utilized by E. J. Marey (*Le mouvement*, 1894) and by Eadweard Muybridge in his atlases of animals and of the nude human figure in motion (1899–1901).

After du Bois Reymond, the most interesting investigations upon the **physiology of nerve** were the discovery of the inhibitory power of the vagus nerve by the Weber brothers (1845); Helmholtz's measurement of the velocity of the nerve current (1850–52), which was avowedly suggested by du Bois Reymond's work; Eduard Pflüger's monograph on electrotonus (1859), in which he first stated the famous laws governing the make and break stimulation of nerve with the galvanic current; the early work on the "excito-secretory system" of Henry Fraser Campbell of Georgia (1857), the Ritter-Rollet phenomenon (1876); Angelo Mosso's investigations of the movements of the brain (1876), his instrument for studying the cerebral pulsations and counting the duration and degree of a sensation transmitted to the brain from without (1876[1]), which won him the prize of the Accademia dei Lincei; the studies of mechanical irritation of nerve by Rudolf Heidenhain (1858), Robert Tigerstedt (1880), and von Uexküll ("nerve-shaker," 1895); Paul Grützner on the effect of chemical stimulation (1893); the investigations of Magnus Blix upon the specific energies of the cutaneous nerves (1884–5), of Alfred Goldscheider upon the temperature nerves (1884–85), and of Henry Head upon the effects of injury and section of peripheral nerves and the mechanism of sensation and cerebration[2] (1905–18). Head's war studies have culminated in the doctrine of the "mass reflex," a diffuse and massive response to stimuli, a primitive defensive reaction against pain, which had seemingly remained dormant until thrown into relief by "shell-shock" and the gross injuries to the spinal cord characteristic of the recent war.

One of the most important experiments was the final demonstration of the indefatigability of nerve (1885[3]) by Henry Pickering **Bowditch** (1840–1911), of Boston, Massachusetts, who founded the first physiological laboratory in the United States (1871), made the first investigation of the staircase phenomenon (*Treppe*) and the "all or none" principle

---

[1] Mosso: Arch. per le sc. med., Turin, 1876–7, i, 252–256.

[2] H. Head and G. Riddoch: Brain, London, 1918, xl, 217–231.

[3] Bowditch: Jour. Physiol., Lond., 1884–5, vi, 133–135.

of contraction in heart muscle (1871), showed that delphine will make the heart beat rhythmically (1871), did important work upon re-enforcement of the knee-jerk (1890), and was a pioneer in investigating the growth of children (1877–90), particularly the dependence of growth upon optimum nutrition rather than race, and arrest of development in a growing child as a warning signal of acute disease or of general decline of health.

Bowditch's proof that nerve cannot be tired out was accomplished by paralyzing the motor nerve-endings in the muscle with curare, the first experiment in producing a functional nerve-block with a drug.

Bernstein had found that a nerve-muscle preparation can be tetanized in ten to fifteen minutes (1877), whence he inferred from other data, that the nerve itself

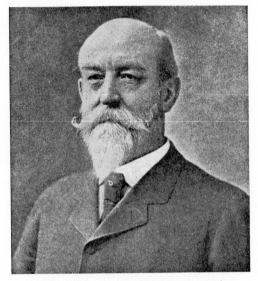

Henry Pickering Bowditch (1840–1911).

is exhausted in the process, but Wedensky (1844) got responses after one to nine hours stimulation, by blocking the nerve from the muscle by cross application of a weak galvanic current to the region between the point of stimulus and the muscle.[1] Maschek got similar results by etherizing the region (1887). Bowditch got muscular twitchings after one to four hours' stimulation under artificial respiration, after the effect of the curare had worn off.

Thus Bowditch's initial experiment in functional nerve blocking led in time to the conduction anesthesia of Halsted and Cushing, the shockless surgery of Crile and even to auto-surgery, in which an operation may be performed upon oneself in front of a mirror.

The whole subject of muscle-nerve preparations was exhaustively treated in the *Electrophysiologie* (1895) of Wilhelm Biedermann (1854–   ), and du Bois Reymond's studies upon electrical fishes were continued by Gustav Theodor Fritsch (1887–90), Karl Schönlein, and the late Sir Francis Gotch (1887–95). The chemical

---

[1] Wedensky: Centralbl. f. d. med. Wissensch., Berl., 1884, xxii, 65–68.

side of nervous activity has been investigated by William D. Halliburton (London, 1901), A. B. Macallum, and Menten (1906).

The starting-point of the neuron theory was the epoch-making experiment of Augustus Volney **Waller** (1816–70), of Elverton Farm, Kent. He showed that when a nerve is cut, the distal stump (the axis-cylinders, severed from the nerve-cells) will soon degenerate, while the proximal stump remains relatively intact (1850), from which he inferred that the nerve-cells nourish the nerve-fibers. By the same method, Waller showed that if an anterior spinal nerve-root is severed, the degenerative changes indicate that the nutritive centers of the motor fibers must lie in the spinal cord, while, in the case of section of the posterior (sensory) roots, they are seen to lie in the posterior root ganglia. These experiments won for Waller the Montyon Prize of the French Academy of Sciences (2000 francs) in 1856, and they have been repeatedly confirmed by the observations of the histologists who worked on the neuron theory. Some important observations on old amputations, made by the late William Howship Dickinson (1832–1913), of Brighton, England, in 1865, demonstrated that the proximal stump of a severed nerve eventually undergoes atrophy.[1]

The theory that the functions of the brain can be localized in the cerebral cortex was introduced in somewhat fantastic form by Franz Joseph **Gall** (1757–1828) as organology or cranioscopy, and by his pupil, Johann Caspar **Spurzheim** (1776–1832), as **phrenology,** their joint researches appearing as a four-volume treatise, with atlas, in 1810–19.[2]

This contained many really important additions to cerebral anatomy and also the theory that the brain is a bundle of some 27 (later 37) separate "organs," presiding over the different moral, sexual, and intellectual traits of the individual, their size being proportional to the preponderance of these traits and manifested on the surface of the skull as protuberances. Gall's theory drove him out of Vienna, but two medals were struck off in his honor in Berlin, and, like Hahnemann, he died rich in Paris. Spurzheim's propagandism led to the formation of secret phrenological societies and phrenological journals in Great Britain and the United States. The theory attracted the favorable notice of Goethe, who shrewdly pointed out that the secret of its hold upon the popular mind lay in the fact that it dealt with particulars rather than general propositions; in other words, the folk-mind, even in fashionable people, as being incapable of dealing with ideas, was not unnaturally preoccupied with the various cranial "bumps" which located the specific amativeness, combativeness, philoprogenetiveness, etc., of the person in question. Exploited by quacks and charlatans, phrenology soon became an object of derision among scientific men.

The first real advance, after the experiments of Flourens and Legallois, was also the most important one, viz., the work of Gustav **Fritsch** (1838–97) and Eduard **Hitzig** (1838–1907), establishing the electric excitability of the brain (1870[3]), which had been doubted since the time of Flourens.

---

[1] Dickinson: Jour. Anat. & Physiol., Lond., 1869, iii, 88–96, 1 pl.

[2] Gall and Spurzheim: Anatomie et physiologie du système nerveux, Paris, 1810–19.

[3] Fritsch and Hitzig: Arch. f. Anat., Physiol. u. wissensch. Med., Berl., 1870, 300–332.

Motor aphasia from injuries or lesions in the region of the third left frontal (Broca's) convolution had, indeed, been established by Bouillaud (1825) and Broca (1861), and localized, epileptiform spasms from definite cerebral lesions had been described by Richard Bright (1836) and Hughlings Jackson (1875); but the experiments of Fritsch and Hitzig upon the dog's brain were the first to show that local bodily movements and convulsions can be produced by stimulation of definite areas in the brain, always identical in different animals of the same species, and that, *per contra*, removal of these areas will produce paralysis or loss of function of the corresponding parts of the body.

These observations were verified and greatly extended by the work of Sir David **Ferrier** (1843–   ), upon mammals, birds, frogs, fishes, and other creatures (1872–76[1]); and the subsequent recharting of the areas.

Horsley and Schäfer (1884–8) and Beevor and Horsley (1887–94) have tended to confirm Ferrier's inference that the motor area of the cerebral cortex is around the central sulcus of Rolando. The special motor and sensory, as well as the "silent" or inexcitable, areas were mapped out by the labors of Flechsig (1876), Munk (1877–89), Bechtereff (1887), François Franck (1887), Gudden (collected in 1889), Henschen (1890–4), and Monakow (1891–2). The main themata were most carefully confirmed on the clinical and pathologic side by Charcot and Pitres (1895).

The subject of the total functions of the cerebral hemispheres and the spinal cord will always be associated with the name of Friedrich Leopold **Goltz** (1834–1902), of Posen, one of Helmholtz's pupils, who became professor of physiology at Halle (1870–2) and Strassburg (1872–1902). Goltz did important work upon cardiac pressure, the mechanism of shock (*Klopfversuch*, 1862[2]), and the functions of the semicircular canals (1870), but his most telling experiments were those upon the effect of excision of the brain and spinal cord in the frog (1869–72[3]) and the dog (1874–96[4]). He showed how the decerebrated or "spinal" frog will hop, swim, jump out of boiling water, croak like the frogs in Aristophanes, and adjust itself mechanically to every stimulation, but will otherwise sit like a mummy and, though surrounded with food, die of starvation, because it is a spinal machine, devoid of volition, memory, or intelligence. If the optic thalami remain intact, the animal will show some intelligence in regard to its own nu‑ trition and sexual instinct; but ablation of the cerebral hemispheres in the dog is followed by restless movements, unintelligent response to stimuli, and inability to feed itself or to swallow. Similar experiments had already been made upon fish, pigeons, and smaller mammals by Rolando, Flourens, Longet, and Vulpian, but no one ever described the phenomena so carefully and graphically as Goltz, who brought out the important fact that the effects of decerebration are the more profound, the higher the animal, as evidenced by amentia in man. The

---

[1] Ferrier: West Riding Lun. Asyl. Rep., Lond., 1872, iii. Functions of the Brain, London, 1876.

[2] Goltz: Königsb. med. Jahrb., 1862, iii, 271–274.

[3] Goltz: Beiträge zur Lehre von den Functionen der Nervencentren des Frosches Berlin, 1869; and Arch. f. d. ges. Physiol., Bonn., 1872, v, 53.

[4] Goltz: *Ibid.*, 1874, viii, 460; 1892, li, 460; 1896, lxiii, 362.

other experiment (excising the spinal cord) had to be performed with the greatest delicacy and care if the animal was to live. Goltz's data showed that, under these conditions, the muscles supplied by spinal nerves are totally paralyzed, with a complete loss of sensation in the corresponding parts; the viscera and blood-vessels lose their tone, the power of adaptability to temperature and other environmental changes is lessened, and perspiration abolished, although pregnancy, labor, and lactation can occur. Goltz's exposition of the "spinal" animal as a brainless mechanism which, in Bernard Shaw's phrase, "blunders into death," and of the animal deprived of its spinal cord as a conscious intelligence with lessened power of coördination and adaptation, initiated much of the work of recent times upon the complex reflexes of the body.

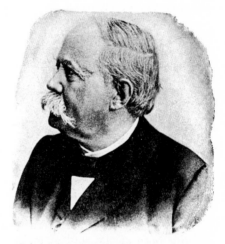

Friedrich Leopold Goltz (1834–1902).

While du Verney had successfully excised the cerebrum and **cerebellum** (1697), the earliest investigation of the cerebellar functions was Rolando's *Saggio* of 1809. This was followed by Flourens' classical experiments on the pigeon (1822) and those of Luigi Luciani (1840–1921) upon the dog (1882–91), which brought out the ataxic incoördination. Experimental excisions of fractional parts were made by a host of observers, from Rolando and Magendie on. Rolando likened the cerebellum to the Voltaic pile, in that it augments and reënforces the voluntary movements initiated by the cerebrum, a view which was reiterated and emphasized by Weir Mitchell (1869). Flourens introduced the idea of nervous coördination, which was again emphasized by John Call Dalton (1861). Hughlings Jackson regarded the cerebellum as the center for continuous movements, the cerebrum as the center for changing movements. The effect of excision of the medulla oblongata and pons Varolii was investigated by Schrader (1887). Robert Whytt found that removal of the anterior part of the corpora quadrigemina abolishes reflex contraction of the pupil to light (1768), Ivan Michailovich Setchenoff thought it contained an inhibitory center for the spinal reflexes (1863), and Charles S. Sherrington showed that a condition of "decerebrate rigidity" obtains upon complete transection (1896–97). The relation of the optic thalamus to opposite-sided sensation, especially in the eye, was noted simultaneously by Panizza and Joseph Swan (1856), and brought out, on the clinical and pathologic side, in an important postmortem by Hughlings Jackson (1875[1]). The sympathetic system was investigated by Friedrich Wilhelm Bidder (1810–94) and Alfred Wilhelm Volkmann (1800–77), who showed that it is largely made up of small, medullated fibers originating from the sympathetic and spinal ganglia (1842[2]); by Claude Bernard, Brown-Séquard, Waller, and Budge, who demonstrated the effect of section and stimulation of the cervical sympathetic (1852–53); by Kölliker (1889) and other modern histologists, who studied the structure of sympathetic cells by improved staining methods; by W. H. Gaskell, who studied visceral and vascular innervation (1886); by J. N. Langley, who studied reflexes from sympathetic ganglia

---

[1] Jackson: London Hosp. Rep., 1875, viii.

[2] Bidder and Volkmann: Die Selbstständigkeit des Nervensystems, Leipzig, 1842.

(1894[1]) and defined the "autonomic system" (1900); and latterly by Henry Head. Of special nerves, the vagus was investigated by the Webers (1845), Schmiedeberg (1871), and Gaskell (1882), the nerves of the heart and chorda tympani by Carl Ludwig, the vasoconstrictors and vasodilators by Claude Bernard (1858), the dilator nerves of the peripheral vessels by Carl Ludwig (1866), the intestinal plexuses by Auerbach and Meissner (1862), the secretory and trophic nerves of glands by Heidenhain (1878), the temperature nerves (1884) and nerves of cutaneous sensation (1885) by Alfred Goldscheider, the distributory fibers of the cranial nerves by Vulpian (1885), the erector mechanism by Eckhard (1863) and Gaskell (1887), the endorgan of the eighth nerve by Julius Ewald (1892), the pilomotor nerves by J. N. Langley (1893), and the nerve-endings for painful sensations by Max von Frey (1896).

The modern concept of **reflex action** was an outgrowth of the cell theory and (its most important corollary) the neuron theory; for it was through the labors of the different histologists and experimenters who worked on the neurons (from Deiters to Harrison), that the complex paths for transmitting impulses from nerve-cell to nerve-cell were traced out and their morphological continuity demonstrated. The initial data were the Bell-Magendie law of the spinal nerve-roots, the law of Wallerian degeneration of nerve-fibers after section, and Goltz's work on the effects of the excision of large segments of the central nervous system. **Türck's** investigations of the cutaneous distribution of the separate pairs of spinal nerves (1858–68) were of capital importance, as also the discovery of the cerebral inhibition of spinal reflexes by Setchenoff (1863[2]), and the investigation of such localized reflexes as the knee-jerk or the mechanism of deglutition. Under the neuron theory, the simple reflex mechanism of external stimulus, afferent path, nerve-center, and efferent path became converted into a "reflex arc," requiring a sensory neuron centered in the ganglia of the posterior spinal roots or the cranial nerves and a motor neuron in the anterior horn of the cord or in the motor nucleus of a cranial nerve. Even this complex was soon perceived to be only an abstraction, since an isolated system of nerve-cells, functionating apart, is unthinkable. It became clear that most reflexes are compounded or coördinated, and that the nervous system functionates as a whole. This idea was specially developed by Charles Scott **Sherrington,** who did a large amount of experimental work on all phases of the subject. Sherrington was the first to investigate the phenomena of "decerebrate rigidity" produced by transection between the corpora quadrigemina and the thalamus opticus (1896–98[3]), and of "reciprocal innervation" and reciprocal inhibition, in virtue of which antagonistic muscles, e. g., flexors and extensors, when under reflex stimulation, are so related that excitation of one center is simultaneous with inhibition of the other (1893–98[4]). Sherrington expanded the theoretical concept of the

---

[1] J. N. Langley: Jour. Physiol., Lond., 1894, xvi, 410–440.

[2] I. M. Setchenoff: Physiologische Studien über die Hemmungsmechanismen für die Reflexthätigkeit des Rückenmarks im Gehirn des Frosches, Berlin, 1863.

[3] C. S. Sherrington: Proc. Roy. Soc. Lond., 1896, lx, 415; and Jour. Physiol., Lond., 1898, xxii, 379.

[4] Proc. Roy. Soc. Lond., 1892–3, lii, 556–564.

"synapse," the separating surface which Foster postulated to exist between two neurons or their terminations, to complete the circuit in the reflex arc; and he did much to develop the knowledge of reënforcement and antagonism in simple and compound reflexes and of coördination in successive (chain) reflexes. The whole trend of his teaching is to the effect that a reflex action is seldom an isolated phenomenon, but one in which several reflex arcs are concerned, so that the true function of the nervous system is to integrate the organism, in the sense of giving it an individuality which is not possessed by a mere collection of cells or organs.[1] No one has handled this abstruse subject with more ability than Sherrington.

In connection with his work, it is proper to mention the important experiments of Erb and Westphal (1875), Jendrassik (1885), Weir Mitchell and Morris J. Lewis (1886), Lombard (1889), Bowditch and Warren (1890), on reënforcement and inhibition of the knee-jerk, of Sigmund Exner (1846–1926) on reënforcement (*Bahnung*) of reflexes (1882), of Jacques Loeb on "chain-reflexes" (1899), and of Pavloff on conditional reflexes (1912).

Experimental **psychology** began in Ernst Heinrich Weber's laboratory, and its modern phases are principally the work of Lotze, Fechner, and Wundt.

Rudolph Hermann **Lotze** (1817–81), of Bautzen, a medical graduate who went over to metaphysics and philosophy, was the author of many important works on analytic psychology, in particular his *Medicinische Psychologie*, or Psychology of the Soul (1852). He was a pioneer in the investigation of space perception and in the scientific exploration of the subconscious states. The elaborate analytics of Jung and Freudian school are foreshadowed in such works as J. C. A. Heinroth's treatise on lying (1834), in which the concept of "pathologic lying" was, in effect, introduced, and Kussmaul's investigations of the psychic life of the newborn child (1859).

Gustav Theodor **Fechner** (1801–87), professor of physics at Leipzig (1839–75), who did much experimental and editorial work in physics and chemistry, was perhaps the first after Weber to apply mathematical physics to the physiology of sensation, and wrote the first treatise on psychophysics (1860[2]). He made extended experimental studies of cutaneous sensation and muscular sense, for example, his record of 24,576 separate judgments of weights; he pointed out the personal or egotistic nature of painful sensation, he followed Weber in his investigations of the threshold limits of sensation, and stated Weber's law in its modern form. In 1838 he first investigated the color phenomena produced by rotating disks with black and white sectors, and mention can only be made of such optical novelties as his "side-window experiment" and his "paradoxical experiment."

Wilhelm **Wundt** (1832–1920), of Neckarau, Baden, was professor of physiology at Heidelberg (1864), Zürich (1874), and Leipzig (1875) and founded the Institute for Experimental Psychology in the latter city (1878). He wrote a text-book of physiology (1865), and three enduring memoirs on muscular motion (1858[3]), sensory perception (1862[4]), and the mechanics of the nerves and nerve-centers (1871–76[5]), which were the foundation of his future work. The first of these is memorable for the famous "isotonic curves" produced by muscle under continuous and constant (amounting to continual) excitation, which, as Burdon Sanderson says, have been copied into every text-book. It also contains valuable researches on muscular action under

---

[1] Sherrington: The Integrative Action of the Nervous System, New York, 1906.

[2] Fechner: Elemente der Psychophysik, Leipzig, 1860.

[3] Wundt: Die Lehre von der Muskelbewegung, Braunschweig, 1858.

[4] Beiträge zur Theorie von der Sinneswahrnehmung, Leipzig, 1862.

[5] Untersuchungen zur Mechanik der Nerven und Nervencentren, Erlangen, 1871–76.

drugs and after transection of the nerves and spinal cord. The book on the nervous mechanism deals with such matters as reaction time and reflex time through the spinal cord and ganglia, and muscle sense. Wundt's contributions to psychology proper are a long list, and include his Elements of Physiological Psychology (1874[1]), Logic (1880–83), Ethics (1886), and his Ethnic Psychology (1904–10[2]). In 1883 he founded the *Philosophische Studien*, a serial devoted to experimental psychology and epistemology.

Other noteworthy contributions to psychology are the measurement of the velocity of the psychic impulse by Donders (1868[3]), the monographs of Duchenne (1862) and Darwin (1873) on the expression of the passions and emotions, Granville Stanley Hall's (1846–1924) study of Laura Bridgman (1879[4]) and his later book on *Adolescence* (1904), Angelo Mosso's book on fear (*La paura*, 1884), the work of G. J. Romanes, Jacques Loeb, C. Lloyd Morgan, H. S. Jennings (*Behaviour of the Lower Organisms*, 1906), Robert M. Yerkes (*The Dancing Mouse*, 1907), and others on comparative psychology, of J. McKeen Cattell, Hugo Münsterberg, J. Mark Baldwin, and others on experimental psychology, and of Krafft-Ebing, Havelock Ellis, and Freud on morbid sexual psychology.

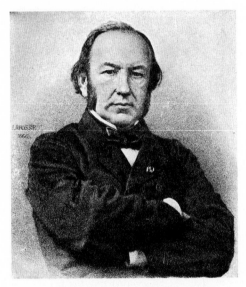

Claude Bernard (1813–78).

Much of our knowledge of the digestive and vasomotor systems was developed by **Claude Bernard** (1813–78), the greatest physiologist of modern France, who was born in the village of Saint Julien (Rhône), where his father was one of the many vine-growers and wine-makers of the region. A chorister and pupil of the Jesuits of the college at Villefranche, young Bernard was driven by straightened family circumstances to become a pharmacist's assistant at Lyons. Sharing the romantic aspirations of the youth of his time, he turned his attention to literature and wrote "La Rose du Rhône," a vaudeville comedy, which was produced with some success, and "Arthur de Bretagne," a five-act tragedy which was long afterward handsomely printed (1886). With this play in hand, he went up to Paris to consult the critic Saint-Marc Girardin, who saw the merits of his work as a dramatic poet, but shrewdly advised him to study medicine as a surer means of gaining a livelihood. This advice was the turning-point in Bernard's career, for it brought him into close contact with Magendie, who directed his genius into its proper channels. Magendie, after three or four demon-

[1] Wundt: Grundzüge der physiologischen Psychologie, Leipzig, 1873–74.

[2] Völkerpsychologie, Leipzig, 1904–10.

[3] Donders: Arch. f. Anat., Physiol. u. wissensch. Med., Leipz., 1868, 657–681.

[4] Hall: Mind, Lond., 1879, iv, 149–172.

strations of Bernard's superb talents, announced, with characteristic generosity, "You are a better man than I." As compared with Magendie, who often experimented at haphazard, like one groping in the dark, Bernard's attitude toward scientific investigation is best summed up in his own words:

"Put off your imagination, as you take off your overcoat, when you enter the laboratory; but put it on again, as you do your overcoat, when you leave the laboratory. Before the experiment and between whiles, let your imagination wrap you round; put it right away from you during the experiment itself lest it hinder your observing power."

All of Bernard's greatest discoveries were based upon accidentally discovered facts, which he used as clues to larger results through his wonderful power of thinking physiologically. It came to be said of him that he was no mere physiologic experimenter, but "physiology itself."[1] Like Magendie and Johannes Müller, he made his bow to "vitalism," but he gave it the widest possible berth. Where Magendie had left medicine *"une science à faire,"* Bernard boldly advanced to the position that the chief aim of physiologic experimentation is to throw light upon morbid conditions. He is the founder of experimental medicine, i. e., the artificial production of disease by means of chemical and physical manipulation.

In 1843, he discovered that cane-sugar, when injected into the veins, appears in the urine, but not if treated with gastric juice prior to the injection. This was the starting-point of his investigation of the **glycogenic function of the liver.** He arrived at this by the accidental discovery of sugar in the hepatic vein of a dog fed upon sugar, whence he proceeded to experiment with a dog[2] fed upon meat, with the same results, and published his papers in 1848–50. By 1857, he had, through a number of ingenious experiments, established the glycogenic function of the liver upon a permanent basis, and had succeeded in isolating glycogen.[3] The fact that this substance could be obtained, seen as such and experimented with was more potent even than Wöhler's work in establishing the fact that the animal body can build up chemical substances as well as break them down. Furthermore, Bernard made it clear that the glycogenic function of the liver is in the nature of an "internal secretion," a term of his invention. Thereafter, as Foster says, "there was an end of the older physiology of the animal body as a bundle of organs, each with its appropriate functions." In 1849, Bernard made his celebrated discovery that a puncture (*piqûre*) of the fourth ventricle of the brain in dogs produces temporary diabetes.[4] Equally important for the physiology of the digestive system was his work on the **pancreatic juice** (1849–56[5]). Up to the time of Bernard, gastric digestion was the whole of digestive physiology. Eberle (1834) suggested that the pancreatic juice emulsifies fats, and Valentin (1844) showed that it acts upon starch, but this was all that had been done and even this was not generally known. Bernard cleared up the whole subject. He showed that "gastric digestion is only a preparatory act," that the pancreatic juice emulsifies the fatty foods passing through the intestines, splitting them up into fatty acids and glycerin; and he demonstrated its power of converting starch

---

[1] "Ce n'est pas un grand physiologiste: c'est la physiologie même." J.-B. Dumas.

[2] Bernard: Compt. rend. Acad. d. sc., Paris, 1848, xxvii, 514; 1850, xxi, 571. Arch. gén. de méd., Par., 1848, 4. s., xviii, 303–319.

[3] *Ibid.*, 1855, xli, 461–469; 1857, xliv, 578, 1325.

[4] Compt. rend. Soc. de biol., 1849, Paris, 1850, i, 60.

[5] Arch. gén. de méd., Paris, 1849, i, 60–61. Compt. rend. Acad. d. sc., Paris 1849, xxviii, 249–253; 1856, suppl., 379–563, 9 pl.

into sugar and its solvent action upon the proteids undissolved by the stomach. Bernard put the experimental pancreatic fistula upon a working basis. His third great achievement was his exposition of the **vasomotor mechanism** (1851–53[1]). Henle, as we have seen, demonstrated the existence of smooth muscle in the endothelium of the smaller arteries (1840); and Kölliker showed that such involuntary muscles are made up of small, spindle-shaped cells (1846). The term "vasomotor" was first employed by Benedikt Stilling (1840) as a hypothetic designation of the nerve filaments supplying the blood-vessels. Bernard started out with the idea that the nervous system sets up chemical changes producing animal heat. On dividing a rabbit's cervical sympathetic nerve (1851), he found, instead of the expected fall in temperature, a sensible rise (4°–6° C.) and a marked increase in vascularity of the ear, but he left it an open question whether the congestion was the cause or the effect of the increased temperature. In August, 1852,[2] Brown-Séquard, then residing in America, showed that galvanism applied to the superior part of the divided sympathetic really causes contraction of the blood-vessels and a fall of the temperature on that side; whence he inferred that the effect of section of the sympathetic was to paralyze and dilate the blood-vessels. Bernard performed the same experiment independently (November, 1852), and similar results were obtained by Waller and Budge (1853). In 1853, Bernard shut off the circulation in the ear by ligating two of its veins, and, finding the same rise of temperature upon section of the sympathetic, argued that the sympathetic controls temperature relations, a view which he held to the end of his life. In 1858, he demonstrated that the sympathetic is the constrictor nerve and the chorda tympani the dilator of the blood-vessels. The discovery of vasodilator and vasoconstrictor nerves[3] completes his work on the circulation. Among his lesser achievements are his experiments with curare (1850–56[4]), in which, by paralyzing the nerve, he demonstrated the independent excitability of muscle, and thus furnished the classical proof of Haller's doctrine of specific irritability; his investigations of carbon monoxide poison (1853–58[5]), showing that it displaces the oxygen in the red blood-corpuscles; and his studies of the "paralytic secretions" occasioned by section of glandular nerves (1864[6]). In the Army Medical Museum at Washington may be seen the historic table upon which Magendie and Bernard performed their experiments.

During the later years of his life, Bernard expounded and extended his doctrines by means of courses of lectures at the Collège de France and the Sorbonne, in particular those on experimental physiology (1855), the effect of poisonous substances and drugs (1857), the physiology and pathology of the nervous system (1858), the liquids of the organism (1859), experimental pathology (1872), anesthetics and asphyxia (1875), and operative physiology (1879). The last of these reveal the unapproachable master in the technic of experimental procedure, and all of them the accomplished man of letters, who began his career as a poet and dramatist. His writings sparkle with luminous aphorisms, which are to medicine what the "Pensées" of Vauvenargues and Joubert are to literature, in that they deal, as never before, with the high calling, the honorable aims and aspirations of the scientific physician. In the early days, Bernard was looked upon askance as a mere vivisector of animals, and he relates that he owed much immunity from persecution to an accidental friendship with a police-

---

[1] Bernard: Compt. rend. Soc. de biol., Paris, 1851, xxxiii, 163; 1852, xxxiv, 472; xxxv, 168; 1853, xxxvi, 378.

[2] Brown-Séquard: Med. Exam., Phila., 1852, viii, 481–504.

[3] Bernard: Compt. rend. Acad. d. sc., Paris, 1858, xlviii, 245, 393.

[4] Compt. rend. Acad. d. sc., Paris, 1850, xxxi, 533; 1856, xliii, 825.

[5] Compt. rend. Acad. d. sc., 1858, xlvii, 393.

[6] J. de l'anat. et physiol., Paris, 1864, i, 507–513.

commissioner, in whose district he was afterward careful to pitch his tent. For the same reason, he was not happy in his married life. Even his daughters became estranged from him through his wife, who had no sympathy with his genius, and was soured by the fact that he did not become a successful practitioner. But honors came in due course. A special chair of general physiology was created for him at the Sorbonne during Magendie's lifetime; and, in 1855, he succeeded the latter as full professor of physiology at the Collège de France, and was admitted to the Académie Française in 1868. Napoleon III was so fascinated with his personality that he gave him two fine laboratories (at the Sorbonne and the Muséum d'Historie Naturelle) and made him a senator (1869). Among his friends were Duruy, Gambetta,

Pasteur, Rayer, Davaine, St. Claire Deville, Berthelot and Renan, who succeeded to his *fauteuil* in the French Academy. Claude Bernard was tall and imposing in presence, with a noble brow and a countenance expressing depth of thought and kindliness of feeling. "As he walked the streets, passersby might be heard to say, 'I wonder who that is? He must be some distinguished man.'"

Of Bernard's pupils, Willy **Kühne** (1837–1900), of Hamburg, professor of physiology at Amsterdam (1868–71), and Heidelberg (1871–1900), is memorable for his investigation of the peripheral end-organs of

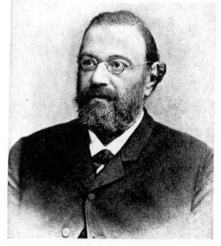

Willy Kühne (1837–1900). (Boston Medical Library.)

the motor nerves (1862), of hemoglobin (1865), of the digestion of proteids by the pancreatic juice (1867[1]), of the proteolytic enzyme in the pancreas, which he called trypsin (1876[2]), of the cleavage of the albumens in gastric and tryptic digestion (1877[3]), of rhodopsin, or "visual purple," and the "chromophanes" of the retina (1877[4]); of the electrical storms in a muscle stimulated under pressure, and its power to excite another muscle compressed with it (1888[5]), and particularly the remarkable series of chemical studies of the intermediate products of peptic and intestinal digestion which he carried on with his pupil, Russell Henry **Chittenden** (1856–   ), of New Haven, Connecticut.

---

[1] Kühne: Virchow's Arch., Berl., 1867, xxxix, 130–174.
[2] Verhandl. d. naturh.-med. Ver. zu Heidelb., 1874–77, n. F., i, 194; 233.
[3] *Ibid.*, 236.
[4] Untersuch. a. d. physiol. Inst., Heidelb., 1877, i, 15, 105, 109, 119, 455.
[5] Ztschr. f. Biol., Munich, 1888, xxiv, 383–422.

Many new substances being isolated and named for the first time by the two investigators (1883–88[1]). Kühne was a man of infinite resource in experimentation, notably in his "optograms," or photographs made directly on an excised retina, and his use of pancreatic ferments as a reagent in histology.

Paul Bert (1830–86), of Auxerre, Bernard's favorite pupil and his successor at the Sorbonne (1868), spoiled a brilliant scientific career by mixing in politics. He was fiercely radical and anticlerical, and, being sent by Gambetta as consul general to Tonkin in 1886, died there of dysentery shortly after. He discovered an unanalyzed substance in the mammary gland (1879), but his best work was La Pression Barometrique (1878), a bundle of scattered essays dealing with the gases of the blood, caisson disease, and particularly with the toxic effects of oxygen at high pressure. In prosecuting these experiments, Bert induced three balloonists to make a high ascension (7500 metres at 300 mm. barometric pressure) armed with bags of oxygen, and only one, Tissandier, survived the attempt. He lived to describe the torpor and the peculiar euphoria which precedes loss of consciousness and death.

In connection with the work of Bernard, we may follow the modern developments of the **physiology of digestion,** of metabolism, and of the ductless glands.

The classical account of the mechanism of the act of deglutition was that of Magendie (1817[2]), who described the three stages in the passage of food through the mouth, pharynx, and esophagus. He thought that the principal coefficients of the motor power were the constrictor muscles of the pharynx, but it was afterward shown by Kronecker and Meltzer that the swallowing reflex is a complex coördinated mechanism, depending mainly upon the mylohyoid and hyoglossal muscles (1880–83[3]). The essential reflex character of the act was demonstrated by Angelo Mosso (1846–1910), of Turin, who showed that, even after section or ligation of the esophagus, the peristaltic wave from the pharynx will, in time, be taken up on the lower side of the gap by means of the nerve-supply and pass to the stomach, while section of the nerves will abolish the reflex completely (1876[4]). The movements of the stomach were first studied in situ by William Beaumont (1825–33) and more accurately by Walter Bradford **Cannon**[5] (1871–   ), of Wisconsin, who studied them with the Roentgen rays, after ingestion of bismuth (1898). That the stomach is, like the heart, an automatic motor mechanism, independent of the nervous mechanism which adjusts its function, was shown by the observations of Hofmeister and Schütz upon the movements of an excised stomach kept warm (1886); by Rud. Heidenhain; by W. B. Cannon, at Harvard (1906), who proved that the gastric movements and secretions continue unabated after section of the extrinsic fibers of the vagus and splanchnic nerves; and latterly in the "visceral organism" which Alexis Carrel has kept alive in an extravital culture-medium (1912). Cannon has also studied the mechanics of digestion in surgical conditions and after surgical operations (1905–9). The mechanism of vomiting was first described by Magendie (1813), who thought that the sole agent was the contraction of the abdominal muscles. Later investigations have shown that he was only half right, the act being a complicated reflex in which the walls of the stomach play an equal part. After the time of Prout and Beaumont, it was contended by Claude Bernard and Barreswil, Lehmann, and others, that the free acid of the gastric juice was, in reality, lactic acid, but this was finally set at rest by the laborious analyses of Bidder and Schmidt (1852), which proved that normally the gastric juice always contains hydrochloric acid in excess. Brücke (1872)

---

[1] Kühne and Chittenden: Zeitschr. f. Biol., Munich, 1883, xix, 160; 1884, xx, 11; 1886, xxii, 409, 423; 1888, xxv, 358.

[2] Magendie: Précis élémentaire de physiologie, Paris, 1817, ii, 58–67.

[3] Kronecker and Meltzer: Arch. f. Physiol., Leipz., 1880, 299, 446; 1883, Suppl.-Bd., 328.

[4] Mosso, in Moleschott's Untersuch. z. Naturlehre (etc.), Frankf., 1876, xi, 331–349.   [5] Cannon: Am. Jour. Physiol., Bost., 1898, i, 359–382.

and others had shown, however, that during carbohydrate digestion, starch can be converted directly into lactic acid in the stomach, probably through the action of the lactic-acid bacillus. The hydrochloric acid in the stomach was shown by Voit (1869) and Cahn (1886) to be derived from the chlorides in the blood-plasma. In regard to the mechanism of its formation, the different theories advanced by Maly, Gamgee, and others are still *sub judice.* The histologic changes in the gastric glands during secretion were studied by Heidenhain (1878), and intravitally by J. N. Langley (1880). The stages of conversion of proteids into peptones in the stomach were first described by Meissner (1859–62), and more exhaustively and finally by Willy Kühne (1877).

The movements of the intestines were studied by Carl Ludwig (1861[1]), who described the swaying motions (*Pendelbewegungen*) between the intervals of peristalsis; by W. B. Cannon, who observed the latter by means of the Roentgen rays (1902[2]), and by Bayliss and Starling, who described peristalsis as a reflex through the intrinsic ganglia (1899[3]). That the peristaltic wave is in one direction and due to some definite arrangement in the intestinal walls was proved by Franklin P. Mall, who cut out a piece of the gut and reversed it *in situ*, producing intestinal obstruction from accumulation of food above the section (1896[4]). In 1912–13, Roger Glénard made cinematographic studies of the intestinal movements, normally and under the action of purgatives, by isolating the entire tract, excised from a rabbit, and keeping it active in a constant perfusion of Locke's solution.[5] The intrinsic nerve plexuses were described by Auerbach and Meissner (1862). Pflüger (1857[6]) showed that stimulation of the splanchnic nerves inhibits the intestinal movements. The net result of investigation goes to show that the intestines, like the stomach, are an automatic mechanism which is regulated by, but not dependent upon, the extrinsic nerves. Similar conclusions in regard to the rectal functions have been reached through the experiments of Goltz upon dogs deprived of the spinal cord (1874), and the skiagraphic observations of Hertz (1907). In 1895, it was shown, by G. H. F. Nuttall and H. Thierfelder, that healthy animal life and perfect digestion are possible without the presence of bacteria in the alimentary canal. Harvey Cushing showed that, above and below the ileum, the intestines are relatively free from bacteria, and that the intestinal tract can be sterilized by fasting (Welch-Festschrift, 1900). Our knowledge of the chemistry and histology of intestinal absorption is largely due to the work of Kühne (1877), Heidenhain (1888–94), and Pavloff and his pupils (1897). What we know of the functions of the liver and pancreas will always be associated with the great name of Claude Bernard. His pupil, Willy Kühne, as we have seen, worked out the cleavage changes of the proteins in the stomach and intestines (1867–77), but, before him, Purkinje and Pappenheim had noticed the proteolytic power of pancreatic extracts (1836), and Lucien Corvisart, in a long series of researches (1857–63[7]), had shown that proteids are converted by the pancreatic juice into the ordinary digestive products, at the temperature of the body, and in alkaline, acid, or neutral media. This corrected the error of Claude Bernard, who supposed that pancreatic proteolysis cannot take place without the previous action of bile. The sugar-forming ferments of the salivary glands and pancreas were investigated by the pathologist, Julius Cohnheim (1863[8]). Ptyalin was isolated by Mialhe (1845[9]), trypsin by Kühne (1876[10]). The derivatives of bile were studied by Thénard (1809), Gmelin (1826), Plattner, who first obtained "crystallized bile",

---

[1] Ludwig: Lehrbuch der Physiologie, 2. Aufl., 1861, ii, 615.

[2] Cannon: Am. Jour. Physiol., Bost., 1901–2, vi, 251–277. Also, "The Mechanical Factors of Digestion," London, 1911.

[3] W. M. Bayliss and E. H. Starling: Jour. Physiol., Lond., 1899, xxiv, 99.

[4] Mall: Johns Hopkins Hosp. Rep., Balt., 1896, i, 93.

[5] Glénard: Les mouvements de l'intestin en circulation artificielle, Paris thesis (Faculté des sciences), 1913.

[6] Pflüger: Ueber das Hemmungsnervensystem für die peristaltischen Bewegungen der Gedärme, Berlin, 1857.

[7] L. Corvisart: Collection de mémoires sur une fonction peu connue du pancréas, Paris, 1857–63.

[8] Cohnheim: Arch. f. path. Anat., Berl., 1863, xxviii, 241–253.

[9] Mialhe: Compt. rend. Acad. d. sc., Paris, 1845, xx, 654, 1483.

[10] Kühne: Verhandl. d. naturh.-med. Ver. zu Heidelb., 1876, n. F., i, 190.

(1844), and particularly by Adolf Strecker (1822–71), who showed that Platner's crystals were a mixture of the sodium salts of glycocholic and taurocholic acids, which, treated with acids, yield the amino-acids, glycocoll and taurine, with cholic acid as a common product (1848–49[1]). Bilirubin was first isolated by Heintz (1851); biliverdin, by Berzelius (1840), who confused it with chlorophyll, and by Valentiner, who first obtained it in crystalline form (1859). Urobilin was discovered in the urine by Max Jaffé (1840–1911) in 1868. Austin Flint, Jr. (1836–1915) claimed that cholesterin is removed from the blood by the liver and discharged from the body as stercorin (1862), but Naunyn and his pupils have assumed it to be a produce of the gall-bladder and ducts and not of the liver-cells (1892). The common bile-tests were introduced by Gmelin (1826), Pettenkofer (1844), Ottomar Rosenbach (1876), and Paul Ehrlich (1883).

The scientific study of **metabolism** has been divided by von Noorden into three stages: First, the qualitative period, inaugurated by Liebig and Wöhler, in which the end-products of animal metabolism and the conditions of their formation were determined. Second, the quantitative period of von Voit and von Pettenkofer, in which food values were carefully studied in dietetic tables and the balance of nutrition determined, after which the thermodynamic relations of metabolic processes were calculated in terms of heat and energy units. Third, the recent era of the study of the intermediate products of metabolism, which is again qualitative, but already in process of becoming quantitative. The earlier experiments were concerned mainly with urinalysis and measurement of intake and output; now they are concentrated upon interpretation of tissue activities in terms of calorimetry and respiratory (basal) metabolism or gas interchange (Du Bois). The initial experiments in metabolism were all quantitative, viz., Sanctorius' efforts to measure his own "insensible perspiration" on the steel-yard, and the attempt of Lavoisier and Laplace to establish an equation between the quantities of heat formed in the body of a mammal and in a burning candle, assuming the quantities of carbon dioxide formed to be the same in both cases (1780). The latter has been signalized by Jacques Loeb as the foundation of scientific biology.[2] All of Lavoisier's work on the exchange of gases in the lungs belongs, in fact, to the subject of metabolism, in the strict modern sense.

During the early period, Magendie was the first to emphasize the importance of the nitrogenous substances in the organism. Prout divided food-stuffs into the saccharine, oily, and albuminous, from the fact that milk, nature's ready-made perfect food, is made up of these ingredients. Next came the work of Liebig and Wöhler on urea and uric-acid compounds, in particular Wöhler's syntheses of urea (1828) and hippuric acid (1842). Liebig was the first to classify the organic food-stuffs and the processes of nutrition (1842). He held that oxygen is the principal chemical co-efficient in living processes, that muscular work is done at the expense of albumen, that fat can be formed in the body from albumen or sugar, and, like Claude Bernard, he believed that food-stuffs have to be changed into physiologic albumen before they can be utilized in the body. The embryologist Theodor Ludwig Wilhelm **Bischoff** (1807–1882), of Hannover, was the first to demonstrate the presence of free CO_2 and oxygen in the blood (1837), studied the urea as a measure of metabolism (1842), and (with Voit) the laws of nutrition and inanition in carnivora (1860). The Alsatian chemist, Boussingault, first attempted to tabulate the metabolic intake and output in different animals (1835–40), and (with Dumas) defined an animal as an

---

[1] Strecker: Ann. d. Chem. u. Pharm., Heidelb., 1848, lxv, 1; lxvii, 1; 1849, lxx, 149.   [2] J. Loeb: The Mechanistic Conception of Life, Chicago, 1912, pp. 4, 5.

oxidizing, a plant as a reducing, apparatus (1844). Bischoff's assistant, Carl von Voit (1831–1908), of Amberg, made many interesting studies on dietetics, particularly in his Handbook of the Physiology of Metabolism in Nutrition (1881), which introduced new methods of determining the intake and outgo in the balance of nutrition and the amount of proteid necessary in foods. In collaboration with the Bavarian hygienist, Max von Pettenkofer (1818–1901), Voit first estimated the amounts of proteins, fat, or carbohydrates broken down in the body (from the total nitrogen and CO_2 eliminated) by means of a special respiration apparatus, constructed at the expense of King Maximilian II of Bavaria (1861), which was further elaborated and improved by Voit himself. Voit and Pettenkofer also demonstrated that fats are formed from the food proteids (1862–81), but, later, this view was not exclusively held to, even by Voit (1886), and was absolutely denied by Pflüger (1892). Voit distinguished between organized or tissue-proteids and unorganized or circulating proteids (1881), and held that the food carbohydrates and proteids are directly consumed in the body (1881), in opposition to the Liebig-Bernard-Pflüger hypothesis, that they have first to be changed into body-substance. Pettenkofer introduced the well-known test for bile (1844), and a new method of estimating the CO_2 in the air (1858). The estimate of the nitrogen content in metabolism was rendered relatively easy by the method introduced by J. Kjeldahl in 1883.

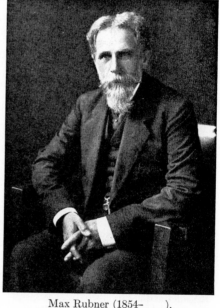

Max Rubner (1854–   ).

Max **Rubner** (1854–   ), of Munich, a pupil of Ludwig and Voit, professor of hygiene and director of the Hygienic Institute at Berlin (1891), discovered that the metabolism is proportional to the surface area of the body (1883), that the specific dynamic action of foods on metabolism is greatest for protein and least for carbohydrates (1902), and was one of the first to investigate metabolic changes in terms of heat and energy units by means of the calorimeter, or by using the animal body as a calorimeter (1891).

The heat relations of the body were first investigated by Lavoisier and Laplace (1780), Crawford (1788), and Scharling (1849), who used ice, water, and air calorimeters respectively. In recent times, many remarkable calorimeters have been invented, e. g., those of Rubner (1896), Steyrer (1907), Möllgard-Anderson (1917), all of the Pettenkofer-Voit type, and such instruments as d'Arsonval's differential air calorimeter (1886), the respiration calorimeters of Haldane (1892), Atwater and Rosa (1897), Atwater and Benedict (1905), Benedict and Higgins (1910), Sonden (1895), Jacquet (1903), Tigerstedt (1906), Grafe (1910), Rolly (1911), H. B. Williams (1912), Riche and Söderstrom (Sage calorimeter, 1913) Benedict (1918), Krogh-Lindhard (1920) and Capstick (1921). With this apparatus, the heat production of the body can be measured directly and also indirectly by calculating it from the respiratory quotient (liters O consumed into liters CO_2 produced) and the nitrogen output in the urine, one method serving as a check upon the other. The value of quantitative work by improved means has been especially shown in such researches as those of Nathan Zuntz (1847–1920) on the blood gases and respiratory metabolism,

Pavy and Moleschott on dietetics, Loewy (1890), Edsall and Means (1914–15) on the effect of drugs on heat production, Atwater and Langworthy on the balance of nutrition (1898), Max Rubner on the isodynamics of nutrition (1902), Chittenden on the minimum nutritive requirements of the body in relation to its capacity for work and nitrogenous equilibrium (1904), F. G. Benedict on the influence of inanition of metabolism (1907), Carpenter and Murlin on metabolism in women before and after childbirth (1911), and Graham Lusk on animal calorimetry (1912–15). In 1899, Magnus Levy and Falk demonstrated that metabolism is high in childhood and low in old age. Metabolism in infancy has been studied by John Howland (1873–1926) (1911), Benedict and Talbot (1914), and others. These results, supplemented by the studies of E. F. Du Bois on boy scouts (1915–16), show that metabolism is very low in the newborn, 50 per cent. above the adult level at the end of the first year, rising to a maximum in the unexplored period between two and six years, after which it falls rapidly up to the age of twenty, with much slower decrease thereafter. The estimation of metabolism in disease is effected by comparing the heat production of the patient at complete rest some fourteen hours after the last meal (basal metabolism) with the normal controls. The extreme variations in the latter have been largely obviated by the improved "linear formula" of Delafield Du Bois for calculating the surface area of the body (1915), to which the metabolism of individuals between twenty and fifty is proportional. This formula gives a normal average basal metabolism of 39.7 calories per square meter. Friedrich von Müller first noted the striking increase of metabolism in exophthalmic goiter (1893). Magnus Levy found the gaseous interchanges very high in Graves' disease (1895–7), very low in myxedema (1904), which results have been amply confirmed, particularly by the work of E. F. Du Bois with the Sage calorimeter (1915–16). The abnormal heat production elucidates the semeiology of the disease and has important dietetic bearings. That the increase of metabolism in typhoid fever is proportional to the rise in temperature has been shown by many investigators. The effect of the starvation factor has been abolished by the high calory diet of Shaffer and Coleman (1909), The respiratory metabolism in the different anemias has been studied by Magnus Levy (1906), Meyer and Du Bois (1916), and others. The latter observers (with Peabody) have investigated metabolism in cardio-renal disease (1916). Grafe found an increase in cancer, and only a moderate increase in low-grade fevers (1904). Varying results in pituitary disease, notably a slight rise of heat production in acromegaly, have been obtained by Falta (1913), Du Bois (1914), and Means (1915[1]). The pathology and treatment of diabetes have been rendered purely chemical problems through such advances as Petters' discovery of acetone in diabetic urine (1857); the work of Kussmaul on acetonemia (1874); of Stadelmann (1883), Külz (1884–87), Minkowski (1884), and Magnus-Levy (1899–1909) on β-oxybutyric ac d in relation to diabetic coma, von Mering's experimental production of diabetes by exhibition of phlorizin (1886); the dietetic studies of Carl von Noorden (1895–1911), the important and extensive studies of Graham Lusk (1898–1915), F. G. Benedict and Joslin (1910–15), the fasting treatment of F. M. Allen (1915) and the discovery of insulin by Banting and Best (1922). Lusk's original observation that a completely diabetic patient will excrete not only all the ingested carbohydrate, but the sugar equivalent of half the protein molecule (1906), has been confirmed by Allen and Du Bois (1916). The true metabolic relations of uric acid, first isolated from the urine by Scheele (1776) and found in gouty and urinary concretions by Wollaston (1797), have been a matter of keen controversy. Important landmarks in its history are Marcet's discovery of xanthin (1819); Strecker's demonstration of xanthin in the urine (1857); Kossel's proof that xanthin bases are derivatives of the urine (1879); the discovery of nuclein in pus-cells (1868) and spermatozoa (1874) by Miescher; the determination of the empirical formula of nucleic acid by Schmiedeberg (1896) of the animal and vegetable nucleic acids by Levene (1912–25) and Jones (1923–5); the "nucleal (microscopic) test" for nucleic acid of Feulgen (1922–4); Kossel's and Hoppe-Seyler's classifications of the nucleins; Horbaczewski's synthesis of uric acid in vitro (1882), and his proof that it is derivable from nuclein (1889); Minkowski's discovery that a diet of xanthin bases will increase uric-acid excretion (1886), and that, in birds, the latter is synthetized in the liver through the influence of lactic acid (1886); and Emil Fischer's family tree of gout, based upon the idea that uric acid and the xanthin bases have a common purin-nucleus (1895). The relation of the liver to metabolism was studied to advantage through a method introduced by

---

[1] See E. F. Du Bois: Am. Jour. Med. Sc., Phila., 1916, cli, 781–799.

the Russian physiologist, Nikolai Vladimirovich **Eck** (1847–   ) in 1877. This consists in establishing a permanent communication between the portal vein and the inferior vena cava (Eck's fistula), abolishing the portal circulation by ligation of the portal vein, so that ligation of the hepatic artery under these conditions is equivalent to excising or excluding the liver.

The name of Rudolph **Heidenhain** (1834–97), professor of physiology at Breslau (1859–97), is intimately associated with the interpretation of all secretory phenomena as intracellular, rather than mechanical, processes.

He investigated the histologic changes in the cells concerned in the secretion of saliva, milk, the gastric and intestinal juices, and the pancreatic ferments, and opposed Ludwig's filtration theory of the formation of lymph and urine on the same grounds, describing lymph as a secretion from the cells forming the walls of the capillaries, and urine as a product of the renal glomeruli, so far as water and inorganic salts are concerned, urea and uric acid being regarded as secretions of the epithelial cells in the convoluted tubes. Most of these theories are contained in his memoir on secretions in Hermann's Handbuch der Physiologie (1880, v). He also investigated the action of poisons on the nerves of the submaxillary gland (1872), the trophic and secretory fibers of the secretory nerves (1878), and the phenomena of intestinal absorption (1888–94). Under du Bois Reymond, he began his studies of the mechanics, metabolism, and heat production of muscular activity (1864) leading to the construction of a "tetanomotor." With Bürger, he made some experimental investigations in hypnotism, but his most striking work was undoubtedly his method of staining the kidney-cells by the injection of indigo-carmin into the blood, which, whatever his hypotheses, shows him to have been an investigator of unique talent.

The beginnings of the theory of the correlation of **ductless glands and internal secretions** were Claude Bernard's work on glycogen (1848–57), the pancreatic functions (1849–56), his fourth ventricle *piqûre* (1849), Addison's account of the suprarenal syndrome (1849–56), and the experiments of Brown-Séquard and Schiff.

Charles-Edouard **Brown-Séquard** (1817–94), a native of Mauritius, was the son of an American father and a French mother, but his lifework was mainly associated with French medicine.

He led a roving existence, posting from one country to another at intervals, and, whether in London, Paris, or New York, he could have attained almost any eminence by continuous effort. He succeeded Claude Bernard as professor of experimental medicine in the Collège de France (1878), and he was successively a professor in the Harvard and Paris medical faculties. In 1852, he confirmed Bernard's work on the sympathetic, having previously made his mark by his experimental transections and hemisections of the spinal cord (1849); his description of hemiplegia with crossed anesthesia (1850[1]) of which he gave an incorrect physiological explanation. There followed his investigations of the associated pains of visceral disease (1857); the effect of tropical heat on the temperature of the body (1859); the "tremospasm" feature of the knee-jerk (1858); the experimental production of epilepsy (1869–70); the experimental production of vasomotor changes in the pulmonary circulation (1872); and the vasodilator effect produced by heat stimulation of the cerebral cortex (1887). Brown-Séquard is, with Claude Bernard, the principal founder of the doctrine of the internal secretions, through his experimental production of an exaggerated Addison's disease in animals by excision of the suprarenal capsules (1856–58[2]), his use of the testicular and other organic juices as remedies

---

[1] Brown-Séquard: Compt. rend. Soc. de biol., 1850, Paris, 1851, ii, 70–73.

[2] Compt. rend. Acad. d. sc., Paris, 1856, xliii, pt. 2, 422, 542. Jour. de la physiol. de l'homme, Paris, 1858, i, 160–173.

(1889–91[1]), his theory that the kidney has an internal secretion (1892[2]), and his treatment of acromegaly by animal extracts (1893[3]). He was founder and editor of the *Journal de la physiologie de l'homme et des animaux* (1858–63), and, with Charcot and Vulpian, of the *Archives de physiologie normale et pathologique* (1868–94).

Moritz **Schiff** (1823–96), of Frankfort on the Main, a pupil of Magendie and Longet, was professor of comparative anatomy at Berne (1854–63), and of physiology at Florence, Italy (1863–76), and Geneva (1876–96). He was a zoölogist by training, attaining particular eminence in ornithology, and there are few aspects of physiology which he did not investigate. Schiff's work was characterized by great originality in the minutiæ of experimental procedure, displaying an almost prophetic insight into many things of present moment. He liked to cross swords with contemporary theorists, and the fact that he sometimes abandoned his own theories, or that some of them have been abandoned by others, has tended to obscure his very solid merits.

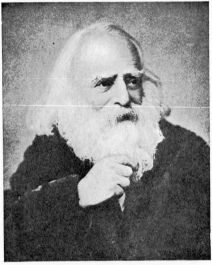

Moritz Schiff (1823–96).

Thus, in 1849, he took the somewhat arbitrary standpoint that the vagus is the motor, rather than the inhibitory, nerve of the heart, from his results on stimulation of the terminal motor fibers, which anticipated the discovery of the accelerator vagus fibers by Ludwig and Schmiedeberg in 1870. He noticed that the ventricle of a dying heart sometimes beats more slowly than the auricle, which vitiated Haller's concept of a peristaltic, muscular wave passing from the great veins through the heart to the aorta, until Gaskell showed the phenomenon to be a simple case of block. He believed that the localized "idiopathic" muscular contractions at the outset of rigor mortis are due to a special chemical stimulus (hormone) formed at death. In 1856, he made experiments which foreshadowed the existence of the vasodilator nerves discovered by Bernard in 1858. In 1867, in anticipation of Pavloff's pupils, he noted that the reflex flow of saliva in a dog with a parotid fistula varies with the methods and substances employed in stimulation. He was one of the earliest to study the effects of removal of the cerebellum, hemisection of the cord, and transection of the cerebral peduncles and spinal nerve-roots (1858); he was the first to notice the effect of excitation of the cerebral cortex upon the circulation; first described the vasoconstrictor function of the great auricular nerve and the inhibitory effect of section of the small superficial petrosal upon reflex salivary secretion; and first regarded the Rolandic area as sensory, although he later abandoned this view. His epoch-making experiments on the effects of excision of the thyroid in dogs, their prevention by thyroid grafts and by the injection or ingestion of thyroid juices (1856–84[4]),

---

[1] Arch. de physiol. norm. et path., Paris, 1889, 5. s., i, 739; 1890, ii, 201, 443, 646; 1891, iii, 746.   [2] Arch. de physiol. norm. et path., Paris, 1892, 5. s., v, 778–786.

[3] Compt. rend. Soc. de biol., Paris, 1893, xlv, 527.

[4] Schiff: Untersuchungen über die Zuckerbildung in der Leber, Würzburg, 1859, pp. 61–63. Rev. méd. de la Suisse Rom., Geneva, 1884, iv, 65–75.

which will be described under 20th century medicine, make him a pioneer of the doctrine of internal secretions and a prophet of thyroid therapy. To this field belong also his experiments on artificial diabetes (1856) and the relation of the nervous system to its production (1859).

"More than to any one else since the time of Harvey," says Sir Lauder Brunton, "do we owe our present knowledge of the **circulation** to Carl Ludwig. . . . Like the great architects of the Middle Ages, who built the wonderful cathedrals, which we all admire, and whose builder's name no man knows, Ludwig has been content to sink his own name in his anxiety for the progress of his work, and in his desire to aid his pupils." **Carl Ludwig** (1816–95) was a native of Witzenhausen, Hesse, a Marburg graduate (1840), professor of anatomy at the latter university (1846–49), professor of anatomy and physiology at Zürich (1849–55), professor of physiology and zoölogy in the Josephinum at Vienna (1855–64), and finally professor of physiology at Leipzig (1865–95), where he founded the Physiological Institute in which so much of his work was done. Ludwig was perhaps the greatest teacher of physiology who ever lived. He had over 200 pupils of all nationalities, and most of the younger generation of investigators in his science were trained by him. Beyond a text-book of physiology (1852–56), two inaugural addresses on the mechanism of urinary secretion (1843) and on blood-

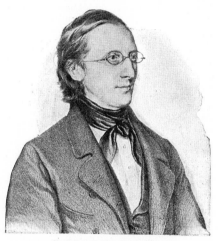

Carl Ludwig (1816–95).

pressure (1865), and a few minor essays, he did but little independent writing. Most of his important discoveries were published under the names of his pupils, some of whom, as von Kries relates, merely sat on the window-sill, while Ludwig and his faithful assistant, Salvenmoser, did all the work. He had a wonderful capacity for selecting themes which would make the pupil find himself. His object was to form capable investigators, while carrying out his own ideas, and, to this end, he always mapped out the experimental problem himself, including its technical details, and usually wrote out the final draft of the paper also.[1]

---

[1] These monographs were published simultaneously, under the pupils' names, in the "Berichte" of the Saxon Academy of Sciences, and in the famous *Arbeiten aus der physiologischen Anstalt zu Leipzig* (1866–77), but, after 1877, in du Bois Reymond's *Archiv*. They cover every aspect of the subject except the physiology of the brain, and reveal, at every turn, the master experimenter, the man of infinite resource in investigation.

Ludwig's principal contributions to physiology are the introduction of the graphic method (1847), with new instruments, like the kymograph, blood-pump, and Stromuhr; perfusion of excised organs (1865-67), his theories of the mechanism of urinary secretion and lymph-formation, his discovery of the innervation of the salivary glands, and his many excursions into the physiology of the circulation. Nearly all these things were done before Ludwig came to Leipzig.

To the Marburg period belongs the mechanical theory of the secretion of urine by osmosis. In 1842,[1] Sir William Bowman, in describing the capsule around the glomeruli and the urinary tubules, advanced the theory that the proximal principles of the urine are secreted in solid form from the epithelium of the venous tubules, solution being effected by water discharged from the glomerulus. Ludwig's theory (1843-44[2]) starts with the idea that the secretion of urine depends upon the beating of the heart, the blood-pressure causing the urinary constituents to pass from the blood through the capillary walls as a dilute liquid, which becomes concentrated, as it passes through the tubules, by osmosis of water to the more concentrated lymph outside. Bowman and Heidenhain treated the glomerular epithelium as a secreting gland. Ludwig regarded it as a passive filter. Ludwig's theory has been accepted by most physiologists, although strong objections to it have been made by Heidenhain[3] and others. In 1869-70, as Brunton points out,[4] Ludwig himself, in collaboration with his pupil, Ustimovitch, performed an experiment which forced him to modify his views somewhat.[5] This consisted in dividing the medulla in the neck of a dog, causing the blood-pressure to fall, and stopping the urinary secretion. Subsequent injection of urea into the veins caused a renewal of the urinary secretion and forced Ludwig to conclude that the effect of pressure was dependent upon the chemical constituents in the blood; in other words, upon osmosis through a selective, semipermeable membrane. In 1847, Ludwig changed Poiseuille's mercury manometer into the kymograph.[6] In 1848 he discovered the ganglionic cells in the interauricular septum.[7] During the Zürich period, he stated, through his pupil, F. W. Noll, the theory that lymph is formed by the diffusion of fluids from the blood through the vessel walls into the surrounding tissues, the motor power being the capillary blood-pressure (1850[8]). In 1851, Ludwig (with Becher and Rahn) discovered the innervation of the submaxillary glands,[9] and, in 1856, he showed that the stimulation of the sympathetic nerve will cause secretion by the submaxillary gland.[10] During the Viennese period, his pupil, Lothar Meyer, investigated the gases of the blood (1857-58); Cloetta discovered inosite, taurin, leucin, and uric acid in the animal body (1855); and Ludwig himself collaborated with the physicist Stephan in a hydrodynamic investigation of the pressure exerted by flowing water in a plane perpendicular to its direction (1858). In 1864, he studied, with Thiry, the effect of the spinal cord upon the blood current.[11] His Leipzig inaugural address (1865) introduced the idea of keeping excised portions of an organism (*überlebende Organe*) active by an artificial circulation or "perfusion." During the Leipzig period, research was varied, but the main objects of study were the heart and the circulation. Thus, in 1866, we find Ludwig with Elie von Cyon, investigating the effect of temperature on heart-beat, and in the same year he discovered the depressor nerve of the heart, and the "nervi erigentes" of the peripheral vessels (1866[12]). With Dogiel, he invented the *Stromuhr* for measuring the amount of blood passing in unit

---

[1] Bowman: Phil. Tr., Lond., 1842, 57-80.

[2] Ludwig: Beiträge zur Lehre vom Mechanismus der Harnsecretion, Marburg, 1843, and Wagner's Handwörterb. d. Physiol., 1844, ii, 637.

[3] Heidenhain: Arch. f. path. Anat., Berl., 1866, xxxv, 158.

[4] Brunton: Proc. Roy. Soc. Med., Lond., 1912, v, Therap. Sect., 139-151.

[5] C. Ustimovitch: Arb. a. d. physiol. Anst. zu Leipz., 1870, v, 217.

[6] Ludwig: Arch. f. Anat., Physiol. u. wissensch. Med., Berl., 1847, 241-302.

[7] Ludwig: Müller's Arch., Berl., 1848, 139-143, 1 pl.

[8] Ludwig and Noll: Zeitschr. f. rat. Med., Heidelb., 1850, ix, 52.

[9] Ludwig, Becher and Rahn: *Ibid.*, 1851, n. F., i, 225-292.

[10] According to his pupil, Czermak.

[11] Ludwig and Thiry: Sitzungs b. d. k.Akad. d. Wissensch., Med.-naturw. Cl., Vienna, 1864, xlix, 2. Abth., 421-454.

[12] Ludwig's Arbeiten (1866), Leipz., 1867, i, 128-149.

time (1867[1]). In 1868, with the same pupil, he found, upon auscultating the heart after ligation of the vena cava, pulmonary artery and vein, and aorta, that the first (systolic) sound is not of valvular origin entirely, but is partly produced by the cardiac muscle.[2] In 1869–70, Lauder Brunton and O. Schmiedeberg began to study the effects of drugs upon the circulation; and in 1871, Schmiedeberg traced the accelerator fibers of the vagus nerve in the dog.[3] In 1871, H. P. Bowditch, experimenting with an excised heart and a frog manometer, showed that the heart muscle always gives a maximal contraction or none at all ("all or nothing"); and Kronecker, investigating fatigue and recovery of muscle, showed that heart muscle cannot be tetanized. In 1871–73, Ludwig, with Dittmar, was the first to localize a vasomotor center (in the medulla oblongata[4]). With Mosso, he made plethysmographic studies on the blood-vessels of the excised kidney (1874); with von Kries, he measured the blood-pressure in the capillaries (1875[5]); with Schmidt-Mülheim, he began to experiment with the injection of peptones into the blood (1880[6]). In 1883, Wooldridge made his important studies on the chemistry of coagulation of the blood, and Conrad Gompertz investigated the arrangement of muscular fibers in the heart (1884). Other important investigations from Ludwig's laboratory were his monograph on the lymphatics (with Schweigger-Seidel, 1872–74[7]); introducing the puncture mode of injection in physiology; Flechsig's investigations of medullated nerve-fibers (1876); Ludwig's study of the digestion of proteids after excision or exclusion of the stomach (with Ogata, 1883[8]), and Bowditch's proof of the non-fatigability of nerve (1890).

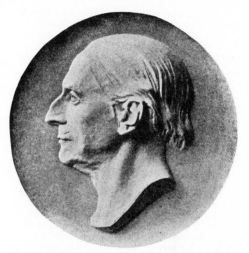

The titles listed give but a faint idea of the immense amount of valuable work done in the Leipzig laboratory, where not a few students, as Burdon Sanderson tells us, "for the first time in their lives came into personal relation with a man who was utterly free from selfish aims and vain ambitions, who was scrupulously conscientious in all that he said and did, who was what he seemed to be and seemed what he was, and who had no other aim than the advancement of his science." "All who met Ludwig," says Kronecker, "came under the influence of his enchanting personality." He lived with his pupils in a "*schöne Gemeinsamkeit*," and was, indeed, in some respects, the personification

Carl Ludwig (medallion). (Courtesy of Professor William Stirling, Manchester, England.

[1] Ludwig's Arbeiten (1866), Leipz., 1867, ii, 196–271.

[2] Ber. d. k. sächs. Gesellsch. d. Wissensch., Leipz., 1868, xx, 89.

[3] Ludwig and Schmiedeberg: *Ibid.*, 1871, xxiii, 148–170.

[4] Ludwig and Dittmar: Ber. d. k. sächs. Gesellsch. d. Wissensch., Leipz., 1871, 135; 1873, 460.

[5] Von Kries: *Ibid.*, 1875, 148.

[6] Arch. f. Physiol., Leipz., 1880, 333.

[7] Die Lymphgefässe der Fascien und Sehnen, Leipz., 1872.

[8] Ludwig and Ogata: Arch. f. Anat. u. Physiol., Leipz., 1883, 89.

of Browning's hawk-nosed, high-cheek-boned, blue-eyed German professor, absolutely sincere and unpretentious, and, however rigorous and
exact in method, captivating every one by his warmth of heart, his
genial sympathy, and the simplicity of his life and aims. Ludwig
was a splendid draftsman, and his mind was of the purely plastic kind,
which visualizes everything as a material phenomenon. For this
reason, he had little use for mathematics, psychology, or any of the
sciences which repose upon a metaphysical basis. He was devoted to
music, however, a great patron of the *Gewandhaus* concerts, and often
had chamber music at his house. The charm of his personality has
been admirably conveyed in the reminiscences of his old pupils,
Kronecker, von Kries, Burdon Sanderson, and William Stirling.

The innervation of the heart was investigated by Henle (1841); by Friedrich
Bidder, who discovered the ganglionic cells at the junction of the auricles and ventricles (1852[1]); by Albert **von Bezold,** who demonstrated the accelerator nerves of
the heart and their origin in the spinal cord (1862); and by Walter Holbrook **Gaskell,**
who showed that the innervation of the heart is the same in cold-blooded and warm-
blooded animals, and that the vagus nerve weakens the heart as well as slows it
(1882–84). A striking experiment upon the heart-beat was made by Hermann
Stannius (1808–83), of Hamburg, who, by placing a ligature at the junction of the
auricle and the sinus venosus, brought the heart to a standstill, while a second ligature, applied to the auriculo-ventricular groove, caused the ventricle to beat again
(1852[2]). In the early days of the neurogenic theory of the heart's action, the effect
of the Stannius ligatures was supposed to be due to inhibition of the ganglia of
Bidder and Remak, but the subject took on a new light with the discovery of the
auriculo-ventricular bundle of His. The pulse was specially studied by Étienne-
Jules **Marey** (1830–1904), who invented the sphygmograph, although the graphic
method in pulse-examination had already been introduced by Karl Vierordt (1855).
Other studies of the pulse were made by Landois, von Kries, and von Frey. Blood-
pressure was especially investigated in Alfred Wilhelm Volkmann's *Die Hæmo-
dynamik nach Versuchen* (1850), by Ludwig Traube (1818–76), who first described
the rhythmic variations in the tone of the vasoconstrictor center (Traube-Hering
waves) in 1865, and by Roy and Adami (1892).

Coagulation of the blood was investigated by Andrew Buchanan, who extracted
the fibrin ferment (1845); and by Alexander Schmidt (1831–94), who gave it its name,
but supposed that coagulation was due to the combination of fibrinogen and serum-
globulin. This error was corrected by Olof Hammarsten (1841–   ), who showed
that coagulation is accomplished by splitting up of the fibrinogen into fibrin and
other substances (1875).

Some of the best modern work on the circulation came from the
Cambridge School of Physiologists, who were all pupils of Sir Michael
Foster (1836–1907). On Huxley's recommendation, Foster became
prælector of physiology at Cambridge in 1870, succeeding to the professorship created in 1883. Here, after a tour of the German laboratories with Sharpey, he made an epoch in teaching which was only excelled
by Ludwig's, and through an unrivaled group of pupils in all branches
of biological science—Balfour (embryology), Liversidge (chemistry),
Milnes Marshall (zoölogy), Sidgwick (animal morphology), Ray (pathology), Francis Darwin (vegetable morphology), Vines (experimental
botany)—apart from the physiological group. Foster collaborated

---

[1] Bidder: Müller's Arch., Berl,. 1852, 163–177.
[2] Stannius: *Ibid.*, 85–100.

with Balfour in "Elements of Embryology" (1874), with J. N. Langley in a book of practical physiology (1876), and in the same year produced his own Text-Book of Physiology, which passed through seven editions and was translated into German, Italian, and Russian. To medical history he contributed his beautiful memoir of Claude Bernard (1899) and the inspiring Lane Lectures on the History of Physiology (1900). His own experimental work was entirely on the heart, in particular his observations on the snail's heart (1859), that any part, separated from the rest will beat rhythmically, and that the heart-beat must be a specific property of general cardiac tissue and not the result of any localized mechanism. Foster's talents as an organizer gradually drew him into an incessant round of public activities. With his entry into Parliament his scientific work ended and he lived forward in his pupils.

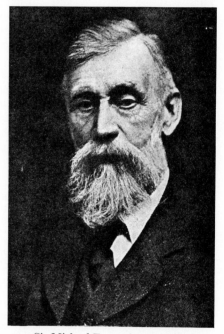

Sir Michael Foster (1836–1907).

Foster's pupils include the embryologist Balfour, Gaskell and Langley, Sherrington, Henry Head, and Charles Scot **Roy** (1854–97), of Arbroath, Scotland, who invented many unique instruments, made important researches on the renal circulation (with Cohnheim), on the extensibility and elasticity of blood-vessels, discovered an automatic rhythmic tonus in the mammalian spleen, devised a successful preventive inoculation against a cattle disease in Argentina, and achieved a great memoir on the mammalian heart (1892) with John George **Adami** (1862–1926), of Manchester, England, another Foster pupil, eminent as the leading pathologist of Canada, and author of important works on cancer, heredity, classification of tumors, and widely known text-books of pathology (1908–12). Among other Foster pupils, A. G. **Dew Smith**, a man of wealth, financed the *Journal of Physiology*, founded by Foster in 1878, and established the Cambridge Scientific Instrument Company, which made the laboratory apparatus.

Henry Newell **Martin** (1848–96), of Newry, Ireland, professor of biology at the Johns Hopkins University (1876–93), carried Foster's methods of teaching into the United States, collaborated with Huxley in his *Elementary Biology* (1875), devised (with W. T. Sedgwick) a method of isolating the mammalian heart for experimentation (1880), studied the effect of variations of blood-pressure and temperature upon the rate of beat of the mammalian heart (1882–83). Martin's pupil and successor, William Henry **Howell** (1860–   ), of Baltimore, Maryland, has investigated such problems as the accelerating effect of increased venous pressure on the heart (1881), the life-history of the blood-corpuscles (1890), blood-serum deprived of proteids as an improvement on Ringer's solution (1893), and the rôle of the "hormones," antithrombin and thromboplastin, in the coagulation of the blood (1911).

The art of keeping animal tissues active extravitally was introduced by Carl Ludwig in his perfusion experiments (Bowditch, 1871), and was perfected by Sydney **Ringer** (1835–1910), of Norwich, England who showed that a frog's heart can be kept beating for long periods of time in a mixture of the chlorides of sodium, potassium, and calcium. This was afterward shown to be equally true of the mammalian heart.[1] Ringer's work signalized the importance of the calcium salts in maintaining tissue activity, and "Ringer's solution," so widely used in physiological experiments, was the culture-medium in which Carrel latterly grew his "visceral organism."

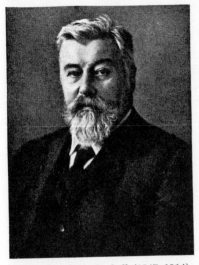

Walter Holbrook **Gaskell** (1847–1914), perhaps Foster's greatest pupil, did the most important work on the heart after Ludwig, and laid the histologic foundations of the modern study of the autonomic nervous system.

During his Cambridge period, Gaskell worked for a while in Ludwig's laboratory (1874) and produced an important paper on the vasomotor nerves of striated muscle (1877[2]). In 1881, he produced his great memoir on the musculature and innervation of the heart,[3] in which it is shown that the motor influences from the nerve ganglia in the sinus venosus influence the rhythm (rate and force) of the heart, but do not originate its movements or beat, which are due to the automatic rhythmic contractile

Walter Holbrook Gaskell (1847–1914). power of the heart-muscle itself and to the peristaltic contraction wave which proceeds from sinus venosus to bulbus arteriosus and from muscle-fiber to muscle-fiber. Following Romanes' experiments upon the bell of Medusa (1875[4]) the zigzag incisions of Gaskell and Engelmann upon extra-vital hearts and isolated strips of heart muscle, containing no nerve tissue, demonstrated the continuity of the rhythmic wave. Gaskell showed it to be reversible by stimulating the ventricle after the second Stannius ligature, proving that the normal peristaltic wave could not have proceeded from the cardiac ganglia. Gaskell introduced the term "heart-block" (from an expression of Romanes) and produced it experimentally, as also fibrillation of the heart and the two-, three-, and four-time gallops of the clinics. These, as also the effects of the Stannius ligatures, and Schiff's observation that the ventricle of a dying heart beats slower than the auricle, Gaskell showed to be simple cases of block. He was the first to investigate the electrical condition of the heart with a galvanometer. Schmiedeberg's observation that stimulation of the vagus after administration of nicotine will hasten the heart (1871), he showed to be a simple case of nicotining the preganglionic inhibitory fibers of the vagus, the switchboard effect across the synapse

---

[1] Ringer: Jour. Physiol., Lond., 1880–87, iii–vii, *passim*.

[2] Gaskell: Proc. Roy. Soc. Lond., 1876–7, xxv, 439–445.

[3] Phil. Tr., Lond., 1882, clxxiii, 933–1033.

[4] Romanes: Phil. Tr., Lond., 1875–6, clxvi, 269–313.

being abolished, and the post-ganglionic accelerator fibers being unaffected by the poison. Thus the true function of the vagus is not inhibitory, but quiescent, integrative, regulative, the nerve acting as whip and bridle, spur and snaffle. In 1886[1] Gaskell produced another vast research on the comparative histology of the nerve-supply of the vascular and visceral systems, mapping out a large part of what Langley more clearly defined as the autonomic or self-governing system. The sympathetic fibers were shown to originate only from the thoracic and lumbar regions of the cord. In 1893, he showed that chloroform lowers blood-pressure by acting directly upon the heart and not on the vasomotor center.[2] The rest of Gaskell's life was devoted to his theory that the central canal of the nervous system was originally the lumen of a primitive gut (1908[3]). His posthumous memoir on *The Involuntary Nervous System* (1916) sums up his lifework.

John Newport **Langley** (1852–1925), of Newbury, who succeeded Foster as professor of physiology at Cambridge (1903), made important investigations on the effects of pilocarpine (1874), and on every aspect of cell changes in secretion (1874–90), showing, in confutation of Heidenhain, that in the process, gland cells do not become more granular, but eliminate some of the granules. In 1889 (with W. L. Dickinson[4]), he showed that upon painting a sympathetic nerve ganglion (Foster's synapse) with nicotine, the passage of nervous impulses across it will be blocked. This was followed by a brilliant series of experiments (1890–1919[5]), which overthrew many current conceptions in regard to the involuntary nervous system, showing that the visceral (oro-anal) system is different in origin from the sympathetic and leading to the classification of the sympathetic and cranio-sacral systems of spinal nerves as "autonomics" for the redistribution of all efferent impulses terminating in smooth (involuntary) muscle. The pupils of Gaskell and Langley include Gowland Hopkins, Elliot Smith, Sir Walter Fletcher, A. V. Hill, Barcroft, Anderson, Rivers, Dale, Lucas, Adrian and Elliott.

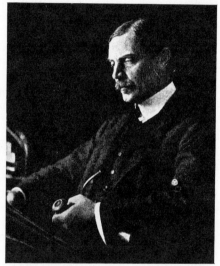

John Newport Langley (1852–1925).

Sir Walter Morley **Fletcher** (1873–   ), of Liverpool, lecturer on natural sciences at Cambridge University (1900–14) and prime mover of many important investigations made in England during the war, is

[1] Jour. Physiol., Lond., 1886, vii, 1–80.

[2] Lancet, Lond., 1893, i, 386.

[3] Gaskell: The Origin of Vertebrates, London, 1908.

[4] Langley and Dickinson: Proc. Roy. Soc. Lond., 1889, xlvi, 423; 1890, xlvii, 379.

[5] See Langley: Lancet, Lond., 1919, i, 951.

36

memorable for his work on intramuscular metabolism (1902–17), particularly lactic-acid formation under anaërobic conditions (with Hopkins, 1907).

Sir Frederick Gowland **Hopkins** (1861–   ), professor of biochemistry in the University of Cambridge (1914), devised a well known method of estimating uric acid in the urine (1892), analyzed tryptophan (with Cole, 1901) and isolated pure glutathione (1921), the nucleus of auto-oxidation in the cell. Experimenting with zein, which contains no tryptophan, he discovered (with Wilcox) that mice will not live long on a diet of zein, carbohydrates and fat, but will continually improve if tryptophan is added (1906). In 1912, he found that a trace of milk added to a deficient diet, ultimately fatal to rats, will immediately bring them up to normal. From findings of this kind, Hopkins argued that certain "accessory factors" in food are necessary to sustain life (1912), the starting-point of subsequent work on vitamine requirements.

John Scott **Haldane** (1860–   ), of Edinburgh, devised the standard apparatus and methods commonly used in gas analysis, gasometry of the blood and estimation of basal metabolism (1892–1918). As director of the Mining Research Laboratory of the University of Birmingham, his investigations of mine explosions, factory ventilation, the cell-storage and expulsion of dusts and the retention of siliceous dust (pneumonokoniosis), have been of great moment to industrial hygiene. His important studies on the chemical regulation of respiration culminated in his expedition to Pike's Peak (1913) in quest of a vitalistic explanation. A staunch and determined vitalist, believing that "life is just life," he was, at the same time, a prime-mover in investigating physiological phenomena by purely chemical means.

Joseph **Barcroft** (1872), of Newry, Ireland, author of an important memoir on the respiratory function of the blood (1914), investigated oxygen consumption in all the tissues (1908–14) and made experiments of fundamental importance on the effects of *mountain sickness* (Cerro de Pasco, 1914) and oxygen deficiency (1920).

Archibald Vivian **Hill** (1886–   ), lecturer on physiology at Cambridge (1919–20) and professor at Manchester (1919–23), has done remarkable work on the thermodynamics of muscle (1909–27), particularly in the invention of instruments (1920–23), estimates of heat production (1911–26), the isometric twitch (with Hartree, 1920–24) and other phases, summarized in his recent book, *Living Machinery* (1927). Recent knowledge of the chemodynamics of muscular contraction is largely due to Embden, Hill and Meyerhof, and to Otto Warburg's quantitative studies of tissue-respiration under aërobic and anaërobic conditions (1908–24). In this field, Keith Lucas (1904–17), Edgar Douglas Adrian (1913–26), W. Hartree (1921–5), and John F. Fulton (1924–6) have also done effective work.

Sir Leonard Erskine **Hill** (1866–   ) has distinguished himself by his work on the cerebral circulation (1896), caisson disease (1912), the effects of humid heat and stuffiness (1910–23) and the physiologic effects of light (1923–7). He is a talented painter and an exhibition of his work was held in London in 1927.

Among Americans who have worked on the circulation are Howell, William Townsend **Porter** (1862–   ), of Plymouth, Ohio, professor of comparative physiology at Harvard University (1906), who helped to found and financed the *American Journal of Physiology* (1898–1915), and is author of a very practical laboratory manual (1900), and of researches on the growth of children (1893–96), the coronary arteries (1893–96), etc.; Henry **Sewall** (1855– .   ), of Winchester, Va., one of Newell Martin's pupils, later professor of medicine in the University of Colorado (1911); Russell **Burton-Opitz** (1875–   ), of Fort Wayne, Ind., who studied the viscosity of the blood (1914), and George Neil **Stewart** (1860–   ), of London, Canada, professor of experimental medicine in the Western Reserve University of Cleveland, Ohio (1907), author of a manual of physiology (1896) and of valuable studies from the H. K. Cushing Laboratory.

One of the greatest physiologists of France was the veterinarian Auguste **Chauveau** (1827–1917), a graduate of the École vétérinaire at Alfort (1839), subsequently director of the Lyons School (1875), where a monument was erected in his memory in 1926. Apart from his treatise on the comparative anatomy of domestic animals (1855–7), his work on the physiology of the heart (with Marey, 1856–64), the thermodynamics of muscular work (1888–91), the cycle of energetic changes in the body (1894), he was abreast of Pasteur in his conception of the nature of pathogenic viruses (1868) and their attenuation (1883–4), and, in detail, attacked all manner of physiological and pathological problems. He was a man of imposing height and presence, not unlike the great novelist Flaubert in appearance.

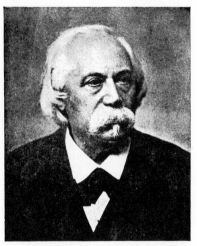

Auguste Chauveau (1827–1917).

Charles **Richet** (1850–   ), of Paris, professor of physiology in the Paris Faculty, introduced the term "anaphylaxis" (1909), and is known for his researches on the gastric juice (1878), the diuretic action of milk and all sugars (1881), the modalities of muscular contraction (1882–3), regulation of animal heat by polypnea (1884–93), his therapeutic innovations of hematotherapy (1888), chloralose (1893), deprivation of chlorides in epilepsy (1900), and zomotherapy (1900), and his dictionary of physiology (1895–1907).

Eugène **Gley** (1857–   ), of Épinal, professor of physiology in the Paris Faculty (1889), demonstrated the existence of iodine in the thyroid gland and the blood, and has done valuable work on the heart muscle (1888), the coagulation of the blood, the effect of drugs, the internal secretions and the pathology of the thyroid gland.

The most important work on **respiration** was done by Eduard

F. W. **Pflüger** (1829–1910), of Hanau-am-Main, a pupil of Johannes Müller and du Bois Reymond, who succeeded Helmholtz as professor of physiology at Bonn in 1859, and held the chair the rest of his life. Under Pflüger, the new Institute of Physiology at Bonn was opened in 1878. In 1868, he founded the famous *Archiv für die gesamte Physiologie* (Pflüger's Archiv), which ran through 130 volumes under his direction, and became the most popular journal of physiology in Germany.

Pflüger early made his mark as a master investigator by his monograph on electrotonus (1859[1]). By his experiments in crossing species (1883) he became the founder of experimental embryology. In his work on metabolism, he opposed the view of Voit that organized (tissue) proteid, in order to undergo metabolism, must first be converted into unorganized (circulating) proteid, maintaining just the opposite view, viz., that proteids can never undergo metabolism or assimilation except in the organized or stationary form; in other words, that proteid metabolism cannot take place until the material is built up into protoplasm. All this turned upon Pflüger's criterion for a proteid, viz., the capacity to maintain life and to enter into the composition of protoplasm, which would, of course, exclude the polypeptides, proteoses, protamins, and the poisonous proteids. Pflüger also made laborious researches to prove that glycogen does not originate from protein material, and, like Pavy, he was forced to surrender his position toward the end of his life. The most effective work of Pflüger and his pupils is the proof that the essential seat of respiration is not in the blood, but in the tissues. This was accomplished in his important memoirs on the gasometry of the blood (1866[2]), on the cause of dyspnea, apnea, and the mechanism of respiration (1868[3]), on the origin and rationale of the oxidative process in the animal organism (1872[4]), and on the heat production and oxidation of living matter (1878[5]). He proved his thesis by showing that frogs, the blood of which had been entirely replaced by normal salt solution, gave off just as much CO_2 and took in just as much oxygen as normal control animals.[6] He invented new physiological instruments, such as the improved mercurial gas-pump (1865), the lung catheter (1872), the aërotonometer (1872), and the pneumonometer (1882).

Pflüger was of a combative disposition, fond of arguing for the sake of argument, and actually believing that science is advanced by vigorous controversy. This has been held to explain his somewhat unreasonable and ill-advised attacks on the neuron theory and on the work of Emil Fischer. He seems to have led the uneventful life of a man devoted exclusively to scientific research. It is said that he spent his last days in bed, correcting the proof-sheets of papers sent to his Archiv.

Lavoisier, as we have seen, showed that respiration and combustion are analogous, and that both are essentially an oxidation with water and carbon dioxide as by-products (1771–80). Hassenfratz showed that the oxygen of the inspired air, being dissolved in the blood, takes up carbon and hydrogen from the tissues. The fact of tissue respiration was demonstrated by Gustav Magnus in 1837, who extracted oxygen and carbon dioxide from both arterial and venous blood by means of a mercurial pump, from which he inferred that these gases are simply dissolved in the blood. Lothar Meyer, working in Ludwig's laboratory (1857) obtained these results

---

[1] Pflüger: Untersuchungen über die Physiologie des Electrotonus, Berlin, 1859.

[2] Centralbl. f. d. med. Wissensch., Berl., 1866, iv, 305–308.

[3] Arch. f. d. ges. Physiol., Bonn., 1868, i, 61–106.

[4] *Ibid.*, 1872, vi, 43, 190.

[5] *Ibid.*, 1878, xviii, 247–380.

[6] *Ibid.*, 1875, x, 251–367.

by the more refined method of heating the blood to extract the gases, and arrived at similar conclusions. Liebig, however, had pointed out (1851) that the blood gases were probably in loose combination with some unknown substance, and this substance Hoppe-Seyler subsequently obtained in crystalline form as hemoglobin (1862–64). The discovery of Sir George Gabriel Stokes that oxygen can be removed from hemoglobin by reducing agents proved that the latter is the agent of combination (1864). The combining agency of the CO_2 is still obscure. The extraction of gases from the blood has been further refined by means of the improved mercurial gas-pumps of Ludwig and Setchenoff (1859), Pflüger (1865), Grehant, and Leonard Hill (1895). The other gas of the blood, nitrogen, was shown to be in a state of simple solution by Lothar Meyer (1857), Pflüger (1864–68), and Paul Bert (1878). The spirometer was invented by John Hutchinson of Newcastle-on-Tyne in 1844.[1] The difficult subject of the metabolism in respiration was investigated by Pettenkofer and Voit (1863), Zuntz (1880), Atwater and Rosa (1899), and Atwater and Benedict (1905). Angelo **Mosso** introduced the concept acapnia (1897) and studied the physiology of respiration in man (1903), at Monte Rosa (1897). At his Institute on the Colle d'Olen (1908), he studied the physiology of respiration at altitudes above the snow line. The proof of Paul Bert that high altitude symptoms are due to imperfect oxygenation of the blood (1878) was apparently contravened by Mosso's acapnia theory (deficiency of CO_2 in the blood), but was finally reëstablished by E. Rippstein's experiments in Kronecker's laboratory (1917) and by subsequent work on oxygen requirements of aviators.

The action of the intercostal muscles in respiration was first investigated by Haller, and, in geometric manner, by G. E. Hamberger (1748). The latter's view was confirmed experimentally by Henry Newell Martin and Edward M. Hartwell at the Johns Hopkins University (1879). The action of the vagus on respiration was first investigated by Isidor Rosenthal (1864), who showed that section of both vagi is always followed by deeper, slower breathing, while the amount of air taken in in unit time is the same as before. He held that the vagus contains two sets of fibers —one to contract the diaphragm, the other to relax it. In 1868, Ewald Hering and Breuer showed, by alternate closure of the trachea at the end of inspiration and expiration, that the mechanism of breathing is automatic and self-regulative, the distention and contraction of the lungs being, in themselves, a normal stimulus of the vagi, the effect which Rosenthal had obtained by stimulation of the divided nerve.

In 1889,[2] Henry **Head,** of London, working in Hering's laboratory at Prague, carried these experiments much further by such novel means as freezing the nerve or etherizing it inside a rubber tube. The sense of his investigations is that the vagus acts like the governor of a steam engine in economizing the energies of respiration, preventing the center in the medulla from wearing itself out. This was shown by section of the vagi, which produced a condition of "spendthrift activity" in the respiratory center.

Normally, each inspiration stimulates the fibers which eventually inhibit it, and, at each expiration, the collapse of the lungs stimulates the inspiratory fibers, thus keeping up a steady automatic rate of respiration, which is largely due to the inhibitory fibers in the vagus. Head, the present editor of *Brain*, has also done most important work on the cutaneous distribution of pain and tenderness in visceral disease (1893–96[3]), showing that the segmentation of the cutaneous areas affected by the different viscera (Head's zones) corresponds strikingly with those belonging to the root ganglia of the spinal nerves. With A. W. Campbell, he showed that herpes zoster is a hemorrhagic inflammation of the posterior nerve-roots and the homologous cranial ganglia (1900[4]). In April, 1903,[5] he submitted to the unique experiment of

---

[1] Hutchinson: Lancet, Lond., 1844, i, 390, 567. Also, Med.-Chir. Tr., Lond., 1845–6, xxix, 234–238, giving three cuts of the spirometer.

[2] Head: J. Physiol., Lond., 1889, x, 1, 279.

[3] Brain: Lond., 1893, xvi, 1; 1894, xvii, 339; 1896, xix, 153.

[4] *Ibid.*, 1900, xxiii, 353–523, 17 pl.

[5] *Ibid.*, 1908, xxxi, 323–450.

division of his own left radial and external cutaneous nerves, in order to study the loss and restoration of sensation, which led to a new classification of the sensory paths. Subsequent studies (1905–18[1]) cover the whole mechanism of sensation from the peripheral nerves inward to the brain, including the classification of peripheral afferent fibers, as to sensation, the grouping of afferent impulses within the cord, the "mass reflex" on complete section of the cord, the termination of secondary paths of sensation in the optic thalamus, and the limitations of sensation when these impulses are redistributed to the cortex.

The ventilatory functions of the diaphragm have been investigated by Charles F. Hoover (1865–1927), of Cleveland, Ohio (1913–17).

Even before Pflüger, respiration of the tissues had been carefully investigated by Felix **Hoppe-Seyler** (1825–95), of Freiburg (Saxony), who is the greatest physiological chemist between Liebig and Emil Fischer.

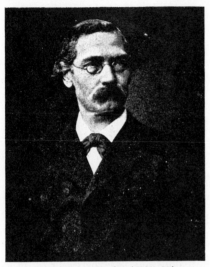

Hoppe-Seyler studied under the three Webers, Skoda, and Virchow, was Virchow's assistant in the Pathological Institute at Berlin (1856–64), professor of applied chemistry at Tübingen (1864–72), and professor of physiological chemistry at Strassburg (1872–95). He was founder of the *Zeitschrift für physiologische Chemie* (1877–95); also the author of a handbook of chemical analysis applied to physiology and pathology (1858), and an epoch-making treatise on physiological chemistry (1877–81). In 1854, he made investigations of the physics of percussion and auscultation, correcting certain errors of Skoda, and he also did some important work in inorganic chemistry and mineralogy.

Felix Hoppe-Seyler (1825–95).

Hoppe-Seyler is particularly remembered by his studies on the blood (1857–91), of which he made analyses for over thirty years. He first obtained hemoglobin in crystalline form, described the spectrum of oxyhemoglobin (1862), first ascertained the formulas of hemin, hematin, and hematoporphyrin (1863), discovered hemochromogen and methemoglobin (1864), and showed that hemoglobin is loosely combined with oxygen, but cannot be separated from CO_2. He also made studies in metabolism, and constructed an apparatus for measuring gaseous interchanges. He was the first to observe the appearance of gas in the blood following a sharp and sudden fall of the atmospheric pressure. His investigations of pus and of pathological transudates led to the discovery of nuclein by his pupil Miescher, and of paranuclein by Lubavin. He first obtained lecithin in the pure state, and introduced the term "proteids." He investigated the chemistry of cartilage, and, in his laboratory, glycosamin was discovered by Ledderhose (1876) and chitosan by himself. He made important analyses of milk, bile,

---

[1] H. Head (*et al.*): Studies in Neurology, London, 1920.

and urine, investigated the chemical products of fermentation, especially in yeast, and his study of chlorophyll was the starting-point of Ehrlich's work on the dynamics of the cell periphery. Personally, he seems to have been an attractive man, of happy, genial disposition.

Of his many pupils, Albrecht **Kossel** (1853–1927), of Rostock, professor of physiology at Marburg (1892–1901) and at Heidelberg (1901–1927), is to be remembered for his important work on the chemistry of the cell and its nucleus (1882–96), on nucleinic acid (1893), on albuminoids (1898), the discovery of adenin (1885), thymin (1894), thymic acid, histidin (1896), and agmatin, for his classification of the proteids, his studies of the fundamental units (*Bausteine*), of the protein molecule, and of the substitution products of albuminoids. He made important investigations in the chemistry of metabolism, and received the Nobel prize for medicine in 1910.

Ernst **Salkowski** (1844–1923), of Königsberg, professor of medical chemistry at Berlin (1874), author of a treatise on the urine (with W. Leube) and a laboratory manual of physiological and pathological chemistry (1893), made the important discoveries of pathological excretion of phenol (1876), pentosuria (1892–5), peptonuria (1897), a quantitative test for oxaluria (1899), employed the antiseptic properties of chloroform in studying fermentation (1888), used his discovery of phytosterin in vegetable fat in detecting adulteration of animal

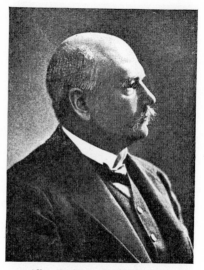

Albrecht Kossel (1853–1927).

fat, and made memorable investigations in digestion, the oxidizing power of the blood, putrefaction, and urinary chemistry.

The **physiological chemistry** of the 19th century was rich in the discovery of new compounds, notably in the analysis and formulation of the decomposition products of proteids at the hands of Paul Schützenberger and others.

After Kirchhoff had effected the hydrolysis of starch by diastase (1815), Braconnot (1820) first hydrolyzed proteins by acids and discovered glycin, the simplest form of proteid. Of the amino-acid constituents of proteins (Kossel's *Bausteine*), cystin was found in calculi by Wollaston (1810), and shown to be a decomposition product of protein by K. A. H. Mörner (1899); tyrosin was discovered by Liebig (1846) and Hinterberger (1849), glycocoll (1848) and alanin (1849) by Strecker, serin by Cramer (1865), phenylalanin by Schulze and Barbieri (1879–81), histidin by Kossel (1896), while tryptophan was named as a hypothetical product by Neumeister (1890), and isolated by Gowland Hopkins and Cole (1901). Leucin was discovered in putrefying cheese by Proust (1818), named by Braconnot (1820), and isolated by Hinterberger (1849). Both leucin and tyrosin were found in the pancreas after death by Virchow (1853), and in the living body by Frerichs (1855). Glutamic acid was isolated by Ritthausen (1866) and Kreutzer (1871), aspartic acid by Kreusler (1869), Radziejewski and Salkowski (1873), ornithin by Jaffé (1877), glutaminic acid by Horbaczewski (1879) and Fränkel (1913), arginin by Schulze and Steiger (1886) and Hedin (1895), lysin by Drechsel (1889), prolin by Willstätter (1900) and Emil Fischer (1901), cysteine by Embden (1901), diaminobutyric acid (1901), oxyprolin (1902), serin (1902) and valin (1906) by Emil Fischer (1901–02), isoleucin by F. Ehrlich (1903), norleucine by Abderhalden and Weil (1913), hydroxylglutaminic acid by Dakin (1918), hydroxylysine and oxyvalin by Schryver and Buston (1925).

The effect of animal enzymes on proteids was studied by Willy Kühne, Kossel, Drechsel, and others. Schulze investigated the effect of vegetable enzymes. Drechsel discovered that the protein molecule contains di- as well as mono-amino acids, and these were investigated by Kossel, Kutscher, and Emil Fischer. In 1881, Schmiedeberg extracted histozyme, a ferment which will disintegrate or synthetize hippuric acid. The nucleins were investigated by Worm Müller (1873) and Miescher (1874); the nucleic acids by Kossel (1893), Altmann (1889), Abderhalden, and Schittenhelm (1906); the albuminoids by Kossel (1898), Drechsel (1891), and Abderhalden (1905). β-oxybutyric acid was isolated by Eduard Külz (1884–87), and investigated in relation to diabetes by Ernst Stadelmann (1883) and Adolf Magnus-Levy (1899–1909). Acetone was discovered in diabetic urine by Wilhelm Petters (1857), and investigated by Carl Gerhardt (1865), Rudolf von Jaksch (1885), and, in the blood, by Adolf Kussmaul (1874). Max Jaffé (1841–1911) discovered urobilin in the intestinal contents (1871) and indican in the urine (1877). Ehrlich introduced his diazo-reaction in 1882. Cryoscopy of the urine was introduced by Sandor Korányi in 1894. Myelopathic albumosuria (proteinuria) was described by Henry Bence-Jones in 1848; acetonuria and diaceturia by von Jaksch (1885), and pentosuria by Ernst Salkowski (1895). The tests of Johann Kjeldahl for estimation of nitrogen in organic matter (1883), of Otto Folin for estimating urea and uric acid, of Gowland Hopkins for urea, of Franz Soxhlet for fats in milk, have all proved of great practical value. The ptomaines were investigated by Selmi, Gautier, Brieger,

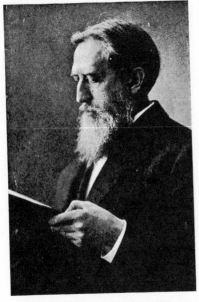

Ernst Salkowski (1844–1923).

Vaughan and Novy. Naegeli's great memoir on the starches (1874), classifying some 200, was followed by the remarkable monographs of Edward T. Reichert on hemoglobin (1911) and starches (1915) as a basis for investigation of biochemical problems (1919). The theory of the open carbon chain and the closed benzene ring was stated by August Kekulé in 1865,[1] developed by van't Hoff and LeBel, and brilliantly applied to the structural theory of chlorophyll by Hoppe-Seyler, and to the "side-chain" theory of immunity by Paul Ehrlich.

The laws of physical chemistry were applied to the physiology of muscles by Julius Bernstein (1902–08), to the question of surface tension by Isidor Traube (1910–11) and Macallum (1910–11), and to various biologic problems by Jacques Loeb. The theory of osmosis and of semi-permeable membranes was investigated by Dutrochet (1827–35), Graham (1854–61), Moritz Traube (1867), Willard Gibbs (1876), van't Hoff and Arrhenius (1887), and H. J. Hamburger (1902–04), and colloids were studied by Graham, Siedentopf, and Zsigmondy.

Almost every great teacher of the subject has written a treatise on physiology. To the early period belong those of Magendie (1816–17), H. Mayo (1827), Joh.

---

[1] For the history of benzol, see A. F. Hollemann: Janus, Amst., 1915, xx, 459–488.

Müller (1834–40), Rudolf Wagner (1838–42), W. B. Carpenter (1842), G. Valentin (1844, 1846), the many editions of Senhouse Kirke's *Handbook* (1848), F. C. Donders (1850), F. A. Longet (1850), and Wagner's *Handwörterbuch* (1842–53). In the second half of the century, we have those of Carl Ludwig (1852–56), J. C. Dalton (1859), W. Wundt (1865), T. H. Huxley (1866), Austin Flint, Jr. (1866–74), Sir Michael Foster (1877), L. Landois (1879–80), W. Stirling (1888), A. D. Waller (1891), E. H. Starling (1892), Max Verworn (1863–1921) (1895), G. N. Stewart (1896), Robert Tigerstedt (1898), L. Luciani (1898–1903), W. H. Howell (1905), M. Duval and E. Gley (1906), H. Zwaardemaker (1910), M. von Frey (1911), and Russell Burton-Opitz (1920). Foster's book is a masterpiece. The "Textbook" edited by Sir Edward Schäfer on the coöperative plan (London, 1898), is remarkable for its wonderful assemblage of historical data, in respect of which it has been likened to Haller's great *Elementa* of 1757–66. The treatise of the late Luigi Luciani (1840–1919), Englished in 1811–17, is also valuable for its historical quality. Of American treatises, that of William H. Howell (1905) is incomparably the best, on account of its clean-cut, lucid presentation of what is known. The recent treatise on general physiology of W. M. Bayliss (1916, 4 ed., 1924) is conceived from the viewpoint of physical chemistry and, with its pleasant, pottering manner and its superb bibliography, is, at the same time, one of the best historical presentations of recent physiology as yet published.

The rise of modern medicine is inseparably connected with the name of Rudolf **Virchow** (1821–1902), the founder of **cellular pathology.** A native of Schievelbein in Pomerania, Virchow graduated at Berlin in 1843, became Froriep's prosector at the Charité in 1845, full prosector in 1846, and, in 1847, founded the *Archiv für pathologische Anatomie*, known everywhere as Virchow's Archiv. His first paper in this periodical advanced the idea that an unproved hypothesis of any kind is a very leaky bottom for practical med-

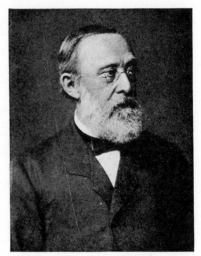

Rudolf Virchow (1821–1902). (Courtesy of Dr. George M. Kober.)

icine to sail or trade upon, and scouted the notion that any one man is infallible in respect of judgment or knowledge. It is one of the strongest manifestos of the modern spirit in recent medicine. In 1848, Virchow was sent by the Prussian government to investigate the epidemic of typhus or "famine" fever then raging among the weavers of Upper Silesia. His exhaustive account of what he saw reminds us of the piling up of horrors in Gerhart Hauptmann's social drama of "Die Weber," and his recommendations included not only hygienic measures and a large charity for these unfortunates, but filed an actual brief for democracy and freedom (*"volle und unumschränkte Demokratie . . . Bildung mit ihren Töchtern, Freiheit und Wohlstand"*). This bold pronouncement, along with the tendencies of his semipolitical periodical, *Die medizinische Reform* (1848–9), soon got Virchow into trouble with the governmental authorities, and, in 1849, he was deprived of his prosectorship, obtaining, at the same time, through the offices of the obstetrician Scanzoni, the chair of pathologic anatomy at Würzburg. Seven years later, after making a brilliant record as lecturer and teacher, he was asked to come back to Berlin upon honorable terms, and, in 1856, was duly installed as professor of pathology at that University, at the same time assuming the directorship of the Pathological Institute, which had been erected for him. Here he entered upon a career of almost unparalleled activity in many directions. He was a man of wide culture and deepest human interests, and he soon became known everywhere as anatomist and pathologist, epidemiologist and sanitarian, anthropologist and archeologist, editor and teacher, social reformer and "old parliamentary hand." He joined the Prussian Lower House in 1862, and from 1880 until 1893 he served in the Reichstag as a faithful and reliable representative of the rights of the people. During the Franco-Prussian War, he organized the Prussian Ambulance Corps and superintended the erection of the army hospital on the Tempelhof. He had much to do with securing a good sewage system for Berlin, and, as president of many different societies, he became easily the most influential medical personality in the Prussian capital. As he grew older, honors came to him from all quarters, and, in 1899, he dedicated the Pathological Museum, to which he gave his private collection of 23,066 preparations; each of which had been prepared, labeled, and placed upon the shelves by his own hand. On his eightiest birthday he received a purse of 50,000 marks from his German colleagues, in aid of the Virchow Institute, with a unique gold medal from the Emperor, and shortly before his death he saw the completion of the splendid municipal hospital in Berlin (January 15, 1902) which is now called by his name.

Virchow derived the inspiration for his life-work from Johannes Müller, and what he accomplished was in every way worthy of his great teacher. In pathology, he had only Morgagni as a possible competitor before him and no one after him. His *Cellular-Pathologie* (1858) set in motion a new way of looking at the body as "a cell-state in which every cell is a citizen," disease being "merely a conflict of citizens in this state, brought about by the action of external forces." Virchow's aphorism *Omnis cellula e cellula*, means that cell development is not discontinuous (as Schleiden and Schwann had supposed), and that there are no specific cells in disease, but only modifications of physiologic types. In other words, "A new growth of cells presupposes already existing cells." This morphologic view is the basis of his work on tumors (1863–67[1]), which treats of these formations as physiologically independent new-growths of either histioid or cellular structure. The two most prominent errors in the cellular pathology were the theories that the cell-contents are the controlling feature of the whole organism, and that there can be no diapedesis of blood-cells, which was afterward disproved by Cohnheim.

---

[1] Virchow: Die krankhaften Geschwülste, Berlin, 1863–67.

Virchow was the first to observe and define leukocytosis, and in 1845, simultaneously with the clinical record of John Hughes Bennett, he described leukemia as "white blood,"[1] In 1846, he separated pyemia from septicemia, and between the years 1846 and 1856 created the doctrine of embolism,[2] his greatest single achievement in pathology, and one which is, in every sense, his very own. Before Virchow, as we have seen, both John Hunter and Cruveilhier saw thrombosis and pyemia as a sequel of phlebitis. Virchow revolutionized existing knowledge by showing that a thrombus is the essential primary condition in phlebitis. His studies of embolism were based upon experiment, and he was the first to recognize the cerebral and pulmonary varieties. In 1856, he demonstrated the embolic nature of the arterial plugs in malignant endocarditis, and attributed the condition to parasites. As a parasitologist, he also did good work on trichinosis (1859–70), and discovered the sarcinic and aspergillic forms of mycosis in the lungs and bronchial tubes. He also pointed out the true relationship between lupus and tuberculosis, introduced new pathological concepts such as agenesia, heteropopia, ochronosis, and first described leontiasis ossea, hematoma of the dura mater, the aortic hypoplasia with contracted heart in chlorotic maidens (1872) and spina bifida occulta (1875). In 1861, he gave the name "arthritis deformans" to rheumatic gout. In histology, he made two important discoveries—the neuroglia (1846[3]) and the special lymphatic sheaths of the cerebral arteries (1851). He made hundreds of contributions to anthropology (his special hobby), from the great atlas of *Crania Ethnica Americana*, prepared "in memory of Columbus and the Discovery of America" (1892), to well-known papers upon racial characters and abnormities, anthropometry, physical anthropology of the Germans, prehistoric finds, prehistoric syphilis, tattooing, and relics of the Trojan War. To medical history he contributed valuable monographs on the leprosoria and other hospitals in the Middle Ages, biographical studies of Morgagni, Johannes Müller, and Schönlein, and he was the first to write upon medicine in relation to the fine arts (1861[4]), but this tiny contribution was surpassed in the same year by the exhaustive monograph of K. F. H. Marx, in which nearly all the important pictures relating to medicine are already classified and listed.[5]

Personally, Virchow was a small, elastic, professorial figure, with snappy, black eyes, quick in mind and body, with a touch of the Slav, something of a martinet in the morgue or lecture-room, often transfixing inattention or incompetence with a flash of sarcasm. Yet he was generous, whole-souled, and broad-minded withal, and none who "made good" was ever lost from sight or memory.[6] In extreme old age, Virchow, always "liberal in politics," became "reactionary in science"; but love of truth, generosity in word and deed, were the essence of his youth and mature manhood. All his life he had been keen and ardent in controversy. He began his career by giving Rokitansky's theory of "crases" a wholesale slashing, with the result that the Viennese pathologist withdrew all reference to the matter from the second edition of his book and never afterward referred to it again. Yet there is no finer tribute in literature to the best features of Rokitansky's work than Virchow's. Then came his disputes with Hughes Bennett about leukemia, and his destruction of the Cruveilhier

---

[1] Froriep's Neue Notizen a. d. Geb. d. Nat. u. Heilk., Weimar, 1845, xxxvi, 151–155.

[2] Beitr. z. exper. Path. (Traube), Berl., 1846, ii, 227–380, and Virchow: Ges. Abhandl., Frankf. a. M., 1856, 219–732.

[3] Virchow's Arch. f. path. Anat., Berl., 1854, vi, 135–138.

[4] Virchow's Arch., Berl., 1861, xxii, 190–192.

[5] Marx: Ueber die Beziehungen der darstellenden Kunst zur Heilkunst. Abhandl. d. k. Gesellsch. d. Wissensch. zu Göttingen, 1861-2, x, 3–74.

[6] Virchow's pupils include Cohnheim, Recklinghausen, Johann Orth (1847–1923).

dogma that phlebitis is the whole of pathology. At the same time, he was cheerfully encouraging Cohnheim to combat the Virchow hypothesis of the non-migration of blood-cells. Believing that the nervous system is not the center of life and does not control the nutrition of peripheral parts, Virchow declined to see anything in Charcot's ataxic joint symptoms but a simple local lesion. He believed in the duality of tuberculosis. He opposed the Darwinian theory; and the new views of Koch and Behring about toxins and antitoxins were hardly acceptable to one who had obliterated the humoral pathology. The peculiarities of the Neanderthal skull were wrongly attributed by Virchow to the

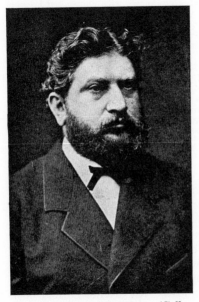

Julius Cohnheim (1839–84). (Collection of A. C. Klebs.)

effects of disease. An accidental shelling of the Muséum d'histoire naturelle in Paris, during the war of 1870–71, led Quatrefages to write an indignant pamphlet stating that the Prussians were not a Germanic, but a barbaric, destructive Mongol race. This stirred Virchow's patriotism to the extent of instigating a colossal public census of the color of the hair and eyes in 6,000,000 German school-children, the solemn official character of which frightened some of the children out of their wits. The sight of a copy of Grimmelshausen's "Simplicissimus" is said to have caused him the same moral indignation which Wordsworth experienced when he saw the first line of Keats' "Ode to a Grecian Urn." These vagaries may be set off by the generosity of his touching defense of Pasteur, his discriminating tribute to the American Army Medical Department, or the laurel-wreaths of praise which he has laid upon the tombs of so many of his predecessors and contemporaries. Above all, he was, in respect of civic courage, an ideal modern man. He did not believe in a characterless, stock-jobbing bourgeoisie, but warmly espoused the cause of those who labor for the common good of all. His lifelong championship of the rights of industrial humanity, valiantly upheld in the very stronghold of the Prussian military government, shows the kind of fiber he was made of.

Of Virchow's pupils, the most eminent was Julius **Cohnheim** (1839–84), of Demmin, Pomerania, who, after serving as a Prussian army surgeon in the Austrian War (1864–65), became an assistant in the Pathological Institute, and was subsequently professor of pathology at Kiel (1868–72), Breslau (1872–78), and Leipzig (1878–84). Under

Willy Kühne, Cohnheim made an important investigation on the sugar-forming ferments (1863[1]), but his inaugural dissertation on the inflammation of serous membranes (1861) marks his bent as a pioneer in experimental histology and pathology.

He introduced the method of freezing fresh preparations in microscopical work, investigated the nerve-endings in muscle by means of silver salts (1863–65), discovered the mosaic fields in cross-sections of muscle which bear his name (1865), and first used gold salts, with brilliant results, in his studies of the sensory nerve-endings in the cornea (1867). His monographs on inflammation and suppuration (1867–73[2]) revolutionized pathology, showing, in direct opposition to the teaching of Virchow, that the essential feature of inflammation is the passage of white blood-cells through the walls of the capillaries, and that pus and pus-cells are formed in this way from the blood. Diapedesis had already been described by Addison (Goulstonian lectures, 1849), but Cohnheim's experiments traced the direct migration of the stained leukocytes to a center of inflammation in the cornea. Valuable papers on venous stasis (1867) and on the relation of the terminal arteries to embolic processes (1872) followed.

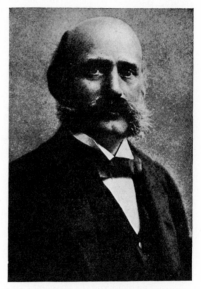

Carl Weigert (1845–1904).

The summit of Cohnheim's experimental achievement was his successful inoculation of tuberculosis in the anterior chamber of the eye of the rabbit (1877[3]), which Weigert wittily described as a demonstration *"in oculo ad oculos."* Two years before, Robert Koch had demonstrated his cultures of anthrax bacillus, and Cohnheim made the prophetic statement that Koch would surpass all others in this field. The last years of Cohnheim's life were clouded by severe complications of gout, an old enemy, and his brilliant career was cut short at the early age of forty-five. He is described as a man of robust, cheerful, energetic disposition, swift and sure of speech, with great powers of wit and sarcasm. Among his pupils were Heidenhain, Litten, Lichtheim, Welch, Ehrlich, Neisser, and Weigert at Breslau, and, at Leipzig, Roy and Councilman.

Carl **Weigert** (1845–1904), of Münsterberg, Silesia, is memorable for his investigations of the pathological anatomy of smallpox (1874–75[4]), and Bright's disease (1879[5]), and by the fact that he was the first

---

[1] Cohnheim: Arch. f. path. Anat. (etc.), Berl., 1863, xxvii, 241–253.

[2] Cohnheim: Neue Untersuchungen über die Entzündung, Berlin, 1873.

[3] Die Tuberkulose vom Standpunkte der Infektionslehre, Leipzig, 1880.

[4] Weigert: Anatomische Beiträge zur Lehre von den Pocken, Breslau, 1874–75.

[5] Weigert: Samml. klin. Vorträge, Leipz., 1879, Nos. 162, 163 (Innere Med., No. 55, 1411–1460).

to stain bacteria (1871[1]), in which he later had great success with anilin colors (1875[2]). He introduced many improvements in the differential staining of the nervous system, notably with acid fuchsin (1882). He also made investigations of the neuroglia (1890–95), and of coagulation-necrosis (1880), described tuberculosis of the veins (1882), and stated the well-known quantitative "law" that the amount of repair in an injured tissue is always in excess of what is needed.

Among the special pathological studies of the period were those of Ludwig Traube (1855), Hermann Senator (1873), Carl von Liebermeister (1875), and Ernst von Leyden (1870–79) on the pathology of fever, Peter Ludwig **Panum** (1820–85) on the experimental pathology of embolism (1863–64), Thomas Bevill **Peacock** on malformations of the human heart (1866), Carl Thiersch on phosphoric necrosis of bones (1867), Wilhelm Waldeyer on the development of cancer (1867–72), F. D. von **Recklinghausen** on adenomyoma and neurofibroma (1882), Paul **Grawitz** on the origin of renal tumors from suprarenal tissues (1884), Julius **Wolff** on the law of transformation in bones (1892), Paul Ehrlich and Adolf Lazarus on anemia (1898). Among Americans, William Pepper (1843–98), described the changes in the bone-marrow in pernicious anemia (1875), William Henry **Welch** (1850–   ) investigated acute edema of the lungs (1877) and embolism and thrombosis (1899), Reginald Heber **Fitz** (1843–1913), gave conclusive demonstrations of the pathology of perforating inflammation of the vermiform appendix (1886), hemorrhagic pancreatitis with fat necrosis (1889), and described intrapleural lipoma of the mediastinum; Francis **Delafield** (1841–1915), of New York, author of a handbook of pathology (1872), *Studies in Pathological Anatomy* (1878–91), and (with T. Mitchell **Prudden**) of a text-book of pathology (1885), which passed through ten editions, made special studies of the pathologic histology of nephritis and pneumonia. Martin H. **Fischer** (1879–   ), of Cincinnati, has made experimental studies of edema (1910) and nephritis (1912).

Following the 18th-century works of Astruc (1743), Gaub (1758), Morgagni (1761), Matthew Baillie (1791), and Kurt Sprengel (1795–97), pathology was the subject of special treatises by Carl Friedrich Burdach (1808), J. W. H. Conradi (1811), A.-F. Chomel (1817), E. D. A. Bartels (1819), J. C. C. F. M. Lobstein (1829–33), Herbert Mayo (1836), and Thomas Hodgkin (1836–40). The first exhaustive treatise on pathology in English was that of Samuel David Gross (Boston, 1839), which was followed by the treatises of Rokitansky (1842–46), Jacob Henle (1846–51), Alfred Stillé (1848), Salvatore De Renzi (1856), Virchow (1858), Samuel Wilks (1859), P. Uhle and E. Wagner (1862), Eduard Rindfleisch (1867–69), Victor Cornil and L. Ranvier (1869–76), T. H. Green (1871), F. V. Birch-Hirschfeld (1876), Cohnheim (1877–80), Ernst Ziegler (1881), Sims Woodhead (1883), Henri Hallopeau (1884), Francis Delafield and T. Mitchell Prudden (1885), Edwin Klebs (1887), D. J. Hamilton (1889–94), V. V. Podwyssotsky (1891–94), Anton Weichselbaum (1892), Ludolf Krehl (1893), Otto Bollinger (1896–97), Alfred Stengel (1898), Harvey R. Gaylord and Ludwig Aschoff (1901), Ludwig Hektoen and David Riesman (1901–02), Guido Banti (1905–07), and John George Adami (1908–12). Noteworthy atlases of pathological illustration are those of Johann Friedrich Meckel (1817–26), Jean Cruveilhier (1829–42), Alexander Auvert (1856), F. A. Thierfelder (1872–81), The Sydenham Society (1877–1906), Alfred Kast and Theodor Rumpel (1892–97), and Paul Grawitz (1893). The outstanding treatise in this list is the text-book (1881) of Ernst Ziegler (1849–1905), which has passed through many revised editions and translations. Ziegler founded the famous *Beiträge zur pathologischen Anatomie* (Jena, 1886) and a *Centralblatt* (Jena, 1890). After his death, Ziegler's *Beiträge* was edited by Felix Marchand and Ludwig Aschoff (1905–28) and became the leading repository of full length *Arbeiten* in Germany. It was followed by the *Journal of Pathology and Bacteriology* (Edinburgh, 1892) founded by Sir German Sims Woodhead (1855–1921), the *Frankfurter Zeitschrift für Pathologie* (Munich, 1907) founded by Eugen Albrecht (1872–1908) in memory of Senckenburg and the Genoese *Pathologica* (1908). Important works on experimental pathology are those of Ludwig Traube (1871–78), Claude Bernard (1872), Salomon Stricker (1877), Victor Paschutin (1885), and Paul

---

[1] Centralbl. f. d. med. Wissensch., Berl., 1871, ix, 609–611.

[2] Jahresb. d. schles. Gesellsch. f. vaterl. Cultur, 1875, Bresl., 1876, liii, 229.

Ehrlich (1909). The monographs of August Hirsch (1860–64), Andrew Davidson (1892), and Frank G. Clemow (1903) on geographical pathology, John William Ballantyne (1861–1923) on fetal pathology (1902–4), F. B. Mallory and J. H. Wright on pathological technic (1897) deserve mention.

The founders of **bacteriology** were Louis Pasteur and Robert Koch, the former being also the pioneer of modern preventive inoculation against disease, while to the latter we owe the development of the correct theory of specific infectious diseases.

Before the time of Pasteur, Leeuwenhoek had seen protozoa (1675) and bacteria (1687) under the microscope. Agostino Bassi (1773–1856) showed that silkworm disease is due to the presence of microörganisms (1836), John Goodsir described sarcinæ in the stomach (1842) and Otto Friedrik Müller was the first to classify bacteria (1773) and protozoa (1786), which Linnæus had lumped together under the vague genus Chaos (1758). C. F. von Gleichen first attempted to stain them with indigo and carmine (1778), which method was pursued by C. G. Ehrenberg (1795–1876), in his great atlas, *Die Infusionsthierchen* (1838), with a more elaborated classification, which included *Vibrio, Spirillum* and *Spirochæta*. This was modified by F. Dujardin (1841) who set up the three genera, *Bacterium, Vibrio* and *Spirillum*. C. W. von Nägeli put all the colorless forms into the group *Schizomycete* (1849). Cultivation on solid media (potato) was first employed by Fresenius (1863), Hoffmann (1869), and Schröter (1875), who first identified bacteria by their cultural characteristics. Ferdinand Julius **Cohn** (1828–98) introduced the first morphological classification of bacteria (1870–75), which held the field for a long time. His discovery of spores in Bacillus subtilis (1876) was followed by Koch's work on anthrax (1876), preceded by that of Casimir Davaine (1863). Before the time of Koch, Kircher (1658), Plenciz (1762), and Henle (1840) had announced the theory of a

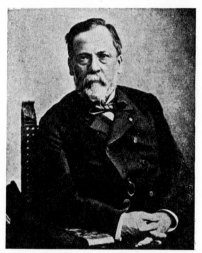

Louis Pasteur (1822–95).

contagium animatum, Hermann Klencke had shown that tuberculosis may be transmitted by cow's milk (1846), Jean-Antoine Villemin (1827–92) had demonstrated that the tubercular virus is specific and inoculable, in a series of masterly experiments (1868) which were confirmed by the further investigations of Edwin Klebs (1873), L.-A. Thaon and J.-J. Grancher (1873), and Julius Cohnheim (1880).

Louis **Pasteur** (1822–95) was born at Dôle (Jura), where his father, one of Napoleon's old soldiers, was a local tanner. As a youth, Pasteur was remarkably good at portrait sketching, but was otherwise only a harmless, enthusiastic fisherman. Awakening to the call of duty, he went to study at Besancon, where he acquired his interest in chemistry, and graduated at the Ecole normale at Paris in 1847.

After this he was successively professor of physics at the Lyceum at Dijon (1848), professor of chemistry (1852–54) at the University of Strassburg, dean and professor of chemistry in the Faculty of Sciences at Lille (1854–57), director [of scientific studies at the École normale at Paris (1857–63), professor of geology and chemistry at the École des beaux-arts (1863–67), professor of chemistry at the Sorbonne (1867–89), and director of the Institut Pasteur (1889–95).

As set forth in the inscriptions on the arches over his tomb, Pasteur is memorable for his work on molecular dyssymmetry (1848), fermentation (1857), spontaneous generation (1862), diseases of wine (1863), diseases of silkworms (1865), microörganisms in beer (1871), virulent diseases (anthrax, chicken cholera) (1877), and preventive vaccinations (1880), particularly of hydrophobia (1885).

The first of these, his classic investigations of the conversion of dextrotartaric acid into the inactive forms (racemic and mesotartaric acids), and his discovery of the splitting up of racemic acid into right- and left-handed tartaric acid by means of optically active substances, gained him the Rumford medal of the Royal Society (1856), and undoubtedly led to the work of van't Hoff and Le Bel on stereochemistry or chemistry in space. They also led Pasteur to the study of ferments and microörganisms through his initial experiment of inducing fermentation in racemic acid by means of albumen, causing the destruction of the dextro-rotatory product by fermentative microorganisms. From this he proceeded to those studies of beer yeasts and lactic-acid fermentation which resulted in the discovery of lactic-acid bacteria, and confuted the errors which Liebig and even Helmholtz had made in regard to the significance of fermentation. He next discovered the anaërobic character of the bacteria of butyric fermentation, introducing the concepts "aërobism" and "anaërobism." A comparison of flasks of yeast in nutrient media, one of which had been sterilized, demonstrated the rôle of microörganisms in changing atmospheric oxygen into CO_2 (1861). His dispute with Pouchet about spontaneous generation was obscured by the fact that Pouchet's hay infusion was more difficult to sterilize than the yeast infusion employed by Pasteur, but the latter prevailed in his contention,[1] winning a prize and membership in the Academy of Sciences. About this time, he discovered that the pellicle so necessary to the formation of vinegar from wine consists of minute, rod-like microörganisms (*Mycoderma aceti*). The investigation of acetic fermentation[2] confuted Liebig's mechanical theory of fermentation and led Pasteur to study the causes detrimental to the three great industries of his country, those of wine, silk, and wool. In 1867, the wine industry of France was worth 500,000,000 francs to the nation. This gain was due to Pasteur's discovery that the spoiling of wine by microörganisms can be prevented by partial heat sterilization (Pasteurization) at a temperature of 55° to 60° C., without any alteration of the taste or bouquet of the vintage (1863–65). This process is now applied to all perishable foods, and is of inestimable importance in the nutrition of infants. In 1849, the silkworm industry of France began to be crippled by the disease *pébrine*. By 1861, the annual revenue from this source had sunk from 130,000,000 to 8,000,000 francs, and enormous sums were spent in importing healthy silkworm eggs from Spain, Italy, and Japan. The mulberry plantations in the Cevennes were abandoned, and the state was petitioned, in 1865, to remedy the evil. In a little house near Alais, Pasteur and his assistants worked for five years on an apparently insoluble problem, and even after he had discovered the cause and prevention of pébrine there came his burst of despair: "*Il y a deux maladies!*" The second disease, *flâcherie*, was conquered in time,[3] but at a terrible cost. The death of one of his daughters and the worry incident to harsh criticism of his failures brought on a severe attack of paralysis. Even his pleasure in such tokens of recognition as a degree of M. D. from Bonn, a prize from the Austrian government, membership in the Royal Society, and a nomination as senator, was spoiled by the outbreak of the Franco-Prussian War. He returned the Bonn diploma and took up the study of the spoiling of beer by microörganisms, again showing the advantages of Pasteurization.[4] About this time, his definition of a ferment as "a living form which originates from a germ," was contested in a posthumous essay of Claude Bernard's,[5] but, in 1874, Lister had sent him the celebrated letter acknowledging the value of his work in relation to antiseptic surgery. Thus Pasteur was

---

[1] Pasteur: Compt. rend. Acad. d. sc., Paris, 1860, l, 303, 849; li, 348, 675; 1864, lviii, 21; 1865, lxi, 1091.

[2] Études sur le vin, Paris, 1866.

[3] Études sur les maladies des vers a soie, Paris, 1870.

[4] Pasteur: Études sur la bière, Paris, 1876.

[5] Bernard: Rev. scient., Paris, 1879, xv, 49–56.

virtually transformed from a chemist to a medical man, particularly in his mode of attacking the problem of infectious diseases. In his studies on anthrax, he was preceded by Davaine, who discovered the bacillus and showed that the virulence of the disease was in proportion to the number of bacteria present (1850–65); by Klebs, who indicated that anthrax virus is non-filterable, since the filtrate will not produce the disease (1871), and by Koch, who first cultivated pure cultures of anthrax bacilli, described their full life-history and their relation to the disease (1877). Pasteur confirmed Koch's results, and disposed of the controversial question of a separate virus by carrying the bacilli through a hundred generations and producing anthrax from the term of the series.[1] At the same time, he discovered, with Joubert and Chamberland, the bacillus of malignant edema (*vibrion septique*), the first find of an anaërobic microörganism of a pathogenic character; and he showed the relation of animal heat to bacterial virulence. As he cared nothing for the taxonomic aspects of bacteriology, it is sometimes forgotten that he discovered the Staphylococcus pyogenes in boils as "*microbe en amas de grains*," and the Streptococcus pyogenes in puerperal septicemia as "*microbe en chapelet de grains*" (1878–9[2]). His discovery of preventive inoculation was due to the accidental fact that virulent cultures of chicken cholera virus, during a vacation from the laboratory, became sterile or inactive, and, when injected, were found to act as preventive vaccines against a subsequent injection of a virulent character. The attenuated virus could be carried through several generations and still maintain its immunizing property. In 1881, he succeeded in producing a vaccine against anthrax, injection of which lowered the mortality-rate to 1 per cent. in sheep and to 0.34 per cent. in horned cattle. Experiments with the viruses of anthrax, chicken cholera, and swine measles (*rouget des porcs*) brought out the principle that the pathogenic properties of a virus can be attenuated or heightened by successive passages through the bodies of appropriate animals, and led to one of the most luminous thoughts in the history of science—that the origin or extinction of infectious disease in the past (syphilis, for instance) may be simply due to the strengthening or weakening of its virus by external conditions, or in some such way as the above. This principle was applied with success against anthrax in the sheep-folds near Chartres, and in preventive vaccinations against hydrophobia, the culture-medium being the spinal marrow of the infected animal.[3] Pasteur's first patient was Joseph Meister, an Alsatian boy, bitten all over by a rabid dog, who was treated with success in July, 1885. Shortly afterward, the Pasteur Institute was opened, and special institutes for hydrophobia inoculations were founded all over the world. Here Pasteur labored almost to the end of his life, with such brilliant pupils as Metchnikoff, Roux, Yersin, Calmette, Chantemesse, Chamberland, and Pottevin. With Ch. Chamberland, he devised the celebrated filter which is called by his name, while Émile Roux did epoch-making work on the diphtheria antitoxin, Metchnikoff on phagocytosis and the lactic-acid bacillus, Alexandre Yersin on the plague bacillus, and Albert Calmette on preventive inoculations against snake-bites.

Pasteur's last years were crowded with honors from all parts of the world, and, after his death, an appropriate mausoleum for his remains, copied from the tomb of Galla Placidia at Ravenna, was built in the Pasteur Institute by his family. Deeply religious, intensely serious, endowed with a mind the quality of which Roux has compared to the action of a blow-pipe flame, Pasteur was a *sensitif*, who suffered unduly all his life from the captious cavillings of lesser men. His return of the diploma from the genial Rhineland University of Bonn can be excused only by his child-like, high-strung devotion to his native land. Literary snobbery has descanted sufficiently upon his "peasant origin," but the man himself was a gentleman of the type described by Wordsworth and Cardinal Newman, one who never inflicts wanton or needless pain upon others. His sympathy with the sufferings of dumb

---

[1] Pasteur: Compt. rend. Acad. d. sc., Paris, 1880, xci, 86, 455, 697; 1881, xcii, 209.

[2] *Ibid.*, 1880, xc, 1033–1044.

[3] Compt. rend. Acad. d. sc., Par., 1885, ci, 765; 1886, cii, 459, 835; ciii, 777.

animals was of a kind which, said Roux, might have seemed comic had it not been touching. We have the testimony of his pupils as to his power of establishing an immediate sympathetic relation between himself and any one sincerely interested in his work, and his sympathies extended, circle-wise, as in Emerson's parable, from the intimate group of his family and pupils, to embrace the people (even the animals) of his native land and the entire human race.[1] His humanity was of that rare and noble kind which, in Emerson's words, "approves itself no mortal, but a native of the deeps of absolute and inextinguishable being."

Robert **Koch** (1843–1910), of Klausthal, Hannover, was educated in the gymnasium of his native town, and took his medical degree at Göttingen (1866), where he was profoundly influenced by the teachings

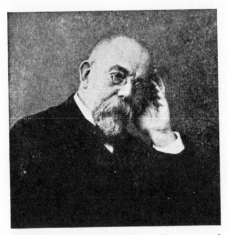

of Jacob Henle, whose theory of contagion (1840) may have started Koch upon his life-work in science. After serving in the Franco-Prussian War, he became district physician (*Kreisphysicus*) at Wollstein, where he varied the monotomy of long journeyings over rough country roads by private microscopic studies. He began with anthrax, and, in April, 1876, reported to the eminent botanist Ferdinand Cohn at Breslau that he had worked out the complete life-history and sporulation of the anthrax bacillus. About a week later, at Cohn's invitation, he gave

Robert Koch (1843–1910). (Courtesy of Captain Henry J. Nichols, U. S. Army.)

a three-day demonstration of his culture methods and results at the Botanical Institute (Breslau), in the presence of Cohn, Weigert, Auerbach, Traube, and Cohnheim, who declared that Koch's was the greatest bacteriological discovery yet made. Cohn immediately published Koch's memoir demonstrating that the anthrax bacillus is the cause of the disease, and that a pure culture grown through several generations outside the body can produce it in various animals (1876[2]). Koch's results were violently opposed by Paul Bert, but completely confirmed by Pasteur. In November, 1877, Koch published his methods of fixing and drying bacterial films on cover-slips, of staining them with Weigert's anilin dyes, of staining flagellæ, and of photographing bacteria for identification and comparison.[3] In 1878 appeared his

---

[1] The writer once had the privilege of hearing an account of Pasteur in which these qualities were very strikingly set forth by one of his pupils.

[2] Koch: Cohn's Beitr. z. Morphol. d. Pflanzen, Bresl., 1876–7, ii, 277–310, 1 pl.

[3] *Ibid.*, 399–434, 3 pl.

great memoir on the etiology of traumatic infectious diseases,[1] in which the bacteria of six different kinds of surgical infection are described, with the pathological findings, each microöorganism breeding true through many generations *in vitro* or in animals. These three memoirs elevated Koch to the front rank in medical science, and, through Cohnheim's influence, he was appointed to a vacancy in the Imperial Health Department (*Kaiserliches Gesundheitsamt*), with Löffler and Gaffky as assistants, in 1880. Here, in 1881, he produced his important paper upon the method of obtaining pure cultures of organisms by spreading liquid gelatin with meat infusion upon glass plates, forming a solid coagulum.[2] When Koch demonstrated his plate cultures at the International Medical Congress in London, Pasteur is said to have rushed forward with the exclamation: *C'est un grand progrès!* and so it proved. The year 1882 was marked by the discovery of the tubercle bacillus by special culture and staining methods. This paper[3] contains the first statement of "Koch's postulates," establishing the pathogenic character of a given microörganism, which had already been adumbrated by Henle[4] and Edwin Klebs.[5] About the same time, Koch and his assistants perfected Merke's idea of steam sterilization (1881). In 1883, Koch, at the head of the German Cholera Commission, visited Egypt and India, discovered the cholera vibrio,[6] its transmission by drinking-water, food, and clothing, and incidentally found the microöorganisms of Egyptian ophthalmia or infectious conjunctivitis (Koch-Weeks bacillus, 1883[7]), for which results he received a donation of 100,000 marks from the Prussian State. In 1885, he was appointed professor of hygiene and bacteriology at the University of Berlin, where his laboratories were crowded with bright pupils from all over the world, among whom were Gaffky, Löffler, Pfeiffer, Welch, and Kitasato.

At the tenth International Medical Congress at Berlin, in 1890, Koch announced his belief that he had found a remedy for tuberculosis. The introduction of tuberculin,[8] his one mistake, in that it was prematurely considered, was hailed all over the world as an event of the greatest scientific moment, and honors and felicitations of all kinds were showered upon Koch from all sides. Although he himself had limited his claims to the possible cure of early cases of phthisis, the great hopes which had been entertained of the remedy were not realized in time, and the number of failures and fatal cases impaired the confidence of the profession, but abated little of his

---

[1] Koch: Untersuchungen über die Aetiologie der Wundinfektionskrankheiten, Berlin, 1878.

[2] Mitth. a. d. kaiserl. Gesundheitsamte, Berl., 1881, i, 1–48, 14 pl.

[3] Berl. klin. Wochenschr., 1882, xix, 221–230. The bacillus was probably seen, though not positively identified in a causal relation, by Aufrecht (1881) and Baumgarten (1882).

[4] Henle: Pathologische Untersuchungen, Berlin, 1840, 43.

[5] Klebs: Amtl. Ber. d. 50. Versamml. deutsch. Naturf. u. Aertze, München, 1877, 49, at bottom.

[6] Koch: Deutsche med. Wochenschr., Berl., 1884, x, 725–728.

[7] Wien. med. Wochenschr., 1883, xxxiii, 1550; also described by John E. Weeks, in Arch. Ophthal., N. Y., 1886, xv, 441–451.

[8] Deutsche med. Wochenschr., Leipz. u. Berl., 1890, xvi, 1029; 1891, xvii, 101, 1189.

great reputation, especially after the discovery that tuberculin is the most reliable means of diagnosis. In 1891, the Institute for Infectious Diseases was founded in Berlin, and remained under Koch's direction until he resigned in 1904, in favor of his pupil Gaffky. In 1892, his ideas were applied in fighting the cholera epidemic at Hamburg, and in 1893 he wrote an important paper on water-borne epidemics, showing how they may be largely prevented by proper filtration.[1] In 1896, he investigated Rinderpest in South Africa at the request of the English government, devised a method of preventive inoculation, and made valuable studies of Texas fever, blackwater fever, tropical malaria, surra, and plague.[2] In 1897, he produced his new tuberculin (T. R.), and in 1898 he investigated malarial fever in Italy. At the London Tuberculosis Congress (1900), Koch announced his view that the bacilli of bovine and human tuberculosis, which had been separated and studied by Theobald Smith in 1898, are not identical, claiming that there is little danger of transmission of the bovine type to man. These views were reiterated at the Washington Congress of 1908, and on both occasions aroused violent controversy, the general trend of opinion at present being provisionally in favor of Koch. In 1902, he studied Rhodesian redwater fever (*Küstenfieber*), horse-sickness, trypanosomiasis, and recurrent fever in German East Africa, and, in the same year, established methods of controlling typhoid which have been adopted almost everywhere.

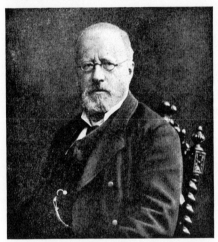

Edwin Klebs (1834–1913). (Surgeon-General's Library.)

Koch received the Nobel Prize in 1905. In 1906, he visited Africa again, at the head of the Sleeping Sickness Commission, introducing atoxyl for the treatment of the disease. Although he was honored by a membership in the Prussian Academy of Sciences and the title of *Excellenz*, he was not happy in the later years of his life. Changes in his domestic arrangements estranged many of his friends, and subjected him to harsh criticism, which he bore with stoicism and dignity, but which told upon him in the end. He died of heart-failure on May 27, 1910, at the age of sixty-seven. His body was cremated at his own request, and his ashes deposited in the Institute which he had founded. In appearance, Koch was a typical German savant of Prussian cast, in character dignified, modest, and fair-minded, altogether one of the greatest men of science his country has produced.

Edwin **Klebs** (1834–1913), of Königsberg, East Prussia, one of the earlier assistants of Virchow at Berlin (1861–66), was professor of pathology at Bern (1866), Würzburg (1871), Prague (1873), Zürich (1882), and Chicago (Rush Medical College, 1896). With Pasteur, he was perhaps the most important precursor in the bacterial theory of infection; indeed, did most to win the pathologists over to this view.

---

[1] Koch: Ztschr. f. Hyg. u. Infektionskr., Leipz., 1893, xiv, 393–426.
[2] Reiseberichte über Rinderpest (etc.), Berlin, 1898.

A man of irascible, precipitate disposition, Klebs was unfortunate in not following up his discoveries with good generalship, but he was undoubtedly a great pioneer in all phases of bacteriology, to whom Koch himself owed much.

He saw the typhoid bacillus before Eberth (1881[1]), the diphtheria bacillus before Löffler (1883[2]), used solid cultures of sturgeon's glue (1872), and investigated the pathology of traumatic infections before Koch (1871[3]). The priority of his inoculations of syphilis in monkeys was recognized by Metchnikoff (1878[4]), and, in his experiments on anthrax (1871[5]) and other diseases, he was the first to filter bacteria and to experiment with the filtrates. In 1874, he invented the fractional method of obtaining pure cultures of bacteria known as "Darwinizing," i. e., killing off the competing germs in the impure culture by successive transfers through a series of fresh media, which was followed by Lister's method of dilution (1877) and prepared the ground for Koch's work. In 1877, Klebs concluded that knowledge of the specific viruses (toxins) of pathogenic bacteria would be essential for further progress. He wrote two text-books on pathology (1869–76, 1887–89), monographs on the bacteriology of gunshot wounds, based upon his experiences in the Franco-Prussian War (1872), on tumors (1877), and gigantism (1884), made many investigations on tuberculosis, and he was, with Gerlach, the first to produce bovine infection or Perlsucht by feeding with milk (1873[6]). In his studies on gunshot wounds (1872) he showed that the filtrate of the wound-discharges is non-infectious, whence he reasoned that traumatic septicemia is of bacterial origin. In 1870, he recognized hemorrhagic pancreatitis as a cause of sudden death, produced valvular disease of the heart experimentally (1876) and investigated the genesis of endocarditis (1878). His studies on malarial fever (with Tommasi Crudeli, 1879) were translated for the Sydenham Society. He experimented with various products for the treatment of tuberculosis, and was the first to experiment with the therapeutic possibilities of the tubercle bacilli of cold-blooded animals (1900).

Friedrich **Löffler** (1852–1915), of Frankfort on the Oder, was for many years a Prussian army surgeon, and eventually became professor of hygiene at Greifswald (1888).

He discovered the bacteria of swine-erysipelas (1882–83[7]), and glanders (1882[8]); established the causal relation of the diphtheria bacillus (1884[9]), differentiating it from the pseudo-diphtheritic organisms, pathogenic to doves and calves (1884–7); eradicated the field-mouse plague in Thessaly by means of the Bacillus typhi murium (1892); and, in his investigations of the foot-and-mouth disease (1898[10]), he was able to prove experimentally that the latter is caused by a filterable virus, establishing this concept and introducing a preventive inoculation against the disease (1899). He wrote an admirable history of bacteriology (1887), left unfinished.

Georg **Gaffky** (1850–1918), of Hannover, also a Prussian army surgeon, became associated with Koch in Berlin, and succeeded him as director of the Hygienic Institute. He discovered the bacillus of rabbit septicæmia, which he obtained in pure culture (1881), investigated cholera, and anthrax, and first obtained a pure culture of the typhoid bacillus, which he then showed to be the true activator of the disease (1884) Ferdinand **Hueppe** (1852–   ), also a Prussian army surgeon, and later chief sani-

[1] Klebs: Arch. f. exper. Path. u. Pharmakol., Leipzig, 1880, xii, 231; 1881, xiii, 381, 3 pl.

[2] Verhandl. d. Cong. f. innere Med., Wiesbaden, 1883, 139–174.

[3] Cor.-Bl. f. schweiz. Aerzte, Bern, 1871, i, 241–246.

[4] Arch. f. exper. Path. u. Pharmakol., Leipzig, 1878–79, x, 161–221, 4 col. pl.

[5] Klebs: Cor.-Bl. f. schweiz. Aerzte, Bern, 1871, i, 279 (Nachschrift).

[6] Arch. f. exper. Path. u. Pharmakol., Leipzig, 1873, i, 163–180.

[7] Löffler: Arb. a. d. k. Gesundheitsamte, Berlin, 1885, i, 46–55.

[8] Deutsche med. Wochenschr., Leipzig u. Berlin, 1882, viii, 407.

[9] Mitth. a. d. k. Gesundheitsamte, Berlin, 1884, ii, 451–499.

[10] Centralbl. f. Bakteriol., 1. Abt., Jena, 1898, xxiii, 371–391.

tarian to the Army of the East in 1914–15, also collaborated with Koch, introduced several important wrinkles in bacteriologic technic, and applied his knowledge directly to the advancement of experimental hygiene, the chief glory of Koch's Institute. He did important work on fermentation (1883), the bacteriology of milk (1884–1912), chlorophyll (1887–1905), water supply (1887–9), disinfectants (1886–91), cholera (1887 –92), racial and social hygiene (1895), wrote a well-known manual on bacteriological methods (1885), and, like Pettenkofer, held strong views on the multiplex causation of infectious disease, as against the rigid dogma of specificity of germs maintained by Henle, Cohn, and Koch. He was master of an admirable literary style.

Equally remarkable was Carl **Flügge** (1847–1923), of Hannover, who after serving as army surgeon in the campaign of 1870–71, qualified as privat docent in hygiene and eventually found himself in Koch's Institute (1909). He wrote two well-known books on microörganisms (1886) and hygiene (1889), discovered and described many bacteria, showed the inadequacy of sterilization in the milk of commerce, the contamination of the atmosphere by the spraying of infected sputum and mucus from mouth and nose (1897), and that the ill-effects of vitiated air are due not to CO_2, but to the stuffiness resulting from humid heat (1905).

The work of these men led to a wonderful output of epoch-making discoveries in bacteriology and parasitology,[1] which went to the creation of the newer public hygiene and the virtual annihilation of most of the communicable diseases.

These are the discovery of the bacteria of leprosy in 1871–4 by Armauer Hansen (1841–1912), of gonorrhea in 1879 by Albert Neisser (1855–1916), of typhoid fever by Carl Joseph Eberth (1880), of lobar pneumonia by Pasteur (1880–81), George Miller Sternberg (1880–81), Albert Fränkel (1884), and Carl Friedländer (1883), of glanders by Friedrich Löffler (1882–86), of erysipelas by Friedrich Fehleisen (1883), of swine erysipelas by Löffler (1882–86), of diphtheria by Edwin Klebs (1883) and Friedrich Löffler (1883–84), of tetanus by Arthur Nicolaier (1884), of Bacillus coli infection by Theodor Escherich (1886), of Malta fever by Sir David Bruce (1887), of cerebrospinal meningitis (1887) by Anton Weichselbaum (1845–1920), of fibrinous pneumonia by Nicolaus Gamaleia (1888), of chancroid by Auguste Ducrey (1889), of influenza by Richard Pfeiffer (1892), of Bacillus aërogenes infection by William Henry Welch and George H. F. Nuttall (1892), of bubonic plague by Shibasaburo Kitasato and A. Yersin (1894), of dysentery by Kiyoshi Shiga (1897), of bovine peripneumonia by Edmond Nocard and Émile Roux (1898) and of whooping-cough by Jules Bordet and Octave Gengou (1906). The microörganisms of the surgical and puerperal infections were discovered and investigated by Pasteur (1878–9), Koch (1878), Gaffky (1881), and Welch (1892). Toxins were first isolated and named (typhotoxine and tetanine) by Ludwig Brieger in 1888. The bactericidal effect of blood-serum was discovered by Hans Buchner (1889), bacteriolysis by Richard Pfeiffer (1894), bacterial hemolysis by Jules Bordet (1898). L. Landois, in 1875, made the important discovery that animal serum will hemolyze human blood. The subsequent discoveries of Maragliano (1892), Landsteiner (1902), and Eisenberg (1901), that the sera of diseased and even of normal donors, will hemolyze alien blood, have revolutionized the whole subject of transfusion. Anaphylaxis was discovered by Edward Jenner (1798) and François Magendie (1839), and investigated by Simon Flexner (1894), C. Richet and Héricourt (1898–1903), Theobald Smith (1903), Rosenau and Anderson (1906), and von Pirquet (1907). Bacterial agglutination was discovered by Max Gruber and Fernand Widal (1896). Opsonins were investigated by Denys and Leclef (1893) and by Wright and Douglas (1903). **Parasitology** was greatly advanced by such monumental treatises as those of K. A. Rudolphi on entozoa (1808–10), G. F. H. Küchenmeister on cestodes (1853) and parasites in man (1855), Carl Theodor von Seibold on teniæ and hydatids (1854), Casimir Davaine on entozoa in man and animals (1860), Thomas Spencer Cobbold on entozoa (1864), Rudolf Leuckart (1822–98) on human parasites (1867), and Raphael Blanchard on medical zoölogy (1886–90). Of parasites producing disease, that of favus was discovered by Schönlein (1839), of psorospermosis by Johannes Müller (1841), of tinea favosa (alopecia) by David Grüby (1841–44), of anchylos-

---

[1] For bibliographical references to these discoveries see Index Catalogue, Surgeon-General's Library, 1912, 2. series, xvii, pp. 135–139.

tomiasis by Angelo Dubini (1843), of recurrent fever by Otto Obermeier (1873), of malarial fever by Alphonse Laveran (1880), of parasitic hemoptysis (paragonomiasis) by Erwin Baelz (1880), of Texas fever (piroplasmosis) by Theobald Smith (1889[1]). The parasite of aspergillosis was discovered and described by Bennett in 1842; the ray fungus (actinomycosis) in man by von Langenbeck (1848) and James Israel (1878), in cattle by Otto Bollinger (1876), the identity of both being established by Emil Ponfick (1844–1913) in 1880; that of nocardiosis by Edmond Nocard (1888–93), that of blastomycosis by Thomas Casper Gilchrist (1896), and that of sporotrichosis by Benjamin R. Schenck (1898). The two last discoveries were made in the Johns Hopkins Hospital.

The theory that mosquitos can transmit malarial fever was indicated even in the Sanskrit Susruta,[2] and the same theory was advanced for yellow fever by Josiah Clark Nott, of South Carolina (1848[3]), and Louis Daniel Beauperthuy (1854[4]). The hypothesis was more definitely stated for yellow fever by Carlos Juan Finlay (1833–1915), of Cuba (1881[5]), and for malarial fever by Albert F. A. King (1883[6]). In the meantime Sir Patrick Manson (1844–1923) had proved that the mosquito is a vector of Filaria sanguinis hominis (1877[7]), and the plasmodium of malarial fever had been discovered by Alphonse Laveran (1845–   ), a French army surgeon, in 1880.[8] These hemocytozoa were accurately described by Ettore Marchiafava and Angelo Celli (1885), and it was shown by Camillo Golgi (1844–1926), the histologist, that malarial paroxysms are coincident with sporulation of parasites (1886), and that the parasite of quartan fever differs from that of tertian (1889). In 1889, Marchiafava and Celli showed that the organisms of the pernicious and the tertian and quartan forms are different; B. Grassi and R. Feletti studied the parasites in birds (1891), D. L. Romanovsky devised a special stain for them (1890), and Ronald Ross, in India, demonstrated the infection of birds by means of the mosquito (1897–98). W. G. MacCallum and E. L. Opie demonstrated sexual conjugation in the flagellated forms (1897–98), and Grassi and A. Bignami showed that the parasites develop only in the Anopheles mosquito (1899). Intracorpuscular conjugation in the parasite as a cause of latency and relapse was demonstrated by Charles F. Craig (1907), also the possibility of malaria carriers. That flies can transmit disease is one of the most ancient of folk-intuitions, implicit in the flea- and fly-amulets of the ancient Egyptians, in the cylinder-seal of Nergal, the Mesopotamian god of disease and darkness (in Pierpont Morgan's collection), in the Biblical references to the "plague of flies" visited upon the Egyptians and the iatromantic power ascribed to Beelzebub, the Fly-god (2 Kings I, 2–6) and in Pliny's ironical recipe of ashes of flies for alopecia, (XXIX, 34), since these represented the god Myiagros or Myiodes, who drove flies away, to the comfort of the bald. Ambroise Paré noticed that flies are disease-carriers at the battle of St. Quentin (1557), Joseph Leidy called attention to the fact in his hospital work during the Civil War (1861–65), A. Raimbert demonstrated the transmission of anthrax by flies (1869), G. E. Nicholas, R. N., noticed that flies and cholera appeared and disappeared together on board ship during the Levantine epidemic of 1850 (1873). The agency of flies in the transmission of cholera was demonstrated by G. Tizzoni and G. Cattani (1886); the life-history of the fly was investigated by A. T. Packard (1874) and L. O. Howard (1909); Battista Grassi showed that flies can carry the eggs of intestinal worms (1883), Angelo Celli showed that they may transmit tuberculosis (1888), and that the bacilli of anthrax, tuberculosis, and typhoid fever retain their virulence and reproductive power after passing through the intestines of flies (1888[9]). In 1892,[10] George M. Kober empha-

---

[1] Smith: Med. News. Phila., 1889, lv, 689–693.

[2] Sir H. A. Blake: J. Ceylon Branch, Brit. Med. Ass., Colombo, 1905, ii, 9.

[3] Nott: New Orleans Med. & Surg. Jour., 1848, iv, 563, 601.

[4] Gaz. offic. de Cumana, 1854, No. 57.

[5] Finlay: An. r. Acad. de cien. med. . . . de la Habana, 1881–2, xviii, 147–169.

[6] King: Pop. Sc. Month., N. Y., 1883, xxiii, 644–658.

[7] Manson: J. Linnæan Soc., Lond., 1879, xiv, 304–311.

[8] Laveran: Compt. rend. Acad. d. sc., Paris, 1880, xciii, 627.

[9] A. Celli: Boll. d. Soc. lancisiana d. osp. di Roma, 1888, viii, 5–8.

[10] G. M. Kober: Rep. Health Officer D. C., Wash., 1895, 258, 260, 266, 270, 280, 281.

sized the importance of flies as disease transmitters and, in his report on typhoid fever in the District of Columbia (1895), definitely located them as such, in connection with a house-epidemic of typhoid from box-privies. In Circular No. 1, Surgeon-General's Office (April 25, 1898), George M. Sternberg brought out the same point. The report of Walter Reed, V. C. Vaughan and E. O. Shakespeare on typhoid in the Spanish-American War (1898) settled the matter by inductive proof.[1]

About 1890, Pasteur's theory of attenuated viruses was extended to the science of toxins and antitoxins by Emil **von Behring** (1854–1917), a Prussian army surgeon who became professor of hygiene at Halle (1894) and Marburg (1895). In his studies on chicken cholera, Pasteur had already noticed the pathogenic effects of a clear filtrate on the specific organism. In 1888, his pupils, Roux and Yersin, got the same results from diphtheria filtrates.[2] Hans Buchner, in 1889,

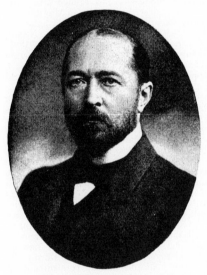

had established the bactericidal effect of blood-serum.[3] While working in Koch's Institute with Kitasato, Behring demonstrated that the serum of animals immunized against attenuated diphtheria toxins can be used as a preventive or therapeutic inoculation against diphtheria in other animals, through a specific neutralization of the toxin of the disease (1890–93[4]). After trying out the remedy in man, Behring began to produce it upon a grand scale (1894). It soon became recognized as the specific treatment for diphtheria. The success of diphtheria antitoxin led to many attempts to treat other specific infections by immune sera, but, except in the case of tetanus and

Emil von Behring (1854–1917).

serpent-poisoning, these have not been uniformly successful. Meanwhile the subject of immunity was developed on the solidist or cellular side by Elie **Metchnikoff** (1845–1916), the eminent Russian biologist, who, in his studies of *Daphnia* (1884), showed how ameboid cells in the connective tissues and the blood engulf solid particles and bacteria, destroying bacteria by absorbing them (phagocytosis). He called these cells "phagocytes," showed their function as scavengers, developed the doctrine of inflammation as the effect of the determination of swarms of

---

[1] For references to fly transmission see the exhaustive history of H. G. Beyer: New York Med. Jour., 1910, xci, 677–685.

[2] Roux and Yersin: Ann. de l'Inst. Pasteur, Paris, 188, ii, 629; 1889, iii, 273.

[3] Buchner: Centralbl. f. Bakteriol., Jena, 1889, v, 817; vi, 1.

[4] Behring: Deutsche med. Wochenschr., Leipz. & Berl., 1890, xvi, 1113, 1145; 1893, xix, 389, 415.

phagocytes to the site of injury by chemiotaxis and upheld the solidist theory of immunity as phygocytosis. This theory, in the hands of Sir Almroth Wright and others, led to vaccinotherapy. During 1892–1901, in fact, Metchnikoff developed the essential locus and functions of the reticulo-endothelial system. Metchnikoff also demonstrated that Pfeiffer's phenomenon (bacteriolysis) can take place in vitro (1895[1]). With Roux, he showed that the higher apes can be inoculated with syphilis (1903–4[2]). His theory as to the effect of lactic acid on bacteria in counteracting the intestinal poisons and prolonging life (1906) has attracted much attention. His best works are his books on the comparative pathology of inflammation (1892), on immunity in infectious diseases (1901) and on "The Nature of Man" (1903), which gives his views on intestinal auto-intoxication. He received the Nobel Prize in 1908.

Hans **Much** (1880–   ), of Zechlin, director of the Immunity and Tuberculosis Institutes at Hamburg, is memorable for his work on leprosy (nastin reaction 1909–10), partigens (1914–20), stimulotherapy (1919–22), unspecific immunity, his novels and poems and his book on Hippocrates (1926).

Sir Almroth Edward **Wright** (1861–   ), of Dublin, Ireland, professor of pathology in the Army Medical School at Netley (1892–1902), was

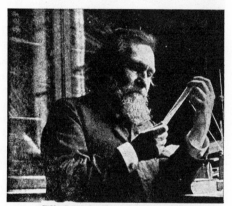

Elie Metchnikoff (1845–1916).

the first to point out the rôle of calcium salts in the coagulation of the blood (1891) and devised a coagulometer for estimating coagulation-time. He made typhoid vaccination practicable (1896–7), having inoculated over 3000 soldiers in India (1898–1900), and the entire British forces in the South African War. Through this work, he originated general vaccinotherapy (1902–7), with the superadded feature of measuring the protective substances in the blood by means of the opsonic index (1903). He is the author of treatises on anti-typhoid inoculation (1904) and immunization (1909), and during the European War investigated wound infection.

[1] Metchnikoff: Ann. de l'Inst. Pasteur, Paris, 1895, ix, 433–461, 1 pl.

[2] *Ibid.*, 1903, xvii, 809; 1904, xviii, 1. The experimental inoculability of syphilis was demonstrated, contrary to the views of Ricord, by Julius Bettinger (1802–87) in anonymous protocols presented to the Society of Physicians of the Palatinate in September, 1855 (Aerztl. Int.-Bl., München, 1856, iii, 426–428). Bettinger carefully kept the authorship of these human inoculations a secret all his life. His findings were subsequently unearthed by Erich Hoffmann (Deutsche med. Wochenschr., 1906, xxxii, 497) and the identity of the "anonymus Palatinus" also established (Dermat. Ztschr., Berl., 1912, xix, 1043; 1913, xx, 220).

Fernand **Widal** (1862–   ), a native of Algiers and professor in
the Paris Faculty, collaborated with Chantemesse in his early work on
preventive vaccinations against typhoid fever (1888), made his mark
by his discovery of bacterial agglutination (1895) and its application
in the diagnosis of typhoid (1896), and described non-congenital hemolytic jaundice (1907).

Bacteriology and pathology have been specially advanced in America
by William Henry **Welch** (1850–   ), of Norfolk, Connecticut, a
pupil of Cohnheim's, who was successively professor of pathology at
Bellevue Hospital Medical College (1879–84) and Johns Hopkins
University (1884), and latterly director of the School of Hygiene
(1916–26) in which chairs he turned
out a long line of worthy pupils.
Welch investigated acute edema of
the lungs in Cohnheim's laboratory
(1877), discovered the Staphylococcus epidermidis albus and its relation to wound infection (1892[1]),
also the Bacillus aërogenes cap-
sulatus (1892[2]), grouping the diseases caused by it (1900[3]). He also
made important studies of embolism
and thrombosis (1899) and, with
Flexner, demonstrated the pathological changes produced by experimental injection of the toxins
of diphtheria (1891–92[4]), simultaneously with von Behring. In 1926,
he was called to the new chair of
medical history in the Johns Hopkins
University.

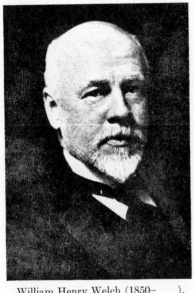

William Henry Welch (1850–   ).

Simon **Flexner** (1863–   ), of
Louisville, Kentucky, now director
of the Rockefeller Institute for Medical Research (1903), has distinguished himself by his work on terminal infections, his experimental
work on venoms (1901), the etiology and therapy of cerebrospinal
meningitis (1909) and infantile poliomyelitis (1910–13) and latterly
on encephalitis and herpes (1920–3) and experimental epidemiology
(1921–4).

Victor Clarence **Vaughan** (1851–   ), of Mount Airy, Missouri, professor of hygiene and director of the Hygienic Laboratory at the University of Michigan (1887–1909), was the first after Panum (1856) and
Selmi (1878) to investigate the poisonous alkaloids and proteins, in

[1] Welch: Tr. Cong. Am. Phys. & Surg., New Haven, 1892, ii, 1–28.
[2] Johns Hopkins Hosp. Bull., Balt., 1892, iii, 81–91, with G. H. F. Nuttall.
[3] *Ibid.*, 1900, xi, 185–204.
[4] *Ibid.*, 1891, ii, 107; 1892, iii, 17.

particular tyrotoxicon (1885), ptomaines and leucomaines (with F. G. Novy, 1888), the bacterial proteids or cellular toxins (1891–1913), and the protein split products (1913). In 1896, he found the poison-producing bacillus in ice-cream and cheese.

His general theory is that bacteria are not plants, but particulate, specific proteins (nucleo-proteins); that all true proteins contain a poisonous molecular nucleus; that the pathogenicity of bacteria depend upon their reproductive power or mass action within the body; that specific infectious diseases result from parenteral protein digestion; that protein sensitization and bacterial immunity are identical; that vaccines are protein sensitizers, but toxin immunity and bacterial immunity are radically different, since the protein poison is not specific but common to all proteins, and these elaborate no antibodies, but, through their secondary groups, develop specific proteolytic ferments capable of digesting the protein which created them.

Vaughan's colleague, Frederick George **Novy** (1864–), of Chicago, professor of bacteriology at Ann Arbor (1902), collaborated with him in his book on ptomaines and leucomaines (1888), has made culture investigations of the trypanosomes, and (with Knapp) discovered the special spirochæte of the American variety of relapsing fever (1906).

Ludvig **Hektoen** (1863–), of Westby, Wisconsin, professor of pathology in Rush Medical College, Chicago (1895), and director of the John McCormick Institute for Infectious Diseases (1902), is one of the most eminent pathologists and bacteriologists in our country. He was the teacher of many of the promising younger people, notably Ricketts, H. G. Wells, Rosenow, Irons, Alice Hamilton, and Morris Fishbein.

He has done much valuable work in experimental medicine, notably on vascular changes in tuberculous meningitis (1896), blastomycosis and sporotrichosis (1899–1907), experimental bacillary cirrhosis of the liver (1901), blood-cultures during life (1903), experimental measles by blood-injections (1905–19), phagocytosis (1905–8) and anti-bodies (1909–18). He first pointed out the possible danger from iso-agglutination in transfusion of blood (1907).

George H. F. **Nuttall** (1862–), of San Francisco, professor of biology at the University of Cambridge (1906), editor and founder of the *Journal of Hygiene* (1901) and of *Parasitology* (1908), first summarized the rôle of insects, arachnids, and myriapods as transmitters of bacterial and parasitic diseases (1899), and his monograph on *Blood Immunity and Blood Relationship* (1904) establishes the identification of different kinds of blood by the precipitin test.

Theobald **Smith** (1859–), of Albany, New York, professor of comparative pathology in Harvard University (1896), has been one of the pioneers in the theory of infectious diseases. In 1886, working with D. E. Salmon, he demonstrated that immunity from hog cholera can be secured by injection of the filtered products of the specific organisms. This was the first experiment in immunization, and was soon followed by the work of Behring, Roux, and others. Smith's demonstration of the parasite of Texas fever (*Pyrosoma bigeminum*) (1889[1]), and his work (with F. L. Kilborne) in tracing its transmission by the cattle

---

[1] Smith: Med. News, Phila., 1889, lv, 689–693.

tick (Boöphilus bovis), was a great advance in the science of protozoan disease (1893). He also demonstrated anaphylaxis (Richet, 1909) from the bacterial products of diphtheria prior to 1903, a discovery which Ehrlich called the "Theobald Smith phenomenon." He made the first clear differentiation between the bovine and human types of tubercle bacilli (1898[1]), his work having been substantiated by Koch, Spengler, and others, and has made many other discoveries in bacteriology, notably the first observation of pleomorphism in bacteria.

Hideyo **Noguchi** (1876–1928), of Japan, a member of the Rockefeller Institute (1914), introduced the luetin (cutaneous) test for syphilis (1911), first obtained a pure culture of *Treponema pallidum* and other treponemata (1913), cultivated the microörganisms of infantile paralysis and rabies (1913), devised a method for obtaining a sterile (bacteria-free) vaccine against smallpox (1915), isolated and cultivated *Leptospira interrogans*, with a preventive vaccine and curative serum for yellow fever (1918–24), cultivated *Bartonella bacilliformis* from Oroya fever and verruga peruana (1926–7) and *Bacterium granulosis* from trachoma (1927).

Edward Carl **Rosenow** (1875–   ), of Alma, Wisconsin, now of the Mayo Clinic, has been the main protagonist of the doctrine of variability of bacteria, notably of streptococci in the production of focal and local infections (1914–16) and of poliomyelitis (1916).

William Hallock **Park** (1863–   ), of New York, author of text-books on bacteriology (1899) and microörganisms, is remarkable for his work on the bacteriology and serology of diphtheria (1892–1906).

Hans **Zinsser** (1878–   ), of New York, professor of bacteriology in Columbia University (1913), is the author of sterling text-books on bacteriology (1911) and infection (1914) and of experimental researches on the *Treponema pallidum*.

Among women, Ruth Tunnicliff, of Chicago, is remarkable for her discovery of a diplococcus in measles (1917), with production of the disease in animals (1922) and successful serum-therapy (1927), her separation of the hemolytic streptococci of scarlatina and erysipelas (1920–27), studies of pleomorphism in fusiform bacilli (1906–23) and of anaërobic organisms isolated from colds (1913–26); Gladys Dick for work on the bacteriology and serology of scarlatina (1921–7); Alice C. Evans for her synthesis of the Brucella group (1923); Anna Wessels Williams for isolation of the No. 8 diphtheria bacillus used in toxin production (1895), and Louise G. Robinovitch for work on thermophilic bacteria (1895).

While Pasteur was investigating fermentation and putrefaction, the most important application of this work was in process of development at the hands of Joseph Lister, a young English surgeon who was destined to make his art a science in the same sense in which the mathematician Cayley defined bookkeeping as a perfect science. **Lord Lister**

---

[1] Smith: Jour. Exper. Med., N. Y., 1898, iii, 451–511.

(1827–1912), the last and greatest of the interesting line of English Quaker physicians, was born at Upton, Essex (April 5th). His father, Joseph Jackson Lister, a London wine merchant, who devoted his leisure hours to optical problems, was, in a sense, the founder of modern microscopy through his epoch-making improvements in the achromatic lenses of the instrument (1830). His special bent was not without its influence upon his son, who, after graduating in medicine from the University of London (1852), produced a number of papers on the histology of muscle, illustrated by delicate drawings of his own. Two of Lister's teachers, William Sharpey and Thomas Graham, were Scots, and it was upon their advice that he went up to Edinburgh to follow surgery under Syme, who made him his house surgeon (1854), and whose eldest daughter afterward became Lister's wife. In 1860, Lister became professor of surgery in the University of Glasgow. It was during the latter years of his residence there that his greatest contribution to the science was made. Meanwhile, he had shown that the contractile tissues of the iris consist of smooth muscle, the first correct account of the mechanism of dilating the pupil (1852[1]); he had studied the early stages of inflammation (1857), he had overthrown the current theory that coagulation of the blood is due to liberation of ammonia, showing that, in the blood-vessels, it depends upon their injury (1851–63[2]); and he had made his mark in surgery by his classical paper on excision of the wrist for caries (1865[3]). Early in his hospital experience, Lister had been deeply impressed with the high mortality from such surgical pests as septicemia, pyemia, erysipelas, tetanus, and hospital gangrene. In his own statistics of amputation (1864–66), he found 45 per cent. of fatal cases, although he had constantly followed Syme's plan of keeping the wound clean by silver wire sutures, drainage, frequent change of dressings, and scrupulous cleanliness. These were the days of "laudable pus," yet Lister had already begun to think of the old Hippocratic healing by first intention as the surgeon's ideal.

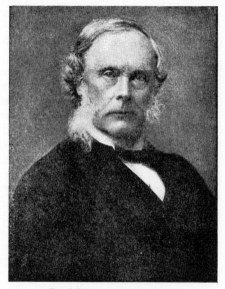

Lord Lister (1827–1912).

---

[1] Lister: Quart. Jour. Micr. Sc., Lond., 1853, i, p. 8 et seq.

[2] Lister: Edinb. Med. Jour., 1859–60, v, 536–540; and Croonian lecture, Proc. Roy. Soc., Lond., 1862–3, xii, 580–611.

[3] Lancet: Lond., 1865, i, 308, 335, 362.

Noticing that, when attainable, this was always dissociated from putrefaction, his attention was accidentally drawn to Pasteur's work, and, grasping its tendency, he set out definitely to prevent the development of microörganisms in wounds. Perceiving that Pasteur's heat sterilizations would avail nothing here, he turned to chemical antiseptics. After trying out zinc chlorid and the sulphites, he hit, by lucky chance, upon carbolic acid, which had been employed, a short while before, in the disinfection of sewage at Carlisle.[1] On August 12, 1865, he employed it in a case of compound fracture with complete success, and, in 1867, published the results of two years' work in two papers,[2] the second of which bears the significant title, On the Antiseptic Principle in the Practice of Surgery. The criticisms which were heaped upon this paper turned upon such non-essentials as the question of priority in the use of carbolic acid, or the character of Lister's dressings, which, complex at the start, were only accidental features of the great surgical principle with which they were confused. Undisturbed by these attacks, Lister proceeded to develop his thesis in the broadest and most scientific manner by original investigation of lactic-acid fermentation, of the relation of bacteria to inflammation, and of the antiseptic healing of wounds. In 1877, he developed a highly ingenious method of obtaining pure cultures of the lactic acid bacillus by gradual isolation of a single bacterial cell with a clever syringe of his invention, the only method of consequence between Klebs (1874) and Koch (1877). In steadfast capacity to deal with ideas, and therefore to profit by mistakes, Lister was perhaps the greatest of the scientific surgeons. All his life, he labored constantly to improve his dressings, from the earlier devices of putty, block tin, layers of oiled silk or gauze, and the carbolic acid spray, to his later experiments with the double cyanides of mercury and zinc and his great innovation of catgut ligatures in the surgery of the vascular system (1880[3]). He boldly applied the antiseptic principle to such conditions as abscesses in the spine and the joints,[4] wiring a fractured patella (1877–83), excision of the knee-joint (1878), operations on the breast (1881), and all manner of operations on the locomotor system, in fact, did as much to extend the domain of surgery as any man of his time. Modern surgery, it is true, has become almost entirely aseptic, in the sense of discarding strong antiseptics in the dressing of wounds, but in both the Listerian ideal of avoiding sepsis remains the same. In 1869, Lister succeeded Syme at Edinburgh, and, in 1877, accepted the chair of surgery at Kings College, London, retiring from practice in 1896. Meanwhile, his fame had long since become international. He was president of the Royal Society during 1895–1900, received his baronetcy in 1883, and was the first medical

---

[1] This substance had already been recommended by the chemist, François-Jules Lemaire (1860), but Lister had heard of neither Lemaire nor Semmelweis.

[2] Lister: Lancet, Lond., 1867, ii, 95, 353, 668.

[3] Lister: Tr. Clin. Soc., Lond., 1880–81, xiv, pp. xliii–lxiii.

[4] See, also: G. M. Kober: Am. Jour. Med. Sc., Phila., 1876, n. .s, lxxii, 427–431.

man to be raised to the peerage (1897). At Pasteur's jubilee, in 1892, Lister paid a feeling tribute to the man whose work he had been first to appreciate. In France, his ideas were defended by J.-M. Lucas-Championnière (1843–1913), who pointed out that asepsis, the Listerian ideal, must always be preceded by antisepsis, and that even heat sterilization is, in the truest sense, antiseptic. This was the weak point of Lawson Tait's argument against Listerism, for the Birmingham gynecologist, who denied that bacteria are pathogenic, would not admit that his own success in ovariotomy was due to those housewifely antiseptics, soap and hot water.[1] Koeberlé washed and scrubbed his own instruments personally, afterward heating them in an alcohol flame. Von Bergmann gradually merged the corrosive sublimate method into steam sterilization (1886) and the elaborate ritual of general asepsis (1891). The military applications of antisepsis, which Lister suggested in 1870,[2] were not taken up until late in the Franco-Prussian War, but his methods were soon grasped by von Volkmann, Thiersch, Mikulicz, and others, and his tour through Germany (1875) was in the nature of a triumphal progress. It was during the World War that Listerism attained its final vindication. On the germ-ridden battlefields of France, the surgeons were driven back to plain antisepsis. Upon hearing of Semmelweis, in 1883, Lister generously declared him to be his forerunner. In the obstetrician's hands, Listerism is now the main safeguard of the woman in childbed. To Listerism are due all modern developments of the surgery of the hollow cavities of the body, including the cranium, chest, abdomen, the joints, and the male and female pelvic viscera. Even the modern sterilizable kitchens, hospital wards and barber shops in white enamel illustrate the Listerian principle of surgical cleanliness. As an operator Lister was not brilliant, but deliberate and careful, aiming, like Kocher or Halsted, to make the recovery of patients a mathematical certainty. In Lister's day the abdomen and the chest, like the joints, were "sacrosanct spaces,"[3] and he did not invade them. His Quaker sobriety, his severe and austere ideals, were not the traits that make for rapid and showy success. His progress was slow; he left no school; but, before he died, the entire guild of surgeons "lived in his mild and magnificent eye." When his body was laid at rest in West Hampstead Cemetery, England had buried her greatest surgeon.

The character of Lister, like his grave and gentle face, was one of rare nobility. As the Quaker is the Puritan transposed into a softer and more grateful key, so his nature had those elements of sweetness which proverbially can come only out of strength. Neglect and opposition he endured with the serene fortitude and dignity of those

---

[1] The cavillings of von Bruns ("*Fort mildem Spray!*"), Tait, and Bantock have, in the end, proved to be of little moment, so far as the generic idea of surgical cleanliness is concerned.

[2] Brit. Med. Jour., Lond., 1870, ii, 243.

[3] Sir St. Clair Thomson: Lancet, Lond., 1927, i, 775.

who are born to the purple, and honors could not spoil him. Of his self-possession in the face of stabs and sneers, his pupil, Sir St. Clair Thomson, relates that he "exhibited no resentment, never retaliated, and only showed how he felt it by the little gasping sigh we all learned to know and to respect as his only sign of sorrow or annoyance." In relation to the ethical side of bedside practice, Lister belongs in the great Hippocratic tradition. His surgical achievement places him at the very head and forefront of English medicine in our time.

Of the surgeons of Lister's time, who developed his ideas in new fields, perhaps the first place belongs to Theodor **Billroth** (1829–94), the pioneer of **visceral surgery.** Born on the island of Rügen, a Berlin

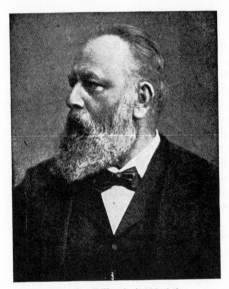

graduate of 1852, Billroth became an assistant in Langenbeck's clinic, and subsequently professor of surgery at Zürich (1860–67) and Vienna (1867–94). Billroth was early interested in wound infections, and, in his "coccobacteria septica," he had undoubtedly grasped the causal idea, but regarded one generic group of bacteria as the cause of a whole family of affections. He wrote an admirable volume of lectures on surgical pathology and therapeutics (1863[1]), which was translated into almost every modern language, but he is especially remembered as the surgeon of the alimentary tract. In 1872, he made the first resec-

Theodor Billroth (1829–94).   tion of the esophagus,[2] and, in 1881, the first resection of the pylorus for cancer, which was successful.[3] He also made the first complete excision of the larynx (1873[4]), is said to have been the first to perform the "interilio-abdominal amputation" (1891[5]), and did a large number of intestinal resections and enterorrhaphies (1878–83[6]). All these operations upon the gastro-intestinal tract did much to elucidate the pathology of those regions; they were, in Naunyn's phrase, "autopsies *in vivo.*"

---

[1] Billroth: Die allgemeine chirurgische Pathologie und Therapie, Berlin, 1863.

[2] Arch. f. klin. Chir., Berl., 1872, xiii, 65–69, 1 pl.

[3] Wien. med. Wochenschr., 1881, xxxi, 162–165.

[4] Arch. f. klin. Chir., Berl., 1874, xvii, 343–356, 1 pl.

[5] Billroth did not report upon an unsuccessful operation, said to have been performed about 1891, so that, by the law of priority, credit is given to Mathieu Jaboulay, who published the first paper in Lyon méd., 1894, lxxv, 507–510.

[6] Zeitschr. f. Heilk., Prague, 1884, v, 83–108.

Billroth, a man of charming, genial personality, had a strong artistic bent, delicately revealed in the few specimens of verse and music which he left, and in his delightful *Briefe*, in some sort, a memorial of his life-long friendship with the great North German composer, Johannes Brahms.

Billroth's most prominent pupils were Mikulicz, Czerny, Wölfler, and Gersuny, all Slavs, and von Eiselsberg, an Austrian.

Johann **von Mikulicz-Radecki** (1850–1905), of Czernowitz, Poland, was Billroth's assistant up to 1881, and professor of surgery at Königsburg (1887) and Breslau (1890).

He did much to improve antiseptic methods, introduced the present modes of exploring the esophagus and the stomach (1881[1]), first treated cancer of the esophagus by resection and plastic transplantation (1886[2]), introduced lateral pharyngotomy in excising malignant tumors of the tonsillar region (1886[3]), described symmetrical inflammation of the lacrimal and salivary glands, Mikulicz's disease (1892[4]), greatly extended the operative surgery of the stomach and the joints, and collaborated in an atlas (1892) and a treatise (1898) on diseases of the mouth. He was one of the first to wear gloves on operative work, but the cotton gloves he used were soon superseded by those of rubber, introduced by Halsted in Baltimore (1890–91), and in Germany (1897) by Werner Zoege-Manteuffel (1857–1926).

Anton **Wölfler** (1850–1917), of Kopezen, Bohemia, professor of surgery at Graz (1886) and Prague (1895), introduced gastro-enterostomy (1881[5]), and devoted special attention to the surgical treatment of goiter (1887–91).

Robert **Gersuny** (1844–   ), of Teplitz, Bohemia, who succeeded Billroth as director of the Rudolfinerhaus (1894), is now best remembered for the introduction of prosthetic paraffin injections (1900).

Vincenz **Czerny** (1842–1916), of Trautenau, Bohemia professor of surgery at Freiburg (1871) and Heidelberg (1887), introduced the enucleation of subperitoneal uterine fibroids by the vaginal route (1881[6]), and extended Billroth's work on the excision of the larynx, the esophagus, the kidneys, and general visceral surgery. His later days were devoted to cancer research, culminating in the opening of the Heidelberg Samariterhaus (1906) under his direction.

Karl **Thiersch** (1822–95), of Munich, one of Stromeyer's pupils, who became professor of surgery at Erlangen (1854) and Leipzig (1887), was a great pioneer of Listerism, and through his studies of epithelial cancer (1865[7]), phosphoric necrosis of the jaws (1867[8]), the healing of wounds (1867[9]), and his improvement in skin-grafting (1874[10]) was a prominent contributor to surgical pathology.

Richard **von Volkmann** (1830–89), of Leipzig, son of the well-known Halle physiologist, and professor of surgery in the latter city (1867–89), also did much to introduce antisepsis after the Franco-Prussian War,

---

[1] Mikulicz: Wien. med. Presse, 1881, xxii, 1405 *et seq.*
[2] Prag. med. Wochenschr., 1886, ix, 93.   [3] Przegl. lek., Krakow, 1886, xxv, 173.
[4] Billroth Festschrift (Beiträge zur Chirurgie), Stuttg., 1892, 610–630, 1 pl.
[5] Wölfler: Centralbl. f. Chir., Leipz., 1881, viii, 705–708.
[6] Czerny: Wien. med. Wochenschr., 1881, xxxi, 501, 525.
[7] Thiersch: Der Epithelialkrebs, Leipzig, 1865.
[8] Thiersch: De maxillarum necrosi phosphorica, Leipzig, 1867.
[9] Handb. d. allg. u. spez. Chir. (Pitha-Billroth), 1867, i, 2. Abth., No. 3.
[10] Verhandl. d. deutsch. Gesellsch. f. Chir., Berl., 1874, iii, 69–75.

was the first to excise the rectum for cancer (1878[1]), described the so-called ischemic contractures or paralyses (1881[2]), and cancer in paraffin-workers, and founded the well-known *Sammlung klinischer Vorträge* (1870), which contains some of the most valuable monographs of recent times. He was a man of aristocratic appearance, a poet ("Richard Leander"), and his "Dreams by French Firesides"[3] is a charming book.

Friedrich **von Esmarch** (1823–1908), of Tönning, Schleswig-Holstein, a pupil of Stromeyer and Langenbeck, who became professor at Kiel (1857–99), was a great military surgeon, having served through the campaigns of 1848–50, 1864–66, and 1870–71. He is most memorable

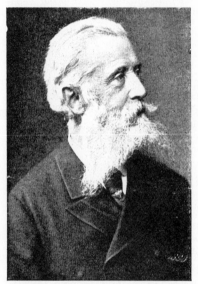

for his introduction of the first-aid bandage on the battle-field (1869–70[4]), and for standardizing surgical hemostasis by the "Esmarch bandage" (1873[5]). He did much to improve the status of military surgery through his contributions on resection after gunshot wounds (1851), the proper locale for field hospitals and bandaging stations (1861), surgical technics (1871), first aid to the wounded (1875), and on first aid in accidents (1882). Esmarch was the pioneer and founder of the so-called *Samariterwesen*, for military nursing, in Germany. Through his marriage with a royal princess, he became an uncle of Emperor Wilhelm II.

Ernst **von Bergmann** (1836–1907), of Riga, Russia, graduated at Dorpat in 1860, served in the Prussian army in the wars of 1866 and

Friedrich von Esmarch (1823–1908). (Collection of A. C. Klebs.)

1870–71, and on the Russian side in the war of 1877–78, after which he became a prominent figure in German medicine. He was called to the chair at Würzburg in 1878, and succeeded Langenbeck at Berlin (1882), where he remained for the rest of his life.

He greatly advanced cranial surgery in his memoirs on head injuries (1873[6]) and surgical treatment of cerebral diseases (1888[7]), and is also notable for his works

---

[1] Volkmann: Samml. klin. Vortr., Leipz., 1878, No. 131 (Chir. No. 42), 1113–1128.   [2] Centralbl. f. Chir., Leipz., 1881, viii, 801–803.

[3] Volkmann: Träumereien an französischen Kaminen, Leipzig, 1871.

[4] Esmarch: Der erste Verband auf dem Schlachtfelde, Kiel, 1869.

[5] Samml. klin. Vortr., Leipz., 1873, No. 58 (Chir. No. 19), 373–384.

[6] Bergmann: Handb. d. allg. u. spez. Chir. (Pitha-Billroth), Erlangen, 1873, iii, 1. Abth., 1. Abschn.

[7] Bergmann: Die chirurgische Behandlung bei Hirnkrankheiten, Berlin, 1888.

on fatty embolism (1863), the surgery of the joints (1872–78), ligation of the femoral vein (1882), diseases of the lymphatic glands (1881), and his various contributions to surgical pathology. He introduced steam-sterilization in surgery (1886), and established the present standardized aseptic ritual (1891). His letters of 1866–77 were edited by A. Buchholz (1911).

Ernst Julius **Gurlt** (1825–99), of Berlin, where he became professor in 1862, took part in all the German wars of the period, wrote with ability on a great variety of themes, and holds a high place in medical literature as the historian of surgery *par excellence*. He was one of the most learned surgeons of his time. His *Geschichte der Chirurgie* (1898), dealing with the history of the subject down to the Renaissance period, is to surgery what Haeser is to medicine, unrivaled for scholarship, exhaustive treatment, and accurate bibliography. It is a work which stands quite apart as one of the greatest monuments of German thoroughness.

In **orthopedics,** especial distinction was attained by the **Heine family,** all of whom were expert mechanicians, in particular Jacob von Heine (1799–1879), of Cannstatt, who first described poliomyelitic deformities (1840) and wrote an important treatise on dislocations (1842); Gustav Simon (1868); Adolf Lorenz (1854–   ), of Weidenau, Silesia, who introduced the bloodless method of reducing congenital dislocations of the hip-joint by forcible manipulation; Julius Wolff (1836–1902), of West Prussia, author of a great monograph on the law governing the pathological transformations of bones (1892), and Albert Hoffa (1859–1908), who introduced a well-known operation for congenital hip dislocations (1890), and was founder and editor of the *Zeitschrift für orthopädische Chirurgie* (1891).

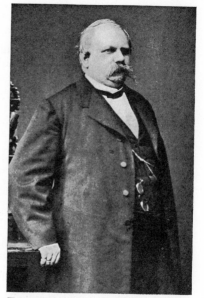

Ernst Julius Gurlt (1825–99). (Courtesy of Dr. George M. Kober.)

Of original operations by German surgeons of the 19th century, we may mention those of the first nephropexy by Eugen Hahn (1881), the first excision of the gall-bladder by Carl Langenbuch (1882), the first colostomy by Karl Maydl (1888), thoracotomy for empyema by Ernst Küster (1889), resection of the rectum by Paul Kraske (1891), excision of the Gasserian ganglion by Fedor Krause (1893), and excision of the stomach by Carl Schlatter (1897). The introduction of the cystoscope (1877–78) by Max Nitze (1848–1906) vastly improved the surgery of the bladder.

Of the French surgeons of the period, Aristide-Auguste **Verneuil** (1823–95), of Paris, who held many hospital appointments and trained many good pupils, made no original discoveries, but is remembered by such procedures as forcipressure in hemorrhage (1875), dry bandaging, treatment of abscesses with iodoform, and by the *Revue de chirurgie* (1881), of which he was one of the founders and editors. He wrote no large monographs, and his works are all contained in the six volumes of his *Mémoires de chirurgie* (1877–88).

Édouard **Nicaise** (1838–96), surgeon at the Laennec Hospital (1880–96), was, like Malgaigne, especially learned in the history of his subject, issued superb modern editions of Guy de Chauliac (1890), Henri de Mondeville (1893), and Pierre Franco (1895), and wrote many fascinating essays.

Jacques-Gilles **Maisonneuve** (1809–97), of Nantes, a pupil of Dupuytren and

Récamier, was one of the most enterprising and versatile of French operators, particularly in surgery of the bones, the intestines and in gynecology. He was surgeon at the Hôtel Dieu from 1862 on, but spent the last years of his long life in retirement. Just **Lucas-Championnière** (1843–1913), who before his graduation (1870) entered Lister's service at Glasgow, did most for the establishment of antiseptics in France. He wrote a *Manuel de chirurgie antiseptique* (1876), and, as a pupil of Broca, did much for trephining, also for the surgery of the osseous system generally.

Félix **Guyon** (1831–1920), a native of the Island of Réunion, professor of genito-urinary surgery at the Paris Faculty (1890), was one of the great teachers of this specialty in his time. His clinics at Necker were followed by students from all over the world. His lectures on genito-urinary diseases (1881) and surgical diseases of the bladder and the prostate (1888) are his most important works. Bigelow's litholapaxy was perfected by Thomson and by Guyon, who was succeeded, and perhaps surpassed, by his brilliant pupil, Joaquin **Albarran** (1860–1912), another exotic, born at Sagua la Grande, Cuba who was twice a gold medalist of the Paris Faculty (1888–89), and professeur agrégé in 1892. In his short life, he became a star of the first magnitude as a teacher and through his many valuable innovations in the diagnosis of intrapelvic conditions by the urine. His works on exploration of the renal functions (1905) and surgery of the urinary passages (1909) are his masterpieces.

Other French surgeons of note were Charles Sédillot (1804–83), who performed the first gastrostomy (1849); Paul Berger (1845–1908), who wrote an exhaustive monograph on the interscapulo-thoracic amputation (1887); Mathieu Jaboulay, who first described the interilio-abdominal amputation (1894), and wrote an authoritative monograph on the surgery of the sympathetic system and of the thyroid gland (1900), in which he was associated with Antonin Poncet (1849–1913); Edmond Delorme (1847–　　), who introduced the operation of decortication of the lungs for chronic empyema (1894–1901); Ulysse Trélat (1828–93), professor at the Hôpital Necker; Louis-Félix Terrier (1837–1908), and Louis-X.-E.-L. Ollier (1825–1900). The Italian surgeons did some bold operating on the heart, the first in this field being Guido Farina, who sutured the right ventricle on June 8, 1896.[1] The first successful suture of the heart was done by L. Rehn at Frankfort on the Main in 1896.[2] Cardiolysis was proposed by Brauer in 1902. Of the Swiss surgeons, Jacques-Louis Reverdin (1842–　　) and Theodor Kocher are memorable for their operations on the thyroid gland, and August Socin (1837–99) for his work in military surgery (1872) and surgical diseases of the prostate (1875). Among the Italians, Luigi Porta (1800–75), Scarpa's successor at Pavia, was notable for his work on the surgery of the thyroid gland and the vascular system.

Sir James **Paget** (1814–99), of Great Yarmouth, England, graduated from St. Bartholomew's Hospital, with which he was all his life associated, and was serjeant surgeon to the Queen, receiving his baronetcy in 1871. A warm friend of Virchow, Paget was, like Brodie, a great surgical pathologist.

His best works are his *Lectures on Tumours* (1851), *Surgical Pathology* (1863), *Clinical Lectures and Essays* (1875), the catalogue of the Pathological Museum of the

---

[1] Farina: Bull. d. r. Accad. di med. di Roma, 1896–7, xxiii, 248.

[2] L. Rehn: Arch. f. klin. Chir., Berl., 1907, lxxxiii, 723–778; Rehn's case was alive when he wrote this paper, over ten years after the operation had been performed.

Royal College of Surgeons (1882), of which he was president (1875), and his original descriptions of eczema of the nipple, with subsequent mammary cancer (1874[1]), and the trophic disorder, osteitis deformans (1877–82[2]). He also made an early note of erythromelalgia (Weir Mitchell's disease), and his life-work illustrates how the surgeon proper can be a good clinical observer.

Sir Jonathan **Hutchinson** (1828–1913), of Selby, Yorkshire, also a St. Bartholomew's man, surgeon to the London Hospital (1859–83), and professor of surgery at the Royal College of Surgeons (1879–83), was another able surgical pathologist, and is especially memorable for his description of the notched, peg-shaped incisor teeth (Hutchinson's teeth) in congenital syphilis (1861[3]), of varicella gangrenosa (1882[4]) and other skin diseases, and for his views of the causation of leprosy, which he attributed to eating fish. His name is further associated with the eponyms "Hutchinson's facies" in ophthalmoplegia, "Hutchinson's mask" in tabes, the unequal pupils in meningeal hemorrhage, and "Hutchinson's triad" (interstitial keratitis, notched teeth, labyrinthine disease) in syphilis, of which he saw over a million cases. His *Archives* of *Surgery* (1889–99) in ten volumes, entirely written by himself, forms a great storehouse of original observations on disease, which will some day be studied like the works of John Hunter.

Sir Victor **Horsley** (1857–1916), of Kensington, England, was a pioneer in experimental and neurological surgery, particularly in his operations on the ductless glands

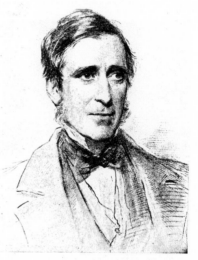

Sir James Paget (1814–99). (From a portrait by George Richmond.)

(1884–86), the brain (1886–90), and in his initial operation for a tumor of the spinal cord (diagnosed by Gowers, 1888[5]), after which, as Cushing says, "certain neurologists began to do their own surgery."

Horsley produced artificial myxedema in the monkey by thyroidectomy (1884), was one of the earliest operators for hypophyseal tumors, and standardized the operations of laminectomy, craniotomy, and intradural division of the nerve in trigeminal neuralgia. With Schäfer, Beevor, and others he charted the areas of the cerebral cortex (1884–94) and, with Gotsch, produced experimental degenerations of the spinal tracts and of currents in the cord (1891). His suggestion that muzzling would stamp out rabies proved effective, and under his inspiration, L. C. Wooldridge made those experiments on saline blood coagulation which led to the use of the normal salt solution.

[1] Paget: St. Barth. Hosp. Rep., Lond., 1874, x, 87–89.

[2] Paget: Med.-Chir. Tr., Lond., 1876–7, lx, 37; 1881–2, lxv, 225.

[3] Hutchinson: Brit. Med. Jour., Lond., 1861, i, 515–519.

[4] Med.-Chir. Tr., Lond., 1881–2, lxv, pp. i–ii.

[5] Sir W. R. Gowers and Horsley: Med. Chir. Tr., Lond., 1887–8, lxxi, 377–430.

Horsley, who came of a family of artists, was a man of aggressive, chivalrous temperament, and with a mind intensely alive. In politics he was dogmatic, self-centered, sometimes inconsistent, with no notion of compromise. His opposition to the use of alcohol and tobacco was based upon isolated observations and experiences, and, although peremptory with his nurses, he was yet ardent for woman-suffrage. He died for his country, having served in Egypt and Gallipoli, succumbing to heat-stroke in Mesopotamia.

Hugh Owen **Thomas** (1834–91), a gifted orthopedist, of Liverpool, wrote much on fractures and deformities (1876–90), invented the extension splint which proved so valuable during the World War, devised the method of treating delayed union of fractures by passive congestion ("damming the circulation"), later revived by Bier, and did much for the after-treatment of motor-nerve injuries.

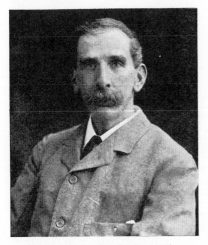

Sir Victor Horsley (1857–1916).

Sir William **MacEwen** (1848–1924), of Rothesay, Scotland, professor of surgery at the University of Glasgow (1892), is notable for his methods of osteotomy for genu valgum (1881), radical cure of oblique inguinal hernia (1887), treatment of aneurysm by acupuncture (1890), and his monograph on *Pyogenic Infective Diseases of the Brain* (1893), which sums up his brilliant work on the surgery of the brain and spinal cord.

Sir William **MacCormac** (1836–1901), of Belfast, Ireland, saw a great deal of military surgery in the Franco-Prussian and Turco-Servian Wars, and early applied Listerian principles with success to the surgery of the joints and the abdomen, particularly in his pioneer operations for intraperitoneal rupture of the bladder (1886[1]).

Sir Frederick **Treves** (1853–1923), of Dorchester, England, is widely known for his works on surgical anatomy (1883), intestinal obstruction (1884), appendicitis, and peritonitis, his System of Surgery (1895), and (with Lang) a very valuable dictionary of German medical terms (1890). He played an important part in the Transvaal War, has written some charming travel sketches, and performed the operation upon King Edward VII in 1902.

Two American surgeons whose life-work extended over into the Listerian period were Bigelow and Gross.

Henry Jacob **Bigelow** (1816–90), of Boston, Massachusetts, who became surgeon to the Massachusetts General Hospital (1846) and professor of surgery in the Harvard Medical School, was the leading surgeon of New England during his life-time. He was the first to excise the hip-joint in America (1852[2]), and, in his monograph on dislocation and fracture of the hip (1869[3]), he first described the mechanism of the iliofemoral or Y-ligament, emphasizing its importance in reducing dislocation by the flexion method. He also introduced the

---

[1] MacCormac: Lancet, Lond., 1886, ii, 1118–1122.

[2] Bigelow: Am. Jour. Med. Sc., Phila., 1852, xxiv, 90.

[3] Bigelow: The Mechanism of Dislocation and Fracture of the Hip, Phila., 1869.

surgical procedure of litholapaxy or lithotrity for rapid evacuation of vesical calculus (1878[1]).

Samuel David **Gross** (1805–84), of Easton, Pennsylvania, professor of surgery at Louisville, Kentucky (1840–56), and at the Jefferson Medical College, Philadelphia (1856–82), was the greatest American surgeon of his time.

He wrote the first exhaustive treatise on pathological anatomy in English (1839[2]), which passed through three editions and was highly thought of, even by Virchow. He also wrote an authoritative treatise on diseases of the genito-urinary organs (1851), containing the first account of the distribution of urinary calculus; the first systematic treatise on foreign bodies in the air-passages (1854), and an important two-volume system of surgery (1859). Gross invented many new instruments, made original experiments upon the effects of manual strangulation (1836) and wounds of the intestines (1843) in animals, dissected and described specimens of molar pregnancy (1839), introduced deep stitches in wounds of the abdominal wall, performed laparotomy for rupture of the bladder, myotomy for wry-neck (1873), and first described prostatorrhea (1860). He knew the literature of his subject well, and his histories of Kentucky surgery (1851) and of American surgery down to the year 1876 are authoritative and accurate monographs. His biographies of Drake, McDowell, John Hunter, Richter, Paré, Mott, and others are all attractive reading.

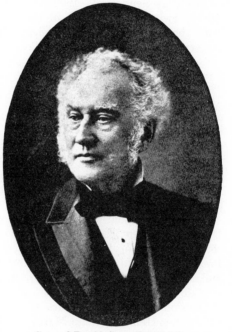

Samuel David Gross (1805–84).

Gross was a strong personality, a stalwart figure, with a beautiful, benignant countenance. His works were crowned, as the inscription of his funeral urn reads, by "the milk-white flower of a stainless life." His statue stands by the Army Medical Museum, Washington, D. C. He was the greatest of the German-American physicians.

William Williams **Keen** (1837–   ), of Philadelphia, professor of surgery at the Jefferson Medical College (1889–1907), is the author of an important work on the surgical complications and sequels of typhoid fever (1898), and has been a brilliant and skilful operator, particularly in diseases of the brain. He was the first to tap the ventricles (1889), did one of the first successful operations for meningioma (1888), with survival of the patient for thirty years (1918) and was a pioneer in linear craniotomy (1891) and the inter-ilioabdominal operation (1904).

---

[1] Bigelow: Am. Jour. Med. Sc., Phila., 1878, lxxv, 117–134.

[2] Gross: Elements of Pathologic Anatomy, Boston, 1839.

He is well known by his American Text-book (1899–1903) and his System of Surgery (1905–21), which are probably the best American works of their kind. Among his historical essays, his *Early History of Practical Anatomy* (1870) is most valuable for its accuracy and thoroughness.

Christian **Fenger** (1840–1902), of Chicago, was the first teacher of pathology in the Middle West, and did notable work on cancer of the stomach, basal hernia of the brain, the ball-valve action of floating gall-stones, and, as a pioneer surgeon, in the operative approaches to brain abscesses, the ureters, and the bile-ducts.

Nicholas **Senn** (1844–1909), a highly trained scientific surgeon, of Buchs, Switzerland, settled in the United States in 1852, graduated from the Chicago Medical College (1868), and became professor of surgery at the Rush Medical College.

Senn made valuable experimental contributions to the study of air embolism (1885), the surgery of the pancreas (1886), gunshot wounds, and intestinal anastomosis, in which he introduced the use of decalcified bone-plates. He was, in fact, a great master of intestinal surgery, especially in the treatment of appendicitis. He devised a method of detecting intestinal perforation by means of inflation with hydrogen gas (1888), and was the first to use the Roentgen rays in the treatment of leukemia (1903).

Senn played an important part in the Spanish-American War, founded the Association of Military Surgeons of the United States (1891), and, at his death, left a fine collection of medical books to the Newberry Library, and other handsome bequests to the city of his adoption.

Other prominent American surgeons of the Listerian period[1] are D. Hayes **Agnew** (1818–92), of Philadelphia, professor of surgery at the University of Pennsylvania, who was prominent in the case of President Garfield, and one of the few surgeons who practised medicine and surgery together; John Thompson **Hodgen** (1826–82), of Kentucky, who devised many instruments and apparatus, in particular, his wire suspension splints for fracture of the femur and forearm, which are still in use; Henry Orlando **Marcy** (1837–   ), of Otis, Massachusetts, who introduced antiseptic ligatures in the radical cure of hernia (1878), and wrote important treatises on hernia (1889) and the surgery of the perineum (1889); Robert Fulton **Weir** (1838–1927), of New York, who has done much in visceral and articular surgery; Charles **McBurney** (1845–1913), of Roxbury, Massachusetts, who discovered "McBurney's point" as a sign for operative intervention in appendicitis (1889); Lewis Atterbury **Stimson** (1844–1917), of Paterson, N. J., author of treatises on fractures and dislocations (1899), operative surgery (1900), and of improvements in gynecological surgery; Lewis Stephen **Pilcher** (1845–   ), of Adrian, Michigan, editor of *Annals of Surgery* (1885); Robert **Abbe** (1851–1928), of New York City, who introduced catgut rings in intestinal anastomosis and suturing (1892); Frank **Hartley** (1856–1913),

[1] See, also, the series: Master-Surgeons of America in Surg., Gynec., & Obst., Chicago, 1922–8, xxxv–xlv, *passim.*

of Washington, who originated intracranial neurectomy of the second and third divisions of the fifth nerve for facial neuralgia (1892); George Michael **Edebohls** (1853–1908), of New York, who introduced the operation of renal decapsulation in the treatment of chronic nephritis and puerperal eclampsia (1901); George Ryerson **Fowler** (1848–1906), who first performed thoracoplasty (1893); Arpad G. **Gerster** (1848–1923), of Kassa, Hungary, author of an early treatise on aseptic and antiseptic surgery (1888); Roswell **Park** (1852–1914), of Pomfret, Connecticut, prominent in connection with President McKinley's case, and author of a text-book of surgery (1896) and an attractive history of medicine (1897); Robert T. **Morris** (1857–   ), of Seymour, Connecticut, author of many technical improvements and original ideas; William B. **Coley** (1862–   ), of Westport, Connecticut, who introduced the treatment of inoperable sarcoma with the mixed toxins of erysipelas and Bacillus prodigiosus (1891–1911), and the brothers, Charles Horace and William James **Mayo,** of Minnesota, authors of many accepted improvements in visceral surgery, whose genius for method and system at the hospital at Rochester, Minn., has made Listerian surgery almost as reliable a science as bookkeeping.

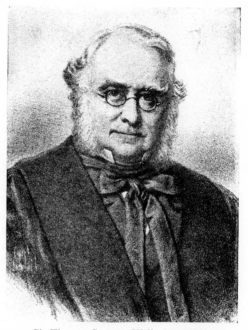

Sir Thomas Spencer Wells (1818–97).

Prominent in orthopedic and plastic surgery were Frank Hastings **Hamilton** (1813–86), of Wilmington, Vermont, who was a pioneer in skin-grafting for ulcers (1854), and wrote an important treatise on fractures and dislocations (1860); and Louis Albert **Sayre** (1820–1900), of New Jersey, who performed the second excision of the hip-joint in America (1855) and introduced the method of suspension in a plaster-of-Paris jacket for Pott's disease (1877).

The **gynecology** of the post-Listerian period was, in the main, a brilliant development of the operative principles which had been established by McDowell, Sims, Emmett, and Battey in America, Koeberlé in France, Gustav Simon in Germany, and Sir Thomas **Spencer Wells** (1818–97) in England. Wells, one of the greatest of the ovariotomists, was a native of Saint Albans, Hertfordshire, a pupil

of Stokes and Graves in Dublin, and of Travers in London.   After
serving seven years as surgeon in the Royal Navy (1841–48), including
an experience in the Crimean War, he settled in London, and, in 1858,
performed his first successful ovariotomy, which was followed by a
large number of favorable experiences with the same operation.   Phenomenal luck attended all his improvements in technic.   In a few
years, he was known to his colleagues and sought by patients all over
the world as an absolutely safe operator in ovarian conditions.   His
work was summed up in his treatise on *Diseases of the Ovaries* (1865–
72).   He was professor of surgery and pathological anatomy and president of the Royal College of
Surgeons, and surgeon to the
Queen's household, receiving his
baronetcy in 1883.

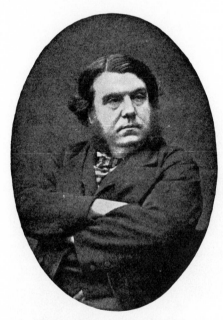

A gynecologist of wider scope
and even greater success was
Robert **Lawson Tait** (1845–99),
of Edinburgh, who settled in
Birmingham in 1871, and made
that city another Mecca for
female patients seeking operative relief.   Tait's success in
operating, as judged by his
statistics, was marvelous.   He
rolled up ovariotomies and other
abdominal sections seemingly
by the thousands, with scarce
a death, yet, strange to say, he
was a violent and even truculent
opponent of Lister.   He declined
to see any causal relation between bacteria and disease, and
pointed, with exaggerated scorn,
to the fact that he never used

Robert Lawson Tait (1845–99).

any antiseptic precautions in his operations beyond simple cleanliness.
The secret of his success was undoubtedly his wonderful skill, plus the
use of warm or boiled water to flush out the abdomen, which was, of
course, asepsis.

Tait performed his first ovariotomy, July 29, 1868; removed an ovary for abscess, February 2, 1872; excised the uterine appendages to arrest the growth of a
bleeding myoma, August 1, 1872; performed his first hysterectomy for myoma in
1873; removed a hematosalpinx, June 21, 1876; performed his first cholecystotomy,
and removed his first pyosalpinx and hydrosalpinx, in 1879; and did the first successful operation for ruptured tubal pregnancy, January 17, 1883.   He was thus a
pioneer in all phases of operative gynecology, was the first to work out the pathology and treatment of pelvic hematocele, and, in his *Lectures* on these subjects
(1888[1]), he points out that the first authoritative treatise on extra-uterine pregnancy

---

[1] Tait: Lectures on Ectopic Pregnancy and Pelvic Hæmatocele, Birmingham,
1888.

was written by John S. Parry (1843–76), of Philadelphia (1876). In 1879 Tait excised the normal ovaries,[1] along the lines laid down by Battey (1872–73), but claimed that in none of his cases were the uterine appendages normal. This, with the similar operation of Alfred Hegar (1830–1914) in 1877, developed "the whole field of pelvic operations for diseases of the organs other than gross ovarian and fibroid tumors" (Kelly). "The peri-uterine phlegmons of Emmet and Thomas became recognized as tubal inflammations and abscesses." In 1879, Tait introduced, among other novelties, his methods of dilating the cèrvix and of replacing the inverted uterus. In 1880, he introduced hepatotomy, and, in 1881, devised the special operation for excision of the uterine appendages by securing the pedicle with a silk ligature, tied by means of his invention, the "Staffordshire knot."[2] His method of "flapsplitting" in plastic repair of the perineum was a valuable innovation (1879[3]), but it was not taken up in America for a long time.

Tait left interesting summaries of conclusions from his operative statistics, treatises on diseases of the ovaries (1873) and diseases of women (1879–89), and pungent essays on rape and other subjects connected with medical jurisprudence. In all these productions, he is a forcible, effective, frequently coarse, not entirely truthful, but always amusing, writer.

Of prominent innovations in operative gynecology, we may mention the different methods of excising or enucleating uterine tumors, introduced by Eugène Koeberlé (1864), August Martin (1876), Karl Schröder (1878–84), and Vincenz Czerny (1881); of excising the uterus, by Wilhelm Alexander Freund (1878), Vincenz Czerny (1878), Benjamin Franklin Baer (1892), Fernand Henrotin (1892), Jean-Louis Faure (1897) and by Ernst Wertheim (1864–1920) in 1900; the improvements in myomectomy by Henry O. Marcy (1881), Joseph Price (1886), Lewis A. Stimson (1889), Joseph R. Eastman (1889), William M. Polk (1889), Florian Krug (1894); of treating uterine displacements, by James Alexander Adams and William Alexander (1882), Robert Olshausen (1886), Howard A. Kelly (1887), and George Michael Edebohls (1901). The introduction of the standard hemostatic forceps by Eugène Koeberlé (1865), his methods of liberating adhesions, of *morcellement* in enucleating fibroids (1865), of constricting the pedicle in ovarian cysts (*pédicule perdu*), of pelvic drainage, were all great advances in operative technique. The surgical posture (elevation of the pelvis) introduced by Friedrich Trendelenburg (1890) was another valuable device. The technic of Cesarean section was improved by Ferdinand Adolph Kehrer (1882), particularly by Max Sänger (1882), by Edoardo Porro (1876), who first performed Cesarean section with excision of the uterus and adnexa (1876), and by Alfred Dührssen, who introduced the vaginal operation (1898). Excision of the vagina was introduced in 1895 by Robert Olshausen (1835–1915), the plastic reformation of the vagina by Alwin Karl Mackenrodt (1896), and a flap operation for atresia of the vagina by George Henry Noble (1900). Cesarean section in puerperal convulsions was introduced by Tjalling Halbertsma (1889). Pubiotomy as a substitute for symphysiotomy is associated with the name of Leonardo Gigli (1902). Extrauterine pregnancy was studied by John S. Parry (1876); by Lawson Tait, who performed the first successful tubal operation (1883), by Richard Werth (1850–1919) in 1887, Joseph Eastman (1888) Joseph Price (1853–1911) in 1890, John Clarence Webster (1892), and B. J. Kouwer, who first described ovarian pregnancy (1897). Much of the history of gynecology up to recent times has been described by Priestley[4] as a series of "crazes," a tendency to follow prevailing fashions. First of all came the uterine displacement craze, when Graily Hewitt in England, Velpeau in France, Hodge in America, championed the cause of the pessary for the treatment of backache or pelvic pain, and every gynecologist felt himself called upon to invent one or

---

[1] Tait: Brit. Med. Jour., Lond., 1879, i, 813.

[2] Tait: Brit. Med. Jour., Lond., 1881, i, 766.

[3] Tait: Obst. Jour. Gr. Brit., Lond., 1879–80, vii, 585–588. Brit. Gynæc. Jour., Lond., 1887–8, iii, 366; 1892, vii, 195.

[4] Sir. W. O. Priestley: On over-operating in gynecology. Brit. Med. Jour., Lond., 1895, ii, 284–287.

to modify some one else's; the unfortunate uterus all the while being, as Allbutt says, either "impaled on a stem or perched on a twig." The pelvic cellulitis craze had its origin in the fact that, in 1857, Gustave Bernutz found a case of peri-uterine abscess due to inflammation of the pelvic cellular tissue, after wihich Bernutz and Goupil published their famous memoir on pelvic cellulitis (1862). This view of pelvic pathology was widely taken up until Gaillard Thomas exploded it in 1880, by showing that much of alleged cellulitis is really peritonitis, and that the former condition is rare in virgins. In like manner oöphorectomy, clitoridectomy, inflammation of the os and cervix uteri, excision of the uterus and its appendages, operations for extrauterine pregnancy, and Cæsarean section all had their day, according to the dictates of fashion. Meanwhile very substantial work was done on the pathological side by Carl Arnold Ruge (1846–1926) and Johann Veit (1852–1917), who described erosions of the cervix uteri (1877), by A. J. Skene on the para-urethral glands (1880), by August Briesky on kraurosis vulvæ (1885), by Max Sänger on decidual sarcoma of the uterus and other decidual tumors (1889–93), by J. Whitridge Williams on papillary cystoma of the ovary (1891) and deciduoma malignum (1895), by Thomas S. Cullen on hydrosalpinx (1895), cancer of the uterus (1900), adenomyoma of the uterus (1908), and diseases of the umbilicus (1916), and by Georg Winter on gynecological diagnosis (1896). The importance of latent gonorrhea in women was first emphasized in 1872 by Emil Noeggerath (1827–95), the general subject developed by Ernst von Bumm (1885), Max Sänger (1889), and the uterine and vesical phases (1895–6) by Ernst Wertheim (1864–1920). The treatment of uterine tumors by galvanism was introduced by Ephraim Cutter (1874) and faradization was first employed by Georges Apostoli (1884[1]).

Samuel Jean **Pozzi** (1846–1918), of Paris, a highly skilled general surgeon, author of many papers on anatomy and abnormities, and deviser of many technical procedures, did most to make gynecology a going concern in France.

Howard Atwood **Kelly** (1858–   ), of Philadelphia,[2] professor of gynecology in the University of Pennsylvania (1888) and the Johns Hopkins University (1889), and founder of the Kensington Hospital in Philadelphia (1883), is a recognized leader of his science in America.

He was a pioneer in the use of cocaine anesthesia (1884), in the treatment of retroflexion of the uterus by suspension (1887), in the introduction of the operations of nephro-ureterectomy, nephro-uretero-cystectomy, vertical bisection of the uterus in hysterectomy, bisection of fibroid or ovarian tumors, horizontal bisection of the cervix for tumors and inflammation, and ideal appendicectomy; the procedures of aëroscopic examination of the bladder and catheterization of the ureters, exploration of the rectum and sigmoid flexure, diagnosis of ureteral and renal calculi by waxtipped bougies, diagnosis of hydronephrosis by injection and measurement of the capacity of the renal pelvis, operating on the kidney by the superior lumbar triangle, treatment of malignant tumors by radium, and various improvements in the treatment of vesicovaginal fistulæ.[3] He is the inventor of the Kelly pad, new rectal and vesical specula, and his *Operative Gynecology* (1898) and *Medical Gynecology* (1908), both illustrated with Max Brödel's drawings, are full of improvements in his science which have made these books among the best American treatises of the time. Kelly is also known by his valuable historical contributions on hypnotism, American gynecology, appendicitis, vesico-vaginal fistula, medical botanists, medical illustration, and American medical biography (1912, 2d ed., 1920). His *Stereo-Clinic* (1910–13) is a permanent photographic record of surgical procedures of the time.

Although antisepsis, and even asepsis, had been employed in **obstetrics** before the time of Lister, the principle did not take hold until

---

[1] For bibliographical references to modern gynecology, see Index Catalogue, Surgeon-General's Library, 1912, 2. series, xvii, 163–166.

[2] Born at Camden, New Jersey.

[3] For references, see the bibliography of Kelly by Miss Minnie W. Blogg, in Bull. Johns Hopkins Hosp., Balt., 1919, xxx, 293–302.

surgeon and obstetrician alike began to cleanse their hands in carbolic or bichloride solutions. The first to employ the carbolic acid solution in obstetrics was Étienne **Tarnier** of Paris (1881[1]), the inventor of the well-known axis-traction forceps (1877[2]) and the introducer of milk-diet in pregnancy.

Important features of the pre-antiseptic period were the artificial induction of premature labor by Carl Wenzel (1804), the use of ergot by John Stearns, of Massachusetts (1808), the suggestion of chlorine water to prevent infantile conjunctivitis by Gottfried Eisenmann (1830), the establishment of the contagiousness of puerperal fever by Holmes (1843) and Semmelweis (1847–61), the first findings of albuminous urine in connection with puerperal convulsions by John C. W. Lever, of Guy's Hospital (1843[3]), Credé's *Handgriff* (1854), the introduction of combined cephalic version by Marmaduke Burr Wright, of Ohio (1854), and of combined podalic version by Braxton Hicks in 1864. In the early part of the century, the two French midwives, Mme. Boivin (1773–1841) and Mme. LaChapelle (1769–1821), published noteworthy treatises on obstetrics (1812 and 1821–25). Mme. LaChapelle's book, with its statistical deductions from 40,000 labor cases, had a good deal to do with the establishment of a proper norm or canon of obstetric procedure at the time. It was followed by such works as those of Velpeau (1829), Cazeaux (1840), and Dubois (1849) in France; Caspar von Siebold (1841), Michaëlis (1842), Kiwisch (1842), Scanzoni (1852), and Carl Braun von Fernwald (1857), Otto Spiegelberg (1858), in Germany and Austria; Fleetwood Churchill (1834) and Francis Henry Ramsbotham (1841) in England; W. P. Dewees (1824), Charles D. Meigs (1849), Hugh L. Hodge (1864), and W. T. Lusk (1882) in America. The best recent American treatise is that of John Whitridge Williams (1903).

Morphological study of the deformed pelvis and of spinal deformity in relation to difficult labor has been almost exclusively in the hands of the German obstetricians. The obliquely contracted pelvis (Naegele pelvis) was first described by Franz Carl

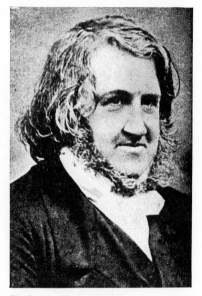

Sir James Young Simpson (1811–70).

Naegele (1839), and the oblique ovoid pelvis including the coxalgic, scoliotic, and kyphoscoliotic forms by Carl C. T. Litzmann in 1853. The straight narrow pelvis, due to defective development of the sacrum, was described by Robert (1842). The osteomalacic pelvis was first observed by William Hunter and described by the younger Stein. The rachitic or pseudo-osteomalacic type was described by Smellie, Sandifort, and the younger Stein, and named by Michaëlis (1851). The spondylolisthetic pelvis was described by Rokitansky (1839) and carefully studied by Kilian as "pelvis obtecta" (1854). Rokitansky also introduced the term "kyphotic pelvis." Baudelocque was the first to observe and describe the funnel-shaped pelvis. The spinous pelvis (pelvis spinosa) was described and figured by Kilian (1854), while Michaëlis and Litzmann first studied the flat pelvis (pelvis plana Deventeri) and its rachitic variety. Congenital cleft of the symphysis pubis was observed by Bonnet (1724) and Creve (1795), and described by Litzmann (1861). All these different varieties were carefully described by Gustav Adolf **Michaëlis** (1798–1848)

---

[1] Tarnier: Tr. Internat. Med. Cong., Lond., 1881, iv, 390.

[2] Tarnier: Ann. de gynéc., Paris, 1877, vii, 241–261.

[3] Lever: Guy's Hosp. Rep., Lond., 1843, 2. s., i, 495–519.

in *Das enge Becken* (1851) and in *Die Formen des Beckens* (1861), by Carl Conrad Theodor Litzmann.

After Semmelweis, the most prominent obstetricians of modern times were Simpson, Credé, and Braxton Hicks.

Sir James Young **Simpson** (1811–70), of Bathgate, Scotland, became professor of obstetrics at Edinburgh in 1840, and soon acquired an enormous practice through his great ability and fascinating personality. As the first to employ chloroform in obstetrics and labor (1847), he made a great name for himself in the history of his science.

Although not without a certain touch of religious fanaticism, which may account for his somewhat bigoted opposition to Lister, he exerted a wonderful influence over his patients, and was, all in all, one of the most remarkable personalities of his time.

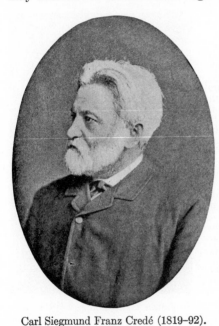

Simpson introduced iron wire sutures (1858), the long obstetric forceps, acupressure (1850–64), and many new "wrinkles" in gynecology and obstetrics, such as the uterine sound (1843), the sponge tent, dilatation of the cervix uteri in diagnosis, "Simpson's pains" in uterine cancer (1863), version in deformed pelves. His memoirs on fetal pathology and hermaphroditism are noteworthy; and he also made valuable contributions to archeology and medical history, particularly on leprosy in Scotland (1841–42). He introduced village or pavilion hospitals, and, by his statistical investigations of the results of major operations (Hospitalism, 1869), did much to improve hospital administration.

Carl Siegmund Franz **Credé** (1819–92), of Berlin, director of the obstetric and gynecologic wards of the Charité (1852), and

Carl Siegmund Franz Credé (1819–92).

professor of obstetrics at Leipzig, introduced two things of capital importance in obstetric procedure—his methods of removing the placenta by external manual expression (1854–60[1]), and of preventing infantile (gonorrheal) conjunctivitis by instillation of silver nitrate solution into the eyes of the newborn (1884[2]). He was editor of the *Monatsschrift für Geburtskunde* (1853–69) and of the *Archiv für Gynäkologie* (1870–92). He was an admirable teacher and a good organizer, having founded the obstetric and gynecologic polyclinic at Leipzig. The two innovations associated with his name entitle him to the permanent gratitude of mankind.

---

[1] Credé: Klin. Vortr. über Geburtschülfe, Berl., 1854, 599–603.

[2] Die Verhütung der Augenentzündung der Neugeborenen, etc., Berlin, 1884. Preceded by Gottfried Eisenmann's recommendation of chlorine water in 1830 (Jacobi).

John Braxton **Hicks** (1825–97), of London, a famous teacher who
held many honorable places, made an epoch in the history of obstetric
procedure by the introduction of podalic version by combined external
and internal manipulation (1863[1]), which forms a connecting link
across the ages with Ambroïse Paré's famous paper. Hick's priority
has been disputed in favor of Marmaduke Burr Wright, who, however,
employed or recommended external handling in *cephalic* version (1854).
Hick's observations on the condition of the uterus in obstructed labor
(1867[2]), and on accidental concealed hemorrhage (1872[3]), are also highly
esteemed by the practitioners of his art.

In the post-antiseptic period, Adolf Gusserow (1836–1906) described pernicious
anemia in pregnancy (1871), Christian Wilhelm Braune (1831–92) studied pregnancy in frozen sections (1872), Gustav
Adolf Walcher (1856–   ) introduced the
hanging posture (*Hängelage*) in the conduct of normal labor (1889), Luigi Maria
Bossi (1859–1919) originated the induction
of premature labor by forced dilatation of
the cervix (1892), Albert Döderlein (1860–
1919) studied the relation of the vaginal
secretions to puerperal fever (1892), Fritz
Momburg (1870–   ) and Felice La
Torre (1846–1923) introduced the use of
the abdominal ligature to prevent uterine
hemorrhage (1908), and C. J. Gauss and
Bernard Krönig (1863–1918), twilight sleep
(1906–15).

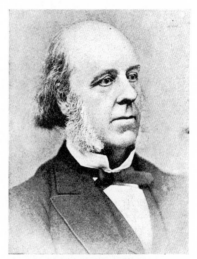

John Braxton Hicks (1825–97). (Boston Medical Library.)

Ophthalmology and the surgery
of the eye were put upon a scientific basis mainly through the
labors of three men, Helmholtz,
Albrecht von Graefe, and Donders.
When the ophthalmoscope was
invented, von Graefe exclaimed:
"Helmholtz has opened out a new
world to us" (*Helmholtz hat uns
eine neue Welt erschlossen*), and the usefulness of the instrument
is sufficiently indicated by the fact that nearly every prominent
eye specialist of recent times has tried to add some improvement
to it. Not only did it elucidate the disorders of the uveal tract, but
even such obscure diseases as those of the brain, the kidneys, and
the pituitary body. Bouchut, in 1893, called the process "cerebroscopy."

Before the time of von Graefe, the infectious forms of granular conjunctivitis
had been described by Baron Larrey (1802), John Vetch (1807), and Jacob Christian
Bendz (1855); William Hyde Wollaston had invented periscopic spectacles (1803)
and the camera lucida (1807); Benjamin Gibson had demonstrated that ophthalmia
neonatorum is due to the vaginal secretions (1807[4]) and the possibility of couching

[1] Hicks: Tr. Obst. Soc. Lond. (1863), 1864, v, 219–259 (Appendix), 265.

[2] *Ibid.* (1867), 1868, ix, 207–227 (Appendix), 229–239.

[3] Brit. Med. Jour. Lond., 1872, i, 207.

[4] Gibson: Edinb. Med. & Surg. Jour., 1807, iii, 159–161.

cataract in the new-born (1811[1]); hyoscyamin and atropin had been used in examination by Franz Reisinger (1825); Sir George Airy had described astigmatism (named by Whewell) and fitted cylindrical lenses for the condition; test-readings of print at a distance had been employed by J. Ayscough (1752), J. G. A. Chevallier (1805), G. Tauber (1816), F. Holke (1830), F. Cunier (1841), and K. Himly (1843); test-types were introduced by Heinrich Küchler (*Schriftnummerprobe*, 1843), Eduard Jaeger von Jaxtthal (1854), C. Stellwag von Carion (1855), Graefe and Donders (1860–62), Hermann Snellen (1862), Ezra Dyer (1862), Giraud-Teulon (1862), and J. Green (1866–8); Kussmaul had described the color phenomena in the fundus (1845); J. Mery (1704), Purkinje (1823), William Cumming (1846), and Ernst Brücke (1847) had considered the significance of luminosity of the eye in vertebrates and man; Philipp Franz von Walther had described corneal opacity (1845); Sichel had published his book on spectacles (1848); the mechanism of vision had been studied by Thomas Young (1801), W. H. Wollaston (1802), Sir Charles Wheatstone (1838–52), Sir David Brewster (1842), William Mackenzie (1845), Johann Benedict Listing (1845), and Helmholtz; and good treatises on eye diseases had been written by Antonio Scarpa (1801), James Wardrop (1808), Georg Joseph Beer (1813–17), Benjamin Travers (1820), John Vetch (1820), George Frick (Baltimore, 1824), William Mackenzie (1830), Sir William Lawrence (1833), Squier Littell (Philadelphia, 1836), C.-J.-F. Carron du Villards (1838), Friedrich August von Ammon (1838–41), the Canadian Henry Howard (1850), Karl Himly (1843), Louis-Auguste Desmarres (1847), Carl Stellwag von Carion (1853–8), and Carl Ferdinand von Arlt (1854–6). The surgery of the eye had been advanced by George James Guthrie (1823), J. F. Dieffenbach (strabismus, 1842), Thomas Wharton Jones (1847), L.-A. Desmarres (1850), and particularly by Sir William Bowman (artificial pupil, 1852; lacrimal obstruction, 1857). In 1820, Captain Charles **Barbier** laid before the Académie des Sciences a monograph on teaching the blind to read and write by a system of combinations of six elevated points, instead of embossed lines. The Barbier six-point system was introduced in Paris by Louis **Braille,** a blind teacher of the blind, in 1829, and in 1836, Braille introduced his system of musical notation for the blind. He acknowledged his indebtedness to Barbier in the preface to his book (1837[2]). In 1845–7, William Moon, of Brighton, England, introduced the Roman line types which are still used, but by 1879, the Barbier-Braille types had become a world-alphabet for the blind.

Albrecht von Graefe (1828–70), of Berlin, the creator of the modern surgery of the eye, and indeed the greatest of all eye surgeons, was the son of Carl Ferdinand von Graefe. After graduating in Berlin in 1847, he was urged to specialize in ophthalmology by Arlt in Prague, and, having followed the clinics of Sichel and Desmarres in Paris, the Jaegers in Vienna, Bowman and Critchett in London, he soon obtained phenomenal success in his native city, becoming professor at the University in 1857. In 1854, he founded the *Archiv fur Ophthalmologie*, which contains most of his important discoveries and inventions and has remained the leading organ of his specialty to date. The first volume alone contains his papers on the disorders of the oblique eye muscles, the nature of glaucoma, keratoconus, mydriasis, diphtheritic conjunctivitis, and on double vision after strabismus operations.

Von Graefe introduced the operation of iridectomy in the treatment of iritis, iridochoroiditis, and glaucoma (1855–62[3]), made the operation for strabismus viable (1857[4]), and improved the treatment of cataract by the modified linear extraction

---

[1] Gibson: Edinb. Med. & Surg. Jour., 1811, vii, 394–400.

[2] L. Braille: Procédé pour écrire au moyen des points, Paris, 1837.

[3] Graefe: Arch. f. Ophth., Berl., 1855–6, ii, 2. Abth., 202; 1857, iii, 2. Abth., 456; 1858, iv, 2. Abth., 127; 1862, viii, 2. Abth., 242.

[4] *Ibid.*, 1857, iii, 1. Abth., 177–386.

(1865–68[1]), which reduced the loss of the eye from 10 to 2.3 per cent. He applied the ophthalmoscope to the study of the amblyopias in functional disorders with extraordinary success; made a brilliant diagnosis of embolism of the retinal artery as the cause of a case of sudden blindness (1859[2]), and proceeded to point out that most cases of blindness and impaired vision connected with cerebral disorders are traceable to optic neuritis rather than to paralysis of the optic nerve (1860[3]), the view maintained before his time. Graefe was also the founder of modern knowledge of sympathetic ophthalmia (1866[4]) and the semeiology of ocular paralyses (1866[5]), described conical cornea, or "keratoconus" (1854[6]), and first noted the stationary condition of the upper eyelid, when the eyeball is rolled up or down, in exophthalmic goiter (Graefe's sign, 1864[7]).

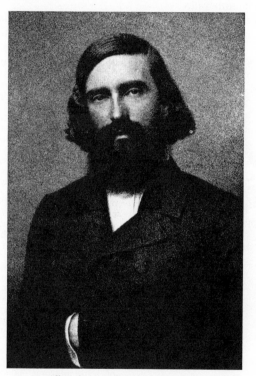

Albrecht von Graefe (1828–70).

Graefe's clinic became famous all over the world, and was followed, not so much by students as by practising physicians, who had come to Berlin to learn about the eye from its greatest master. His pupils included nearly all the greater ophthalmologists of the 19th century,

---

[1] Graefe: Arch. f. Ophth., Berl., 1865, xi, 3. Abth., 1; 1866, xii, 1. Abth., 150; 1868, xiv, 3. Abth., 106.

[2] *Ibid.*, 1859, v, 1. Abth., 136–157.

[3] *Ibid.*, 1860, vii, 2. Abth., 58–71.

[4] *Ibid.*, 1866, xii, 2. Abth., 149–174.

[5] Symptomenlehre der Augenmuskellähmungen, Berlin, 1867.

[6] Arch. f. Ophth., Verl., 1854–5, i, 1. Abth., 297–306.

[7] Deutsche Klinik, Berl., 1864, xvi, 158.

notably Forster, Saemisch, Lieberich, Pagenstecher, Alfred Graefe, Jacobson, and Horner of Zürich, who described the sympathetic syndrome (Horner's triad, 1864[1]), also associated with the name of Claude Bernard. Graefe was a man of refined, spirituel type, a *Johanniskopf*, as the Germans say, whose health did not long withstand the strain of such tremendous work as he accomplished in so short a life. Graefe was fond of pranks and practical jokes, even after his youthful days were over, and many pungent witticisms attributed to him are still quoted and remembered.

Frans Cornelius **Donders** (1818–89), of Tilburg, Holland, was educated as an army surgeon, but became a professor in the Utrecht Faculty in 1848, and, after 1862, devoted himself exclusively to ophthalmology.

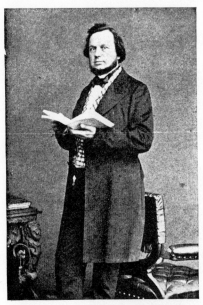

Frans Cornelius Donders (1818–89).

To this field belong his studies of the muscæ volitantes (1847), the use of prismatic glasses in strabismus (1848), the relation between convergence of visual axes and accommodation (1848), regeneration of the cornea (1848), hypermetropia (1858–60), ametropia and its sequels (1860), astigmatism (1862–3), anomalies of refraction as a cause of strabismus (1863), the invention of the ophthalmotonometer (1863), and, above all, his great work on *The Anomalies of Refraction and Accommodation,* which was published, not in Dutch, but in English, by the New Sydenham Society (1864). As a contribution to physiological optics, this book ranks with the labors of Helmholtz. It contains Donders' explanation of astigmatism, his definitions of aphakia and hypermetropia, his sharp distinctions between myopia and hypermetropia (as errors of refraction) and presbyopia (as senile change with diminished accommodation), his views of myopia as the result of excessive convergence and the cause of genuine divergent strabismus, of hypermetropia as the cause of convergent strabismus, of the ciliary muscle as the only muscle used in accommodation and its action in bulging the anterior surface of the lens, and of asthenopia (eye-strain) as the result of anomalies of refraction, muscular insufficiency or astigmatism.

Donders' work has been the main source of knowledge on the improvement of disorders of vision by spectacles up to the time of Gullstrand. It is said that, while impatiently waiting for one of Helmholtz's ophthalmoscopes, he contrived one for himself in which the silvered mirror with central perforation, now in use, was substituted for the superimposed glass plates of the Berlin master's instrument. In 1845, Donders became editor of the *Nederlandsch Lancet,* and in 1851 he established the Netherlandish Hospital for Diseases of the Eye (*Neder-*

---

[1] Horner: Klin. Monatsbl. f. Augenheilk., Stuttg., 1869, vii, 193–198.

landsch Gasthuis voor Oogleiden); but his labors were not entirely confined to the eye. In 1863, he succeeded Schroeder van der Kolk as professor of physiology at Utrecht, and established the New Physiological Laboratory in the same city (1866). His most important contribution to physiology was the first measurement of the reaction time of a psychical process (1868[1]). In 1845, he wrote on metabolism as the source of heat in animals and plants, and his contributions on the physiology of speech (1864–70[2]) are of great importance. Donders was highly accomplished, speaking English, French, and German like a native, yet modest to the point of diffidence. His earlier military avocations gave him a polished *tenue* which, with his natural personal charm, made him known all over Europe as one of the most attractive specialists of his time.

Prominent among von Graefe's pupils were his nephew, **Alfred Karl Graefe** (1830–99), who made a clinical analysis of disordered movements of the eye (1858), invented a special "localization ophthalmoscope" for extracting deep-lying cysticerci, wrote a monograph on the treatment of infantile conjunctivitis by caustics and antiseptics (1881), and, with Saemisch, edited the well-known Graefe-Saemisch *Handbuch der Ophthalmologie* (1874–80); Julius **Jacobson** (1828–89), of Königsberg, who made a great improvement in the operative treatment of cataract by his peripheral incision under chloroform anesthesia (1863), reducing the loss of the eye from 10 to 2 per cent., and further improving the operation by extraction within the capsule (1888), originated the operative treatment of trachoma and trichiasis (1887), wrote a fine memoir on the work of his friend von Graefe (1885), and enjoyed the largest consulting practice in eastern Europe, patients streaming in even from Russia; the brothers Alexander (1828–79) and Hermann **Pagenstecher** (1844–1918), the former of whom made his mark in the history of cataract by the extraction of the lens in the closed capsule through a scleral incision (1866); Edwin Theodor **Saemisch** (1833–1909), of Luckau, who first described serpiginous ulcer of the cornea and its treatment (1870) and vernal conjunctivitis or *Frühjahrskatarrh* (1876), and edited the above-mentioned Handbuch with the younger Graefe; Julius **Hirschberg** (1843–1925), of Potsdam, whose name is associated with the introduction of the electromagnet into ophthalmology (1885), with a dictionary of ophthalmology (1887), with the editing of the Arabic texts (1905), and with the most complete and scholarly history of his science which has ever been written (1899–1911); Theodor **Leber** (1840–1917), who studied the diabetic disorders of the eye (1875) and the disorders of circulation and nutrition of the eye (1876); Ludwig **Laqueur** (1839–1909), who introduced the use of physostigmin in glaucoma (1876); Richard **Liebreich** (1830–1917), of Königsberg, who introduced lateral illumination in microscopic investigation of the living eye (1855), and published the first atlas of ophthalmoscopy (1863), in which he was followed by Jaeger von Jaxtthal (1869); and Hermann Jakob **Knapp** (1832–1911), of Dauborn, Hesse-Nassau, who became one of the leading ophthalmologists of New York City, founded the *Archives of Ophthalmology and Otology* (New York, 1869), and wrote valuable memoirs on curvature of the cornea (1859) and intra-ocular tumors (1869), and other subjects.

On the didactic side, the most eminent living ophthalmologist is Ernst **Fuchs** (1851–   ), of Vienna, a pupil of Brüke and Billroth, Arlt's assistant (1876–80), professor of ophthalmology at Liège (1880–85) and Vienna (1885). He is the author of important monographs on sarcoma of the uveal tract (1882), blindness (1885), and the histopathology of sympathetic ophthalmia (1905), of improvements of Jaeger's test-types (*Leseproben für die Nahe*, 1895), and of the out-

---

[1] Donders: Arch. f. Anat., Physiol. u. wissensch. Med., Berl., 1868, 657–681.
[2] Donders: De physiologie der spraakklanken, Utrecht, 1870.

standing German treatise on eye diseases (1889), which has passed through 12 editions and many translations, including the Japanese.

Of works relating to the normal eye, we may mention Henry Gray's memoir on the optic nerves (1849), Max Schultze's memoir on the anatomy and physiology of the retina (1866); the theories of vision of Helmholtz (1867), Ewald Hering (1872–75) and Christine Ladd Franklin (1892); Willy Kühne's investigations of visual purple (1877), and the memoirs of Ramón y Cajal on the vertebrate retina (1892) and of Johannes von Kries (1853–   ), on the function of the retinal rods (1895). The examination of the eye was furthered by such inventions as the astigmometer (1867) of Emile **Javal** (1839–1907), of Paris; by the Javal-Schiötz ophthalmometer (1881); by the method of retinoscopy introduced by Ferdinand Cuignet (1873), and by the keratoscope invented by A. Placido (1882). Color-blindness was investigated by the Swedish physiologist Alarik Frithiof **Holmgren** (1831–97), who introduced the wool-skein test (1874) and gave special consideration to color-blindness under railway and maritime conditions (1878). The relation of eye-strain (asthenopia) and astigmatism to headaches and other neurotic symptoms was first noted by S. Weir Mitchell (1874) and William Thomson (1879), and applied extensively to morbid psychology (1888) by George Milbry **Gould** (1847–1922), who showed that a very minute error of refraction, discoverable only after paralysis of accommodation by cycloplegics, may suffice to lower resistance to disease by profound nervous irritation and mental misery. The presbyopia which connotes eye-strain may be due to congenital malformation of the sclera (Arthur Keith). The work of Alexander Duane (1858–1926) on accommodation and on evolution of squint and of James **Thorington** (1858–   ) on refraction (1916) has taught much. The relation of eye diseases to general and organic diseases of the body was especially treated by Richard Förster (1877) and in 1898 by Hermann **Schmidt-Rimpler** (1838–1915), who was also, with Hermann **Cohn** (1838–1906), a pioneer in the examination of the eyes of school-children.

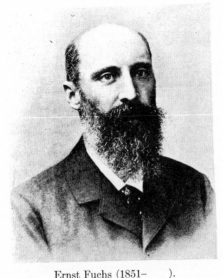

Ernst Fuchs (1851–   ).

The semeiology of the eye in nervous diseases was treated in extenso by Hermann Wilbrandt and Alfred Sänger (1900–1913). The bacteriology of the eye was especially advanced by Robert Koch, who discovered the bacilli of two different forms of Egyptian conjunctivitis (1883); by John E. Weeks, who found the same organism as the cause of "pink-eye" (1886); by Henri **Parinaud** (1844–1905), of Paris, who described an infectious tubercular conjunctivitis transmissible from animals to man (1889), and a lacrimal pneumococcic conjunctivitis in new-born infants (1894), both associated with his name; and by Victor Morax and Theodor Axenfeld, who simultaneously described the diplobacillary form of chronic conjunctivitis (1896–97). In 1894, Axenfeld described in masterly style the pyemic or metastatic ophthalmia, first noted by J. H. Meckel in 1854. Apart from the Graefe-Saemisch Handbuch, the best modern works on ophthalmology are the monumental treatises of Ernst Fuchs (1889, 12 ed., 1910) and Edmond Landolt (1846–1926), published 1880–89. Another good work is that of the Greek, Photinos Panas (1894), whose name is especially associated with an operation for congenital and paralytic ptosis (1886). Besides the Americans already referred to, we may mention Henry Willard Williams (1821–1895), who introduced the treatment of iritis without mercury (1856) and a method of suturing the flap after cataract extraction (1866); Cornelius Rea Agnew (1830–88), who described a method of operating for divergent squint (1866); Henry Drury Noyes (1832–1900), who first investigated retinitis in glycosuria (1867); Lucien Howe (1848), author of *The Muscles of the Eye* (1907); Casey A. Wood (1856–   ), editor of the *American Encyclopedia of Ophthalmology* (1913–21), notable for work on alcoholic amblyopia (1904) and a monograph on the fundus oculi in birds (1917); Edward Jackson (1856–   ), editor of the *American Journal of Ophthalmology* (1898), author of a valuable work on skiascopy (1895); George E. de Schweinitz (1858–   ), author of a sterling text-book (1892), who has done much valuable work on the toxic amblyopias (1896); and the work of E. Dyer on asthenopia (1865), George T. Stevens on classification of the heterophorias (1886), G. C. Savage on functions of the oblique muscles (1893), and William H. Wilmer on eye conditions in aviators (1918). Many instruments and test types have been invented, notably the electric light ophthalmoscope of W. S. Dennett, F. Buller's shield for ophthalmia neonatorum (1874), and the tangent-plane of Alexander Duane. Aside from the great work of Julius Hirschberg (1899–1911), good histories of ophthalmology have been written by August Hirsch (1877), P. Pansier (1903), and Carl Horstmann (1905).

Laryngology and **rhinology** were specially advanced by the introduction of laryngoscopy by Benjamin Babington (1829), Robert Liston (1837), Manuel Garcia (1855), Ludwig Türck (1858–60), and Johann Czermak (1858); of rhinoscopy by Philipp Bozzini (1773–1809), in 1807, and (successfully) by Czermak (1859); of autoscopy of the larynx and trachea without the mirror by Alfred Kirstein (1863–   ), of Berlin (1895), and of direct bronchoscopy by Gustav Killian (1860–1921), of Mainz (1898). Laryngoscopy was introduced in New York in 1858 by Ernest Krakowizer of Vienna, who was the first physician in America to demonstrate the vocal cords. In 1858 also, Ephraim Cutter, of Massachusetts, devised a laryngoscope with two tubes, one for observation, one for illumination. Suspension-laryngoscopy (*Schwebelaryngoskopie*) was introduced by Killian (1912). The anatomy of the larynx and the physiology of the voice and speech were investigated by Johannes Müller (1839), Ernst von Brücke (1856), F. C. Donders (1870), Hubert von Luschka (1873), and Carl Ludwig Merkel (*Anthropophonik*, 1876). Max Schultze investigated the histology and nerve-endings of the Schneiderian membrane (1863), Emil Zuckerkandl (1861–1921), the anatomy and pathology of the accessory sinuses (1882–92), and Hendrik Zwaardemaker (1857–   ) the physiology of smell (1895). A perfected method of photographing the larynx was devised by Thomas Rushmore French (1884). Important early treatises on laryngology were those of John Cheyne (1777–1836) on the *Pathology of the Membrane of the Larynx and Bronchia* (1809), William Henry Porter (1790–1861) on the surgical pathology of the larynx and trachea (1826), Armand Trousseau and Hippolyte Belloc on laryngeal phthisis, chronic laryngitis, and disorders of the voice (1837), Horace Green (1802–66) on diseases of the air-passages (1846), Samuel D. Gross on foreign bodies in the air-passages (1854) and Sir Morell Mackenzie on laryngeal tumors (1871). As Bryson Delavan says,[1] the sciences of laryngology and rhinology were placed upon a firm literary basis through the three treatises of J. Solis Cohen (1872), Sir Morell Mackenzie (1880) and Francke Huntington Bosworth (1881). Intubation of the larynx in croup was introduced by Eugène Bouchut (1818–91) in 1856–8, first done in Paris in connection with tracheotomy by Trousseau (1851–59), and perfected through the conscientious labors (1885–88) of the self-sacrificing Joseph P. **O'Dwyer** (1841–98), of Cleveland, Ohio, whose name stands with those of Semmelweis and Credé as one of the great benefactors of infant life. **Horace Green** (1802–66), of Crittenden, Vermont, a friend of Trousseau, was the pioneer of laryngology in the United States, the first to treat diseases of the throat by local applications (1838), the first to describe cystic and malignant laryngeal growths (1851–2), and the author of important works on croup (1849) and the surgical treatment of polyps of the larynx (1852). In 1873, Clinton Wagner organized the Laryngological Society of New York, the earliest association of its kind. Elsberg, J. Solis Cohen, Knight, and Lefferts founded the *Archives of Laryngology* (New York, 1880–83). As to instrumentation, the ancient Icelanders used a ring-knife uvulotome, the tonsillotome was invented by P. S. Physick (1828), and the ring-knife tonsillotome by Fahnestock (1832). Charles Henri Ehrmann (1792–1878) was the first to remove a laryngeal polyp (1844). Victor von Bruns (1812–13) first enucleated a laryngeal polyp by the bloodless method (1862), and was the pioneer of laryngoscopic surgery (1865). Rudolph Voltolini (1819–89) first employed the galvanocautery in laryngeal surgery (1867) and performed the first laryngeal operation through the mouth with external illumination (1889). Paralysis of the

---

[1] See his excellent historical sketch in Howard Kelly's "Cyclopedia of American Medical Biography," Philadelphia, 1912, pp. lxiii–lxxi.

vocal cords was first carefully studied by Carl Gerhardt in 1863–72. Ottomar Rosenbach (1880) and later Sir Felix Semon (1848–1925) stated the law governing the site of immobilization of the vocal cords in complete and incomplete paralysis of the recurrent laryngeal nerve. The first important treatises on diseases of the nose were the Paris thesis of Jacques-Louis Deschamps *fils* (1804) and the *Ophrésiologie* (1821) of Hippolyte Cloquet (1787–1840), which were followed by such books on rhino-laryngology as those of Horace Green (1846), Carl Seiler (1879), M. Bresgen (1881), E. F. Ingals (1881), Sir Morell Mackenzie (1880–84), C. E. Sajous (1885), Ottokar von Chiari (1887), R. Voltolini (1888), Lenox Browne (1890), and F. H. Bosworth (1890–92). In 1832, the explorer, George Catlin, published his classic on *Mouth Breathing*, based upon his observations of nasal obstruction in North American Indians. Benjamin Löwenberg was the first to consider the nature and treatment of ozena (1885), and Ludwig Grünwald (1863–   ) the surgical treatment of nasal suppuration and disease of the ethmoid and sphenoid (1893). Ephraim Fletcher Ingals (1848–1918), of Lee Centre, Illinois, treated deflections of the nasal septum by partial excision in 1882, and this operation was finally perfected by Robert Krieg (1889), Otto T. Freer (1902), and Gustav Killian (1904). Killian also originated the radical operation for chronic inflammation of the frontal sinus (1903). The best histories of laryngology and rhinology are those of Louis Elsberg (1879–80), Gordon Holmes (1887), Jonathan Wright (1898, 1914), and the monumental work of C. Chauveau on the history of diseases of the pharynx (Paris, 1901–06[1]).

The foundations of **otology** were the catheterization of the Eustachian tubes through the mouth by Guyot (1724) and Cleland (1741), the mastoid operations of Petit (1774) and Jasser (1776), Cooper's perforation of the tympanic membrane for deafness (1800), and the monographs of Valsalva, Cotugno, Scarpa, and others. The first treatise on diseases of the ear was written by Jean-Marc-Gaspard Itard (1775–1838), of Oraison (Provence), in 1821, and this important work was followed by such treatises as those of Joseph Toynbee (1860), Anton Friedrich von Tröltsch (1866), Lawrence Turnbull (1872), Sir William B. Dalby (1873), St. John Roosa (1873), Adam Politzer (1878–82), Victor Urbantschitsch (1847–1921) (1880), and Friedrich Bezold (1906). Max Schultze described the nerve-endings in the labyrinth (1858), Helmholtz the mechanics of the ossicles and membrana tympani (1869), Goltz the physiological significance of the semicircular canals (1870). The younger [Magnus Christian] Retzius wrote an important monograph on the vertebrate ear (1884), Julius Richard Ewald (1856–   ) studied audition in birds deprived of the labyrinths (1892) and Stanislav Stein the functions of separate parts of the labyrinth (1894). Adam **Politzer** (1835–1920), of Alberti, Hungary, was the first to obtain pictures of the membrana tympani by illumination (1865), which he afterward illustrated in an atlas of 14 plates and 392 pictures (1896). The transmission of sounds through the cranial bones in diagnosis of aural diseases was first studied by Johann C. A. Lucae (1870), and great advances in exploration were made by Friedrich **Bezold** (1842–1908), of Rothenburg ob der Tauber, who gave the first clear description of mastoiditis (1877), introduced new tests for audition in deaf-mutism (1896) and in unilateral deafness (1897). Among other advances were the Weber and Rinné tests, Hartmann's diapasons, and Sir Francis Galton's whistle for determining the superior limits of audition. The pioneers of aural surgery in the 19th century were Sir Astley Cooper (1801) and Sir William Wilde (1843–53), and after their time the most important English work on the subject was that of James Hinton (1827–75), of Guy's Hospital (1874). The modern surgery of the ear and mastoid has been mainly the work of the Germans. In 1873, Hermann **Schwartze** (1837–1910) and Adolph **Eysell** described the method of opening the mastoid by chiseling (*typische Aufmeisselung*). This operation was further improved by Emanuel **Zaufal** (1884) and Ernst **Küster** (1889), while Ludwig. **Stacke** (1859–1918) introduced excision of the ossicles (1890) and greatly improved the surgery of the middle ear (1892–97). Aural vertigo was first described by Prosper **Ménière** (1799–1862) in 1861, was again noted by Charcot as "vertigo ab aure læsa" (1874), while the relations between nystagmus and vestibular or cerebellar disease had been noted by Purkinje and Flourens, and have been developed, in the 20th century, by Robert Bárány. The authoritative history of otology by Adam **Politzer** (1835–1920) is now completed (1907–13[2]).

---

[1] For bibliographic references to this section, see Surgeon-General's Catalogue, 1912, 2. s., xvii, pp. 171, 172.

[2] For bibliographic references to this section, see Surgeon-General's Catalogue, 1912, 2. s., xvii, pp. 172, 173.

Modern **dentistry,** since the days of Fauchard, Pfaff and Hunter, has been largely developed by Americans.[1] On the technical side, the hand mallet (E. Merrit, 1838), vulcanite artificial dentures (Charles Goodyear, Jr., 1855), the rubber dam (S. C. Barnum, 1864), the Morrison and Bonwill dental engines (1870–71), crown and bridge work (C. M. Richmond, 1878), the use of amalgams and porcelain inlays and other devices are nearly all of American origin. The science of malocclusion and its treatment by orthodontal procedure originated with Fauchard (1728) and John Hunter (1771) and has had a lengthy and complex history, culminating in the epochal work of Edwin Hartley **Angle,** who, since 1887, has devoted over thirty years to the classification of the different modes of malocclusion, their treatment by the many technical appliances of his invention[2] and to the organization of a School of Orthodontia (1900) and a Society of Orthodontists (1901). Dental bacteriology, upon which aseptic and antiseptic dentistry is based, was developed by Willoughby Dayton Miller (1853–1907), an American professor in Berlin (1890[3]). The treatment of pyorrhea alveolaris by scraping was introduced by John M. Riggs (1876). The first American books on dentistry were those of R. C. Skinner (1801) and B. T. Longbothom (1802[4]). The most important book is that of Chapin A. Harris (1839[5]). Modern maxillo-facial surgery, which made such a remarkable record in the European War, owes much to Simon P. Hullihen, James Edmund Garretson (1828–95), Norman W. Kingsley (1829–1913), Truman W. Brophy, Thomas Fillebrown (1836–1908), Matthew H. Cryer, John S. Marshall, Thomas L. Gilmer (1849–   ), Vilray Papin Blair (1871–   ), and other Americans, and latterly to such European surgeons as Pierre Sebileau, A. C. Valadier and H. D. Gilles (*Plastic Surgery of the Face,* 1920). In England dentistry was lifted from the status of a trade to that of a science by Sir John Tomes (1815–95), a surgeon, who early made his mark by his studies on the histology of bone and teeth (1849–56), invented a practicable dental forceps (1839–40), wrote a well-known *System of Dental Surgery* (1859), was one of the founders of the Odontological Society (1856) and the Dental Hospital (1858), and was instrumental in securing passage of the Dental Act (1878), for the compulsory education and registration of dentists.

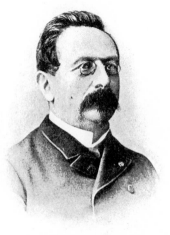

Jean-Antoine Villemin (1827–92).

Neither the English nor the French **clinical medicine** of this period had the rigorous scientific tendency which characterized the German. In England, pathology was little studied after the time of Bright, Hodgkin, and Addison, although the English talent for careful clinical observation was amply illustrated. The brightest phase of French medicine in the second half of the 19th century was its neurology. With the exception of Charcot, most of the French clinicians of the time were brilliant and elegant expositors of internal medicine, as Helmholtz has

---

[1] See Dental Cosmos, Phila., 1920, lxii, 1–73.

[2] E. H. Angle: Malocclusion of the Teeth, Philadelphia, 1887, (7. ed., 1907). For the history of orthodontia, see B. W. Weinberger: Orthodontics, St. Louis, 1926.

[3] W. D. Miller: The Microörganisms of the Human Mouth, Philadelphia, 1890.

[4] R. C. Skinner: A Treatise on the Human Teeth, New York, 1801; B. C. Longbothom: Treatise on Dentistry, Baltimore, 1802.

[5] C. A. Harris: The Dental Art, 1839.

described them, rather than original workers in pathology. Indeed, as we shall see, there are no professional pathologists in French medical schools, their places being supplied by physicians practising in hospital.

In experimental medicine, Jean-Antoine **Villemin** (1827–92), of Prey (Vosges), a medical graduate of Strassburg (1852), and professor at Val de Grâce, achieved an undying reputation by his proof that tuberculosis is a specific infection, due to an invisible, inoculable agent and transmissible by inoculation from man to the lower animals (1865–69). Before the advent of Pasteur, these ideas could gain no credence, although Villemin did what he could to spread the doctrine of contagious phthisis. In 1870, he told his aids at Val de Grâce that "the phthisical soldier is to his messmate what the glandered horse is to its yokefellow."

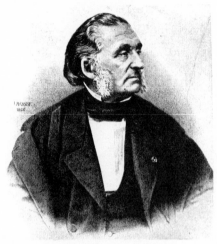

Armand Trousseau (1801–67).

Of the French clinicians, Armand **Trousseau** (1801–67), of Tours, a pupil of Bretonneau, professor in the Paris Faculty (1850) and physician at the Hôpital St. Antoine (1839) and the Hôtel Dieu (1850), occupied about the same position in French medicine as Bright and Addison, Stokes and Graves over the Channel. He received the prize of the Academy of Medicine for his classical treatise on laryngeal phthisis (1837), was the first to perform tracheotomy in Paris (1831[1]), and was a pioneer in the introduction of thoracentesis (1843) and intubation (1851). He first described gastric vertigo and a diagnostic sign of infantile tetany, consisting of the voluntary reproduction of the paroxysms during the attack by compressing the affected parts. His *Clinique médicale de l'Hôtel Dieu* (1861), which passed through three editions, contains his best work, much of which has silently taken its place in the text-books. He was a man of big personality, a great master of clinical delineation, and a generous interpreter of the ideas of other men, particularly of the diseases described by Bretonneau, Addison, Hodgson, Corrigan, and Duchenne of Boulogne. His best pupils were Dieulafoy and DaCosta.

Georges **Dieulafoy** (1839–1911), of Toulouse, who wrote the most readable French treatise on internal medicine in his day (1880–84[2]), and is otherwise remembered by his employment of the trocar in the

---

[1] Trousseau: Jour. de conn. méd.-chir., Paris, 1833–34, i, 5; 41.

[2] Dieulafoy: Manuel de pathologie interne, Paris, 1880–84.

treatment of pleurisy, hydatids, etc. (1869–72[1]), was a fiery clinical orator of the meridional type, who never bothered himself about scientific speculations, but built up a large clientèle and as a wise humane physician, enjoyed the expression or exploitation of his personality in the clinics. Handsome and gay (*le beau Dieulafoy*), he was gifted with great powers of elocution and mimicry, a natural born actor, with the gestures and intonations of an Italian tenor—*des gestes qui implorent et qui caressent*—and he always succeeded in posing his diagnosis in a way to excite the greatest admiration. At the bedside, Dieulafoy was ideal. A physician of alert intelligence and fascinating personality, who at least endeavored to make his teaching anything but dull, his passion was to show his pupils how to get good answers by asking the right questions, without offending or tiring the patients. The patient he held to be entitled to the highest consideration and sympathy. He had an excellent classical education and first attracted Trousseau's attention by helping him out with a citation from Ovid. He did good work in separating out the complications of appendicitis and other minutiæ. In his spirited clinical improvisations, he excelled in coining such expressions as "*le foie appendiculaire*," which illustrate his virtuosity in the use of the French language, but convey nothing

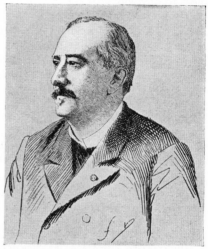

Jean-Alfred Fournier (1832–1914).

very definite to the mind. A tablet to his memory was set in the walls of the Ampithéâtre Trousseau in 1914.

Sigismond **Jaccoud** (1830–1913), of Geneva, was another prominent Parisian internist, whose treatise on practice (1871) and clinical lectures (1867–88) enjoyed about the same reputation as Dieulafoy's.

Jean-Alfred **Fournier** (1832–1914), of Paris, professor in the Paris Faculty, whose name is associated with the great venereal clinic at the Hôpital St. Louis, was reputed as a teacher of great power, possessed of a clear, harmonious voice, full of the finest delicacy and courtesy to patients or pupils, universally liked, and penetrating even the dullest minds by his luminous intelligence and clear, effective mode of expression. With Diday, of Lyons, Fournier did most to develop the subject of congenital syphilis, in which he brought "order out of chaos." Practically all his life had been devoted to the study of this disease, to every phase of which he added something of clinical importance, as

---

[1] Dieulafoy: De l'aspiration pneumatique sous-cutanée, Paris, 1870.

also to its social aspects (*Syphilis et Mariage*, 1890). He introduced the concept "parasyphilis" and his statistics on the causal relation of lues to ataxia and paresis (1876–94[1]) are, with those of Erb, the most important contributions to the subject. In March, 1901, he founded the Society of Sanitary and Moral Prophylaxis. Fournier is described as a keen-eyed, close-cropped military figure, looking like an old artillery officer.

Henri **Huchard** (1844–1910), of Auxon (Aube), was a clinician of the same effective type. He is especially remembered for his studies in therapeutics, his *Traité des névroses* (with Axenfeld, 1883), his great monograph on disorders of the circulation (1889), and particularly by his work on the clinical forms of arteriosclerosis (1909), which he did most to develop.

Charles-Jacques **Bouchard** (1837–1915), late dean of the Paris Faculty, a masterful, dominant figure, described the fulgurant pains of ataxia with Charcot (1866), was the first to call attention to auto-intoxication (1887) and to diseases caused by diminished nutrition (1879–80), and wrote a treatise on general pathology (1899), which was a popular students' text-book.

Georges **Hayem** (1841–   ), of Paris, was professor of therapeutics (1879–93) and clinical medicine (1893–1911) in the Paris Faculty, and planned the Hôpital St. Antoine, where he held his clinics. He made his mark by his work on transfusion of artificial serum (1881), cholera (1885), his books on diseases of the stomach (1897) and digestion (1907), and particularly by his great work on the blood (*Du Sang*, 1889) and its pendant on blood diseases (1900). He was the father and founder of hematology, which was almost unknown when he took it up in 1875.

In 1877, he discovered the hematoblasts (Osler, 1873) or thrombocytes of Deetjen and Dekhuyzen (1901) and elucidated the rôle of these third corpuscles as fibrin formers in coagulation (1883). He devised various chemical methods of examining the gastric juice, now displaced by Röntgenoscopy, noted the infectious myocarditis of typhoid, the spinal complications of gonorrhea, the bulbar form of tabes, and, in 1897–8, described the chronic splenomegalic jaundice which is identical with the congenital hemolytic jaundice of Minkowski and Chauffard (1900).

Among the original contributions of French clinicians are J.-A. Villemin's proof of the inoculability of tuberculosis (1868), the theses of L.-A. Thaon and Jacques-Joseph Grancher (1843–1907) on the unity of phthisis (1873), Joseph Dumoutier's account of sleeping sickness (1868), Paul Lorain's delineation of sexual infantilism (1871), the descriptions of chronic interstitial hepatitis (1874) by Georges Hayem (1841–   ), of cirrhotic jaundice (1875) by Victor-Charles Hanot (1844–96), of primary endotheliomatous hypertrophy of the spleen (1882) by Ernest Gaucher (1855–1918), of enteroptosis and gastroptosis by Frantz Glénard (1885), of paralytic vertigo (kubisagari) by F. Gerlier (1886), of primitive cancer of the pancreas by Louis Bard and Adrien Pic (1888), of cyanotic polycythemia by Henri Vaquez (1892); Ch. Bouchard (1887) and A. Combe (1907) on auto-intoxication; the definition of the concept "acetonemic vomiting" (1905) by B.-J.-A. Marfan and others; and the pediatric treatises of Charles-Michel Billard (1828–33); and of F. Rilliet and A.-C.-E. Barthez (1838–43), which contains an early account of poliomyelitis. Of later French pediatricians, Jacques-Joseph Grancher (1843–1907), Jules Comby (1853–   ), and B.-J.-A. Marfan (1858–   ) are prominent as authors of treatises and monographs and editors of pediatric journals.

---

[1] Fournier: Les affections parasyphilitiques, Paris, 1894.

German clinical medicine in the second half of the 19th century includes such names as Frerichs, Traube, Kussmaul, Gerhardt, Ziemssen, Leyden, Senator, Naunyn, and Friedrich Müller.

Friedrich Theodor von **Frerichs** (1819–85), of Aurich, graduated at Göttingen in 1841, and soon achieved a reputation as an ophthalmologist, but afterward went over to scientific and internal medicine and became one of the founders of experimental pathology. He received his professorship at Göttingen in 1848, afterward holding chairs at Kiel (1850) and Breslau (1852), succeeding Schölein at Berlin in 1859. Frerichs

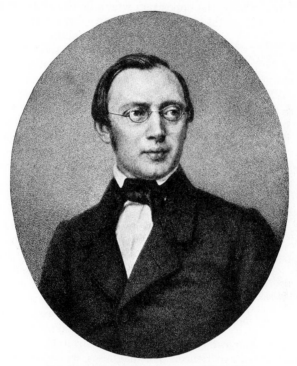

Friedrich Theodor von Frerichs (1819–85).

seems to have attained the summit of his profession in a surprisingly short while, and his course from Göttingen to Berlin has been likened by Naunyn to a triumphal progress. Students hung upon his lips, and his colleagues revered his wonderful precision in diagnosis. At forty, he had already done his best work, his great monograph on digestion in Wagner's Dictionary of Physiology, his discovery of leucin and tyrosin in the urine of acute yellow atrophy of the liver (1855[1]), his pathological studies of cirrhosis of the liver, pernicious malarial fever, and melanemia, and his books on Bright's disease (1851[2]) and diseases of

[1] Frerichs: Deutsche Klinik, Berl., 1855, vii, 341–343.
[2] Frerichs: Die Bright'sche Nierenkrankheit, Braunschweig, 1851.

the liver (1858[1]). Yet, at Berlin, as his pupil, Naunyn, tells us, Frerichs seemed, at the height of his reputation, to undergo a kind of spiritual and intellectual blight. Apart from his students, of whom he had always a large following, he became secluded, reserved, and querulous, and wrote little. The second volume of his work on diseases of the liver (1868) is said to show a distinct falling off in talent, although his lectures were always highly esteemed for their beautiful concision and accuracy, and he enjoyed an enormous consulting practice. This change in Frerich's personality was due, Naunyn thinks, to his extreme sensitiveness to criticism; to the opposition which he encountered in Berlin, especially from his mistakes about the origin of the bile-pigments and

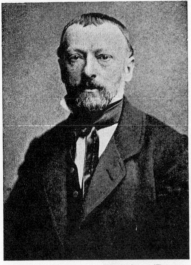

acids; to his falling out with Traube, his colleague at the Charité, and to the aggressive enmity which he encountered at the hands of Virchow. So strong was Virchow's personality that even Graefe and Langenbeck lined up with him in official opposition to Frerichs, whose productiveness was soon sterilized by this professional jealousy. It was under the sympathetic influence of Leyden, who came on at the Charité in 1876 and eventually succeeded him, that he brightened up again and produced a monograph worthy of his fame, his work on diabetes (1884[2]), based upon 400 cases and 55 autopsies. The clinical lectures of Frerichs, which he delivered offhand, are described by Naunyn as of classic perfection of phrase, clear and plastic in the delin-

Ludwig Traube (1818–76). (Boston Medical Library.)

eation of disease, and as having a rare freshness from the number of facts drawn from his own experience. His diagnoses, which he made offhand, directly upon seeing the cases, were usually intuitive, always developed as a disturbance of physiological function, and never admitted to be wrong. Like Skoda, Frerichs was indifferent to patients, even to students, caring only for the scientific aspects of the disease itself, although he always condescended to outline a course of treatment, including a prescription. In person he was tall and ungainly, yet imposing through his style of delivery, which was frequently dramatic. The interests of Frerichs is that he developed scientific clinical teaching in Germany. His pupils include some of the brightest spirits of modern times, such men as Ehrlich, Naunyn, Leyden, and von Mering.

---

[1] Frerichs: Klinik der Leberkrankheiten, Braunschweig, 1858.
[2] Frerichs: Ueber den Diabetes, Berlin, 1884.

Ludwig **Traube** (1818–76), of Ratibor, Silesia, was a pupil of Purkinje, Johannes Müller, Skoda, Rokitansky, and Schönlein, becoming the latter's assistant in 1849 and professor at Berlin in 1857. Traube early made his mark as the founder of experimental pathology in Germany.[1]

He investigated the pulmonary disorders occasioned by section of the vagus nerve (1846). This was followed by studies of suffocation (1847), crises and critical days (1850), the pathology of fever, the effects of digitalis and other drugs, the relation of cardiac and renal disorders, and particularly by his *Gesammelte Beiträge zur experimentellen Pathologie* (1871–78), which gave him a wide reputation. He introduced the thermometer in his clinic about 1850.

Traube was one of the first of the Jewish physicians to receive official recognition after the events of 1848. His clinics at the Charité soon became very popular on account of his exact methods and his honest, sincere attitude toward his patients. His countenance, like Carlyle's or Ehrlich's, has about it that indefinable something which we associate with the honest man. His long-standing difference with Frerichs was due to the usual disputes about clinical material, of which the latter, as physician-in-chief, had the lion's share.

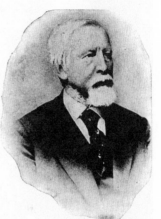

Adolf **Kussmaul** (1822–1902), of Graben, near Karlsruhe, began as an army surgeon, becoming later professor at Heidelberg (1857), Erlangen (1859), Freiburg (1863), and Strassburg (1876).

His earlier studies were upon the changes of color in the eye (1845), the effect of the circulation upon the movements of the iris (1856), the relation between anemia and epileptiform convulsions (1857). Of greater importance were his monographs

Adolf Kussmaul (1822–1902).

on the psychology of the new-born infant (1859), on mercurial salivation and its relation to constitutional syphilis (1861), and on disorders of speech (1877). He was the first to describe "periarteriitis nodosa" (1866[2]), progressive bulbar paralysis (1873), and diabetic coma with acetonemia, and the peculiar type of breathing ("air hunger") associated with the condition (1874[3]). He added much to the knowledge of tetany and osteomyelitis. Equally brilliant were his contributions to diagnosis and therapeutics. He introduced the concept of "pulsus paradoxus" (1873[4]), was the first to diagnose mesenteric embolism in the living subject (1864), the first to attempt esophagoscopy and gastroscopy (1869[5]), the first to wash out the stomach with the stomach-tube for gastric dilatation (1867–69), to treat gastric ulcer with large doses of bismuth, and to employ thoracentesis (1868[6]).

---

[1] See A. Boruttau: Ztschr. f. exper. Path., Berl., 1919, xx, 144–148.

[2] With Rudolf Maier: Deutsches Arch. f. klin. Med., Leipz., 1866, i, 484–518.

[3] *Ibid.*, 1874, xiv, 1–46.

[4] Kussmaul: Samml. klin. Vortr., Leipz., 1873, No. 54 (Innere Med., No. 62), 1637–74.

[5] Deutsche Ztschr. f. Chir., Leipz., 1900–1901, lviii, 500–507, 1 pl. (Communicated by G. Killian).

[6] For references to these and other contributions of Kussmaul, see Deutsches Arch. f. klin. Med., Leipz., 1902, lxxiii, 1–89.

Kussmaul's *Jugenderinnerungen* (1899) is one of the best of medical autobiographies, containing interesting sidelights on the palmy days of the New Vienna School. On Christmas Day, 1893, he distributed among his friends a volume of poems, privately printed under the pseudonym "Dr. Oribasius."

Hugo **von Ziemssen** (1829–1902), one of Virchow's pupils, was professor of clinical medicine at Erlangen (1863), and (after serving in the Franco-Prussian War) at Munich (1874), where he directed the city hospital and founded the first clinical institute for instruction in the specialties (1877). Ziemssen was one of the great medical encyclo-

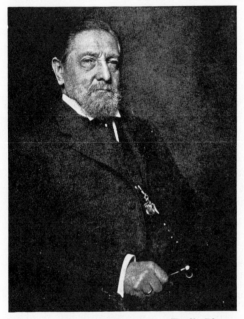

pedists, whose fame rests largely today upon his Handbook of Special Pathology and Therapeutics in seventeen volumes (1875–85). He edited handbooks of therapeutics (1880–84), hygiene (1882–86), and skin diseases (1883–84), and made innumerable contributions to many different subjects.

Ernst **von Leyden** (1832–1910), of Danzig, a pupil of Schönlein and Traube, succeeded the latter at Berlin in 1876, and also succeeded to Frerichs' clinic upon his death (1885). In 1894, he was called to the Russian court to treat Czar Alexander, for which he received a patent of nobility in 1895. In 1879 he founded, with Frerichs, the *Zeitschrift für klinische Medizin*, and, in

Ernst von Leyden (1832–1910). (Berlin Photographic Company.)

the later years of his life, was an active co-editor of several other journals. He did most to promote the movement for hospitalization of phthisical patients in Germany.

He acquired a great reputation in Berlin and specialized in neurology, his most famous work being his clinical studies of tabes dorsalis (1863–1901), respiration in fever (1870), diseases of the spinal cord (1874–76), poliomyelitis and neuritis (1880), periodic vomiting (1882), and prognosis in heart disease (1889).

Hermann **Nothnagel** (1841–1905), a pupil of Traube and Virchow, Leyden's assistant at Königsberg (1865–68), and professor at Freiburg (1872), Jena (1874), and Vienna (1882–1905), wrote an authoritative treatise on therapeutics (1870), made many excellent contributions to neurology. He was a gifted orator, an impressive lecturer, and a man of high ideals. A victim of angina pectoris, he stoically set down his own symptoms in writing just before his end.[1]

Nothnagel is especially memorable for his encyclopedic Handbook of Special Pathology and Therapeutics in 24 volumes (1894–1905). He first described universal anesthesia or absence of all sensation in the body (*Seelenlähmung*) in 1887. His favorite clinical themes were the diagnosis of cerebral diseases (in which he separated disease of the optic thalamus) and diseases of the intestines and peritoneum, on which he wrote a classic monograph (1898).

Hermann **Senator** (1834–1911), of Gnesen, Polish Prussia, a pupil of Müller, Schönlein, and Traube, became one of the directors of the Charité in 1881, and after Frerichs'

death he was given a separate medical clinic and the University polyclinic (1888).

He made his reputation by his investigations of the pathology of fever and its treatment (1873), diabetes (1879), albuminuria in health and disease (1882), which was translated for the New Sydenham Society (1890), and diseases of the kidneys (1896). He also described infectious peripharyngeal phlegmon (1888).

Carl **Gerhardt** (1833–1902), of Speyer, professor at Jena (1861), Würzburg (1872) and Berlin (1885), devoted himself mainly to internal medicine, pediatrics, and laryngology.

He made important contributions on laryngeal croup (1859), paralysis of the vocal cords (1863–72), laryngeal tumors (1896), syphilis of the larynx and trachea (1898), and was the author of treatises on auscultation and percussion (1890), diseases of children (1880), and the editor of a great handbook of pediatrics (1877–96).

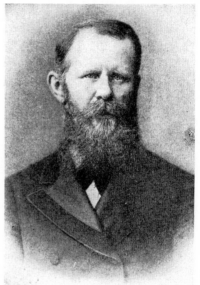

Hermann Nothnagel (1841–1905). (Boston Medical Library.)

In 1865, following Wilhelm Petters' discovery of acetone in diabetes (1857), he introduced his iron-chloride reaction for aceto-acetic ether in acetonemic urine.

Along with Gerhardt, the principal German contributors to **pediatrics** were Eduard Heinrich **Henoch** (1820–1910), of Berlin, a pupil of Schönlein and nephew of Romberg, who wrote a Clinic of Abdominal Diseases (1852–58), a masterly series of essays on children's diseases (1861–68), lectures on pediatrics (1881), and described Henoch's purpura (1874[2]) and dyspeptic asthma (1876[3]); the Viennese, Alois **Bednar** (of Bednar's aphthæ), whose treatise on diseases of infants (1850–53) is equally well known; Theodor **Escherich** (1857–   ), of Munich, whose treatise on

---

[1] Nothnagel: Deutsche med. Wochenschr., Leipz. & Berl., 1905, xxxi, 1564.

[2] Henoch: Berl. klin. Wochenschr., 1874, xi, 641–643.

[3] *Ibid.*, 1876, xiii, 241–243.

the intestinal bacteria of infants (1886[1]), contains the first account of
Bacillus coli infections; Adolf **Baginsky** (1843–1918), of Berlin, author
of a handbook of school hygiene (1876), a text-book of pediatrics
(1882) and many separate studies; and the Galician, Adalbert **Czerny**
(1863–   ), who introduced the concept "exudative diathesis" (1907[2]),
and with Arthur Keller (1906) wrote a great treatise on the disorders
of infantile nutrition, in which the digestive diseases of infants and
children are separated and classified according to metabolic relations.

The subject of scientific infant feeding was inaugurated by Philipp
Biedert (1847–   ), who wrote the first important treatise (1880),

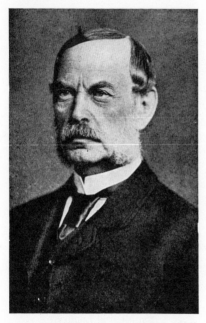

Eduard Heinrich Henoch (1820–1910).
(Collection of A. C. Klebs.)

giving a minute classification of
gastro-intestinal diseases in infancy. This was followed by the
treatise on the metabolism of infancy and childhood (1894) of
Wilhelm Camerer (1842–   ), and
the joint treatises on infant nutrition and its disorders by Adalbert
Czerny and Arthur Keller (1906),
Leo Langstein and Ludwig F.
Meyer (1910), Ludwig Tobler and
G. Bessau (1914).

Of recent German pediatrists,
the greatest was Otto **Heubner**
(1843–1926), a pupil of Wunderlich
and after 1913, professor at Berlin,
author of treatises on disorders
of infant nutrition (1894), diseases
of children (1903–6), and originator of the method of caloric
feeding. In 1898–9, he made,
with Max Rubner, the important investigations of the food
requirements of the normal and
atrophic infant, which have been
the basis of all subsequent work in infant metabolism. His pupil,
Heinrich **Finkelstein** (1865–   ), of Leipzig, originally a geologist,
succeeded Heubner as professor at Berlin, and in 1905–12, produced a
remarkable treatise on diseases of nurslings. In 1906–10, he introduced
his theory of salt and sugar intoxication (alimentary fever) as the basis
of infantile nutritive disorders, with a special "albumen milk" (*Eiweiss-
milch*) to relieve the condition; in opposition to the theories of Biedert
that casein is harmful, of A. Czerny that fats are harmful, of Escherich
that intestinal bacteria are harmful, of Rotch that proteids are harmful

---

[1] Escherich: Die Darmbakterien des Säuglings, Stuttgart, 1886.
[2] A. Czerny: Monatschr. f. Kinderheilk., Leipz. & Wien., 1807–8, vi, 1–9.

(percentage feeding). This theory of Finkelstein, latterly abandoned in part by himself, was the storm-center of controversy for a full decade.

Arthur **Schlossmann** (1867–   ), of Dresden, author of important works on infant hygiene (1907) and stall hygiene (1909), collaborated with Meinhard Pfaundler in a massive pediatric handbook (1906). In 1908–14, with H. Murschhauser, he showed the marked effect of muscular activity on heat production during the estimation of basal metabolism; and in 1913, investigated the fasting metabolism of infants. He organized the recent hygienic exhibit (*Gesolei*) at Dusseldorf (1926).

Bernard **Naunyn** (1839–   ), son of a burgomaster of Berlin, was Frerichs' clinical assistant for seven years, afterward professor of clinical medicine at Dorpat (1859), Bern (1872), and Königsberg (1872), finally succeeding Kussmaul at Strassburg in 1888.

Of all Frerichs' pupils, Naunyn and Ehrlich have best followed the master's bent in experimental pathology and pathological chemistry. Aside from his earlier investigations of hydatids and the chemistry of the transudates, Naunyn has devoted his whole life to the study of metabolism in diabetes and in diseases of the liver and the pancreas.

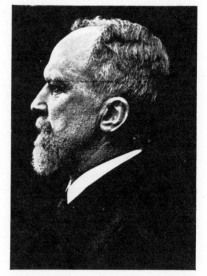

Bernard Naunyn (1839–   ). (Surgeon-General's Library.)

With Klebs and Schmiedeberg, he founded the *Archiv für experimentelle Pathologie und Pharmakologie* in 1872, and, with Mikulicz, the *Mittheilungen aus den Grenzgebieten der Medizin und Chirurgie* (1896). His most important works are his clinical study of gall-stones (1892[1]) and his monograph on diabetes (1898[2]).

In the book on biliary calculus, he introduced the new concept of "cholangitis" as an inflammation of the lining membrane of the smallest bile-ducts causing obliteration of their lumina, explaining catarrhal jaundice and syphilitic hepatitis as primary and secondary forms of infectious cholangitis and regarding biliary calculi as the effect rather than the cause of the same disease. His treatment of the condition by drainage of the bile tract shows how the modern clinician may think surgically as the surgeon clinically. He opposed Flint's idea that cholesterin is a specific product of the liver secretions or of metabolism. In 1883, his pupil, E. Stadelmann, discovered β-oxybutyric acid and Naunyn introduced the term "acidosis" (1906) to define the metabolic condition of acid formation in diabetic coma.

When Naunyn went to Strassburg, his rigorous Prussian temperament excited a great deal of prejudice and opposition among the Alsatian population, and it took him thirteen years to succeed, where even the suave Kussmaul had failed, in having the ancient city hospital (built

---

[1] Naunyn: Klinik der Cholelithiasis, Leipzig, 1892.

[2] Der Diabetes mellitus, Vienna, 1898.

40

1718) converted into the splendid new building (1901). In spite of an attractive call to Vienna, he fought it out in Alsace, where his splendid clinical abilities, his stern fidelity to duty, his love of truth, his polished wit and sarcasm, did not fail of recognition in the end. On the social side, he was known as a man of widest culture, especially in music. His volume of Memoirs (1925[1]) is one of the most interesting books in its class.

Naunyn's pupils number such distinguished pathological chemists as **Ernst Stadelmann** (1853–   ), of Insterburg, who investigated the relation of β-oxybutyric acid to diabetic coma (1883), the effect of alkalies on metabolism (1890), discovered tryptophan (1890), described pentosuria (1894), and, with M. Afanassyeff (1883), worked out the experimental pathology of toxemic and hemolytic jaundice (1891[2]); Oscar **Minkowski** (1858–   ), of Alexoten, Russia, who described congenital acholuric jaundice with splenomegaly and urobilinuria (1900[3]), studied the presence of oxybutyric acid in diabetic urine (1884), the effect of excision of the liver on metabolism (1885), and, with Joseph von Mering, the production of diabetes by excision of the pancreas (1889–93); Max **Schrader** (1860–   ), who made valuable studies on the inhibitory center of the heart (1886) and the comparative physiology of the brain, and Adolf **Magnus Levy** (1865–   ), whose name is particularly associated with diabetic coma and its treatment (1899–1909). Naunyn and his pupils did the best recent work in chemical and experimental pathology. Joseph von **Mering** (1849–   ), of Cologne, a pupil of Frerichs and Hoppe-Seyler, investigated phlorizin diabetes (1886) and collaborated with Minkowski in his experimental work on pancreatic diabetes (1889).

Carl von **Noorden** (1858–   ), of Bonn, professor at Frankfurt (1893) and Nothnagel's successor at Vienna (1906), has made important studies of albuminuria in health (1885), disorders of metabolism (1892–95), and the treatment of the same (1909). His pupils, H. Eppinger, W. Falta, and C. Rüdinger, have done much to develop the doctrine of the correlation of the internal secretions of the ductless glands (1908–9).

Friedrich von **Müller** (1858–   ), of Augsburg, a pupil of Voit and Gerhardt, succeeded Biermer at Breslau (1890), and has held chairs at Marburg (1892), Basel (1899), and at Munich (1902), where his clinic is now one of the most largely frequented in Europe. He first noted the increased metabolism in exophthalmic goiter (1893), and is perhaps the most scientific teacher of internal medicine today.

Karl Friedrich **Wenckebach** (1864–   ), of Vienna, is notable for his work on cardiac disorders, particularly the arrhythmias (1903, 1914).

Hermann **Sahli** (1856–   ), of Bern, director of the University Clinic there, is widely known for his books on percussion in children (1882) and methods of clinical investigation (1894).

He introduced observation of gastric acidity in tabetic crises (1885), the glutoid-capsule test of pancreatic function (1897) test breakfasts of soup (1902), a desmoid test for pepsin digestion (1905), a method of estimating free acid (pH) in the gastric juice by titration of the indicator (1924) a hemometer (1902) and a portable mercury manometer (1904), sphygmobolometry (1907–25), along with salol (1885), guaiacol

[1] Naunyn: Erinnerungen, Gedanken und Meinungen, Berlin, 1925.

[2] Stadelmann: Der Icterus (etc.), Stuttgart, 1891.

[3] Minkowski: Verhandl. d. Cong. f. inn. Med., Wiesb., 1900, xviii, 316. A non-congenital hemolytic icterus was described by F. Widal and P. Abrami (1907).

in phthisis (1887), mild dosage of tuberculin (1906), pantopon (1909), and other therapeutic wrinkles. In 1892, he described acute rheumatism as an attenuated staphylococcic pyemia, and has maintained strong views of his own upon hemophilia (1905), the influenza virus (1919), antibodies (1920–21) and other moot points of medical theorizing.

Carl Anton **Ewald** (1845–1915), of Berlin, an assistant of Frerichs and Senator's successor at the Augusta Hospital (1886), is known everywhere for his great work in disorders of digestion (1879–88), his use of intubation in exploring the contents of the stomach (1875), and his "test-breakfast," which he devised (1885) with his pupil, Ismar **Boas** (1858–   ), of Exin, Posen, author of diseases of the stomach (1890–93) and the intestines (1899) are also highly esteemed. Boas founded the first polyclinic for gastro-intestinal diseases in Germany (Berlin, 1886). Ewald was editor of the *Berliner klinische Wochenschrift* (1881–1907), librarian of the Berlin Medical Society and an authority on forestry.

Ernst **Finger** (1856–   ), of Vienna; Hermann von **Zeissl** (1817–84), of Zwittau, Moravia, and his son Maximilian von Zeissl (1853–   ), of Vienna, have distinguished themselves in the field of genito-urinary and venereal diseases.

The most prominent clinicians and pathologists at Guy's Hospital during the later period were Gull, Wilks, and Hilton Fagge. Sir William Withey Gull (1816–90), of Colchester, England, graduated in medicine from the University of London (1846) and soon became associated with Guy's, where he taught medicine for the rest of his life.

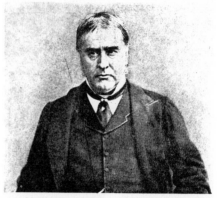

Sir William Withey Gull (1816–90).

He was one of the first to note the posterior spinal lesions in locomotor ataxia (1856–58[1]), described intermittent hemoglobinuria (1866[2]), myxedema (1873[3]), and, with Sutton, the "arteriocapillary fibrosis" in chronic nephritis (1872[4]), which showed that the concept "Bright's disease" is something more than a local renal affection. He also wrote upon vascular obstructions, cerebral abscess, "anorexia nervosa," factitious urticaria, and described, with Addison, "vitiligoidea" or xanthelasma (1851–52[5]). He was one of the pioneers in the use of male fern in tenia (1855) and of static electricity in the treatment of nervous diseases (1852[6]).

Gull was one of the greatest practitioners of his time, Napoleonic in appearance, witty, genial, attractive, and a beautiful lecturer. He

[1] Gull: Guy's Hosp. Rep., Lond., 1856, 3. s., 11, 143; 1858, iv, 169.

[2] *Ibid.*, 1866, 3. s., xii, 381–392.

[3] Tr. Clin. Soc. Lond., 1873–74, xii, 180–185.

[4] Med.-Chir. Tr., Lond., 1871–72, lv, 273–326, 2 pl.

[5] Guy's Hosp. Rep., Lond., 1850–51, 2. s., vii, 265, 2 pl.; 1852–3, viii, 149, 1 pl.

[6] *Ibid.*, 1852–53, 2. s., viii, 81.

is said to have fascinated his patients, to whose cases he gave unstinted time and pains, but, although adored by his pupils, he sometimes repelled his colleagues by his magisterial manner and his imperious temper. His clever epigrams, "Savages explain, science investigates" and "You are a healthy man out of health," intended to soothe a troublesome hypochondriac, are often quoted. He defined a neurotic woman as "Mrs. A. multiplied by four," and to another he said, "Madame, you have a tired heart." He opposed surgical anesthesia with similar flippancies, and affected a sort of therapeutic nihilism, although he was, in reality, remarkably skilful with such drugs as he used. "The road to medical education," he said, "is through the Hunterian Museum and

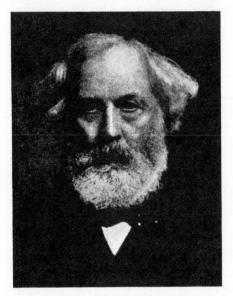

not through an apothecary's shop." He left a fortune of £344,000, almost unprecedented in the history of medicine.

Sir Samuel **Wilks** (1824–1911), of Camberwell, England, was associated with Guy's Hospital all his life, and, in his charming *Biographical Reminiscences* (1911), he appears as its loyal historian, recounting the discoveries of his colleagues with scrupulous fidelity and settling many points of priority. The writings of Wilks really gave the diseases called after Bright, Addison, and Hodgkin their place in English medicine.

Sir Samuel Wilks (1824–1911).

He himself introduced the term "enteric fever," was one of the first to study visceral syphilis (1857–63[1]), left clear accounts of such rare conditions as osteitis deformans (1868[2]), acromegaly (1869[3]), gave a classical account of alcoholic paraplegia (1868[4]), and, as dermatologist, described the "lineæ atrophicæ" on the skin (1861[5]) and the dissecting-room warts (verrucæ necrogenicæ), or subcutaneous tuberculosis of Laennec (1862[6]).

Wilks was a personality of rare kindliness and charm, described by Osler as one of the handsomest men in London in his time, with "a splendid head and merry blue eyes, a man whose yea was yea and

[1] Wilks: Tr. Path. Soc. Lond., 1857–58, ix, 55; 1860–61, xii, 216. Guy's Hosp. Rep., Lond., 1862–63, s., ix, 1–63, 4 pl.

[2] Tr. Path. Soc. Lond., 1868–69, xx, 273–277.

[3] Wilks: Biog. Reminiscences, London, 1911, 198.

[4] Med. Times and Gaz., Lond., 1868, ii, 470.

[5] Guy's Hosp. Rep., Lond., 1861, 3. s., vii, 297–301.

[6] *Ibid.*, 1862, viii, 263–265.

whose nay, nay." His lectures on pathological anatomy (1859, re-edited by Walter Moxon, 1875), and on diseases of the nervous system (1878) were standard sources of knowledge among English students of his time.

Charles Hilton **Fagge** (1838–83), of Hythe, England, editor of the Guy's Hospital Reports, was an able pathologist and clinician, an authority on heart disease, an investigator of cretinism and rickets, and an expert dermatologist. He translated Hebra for the Sydenham Society (1866–68), grouped keloid, morphea and spurious leprosy under the category "scleriasis" (1867), and gave the classical description of gastromesenteric ileus (1869[1]), first noticed by Rokitansky. His *Principles and Practice of Medicine* (1885–86), which was completed by Philip Henry Pye-Smith (1840–1914) and Wilks after his death, is one of the solid books of the time.

Golding **Bird** (1814–54) of Downham, Norfolk, described oxaluria (1842), wrote an important book on *Urinary Deposits* (1844), and was a pioneer in static electrotherapy (1841–49), which he employed with success in amenorrhea.

Frederick William **Pavy** (1829–1911), of Wroughton, Wiltshire, who graduated from the University of London (1850–53) and lectured at Guy's Hospital from 1856 to 1877, had worked with Claud Bernard in 1853, and devoted his whole life to opposing his master's thesis that the liver is a storehouse of available carbohydrates.

By many ingenious arguments based largely upon original experimental work, he showed that the liver does not change glycogen into sugar during life, that oxygen does not destroy sugar in the blood, and that glycogen itself exists in the blood; but, as his knowledge of the subject advanced, his views unconsciously adjusted themselves to those finally held by Bernard. Pavy was undoubtedly right, however, in holding that too much stress has been laid upon the liver as a sugar producer. He was the first to describe cyclic or postural albuminuria (1885) and the typhoidal arthritis known as "Pavy's joint" and is also remembered by his substitution of ammonia for caustic potash in Fehling's solution (Pavy's blue fluid), which, as Pavy's pellets, was one of the first preparations to be made in tabloid form. He had probably the largest practice in London in diabetic cases, in the treatment of which he was particularly successful, and his "Treatise on Food and Dietetics" (1874) is an index of his reputation as an investigator of metabolism.

Sir William **Jenner** (1815–98), of Chatham, England, professor at the University College, London, and physician to Queen Victoria, was Gull's great rival in practice, in which he was so successful that he left behind him a fortune of £375,000. His fame today rests upon the fact that, from a rigid clinical and pathological examination of 36 cases, he separated typhus from typhoid fever (1847[2]), although ten years later than Gerhard in America. Jenner was a short, stout, solid, able-bodied man, yet so averse to exercise that he said he would not even walk from his front door to his brougham if he could get someone to carry him.

Charles **West** (1816–98), of London, was a practitioner of obstetrics, gynecology, and pediatrics, whose *Lectures on Diseases of Children* (1847) was the best English work of his time and was translated into many languages, notably by Henoch into German. He delivered the

---

[1] Fagge: Guy's Hosp. Rep., Lond., 1869, 3. s., xiv, 321–339. Tr. Path. Soc. Lond., 1875–76, xxvii, 157–160.

[2] Jenner: Month. Jour. Med. Sc., Edinb., 1849, ix, 663–680.

Lumleian lectures on nervous disorders in children (1871) and was the main founder of the Hospital for Sick Children in Great Ormond Street, which, under the direction of Still, has now the largest clientèle of children in the world.

Other prominent English practitioners of the time include John Hughes Bennett (1812–75), who described leukemia (1845); Charles J. B. Williams (1805–89), who was, in his day, an authority on consumption and diseases of the chest; Thomas Blizard Curling (1811–88), who first noted myxedema (1850); Sir Alfred Baring Garrod (1819–1907), who introduced the "thread test" in gout (1848–54[1]), and wrote an important treatise on the subject (1859); William Brinton (1823–67), who described plastic linitis, in his work on *Diseases of the Stomach* (1859); Sir Thomas Barlow (1845–   ), who first described infantile scurvy (Barlow's disease, 1876–82[2]), and George Frederick Still (1868–   ), physician to the Great Ormond Street Hospital, who described arthritis deformans in children (Still's disease, 1896[3]).

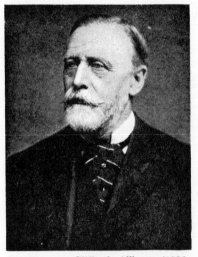

Sir Thomas Clifford Allbutt (1836–1925), Regius Professor of Physic at the University of Cambridge, described the histology of syphilis of the cerebral arteries (1868), gave an early description of the joint symptoms in locomotor ataxia (1869[4]), was the author of the Goulstonian lectures on the visceral neuroses (1884), the Lane lectures on diseases of the heart (1896), and also edited a useful and learned *System of Medicine* (1896–99, 2d ed., 1905–11). His observations on the effect of strain in producing heart disease and aneurysm (1871[5]) are important, in connection with the work of DaCosta and the "effort syndrome" of Lewis. His two-volume treatise on diseases of the arteries (1915) summarizes his own original work on the circulation. His valuable contributions on medieval science (1901) and surgery (1905), Greek medicine in Rome (1909[6]), and Byzantine medicine (1913[7]) give him a unique place among medical historians. Few have approached him in literary style and the power to stimulate thought.

Sir William **Osler** (1849–1919), of Bond Head, Canada, Regius

Sir Thomas Clifford Allbutt (1836–1925).

[1] Garrod: Med.-Chir. Tr., Lond., 1848, xxxi, 83; 1854, xxxvii, 49.

[2] Barlow: *Ibid.*, 1882–83, lxvi, 159–219. Early cases were described by J. O. L. Möller (1856–60), who did not consider the pathology of the condition.

[3] Still: *Ibid.*, 1896–97, lxxx, 47–59.

[4] Allbutt: St. George's Hosp. Rep., Lond., 1868, iii, 55; 1869, iv, 259.

[5] Allbutt: St. George's Hosp. Rep., 1871, v, 23.

[6] Allbutt: Brit. Med. Jour., Lond., 1909, ii, 1449; 1515; 1598.

[7] Allbutt: Glasgow, Med. Jour., 1913, lxxx, 321; 422.

Professor of Medicine at the University of Oxford (1904), was professor at his alma mater, McGill University (1874–84), the University of Pennsylvania (1884–89), and at the Johns Hop'kins University (1889–1904), where he did most to develop the scientific teaching of internal medicine in the hospital wards.

He was one of the earliest investigators of the blood-platelets (1873); described the visceral complications of erythema multiforme (1895), a form of multiple telangiectasis (1901), and chronic cyanosis with polycythemia and enlarged spleen (1903); devoted special monographs to the cerebral palsies of children (1889), chorea (1894), abdominal tumors (1895), angina pectoris (1897), cancer of the stomach (1900), and has done much *Filigranarbeit*, such as the description of the erythematous swellings (Osler's spots) in malignant endocarditis (1908).

Osler's *Principles and Practice of Medicine* (1892, 9th ed., 1920) is the best English text-book on the subject in our time. His essays on *Linacre* (1908), *An Alabama Student* (1908), *Servetus* (1910), and other subjects are among the most attractive of modern contributions to the history of medicine. In this field he is especially memorable for his studies of the work of the earlier American clinicians, whose modern status he has done most to establish. He was the editor of *Modern Medicine* (1910), also founder and editor of the *Quarterly Journal of Medicine* (1908).

When he came to die, Osler was, in a very real sense, the greatest physician of our time. He was one of Nature's chosen. Good looks, distinction, blithe, benignant manners, a sunbright personality, radiant with kind feeling and good will toward his fellow men, an Apollonian poise, swiftness and surety of thought and speech, every gift of the gods was his; and to these were added careful training, unsurpassed clinical ability, the widest knowledge of his subject, the deepest interest in everything human, and a serene hold upon his fellows that was as a seal set upon them. His enthusiasm for his calling was boundless. As Hare says, "Osler went into the postmortem room with the joyous demeanour of the youthful Sophocles leading the chorus of victory after the battle of Salamis." All young English and American physicians who have followed the science and art of medicine in this spirit have been "pupils of Osler." His writings have been aptly described as belonging to the true "literature of power." The loss of his boy, killed in the artillery action about the Ypres salient, broke his heart, but could not bend his resolution to front disaster "with the courage

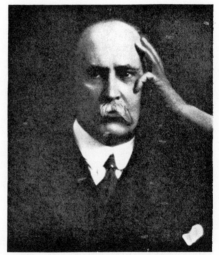

Sir William Osler (1849–1919).

that befits a man." At the last, he took up medical bibliography, and all but achieved his great *Bibliotheca Prima*, a Hallerian catalogue of his wonderful collection of historical texts. Bequeathed to his Alma Mater at McGill, it will stand as a monument of his devotion to his profession—

"The silent organ loudest chants
The master's requiem."

In Osler's clinic at the Johns Hopkins, much important work was done, such as the studies of malarial fever by W. S. Thayer and others (1886–1902), the investigation of amebic dysentery by William T. Councilman and Henri A. Lafleur (1890–91), the finding of the microörganisms in gonorrheal endocarditis and septicemia by W. S. Thayer and George Blumer (1896), the studies of eosinophilia in trichinosis by Thayer and Thomas R. Brown (1897–98), the demonstration of sexual conjugation in the malarial parasites by William G. MacCallum and Eugene L. Opie (1897–98), and the exhaustive study of pneumothorax by Charles P. Emerson (1903).

Lewellys Franklin **Barker** (1867–   ), of Norwich, Ontario, who succeeded Osler as physician-in-chief at the Johns Hopkins Hospital, did much to advance the study of anatomy in America by his works on the nervous system (1899) and anatomical nomenclature (1907), his translation of Spalteholtz's Hand Atlas (1900), and his *Laboratory Manual* (1904), and has added much to the literature of neurology and clinical pathology.

In 1896, he described a unique case of "circumscribed unilateral and elective sensory paralysis," analogous in its bearings to the auto-observation of Henry Head, and with Frederick M. Hanes (1909), the eye signs in chronic nephritis. With F. J. Sladen he has also made interesting clinical and pharmacological studies of the autonomic system (1910–13) and is the author of an exhaustive treatise on diagnosis (1916) and editor of a systematic work on Endocrinology and Metabolism (1922).

William Sydney **Thayer** (1864–   ), of Milton, Massachusetts, professor of clinical medicine at the Johns Hopkins University, has made extensive investigations of malarial fever (1895–97) and typhoid fever (1904), the observations on gonorrheal endocarditis and trichinosis above referred to, and made the first clinical notation of the third sound of the heart (1908).

Of other American practitioners, Henry Ingersoll **Bowditch** (1808–92), of Salem, Massachusetts, a Harvard medical graduate (1832) and a pupil of Louis, is now remembered by his innovation of paracentesis of the chest in pleurisy (1851), his translations from Louis (1836), his books on the stethoscope (1846) and on *Consumption in New England* (1862), his history of Public Hygiene in America (1877), and his work as a student of phthisis, as an activator of public health measures (1869–79), and as an opponent of slavery.

Austin **Flint,** Sr. (1812–86), of Petersham, Massachusetts, was, in his lifetime, an authority on medical practice and auscultation, particularly through his treatises on practice (1866), percussion and auscultation (1876), and medical ethics (1883). His monograph on phthisis (1875) "is still of value today" (Osler). His son, Austin Flint, Jr., was an eminent physiologist.

Alfred L. **Loomis** (1831–95), of Bennington, Vermont, who settled in New York City, wrote the best American text-book on *Physical Diagnosis* (1873), which even today is sometimes consulted.

James **Tyson** (1841–1919), of Philadelphia, professor of pathology (1876–89) and practice (1899–1910) in the University of Pennsylvania, is notable for his works on the cell doctrine (1870), examination of the urine (1875), physical diagnosis (1891), practice (1896), and, in particular, his monograph on Bright's disease and diabetes (1881).

William **Pepper** (1843–98), a native of Philadelphia, described the changes in the bone-marrow in pernicious anemia (1875), wrote many good papers, and edited the first large American *System of Medicine* (1886), but, apart from his great practice, his activities were mainly devoted to the University of Pennsylvania, of which he became provost (1881–94), and where he greatly improved the facilities for medical education.

Jacob M. **DaCosta** (1833–1900), of Philadelphia, the accomplished pupil of Trousseau, wrote a standard treatise on diagnosis (1864), and much upon functional diseases of the heart. He was perhaps the ablest clinical teacher of his time in the Eastern States. His ideas on respiratory percussion were adopted by Friedrich, his views on typhus by Jaccoud. He described irritable heart in soldiers (1862–71), which was also noted by Alfred **Stillé** (1813–1900), who played an important part in establishing the individuality of typhus and typhoid fevers (1838) and was a prominent teacher of pathology.

Edward Gamaliel **Janeway** (1841–1911), of New Brunswick, New Jersey, who succeeded Flint as professor of practice at Bellevue Hospital Medical College, was the first to found an extensive whole-time consultant practice in this country. His *Pathological Reports on Autopsies* (1870), the record of six years of hard work at Bellevue, and his expert skill in microscopy, constituted the basis of his wonderful skill and subtlety in diagnosis. He was in every sense a great bedside physician. He was commissioner of health in New York (1875–81), secured the first hospital for contagious diseases in Manhattan, and first called the attention of the American profession to leukemia (1876), the contagiousness of tuberculosis (1882) and the fever of tertiary syphilis (1898).

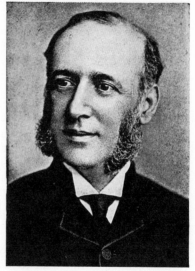

Jacob M. DaCosta (1833–1900).

His son, Theodore Caldwell **Janeway** (1872–1917), professor of medicine at the Johns Hopkins University (1914–17), author of *The Clinical Study of Blood-pressure* (1904), was well known as an advanced clinician at the time of his untimely death.

Henry Leopold **Elsner** (1857–1916), late professor of medicine at the University of Syracuse, summed up the experience of a lifetime in his massive treatise on prognosis (1916), almost the only important work on the subject after Prosper Alpinus (1601).

Nathan Smith **Davis** (1817–1904), of Chicago, perhaps the leading practitioner of that city in his day, was the father of the American

Medical Association, and author of a history of medical education in the United States (1851) and a much better report on the same subject (1877).

Frank **Billings** (1854–   ), of Highland, Wisconsin, professor of medicine in the University of Chicago, edited Frederick Forchheimer's *Therapeusis of Internal Diseases* (1914), and, with E. C. Rosenow and others, developed the doctrine of focal infection from bacteria of the streptococcus pneumococcus group *via* the teeth, tonsils, and other portals (1909–16[1]).

Richard Clarke **Cabot** (1868–   ), of Brookline, Mass., author of various treatises on diagnosis (1896–1901), was an early worker with blood-pressure protocols (1903), challenged the accuracy of most hospital diagnoses as tested by autopsy findings, introduced the idea of **teaching medicine by case-histories,** as exemplified in his own treatise (1906), his "Differential Diagnosis" from 702 cases (1911–15), and in the subsequent collections of James Gregory Mumford (1863–1914) in surgery (1911), E. W. Taylor (1917) in neurology (1911), and John Lovett Morse in pediatrics (1913).

Emanuel **Libman** (1872–   ), of New York, professor of clinical medicine in Columbia University, is remarkable for his original investigations of endocarditis, notably the subacute bacterial, active, and bacteria-free stages (1906–28) and the atypical verrucous phase (with Benjamin Sacks, 1923), streptococcic enteritis (1897), protein precipitation by bacteria (1901), blood-culture and transfusion (1906), lateral sinus thrombosis (1906–17), coronary artery thromboses (1919–28), and for his pupils, Leo Buerger (thrombo-angiitis), A. A. Epstein (lipoid nephroses), A. E. Cohn, Celler, Ottenberg, and others.

Prominent among American specialists in gastro-enterology are John Conrad **Hemmeter** (1864–   ), who was a pioneer in radiography of the stomach (1896) and duodenal intubation, and author of the earliest complete American treatises on diseases of the digestive organs (1896), stomach (1897) and the intestines (1901), a manual of physiology (1913), and *Master Minds in Medicine* (1927); and Max **Einhorn** (1862–   ), of Grodno, Russia, a Berlin graduate and professor in New York, who has invented many ingenious devices and instruments, such as gastro-diaphany (1887), stomach-buckets (1890), duodenal buckets (1908), and is author of well-known treatises on diseases of the stomach (1896), of the intestines (1900) and dietetics (1905).

Abraham **Jacobi** (1830–1919), of Hartum, Westphalia, a graduate of Bonn (1851), was held in detention for his participation in the German revolution of 1848, and settled in New York in 1853, where he became honored and revered as one of the leading practitioners in this country and the Nestor of American pediatrics, a subject which he taught in different medical schools of New York for forty-two years. He played a prominent part in the advancement of American medicine, and wrote

---

[1] Billings: Focal Infection. Lane Lectures, New York, 1916.

discourses, distinguished by quaint wit, varied learning, and true wisdom (Collectanea Jacobi, 1909), including the authoritative monograph on the history of American pediatrics (*Baginsky-Festschrift*, 1913).

In 1857, he began lecturing on pediatrics at the College of Physicians and Surgeons, and thus "pressed the button which set the pediatric clinic in motion" (Adams). It was due to his efforts that the New York Medical College started the first pediatric clinic in this country (1860). He was a founder and editor of the *American Journal of Obstetrics* (1868–71), and the author of works on disorders of dentition (1862), infant diet (1872, 1875), diphtheria (1876, 1880), diseases of the thymus gland (1889), and pediatrics (1896–1903). In 1854, he made a laryngoscope of his own. In 1874, he noted that congenital lipomata are finely lobulated and unencapsulated.

Contemporaneous with Jacobi as a pioneer of pediatrics in America was the modest and unworldly Job Lewis **Smith** (1827–97), of Stafford, N. Y., whose *Treatise on the Diseases of Infancy and Childhood* (1869), based upon his own clinical and pathological findings, passed through eight editions (1869–96).

Of recent American pediatricians, John M. **Keating** (1852–93), of Philadelphia, edited a *Cyclopædia* (1890–91), Louis Starr (1849–1925) of Philadelphia an *American Text-Book* (1894), Henry Koplik (1858–1927), of New York, discovered the spots diagnostic of measles (1898) and published a pediatric treatise (1902). Similar treatises have been written by John Ruhräh (1905), John Lovett Morse (1911), C. G. Kerley (1914) and others. Treatises on the neurotic disorders of childhood were written by Bernhard Sachs (1895) and B. K. Rachford (1905). A translation of the Pfaundler-Schlossmann *Handbuch* was edited by Linnæus E. La Fetra in 1912. A *System of Pediatrics*, edited by Isaac A. Abt (1867–), of Chicago, was published in 1922. John Ruhräh has published an authoritative anthology of the older pediatric texts (1925).

Infant nutrition was first studied in a scientific manner in America by Thomas Morgan **Rotch** (1849–1914), of Philadelphia, a medical graduate of Harvard (1874),

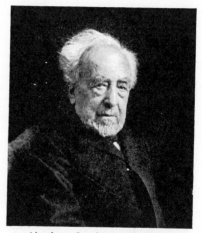

Abraham Jacobi (1830–1919).

who held its first chair of pediatrics (1888). Perceiving that the earlier efforts of Meigs and Pepper to approximate cow's milk to mother's milk by comparative analyses failed through the specific needs of fat, sugar, or protein in different babies, he introduced the method of percentage feeding, in which these elements were employed as needed. He founded the first milk laboratory (Walker-Gordon) in Boston (1891), which was soon followed by one in London, and through his studies of substitute and percentage feeding and the necessity of surveillance of such laboratories, originated the movement for a clean milk-supply. He also established the Infants' Hospital of Boston, and wrote an important pediatric treatise (1896).

Henry Dwight **Chapin** (1857–), of New York, has written treatises on infant feeding (1902) and pediatrics (1909). Chapin and Luther Emmet **Holt** (1855–1924), of Webster, N. Y., author of treatises on infant nutrition (1894–1915) and pediatrics (1897–1916), were the advocates of top-milk, whole-milk, skimmed-milk mixtures, and other modes of home modification of milk which were followed by the cereal decoctions recommended by Jacobi and Chapin, and complete pasteurization or boiling of the milk. Milk commissions to insure a pure supply to large towns originated with Henry Leber Coit (1854–1917). In this country, individual feeding of the individual child, according to its needs, is preferred to the German method of feeding by calories in proportion to the infant's weight originated by Finkelstein.[1]

---

[1] Mixsell: Arch. Pediat., N. Y., 1916, xxxiii, 292.

In recent investigation of infant metabolism, important work has been done by Julius Parker Sedgwick [1876–1923] (1906), John Howland (1910–16), Fritz B. Talbot and F. G. Benedict (1909–16), Bert R. Hoobler (1911–15), John R. Murlin (1910–15), Alfred F. Hess (1912–20), and many others.

Geriatrics, the earliest text of which is Sir John Floyer's *Medicina Gerocomica* (1724), has found modern expression in the writings of Canstatt (1839), Charcot (1881), J. M. Fothergill (1885), Seidel (1890), and the recent treatises of I. L. Nascher (1914) and Malford W. Thewlis (1919).

Much good work has been done in America by such teachers and practitioners as the Jacksons, the Shattucks, the Bowditches, the Minots, James J. Putnam, R. C. Cabot (Boston); Charles L. Dana, L. E. Holt, T. Mitchell Prudden, Frank P. Foster, Joseph Collins, M. Allen Starr (New York); the Mitchells, James M. Anders, Wharton Sinkler, John Herr Musser (1856–1912), Alfred Stengel (Philadelphia); Eugene F. Cordell, Frank Donaldson, Thomas B. Futcher, H. B. Jacobs, Henry M. Thomas, John C. Hemmeter (Baltimore); Samuel C. Busey, W. W. Johnston, D. S. Lamb, S. S. Adams, George M. Kober, J. B. Nichols, W. M. Barton (Washington, D. C.); James B. Herrick, Frank Billings, Henry Baird Favill (Chicago); Charles F. Hoover (Cleveland); George Dock, W. J. Calvert (St. Louis); Christian Rasmus Holmes (1857–1920) (Cincinnati); Joseph Jones, Edmond Souchon, Arthur Washington De Roaldès (laryngology), Isadore Dyer (1865–1920) (leprosy) (New Orleans); Henry Sewall, Walter A. Jayne, Charles D. Spivak (Denver), and, in Canada, by Robert Palmer Howard, F. J. Shepherd, James Bovell, George Ross, A. D. Blackader, Sir James Grant, J. George Adami, J. Playfair McMurrich (anatomy), John McCrae, Fraser Harris, and Maude E. Abbott, to mention only a few names.

Among the many important advances in **diagnostic procedure** were the graphic method of investigating the pulse introduced by Karl Vierordt (1855), A. Stich's suggestion of the use of reflexes in diagnosis (1856), the sphygmograph of Étienne-Jules Marey (1860), the sphygmomanometers of Ritter von Basch (1881), C. Potain (air sphygmomanometer, 1889), Scipione Riva-Rocci (1896–1903) and Leonard Hill (1897), the tonometer of Gustav Gaertner (1899), the oscillometer of V. M. Pachon (1909), for exploring ultra-sensible pulse and blood-pressure, the introduction of esophagoscopy by Kussmaul (1868), cystoscopy, urethroscopy, and rectoscopy by Max Nitze (1877), gastroscopy by Mikulicz (1881), gastrodiaphany by Max Einhorn (1889), autopsy of the air-passages by Alfred Kirstein (1895), direct bronchoscopy and suspension laryngoscopy by Gustav Killian (1898–1912); above all the x-rays (1893) by Wilhelm Konrad von **Roentgen** (1845–1923); Kernig's sign in cerebrospinal meningitis (1884), Henry Koplik's sign in measles (1898), Pietro Grocco's triangle in pleurisy (1902), the differentiation of pericardial pseudocirrhosis of the liver (Pick's disease) by Heinrich von Bamberger (1872) and Filipp Josef Pick (1834–1910) in 1896, J. C. Faget's note of the relation between pulse and temperature in yellow fever (1875[1]), and such phases of urinary analysis as Fehling's test for sugar (1848), Bence Jones' proteid (1848), indicanuria (Max Jaffe, 1877), Salkowski's modification of the Trommer test for grape-sugar in the urine (1879), Wilhelm Ebstein's note of cylindruria in diabetic coma (1881), E. Legal's test for acetonuria (1882), Ehrlich's diazo-reaction (1883), Rudolf von Jaksch on acetonuria and diaceturia (1885), Matthew Hay's test for bile (1886), F. Gowland Hopkins' mode of estimating uric acid (1893), cryoscopy, introduced by Sandor Korányi (1894), Ernst Salkowski on pentosuria (1892–95), and M. Bial's test for the same (1903), the test of Percy John Cammidge in pancreatic disease (1904), Albarran's experimental polyuria (1905), L. Ambard's uremic constant (1910), and the phenolphthalein test in renal disease devised by L. G. Rowntree and Geraghty (1910).

Modern **neurology** is mainly of French extraction and derives from Duchenne, of Boulogne, through Charcot and his pupils.

In the 18th century, Johann Peter Frank had filed a special brief for the study of diseases of the spinal cord (1892); Fothergill had described facial neuralgia (1773); Whytt, tubercular meningitis (1768); Cotugno, sciatica (1770); Pott, pressure paralysis from spinal deformity (1779); Lettsom, the drug habit and alcoholism (1786); Nikolaus Friedreich, facial hemiplegia (1797), and John Haslam, general paralysis (1798). In the early 19th century, cerebral dropsy was described by George Cheyne

---

[1] J. C. Faget: Monographie sur le type et la specificite de la fièvre jaune, Paris and New Orleans, 1875.

(1808), delirium tremens by Thomas Sutton (1813) and John Ware (1831), tetany by J. Clarke (1815), S. L. Steinheim (1830), and J. B. H. Dance (1832); paralysis agitans by Parkinson (1817), softening of the brain by Rostan (1820), alcoholic neuritis by James Jackson (1822), neuroma by W. Wood (1829), and electric chorea by Angelo Dubini (1846). Epilepsy and spinal hemiplegia have been known since the Greeks and chorea since the time of Sydenham. Tabes dorsalis had been vaguely considered by Schelhammer (1691) and Brendel (1749), and was the subject of the dissertations of Ernst Horn's pupils, Loewenhard (1817), von Weidenbach (1817), Schesmer (1819), Gossow (1825), but these last, Max Neuburger thinks, really deal with cases of prostatic neurasthenia. Horn's own view of the disease, faulty as to pathology and semeiology, is given in the dissertation of his son, Wilhelm von Horn (1827). In 1844 Steinthal gave a remarkably exact and complete description of the characteristic gait, the paresthesia, the electric pains, the gastric and vesical crises and the amaurosis, but this was soon forgotten.[1]

The first real advance in the diagnosis of ataxia was made by Moritz Heinrich **Romberg** (1795–1873), of Meiningen, who graduated at Berlin in 1817 (with a classical thesis on achondroplasia), and became professor there in 1838. His *Lehrbuch der Nervenkrankheiten* (1840–46) was the first formal treatise on nervous diseases, and made an epoch by its careful collation of hitherto scattered data, its clear, precise clinical pictures and its attempt to systematize treatment. It contains (p. 795) the well-known "pathognomonic sign" that ataxics cannot stand with their eyes shut (Romberg's sign), and a description of "ciliary neuralgia." Romberg's "propædeutic clinic" at Ber-

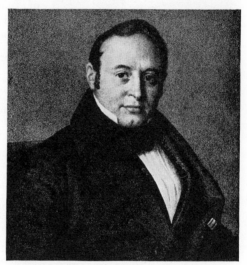

Moritz Heinrich Romberg (1795–1873).

lin, instituted in 1834, was much frequented for the advantages derived from diagnoses made by physical examination.

Guillaume-Benjamin-Amand **Duchenne** (1806–75), who, as Collins says, found neurology "a sprawling infant of unknown parentage which he succored to a lusty youth," was descended from a long line of seafaring people at Boulogne, and it was an inborn love of science which prevented him from complying with his father's wish that he should become a sailor. Coming up to Paris, he studied under Laennec, Dupuytren, Magendie and Cruveilhier, graduated in 1831, and after practising for some years in Boulogne, settled in the capital and devoted the rest of his life to neurology and electrophysiology. His method of prosecuting his studies was peculiar. A strange, sauntering,

---

[1] Martin Steinthal: Jour. f. prakt. Heilk., Berl., 1844, xcviii, 1. St., 1–56; 2. St., 1–84, cited by Neuburger.

mariner-like figure, he haunted all the larger Parisian hospitals from day to day, delving into case-histories, holding offhand arguments with the internes and physicians-in chief, who frequently laughed at him for his pains, and following interesting cases from hospital to hospital, even at his own expense. All this was done in an unconventional and eccentric way, which at first laid him open to suspicion and exposed him to snubs, but the sincerity of the man, his transparent honesty, and his unselfish devotion to science for itself, soon broke down opposition, and, in the end, when his reputation was made, he was greeted everywhere with the warmest welcome. Being timid and inarticulate in relation to public speaking, he was aided by his friend, the fair-minded and generous Trousseau, who, out of fondness for Duchenne, often voiced his ideas with effect in medical societies.

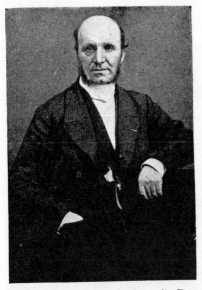

Guillaume-Benjamin-Amand Duchenne, of Boulogne (1806–75). (From a carte de visite photograph in the Surgeon-General's Library.)

Faraday discovered induced currents (1831), and Duchenne employed these in the treatment of paralysis and other nervous disorders. He first set out to classify the electrophysiology of the entire muscular system, studying the functions of isolated muscles in relation to bodily movements, and summarized his results in *De l'électrisation localisée* (1855). He started with the observation that a current from two electrodes applied to the wet skin can stimulate the muscles without affecting the skin. It was his brilliant application of this principle to pathological conditions which brought out so many fine points in the diagnosis of nervous disorders and made him the founder of electrotherapy, in which he was followed by Remak, Ziemssen and Erb. His electrophysiological analysis of the mechanism of facial expression under emotion, illustrated by many striking photographs (1862[1]), is approached only by Darwin's work on the observational side. Duchenne was the first to distinguish between the different forms of lead palsy and of facial paralysis from lesions of the brain or nerves, including the rheumatic and lacrimal forms. But his great field was the spinal cord. In 1840, Jacob von Heine (1800–79), of Canstatt, had described infantile paralysis as a spinal lesion,[2] but in the face of his description, it was usually regarded as an atrophic myasthenia from inactivity. Duchenne pointed out that such a profound disorder of the locomotor system must needs come from a definite lesion, which he located in the anterior horns of the spinal cord (1855). His view was afterward confirmed by Gull, Charcot, Cornil, and Vulpian. He also described anterior poliomyelitis in the adult as due to atrophic lesions of the ganglion cells of the anterior horns, and his name is permanently connected with spinal progressive muscular atrophy of the "Aran-Duchenne type" (1847–61). In 1850, F.-A. Aran, of the Hôpital St. Antoine, published some cases of spinal progressive muscular atrophy which has been worked out by Duchenne.[3] In his exhaustive study of the whole matter, Du-

---

[1] Duchenne: Mécanisme de la physionomie humaine (etc.), Paris, 1862.

[2] Heine: Beobachtungen über Lähmungszustände der unteren Extremitäten (etc.), Stuttgart, 1840.   [3] Aran: Arch. gén. de méd., Paris, 1850, 4. s., xxiv, 4; 172.

chenne at first regarded the disease as a primitive alteration of the muscles, then assumed a lesion in the anterior horn of the spinal cord, finally, under pressure of current opinion, returned to his original view of a primitive muscular atrophy.[1] He described the initial pseudohypertrophies in detail, but did not interpret them, as Erb did. The most definite thing which Duchenne described was the bulbar or glosso-labio-lingual paralysis (1860[2]), which is known by his name, as also the pseudo-hypertrophic form of muscular paralysis (1868[3]). Although the latter is now recognized as one of the many forms of muscular dystrophy, it was Duchenne's careful work in the hospital wards which first opened up the whole subject. In his work on locomotor ataxia. Duchenne labored under one great disadvantage. He cared little for book knowledge, and knew nothing of the work of Steinthal and Romberg, let alone the fact that Edward Stanley had described disease of the posterior columns of the spinal cord in 1839 and Sir William Gull in 1856–58. In 1858–59,[4] Duchenne described the disease at full length, differentiating it from the paralyses, demonstrating the lesion in the cord and pointing out that it is due to lues. When he heard of the work of the German clinicians, he contended that the ataxies observed by them were not the same as those he had seen, and so obscured his subject in controversy.

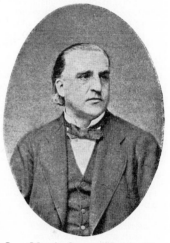

In appearance, Duchenne was a deep-chested, broad-shouldered, sailor-like man, whose ruddy, contented, humorous countenance has been well preserved in the many photographs in his work on physiognomy. He was at once jolly, expansive and absent-minded, brusque yet cordial, disputatious yet tactful, and attributed his success in bearding the lions of the hospitals to his combination of poise and insensitiveness. The last four years of his life were clouded by arteriosclerosis of the brain, and he died forgotten and unhonored, except by a corporal's guard

Jean-Martin Charcot (1825–93).

of old friends at his grave; but he is, with Charcot and Marie, one of the greatest neurologists of France. The best account of him in English is the sympathetic study of Joseph Collins (1908[5]).

Contemporary with Duchenne and far superior in the scope and general accuracy of his work was Jean-Martin **Charcot** (1825–93), of Paris, who graduated in 1853 with a thesis on arthritis nodosa, and in 1862 became physician to the great hospital of the Salpêtrière, with which his name will always be associated. Here, from small beginnings, he created the greatest neurological clinic of modern times, which was followed by enthusiastic students from all parts of the world. His clinics were lessons in visualization, his aim being to teach his pupils

---

[1] Duchenne's final account of the disease is given in his De l'électrisation localisée, 2. éd., Paris, 1861, 437–547.

[2] Duchenne: Arch. gén. de méd., Paris, 1860, 5. s., xvi, 283; 431.

[3] *Ibid.*, 1868, 6. s., xi, 5; 179; 305; 421; 552.

[4] Duchenne: Arch. gén. de méd., Paris, 1858, 5. s., xii, 641: 1859, xiii, 36; 158; 417.

[5] Collins: Med. Record, N. Y., 1908, lxxiii, 50–54.

to detect deviations from the schematic types of nervous disease described in his formal lectures.

Charcot was not only a great neurologist, but early made his mark in his lessons on senile and chronic diseases (1867), diseases of the liver, the biliary passages, and the kidneys (1877). He left memorable descriptions of chronic pneumonia, gout and rheumatism, endocarditis, and of tuberculosis, in the dual nature of which he did not believe. He made important clinical studies of the localization of functions in cerebral disease (1876), and (with Albert Pitres) on the cortical motor centers in man (1895). The five volumes of his lessons on nervous diseases delivered at the Salpêtrière (1872–93) are a good summary of his work, much of which was, as with Ludwig, conveyed through the medium of his pupils. Thus, in 1866, he described, with Henri Bouchard, miliary aneurysms, emphasizing their importance in cerebral hemorrhage; with Georges Delamarre, the gastric crises in locomotor ataxia (1866); with Bouchard, the ataxic *douleurs fulgurantes* (1866); with Alexis Joffry, the lesions in muscular atrophy (1869); with Pierre Marie, the peroneal form of muscular atrophy (1886); and his ideas on hysteria and hystero-epilepsy were set forth in the clinical studies of Richer (1879–85) and Gilles de la Tourette (1891). He defined hysteria as a psychosis superinduced by ideation, the touchstone being the subject's capacity for responding to suggestion. He considered "the phases of the major attack, the innumerable psychic and somatic manifestations, the phenomena of transference on the application of metals, the sensory changes in hemianesthesia and hemianalgesia the motor phenomena of contracture and spasm, the visual features, the relation of hysteria to traumatism, its frequency in the male—these and a score of related problems" (Osler). In muscular atrophy, he differentiated between the ordinary wasting or Aran-Duchenne type and the rarer amyotrophic lateral sclerosis, which the Germans call by his name (1874); and described, with Marie, the progressive neural or peroneal type (1886), which was also described, in a Cambridge graduating dissertation (1886) by Howard Henry Tooth (1856–1926). He differentiated the essential lesions of locomotor ataxia and described both the gastric crises and the joint affections (Charcot's disease). He separated multiple sclerosis from paralysis agitans, although the "intentional tremor" which he signalized as a differential sign had been noted by Bernhard Cohn in 1860. "No writer," says Osler, "has more graphically described the trophic troubles following spinal and cerebral disorders, particularly the acute bedsore." Like Babinski after him, Charcot regarded hypnotism as a neurotic condition, akin to, if not identical with, hysteria, and there was a long-drawn battle between the school of the Salpêtrière and that of Nancy (under Liébeault and Bernheim) as to the part played by suggestion, which, in the hands of the latter, some say, became mere brow-beating. Charcot was not deceived by the feigning of some of his patients, and, in the end, regarded hypnotism as a doubtful therapeutic measure. The soundness of his view is borne out in the modern tendency to merge the procedure into psychotherapy in which he was the pioneer.[1] Charcot was a purely objective investigator, cared little for the special psychology of neurotic patients, and so was saved from some of the subjective exaggerations of the Freudian school. "For purely psychological investigation," says Havelock Ellis, "he had no liking, and probably no aptitude. Any one who was privileged to observe his methods of work at the Salpêtrière will easily recall the great master's towering figure; the disdainful expression, sometimes, even, it seemed, a little sour; the lofty bearing, which enthusiastic admirers called Napoleonic. The questions addressed to the patient were cold, distant, sometimes impatient. Charcot clearly had little faith in the value of any results so attained."

Apart from his clinical work, Charcot was an artist of talent, and the creator of the study of medical history in the graphic and plastic arts. With Paul Richer, he published two fascinating monographs on demonomania in art (1887), and on the deformed and diseased in art (1889), while many valuable studies by his pupils, Henri Meige, Richer, and others appeared in his *Nouvelle Iconographie photographique de la Salpêtriére* (1888–1918), an album *in extenso* of the constitutional

---

[1] Charcot: La foi qui guérit, Paris, 1893.

aspects (facies and habitus) of nervous diseases, which is unique in the history of medicine. Through his wife, who was a lady of wealth, Charcot lived in easy circumstances, but his clinical genius, his keen, clear mind, his poise and dignity, would have made him a commanding figure in any station in life.

Pierre **Marie** (1853–   ), of Paris, Charcot's ablest pupil, graduated in 1883, and became professor in the Paris Faculty in 1889. In 1886, he described, with Charcot, the peroneal type of muscular atrophy,[1] and has made at least four original delineations of new forms of nervous disease.

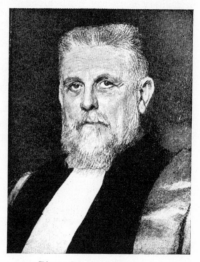

Pierre Marie (1853–   ).

These are his descriptions of acromegaly, pointing out the pituitary lesion (1886[2]), hypertrophic pulmonary osteo-arthropathy (1890[3]), hereditary cerebellar ataxia (1893[4]), and the so-called rhizomelic spondylosis or Strümpell-Marie type of spinal arthritis deformans (1898[5]). He has also made an assault of destructive criticism upon Broca's conception of aphasia, maintaining that the third left frontal convolution has no special rôle in spoken language (1906), and upon the identity of the Aran-Duchenne type of muscular atrophy, which he challenges (1897). During the European War he did most valuable work upon disorders of the peripheral nerves and other effects of gunshot lesions upon the nervous system. He has recently edited a *Traité international de psychopathologie.*

Jules **Dejerine** (1849–1917), of Geneva, took his M.D. at Paris (1879), and was successively chief of clinics at Bicêtre (1882–1901), professor of history of medicine and clinical medicine in the Paris Faculty (1901), and clinical chief at the Salpêtrière (1911–17). In 1890, he married Miss Klumpke, of San Francisco, a Paris graduate of 1889, who collaborated with him in his great work on the anatomy of the nervous centers (1895–1901), and was the *patronne* of his circle of pupils up to her death (1927).

Dejerine is remarkable for his separations of peripheral (neuritic) tabes from medullary tabes (1882–92), and of the scapulo-humeral and fascio-scapulo-humeral types of muscular atrophy (with Landouzy, 1886), for his work on the sclerosis in Friedreich's disease (with Letulle, 1890), his descriptions of hypertrophic progressive, interstitial neuritis (with Sottas, 1893), olivo-ponto-cerebellar atrophy (with Thomas, 1890), the thalamus opticus syndrome (1903), the semeiology of spinal radiculitis (1905), the tabetic muscular atrophies (with Sottas, 1906), the parietal lobe syndrome

---

[1] Marie: Rev. de méd., Paris, 1886, vi, 97–138.

[2] *Ibid.*, 1886, vi, 297–333.

[3] *Ibid.*, 1890, x, 1–36.

[4] Semaine méd., 1893, xiii, 444–447.

[5] Rev. de méd., Paris, 1898, xviii, 285–315.

41

(1914), and his treatise on the semeiology of nervous diseases (1914). Retaining his rank in the army, he spent himself by thirty-one months' exhausting service in the World War.

Of other French neurologists associated with the Salpêtrière tradition Georges Gilles de la Tourette (1857–1904) was remarkable for his description of impulsive tic (1885) and his great treatises on hypnotism (1887) and hysteria (1891–5). Fulgence Raymond (1844–1910), of St. Christophe (Indre-et-Loire), started in life as an army veterinarian, but took his medical degree at Paris in 1876 and became Charcot's chosen successor at the Salpêtrière (1894–1910), where his teaching was of a more dispersed and less dramatic type. He is remarkable for his clinical lectures on neurology (1894–1902), his studies of the spinal scleroses, pseudotabes, diseases of the cauda equina, premature senescence (1910) and two monographs (with Janet) on neuroses and fixed ideas (1898), obsessions and psychasthenia (1903). A monument to his memory was erected at St. Christophe on October 5, 1913. Joseph Babinski (1857–   ) of Paris, once Charcot's clinical chief, now chief at La Pitié, is notable for his elucidation of the toe reflexes (1896, 1903), the pupillary (1899), the defensive (1915) and pilomotor reflexes (1921), the general use of reflexes in diagnosis and in military neurology (with Froment, 1917) and his dismemberment of hysteria as pithiatism (1886–1909). André Thomas (1867–   ) studied the cerebellum (1897–1911) and its wounds (1918). Henri Meige (1866–   ) described hereditary trophedema (1899) and edited the Iconographie. Achille Souques studied feigned hysterical diseases of the spinal cord (1891) and described camptocormy (1916); and Paul Richer (1849–   ), the artist of the Salpêtrière, published treatises on hystero-epilepsy (1879–81), artistic anatomy (1890, 1903, 1906) and physiology (1895), medicine in art (1902) and made a series of statuettes representing paralysis agitans, myxedema, progressive muscular atrophy and glosso-tabio-lingual paralysis.

The ablest German neurologist, after Romberg, is Wilhelm Heinrich Erb (1840–1921), of Winnweiler, Bavaria, a pupil of Nikolaus Friedreich, who became professor at Heidelberg (1880).

In 1868, Erb introduced the method of electrodiagnosis by galvanic and induction currents. He followed Duchenne in the extensive development of electrotherapy (1882), wrote important hand-books on diseases of the cerebrospinal nerves (1874) and of the spinal cord and medulla (1876), and did much to establish the modern theory of the muscular dystrophies, which he described and classified (1891). He also described brachial palsy (1874[1]), syphilitic spinal paralysis (1875[2]), the juvenile type of muscular atrophy (1884[3]), and the so-called asthenic bulbar paralysis or myasthenia gravis (1878[4]), also described by Willis (1685) and by Goldflam in 1893 (Erb-Goldflam symptom-complex). Simultaneously with Westphal (1875), Erb discovered the significance of the knee-jerk in locomotor ataxia[5] and, with Fournier, he did most to establish a statistical causal relation between tabes and syphilis.

Other German neurologists of the period were Nikolaus Friedreich (1825–82), of Würzburg, who described hereditary ataxia (1863–76[6]) and paramyoclonus multiplex (1881[7]), diseases which are sometimes eponymically confused; Carl Friedrich Otto Westphal (1833–90), of Berlin, who described agoraphobia (1871), pseudosclerosis (1883[8]), signalized the knee-jerk in diagnosis (1875[9]) and did important work in psychiatry (1892); Heinrich Quincke (1842–1922), who described angioneurotic edema (1882[10]), which had also been noted by John Laws Milton as giant

[1] Erb: Verhandl. d. naturh.-med. Ver. zu Heidelb., 1874–77, n. F., i, 130–137.

[2] Berl. klin. Wochenschr., 1875, xii, 357–359.

[3] Deutsches Arch. f. klin. Med., Leipz., 1883–84, xxxiv, 467–519.

[4] Erb: Arch. f. Psychiat., Berl., 1878–79, ix, 172.

[5] Arch. f. Psychiat., Berl., 1875, v, 792; 803.

[6] Friedreich: Arch. f. path. Anat. (etc.), Berl., 1863, xxvi, 391; xxvii, 1: 1876, lxviii, 145; lxx, 140.

[7] Ibid., 1881, lxxxvi, 421–430.

[8] Westphal: Arch. f. Psychiat., Berl., 1883, xiv, 87; 767.

[9] Westphal: Ibid., 1875, v, 803–834.

[10] Quincke: Monatsh. f. prakt. Dermat., Hamb. and Leipz., 1882, i, 129–131.

urticaria (1876), and introduced lumbar puncture (1895[1]); Adolf **Strümpell** (1853–1925), of Neu-Autz, Courland, who is well known for his treatise on internal medicine (1883) and who described spondylitis deformans (1897) and pseudosclerosis of the brain (Westphal-Strümpell disease); Paul Julius **Möbius** (1854–1907), of Leipzig, who described dysthyroidism (1886), infantile *Kernschwund* (1892), and akinesia algera, and wrote monographs on the physiological weak-mindedness of women (1900) and the pathology of men of genius (1889–1904); Hermann **Oppenheim** (1858–1919), of Berlin, who first described amyotonia congenita (1900) and "myohypertrophia kymoparalytica" (1914), and is the author of important treatises on the traumatic neuroses (1889), brain tumors (1896), cerebral syphilis (1896), myasthenic paralysis (1901) and neurology (1894), and Max **Lewandowsky** (1876–1918), of Berlin, editor of a great handbook of neurology (1911), left unfinished through his death during the Great War.

The leading English neurologists of the period were John **Hughlings Jackson** (1834–1911), of Yorkshire, who did much to establish the use of the ophthalmoscope in diagnosing brain diseases (1863), made valuable studies of aphasia (1864), described unilateral convulsions or Jacksonian epilepsy (1875[2]), and originated the doctrine of "levels" in the nervous system (1898); Sir William Richard **Gowers** (1845–1915), of London, who is well known for his treatises on diseases of the spinal cord (1880), in which he described Gowers' tract, epilepsy (1881), diseases of the brain (1885) and the nervous system (1886–8), did much to systematize existing knowledge of these conditions. His treatise on medical ophthalmology (1897), beautifully illustrated by his own hand, was of great value in diagnosis. Gowers did good work on the finer anatomy of the nervous system, described ataxic paraplegia, introduced the aluminum chloride treatment of tabes and invented the hemoglobinometer (1878); Henry Charlton **Bastian** (1837–1915), of Truro, one of the founders of English neurology, and author of important books on the brain (1882), the paralyses (1886–93), aphasia (1898), and spontaneous generation (1913); Sir Victor **Horsley** (1857–1916), of Kensington, England, who did admirable work on the physiology of the nervous system, the functions of the ductless glands, and, with Gowers, was the first to remove a tumor of the spinal cord (1888).

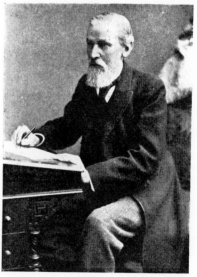

Sir William Richard Gowers (1845–1915).

In America, George Miller Beard introduced the concept of neurasthenia or nervous exhaustion (1869), outlined by Eugene Bouchut as *nervosisme* (1860);

---

[1] Quincke: Berl. klin. Wochenschr., 1895, xxxii, 889–891.

[2] Jackson: Brit. Med. Jour., Lond., 1875, i, 773.

George Huntington described hereditary (Huntington's) chorea (1872); William Alexander Hammond (1828–1900), once Surgeon-General in the United States Army, made his mark with his *Physiological Memoirs* (1863), described athetosis (1873), and wrote a good book on nervous diseases (1871); Francis Xavier Dercum (1856–   ), of Philadelphia, described adiposis dolorosa (1882); Thomas G. Morton described metatarsalgia (1876); Bernhard Sachs (1858–   ), described amaurotic family idiocy (1887–96), the ocular manifestations of which had been noted in 1880 (Tay-Sachs disease) by Waren Tay (1843–1927) and wrote the first American treatise on the nervous diseases of children (1895); Wharton Sinkler isolated the great toe reflex (1888); William F. Milroy, of Omaha, Nebraska, described persistent hereditary edema of the legs, or "Milroy's disease" (1892[1]); Charles Karsner Mills (1845–   ), of Philadelphia, founded the neurological wards in the Philadelphia General Hospital (1877), described unilateral progressive ascending paralysis (1900), unilateral descending paralysis (1906), and macular hemianopsia (1908). Christian Archibald **Herter** (1865–1910), of Glenville, Connecticut, author of studies of experimental myelitis (1889), chemical pathology (1902), intestinal infantilism (1908) or the cœliac disease of Gee (1888), and a text-book on the diagnosis of nervous diseases (1892). He founded the *Journal of Biological Chemistry* (1905), helped to organize the American Society of Biological Chemists (1908) and the Rockefeller Institute (1901), and established the Herter lecture foundations at the Johns Hopkins and Bellevue Hospitals.

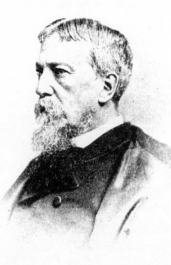

Silas Weir Mitchell (1829–1914). (National Academy of Sciences.)

Charles Loomis **Dana** (1852–   ), of Woodstock, Vermont, author of a *Text-Book of Nervous Diseases* (1892), was, with James Jackson Putnam (1846–1918), of Boston (1891), among the first to differentiate the primary combined scleroses, described acute transverse myelitis with perforating necrosis, lesions of the cortex in chronic myoclonias, serous meningitis or "wet-brain," has done experimental work on the pineal gland, and proposed resection of the posterior spinal nerve-roots within the dura for pain, athetosis, and spastic paralysis, which was performed by Robert Abbe (December 31, 1888).

Silas **Weir Mitchell** (1829–1914), of Philadelphia, the leading American neurologist of his time, was a graduate of the Jefferson Medical College, Philadelphia (1850). In 1851–52, he studied in Paris and came under the influence of Claude Bernard.

In 1859, with Hammond, he investigated the arrow and ordeal poisons, corroval and vao, and he was the first, after the Abbate Fontana and Bonaparte, to investigate serpent venoms (1870–86). With Edward T. Reichert he isolated the diffusible globulins of the venoms: His studies have an important bearing upon the more recent work of Fraser (1896), Calmette (1896), Preston Kyes (1902–3), Flexner and Noguchi (1909). In 1869, he pointed out the coördinating functions of the cerebellum

---

[1] Also described by Nonne (1891) and Henri Meige (trophedema, 1899).

and, with Morris J. Lewis, demonstrated that the knee-jerk can be reënforced by sensory stimulation (1886). During the Civil War, Surgeon-General Hammond created special military hospitals for diseases of the heart, lungs, and nervous system. Mitchell was in charge of Turner's Lane Hospital, Philadelphia, where he established a special ward for nervous patients, and here, with George Reed Morehouse (1829–1905) and William W. Keen, he made those studies of gunshot and other injuries of peripheral nerves (1864) which were afterward expanded in his important work, on *Injuries of Nerves and Their Consequences* (1872). This book contains the earliest distinct accounts of ascending neuritis, the treatment of neuritis by cold and splint-rests, the psychology of the amputated and other data which have been absorbed in the text-books. Mitchell was the first to describe causalgia (1864), erythromelalgia, or red neuralgia (1872–78[1]), and postparalytic chorea (1874[2]), and he was (with William Thomson) the first to emphasize the importance of eye-strain as a cause of headache (1874[3]). In 1875, Mitchell introduced a treatment of nervous disease by prolonged rest in bed, with such adjuvants as optimum feeding, massage, and electricity, the so-called **"rest cure,"** or Weir Mitchell treatment, which is now used everywhere. His ideas on the subject were summed up in his classical monograph, *Fat and Blood* (1877), which has been translated into French, German, Spanish, Italian, and Russian. Mitchell was also the first to study the effect of meteorological changes upon traumatic neuralgias, particularly in old amputation stumps (1877). He made a large number of minor contributions of highly original character, notably those on ailurophobia, phantom limbs, disorders of sleep, *Wear and Tear* (1873) and on freezing his own ulnar nerve. To the history of medicine he contributed an accurate history of instrumental precision (1892) and his memorials of Harvey (1907–12).

In the world of letters, as poet and novelist, Mitchell has a place near Goldsmith and Holmes, not far below Scott and Lamb, the beloved masters of what Owen Wister calls the "Literature of Encouragement." In person, even in his demure choice of quaint phrases, Mitchell was himself a survival of the old-fashioned American gentleman of colonial type. In sobriety and versatility he was like some of the great 18th century physicians, in perception of the fine side of life he suggests Turgenieff, in sense of honor, he was like Bayard or Colonel Newcome. "Who dares draw illness as it is," he makes a physician say, yet, not Balzac, Flaubert, Maupassant or Zola, "knew more of evil and sorrow and pain." "The tone of his books," Wister continues, "is a lesson and a tonic for an age that is sick and weak with literary perverts."

Other innovations in neurology besides those already mentioned were the original descriptions of unilateral paralysis with crossed anesthesia by Brown-Séquard (1851), acute ascending paralysis by Octave Landry (1859), congenital cerebral spastic paraplegia by William John Little (1861), symmetrical gangrene by Maurice Raynaud (1862), disease of the crura cerebri (Weber's syndrome) by Hermann Weber (1862), alcoholic paraplegia by Sir Samuel Wilks (1868), plexiform neurofibroma (*Rankenneuroma*) by Paul von Bruns (1870), myotonia, described in his own person, by Julius Thomsen (1876), syringomyelia with trophic disturbances by Augustin-Marie Morvan (1883), impulsive tic or saltatory spasm (jumping, latah, myriachit) by Georges Gilles de la Tourette (1884), subacute combined degeneration of the spinal cord (1884) by Otto Leichtenstern (1845–1900) and Ludwig Lichtheim (1845–1915), astasia-abasia by Paul Blocq (1888), progressive interstitial hypertrophic neuritis of infants by Joseph-Jules Dejerine (1849–1917) and Jules Sottas (1893), infantile progressive muscular atrophy by Guido Werdnig (1890–94) and Johann Hoffmann (1894), meralgia paræsthetica by Max Bernhardt and Valdimir Karlovich Roth

---

[1] Mitchell: Amer. Jour. Med. Sc., Phila., 1878, n. s., lxxvi, 17–36.

[2] *Ibid.*, 1874, lxviii, 342–352.

[3] Med. and Surg. Reporter, Phila., 1874, xxxi, 67–71.

(1895), and amyotonia congenita by Hermann Oppenheim (1900), the Guillain-Thaon syndrome (transitional cerebrospinal syphilis, 1909), and progressive lenticular degeneration by S. A. Kinnier Wilson (1912), which Gowers had recognized as "tetanoid chorea" (1888) and which Frerichs had also adumbrated in his treatise on diseases of the liver (1884). Herpes zoster was first ascribed to a lesion of the spinal ganglia by Friedrich von Bärensprung (1861–63), and was further localized as an acute hemorrhagic inflammation of the posterior spinal and cranial ganglia by Henry Head and A. W. Campbell (1900). Megrims and all mental disturbances coming under the description of brain-storms or nerve-storms were described by Edward Liveing (1873). The visceral neuroses were investigated by Sir Clifford Allbutt (1884), and the pathology of the cerebral circulation by Leonard Hill (1896). Aphasia first described and localized by Bouillaud (1825[1]), defined as "aphemia" and allocated to the left third frontal convolution by Broca (1861). Hughlings Jackson (1864) introduced the concept "imperception" (Freud's agnosia) and virtually described apraxia (Liepmann, 1900). H. C. Bastian (1869) described what Kussmaul (1877) subsequently termed word-blindness (dyslexia, Rudolf Berlin, 1887) and word-deafness. Agraphia was described by W. Ogle (1867) and asymbolia by F. C. Finkelnburg (1870). The monograph of Fritsch and Hitzig on localization of cerebral functions (1870) engendered a school of "diagram makers," of whom Sir W. H. Broadbent (1879), Bastian (1880–98[2]), Carl Wernicke (1874[3]), and Ludwig Lichtheim (1885) deduced the clinical modalities of aphasia from supposititious lesions of the speech centers or their commissural pathways (Head). Wernicke, in particular, allocated audition to the first temporal speech to the third temporal (Broca's) convolution and aphasic disorders to a general zone in the left temporo-parietal lobe (1874–81). This locus was accepted by Pierre Marie in his iconoclastic papers of 1906,[4] which challenged the restriction of aphasia to Broca's convolution and resolved Broca's aphasia into the sensory aphasia of Wernicke plus anarthria (loss of mechanical capacity for exteriorisation of language), which Liepmann has further differentiated from verbal apraxia and motor aphasia (1913). Confusion was worse confounded by such new phases as Liepmann's subdivisions of apraxia and agnosia (1908[5]), C. von Monakow's concept of diaschisis or loss of functional continuity at the synapses (1909–14), Arnold Pick's aggramatism (1913[6]), and S. E. Henschen's word-hearing and visual centers (1918–24). The delicate casuistry of amnesia, aphasia, and allied disorders of speech is ably discussed by Henry Head (1926[7]), who defines the clinical modalities of aphasia as verbal syntactical, nominal, and semantic (inability to comprehend the meaning of words).

After the time of Pinel and Reil, the **treatment of the insane** without mechanical restraints (open-door method) was advanced by John **Conolly** (1856) and by the Tukes, of whom Daniel Hack **Tuke** (1827–95) collaborated with John Charles Bucknill in a *Manual of Psychological Medicine* (1858), highly esteemed in its day. Another advocate of the no-restraint system was Wilhelm **Griesinger** (1817–68), of Stuttgart, a pupil of Schönlein, a clinical assistant of Wunderlich, and ultimately Romberg's successor at Berlin (1865–67), who, apart from his work in

---

[1] Erich Ebstein points out that cases of aphasia had been described by van Swieten (1753) and Goethe: *Wilhelm Meister*, vii, ch. 6, and *Wanderjahre*, iii, ch. 13 (1796), which had, however, been preceded by the case of Linnæus (1742). Thomas Hood (Phrenol. Tr., 1822, iii), it is said, published a case with autopsy before Bouillaud, who, however, made 700 by 1848, and will always be credited with the classical account of the disease. The term "aphasia" was devised by the celebrated Hellenist, Crisaphis (Trousseau). See Ebstein, Zeitschr. f. d. ges. Neurol., Berl., 1913, xvii, 58–64.

[2] H. C. Bastian: Aphasia and Other Speech Defects, London, 1898.

[3] C. Wernicke: Der aphasische Symptomcomplex, Breslau, 1874.

[4] P. Marie: Semaine méd., Paris, 1906, xxvi, 241; 493; 565.

[5] H. K. Liepmann: Drei Aufsätze aus dem Apraxiegebret, Berlin, 1908.

[6] A. Pick: Die aggramatischen Sprachstörungen, Berlin, 1913.

[7] H. Head: Aphasia, 2. v., Cambridge, 1926.

psychiatry, distinguished himself by his early description of hookworm infection as "tropical chlorosis" (1886), and did much, in Germany at least, to clear up the status of typhus, typhoid, relapsing and malarial fevers, in his monographs on infectious diseases (1857–64). Griesinger's "Pathology and Therapy of Psychic Disorders" (1845) did away with much of the mysticism of the past, gave clear and unmistakable clinical pictures based upon rational psychological analysis, aimed to connect the subject with pathologic anatomy and advocated the open-door and the psychiatrical clinic. Since Griesinger's time, the scientific study of insanity has been mainly in the hands of the Germans.

Theodor **Meynert** (1833–92), of Dresden, professor of neurology and psychiatry at Vienna (1873–92), editor of the *Jahrbücher für Psychiatrie* (1889–92), made many investigations of the anatomy and physiology of the brain (1865–72), described amentia, and wrote on insanity as "Diseases of the Fore-Brain" (1884).

Carl **Wernicke** (1848–1905), of Tarnowitz, Upper Silesia, professor at Berlin (1885) and Breslau (1890), described sensory aphasia, including alexia and agraphia (1874), diseases of the internal capsule (1875), acute hemorrhagic polioencephalitis (1881), and presbyophrenia (1900); wrote treatises on brain diseases (1881–83) and insanity (1894–1900), and issued a splendid atlas of the brain (1897–1904).

Emil **Kraepelin** (1856–1927), of Neustrelitz (Mecklenburg), professor of psychiatry at Dorpat (1886), Heidelberg (1890) and Munich

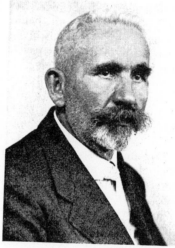

Emil Kraepelin (1856–1927).

(1903), was the pioneer of experimental psychiatry (1896[1]). His *Kompendium* (1883) and thirty lectures on psychiatry (1901) introduced a new and simple classification of insanity, emphasizing the affective, precocious, involutional, katatonic and maniacal forms, introducing the concepts "dementia præcox" and "manic-depressive insanity," and bringing about many simplifications by clever grouping of related varieties. Kraepelin made the classical analysis of the fatigue-curve and the classical investigations on the psychic effects of alcohol (1883–92), which were continued by Raymond Dodge and Francis G. Benedict (1915). He introduced the idea of indeterminate punishment (1880[2]), opposed the use of alcohol. created a museum of the barbarities inflicted upon the insane, and travelled far and wide to investigate the

---

[1] Kraepelin: Psychol. Arb., Leipz., 1896, i, 1–91.
[2] Die Abschaffung des Strafmasses, Stuttgart, 1880.

mentality of primitives and the prevalence of paresis and insanity in
the tropics and among autochthons. The last years of his life (1922–27)
were devoted to the completion of the Deutsche Forschungsunstalt
für Psychiatrie at Munich. A man of sound, positive intelligence and
remorseless logic, Kraepelin was the great systematist of psychiatry,
in which he brought order out of chaos.

Paul Eugen **Bleuler** (1857–   ), of Switzerland, has expanded
Kraepelin's original concept of "dementia præcox" to include a group
of "schizophrenias" (1910) which imply many things not regarded by
Kraepelin, in particular "autism," or the mental life of introverted or
introspective people, who lead shut-in lives. Bleuler also described
"relative idiocy" (1914).

Adolf **Meyer** (1866–   ), Switzerland, professor of psychiatry at
the Johns Hopkins University (1910), has steered and maintained a
middle course between behaviorism and introspection, basing his
psychiatry upon "psychobiology," which makes no sharp division
between physiologic and psychologic data, but envisages mental phenomena as "higher and more complicated (frontal lobe) integrations or
sublimations of the instinctive processes originating in the brain-stem."

Richard von **Krafft-Ebing** (1840–1902), of Mannheim, a pupil of
Friedreich and Griesinger, professor at Strassburg (1872), Graz (1873),
and Vienna (1889), wrote the best German work on forensic psychiatry
(1875), also a treatise on psychiatry based upon clinical experience
(1879), and is especially known for his *Psychopathia sexualis* (1886),
which classifies and describes the various forms of sexual inversion and
perversion, especially in their medicolegal relations. Theodor **Ziehen**
(1862–   ), of Frankfurt, A. M., professor at Jena (1892), is remarkable
for his work on physiological psychology (1891–8), morphology of the
central nervous system (1892–9), and the psychopathology of children
(1902–17). Of the French psychiatrists, Jules **Baillarger** (1809–90) investigated manic-depressive insanity as *folie à double forme* (1853–4)
and cretinism (1873), and founded the *Année médico-psychologique*
(Paris, 1843), now edited by Henri Colin (1921).   Paul Sérieux (1864–
) wrote on reasoned insanity (with Capgras, 1909).   René Semel-
aigne (1855–   ) made a valuable study of the Pinels and the Tukes
(*Aliénistes et philanthropes*, 1912).

Of English psychiatrists, Sir Thomas Smith **Clouston** (1840–1915),
late editor of the *Journal of Mental Science*, wrote a volume of clinical
lectures on mental diseases (1883); Henry Maudsley (1835–1918) was
a prolific writer on psychological themes; Charles Arthur **Mercier** (1852–
1919) was author of a text-book (1902), but his most valuable contributions are those on criminal responsibility (1905), conduct and its disorders
(1911), crime and insanity (1911), and his historical studies of astrology
(1914) and leper houses (1915); John Milne **Bramwell** (1852–   ) has
written much on hypnotism; Sir Frederick Walker **Mott** (1859–1926),
editor of *Archives of Neurology*, was author of the Croonian lectures
on the degeneration of the neuron (1900). L. S. **Forbes Winslow**

(1844–1913) wrote treatises dealing with the legal (1874) and picturesque aspects of lunacy (1898–1912), and entertaining memoirs (1910);
Hugh **Crichton Miller** (1877–   ) has written interestingly on hypnotism. Mention should be made of the Italians, **Sante de Sanctis**
(dementia præcosissima, 1906), Giovanni **Mingazzini** (encephalitis
lethargica, 1921), Eugenio Tanzi (1904), and Leonardo Bianchi (1905),
whose psychiatric treatises have been Englished; of the Russians, Ivan
Pavlovich Merzheyevski (1838–1908), Nikolai Nikolaïevich **Bazhanoff**
(1857–   ), Ivan Alexandrovich **Sikorski** (1845), notable for his work
on physiognomy of the insane (1887–93), Sergiei Sergievich **Korsakoff**
(1853–1900), who described polyneuritic insanity (1887) and wrote a
text-book (1893), and Vladimir Michailovich **Bechtereff** (1857–1927),
author of a classification of insanity (1891), a neurological treatise
(1894–9), and psychiatric lectures (1908); and of the Americans, Edward
Charles Spitzka (1883), Henry J. Berkley (1900), Stewart Paton (1905),
and William A. **White** (1909). As superintendent of the Government
Hospital for the Insane (1903), editor of the *Psychoanalytic Review*,
and author of a treatise on mental mechanisms (1911) White has done
much for recent psychiatry. With Smith Ely **Jelliffe** (1866–   ), of
New York, editor and translator of many things of historic interest
and value, White collaborated in a treatise on diseases of the nervous
system (1915), presenting most advanced views of the nervous and
psychic mechanisms as transformations of energy. Henry Mills **Hurd**
(1843–1927), professor of psychiatry (1889–1906) and superintendent of
the Johns Hopkins Hospital (1889–1911), was editor of *The Institutional
Care of the Insane in the United States and Canada* (1916), which contains his valuable history of American psychiatry.

New methods of psychopathological investigation were introduced by Robert
Sommer (1899). Psycho-analysis was introduced by Sigmund Freud and C. G.
Jung (1893–1909). General paralysis of the insane was described by John Haslam
(1798) and Calmeil (1826), moral insanity by James Cowles Prichard (1835), circular insanity by Jean-Pierre Falret (1854), hebephrenia by Karl Kahlbaum (1863)
and Hecker (1871), katatonia by K. Kahlbaum (1874), psychasthenia by Pierre
Janet (1903), presenile dementia, with plaques in the brain (1911) by Alois Alzheimer
(1864–1915). A valuable contribution is that of Broussais (*De l'irritation et de la
folie*, 1828), who. like Stahl, was at his best in the psychic field (Zillboorg). Paul
Briquet (1796–1881) published a monumental treatise on hysteria (1859). Alcoholic
paraplegia, already noted by James Jackson (1822) and Sir Samuel Wilks (1868),
was described as a polyneuritic psychosis by Sergiei Korsakoff (1887). Heinrich
Laehr (1820–1905), editor of the *Allgemeine Zeitschrift für Psychiatrie* (1858–   ),
made valuable directories of the insane asylums of the Germanic countries (1852–
82), an unrivaled bibliography of the literature of psychiatry, neurology, and psychology from 1459 to 1799 (1900), and a calender of psychiatry (1885) containing,
day by day, all the important events connected with the history of the subject, including the martyrology of physicians and asylum attendants killed by the homicidal
insane. Otto Mönkemöller has written well on the history of psychiatry (1903–10).

The later 19th century marks the scientific or parasitic period of
dermatology, in which many cutaneous diseases were directly traced to
microscopic organisms, especially under the leadership of Sabouraud
and Unna.

Hebra's work was completed and extended by his son, **Hans von Hebra** (1847–1902), of Vienna, who wrote a text-book on skin diseases in relation to diseases of the entire organism (1884), described rhinoscleroma (1870) and rhinophyma (1881), and by his pupil, the Hungarian Moriz **Kaposi** (1837–1902), who completed the elder Hebra's text-book, besides writing one of his own (1879), and described pigmented sarcoma of the skin (1872), diabetic dermatitis (1876), xeroderma pigmentosum (1882), lymphoderma perniciosa (1885), the various forms of lichen ruber (1886–95), and ultimately put Hebra's impetigo herpetiformis upon a definite footing (1887). Isidor Neumann's treatise of 1869 was frequently translated and widely read. Dermatology was also popularized by Sir William James Erasmus **Wilson** (1809–84), who made an early reputation by his *Dissector's Manual* (1838), *Anatomist's Vademecum* (1840), and anatomical plates, his *Diseases of the Skin* (1842), dermatological *Atlas* (1847), and his Royal College of Surgeons lectures on dermatology (1871–78), particularly by his gift of £5000 for founding a chair of dermatology in the latter institution and the extensive collection of dermatological preparations which he made for the same. Wilson classified cutaneous disorders as diseases of the true derma, of the sudoriparous and sebaceous glands, the hair and follicles, and he was the first to describe trichorrhexis nodosa (trichodasis, 1849), erythema nodosum (1857), lichen planus (1869) and dermatitis exfoliativa (1870). He brought Cleopatra's Needle to London and is said to have established the custom of a daily bath. Tilbury Fox (1836–79) author of two treatises (1863, 1865–75), an atlas (1875–77), and a famous book on endemic skin diseases of India (1876), identified the *kerion* of Celsus as ringworm (1862), segregated impetigo contagiosa (1862), with an ammoniated mercury treatment, located epidermolysis bullosa (1879, Goldscheider, 1882) and described lymphangioma, dermatitis herpetiformis, and urticaria pigmentosa. Among the French dermatologists of the earlier period were Alphée Cazenave (1795–1877) who described pemphigus foliaceus and H. E. Schedel, authors of a text-book (1828) which became authoritative; M.-G.-A. Devergie (1798–1879), author of a treatise emphasizing etiology (1857) who described Hebra's lichen ruber as pityriasis rubra pilaris; Antoine-P.-E. Bazin (1807–78), who described mycosis fungoides (1862), acne varioliformis (1862), also keloid acne, erythema induratum, and hydroa vacciniforme. Bazin made a new classification, stressing parasitic etiology, which had been noted by the Arabians, by Cosimo Bonomo, who described the parasite of scabies (1687), by John Hunter, who gave a clinical description of the disease; by Wichmann, of Hamburg, who established its parasitic nature (1786); by Schönlein, who described the achorion fungus of favus (1839); by David **Grüby** (1810–98), who described a contagious tinea sycosis or mentagra (porrigo decalvans or phytoalopecia), due to a fungus (1841–43), and by Carl Eichstedt, who established the relation between pityriasis versicolor and Microsporon furfur (1846). Grüby's work received little attention until the **bacteriologic and parasitologic period,** when it was taken up by Raymond **Sabouraud** (1864–   ), of Paris, who made extensive studies of the different varieties of trichophyton (1894[1]), the etiology of eczema (1899–1900), diseases of the scalp (1902–   ), of pityriasis, and the "pellicular alopecias" (1904[2]). Sabouraud did the best work on the mycotic diseases of the skin. In 1881, Thin had shown that trichophyton is distinct from ordinary fungi. Eczema marginatum of the groin and axilla (dhobie itch) has been traced to the Epidermophyton inguinale, pityriasis versicolor to Microsporon furfur, tropical tinea imbricata to another ringworm fungus. Meanwhile extremely valuable work was done on the pathological, bacteriological, and therapeutic side by Paul Gerson **Unna** (1850–   ), of Hamburg, who was severely wounded as a volunteer in the Franco-Prussian War, and afterward founded a private clinic (1881) and a hospital for skin diseases (1884) in his native city. He published valuable works on the anatomy (1882) and histo-pathology of the skin (1894) and the treatment of skin diseases (1898), founded the *Monatshefte für praktische Dermatologie* (1882) and *Dermatologische Studien* (1886), and edited an international atlas (1889) and a histopathological atlas (1894) of skin diseases. Unna, a most prolific writer, described seborrheic eczema (1887–93), the morococci of eczema (1892–97), the different cocci of favus (1892–99), phlyctænosis streptogenes (1895), pustulosis staphylogenes (1896), described the pathology of leprosy (1910), and introduced ichthyol and resorcin (1886), and specially coated pills for local absorption in the duodenum (1884).

Among the original descriptions of skin diseases in the modern period are those

---

[1] R. Sabouraud: Les trichophyties humaines, Paris, 1894.

[2] Pityriasis et alopécies pelliculaires, Paris, 1904.

of porrigo (1864), dysidrosis (1873), and hydroa (1880) by Tilbury Fox (1836-79), colloid milium by Ernst Wagner (1866), dermatitis exfoliativa by Erasmus Wilson (1870), giant urticaria (angioneurotic edema), by John Laws Milton (1876), angiokeratoma by Wyndham Cottle (1877), infantile exfoliative dermatitis by Ritter von Rittershain (1878), neurofibroma by F. D. von Recklinghausen (1882), epidermolysis bullosa by Alfred Goldscheider (1882), varicella gangrenosa by Sir Jonathan Hutchinson (1882), xeroderma pigmentosum (1882), lymphodermia perniciosa (1885), lichen ruber moniliformis (1886) by Moriz Kaposi (1837-1902), who also established the definite status of impetigo herpetiformis (1887), lichen ruber planus (1895), and pemphigus vegetans (1896); erythema elevatum by Judson S. Bury (1888), follicular psorospermosis by Jean Darier (1889), acanthosis nigricans by Sigmund Pollitzer and V. Janowsky (1890), angiokeratoma (1891), and porokeratosis (1893) by Vittorio Mibelli (1891), hyperkeratosis by Emilio Respighi (1893), benignant sarcoid by Cæsar Boeck (1899), chronic atrophic acrodermatitis by J. Herxheimer and Kuno Hartmann (1902), granulosis rubra nasi by Josef Jadassohn (1901), parapsoriasis by Louis Brocq (1902), lichen nitidus by Felix Pinkus (1907), and precancerous lesions by Bowen (1912) and Darier (1914). Of Americans, Robert William Taylor described idiopathic progressive atrophy of the skin (1876); Louis A. Duhring, dermatitis herpetiformis (1884); Andrew Rose Robinson, hydrocystoma (1884); Thomas Caspar Gilchrist, blastomycetic dermatitis (1896); Benjamin R. Schenck, sporotrichosis (1898); and Jay F. Schamberg, the progressive pigmentary dermatitis which goes by his name (1900-01[1]).

Recent dermatology has profited mainly by the newer views of the skin as a sensitive index of internal disease and a defensive mechanism, by the knowledge gained from cutaneous sensitization tests for infection, and by the extensive use of radiotherapy and ultraviolet light in all manner of cutaneous disorders.

The work of Magendie in experimental **pharmacology** was ably continued by Alexander Crum Brown and Thomas Richard Fraser, who first investigated the relation between the chemical constitutions of substances and their physiological action ("anchoring the molecules") (1867[2]), in which they were followed by Lauder Brunton and J. T. Cash (1884-92), and by Cash and W. R. Dunstan (1893). Friedrich Walter investigated the actions of acids upon the animal organism (1877), Ernst Stadelmann the action of alkalies upon metabolism (1890). Admirable text-books on materia medica and therapeutics were written by such men as Sydney Ringer in England (1869) and H. C. Wood in America (1874), both of whom aimed to establish the status of drugs on the clinical side, while Buchheim, Schmiedeberg, and Binz in Germany, Brunton and Cushny in England, have done brilliant experimental work on animals. The latter names have been particularly associated with the destructive and critical pharmacodynamics of the present time, the aim of which is to apply a rigorous sifting process to the vast numbers of alleged remedies listed in the various formularies and pharmacopeias, on the principle of "Prove all things, hold fast to that which is good." The effect of this destructive criticism has not only been admirable in reducing the gigantic vegetable materia medica of the past to reasonable proportions, but, in the face of the huge output of coal-tar products by the German chemists, initiated by Perkin's

---

[1] For bibliographical references to these diseases, see Index Catalogue (S. G. O.), 1912, 2 s., xvii, 150-152.

[2] Tr. Roy. Soc. Edinb., 1867-9, xxv, 151-203.

discovery of aniline dyes (1856), it became absolutely necessary. "The period of constructive pharmacology," Cushny declares, "has scarcely dawned" and he points out that remedies may now "be numerated in units where they were once counted in scores." The French clinicians Henri Huchard and Charles Fiessinger, for instance, have limited actual drug therapy to some 20 remedies or groups of remedies, viz.: opium, mercury, quinine, nux vomica, digitalis, arsenic, phosphorus, ergot, belladonna, chloral, bismuth, the bromides, the hypnotics, the purgatives, the antiseptics, the anesthetics, the antipyretics, the nitrites, the sera and vaccines, the animal extracts, each of which has a specific therapeutic intention.[1] An International Conference for the unification of the formulæ of heroic remedies was held at Brussels in 1902. The

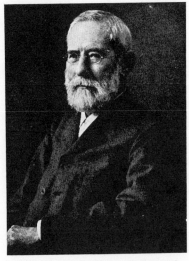

Oswald Schmiedeberg (1838–1921).

whole tendency of recent pharmacology is in the direction of simplification and specificity; but it is rightly contended by the therapeutists of the older school that people are not necessarily rabbits and guinea-pigs of larger growth, since individual drugs have different effects, not only upon different animals, but upon different human beings. The only final test of the reliability of a drug is at the bedside.

The leading pharmacologists of the German school are Rudolf **Buchheim** (1820–79), of Bautzen, professor at Leipzig (1846), Dorpat (1849), and Giessen (1867), who published a text-book of materia medica in 1856 and investigated the action of potassium salts, of purgatives, cod-liver oil, ergot, the mydriatic alkaloids of the Solanaceæ, etc.; his pupil, Oswald **Schmiedeberg** (1838–1921), of Courland, professor at Dorpat (1870) and Strassburg (1872), who first investigated the action of poisons on the frog's heart (in Ludwig's laboratory, 1871), and hippuric acid synthesis in the kidneys (1876), discovered sinistrin (1879) and histozyme (1881), determined the true formula of histamin and nucleic acid from Miescher's posthumous notes (1896), and did a great amount of critical and experimental work on muscarin (1869), ferratin (1893), digitalis and other drugs, the tendency of which is crystallized in his well-known elements of pharmacology (1883). Karl **Binz** (1832–1912), of Bernkastel, was a pupil of Virchow and Frerichs and professor at Bonn (1868), where he founded the Pharmacological Institute of the University (1869). Binz published a text-book on

---

[1] H. Huchard and Ch. Fiessinger: La thérapeutique en vingt médicaments, Paris, 1910.

materia medica (1866) and lectures on pharmacology (1884), made experimental investigations of the action of quinine, alcohol, arsenic, the ethereal oils, the halogen compounds, and the anesthetics, and wrote an admirable history of anesthesia (1896). Georg **Dragendorff** (1836–98), of Rosteck, professor of pharmacy at Dorpat (1864–93), wrote on toxicology (1868), forensic chemistry (1871), and a history of vegetable drugs (1898). Hans **Meyer** (1853–   ), of Insterburg, a pupil of Ludwig and Schmiedeberg, professor at Dorpat (1881), Marburg (1882), and Vienna (1884), and E. Overton, have devoted especial attention to the part played by lipoid solvents in narcosis.

Of French pharmacists and therapists, Jean-Baptiste Alphonse **Chevallier,** Sr. (1793–1879), of Langres, was professor at the École de pharmacie (1835) and author of a dictionary of adulterations (1850) and countless articles; François-L.-M. **Dorvault** (1815–79) edited *L'Officine* (1845) and wrote a treatise on iodine (*Iodognosie,* 1850); Marcellin **Berthelot** (1827–1907) devised a method for liquefying gases (1850), did many feats in synthetic chemistry, notably on animal fats (1853), alcohol (1860), hydrocyanic acid (1867) and benzin (1868), investigated etherification (1853), wines (1863–92), discovered many new sugars (1858–63), and published treatises on synthetic chemistry (1860) and thermochemistry (1879); Émile **Bourquelot** (1851–1921) did remarkable work on soluble ferments in fungi and on the synthesis of glucosides, of which he produced no less than 15 yielding glucose on emulsive hydrolysis (1920). The polyhistorian Adolphe **Burggraeve** (1806–1902), originator of dosimetric therapy (1876), and Georges **Dujardin-Beaumetz** (1833–95) were both of them prolific writers on therapeutics.

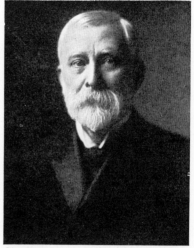

Sir Thomas Lauder Brunton (1844–1916).

Sir Thomas Lauder **Brunton** (1844–1916), of Roxburghshire, Scotland, an Edinburgh graduate (1868), who was assistant physician (1875–97) and full physician (1897–1904) to St. Bartholomew's, studied with Brücke, Kühne and Ludwig, and became a master in the application of the physiological findings of pharmacology to internal medicine.

From the time of his graduating dissertation on digitalis (1868), his special field was the action of drugs on the heart. In 1867, he ascertained that rise of arterial pressure is a feature of angina pectoris and recommended the exhibition of amyl nitrite on physiological grounds.[1] He introduced the vasodilator remedies and,

---

[1] Brunton: Lancet, Lond., 1867, ii, 97.

in 1874, employed raw meat in diabetes in order to supply a glycolytic ferment. He practised medicine as a science, interpreting symptoms as altered physiology rather than as consequences of the end-results of altered structure. He served on the second Chloroform Commission at Hyderabad (1889), was an early and constant advocate of universal physical and military training for "preparedness," was knighted in 1900 and created a baronet in 1908.

Personally Brunton was the "kindly Scot," a mixture of sagacity and simplicity, generous, sportsmanlike, and self-sacrificing. He paid all the expenses and salaries of his pharmacological laboratory at St. Bartholomew's, was a warm personal friend of Billings, and made princely donations to the Surgeon-General's Library.

His works include the well-recognized and frequently translated text-book of pharmacology and therapeutics (1885), the Croonian Lectures upon the relation between chemical structures and physiological action (1892), the popular *Lectures on the Action of Medicines* (1897), monographs on disorders of digestion (1886), disorders of assimilation (1901), and the therapeutics of the circulation (1908), and a vast number of individual papers.

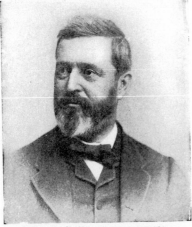

Horatio C. Wood (1841–1920).

Sir Thomas Richard Fraser (1841–1920), of Calcutta, India, a medical graduate of Edinburgh (1852), where he succeeded Sir Robert Christison as professor of materia medica (1877–1917), was one of the pioneers of experimental pharmacology through his original work on physostigmine (1863–7), strophanthus hispidus (1873–95), which he added to the pharmacopœia, and his investigations of arrow-poisons and serpent venoms.

Arthur Robertson Cushny (1866–1926), of Scotland, professor of pharmacology at Ann Arbor (1893–1905) and in the universities of London (1905–18) and Edinburgh (1918–25), was a pupil of Schmiedeberg (1891–3). His text-book of pharmacology and therapeutics (1899) is imbued with the spirit of his master. He did admirable work on the effects of digitalis on heart-muscle (1897–1925), on renal secretion (1901–4), and on the biological relations of optical isomeres (1925). In 1899, he recognized the similarity between clinical delirium cordis and experimental auricular fibrillation (Lewis, 1909).

Horatio C. Wood (1841–1920), of Philadelphia, was professor of botany (1866–76) and therapeutics (1876–1907), also professor of nervous diseases (1875–1901) in the University of Pennsylvania.

He made an important investigation of the pathology of sunstroke (1872), wrote a memoir on *The Fresh-water Algœ of North America* (1872), and a pioneer treatise on therapeutics (1874), in which the effects of the various drugs upon man in small doses were first discussed, then of experimentation upon animals, which, with the evidence of toxicology, was made the rationale of their use in disease. This book also contains a standard classification of drugs. Wood wrote a valuable monograph on fever (1880), investigated amyl nitrite (1871), discovered the physiological and therapeutic properties of hyoscine (1885), introduced atropine to combat the fall of blood-pressure in shock, and first systematized the treatment of accidents in anesthesia (1890). He was editor of the *Philadelphia Medical Times* (1873–80), the *Therapeutic Gazette* (1884–90), the United States Dispensatory (1883–1907), and was author of a book on nervous diseases (1887).

Hobart Amory **Hare** (1862–   ), of Philadelphia, professor of therapeutics in the Jefferson Medical College (1891), editor of the *Therapeutic Gazette* (1891) and other periodicals, is author of well-known text-books on therapeutics (1890), diagnosis (1896), and practice (1907), of monographs on mediastinal disease (1888), epilepsy (1889) and fever (1890), and is editor of a System of Therapeutics (1890–1911).

John Jacob **Abel** (1857–   ), of Cleveland, Ohio, professor of pharmacology at the Johns Hopkins University (1893), is editor of the *Journal of Pharmacology and Therapeutics* (1909). He first isolated epinephrin (1898) and bufagin (1911), investigated the constituent of the suprarenal capsule which raises blood-pressure (1897–1905), the poisons of *Amanita Phelloides* (1909), the convulsant dye-stuffs (1910–11), the presence of histamine in the tissues (1919–20), the secretions of the pituitary gland (1920–23). His pharmacological studies of the phthaleins and their derivatives (1909) led to the universal clinical use of phenolsulphonephthalein as a functional test in renal disease by L. G. Rowntree and J. T. Geraghty (1910) and of phenoltetrachlorphthalein in testing the functional capacity of the liver (Rowntree, Hurwitz, and Bloomfield, 1913). By vividiffusion (1912–14) Abel first obtained amino-acids directly from the blood, has produced a crystallized insulin, with determination of its chemical composition and properties (1925–8), and devised the method of plasmaphæresis (1914).

Among his pupils, Reid Hunt (1870–   ) is known by his studies on experimental alcoholism (1907), the thyroid (1909), and choline derivatives (1911); Leonard G. Rowntree (1883–   ) for the above mentioned functional tests (1910–13); David I. Macht has investigated the opium alkaloids (1915–16) and other substances. Arthur S. Loevenhart (1878–   ) demonstrated the reversibility of lipase (with J. H. Kastle, 1900) and with Samuel J. Crowe discovered that hexamethylenamin (urotropin) is excreted in the cerebrospinal fluid (1909), which led to its extensive use in membranous diseases caused by microörganisms.

The special action of magnesium salts upon tetanus was investigated in America by Samuel James Meltzer and John Auer (1905–6).

Of American pharmacists Joseph Price Remington (1847–1918) published a treatise (1886 and edited the Wood and Bache Dispensatory (1883–1918 ; Edward Robinson Squibb (1819–1900), of Wilmington, Delaware, whose life was spoiled by the mutilations from an ether explosion, founded and edited the *Ephemeris* (1882–1900), and was a pioneer in the insurance of purity in manufactured drugs, in which his name became a symbol of honor; Charles Rice (1841–1901), of Austrian birth, was the most learned and versatile of American pharmacists. Torald Sollmann (1874–   ), author of many investigations and text books, is the prime mover of the Council on Pharmacy of the American Medical Association.

John Uri Lloyd (1849–   ) has made many valuable historical contributions (1900–20), as also Edward Kremers (1865–   ) professor in the University of Wisconsin (1892) and editor of the *Pharmaceutical Review* (1896–1900).

Among the many **new drugs** introduced in recent times are lecithin (Gobley, 1846; Danilevsky, 1896), chloral (1869) by Oscar Liebreich (1838–1908), pyoctanin (E. Merck, 1872), pilocarpin (Hardy and Gerard, 1873), vaseline (R. A. Chesebrough, 1875), antipyrin (Knorr) by W. Filehne (1884), cocaine (as anesthetic) by V. K. Anrep (1879–84[1]), and C. Koller (1884), salipyrin by Riedel (1884), formalin (I. Loew, 1885), creolin (J. Schenkel, 1885), strophanthus hispidus by Sir T. R. Fraser (1885), urethane by R. von Jaksch (1885), ichthyol and resorcin by P. G. Unna (1886), salol by M. von Nencki (1886), acetanilide (antifebrine) by Arnold Cahn and P. P. Hepp (1886), phenacetine (Kast and Hinsberg, 1887), ephedrine (Nagai, 1887), sulphonal (Baumann, 1884) by Alfred Kast (1888), trional and tetronal by Eugen Baumann and Alfred Kast (1888), tropacocaine (Giesel, 1891), thiosinamine (Hebra, 1892), pyramidon (Filehne and Spiro, 1893), hetol (Landerer, 1893), urotropin (Nicolaier, 1894), suprarenal extract by G. Oliver and E. A. Schäfer (1894–95), eucaine by Merling (1896), heroin by Dreser (1898), sodium cacodylate (Gautier, 1899), adrenaline (1901) by Jokichi Takamine (1854–1922), bornyval (Riedel, 1903), digalen (Cloetta, 1904), veronal (1904) and proponal (1905) by Emil Fischer and Joseph von Mering, fibrolysin (Mendel, 1905), novocaine by Alfred Einhorn (1905), scarlet red (Biebrichs, 1882) by B. Fischer (1906), digipuratum (Knoll, 1907), bismuth paste by Emil J. Beck (1908), pantopon by Hermann Sahli (1909), salvarsan ("606") by Ehrlich (1909), optochin by Morgenroth and Levy (1911), sanocrysin by Møllgard (1913), dichloramine-T (Dakin, 1918), and synthalin by E. Frank (1926).

Emetin, introduced by J. L. Bardsley, of Manchester, in 1829, as a remedy for dysentery, was found to be amecibidal by Edward B. Vedder (1910–11) and its use in amebic dysentery was established clinically by Sir Leonard Rogers (1912). Yoghurt, introduced by Metchnikoff (1906), was the starting point of Bacillus bulgaricus and B. acidophilus therapy.

Of other therapeutic measures, **electrotherapy** was modernized by Duchenne of Boulogne (1847–55), Robert Remak (1855–58), Hugo von Ziemssen (1857), Moriz Benedikt (1868–75), and Wilhelm Heinrich Erb (1882). Phototherapy was advanced by Niels Ryberg Finsen (1860–1904). The first definite results of the effect of galvanic electrolysis were obtained in the treatment of urethral stricture by the Swede, Gustav Crusell (1839[2]), who published a monograph on galvanism in the treatment of local disorders in 1841–43. Static electricity was first employed at Guy's Hospital by Thomas Addison, Golding Bird, and Sir William Gull (1837–52); the double faradic current was used against uterine diseases and tumors by Georges Apostoli at Paris (1884); high-frequency currents were introduced by Jacques-Arsène d'Arsonval (1887–92) and employed by Franz Nagelschmidt in electric thermopenetration (diathermy) (1906–8); and electrocoagulation (1910). Ionotherapy (galvanism), suggested by Edison in 1890, was introduced by Stéphan Leduc of Nantes in 1900. The **X-rays,** discovered by Wilhelm Conrad Roentgen in 1895, soon became a most reliable aid in diagnosis, and, in the hands of experts, a useful therapeutic measure, as also radium. Radium therapy, particularly ultra-penetrating radiation, which rendered its action potent for neoplasms, without damaging healthy tissues, was largely developed during 1906–19 by Henri Dominici (1867–1919), an Englishman of Corsican descent.[3]

The **hypodermic syringe** was introduced in Europe by Francis Rynd (1845), Charles-Gabriel Pravaz (1851), and Alexander Wood (1855), and, in America, by Fordyce Barker (1856) and George Thomson Elliott (1858). Tablet triturates for this and other purposes were invented and introduced by Robert M. Fuller, of Philadelphia (1878). Magendie and Gaspard revived experimental intravenous injections of drugs (1823). G. B. Halford, of Melbourne, Australia, reintroduced Fontana's injections of ammonia in snake-bite (1869–73). A. S. Landerer introduced hetol injections in phthisis (1892), Guido Baccelli injections of quinine in malarial fever (1890) and of corrosive sublimate in syphilis (1894), and injections of colloidal metals (collargol, etc.) were introduced by Benno Credé (1901).

In 1895, Carlo Forlanini (1847–1918) introduced the treatment of phthisis by artificial pneumothorax, which had been suggested by Carson (1842), and was introduced in America by John B. Murphy (1898). The principle of employing deep alcohol injections in neuralgia was suggested by Pitres and Vaillard (1887), and first applied by Karl Schloesser (1903).

---

[1] V. K. Anrep: Pflüger's Arch., Bonn, 1879, xxi, 47; Vrach, Petrograd, 1884, v, 773.

[2] G. S. Crusell: Ueber den Galvanismus als chemisches Heilmittel gegen örtliche Krankheiten, St. Petersburg, 1841–43.

[3] See J. Barcat: Arch. Radiol. and Electrotherapy, Lond., 1920, xxiv, 343–345.

Hydrotherapy was popularized by Max Joseph Oertel and the Silesian farmer, Vincenz Priessnitz (1799–1851), whose cold packs and barefoot promenades through dewy meadows were followed up by the Bavarian pastor Kneipp; by C. Munde at Gräfenberg (1839); in England, by James Manby Gully at Malvern (1842); and, in the United States, by Russell Thacher Trall (1844), Joel Shew, and others. Scientific hydrotherapy is especially associated with the names of Ernst **Brand** (1827–97), a practitioner at Stettin, who put Currie's forgotten cold-bath treatment of typhoid fever upon a reliable working basis (1861–63); and Wilhelm **Winternitz** (1835–1917), of Josefstadt, Bohemia, professor at Vienna (1881), director of the hydropathic establishment at Kaltenleutgeben, and founder of the *Blätter für klinische Hydrotherapie* (1890), who wrote the best modern treatise on the subject (1877–80), based upon experimental as well as clinical investigation. Oskar Lassar in Berlin (1883) and Simon Baruch (1840–1921) in New York were the leading propagandists for public baths within the means of the people in large cities.

In 1834 Victor-Théodore Junod (1809–81) investigated the effects of compressed and rarefied air upon the body and its members, which he applied in therapy as "hemospasia" or giant-cupping, summarized in his treatise of 1875. This method consisted in the production of a fainting spell by drawing the blood from the brain to the foot, a species of blood-letting without letting blood, the revulsive effects of which were extraordinarily successful in various diseases and analogous to the results obtained by protein therapy.

Dietetics and regimen were advanced by William Banting (1797–1878), of England, who in his *Letter on Corpulence* (1863), introduced the cure of obesity by the general reduction of food, including the exclusion of fats and carbohydrates (1863), by Liebig, Wöhler, Beaumont, Moleschott, Pavy, Pavloff, Rubner, Chittenden, and the other investigators of nutrition and metabolism, by Boas and Ewald, who introduced test-meals in digestive disorders, by Debove, who originated forced feeding in phthisis, and laterly by Carl von Noorden, who has made a special study of dietetics in disorders of metabolism and introduced the oatmeal diet in diabetes. Special treatments of heart disease were introduced by the laryngologist Max Joseph Oertel (1835–97), of Dillingen, Bavaria, whose method consists in proteid diet with reduction of liquids, free perspiration, and graduated uphill exercises (1884) and by Theodor Schott (1852–), who, at Nauheim, discovered the beneficent effect upon weak hearts of carbonated baths (1883) combined with slow gymnastics, executed by the patient and resisted by the operator. The stomach-pump, for the removal of opium and other poisons (Monro *secundus*), was introduced simultaneously by Edward Jukes and Francis Bush, two English physicians, in 1822.[1] Simple intubation, with lavage, for gastric dilatation from pyloric obstruction, was introduced by Adolf Kussmaul (1867–69).

The scientific applications of **hypnotism** were principally studied by Charcot and his pupils at the Salpêtrière and by the two leaders of the Nancy school, Ambroise-Auguste Liébeault (1823–1904) in his *Le sommeil provoqué* (1889) and *Thérapeutique suggestive* (1891) and Hippolyte-Marie Bernheim (1840–1919) in *De la suggestion dans l'état hypnotique et dans l'état de veille* (1884) and *Hypnotisme, suggestion, psychotherapie* (1891). These titles show the general tendency away from hypnotic suggestion and toward mental and moral suasion or psychotherapy, which was implicit in Charcot's teaching (*la foi qui guérit*). Psychotherapy was put upon a working basis in such works as Paul Dubois' book on the moral treatment of psychoneuroses (1904), and *Isolement et psychothérapie* (1904) by Jean Camus and Philippe Pagniez. The treatment of neurotic persons by suggestion became the word of ambition. It was applied by Rev. Elmwood Worcester at the Emanuel Church at Boston, by Émile Coué (1857–1926) (auto-suggestion) and others, with a suspicious flavor of charlatanry in some instances.

Gymnastics for therapeutic purposes were introduced as "Swedish movements" by Per Henrik Ling (1776–1839) about 1813, and have latterly been elaborated into such methods as mechanotherapy and kinesitherapy, particularly at the Zander Institute. The gospel of life and exercise in the open air, the feeling that external nature has a kindly healing side toward bodily and mental ills, was implicit in the

---

[1] Bush: London Med. & Phys. Jour., 1822, xlviii, 218–220. Jukes: *Ibid.*, 384–389. Jukes claims priority of publication, but does not give the source of his antecedent paper. His priority is, however, acknowledged by Sir Astley Cooper (Lancet, Lond., 1823, i, 223), who says that Jukes originally employed a gum-elastic bottle for suction, the syringe having been suggested by Bush.

teachings of Greek medicine, has been the theme of such modern writers as Thoreau, Walt Whitman, and John Burroughs, and has been applied with success in the treatment of phthisis everywhere and in neurasthenic states, by J. Madison Taylor and other specialists.

The founder of **experimental hygiene** was Max **von Pettenkofer** (1818–1901), of Lichtenheim, Bavaria, a pupil of Liebig and Bischoff, who, from boyhood, had been drawn to chemistry through residence in the house of his uncle, then court apothecary. Dissension with this uncle threw young Pettenkofer upon his own, and he was driven to the stage, playing several rôles at Ratisbon with marked ability. Recon-

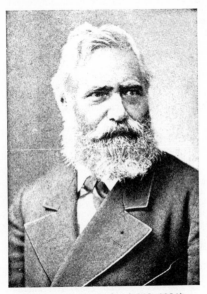

Max von Pettenkofer (1818–1901).
(Boston Medical Library.)

ciliation effected through marriage with his cousin, he resumed his studies and graduated in medicine at Munich in 1843. In 1847, after some political opposition, he was made professor of "dietetic chemistry" at Munich and, in 1853, became professor of hygiene at the same university, where, under his direction, the first Hygienic Institute was opened, in 1879. Pettenkofer was the art-loving, versatile Bavarian, author of a volume of sonnets (1886), and equally distinguished in general and physiological chemistry, metabolism, epidemiology and experimental hygiene. His personal resemblance to Victor Hugo was noted by his friend Welch. At the age of seventy-four, Pettenkofer boldly risked his life in an experiment. Lonely and bereft of wife and children at eighty-three, he made an end of himself by a revolver shot on the night of February 10, 1901.

In 1844 he introduced the well-known test for bile acids and in 1863–83, with Voit, he made his classical investigations of metabolism in respiration. He also demonstrated hippuric acid, creatin, and creatinin in the urine (1844), improved the assaying of gold, silver, and platinum in coins of the Bavarian mint (1846–8), showed that the saliva contains sulphocyanic acid (1846), made lighting by wood gas viable (1857), put Liebig's meat extract into commerce (1862), and even devised a method for restoring the cracked, mildewed paintings of the Munich Pinakothek (1863). From 1855 on he devoted much attention to the etiology of cholera and typhoid fever, the spread of which he attributed to soil and soil-water. He held that cholera will never spread over a foundation of solid rock or concrete; and postulated for infection three factors, viz., a specific germ (x), a moist, porous soil befouled with decaying organic material (y) and a toxic substance (z) produced by the "ripening" of x through contact with y. He further admitted individual predisposition or susceptibility. His *Bodentheorie* is thus not unallied to Pasteur's doctrine that the rise or extinction of epidemics is due to strengthening or weakening of the virus by environmental conditions. Koch's comma bacillus (1883) was accepted by Pettenkofer as x, but he insisted upon the y and z factors to the extent of swallowing a virulent cholera culture from Gaffky's laboratory along with Emmerich, Stricker, Metchnikoff, Ferran, and other pupils. In spite of his somewhat arbitrary views, he all but rid the city of Munich of typhoid through the introduction of a proper system of drainage, a subject which frequently involved him in controversy with Virchow. Pettenkofer's most important contributions to experimental hygiene were his method of estimating carbon dioxide in air and water (1858), his investigations of the ventilation of dwelling houses (1858), and the relation of the atmosphere to clothing, habitations and the soil. He studied the relative advantages of stove and hot-air heating, showed that the soil contains air and CO_2, that air passes through the thickest masonry, and that the atmosphere may be contaminated by gases deep in the earth. He was ennobled in 1883 and became president of the Bavarian Academy of Sciences in 1889. In 1882, Pettenkofer published, with Ziemssen, the *Handbuch der Hygiene*, and he was one of the co-editors of the *Zeitschrift für Biologie* (1865–82) and the *Archiv für Hygiene* (1883–94). Experimental hygiene, as based upon the bacterial theory of infection, took a new start with the work of Koch and his associates in the Hygienic Institute at Berlin.

Perhaps the most important of the earlier treatises on **public hygiene** after the time of Johann Peter Frank were John Roberton's *Medical Police* (Edinburgh, 1808–9) and the treatises of François-Emmanuel Fodéré (1822–24) and Alexandre-J.-B. Parent-Duchâtelet (1836), who also wrote an epoch-making work on prostitution in the city of Paris (1836). David Hosack wrote on the medical police of New York City (1820). In the first half of the century, the subject was extensively cultivated in France. Various treatises were written by Motard (1841), Royer-Collard (1843), Bourdon (1844), Michel Levy (1844–45), Briand (1845), Foy (1845), Boudin (1846), while Parkes's Manual of 1864 set the pace for later works by L. Hirt (1876), E. Fazio (1880–86), G. H. Rohé (1885), Max Rubner (1888), E. Flügge (1889), J. Uffelmann (1889–90), W. Prausnitz (1892), L. Mangin (1892), Ferdinand Hueppe (1899), A. W. Blyth (1900), Charles Harrington (1901), W. T. Sedgwick (1902), Josef Rambousek (1906), and M. J. Rosenau (1913). Pettenkofer's great handbook (1862–94) was followed by similar coöperative works, edited by Thomas Stephenson and Sir Shirley F. Murphy (1892–94), Theodor Weyl (1893–1901) and Max Rubner (1911). **Industrial hygiene** was advanced by Sir Humphry Davy (1779–1829), who invented the well-known safety lamp for coal-miners (1815); by Charles Turner Thackrah (1795–1833), of Leeds, one of Sir Astley Cooper's pupils, who, in his treatise of 1832, first investigated brass-founders' ague, dust diseases, etc.; by Tanquerel des Planches (1809–62), who wrote an important work on diseases in lead workers (1839); by François Melier, who dealt with the hygiene of tobacco manufacturers (1849); by A.-L.-D. Delpech, who investigated the rubber industry (1863), and, with J. B. Hillairet, the diseases of chromium manufacturers (1869–76). In Germany, Ludwig Hirt (1844–   ), of Breslau, wrote a monumental four-volume treatise on occupational diseases (1871–78), which was followed by the *Handbücher* of H. Eulenburg (1876), H. Albrecht (1894–96) and Th. Weyl (1908). In England, Sir Thomas Oliver has paid especial attention to dust diseases, miners' and live-wire accidents (*Dangerous Trades*, London, 1902), and Leonard Hill investigated caisson disease (1912) and the general evils of stuffy atmosphere. In America, the investigations and reports of C. F. W. Doehring (1903), George M. Kober (1908–16), John B. Andrews (1910–16), Frederick L. Hoffman (1908–16), and William C. Hanson (dust and fumes. 1913) have proved of great value. Important monographs are those of Josephine Goldmark on industrial fatigue (1912), George M. Price on the modern factory (1914), W. Gilman Thompson on occupational diseases (1914), the coöperative treatise on the same subject edited by George M. Kober and William C. Hanson (1916), *Industrial Medicine and Surgery* by Harry E. Mock (1919) and the study of industrial poisoning (1925) by **Alice Hamilton,** who now holds the chair of industrial medicine at Harvard (1919). Rudolf Virchow played an important part in the sanitation and sewage disposal of Berlin (1868–73) and was the originator of the modern movement for the hygiene and inspection of school-children (1869), which was ably carried forward by the labors of Edwin Chadwick (1871), Hermann Ludwig Cohn (1887), and a host of workers. School lunches for children, first established by Count Rumford, in 1792, were revived in the *Caisse des écoles* of a French batallion in Paris in 1849. These became permanent *cantines scolaires* by law in 1882. Victor Hugo started a school luncheon movement at Guernsey in 1866. In Germany, the movement began at Munich in 1876, and by 1909 was extended to half the cities of the empire. It began in England in 1902, and in New York City on November 23,

1898.[1] Dental clinics were introduced at Strassburg and Darmstadt in 1902. There are now 120 in Germany. Food chemistry and the detection of adulterants was the subject of special treatises by F. C. Knapp (1848), Moleschott (1850), A. Chevallier (*Dictionnaire*, 1850), F. Artmann (1859), E. Reich (1860), J. König (1878), H. Fleck (1882). The **sanitation of hospitals** was greatly forwarded in the writings of Florence Nightingale (1859), Lord Lister (1870), Sir Douglas Galton (1893), Sir Henry Burdett (1891–93), and by the lessons gained in the construction of such fine modern structures as the Johns Hopkins Hospital in Baltimore (1889), the Hamburg Eppendorf pavilion (1889), or the Rudolf Virchow in Berlin (1906). The hygiene of habitations and the planning of towns is a subject of recent interest among architects and sanitary engineers. In 1874, Lord Kelvin said that there can be no proper hygiene of indoor life until "architecture becomes a branch of scientific engineering."[2]

Public hygiene in England was specially advanced by the reports of Sir James Phillips **Kay-Shuttleworth** (1804–77) on the cotton workers of Manchester (1832), the training of pauper children (1841), and

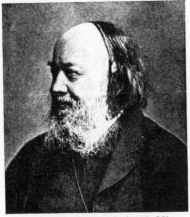

Sir Edwin Chadwick (1800–90).

public education (1852–62); and those of Thomas **Southwood Smith** (1788–1861) to the Poor-Law Commissioners on the physical causes of preventable sickness and mortality among the poor (1838). The reports of the great lawyer sanitarian, Sir Edwin **Chadwick** (1800–90), on poor-law reform (1834–42), health of the laboring classes (1842), and cemeteries (1843–55) gave a definite objective to administrative activities by showing how the census and bills of mortality could be used to diagnose public ailments and thus really initiated the "sanitary era" of public hygiene.[3]

Through Lemuel Shattuck (1850) Chadwick may be said to have started public health activities in the United States, and latterly influenced even Billings (1871–95). **Sir John Simon** (1816–1904), in his famous *Public Health Report* (1887) and *English Sanitary Institutions* (1890), exerted great influence upon modern developments and legislation, and Henry Wyldbore **Rumsey** (1809–76), by sharp criticism, telling evidence before public committees, by his recommendation of university degrees in state medicine (1865), and by the effect of his Essays in state medicine (1865) and on the fallacies of statistics (1875) did yeoman's service in advancing sanitary legislation. The most important English treatise on hygiene is the manual of Edmund Alexander **Parkes** (1819–76), published in 1864, in the preparation of which he

---

[1] New York Med. Jour., 1916, ciii, 1037.

[2] Lord Kelvin: Popular Lectures, London, 1884, ii, 211.

[3] For a stimulating account of Chadwick's work and its far-reaching consequences, see Haven Emerson: Jour. Prev. Med., Baltimore, 1927, i, 401–427.

was aided by **Lord Sidney Herbert** (1810–61), of Lea, who was Secretary for War at the outbreak of the Crimean War (1854) and chairman of the Royal Commission on the sanitary conditions of the army and of military hospitals and barracks. Lord Herbert was in frequent consultation with Parkes as to the formation of the Army Medical School at Fort Pitt, Chatham, in 1860, which was transferred to the Royal Victoria Hospital, Netley, in 1863. It was the friendship of Lord and Lady Herbert for Florence Nightingale which led to the latter's passage to Scutari with forty nurses to look after the soldiers in the Crimean contest. It is said that all the recommendations made by the South African Royal Commission in 1901 had been made by Lord Herbert fifty-five years before. His colleague, Parkes, held the first chair of hygiene in England (at Fort Pitt, 1860), and the Parkes Museum of Hygiene was instituted in his memory, July 18, 1876, and opened on June 28, 1879. Baron Mundy, of Vienna, called Parkes "the founder and best teacher of military hygiene in our day, the friend and benefactor of every soldier."

The epidemiologist, William **Budd** (1811–80), of North Taunton, Devonshire, described by Tyndall as "a man of the highest genius," did the best English work of this time in infectious diseases. His monograph on typhoid fever (1873) demonstrated its contagious nature and the different modes of its transmission. In 1866, he stamped out

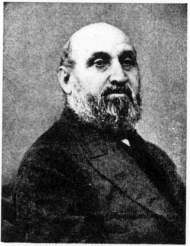

William Farr (1807–83). (Boston Medical Library.)

cholera in Bristol, lowering the mortality to 29 cases as against 1979 in 1849. His famous recipe for the rinderpest epidemic of 1866, "a poleaxe and a pit of quicklime," was ridiculed, but proved to be the true one. George Budd described an atypical cirrhosis of the liver (without jaundice) from auto-intoxication (Budd's disease), and William wrote a famous paper on symmetrical disease (1842). John **Snow** (1813–58), of York, a London medical graduate of 1844, first stated the theory that cholera is water-borne and taken into the system by the mouth (1849), in an essay which was awarded a prize of 30,000 francs by the Institute of France. During a severe London epidemic of cholera in 1854, he told the vestrymen of St. James that the outbreak would cease if the handle of the Broad Street Pump were removed, which proved to be the case. In 1841, he devised a sort of pulmotor for asphyxiated infants and a trocar for thoracentesis. He was a pioneer in anesthesia, having delivered the Queen by chloroform in 1853 and 1857. The second edition of his work on cholera (1852), which contains a remarkable statement of the germ theory, cost him £200 and netted him a few shillings.

The leading English medical statist of his time was William **Farr** (1807–83), of Kenley, Shropshire, who, in 1839, at the instance of Chadwick, gave up medical practice to enter the Registrar General's office, in the reports of which he published his classic letters on the causes of death in England (1839–70). His other papers were collected in the volume *Vital Statistics* (1885), with the exception of his important letter to the Daily News (February 17, 1866[1]), which contains the first statement of "Farr's law," viz., that the curve of an epidemic at first ascends rapidly, then slopes slowly to a maximum, to fall more rapidly than it mounted. He first plotted this curve from the smallpox epidemic of 1840, and from it he predicted, with success, the early subsidence of the devastating cattle-plague of 1865–6. The epidemic curves, subsequently evolved by Brownlee, Ross and others, are usually of the bell-shaped Farr type (Pearson's class iv). Farr devised the scheme of nomenclature and nosology of the Royal College of Physicians, which is still used in the classification of medical literature and medical libraries. He edited the *British Medical Almanack* (1835–39), which contains his valuable medical chronology, his remarkable *Essay on Prognosis* (1838), and a history of the medical profession in England (1893).

In the United States, the leading prime-movers of public hygiene were Lemuel **Shattuck** (1793–1859), of Boston, who, by his famous report to the Massachusetts Sanitary Commission (1850) did for New England what Chadwick, Farr, and Simon had done for England; John Shaw **Billings** (1838–1913), who strove to give their ideas a nation-wide application, while Stephen Smith, Hermann M. Biggs, W. H. Park, S. S. Goldwater in New York, Baker in Michigan, Dixon in Pennsylvania, Welch and Fulton in Maryland, Folsom and Sedgwick in Massachusetts, Joseph Jones in Louisiana, Winslow in Connecticut, Rauch in Illinois, and Kober in the District of Columbia did yeoman service for their several states. Much was done by such organizations as the United States Public Health Service and the American Medical Association. The most accomplished scientific sanitarian of the later period was William Thompson **Sedgwick** (1855–1921), of West Hartford, Connecticut, one of Newell Martin's pupils, who, in collaboration with William Ripley Nichols and Thomas M. Drown, did most important work on sewage experimentation and purification of water, and as director of the Massachusetts Institute of Technology (founded 1861), was the source of inspiration of Whipple, Winslow, Jordan, Calkins, and the younger men. The same influence radiated from Welch to his pupils at the School of Hygiene of the Johns Hopkins University during the decade 1916–26.

---

[1] Reprinted by J. Brownlee in Brit. Med. Jour., Lond., 1915, ii, 250–252.

Perhaps the earliest modern work on **statistics** was the famous *Essay on the Principle of Population* (1798) of Thomas Robert **Malthus** (1766–1834), of Guildford, England, which maintains that food-supply and birth-rate increase in arithmetical and geometrical ratios respectively, so that poverty is the natural result of increased population. It has exerted a profound influence upon the postponement of marriage and the decrease in size of families down to the present time, although it is erroneous to describe methods of preventing conception as "Malthusian," as these (originally suggested by Condorcet) were unequivocally condemned by Malthus. Medical statistics were introduced by Louis (1835). The modern methods of arriving at the mortality of large cities and other data were blocked out by the Hungarian statistician Josef von Körösi (1873); the fallacies and various mathematical relations of vital statistics were studied by Rumsey (1875) and Farr (1885). In America, John Shaw Billings (1838–1913) made valuable contributions, particularly in his Cartwright Lectures (1889) and his special reports on the United States Census. Frederick L. Hoffman has investigated the statistics of cancer (1915) and other diseases. The statistical investigations of Jacques Bertillon (1851–1914) on the depopulation of France (1880–1911[1]) have had their effect upon other countries in which a falling off of the birth-rate is noticeable. Karl Pearson's work belongs to the 20th century. In America, his biometric methods have been applied with telling effect to vital and medical statistics by John S. Fulton, Charles B. Davenport and Raymond Pearl.

In the department of **medical jurisprudence,** the treatises of 1798 (2d. ed., 1812) by François-Emmanuel Fodéré (1764–1835) was the standard source of authority in France in the early part of the century. In Germany, Johann Ludwig Caspar (1796–1864), of Berlin, achieved a wide reputation through his works on medical statistics and state medicine (1825–35), judicial postmortems (1851–53), and his Practical Handbook of Legal Medicine (1856), which remained, for a long time, unsurpassed for its wealth of facts and sound judgments. The first treatises in English were written by the Americans, Theodric Romeyn Beck (1823) and Isaac Ray (1839). William Augustus Guy (1810–85) was the first English writer on the subject (1844). Other American treatises of note were those by Francis Wharton and Moreton Stillé (1855), and John Ordronaux (1869); both deal with forensic medicine from the lawyer's point of view. The four-volume treatise of Witthaus and Becker (1894–96) is a comprehensive modern encyclopedia, written by many hands. Heinroth (1825), Isaac Ray (1839), Krafft-Ebing (1875) and Charles Arthur Mercier (1890) have dealt with the jurisprudence of insanity, Carl Ferdinand von Arlt with the medicolegal aspect of injuries of the eye (1875), M.-J.-B. Orfila (1813–15), Sir Robert Christison (1829), Auguste-Ambroise Tardieu (1867) and Georg Dragendorff (1868–72) with toxicology, Frank Hastings Hamilton with the jurisprudence of deformities after fractures (1855), and Krafft-Ebing with sexual perversion and inversion (1886–7). Theodore George Wormley wrote a sterling work on the microchemistry of poisons (1867), and Virchow's little handbook of postmortem technic (1876) was the *vade mecum* of its day. In recent times, Paul Brouardel (1837–1906), of Paris, is memorable for a number of exhaustive monographs of value, in particular, those on death and sudden death (1895), hanging, strangulation, suffocation and drowning (1897) and infanticide (1897). The precipitin test (Bordet-Uhlenhuth) for blood-stains was introduced in 1901,[2] and a cobra-venom reaction in insanity (Much-Holtzmann) in 1909.[3]

From the time of Haller, the study of **medical history** has been mainly in the hands of German and French writers.

British scholars, such as Francis Adams (1796–1861), of Banchory, Scotland, or William Alexander Greenhill (1814–94), of London, editor of Sydenham, have made valuable translations of the greater Greek and Roman classics. Charming books and essays, with the genuine flavor of letters, have been written by William MacMichael (*The Gold Headed Cane*, 1827), John Brown (*Horæ Subsecivæ*, 1858), J. Cordy Jeaffreson (*A Book About Doctors*, 1860), Wilks and Bettany (*History of Guy's Hospital*, 1892), Sir Benjamin Ward Richardson (*Disciples of Æsculapius*,

---

[1] J. Bertillon: La dépopulation de la France, Paris, 1911.

[2] Uhlenhuth: Deutsche med. Wochenschr., Leipz. & Berl., 1901, xxvii, 86; 260.

[3] Much: Centralbl. f. Bakteriol. (etc.), Beil. zu 1. Abt., Jena, 1909, xlii, 48–50.

1900), particularly by the two Regius professors, Osler and Allbutt; yet no work on
a large scale has been attempted in Great Britain or America which will measure up
with the performances of Haeser or Daremberg, unless it be Charles Creighton's
History of Epidemics in Britain (1894). Thomas Young's Introduction of Medical
Literature (1813), an unfinished history of medicine by Edward Meryon (1861), a
very readable one by Edward T. Withington (1894), the studies of John Flint South
(1886), Sydney Young (1890), and D'Arcy Power (1899), on English surgery, Sir
Clifford Allbutt's studies of medieval science and surgery (1901–05), J. F. Payne on
Anglo-Saxon medicine (1904), L. M. Griffiths on medical philology (1905), Norman
Moore on medical education in Great Britain (1908), Raymond Crawfurd on the
King's Evil (1911), plague and pestilence (1914), Charles A. Mercier on astrology in
medicine (1914) and leper-houses (1915), Charles Singer's studies on the history of
contagion, microscopy and tropical medicine, and the illuminating essays of Sir
William Osler are among the best things that have been done in England.   Until
recently, American contributions have been meager in extent.   Noteworthy are the
essays of Joseph Meredith Toner, George Jackson Fisher, John Call Dalton's Cartwright lectures on the experimental method (1882) and his *Doctrines of the Circulation* (1884), the historical survey entitled "A Century of American Medicine" (1876),
the *Medical Essays* of Oliver Wendell Holmes (1883), Weir Mitchell's history of instrumental precision in medicine (1892) and his Harvey memorials, James J. Walsh's
studies of medieval medicine, the history of nursing by Mary Adelaide Nutting and
Lavinia L. Dock (1907–12), John G. Curtis's study of Harvey (1916), Henry M.
Hurd's history of American psychiatry (1916), Jonathan Wright on ancient medicine,
the studies of Renaissance medicine by Edward C. Streeter, naval medicine by
Frank L. Pleadwell, medical mythology by Walter A. Jayne, Mortimer Frank's
translation of Choulant (1920), John Ruhräh's anthology of pediatrics (1925).   The
English translation of Baas by Henry E. Handerson (1837–1918), of Orange, Ohio,
preserves the humorous flavor of the original and is doubly valuable for the superadded material.   The earliest American histories of medicine were those of Peter
Middleton (1769), Robley Dunglison (1872), and the short history of Roswell Park
(1897); the history of medicine in the United States has been treated by James
Thacher (1828), Francis Randolph Packard (1901) and James Gregory Mumford
(1903); Jewish medicine by Charles D. Spivak, F. T. Haneman (1904), and Harry
Friedenwald; medical folk-lore by Robert Fletcher; medical botanists and medical
illustrators by Howard A. Kelly.   William A. Heidel has made valuable contributions on Greek corpuscular theories (1910) and *Hippocratea* (1914).

The earliest German work of consequence in the 19th century was the *Geschichte
der Heilkunde* of J. F. K. **Hecker** (1795–1850) which was followed by his collective
monograph on the great epidemics of the Middle Ages (1865).   The most scholarly
and thoroughgoing medical history of the period was written by Heinrich **Haeser**
(1811–84), who became professor of medicine at Jena (1839), Greifswald (1849) and
Breslau (1862).   Haeser, the son of a music director at Weimar, was brought up in an
atmosphere of culture and was one of the most learned physicians of his time.   His
earlier works on the history of epidemic diseases (1839–41) and his *Bibliotheca epidemiographica* (1843), with the valuable *Additamenta* by Johann Gottlieb Thierfelder (1843) demonstrate his talents for close investigation.   These came to apt
fruition in his *Lehrbuch der Geschichte der Medizin und der Volkskrankheiten* (1845),
which, in its third edition (1875–82), had become an unrivaled storehouse of knowledge, wonderfully accurate as to dates and citations, and with but few of the usual
slips and errors.   The third volume, on the history of epidemics, contains original
citations of many first-hand descriptions of disease from the old municipal and
monkish chronicles, a field in which Haeser has been equalled only by Sudhoff.
Haeser's masterpiece was followed in Germany by the histories of Wunderlich
(1859), Johann Hermann Baas (1876), Julius Pagel (1898, revised by Sudhoff 1901–6),
Max Neuburger (1906) Paul Diepgen (1913–24), Sudhoff and Meyer-Steineg (1920),
all works of solid and sterling merit.   Russian medicine was handled by Wilhelm
Michael Richter (1813–17), Arabian medicine by Heinrich Ferdinand Wüstenfeld
(1840), and Karl Opitz (1906).   The study of medicine in relation to art was inaugurated by Virchow (1861), blocked out in detail by Marx (1861), placed upon its feet by
the extensive work of Charcot and his pupils and continued in such German works
as *Der Arzt* (1900) by Hermann Peters (1847–1920), Eugen Holländer on medicine
in classical painting (1903), medical caricature and satire (1905) and medicine in the
plastic arts (1912), Robert Müllerheim on the lying-in chamber in art (1904) and
F. Parkes Weber on death in art (1910).   Medicine in ancient India was treated by
Sir Bhagvat Sin Jee (1896) and August F. R. Hoernle (1907), medicine in Mexico

by Francisco A. Flores (1886–8), medicine in Upper Canada by William Canniff (1894), the history of syphilis by Conrad Heinrich Fuchs (1843), Julius Rosenbaum (1845), Iwan Bloch (1901–11), J. K. Proksch (1889–1900), H. F. A. Peypers (*Lues medii aevi*, 1895), Karl Sudhoff (1912–25), K. Dohi (1923), and Gaston Vorberg (1923); the history of medieval leprosy by Virchow (1860–61), German medicine by Heinrich Rohlfs (1875–82) and August Hirsch (1893), the history of therapeutics (1877) and the medical clinic (1889) by the Dane J. J. Petersen (1840–1912), Viennese medicine (1884) and the history of medical education (1889) by Theodor **Puschmann** (1844–99), Thibetan medicine by Heinrich Laufer (1900), cuneiform medicine by Felix von Oefele (1902), Germanic balneology by Alfred Martin (1906), Persian medicine by the Norwegian, Adolf Mauritz Fonahn (1910), and Jewish medicine by Julius Preuss (1911). Apart from Haeser, the history of epidemiology has been followed by Noah Webster (1799–1802), by J.-A.-F. Ozanam (1817–35), Hecker (1865), Alfonso Corradi (1865–86), Charles Creighton (1891–4), and George Sticker (1896–1925). Remarkable medical scholars were Johann Ludwig **Choulant** (1791–1861) of Dresden, author of sterling bibliographies (1828–42) and an unrivalled history of anatomical illustration (1852); Karl Friedrich Heinrich **Marx** (1796–1877) of Göttingen, the first modern to signalize the importance of Leonardo da Vinci in anatomy (1848), the first to list and classify paintings of medical interest (1861) and author of *Origines contagii* (1824–27) and of exhaustive studies of Herophilus (1838), Blumenbach (1840), Paracelsus (1842), Leibnitz (1859), Conring (1872), Paullini (1873) and Schneider (1873); August **Hirsch** (1817–92), author of the monumental Handbook of Historic-Geographic Pathology (1860–64); Gurlt, the historian of surgery; Moritz **Steinschneider** (1817–1907), one of the greatest of medical archivists, who catalogued the Hebrew MSS. in the Bodleian (1857), at Leyden (1858), Parma (1868), Munich (1875), Hamburg (1878) and Berlin (1878–97), made a list of 3014 early Jewish physicians (1896, completed by A. Freimann and L. Lewin, 1914–21), made valuable studies of pseudo-epigraphic literature (1862), the Arabic sources of Constantinus Africanus (1866), Donnolo (1868), Arabian toxicology and quackery (1866), Arabic translations from the Greek (1891), and crowned his labors with his great work on the Hebrew translations of the Middle Ages (1893); Valentin **Rose**

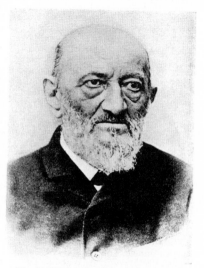

Moritz Steinschneider (1817–1907).

(1829–1916), cataloguer of the Latin MSS. in the Royal Library at Berlin (1893–1905) and editor of *Aristoteles pseudepigraphicus* (1863), *Anecdota græca et græco-latina* (1864–87), Vitruvius (1867–99), medical Pliny (1875), Anthimus (1877), Cassius Felix (1879), Theodorus Priscianus (1882) and Ægidius Corboliensis (1907); Max **Höfler** (1848–1915), author of a dictionary of old German medical terms (1899), J. Berendes, the translator of Dioscorides and Paul of Ægina; and the medical philologists, Hermann Diels, Johannes Ilberg and Max Wellmann, now professor of medical history at Berlin (1920). Julius **Pagel** (1851–1912), a busy practitioner of Berlin, editor of Mondeville (1889–92) and Mesue (1893), wrote a history of medicine in 1897 and issued a capital biographical lexicon (1900), an encyclopedic history of medicine (1901–6), and a useful medical chronology (1908). The work of Karl Sudhoff has a high place in the 20th century. Eminent German historians of pharmacy are Eduard Rudolf Kobert (1888–96), Hermann Peters (1889), Hermann Schelenz (1907), J. Berendes (1907–   ), Theodor Gottfried Husemann, L. Lewin (toxicology); and of military medicine, Franz Hermann Frölich (1839–1900), Emil Knorr (1880), Albert Köhler (1899), and Wilhelm Haberling (1910–17). The ablest medical historian of France was Charles-Victor **Daremberg** (1817–72), of Dijon, who edited and translated Oribasius (1851–76), the Four Masters (1854), select works of Hippocrates (1843), Galen (1854–56) and Celsus (1859), made original investigations of Homeric medicine (1865), Hindu medicine (1867), medicine between Homer and Hippocrates

(1869), and wrote an admirable history of medicine (1870), which is still consulted. Daremberg was a warm friend of Émile **Littré** (1801–81) of Paris, one of the greatest of medical philologists, whose work is noticed below. Other French contributions of value are the medical histories of Eugene Bouchut (1873) and Léon Meunier (1911), the studies of medicine in the Latin poets by Prosper Ménière (1858) and Edmond Dupouy (1885), Maurice Raynaud's book on medicine in the time of Molière (1862), Achille Chéreau's histories of French medical journalism (1867), plague in Paris (1873), Coitier (1861), Mondeville (1862), Guillotin (1873) and the library of the Paris Medical Faculty (1878), the splendid memorials of the Paris Medical Faculty by Auguste Corlieu (1896) and Noé Legrand (1911), Ernest Wickersheimer's study of Renaissance medicine in France (1905) and Raphael Blanchard's *Epigraphie médicale* (1909–15). In Holland, C. Broeckx (1807–69), editor of Yperman's *Cyrurgie* (1863), Franz Zacharias Ermerins (1808–71), editor of a Græco-Latin edition of Hippocrates (1859–64), and Carel Eduard Daniels (1839–   ). H. F. A. Peypers (1853–1904), founder and editor of *Janus* (1895–1904), was succeeded by E. C. van Leersum (1862–   ), editor of Yperman (1913), and J. G. de Lint. In Italy, Francesco Puccinotti (1872–1922) wrote a good history of medicine (1850–66), the Copenhagen manuscripts of the School of Salerno were edited by Salvatore De Renzi (*Collectio Salernitana*, Naples, 1853–59) and Piero Giacosa (1901), De Renzi wrote a five-volume history of Italian medicine (1844–8), Alfonso Corradi (1833–92) a history of Italian epidemics up to 1850 (7 vols., 1865–86), Giuseppe Albertotti (1851–   ) on medieval ophthalmology, and Vincenzo Guerrini a history of dentistry (1909). Latterly, Pietro Capparoni (Rome), Andrea Corsini (Florence), Modestino del Gaizo (Naples), Arturo Castiglioni (Padua), and Domenico Barduzzi (Siena) have done excellent work in original medico-historical investigation. In Spain Anastasio Chinchilla wrote a 4-volume history of Spanish medicine (1841–8), which was followed by the 7-volume bibliographical history of Antonio Hernandez Morejon (1842–72) and, in recent times, by the history of Eduardo Garcia del Rio (1920) and the studies of J. Olmedilla y Puig. Histories of Portuguese medicine (1891) and of medical education in Portugal (1925) were written by Maximiano Lemos. The chair of medical history in the Paris Faculty, has been held intermittently by Goulin (1795–9), Cabanès (1799–1808), Moreau de la Sarthe (1818–22), Daremberg (1870–72), Lorain (1873–5), Parrot (1876–9), Laboulbène (1879–99) and Menetrier (1920). The study of medical history was maintained at Vienna (1869–79) by Franz Romeo Seligmann (1808–92) and his successors, Theodor Puschmann (1844–99) and Max Neuburger; at Berlin by Hecker (1834–50), Hirsch (1863–93), Pagel (1898–1912) and Max Wellmann (1920–28), at Leipzig by Sudhoff, at Glasgow by Comrie, in Baltimore by Billings, Welch, Osler and Cordell. Useful biographical dictionaries of medicine are those of J. A. Dezeimeris (1828–9), Bayle and Thillaye (1855), August Hirsch and E. Gurlt (1884–8) and Pagel (1900). The notices in the *Dictionary of National Biography* (1885–1912) for English physicians; and for American physicians, James Thacher (1828), S. D. Gross (1861), W. B. Atkinson (1878), R. F. Stone (1894), Irving A. Watson (1896) and Howard A. Kelly (1912) are indispensable. Medical geography was handled by F. Schnurrer (1813), V. Isensee (1833), Marshall (1832), C. F. Fuchs (1853), A. Mühry (1856), J. Boudin (1857), A. Hirsch (1860–64), Andrew Davidson (1892) and Frank G. Clemow (1903).

Among the modern periodicals devoted to medical history are Hecker's *Litterarische Annalen der gesammten Heilkunde* (Berlin, 1825–35), Choulant's *Historisch-literarisches Jahrbuch* (Leipzig, 1838–40), *Janus*, edited by A. W. E. Th. Henschel (Breslau, 1846–8) and continued at Gotha (1851–3), H. and G. Rohlf's *Deutsches Archiv für Geschichte der Medizin und medizinische Geographie* (Leipzig, 1878–85), Sir Benjamin Ward Richardson's *Asclepiad* (London, 1885–95), M. Lemos' *Archivos da historia da medicina portugueza* (Oporto, 1887–96, n. s., 1910–14), the *Caledonian Medical Journal* (Glasgow, 1891–1916), Cabanès' *Chronique médical* (Paris, 1894–1928), *Janus* (Amsterdam, 1896–1928), the new series of *La France médicale* (ed. A. Prieur, Paris, 1900–1914), the *Abhandlungen zur Geschichte der Medizin* (Breslau, 1902–6), the *Medical Library and Historical Journal* (Brooklyn and New York, 1903–7), which had a short-lived successor, the *Æsculapian* (Brooklyn, 1908–9), and the *Archiv für Geschichte der Medizin* (Leipzig, 1907–28), founded and edited by Karl Sudhoff. The latter is by far the most important periodical on the subject which has yet appeared, the contents being devoted exclusively to original research. In Holland, apart from *Janus* (1896–1928), many valuable papers have appeared in the *Nederlandsch Tijdschrift voor Geneeskunde* (current). Among the monographic serials are Sudhoff's *Studien zur Geschichte der Medizin* (Leipzig, 1907–15), Theodor Meyer-Steineg's *Jenaer medizin-historische Beiträge* (1912–   ), Wilhelm Maar's *Medi-*

cinisk-historisk Smaaskrifter (Copenhagen, 1912–14), and the *Opuscula selecta neerlandicorum de arte medica* (1907–27), an anthology of Dutch medical classics. Several medical history societies are now publishing transactions, notably the Deutsche Gesellschaft für Geschichte der Medizin und der Naturwissenschaften at Leipzig (*Mitteilungen*, 1902–28), the Charaka Club, New York (*Proceedings*, 1902–28), the Société française d'histoire de la médecine, Paris (*Bulletin*, 1903–28), the Società italiana dell istoria critica delle scienze mediche e naturali, Rome (*Rivista*, 1910–28), the Society of Medical History of Chicago (*Bulletin*, 1911–28) and the Historical Section of the Royal Society of Medicine of London (*Proceedings*, 1912–28). The *Bulletin* of the Johns Hopkins Hospital (1890–1928) is the literary organ of the Hospital Historical Club. The *Annals of Medical History* (1917–28), edited by Francis R. Packard, is now the leading American periodical of the subject. *Medical Life* (New York, 1920–28), edited by Victor Robinson, is remarkable for symposia on special subjects. The careful reviews in the Leipzig *Mitteilungen*, under the direction of Sudhoff, Siegmund Günther, and latterly of Wilhelm Haberling, afford a convenient clearing-house of all recent medico-historical literature. Notable among the periodicals devoted to the history of science, as well as medicine are *Isis* (Brussels, 1913–28), edited by George Sarton, the *Archiv für Geschichte der Naturwissenschaften* (Leipzig, 1908–22), revived 1927–8), and the *Archivio di storia della scienza* (1919–28), edited by Aldo Mieli.

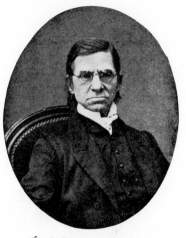

Émile Littré (1801–81).

Medical lexicography in the 19th century attained its stride, both in respect of solid performance and practical utility, in the wake of the gigantic accomplishment of Émile **Littré** (1801–81), whose five-volume dictionary of the French language (1863–72) is authoritative. Littré (Pasteur's laic saint) was so modest in relation to his ideals that he was lacking in initiative. His great bilingual edition of Hippocrates (1839–61) was prepared at the instance of Rayer and Andral. It was paralleled by his edition of Pliny's Natural History (1848–50) and followed by many interesting historical studies (1861–81), notably those on Celsus, Magendie, Cuvier, Buckle, Gil Blas, the great epidemics, historical suicides and poisonings, the pest-carriers, spiritism and the cholera of 1832, which set the pace for Cabanès, and others who have followed this *genre* of historical writing. The medical dictionary of Pierre-Hubert Nysten (1810) was, in its tenth edition (1855), entirely recast and enlarged by Littré and Charles Robin (1821–85), reaching its 21st edition in 1905.

Nysten was followed by a swarm of medical dictionaries in all languages, notably those of A. F. Hecker (1816–22), Robley Dunglison (1833), James Copland (1834–59), R. D. Hoblyn (1835), Otto Roth (1878), the New Sydenham Society (Henry Power and L. W. Sedgwick, 1878–99), Sir Richard Quain (1882), George M. Gould (1890), J. S. Billings (1890), A. L. Garnier and V. Delamare (1900), L. Landouzy and F. Jayle (1902), W. Guttmann (1902), and the *Larousse médical illustré* of E. Galtier-Boissière (1912). In point of scholarship, the best medical dictionary of American origin is the four-volume work (1888–93) by Frank Pierce Foster (1841–1911), which was followed by a number of very practical books in flexible leather by W. A. N. Dorland (1900), H. W. Cattell (1910) and Thomas L. Stedman (1911).

Among dictionaries of special terms are those of Julius Hirschberg for ophthalmology (1887), Charles Richet for physiology (1895–1907), Wilhelm Roux for embryology, and the *Larousse médical de guerre* (Galtier-Boissière, 1917) for military medicine.

As the modern period has been the great age of medical periodicals, so too it has been the age of **medical bibliography.**

In the past, Conrad Gesner did something of the kind as early as 1545. Haller was the leading medical bibliographer of the 18th century, and, in the 19th, Young (1813), Haeser (1862), Ploucquet, Forbes, Atkinson, Watts, and others did good work; but the first attempt to give an indexed author catalogue of an entire period, including the contents of periodicals, was the *Medicinisches Schriftsteller-Lexicon* (33 volumes, 1830–45) of the Danish surgeon, Carl Peter **Callisen** (1787–1866). As a complete conspectus of the medical literature of the last half of the 18th century and the first third of the 19th, this production ranks with Haller's as one of the most

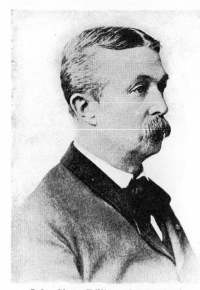

wonderful things ever achieved by a single man. It is invaluable for scope and accuracy. Other works of equal value are the *Handbuch der Bücherkunde* (1828) of Ludwig Choulant (1791–1861), which, in its second edition (1841), is, with the indispensable *Additamenta* of Julius Rosenbaum (1847), the best check list we have of the different editions of the older medical writers.

The opportunity for a unique bibliography of the entire medical literature of the world was afforded by the building up of the Library of the Surgeon-General's Office at Washington, which, at the outbreak of the Civil War, consisted of some 1000 odd volumes and became, in time, the best medical library in the world through the energy, perseverance, and ability of its principal founder, John Shaw

John Shaw Billings (1838–1913).   **Billings** (1838–1913), a native of Indiana, who had been a distinguished army surgeon in the Civil War. In 1876, Billings published a *Specimen Fasciculus* of a combined index catalogue of authors and subjects, arranged in a single alphabet in dictionary order, and, in 1880, he issued the first volume of the *Index Catalogue* of the library, in which he was assisted by Robert **Fletcher** (1823–1912), of Bristol, England.

This work, the most exhaustive piece of medical bibliography ever undertaken, has now reached its forty-fifth volume (third series, ix), and embraces the contents of a medical library of over 800,000 items. The selection of the material and the scientific classification in the first series (1880–95) were made by Billings; the careful proofreading was done by Fletcher; both classification and proofreading of the second series (1896) were done by Fletcher up to the time of his death (1912). This work, and the *Index Medicus*, a monthly bibliography of the world's medical literature, edited in the first series (1879–99) by Billings and Fletcher, and revived, with Fletcher as editor-in-chief, by the Carnegie Institution of Washington (1903–27), are known to all physicians who use medical literature. Apart from his talents as a medical bibliographer, Billings was a man of all-round ability, an able operative surgeon in wartime, an authority on military medicine, public hygiene, sanitary engineering, statistics and hospital construction, the author of the most critical account of American medical literature (1876) and the best history of surgery that has been published in English (1895) and widely known as the designer of the Johns Hopkins and other modern hospitals.

Altogether, Billings did a giant's work for the advancement of American medicine. The crown of his achievement as a civil administrator was the New York Public Library, which he planned with his own hands and brought to its present state of efficiency. Fletcher made many admirable contributions to anthropology and medical history.

The example set by Billings in the Surgeon-General's Library and its Index Catalogue gave an enormous impetus to the growth of **medical libraries** in the United States, of which there are now 200 as against 118 in Europe. The three largest medical libraries in the world are the library of the Paris Medical Faculty (240,000 volumes, 800,000 pamphlets), the Surgeon-General's Library at Washington, D. C. (238,799 volumes, 366,925 pamphlets), and the Library of the Lenin Imperial Medico-Military Academy at Leningrad (180,000 volumes). The Library of the College of Physicians of Philadelphia (founded 1788) has 154,293 volumes, 163,064 pamphlets, 431 manuscripts and 376 incunabula, of which 257 have been made available to the profession, by photostat, by the librarian, Charles Perry Fisher; the Library of the Medical and Chirurgical Faculty of Maryland (founded 1830), 50,000 volumes. The Library of the New York Academy of Medicine (founded 1846) now possesses 149,950 volumes, 112,245 pamphlets, 1570 files of periodicals and has recently acquired a handsome new building on Fifth Avenue (1926). Its present librarian is Archibald Malloch, who succeeded John S. Brownne. The Boston Medical Library, founded August 20, 1875, with Oliver Wendell Holmes as president, James R. Chadwick and Edwin H. Brigham as librarians, has some 145,988 volumes, 96,623 pamphlets and 173 incunabula. The Librarian during 1905–27 was John W. Farlow, succeeded by Charles F. Painter (1928), with James F. Ballard as Director. The Medical Library Association of the United States and Canada (founded 1898) has been represented by the periodicals *Medical Libraries* (1898–1902), edited by Charles D. Spivak (1861–1927), a short-lived *Bulletin* (1902), *The Medical Library and Historical Journal* (1903–7), and the present *Bulletin of the Medical Library Association* (1911), edited by John Ruhräh and Miss Marcia C. Noyes, and latterly by Jean Cameron (Montreal).

THE TWENTIETH CENTURY: THE BEGINNINGS OF ORGAN-
IZED PREVENTIVE MEDICINE

PRIMITIVE medicine, with its Egyptian and Oriental congeners, is essentially a phase of anthropology. Greek medicine was science in the making, with Roman medicine as an offshoot, Byzantium as a cold-storage plant, and Islam as traveling agent. The best side of medieval medicine was the organization of hospitals, sich nursing, medical legislation and education; its reactionary tendencies are mainly of antiquarian interest. The Renaissance Period marks the birth of anatomy as a science, with a corresponding growth of surgery as a handicraft. The best of 17th century medicine was purely scientific. Eighteenth-century medicine was again retrograde in respect of system-making, but has to its credit the beginnings of pathology, refined diagnosis (Auenbrugger), experimental and physiological surgery (John Hunter), and acquires an added social interest in relation to the beginnings of preventive inoculation (Jenner), and the formulation of a definite program of public hygiene (Frank). In the 19th century, the advancement of science was organized and scientific surgery was created. The interest of 20th century medicine is again social.

The most noticeable things about recent medicine have been the trend toward coöperation and international solidarity, and the fact that nearly every important advance which has been made is prophylactic, *i. e.*, comes within the scope of preventing the occurrence, the recurrence, or the spread of the disease. Listerism; the gifts to mankind of Jenner, Pasteur, Semmelweis, Credé, and O'Dwyer; the chemical and bacteriological examination of air, water, food, soils, and drugs; the purification of sewage; cremation; the hygiene of occupations and habitations; the medical inspection and care of school-children and factory children; the Binet-Simon tests; vacation colonies; social surveys and settlement work; town planning; the police surveillance of perverts and criminal characters in great cities like Berlin; the Swedish and American experiments at social control of the use of alcohol; the revival of the old Greek ideal of athletics and personal hygiene; the displacement of the medieval ascetic view of the sexual instinct by the clear-eyed scientific view; social organization against venereal infections; the proposed legal regulation of marriage and sterilization of degenerate stock; the intensive study of alcoholism, the drug habit, syphilis, tuberculosis, and cancer; the use of medical bibliography and statistics to get extensive information as to pathological conditions in space and time; the coöperation of universities, armies, public health services and private endowments in preventing tropical or parasitic diseases; international congresses; the Geneva Convention; even such things as Banting, Bertillonage, Esmarch bandages, or sanitary towels and drinking cups, are all features of preventive medicine or medicine on a grand scale. Misapplication of some of these devices has already led to social slavery worse than that of feudalism, because, as Emerson said, "The race is great, the ideal fair, the men whiffling and unsure." In the hands of corrupt politicians, Johann Peter Frank's concept of a scientific medical police may become a stalking horse for private vindictiveness, in the regulation of marriage, for instance. As Allbutt has wittily said: "The Greek philosopher, like the modern socialist, would sacrifice man to the State; the priest would sacrifice man to the Church; the scientific evolutionist would sacrifice man to the race." In actuality, much of the evil in the recent world has been wrought by the fanaticism of having one's own way, or what Billings ironically termed, "exercising a little judicious supervision over the affairs of our neighbors," set off by the "vocal vanity" of lofty sentiments or the engraving of the same on arch or architrave of public structures.

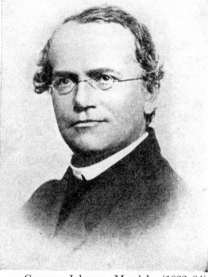

Gregor Johann Mendel (1822–84). (Courtesy of Professor William Bateson, London.)

The tendency in all branches of recent science, even in zoölogy, sociology, therapeutics, internal medicine and surgery, has been to pass out of the descriptive into the experimental stage. The aim of science to predict and control phenomena is sensed in the application of the equation in Mendel's law to the experimental study of heredity (genetics), in Loeb's proof that the fertilization and development of the embryo is a chemical process, in the consideration of the accessory chromosome as the determinant of sex, in the extravital cultivation and rejuvenation of tissues, in the conquest of communicable diseases or the recent developments of Hunterian or physiological surgery.

In 1865,[1] the Augustinian monk, Gregor Johann **Mendel** (1822–84), abbot of Brünn, announced the results of certain experiments on hybridization in peas in the form of a law which has shed much light upon inheritance and the origin of species.

If we agree to represent the generation of hybrids by the mathematical process of squaring, and if a represents a dominant or unchangeable character, and b a recessive or latent character in the parents, then Mendel's law, in its simplest form,

---

[1] Mendel: Versuche über Pflanzen-Hybriden, Verhandl. d. naturf. Ver. in Brünn (1865), 1866, iv, 3–270.

becomes identical with Newton's binomial theorem: $(a+b)^2=a^2+2ab+b^2$; in other words, one-half of the progeny will breed true to the parental characters $(2ab)$, while the other half will be divided equally between offspring possessing only the dominant (a) and the recessive (b) characters. In subsequent generations, the hybrid offspring will breed according to Mendel's law, while the dominants and recessives will breed true to their kinds. Thus if red and white flowering specimens of the plant "four o'clock" are crossed, the offspring will be red, pink and white in the proportion of 1 : 2 : 1 (Correns). If the second generations of two hybrid plants are imbred, the proportion will be 9 : 3 : 3 : 1 in a sliding scale from dominants to recessives. In a trihybrid cross, the same 3 : 1 ratio will be maintained. The unit characters (genes) are thus segregated (redistributed) and independently assorted, without reference to the original parent stocks.

For at least thirty-five years this unique approximation, printed in an obscure periodical, remained unnoticed, but in 1900, Hugo de Vries (1848–   ), C. Correns, and E. Tschermak simultaneously confirmed Mendel's results in every respect, while Francis Galton had arrived at a statistical "law of heredity," based upon his observations on the pedigrees of Basset hounds (1897). From his experiments with the primrose *Œnothera Lamarckiana*, de Vries advanced his hypothesis of **mutation** (1901[1]), or the abrupt or spontaneous origin of species from large discontinuous variations (mutations). William Bateson (1861–1926) did much to focus and elucidate the main points at issue in his great book on *Variation* (1894). Through Mendel's proof that heredity can be understood and dealt with in terms of simple mechanism, biology began to be an experimental rather than a speculative science.

Following the mutation theory of de Vries (1901), developments were rapid. In 1903, the Danish botanist Wilhelm **Johannsen** (1857–1927[2]), experimenting with beans, showed that in self-fertilizing plants, a **pure line** of descendants is maintained indefinitely, in which case natural selection is non-effective. Selection, therefore, depends upon the genetic variability which Mendel found in such a plant as Pisum sativum, or Luther Burbank in the hybrids with which he experimented so successfully. This variability springs from Johannsen's genotype (constellation of genes) and not from the illusory phenotype (group aspect). Cases of extreme variability of inheritance (*e. g.*, in cereals), which seemed an exception to Mendel's law, were brought under it by the "multiple factor" theory of H. **Nilsson-Ehle** (1908), in virtue of which the genes are not only segregated and assorted, but may, in some cases, exert a cumulative effect upon specific characters in the descendants. About this time, Bateson, Punnett, Castle and others began to work in the new science of **genetics** which was put upon its feet mainly through the epoch-making work of Thomas Hunt **Morgan** upon the fruit fly (*Drosophila ampelophila*).[3] With his assistants, Bridges, Sturtevant and Muller, Morgan produced over 200 mutations in Drosophila and discovered the mechanism of heredity, viz., that the Mendelian assortment of genes can be definitely allocated to the behavior of the chromosomes. This long and patient investigation covered the new phenomena of coupling and repulsion (linkage), sex-linked inheritance, criss-cross inheritance, crossing over, double crossing over and the plotting of the locus of genes on chromosome maps. Connected with the counting of the chromosomes in many plants and animals, the discovery of the accessory chromosomes by Henking (1890) and Montgomery (1898), their identification as the determinants of sex by Clarence Erwin McClung (1902),[4] and the phenomena of linkage, first

[1] H. de Vries: Die Mutationstheorie, Leipzig, 1901.

[2] W. Johannsen: Ueber Erblichkeit, Jena, 1903. Elemente der exakten Erblichkeitslehre, Berlin, 1919.

[3] T. H. Morgan, A. H. Sturtevant (*et al.*): The Mechanism of Mendelian Heredity, 2. ed., New York, 1923.

[4] C. E. McClung: Biol. Bull., Bost., 1902, iii, 43–48. T. H. Morgan: Theory of the Gene.

noted by Bateson and Punnett (1906), is the complete elucidation of the mechanical factors involved in the determination of sex. All this has exerted a profound influence upon our present views of the doctrine of natural selection in evolution.

The effect has been to deprive Darwin's idea of the supernatural and ethical attributes which have been read into it by overzealous admirers, but no experiments to date have demonstrated that species originate by mutation alone. Darwin perhaps overemphasized the significance of the *external* factor of environmental stress in the struggle for existence as originating morphological species by long-continued (eventually) "natural" selection. Mendel and his followers located the *internal* biochemical forces at work in bringing about the mathematical permutations and combinations of the determinants in the supposed discontinuous origin of species *de novo* or *per saltum.* But whether evolution proceeds by slow gradations or by leaps and bounds or, what seems most likely, is capable of both continuous and discontinuous processes, the apparently spontaneous results of saltatory (Mendelian) variation must have had, in each case, "a long foreground," in the sense of being the end product of a complex series of physico-chemical changes. Morgan's experiments show that the results obtained in the flowerpot, the milk bottle, and the breeding pen are identical with those occurring in wild nature, some of which are beyond the memory of man. In Cuénot's remarkable mutations in spotted mice (1903), in those of Castle with hooded rats (1914), and in Maude Slye's epoch-making experiments on malignant tumors in mice (1913–27) the changes are, in all probability, due to the cumulative effect of genes and not, as Castle maintains, to alterations in the genes themselves. In the simplest case, that of Johannsen's pure lines, it is seen that self-fertilizing races either become automatically pure (Jennings, Pearl) or were pure to start with. Old Sir Thomas Browne,[1] the first to use the term, said that "mutations, however they began, depend upon durable foundations, and such as many continue forever," which seems the conclusion of the whole matter. The mutations observed in wild nature are only significant for the maintenance of the species, and as wild species differ in many details and are identical in only a few, it is plain, as Morgan points out, that survival was established by modifying and improving the species bit by bit. In place of the older picture of the struggle for existence, the future holds out the possibility of peaceful improvement by the gradual incorporation of characters beneficial to the race. Selection produces nothing new, but only more kinds of favored individuals, a process which Morgan defines as creative evolution in the mechanical sense. From this "sliding scale" in the direction of advantageous selection, we arrive at the notion of **emergent evolution**[2] as Mendelian mutation by discrete steps, each introducing something new. Natural selection and mutation may

---

[1] Pseudodoxia Epidemica, Book vi, ch. x, "Of the Blackness of Negroes" (Bohn's ed., v. ii, p. 188), cited by Punnett.

[2] H. S. Jennings: Emergent Evolution, Science, N. Y., 1927, lxv, 19–25.

43

"explain" the origin of structural adaptations, so that their trans-
mutations can be verified, if need be, in the laboratory, but of the
origin of organic and functional adaptations, such as the regeneration
of tissues, automatic regulation of form, development of embryos from
fractions of the ovum or by chemical activation (parthenogenesis),
these theories tell us nothing, because the "power of adaptation" which
is assigned as a reason is the very thing we are called upon to account
for and explain. Here, perhaps, we may ask "how," but not "why."
At most, we can only explain adaptation by harking back to the old
Hallerian doctrine of the specialized "irritability" of individual protoplasmic tissues, which Ehrlich has declared to be one of the most obscure phases of physiology.

The science of genetics has not only sifted and clarified the vague methods of
stockraisers in the past, but has also afforded the true explanation of such paradoxes
as telegony, atavism or maternal impressions and has already formulated the basic
principles of scientific plant and animal breeding. The remarkable results obtained
by Gowen with cattle, Pearl and Goodale with egg production, Hayes, East and
Jones with tobacco, not to mention Burbank, suggest endless possibilities for conscious improvement of the human stock. It is known that the only way to get at the
validity of the genotype is to study the progeny ("By their fruits ye shall know
them"); that inbreeding is not good for mass production; that hybrid vigor (heterosis)
is most effective en masse, but that both inbred and outbred lines trail off to a dead
level after a number of generations. Thus, Miss H. D. King's experiments with 30,-
000 inbred rats (1918) show that the initial decline in vigor and fertility is illusory,
provided the food be good, while Wright got just the opposite effects in guinea-pigs
(1915-22), and the results of East and Jones with dent corn (1920) afford a good
picture of the effects of consanguinity. The fallacies in Ruffer's reasoning about incest in Egyptian royalty (1921) become self-evident. What is known of Mendelian
dominance of dark eyes over blue, of brachydactyly, stiff joints, webbed fingers, clawed
hands, white forelocks or diabetes insipidus as dominants, of left-handedness, bronchial asthma and hay-fever as recessives, of color-blindness, night blindness, feeble-
mindedness, and hæmophilia as sex-linked, of the genetics of blood-grouping, subjects all these traits to individual, if not social, control. The Mendelian dominance
of dark eyes confirms Schopenhauer's theory that the dark people are the aboriginal and fundamental people, and Charles Reade's observation of the kindness
of blue-eyed women toward dark men, and, vice versa, has been delightfully elucidated
by Anita Loos.

Recent studies of such family groups as those of European royalty, of Jonathan
Edwards, of Galton's 977 interrelated Englishmen of eminence, of the Bachs, of
the defective Jukes, Kallikaks and Nams, lead to the conclusion that environment
has little effect upon strongly individualized people, that the only effect of identical
training upon miscellaneous groups of people is to widen the gulf between the bright
and the dull, and that hereditary endowment will out and is omnipotent as Goethe
believed—

> "Setz' dir Perücken auf von Millionen Locken,
> Setz' deinen Fuss auf ellenhohe Socken,
> Du bleibst doch immer was du bist."[1]

Mendelian doctrine has been vastly forwarded by the new statistical
science of **biometrics**, which is the special creation of Francis Galton
and his brilliant pupil, **Karl Pearson** (1857–   ). The theory of
probabilities was first applied to sociological phenomena by the Belgian
astronomer and statistician, Adolphe Quetelet (1796–1874[2]), but

---

[1] Cited by Robach.

[2] Quetelet: Sur l'homme, Brussels, 1836; Lettre . . . sur la théorie des
probabilités appliquée aux sciences morales et sociales, Brussels, 1846; Loi de pério-
dicité, Brussels, 1879, etc.

Galton's *Natural Inheritance* (1889) introduced the statistical study of biological variation and inheritance. Pearson, an English barrister, now director of the Laboratory for National Eugenics, founded by Galton, has applied the higher mathematics in the most ingenious way to the solution of these problems and has created a rational school of iatromathematics. His fascinating volumes on *The Chances of Death* (1897) opened out many new views as to the meaning of statistics as interpreted by algebraic curves, the significance of correlations, and the use of the same in obtaining accurate data as to the hidden causes of biological and social phenomena which cannot themselves be measured quantitatively.

Galton used the term "regression" to indicate the extent to which an average biological unit is more like the mean or mediocre level of the general stock than like its parent. By correlation, Pearson means the logical opposite, viz., the extent to which the offspring resembles its parents rather than the average unit of the species. If parent and offspring are exactly alike, in respect of the quality under investigation, the correlation curve will be a line making an angle of 45° with the abscissæ or the ordinates. If the filial quality exists to a lesser degree than the parental, the curve will have a more insignificant slope, the degree of slope ("correlation-coefficient") being the tangent of the angle made with the horizontal. If there is no correlation, the curve will be a horizontal line. By this means, Pearson has brought out many new facts and bionomic theorems, most of them in the journal *Biometrika* (1901)[1] and latterly in the *Annals of Eugenics* (1925). He has shown (for example), that, in the case of tuberculosis, it is not the disease but the diathesis which is inherited, not the seed but the soil; that there is no neurotic inheritance from alcoholic parentage unless the stock itself be neurotic; that the death-rate from disease is selective in a large percentage of cases, and that a higher infantile death-rate implies the survival of a stronger and more enduring stock. There is a definite tendency in nature to handicap the first-born, who are weaker than subsequent offspring. Pearson maintains that "to make the first-born 50 per cent. instead of something less than 22 per cent. of the whole number of births," spells degeneracy.[2] Pearson believes that the improvements of medical science and the tendency of nature to insure the survival of the fittest are diametrically opposing forces, and he contends, *e. g.*, from the surprising fertility of successive generations of achondroplasic dwarfs, that the humane tendency of modern medicine to preserve the diseased and deformed is not only detrimental to the human species, but can only be set off or obviated by preventing these defectives from breeding their kind. He has indicated how Galton's law of ancestral inheritance can be improved upon by selective breeding, so that regression, the tendency to revert to a mediocre average, will in a few generations be hardly sensible. He claims that tall women procreate faster than small women, that dark-eyed people are more fertile than the light-eyed, and has established the law of "assortative mating," in virtue of which human beings, in most cases, mate, not as usually believed, with their opposites in stature, complexion, etc., but with their own kind. In this respect, he finds that husband and wife are more nearly alike than uncle and niece or first cousins, in accordance with the French proverb, *Les époux se ressemblent.* The inference is that, according to Galton's law, the like tend to perpetuate and strengthen their kind by mating, biologically speaking, in their own class. It follows that a greater amount of high-grade ability could be produced by selective breeding, since "the average genius we meet is more likely to be an exceptional variation of a mediocre stock than a common variation of an exceptional stock. This accounts for the fact that the sons of geniuses are often so disappointing."

These theories of Galton and Pearson have met with no little opposition, not because they are incorrect, but because they have been taken too literally. According to Weismann's theory, acquired char-

---

[1] Founded, in 1901, by W. F. R. Weldon, Francis Galton, and himself.

[2] Pearson: On the Handicapping of the First-born, London, 1914, p. 66.

acters are not inherited, and the finest moral or mental traits in the parents will not benefit the offspring unless they have the right start in life. Oliver Twist may go to the bad in a den of thieves, and Bill Sykes may have it in him to steal and murder, even with the most careful upbringing. That conduct is reaction to stimuli, that morality is always an inhibition, showing, at least, the importance of "early training" (euthenics), was sensed by the broad-minded Goethe, who declared himself capable of committing any crime. For the weak, "the environment of today is the heredity of tomorrow" (Tredgold). The strong, in an unfavorable environment, get out of it. The studies of the Jukes family by R. L. Dugdale (1877), the Hill Folk, and the Nams show one side of the shield, Galton's investigations of talented families the other, the record of the Kallikak family by H. H. Goddard (1915) and A. H. Estabrook's summary of *The Jukes in 1915*[1] both sides. In 130 years, the five Jukes sisters produced 2094 descendants, 1258 living in 1915, of whom half were feeble-minded, shiftless and immoral, the other half mentally and emotionally normal. Reaction to stimuli (environment), in each case, was weak-charactered or strong-charactered as the inheritance was bad or good. Estabrook's findings show that consanguineous marriages of defectives produce defectives, that licentiousness is hereditary, pauperism and crime resultants of feeble-mindedness, change of environment beneficial to degenerate stock and that sterilization of defectives would interfere less with personal liberty than custodial care. Thus Nature cares nothing for the ways of man, but takes care of her own, be they lewd, thievish, murderous, or even feeble-minded, provided they are sufficiently well-sexed to propagate their kind. As passive agents of social degeneracy, the feeble-minded are as potent as the aggressively criminal. "A flea is as untameable as a hyena."[2]

The work of Bateson, Punnett, of Charles B. Davenport and the experts at the Cold Spring Harbor Station (organized 1910), bears out the Mendelian axiom that, as the individuality of a living organism is established by the presence or absence of certain biological determinants, so qualities may be inherited, but not their absence. As brown eyes are due to the presence, blue eyes to the absence, of a certain pigment in the iris, as dancing mice differ from normal mice in lacking part of the internal ear, so brachydactyly (short fingers), presenile cataract, keratosis, xanthoma, hypotrichosis congenita, diabetes insipidus, night-blindness, and Huntington's chorea indicate the presence of certain factors in the germ-plasm which may interdict the union of two such abnormals; but albinism, deaf-mutism, retinitis pigmentosa, congenital imbecility, and the tendency to respiratory and neurotic disorders are due to an inherent lack of something which may be supplemented by judicious cross-breeding with sound stock,[3] although Pearson contends that it is a waste of good material to employ sound stock for this purpose.

---

[1] A. H. Estabrook: The Jukes in 1915, Washington, 1916.

[2] R. W. Emerson: The point is well brought out in Mrs. Finlayson's study of the Dack Family, as an example of nature's power of perpetuating hereditary lack of emotional control (Eugenics Record Office, Bull. No. 15, Cold Spring Harbor, 1916).

[3] C. B. Davenport: Eugenics, New York, 1910; Heredity (etc.), New York, 1911, *passim*.

Nature's tendency to revert to the mediocre level of the common stock, to Walt Whitman's "divine average," will make the average a very low level indeed if it proceeds downward from poor or faulty material to start with. It is a well-ascertained fact that the thorough-bred animal, with generations of biologically desirable ancestors behind him, is prepotent over the normal animal. But actual selection is often influenced by the bizarre caprices of "the unstable heart of man," and while individual propagandism could be made extremely effective, social control would be difficult of accomplishment without tyrannous espionage and surveillance. In the lower strata of society, marriage laws may not prevent illegitimacy or incest, vasectomy is dubious,[1] and selective pure-line breeding, without some striking quality to start with, might only result in a race of negative prigs. "A far more effective means of restricting bad germ-plasm than placing elaborate marriage laws upon our statute-books is to educate the public sentiment and to foster a public eugenic conscience, in the absence of which the safeguards of the law must forever be largely without avail" (Walter).

In America, the most remarkable work done by the newer statistics is that of Raymond **Pearl** (1879), of Farmington, New Hampshire, a mathematician of unusual ability, who is now professor of biometry and vital statistics in the School of Hygiene of the Johns Hopkins University (1918).

During 1899–1906, he demonstrated the principle of "improvement by practice" in the morphogenesis of Ceratophyllum (1907), the occurrence of assortative mating in Paramecium and made the first biometric analysis of the weight of the human brain. In 1907–17, he demonstrated the Mendelian inheritance of egg production in the domestic fowl, the fact that alcohol has a beneficial selective action upon its germ-cells, with other generalizations as to its reproductive processes, and formulated the mathematical relations of inbreeding and its consequences. In 1917–19, he made a detailed analysis of food production and consumption in the United States. During 1919–27, Pearl was engaged in constructing life-tables for other forms of life than man, in demonstrations of the Mendelian inheritance of longevity, of the beneficial effect of the moderate use of alcohol upon human longevity (1926) and in analyses of the effects of density of population upon natality and mortality (1920–1927), culminating in his most important contribution to biometrics, the logistic curve of population growth (1920). His conclusions are that the higher the density of population the lower the birth-rate, whence the population of any nation or community covering a given area will, in passing through the hunting, pastoral, agricultural and industrial stages, slowly increase up to the point of optimum relation between its density and subsistence resources and thereafter remain stationary (1925).

Huxley's distinction between morphological species and physiological species becomes of moment in recent work on the **determination of sex.**

The trend of opinion indicates that while the mechanism of sex determination may be allocated to the accessory (XY) chromosomes signalized by McClung (1902), the ultimate process of sex differentiation is a much more complex matter. That the XY chromosomes function as determinants of sex is indicated by the peculiarities

---

[1] The undesirable tendencies of mutilated or eunuchoid individuals, let loose upon society, are well known in the Orient and are frequently emphasized in the footnotes of Sir Richard Burton's Arabian Nights.

of their behavior in different animals and by the fact that genes, presiding over sex-linked inheritance, appear to be located in these chromosomes (Morgan). Identical (enzygotic) twins, developed from the same ovum, are always of the same sex. But Goldschmidt has produced intersexes of all degrees in the gypsy moth (*Lymantria*), by crossing the Japanese and European species (1921[1]) and the disturbance of equilibrium between the male and female determinants suggests the interplay of some other forces than assortment and cumulative action of genes. Working with a strain of Drosophila, Bridges got males, females, supermales, superfemales, and intersexed types, the sorting in the chromosome maps indicating that all the chromosomes, and not merely X and Y are involved in the process (1925), but in insects the sex glands play no part. What tips the beam in mammals is suggested by F. R. Lillie's observations on the rôle of sex hormones in the production of free martins (1917) or by Crew's Buff Orpington hen, which, after an exemplary career as a layer of eggs, turned into a male and begot chicks, as a result of destructive ovarian tuberculosis (1923[2]). Many similar cases, German and other, show that the activator, whether endocrine or metabolic, is in all probability chemical. The basic mechanism (morphology) of sex and its physiological development are two entirely different things. Goldschmidt's theory of time sequences (gene velocity) or the view that the female is virtually a male, swamped by female hormones, are, like the archetypal gynandromorph in Plato's Symposium, mere speculation.

Through developments such as these, biology is fast becoming a phase of general physiology. A striking illustration is the almost complete reorganization of **anthropology** by data drawn from physiology and pathology and the effect of this realignment upon recent medicine.[3]

During the period 1850–1900, the solidist (cellular) pathology of Virchow dominated medicine, and, as in all Cnidian phases, consideration of the patient as a whole was lost in the pathological lesion or specimen as the *sedes morbi*. The rise of bacteriology merely transferred this dominance from cell to bacillus, but with the new sciences of serology and endocrinology, the humoral pathology was revived and a new order of things obtained. Signs of the approaching change were Möbius' view of exogenous and endogenous diseases, Hueppe on the relation of the resistance of the body to external forces (1893) and Kraus on fatigue as a measure of the constitution (1897). In 1914, Martius published his important book on *Constitution and Selection*. With the publication of Martin's *Lehrbuch* (1914), the older anthropology ended in a brilliant *fanfare*. With the World War, the doctrine of the **Constitution** took a sudden leap forward, and was further helped out by the development of Mendelian reasoning (genetics) and of endocrinology. Consideration of the soldier as a whole, and of vast outdoor clinics of men *en masse*, tended to revive the general pathology of Hippocrates, just as the pathological lesion and the bacillus forwarded special (local) pathology and specific therapy. The constitution came to be seen as the summation of inherited traits which are basic in resistance, susceptibility and predisposition to disease. The constitution became assimilated to the genotype of Johannsen; the physical habitus and facies to the sometimes illusory phenotype. In the view of Keith (1911), Crookshank (1912), and Paulsen (1920), race is the outward and visible sign of a definite equilibrium of endocrine secretions, and since the constitutional diseases and insanities are imbalanced states or "caricatures of the normal" and independent of race, the typology of the constitution is an inter-ethnic phenomenon. Thus Allbutt's view of health as a diathesis (like scrofula or syphilis), the most useful cycle of the growing human organism, comes into its own and acquires new criteria from a study of the abnormal, even as Freud has illuminated the mechanisms of normal thinking. Salient in this connection is the work of Ernst Kretschmer (1888–   ) on *Constitution and Character* (1921[4]) which signalizes the fat-faced, chesty, well-nourished people (pycnics, extroverts, or cycloids) and the thin-faced, thin-bodied, attenuated El Greco people (leptosomics, introverts, or

[1] R. Goldschmidt: Geschlechtsbestimmung, Berlin, 1921.

[2] F. A. E. Crew: Jour. Hered., Wash., 1923, xiv, 361.

[3] J. Paulsen: Arch. f. Anthrop., Braunschweig, 1925, N. F., xxi, 57–69.

[4] E. Kretschmer: Körperbau und Charakter, Berlin, 1921.

schizoids) as indices of peculiar mentality, tending, at the pathological limits of the series, to the manic-depressive and dementia præcox psychoses of Kraepelin's classification. Cycloids are cheerful, temperamental, well-adjusted to the business world, but liable to sudden alternations of exhilaration and depression. Schizoids are maladjusted, of cloven personality (*amina anceps*), Ishmaelites and victims of shut-in mentality (autism), with its implications of mental childishness, frustrated sexuality and hostility to the world at large. This arrangement seems reasonably true to human nature, has an impressive statistic, and was withal an immense advance upon the military classification of Chaillou and McAuliffe (1912) as muscular (athletic), digestive (pycnic), respiratory (chesty) and cerebral (leptosomic). Other data of constitutional anatomy are derivable from photography (Charcot's *Iconographie*, 1877–1918), endocrinology (Cushing, Biedl, Falta) and anthropometry. A leading exponent of data derivable from measurements is George Draper (1924[1]), who seeks the genotype *via* the phenotype and has already accumulated valuable indiciæ of tendency to pernicious anemia, gastric ulcer, phthisis, etc. The subject has now an immense literature, including a periodical (1914[2]), the treatises of Bauer (1917) and Halban-Seitz (*Biologie der Person*, 1926) and many interesting papers bearing upon the gonadal, gynecologic, pediatric, and neuro-psychiatric phases.

With the publication of the *Allegemeine Rassenkunde* of Walther Scheidt (1925), German anthropology definitely passed over to the study of the individual human being. A more empirical phase, the study of personality (**characterology**), is also represented by a special periodical (1924[3]), but its tendency was already foreshadowed in the pathographies of Möbius (1889–1904) and the post-bellum extravagances of realistic (psycho-sexual) biography. Should the constitution become basic for all branches of medicine, then, medicine (it is argued) becomes a vassal of anthropology. That the doctrine itself is as old as the hills was noted by Sudhoff, who warns that it is largely dependent upon syllogisms and may again "blight the green fields of clinical observation with dialectic mildew." That the constitution is the biological fate of the individual, Schopenhauer's "*arrêt irrévocable* of his destiny," is suggested by an apparently authenticated case of two male (identical) twins, who lived apart under widely different circumstances, to be affected simultaneously with diabetic gangrene and die of uremia at sixty.[4]

The inevitable pother about **materialism** and **vitalism,** started by Driesch, has latterly resolved itself into a reaction toward mysticism, due in part to contradictory findings in laboratory experimentation, lost motion over futilities, the confusional status of medical doctrine, the gigantic and senseless proliferation of meaningless literature, and the general pessimism and scrambling of brains consequent upon the World War. The output of medical literature is now so vast that it has been suggested that it ought to be stopped at intervals, to ascertain its tendency (if any). Never have medical authors been so verbose and to so little purpose! It is coming to be recognized that vitalism, catalysis, tropisms and clinical entities are mere verbiage and

---

[1] G. Draper: Human Constitution, New York, 1924.

[2] Zeitschrift für angewandte Anatomie und Konstitutionslehre, Berlin, 1914.

[3] Jahrbuch für Charakterologie, Berlin, 1924.

[4] R. Michaelis: Arch. f. Rassen- u. Gesellschaftsbiol., Berl., 1904, i, 199–200.

their ultimate nature unintelligible. In this connection, Wright invokes ironically the immobilized God of Aristotle, "The Unmoved Mover behind the demiurge," operating by entelechy or *élan vital.* In other words, it is given us to ask "how?" With reference to the *noumenon* of Kant, we are fools to repeat Galen's mistake and ask "why?" The war has taught us that we can no longer hope to predict the future from the past. Among those who never lost faith in experimentation and the future of science, the first place belongs to our leading exponent of the **general physiology** of Claude Bernard.

Jacques **Loeb** (1859–1924), a medical graduate of Strassburg (1884), sometime professor of biology and physiology at Bryn Mawr (1892–1900), the University of Chicago (1900–1902), University of California (1902–1910), and later head of the department of experimental biology in the Rockefeller Institute, devoted most of his life to the dynamic or chemodynamic study of living processes.

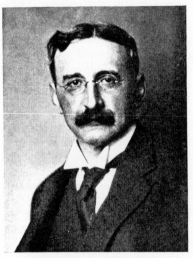

Jacques Loeb (1859–1924).

In his work on the physiology of the brain, he made original researches on the chain reflexes, and overthrew Munk's position that the Rolandic area is made up of cellular "sensory spheres," by showing that the particular paralysis occasioned by each cortical excision will be abolished as soon as the wound is healed. He was one of the first to settle the question: of what order of magnitude is the smallest particle that can show all the phenomena of life? (1893[1]) and the experiments made by himself and pupils upon temperature coefficients have established other important criteria of physiological processes. He made extensive investigations of the effects of electrolytic, thermal, and radiant energy upon living matter, and founded the theory of "tropisms" (1889[2]) as the basis of the psychology of the lower forms of life, purely mechanical and chemical data displacing the old theory of purposeful instinctive reactions. Even for the higher forms, his main position was that all actions of fundamental importance are instinctive, have nothing to do with states of consciousness, and that even these may have a chemical basis. In 1889, he caused the unfertilized eggs of the sea-urchin to develop into the swimming larvæ by treating them with hypertonic sea water (*i. e.*, in which the concentration has been raised by the addition of salt or sugar). Similar results had been published by Tichomiroff (1886), who claimed to have developed unfertilized silkworm eggs by rubbing them gently with a brush or by temporary immersion in concentrated sulphuric acid. Bataillon got similar effects by needle-punctures (1911). Loeb carried his imitation of normal fertilization further by a preliminary treatment with butyric acid, producing an artificial fertilization membrane with complete development, following immersion of the eggs in a hypertonic solution before returning them to normal sea water. The formation of the membrane is supposed to accelerate oxidation, which Loeb regarded as the criterion of a living process. He further showed that the ovum has a selective, specific activating influence on the spermatozoön. In 1916, Loeb stated that he had

[1] Loeb: Arch. f. d. ges. Physiol., Bonn, 1894–95, lix, 379–394.

[2] Der Heliotropismus der Thiere, Würzburg, 1890, and later publications.

seven male parthenogenetic (fatherless) frogs (*Rana pipiens*), over a year old, produced by the Bataillon method of pricking the unfertilized egg.[1]

After rounding up the results of his work in a brilliant series of books (1890–1918), the last years of his life were spent in adapting the data of colloid chemistry to the laws of classical chemistry, as summarized in his work on *Protein Solutions* (1922). He held that, in the light of their measurable acid-base equilibria, "proteins form true ionizable salts with acids and alkalies," but in applying the Donnan equilibria (1910) to the theory of colloid behavior, he vitiated his labors by viewing the ion not as an electrolyte, but as a freely floating electric charge or electron (Armstrong). Loeb was a monist, who believed, with Emerson, that legislators should be specially educated for their duties and that scientific men should have a voice in legislative assemblies. His comment on the World War ("the Simians!") is characteristic of the man.

As Maxwell, Gibbs, or Einstein developed certain phases of mathematics merely to elucidate physical phenomena, so recent advances in **anatomy** turn almost entirely upon collateral investigations in physiology and pathology and sometimes upon new wrinkles in diagnosis and therapeutics. In the newer trend, anatomy is functional, therefore physiological, so much so indeed that it has been falsely dubbed the "dynamics" of the organism, as if usurping the domain of physiology. In such studies as Gaskell's mapping of the sympathetic-autonomic system, the Aschoff-Maximow map of the reticulo-endothelial system and its extension to the neuraxis, the elucidation of the mechanism of the Magnus reflexes or of the cerebrospinal circulation, the physiological anatomy of Leonardo comes into its own. Such structures as the brain-stem, the pallium, the dorsal lip of the blastopore, inspire the feeling voiced by Hertz with reference to Maxwell's six equations expressing the electromagnetic theory of light, viz., that they are "wiser than we are." In this sense, anatomy is truly the statics of the organism. Röntgenology, intravital staining, micro-dissection and other devices afford powerful aids at need (*non eget arce*), and even the graphics of Neugebauer and Dickinson on the uncertain structural variations of the female genital tract, with reference to sexual compatibility, contraception, sterility, and labor, have the inevitable practical tendency of recent medicine.

Galen, founder of neurological anatomy, would rub his eyes over such abstruse monographs as those of Winkler on the octavus motor system (1907–18), Head on the dual mechanism of sensation (1920), Kappers and Fortuyn on the comparative anatomy of the nervous system (1920–21), Economo and Koskinas on the finer anatomy of the cortex (1925), or Brouwer on the cerebral mechanism of vision (1926).

The *Altmeister* of neurological anatomy is Santiago **Ramón y Cajal** (1852–   ), the son of an Aragonese physician and a graduate of

---

[1] Loeb: Proc. Nat. Acad. Sc., Wash., 1916, ii, 314.

Madrid (1883).   After some military service in Cuba (1873–5) he became assistant in anatomy at Zaragosa (1877).   Ramón y Cajal was talented in drawing and painting, and took up histology.   In 1888–9, he improved Golgi's chrome-silver stain (1883), and applied it to the whole nervous system, evolving his doctrine of the neurons toward 1890.   After holding chairs at Valencia (1883) and Barcelona (1887), he settled in Madrid (1892) and produced his great *Textura del Sistema Nervioso* (1897–1904), and founded a *Revista* (1896–1900), continued as *Trabajos* (1901, current).   These vast labors in histology comprise discoveries in all parts of the nervous system, notably the optic chiasm, olfactory lobes, medulla, cerebellum, cerebral nerves, spinal ganglia, and the innervation of the retina.   With Golgi, Cajal was awarded the Nobel Prize in

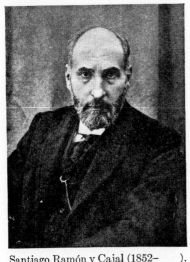

1906.   His later years have been devoted to work on the degeneration and regeneration of nervous tissue (1908–28[1]).   Highly esteemed by Kölliker and all other great histologists, Cajal has lamented the barrier of language which has excluded his total achievement from the knowledge of his profession.   His *Charlas de café* (1920), strongly-tinged with Latin pessimism, reveals the philosophical bent of a noble mind and a distinguished personality.

Of his pupils, the most remarkable are Nicolás Achucárro (1851–1918) and Pio del **Rio Hortega,** who devised a new staining method (1918) and discovered two new types of glia cells,

Santiago Ramón y Cajal (1852–   ).   viz., the mesodermal microglia (1919) and the ectodermal oligodendroglia (1919–21), which are disposed about the neurons in the gray matter, extending tendrils which partly invest the myelin sheaths in the white matter.

The intracranial and intraspinal spaces containing the **cerebrospinal fluid** were investigated by Key and Retzius (1875), their development by Florence Sabin (1902) and Weed (1917), the perivascular channels by Virchow (1851), Robin (1859), Duke (1894) and F. W. Mott (1910). The pathways and portals of the circulation of the fluid, from its origin in the choroid plexus, through the four ventricles into the subarachnoid spaces and the cisternæ *via* the foramina of Magendie and Luschka, to its evacuation by the venous sinuses of the brain and the lymphatics, were mapped out by Lewis H. **Weed** (1886–   ), of Cleveland, Ohio (1914–23).   These studies were beg n in Cushing's clinic, in connection with investigation of hydrocephalus. Walter E. Dandy and Kenneth D. Blackfan demonstrated the origin of the fluid from the choroid plexus by blocking the Sylvian aqueduct and the foramen of Monro for the production of experimental types of internal hydrocephalus (1913–14).   The origin of the meningeal lining of the pathways from the mesenchyme was demonstrated

[1] Ramón y Cajal: Studies on the Degeneration and Regeneration of the Nervous System, 2 v., Oxford, 1928.

experimentally by S. C. Harvey and H. S. Burr (1924–6). Evacuation by the lymphatics was maintained by Goldmann (1913), but was shown to be slight by Weed (1923). Injection of trypan blue into the subarachnoid spaces by Goldmann (1913) and Woollard (1924) indicate that the mesothelial cells of the meningeal pathways may become macrophagic (meningocytes) and thus take on the rôle of scavengers. Thus, Magendie's problem of the origin and locus of the fluid bathing the central nervous system, or what Cushing calls the "Third Circulation" (1925), was worked out by experiment. Another remarkable triumph of experimental anatomy was the demonstration of the structural mechanism of the postural reflexes of Magn s (1924). The proprioceptive mechanism had already been elucidated by Sherrington (1906), that of the red nucleus by C. von Monakow (1910). The rôle of the labyrinth was demonstrated by the effective Leonardine models of H. G. de Burlet of Utrecht (1924), the relations of the auditory (octavus) nerve by C. Winkler (1907–18) and A. Kappers (1920), the rôle of the red nucleus by G. G. J. Rademaker (1926), the localization of cerebellar functions by Elliot Smith (1902), Horsley (1906), I. L. Bolk (1906), Sven Ingvar (1906), L. Luciani (1915), Gordon Holmes (1918), and F. R. Miller (1926). With reference to diseases of the corpus striatum, the physiological anatomy of the extra-pyramidal system was investigated by Elliot Smith (hypopallium, 1910), Kinnier Wilson (1913–14), Monakow (1924), and D. McAlpine (1926). Head's theory of the dual mechanism of cutaneous sensibility and of deeper sensations (1905) has received extensive confirmation through work on the "Edinger fibre system" (1889), B. Brouwer's studies on segmental anatomy (1915) and the comparative data adduced by Parsons (1927). The locus of the projection of retinal sensations on to the optic tract, including the loss of mid-brain connections (monocular vision) in primates has been elucidated by M. Minskowski (1913), Gordon Holmes (1916), B. Brouwer (1923–6) and H. H. Woollard (1926). In the field of X-ray anatomy, such methods of local exploration as pneumoperitoneum (Weber, 1913), ventriculography (Dandy, 1918), and cholecystography (Graham and Cole, 1924) have thrown much light on variations of structure and situs in vivo. The study of anatomy in the living subject, the "art of anatomy" rather than the science, is coming to be an effective device in teaching, whether by fluoroscopy, Röntgenography, reflected light, or the ordinary methods of a physical examination and can be utilized at the same time, for instruction in rudimentary physiology, diagnosis, Röntgenology, and the clinical aspects of the constitution.[1]

Through the newer devices of micro-dissection, micro-injection, and intravital staining experimental cytology and tissue-cultivation have become going sciences.

By such means, the organized structures of the cell have been studied in minute detail, notably the nucleus and chromosomes (Kite and Chambers, 1912–25), the invisible reticulum of Golgi (Gatensby 1919, Parat 1926), and the visible mitochondria by Margaret and Warren Lewis (1914), E. V. Cowdry (1916), and Guillermond (1919). The recent contention of Heringa (1924) and Boeke (1926), that the cells are bound together by protoplasmic bridges and function as a whole, merely revamps one of the outworn phases of the neuron controversy, confuted by R. G. Harrison (1910) and latterly by Robert Chambers (1925). Harrison, who virtually started extravital cultivation of tissues by his proof of the outgrowth of nerve-fibers from ganglion cells (1910), has since demonstrated the origin of the sheath-cells of nerve from the neural (ganglion) crest, the placodes and ultimately the neuroblasts of the medullary tube (1924). Removal of the ganglion crest results in a series of naked axis-cylinders. In the same way, E. Müller and S. Ingvar have shown the origin of the spinal ganglia and the sympathetic nervous system from the ganglion crest (1923). These and other experiments on morphogenesis of nerve elements were made possible by the improved technic of M. T. Burrows (1911), who substituted blood-plasma for lymph in Harrison's initial experiment. Cells in extravital culture will not grow without an espalier (Lewis). Further improvements were the use of embryonic and chicken extract as growth promoters, the trephones of Carrel (1923) and the differential stains (janus green and black) introduced by the Lewises. Pure cultures were first obtained by the methods of A. Fischer (1922) and A. H. Drew. The tedious process of making successive explants is avoided by a special culture flask. By the explanta-

---

[1] E. J. Carey: Bull. Assoc. Am. Med. Coll., 1928, iii, 10–30.

tion method, Carrel kept a culture of fibroblasts growing for twelve years, and has observed the transformation of macrophages into cells resembling fibroblasts (1926). Transformation of mononuclears into macrophages and giant-cells has been studied *in extenso* by the Lewises (1925–7). In 1915–20 Margaret Lewis made an elaborate study of contraction of smooth and striated muscle-cells, the rapid pendulum movements in heart-muscle and other phenomena, showing that they take place in the protoplasm alone.

Recent **embryology** illustrates both sides of the shield in the footless controversy about vitalism: seeming triumph of the mechanists in the wonderful advance of genetics; triumph of the totipotency of protoplasm (Driesch) in studies of organization of growth and regulation of form. Here, facing the very beginnings of organized life, the vitalists are on their own ground and justified of their children.

That the dorsal lip of the blastopore is the center and starting point of cell differentiation and regulation of form in the embryo was first noted by **Warren Lewis** (1907). The discovery was elaborated by Brachet (1921) and Spemann (1923). Spemann showed that if a bit of this dorsal lip be implanted into another embryo (even of different species), it will engender a secondary embryo made up of cells of the implant and the host. Similar effects can be obtained by sectioning the original embryo above the blastopore and a transplant of indifferent tissue on to the dorsal lip will acquire organizing properties. Further experiments on the developing eye by Warren Lewis (1907), Spemann (1913), Fischel (1916), and Peterson (1923) go to show that it is an harmonic equipotential system, with the optic plate and optic vesicle as organizers. Removal of the optic plates by microsurgery results in no eyes. Transplants of a portion of the plate after rotation through 180 degrees result in four eyes. Bits of optic plate or vesicle can produce whole eyes (Lewis). Stockard produced cyclopia by immersion in magnesium salts, even to complete suppression of both eyes. Spemann got similar effects by constriction. The optic nerve is usually absent. Regulation of form in the eye is independent of the nervous system.

The œstrus or sexual cycle was studied in the guinea-pig by C. R. Stockard and Papanicolaou (1917), in the pig (1921) and the monkey (1923) by G. W. Corner, in the rat by Long and Evans (1923). The formation of the corpus luteum was studied by Aschoff and pupils. Parkes' work on the hormone œstrin (1926) shows that œstrus is independent of the corpus luteum. F. Hitschmann and Adler demonstrated the histological changes going on in the uterus throughout the menstrual cycle, Stockard and Papanicolaou those in the vagina (1917). Corner plotted the time relations of the œstrus cycle in the pig (1921) and showed the correspondences of the monkey cycle with that in man (1923). German war data show that human fertility is highest in the week after menstruation, falling gradually to virtual sterility in the week preceding menstruation (Fraenkel and Schroeder, 1914). Fertilization in the intermenstrual period is conditioned by irregular ovulation or survival of spermatozoa. Vaginal smears give no clue to events in the human cycle, although reliable in lower animals (Jessie King, 1926). The interstitial cells of the testes were first investigated by Franz Leydig (1850) and their secretions were held by Ancel and Bouin (1923) to maintain the secondary sexual characters in the absence of spermatogenesis. Astley Cooper believed that ligation of the vas deferens will not cause aspermatogenesis unless there is malposition of the testicle (1830), which was confirmed by Moore (1926). Rejuvenation by transplants of gonads, testes, or ovary into castrated or spayed animals was first essayed by E. Steinach (1920). The studies of intersexuality by Lillie (1917), Goldschmidt (1921) and others led to new views. In hibernating animals, proliferation of the Leydig cells occurs during the rutting season in the marmot, but not in the mole, and is relatively rare in man and rodents, whence the hormone of secondary sexuality may perhaps be sought in the Sertoli cells of the spermatogonia (Woollard[1]).

The fact that the intravital storage of a dye by a cell resembles phagocytosis (H. M. Evans, 1914–15), and the discovery of E. E. Goldmann that the Kupffer cells in the liver are the first to take up intravital stains, (1909) pointed the way into the **reticulo-endothelial system,** adumbrated by Ranvier (1900) and by Metchnikoff, in

---

[1] H. Woollard: Recent Advances in Anatomy, London, 1927.

1892–1901. Metchnikoff described phagocytosis in leukocytes in 1884, located the phagocytic function in the endothelial cells of blood-vessels (1892), the large mono-nuclears or "macrophages," the clasmatocytes (Ranvier), the lymphocytes and other fixed cells found in the spleen, lymph-nodes, connective tissue, neuroglia, and muscle-fiber, describing them as a "digestive system within the tissues" in virtue of their power to absorb red blood-cells, lepra bacilli or dust. To these he attributed the formation of agglutinins, coagulins, and virtual antibodies. Aschoff, who sub-sequently mapped out the system as reticular and endothelial (1913), regards this chapter in Metchnikoff as "the most significant in the whole conception of *defensio*, *i. e.*, the reactive processes of inflammation." The view that the system is endo-thelial and concerned in the production of antibodies was also stressed by H. M. Evans (1915). Kiyono studied the storage of carmine particles by these cells "from mammals to cyclostomes" (1914). The locus of the system was mapped out by Aschoff and Maximow, as made up of cells not necessarily identical in structure, but similar in function and staining reactions. Aschoff regards the histiocyte (macro-phage) as a scavenger, a major coefficient in the formation of granulation tissue, par-ticularly in tubercle, malarial spleen, leproma, kala azar, and an agent in immunity. Mallory and Maximow challenge the origin of these cells from fixed, specialized tissues, but their true interest is functional. Histiocytes change hemoglobin into bilirubin, and this bile-forming function is not confined to the liver cells (McNee, 1913–24), but can take place in the spleen, the bone-marrow, and connective tissues after exclusion of the liver (Whipple, 1913; Mann, 1924–25). These cells can form fibroblasts and change into giant or sarcoma cells, destroy blood-corpuscles, and remove any particles injected into the blood-stream within eighteen minutes. Their rôle in Banti's disease, Gaucher's disease, and glandular fever (mononucleosis) is a new chapter in pathology. The striking differences in the early development of the human ovum from that of any other species have been brought out in G. H. Teacher's implantation experiments (1925) and the study of the Miller ovum (1913), the youngest known human embryo, by George E. Streeter (1927), who has stressed the futility of interpreting the development of all animals in terms of the base-line embryology of the chick, the rabbit and the frog.

Of **physiology,** Huxley said that "its subject-matter is a large moiety of the universe—its position is midway between the physico-chemical and the social sciences"; its value as a discipline is largely "the training and strengthening of common sense." The merit of Jacques Loeb is that he adhered to this noble program and tried to interpret physiology in what Karl Pearson calls "the conceptual short-hand of physics and chemistry." Where he failed was where "mathematical deduction breaks down on the subtlety of Nature and physical induction on her imperceptibility," and here, as Lord Bacon said, "it is easier to evolve truth from error than from confusion." From LaMettrie's *L' Homme Machine* (1748) to Loeb's *The Organism as a Whole* (1916) or the *Living Machinery* (1927) of A. V. Hill, the materialistic hypothesis has served to clarify concepts and to obliterate childish mysticism. Stensen expressed its merits and defects when he said of Descartes that he did not pretend to expound the actual human body but "a machine capable of performing all its functions." Anything else is mere subjective speculation. In the General Physiology of Bayliss (4th ed., 1924), the subject is treated rigorously as a branch of dynamics, a science of "processes rather than structures," in accordance with the dictum of Jennings: "An animal is something that happens." This tendency is everywhere apparent in the physiology of the last quarter-century, and the only danger attaching to it is the merging of the subject into the physical sciences upon which it is based, in which case the physiologist ceases to think physiologically.

Beginning with the **circulation,** the immense amount of investigation of the blood alone has created an independent science of **hematology,** intimately associated with laboratory diagnosis and pathology.

The precursors were Nasse (1835), Andral (1843), Virchow (1845), Schultze (1852), Hayem (1882–89), Ehrlich (1885–98), Metchnikoff (1892). The leading later exponent was Arthur **Pappenheim** (1870–1916), author of *Morphologische Hæmatologie* (1910), and editor of *Folia Hæmatologia* (1904–16). Ehrlich (1898) classified the leukocytes; and stood out for the polyphyletic origin of the blood-corpuscles (from individual stem-cells) confirmed by Florence Sabin (1920–22), as against the monophyletic theory of Pappenheim (1898–1919), Maximow (1902–10), and Ferrata (1918) (from one mother cell). The mapping out of the recitulo-endothelial system by Aschoff and Landau (1913) and by Maximow (1924) is a phase of pathology. The relative volumes of corpuscles and plasma are estimated with the hematocrit of S. G. Hedin (1891). The surface and shape of the corpuscles have been investigated by Bürker (1922) and Gough (1924), the suspension stability (1921) and sedimentation rate of erythrocytes (1918–21) by Fahraeus; the ratio of hemoglobin content to surface area of erythrocytes by Bürker (1922), the causes of agglutination by Linzenmeier (1921). Carbon dioxide carriage is studied by the CO_2 dissociation curves of Christiansen, Douglas, and Haldane (1914[1]). Buffer salts and hydrogen-ion concentration were first investigated by S. P. L. Sørensen (1909). The methods for investigating pH include the formula of K. H. Hasselbalch (1910), the various indicator methods and the dialysis methods of Levy, Rowntree, and Marriott (1915), Dale and Evans (1920), and Cullen (1922). In the nomogram of L. J. Henderson (1921), the statics and dynamics of the blood are charted in a set of six dependent variables, from any two of which the remainder can be predetermined. The methods of estimating the work and output of the **heart** were devised by Adolf Fick (1882), Zuntz and Hagemann (1898), Krogh and Lindhard (1912), and for oxygen utilization by Christiansen *et al* (*supra* 1914), Yandell Henderson and Prince (1917), Barcroft *et al* (1921), Meakins and Davies (1922). Marey's views on regulation of the heart-rate were corrected by Anrep and Starling (1925). Regulation of stroke volume was investigated by Patterson and Starling (1914), regulation of venous return by August Krogh (1912), and others, and the efficiency of the heart by C. L. Evans and Matsuoka (1915–18). Starling's "Law of Heart," viz., the simultaneous increase of diastolic volume and arterial blood-pressure (output) is elucidated in his Linacre Lecture of 1918. The **capillary circulation** was first studied under the microscope by Leeuwenhoek (1686), latterly by Stricker (1865), Roy and Brown (1879), Langley (1911), Schäfer (1912), and Krogh (1919–22), and with the naked eye by Cotton *et al* (1917), Ebbecke (1917), Carrier (1922), Weiss (1923), and Sir Thomas Lewis (1923–4). The existence of the Rouget cells (1873–9) was confirmed by Vimtrup (1922). Heubner's capillary dilator poisons (1907) were studied by H. H. Dale, Laidlaw, and Richards (**histamine,** 1910–19), Krogh (urethane, 1920), and Burn (1922), reactions to stimuli by Hooker (1920), Bayliss (vasodilator supply, 1923) and Doi (1923), capillary pressure by Sir Leonard Hill (1920), with measurements in man by Carrier and Rehburg (1922). Krogh's dialyzing membranes (1919) are used in estimating permeability. The constrictor effect of adrenaline was demonstrated by Dale and Richards (1919), Krogh (1919) and Hooker (1920). A pituitary hormone is regarded as the activator of capillary tonus by Krogh (1920) and Lewis (1923–4), and adrenaline by Dale and Richards (1919). The rôle of the capillaries in urinary secretion is advanced by Richards and Schmidt (1922). The rôle of the capillaries in wound shock and traumatic toxemia, analogous to the effect of histamine (Dale and Laidlaw, 1919), which makes the heart "bleed into its own dilated capillaries" has been the work of Bayliss and Cannon (1918–19), M. N. Keith (1919), and Krogh (1922). The trend of recent thinking in regard to the heart's action is overwhelmingly in favor of the myogenic theory of Gaskell and Engelmann, which received its strongest support from embryology.

By 1883, Gaskell and Engelmann had proved that heart impulses are conducted by muscular pathways. In 1893, Wilhelm His, Jr. (1863–   ), and, a little earlier, Stanley Kent (1892–3), discovered a narrow band of muscle, an embryonic rest between the auricles and ventricles, now called the auriculoventricular bundle of His, which

---

[1] Christiansen [*et al.*]: Jour. Physiol., Lond., 1914, xlviii, 244–271.

acts as a bridge for contractile impulses, in accordance with Gaskell's theory that this phenomenon is due to the inherent contractility of cardiac muscles alone. Later, Arthur Keith and M. Flack (1907) discovered a tissue-rest of fine, pale, faintly striated fibers in the heart wall, supplied with arterioles and connected with the Purkinje fibers and nerve terminals, the so-called Keith-Flack or sino-auricular node, "the pacemaker of the heart" (Thomas Lewis, 1910–13). S. Tawara traced out the muscular ramifications from the His bundle (the ventricular basket-work of cells noted by Purkinje), and discovered another muscular (atrioventricular) node in close relation to it (1906–8). If the His bundle is destroyed in the dog, the contractile impulse will no longer pass from the auricle to the ventricles, and the latter will immediately assume their own autonomy, beating at a much slower rate, while the auricles, controlled by the vagus, will go on as before. This is the condition known as complete heart block or Stokes-Adams disease (1846) which His produced experimentally in 1895. At the Johns Hopkins Hospital, Erlanger, by means of a clamp compressing the His bundle, in the dog, thus blocking the auricular impulse, has, like Gaskell, produced two-time, three-time and four-time rhythms, finally passing into complete heart block. In 1910, E. B. Krumbhaar described a case of complete heart block entirely independent of lesion of the His bundle, and in 1917, impermanent types due to different causes. Further light upon the intimate pathology of cardiac disturbance was thrown by the string galvanometer invented by Willem **Einthoven** (1860–1927) of Leyden in 1902.[1] In 1878,[2] Burdon Sanderson and Page made the first records of the heart-beat with the capillary electrometer. Gaskell's galvanometer studies of the electrical condition of the heart followed in 1881–2. In 1885, Kölliker and H. Müller showed that the action currents of a contracting heart will contract the muscle of a muscle-nerve preparation, if the nerve of the latter be laid across the heart. In 1889,[3] Augustus D. Waller (1856–1922) conceived the idea of measuring and figuring the variation of the action currents in the living heart by leading them off through electrodes placed upon the moist skin, connected with a galvanometer, the curves being obtained by photographing the movements produced by the mercury of a Lippmann electrometer, which was first done by Marey (1876). Owing to the lag or inertia of the mercury meniscus, the curves in Waller's method were not true curves and had to be corrected by mathematical computations. The process was rendered accurate by the sensitive instrument of Einthoven, which consists essentially of an extremely delicate thread of platinum or of silver-coated quartz strung, like a violin-string, midway between the poles of a stationary electromagnet. This reverses the ordinary conditions in galvanometers, in which the magnet is movable and the measurable current passes through stationary coils. When the feeble heart currents pass through the delicate string, the deflections are smaller and shorter, or greater and longer in proportion to its state of tension. These deflections can be screened and photographed as pictures of cardiac excitation. Einthoven called them "electrocardiograms," or telegrams from the heart, in that they give an accurate bulletin of its electromotive condition. Although his instrument is expensive, it has been of material assistance in analyzing and even diagnosing such conditions as valvular disease, heart block, auricular fibrillation, paroxysmal tachycardia, pulsus alternans, pulsus bigeminus, three- and four-time gallops and other rhythmic changes.[4]

The pioneer in the graphic study of cardiac arrhythmias was Sir James **Mackenzie** (1853–1925), of Scone, Perthshire, an Edinburgh graduate of 1878, who first made simultaneous records of the arterial and venous pulses to elucidate the clinical condition of the heart; and by raising the question, "How much work can the heart do?" concentrated future investigation upon the energetics of heart-muscle (1893–94). After practising at Burnley for nearly thirty years (1879–1907), Mackenzie went

[1] Einthoven: K. Akad. v. Wetensch. te Amst. Proc. Sect. Sc., 1903–4, vi, 107–115, 2 pl.

[2] Sanderson and Page: Jour. Physiol., Lond., 1879–80, ii, 384: 1883–4, iv, 347.

[3] A. D. Waller: Phil. Tr., 1889, Lond., 1890, clxxx, B, 169–194.

[4] Some of these arrhythmias were implicit in Vieussen's original description of the irregular pulse in mitral stenosis (1685) and in Bouillaud's *delirium cordis* or *folie du cœur* (1835).

up to London as consultant (1907) and made his mark by his sincere, earnest attitude toward the sick and his sterling books on the pulse (1902), heart disease (1908), semeiology (1909), and angina pectoris (1923). He was knighted in 1915, retired from practice in 1918, and started an Institute for Clinical Research at St. Andrews (1919), to which he gave £10,000 in fees received up to his death. He was one of the greatest of modern bedside physicians, attracting patients from all over the world, and by a strange irony of fate, died of angina pectoris on January 26, 1925. Mackenzie first investigated the multiform arrhythmias, and differentiated "nodal rhythm" (1902–8), which Sir Thomas **Lewis** (1881–   ) defined as "auricular fibrillation" and identified with "pulsus irregularis perpetuus" (H. E. Hering, 1903), producing the con-

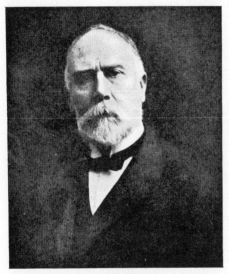

dition experimentally by sewing electrodes into the auricle of an animal (1909). Mackenzie also demonstrated the wonderful efficiency of digitalis in auricular fibrillation (1910), and the use of this drug is now interdicted in the sinus arrhythmias, heart-block, paroxysmal tachycardia, and the pulsus alternans of Traube (1872). Lewis has edited *Heart* (1909–27) and also described "auricular flutter" (1912), and the "effort syndrome" of the Western Front (D. A. H., 1918–19).

Sir James Mackenzie (1853–1925).

Cushny showed the value of the electrocardiogram in checking up the effects of digitalis, which apparently depresses the conductivity of the His bundle (1897–1917). Thus the view of Schmiedeberg, that digitalis not only slows the heart by vagal stimulation, but stimulates the cardiac muscle (1874), has given place to the older, classical view of Bouillaud, that, clinically, digitalis is a true "opium of the heart" (1835). Many other investigations have been made, and the new English periodical, *Heart* (London, 1909), was founded for such studies. In 1906, Einthoven laid wires between the Leyden Hospital and his laboratory and was able to take cardiac tracings from ward patients at a distance of more than a mile. Further, it has been found possible to obtain graphic figurations of the rhythm of the heart-sound (phonocardiograms) by means of a stethoscope and a Marey tambour, the receiver being a microphone or such devices as manometric flames, or the Weiss phonoscope, the receiver of which is a soap-bubble. These records can be placed in juxtaposition with curves of the carotid pulse for comparison. The electrical telephone-stethoscope of S. G. Brown intensifies the heart-sounds 60 times and by connecting this with the long-distance service, heart-sounds in London have been heard distinctly by physicians on the Isle of Wight, a distance of about 100 miles.[1]

---

[1] For a full account of these instruments, with illustrations, see the admirable résumé by Professor L. F. Barker, Johns Hopkins Hosp. Bull., Balt., 1910, xxi, 358–389.

The study of the mechanism of **tissue-oxidation** and its automatic activator (glutathione) is of recent vintage.

The jumping-off place was the classical paper of Sir Walter **Fletcher** and **Gowland Hopkins** showing the accumulation of lactic acid in the tissues (muscle) in the absence of oxygen (1907). This displaced the older theory of storage of available "intramolecular oxygen" in case of need. It was followed by Winterstein's paper on the quantitative relations of oxygen excess during recovery of tissues from anaërobism and the work of Fletcher and Brown on CO_2 production during the anaërobic period (1914). Oxygen-usage is estimated by the microrespirometers of Thunberg (1905) and Winterstein (1907). The discovery of ozone by C. F. Schönbein (1839) started the search for an activator of oxidation within the cell. Oxidation and reduction are reciprocal and reversible (Mansfield Clark, 1923–8). Oxygenase and peroxidase, the enzymes of autoxidation in plants, were discovered by Bach and Chodat (1903–4). The next steps were the isolation of **glutathione** (the philothion or protein hydride of De Rey Pailhade, 1888) in the pure state by Gowland Hopkins (1921), its exact formulation by his pupils (1923), and the synthesis of the racemic and optically active forms by Stewart and Tunnicliffe (1925). The discovery by Hopkins and Dixon of a residual substance in the tissues (Meyerhof, 1918), which promptly reduces glutathione as fast as it is oxidized (1922). established its rôle as a hydrogen acceptor and the probable chemical mechanism of autoxidation in the tissue cells, viz., tissue reduction of glutathione as fast as it is oxidized. The importance of cell-structure in oxidation was stressed by Otto **Warburg** (1914), and is illustrated by his "charcoal model" of cell respiration (1921–3), which turns upon the oxidation of amino-acid solutions when shaken with blood charcoal at room temperatures.

Since the nervous mechanism of the automatic regulation of breathing was elucidated by Hering and Breuer (1868), Head (1889), and Scott (1908), recent study of **respiration,** as the convection of oxygen from the air to the tissues from the lungs by the blood, has been transferred from the lungs to the blood and the tissues.

As indicated above, the older views of oxygen storage and "biogen molecules" have been discarded, for even in such anaërobes as intestinal worms, Spallanzani's snails, or the leech, which can live without oxygen for ten days, CO_2 is given off by methods all their own. Oxygen consumption has been estimated in all the tissues by Barcroft (1908–14), Rhode (1910–13), Evans (1912), Krogh (1919), and others. Oxygen consumption in the lungs has been found to be only $\frac{1}{2}$ the amount taken up by the salivary gland at rest; apart from the erythrocytes, that of the blood is minimal. The iron in the hemoglobin is the key to Warburg's charcoal model (1923). The Verworn view of narcosis as inhibition of oxidation (1912) is discarded. Mosso's acapnia (CO_2 deficiency) is discarded. Oxygen hunger does not affect CO_2 stimulation of the respiratory center until the lowest ebb. Animals may live for weeks with both vagi cut (Schaefer, 1919). The view of Bohr that the alveolar epithelium of the lungs may actively secrete oxygen at need (1909) as in the swimming bladder of fishes, was put to the test by Douglas, Haldane, Henderson, and Schneider on the summit of Pike's Peak, Colorado (1913). and subsequently by Barcroft on Cerro de Pasco (1914). The symptoms of oxygen hunger (mountain sickness) were those of monoxide poisoning and were ascribed by Barcroft to oxygen deficiency in the medulla. Haldane claimed that there is actual oxygen secretion under acclimatation, to make the oxygen tension of arterial blood higher than that of alveolar air. Experiments by Krogh (1910), Hartridge (1912), and Barcroft (1920), who lived six days in a glass box at low oxygen tension (84 mm.), showed no evidence on this point. The regulation of respiration by the CO_2 concentration in arterial blood (i. e., rise = hyperpnea; fall = dyspnea → apnea) was shown by **Haldane** and **Priestley** (1905[1]). That this in turn depends upon hydrogen-ion concentration of the blood was shown. by Winterstein (1911) and Hasselbalch (1912). The various appratus employed in establishing the chemical regulation of respiration were devised by Haldane (1892–1918), Winterstein (1912), and Barcroft (1914).

---

[1] Haldane and Priestley: Jour. Physiol., Lond., 1905, xxxii, 224–266.

44

In the 19th century, the only important contributions to the thermodynamics of **muscular contraction** were those of Helmholtz (1847–8) and Fick (1882) on heat production in muscle.

The suggestion of Gad that contraction is associated with lactic acid formation (1893) was brilliantly demonstrated by Fletcher and Hopkins (1907), and Fletcher had previously shown that the CO_2 output of excised muscle is accelerated by stimulation and onset of rigor mortis and increased in a bath of oxygen (1902[1]). The problem was to show that muscle is a machine for converting chemical energy into mechanical work. The chemical changes in resting and contracting muscle were investigated by Embden and Laquer (lactacidogen, 1914), Meyerhof (1919–23), Krogh and Lindhard (1920). The view that liberation of phosphoric acid accompanies the lactic, producing colloidal swelling under contraction is held by the Frankfort School (Embden, 1913–25), but not generally accepted. The rôle of co-enzymes (Bertrand, 1897) as activators of aërobic and anaërobic muscle, of carbohydrates as sources of lactic-acid formation and contraction (Meyerhof and Himwich, 1924), of fats as a source of fatigue Krogh and Lindhard 1920) are phases of recent work. The potential energy set free and the realizable work are comparable with the intrinsic and available energy of thermodynamic systems. The mechanism has been likened to work done against a stretched spring (Fick, 1882), the lifting of an anchor by a chain and windlass (Fenn, 1923), or by an India-rubber cord about a windlass (Evans, 1925). The realizable work is measured by Fick's *Arbeitsammler* (1882), Blix's muscle indicator diagram (1891), Hill's inertia lever (1920), and inertia flywheel (1922) for maximum work and the bicycle ergometers of Atwater and Benedict (1904), Krogh (1913), and Cathcart (1923). Estimates of heat production by the thermopiles of Hill (1920) and Fenn (1923), have been made by Hill (1911–26), Fenn (1923–24), Slater (1923), and Gasser (1924). The isometric twitch (without shortening) was investigated by Hartree and Hill (1920–24), Sherrington (1921), Adrian (1922), and others; chronaxia or duration of excitation (L. Lapicque, 1909) by L. and M. Lapicque (1909–25). That muscle gives all-or-none responses was demonstrated by Keith-Lucas (1909) and F. H. Pratt (1917–19).

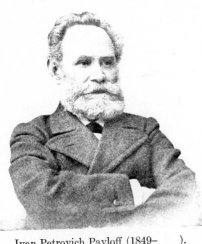

Ivan Petrovich Pavloff (1849–   ).

During the last forty years, a large number of Russian dissertations bearing upon digestion appeared, mainly by pupils of **Pavloff,** who did the most important work of his time, both upon digestion and the science of **conditional reflexes.**

Ivan Petrovich **Pavloff** (1849–   ), the son of a Russian priest, of the Ryazan government, was a pupil of Heidenhain and Ludwig, became director of the Institute for Experimental Medicine at Leningrad (1890), and in 1904 received the Nobel prize for his investigations. The success of Pavloff's early experiments was due to his remarkable skill in operating on laboratory animals. A brilliant, ambidextrous surgeon in his methods of producing gastric and pancreatic fistulæ,

[1] Fletcher: Jour. Physiol., Lond., 1902, xxviii, 474: 1907, xxxv, 247.

the ultimate tendency of his work was, at first, not clearly sensed, as he was concerned mainly with the digestive system.

As early as 1852, Bidder and Schmidt had reported that the sight of food will produce a copious flow of gastric juice in a gastrostomized dog, and Richet (1878) had obtained a similar effect in a patient who had to be fed through a gastric fistula, on account of a strictured esophagus. Heidenhain failed to obtain this result in a fistulized dog, whence it was inferred that he had in some way damaged the nerve connections in preparing his fistula (1880). Pàvloff improved the Heidenhain fistula by keeping the nerve-supply intact, and so standardized it for modern procedure. In addition, he severed the dog's esophagus in such wise that swallowed food might be discharged at the upper opening, and unswallowed food ingested into the stomach at the lower. Three sets of experiments were then possible: The dog might be allowed merely to see or smell the food, a Barmecide feast which Pavloff called "psychical feeding"; or, the animal might chew the food which passed through the esophageal opening, constituting a sham meal; or, a true feeding might be obtained by introducing the food through the lower stoma of the esophagus. In the first two instances, the effect of smell, sight, taste, chewing, and swallowing was such that a copious and continual gastric secretion—as much as 700 c.c. in five or six hours— was obtained without the introduction of any food into the stomach. Pavloff called this effect a "psychical secretion." He next showed that severing the splanchnic nerves does not affect the phenomenon, but section of both vagi will abolish the reflex secretion, and direct stimulation of the peripheral ends of the cut vagi will, after a short interval, revive it. This proved that the gastric secretion is regulated by the vagus. Under the third condition, mere mechanical stimulation of the stomach by the introduction of food through the esophageal opening, while the dog is asleep or inattentive, does not necessarily stimulate secretion, contrary to received opinion. Chischin, Pavloff's pupil, found that, when the psychical stimuli are shut off in this way, the amount of secretion varies with the kind of food, being positive for meats and peptones generally, and negative for other substances, which, when eaten, might cause a psychical secretion (1894[1]). By means of a special pancreatic fistula, Pavloff was able to indicate that the secretory fibers of the pancreas are in the vagus nerve. In 1895, Dolinsky found that the introduction of acids into the duodenum causes a flow of pancreatic juice, from which it is inferred that the acid in the gastric juice sets up this secretion, probably through the production of the hormone which Bayliss and Starling call secretin (1902). Chepovalnikoff, another Pavloff pupil, discovered that pancreatic juice from a fistula acquires a powerful solvent action on proteids from contact with the duodenal membrane or its extract, and the latter Pavloff assumed to contain a special enzyme, "enterokinase," which activates the pancreatic juice (1899[2]). While these researches, summed up in Pavloff's book on *The Work of the Digestive Glands* (1900), are the most important contributions to the physiology of digestion in our time, they merely led up to more important studies in a terrain hitherto unexplored, viz., the functioning of the higher centers of the brain. It had been noticed that, in a spinal (decerebrated) animal, responses to stimuli are always predictable, while in normal animals they are uncertain, sometimes negative or even evoked by no apparent stimuli. Pavloff called the ordinary inherited reflexes (the vague "instincts" of the biologist) *unconditional* and such acquired responses as those of the burnt child or the beaten dog *conditional*. From his experiments, he reasoned that to stimulate a receptor organ, simultaneously with reflex stimulation of an effector, may induce a new reflex. In choosing the parotid of the dog as being an isolated organ with a single response, he revealed his genius for thinking physiologically, for with this step there was an end of subjective readings of cerebration, deriving from the mind of the investigator. Pavloff likened his hungry dog to a telephone exchange (1910), and got salivary responses *via* a smell, the ringing of a bell, quarter-tones on a violin, reaction to pain, discrimination between metronome beats under or over 100 per minute, detection of differences of $\frac{1}{8}$ of a tone and audition of sound vibrations up to 120,000 per second. In 1907, his pupil, Krasnogorsky, discovered conditional reflexes in infants. These were followed up by J. B. Watson (1916), who developed the behavioristic psychology. In 1911, Protopopoff produced the knee-jerk as a conditioned reflex from a light stimulus alone. Experiments in mice indicate that predisposition to particular condi-

---

[1] Chischin: St. Petersburg dissertation, 1894.

[2] N. P. Chepovalnikoff: St. Petersburg dissertation, 1899.

tioned reflexes may be inherited.   The effects of inhibitions, combined reflexes, and
other aspects of this great work will be found in Pavloff's treatises of 1912 and 1923.[1]
In 1911, he acquired the Reflex Tower at Leningrad, a laboratory in which the experimenter can be isolated from his animal, and both from the outside world.   Of
Pavloff's recent pupils, the most remarkable is Leon A. **Orbeli** who, with his pupil,
A. G. Ginetsinsky (1922), has shown that contrary to the view of Langley, the sympathetic nervous system exerts a definite influence upon skeletal muscle (1923–4)
such as hastening the recovery of tetanized muscle, production of a tonomotor effect
upon the muscle of the tongue *via* the lingual nerve, effects of efferent sympathetic
fibers on the spinal reflexes (1925) and other phases of an adaptive regulatory function.   Paralyses produced by stimulation of the lower end of the sympathetic trunk
were first noted by Pavloff (1920) and attributed to the existence of special trophic
nerves, which he believes to control all organs and tissues.   Such nerves had been surmised by clinicians, but were never demonstrated before Pavloff.   A. D. Speransky has
shown the effects of freezing the brain, with a method of immunization against it,
also the fact that toxins of disease can enter the brain from the blood by the cerebrospinal fluid, while the antitoxins cannot pass the barrier between the brain and the
blood either way (1925).

Recent knowledge of **postural reflexes** started with Sherrington's
observations of decerebrate rigidity (1898–1915) and is contained largely
in the monumental *Körperstellung* (Berlin, 1924) of Rudolf **Magnus**
(1872–1927), late professor of pharmacology at Utrecht.

This includes exhaustive experimental consideration of static reflexes
(pose and righting of the body) and the stato-kinetic reactions to rotation, progressive and partial movements.   The effects of unilateral and
bilateral labyrinthectomy are found to correspond with the clinical
data of otology and neurology, as also the behavior in decerebrate
rigidity with intact labyrinth, medulla or thalamus (thalamus-animal).
As Sherrington showed (1898), the cerebellum plays no part in postural
reflexes, which have been allocated to the red nucleus and Deiters'
nucleus.   The mechanism of tonus was allocated to the sympathetic
nerve supply by Boeke (1913) and by Hunter and Royle (experimental
ramisectomy, 1924–5) but surgical applications of the latter procedure
have not been uniformly successful.

The physiology of **nutrition and metabolism** has attained a going
stride in the 20th century.

The starting point of recent knowledge of the **vitamins** or accessory food factors was an experiment of N. Lunin in Bunge's laboratory, showing that a synthetic
milk diet lacks an unknown factor necessary for growth in animals (1880), which
was confirmed by Gowland Hopkin's proof of the beneficial effect of a minute quantity of fresh milk upon an artificial growth-inhibiting diet in rats (1912).   In 1882–6,
Takaki eradicated beriberi from the Japanese Navy by an improved mixed diet,
which led to the experiments of C. Eijkman and Grijns on the effect of a monotone
diet in producing avian beriberi (polyneuritis), and their discovery of an antineurotic
substance in rice-husks and beans (1897–1906).   In 1907, Fraser and Stanton treated
experimental polyneuritis successfully with alcoholic extract of rice polishings.   In
1904, Abderhalden and Rona showed that casein predigested by pepsin or H_2SO_4
will inhibit growth in a casein-sugar diet in mice, while Ethel Wilcock and Hopkins
showed that inhibition of growth in a zein (gliadin) diet is due to lack of lysin and
tryptophan (1907), which latter was destroyed by acid digestion of casein in Abderhalden's initial experiment (1904).   The experiments of Henriques and Hansen on
the ill-effects of a gliadin diet (1905) were explained in the same way.   Similar results were obtained in cattle-fodder by E. V. McCollum, Steenbock and others (1911).
In 1912, Osborne and Mendel showed that rats can live 530 days on protein-free

---

[1] I. P. Pavlov: Conditioned Reflexes, Transl. by G. V. Anrep, Oxford, 1927.

milk and gliadin, but cannot grow for lack of glycin and lysin. Similar results in stopping growth were obtained by experimental deficiency of tyrosin and phenyl-analin (Abderhalden, 1913), cystin (Osborne and Mendel, 1915), arginin and histidin (Ackroyd and Hopkins, 1916), and prolin (Barnett Sure, 1925). Meanwhile, Casimir Funk had introduced the term "vitamine" to denote the missing accessory factor in the polished rice production of beriberi (1911), attempted to isolate it from the pericarp and postulated vitamin deficiency for beriberi, scurvy, pellagra, and rickets. In 1913–16 McCollum, Davis, and Kennedy located a growth-producing substance in butter-fat and eggs (fat-soluble vitamin A) and a water-soluble vitamin B as the missing (antineuritic) factor in a beriberi-producing diet.[1] A water-soluble vitamin C was postulated by Holst and Frölich for the missing factor in diets producing scurvy (1913). A. F. Hess showed it to be abundant in citrus fruits and tomatoes (1914–18). Experimental rickets by dietetic deficiency was produced in puppies by Leonard Findlay (1908), in rats by McCollum and Simmonds (1917), with marked improvement on the addition of cod-liver oil (E. Mellanby, 1919), a phosphorus salt (Sherman and Pappenheimer, 1920), exposure to sunlight (Hess, 1921) or irradiation of food with ultraviolet light (Steenbock and Black, 1924). The effect of the cod-liver oil on deposition of calcium on the bones and increase of phosphorus in the blood was shown by Howland and Park (1920), affording an x-ray check on the new treatment. That the missing vitamin was not vitamin A was shown by Hopkins' initial experiment of destroying the growth-producing power of a heated fat by passage of oxygen through it (1920) and Zucker's production of a concentrated antirachitic derivative of cod-liver oil, free from vitamin A (1921). Cholesterin, the antirachitic substance extracted from cod-liver oil by Windaus (1917), was therefore denominated vitamin D. In 1925, Hess and Weinstock (in May) simultaneously with Steenbock and Black (June) showed that the substance which acquires antirachitic properties upon irradiation is cholesterol (in animal products) or phytosterol (in plants). In a sense, vitamin D is, therefore, an effect of irradiation. A fat-soluble vitamin E, allocated to reproductive power and sterility, was postulated in wheat-germ and lettuce leaves by Evans and Bishop (1922–3). The present classification of vitamins is tentative and perhaps artificial for, as Friedrich Müller observes, deficiency of calcium, magnesium, iron or iodine is as definite in its effects as deficiency of amino-acids or of irradiated cholesterol. Thus as indicated by the remarkable dietetic experiments of Goldberger (1915–20), and those of Chick and Hume on zein feeding in monkeys (1920), pellagra and hunger edema may be due to deficiency of tryptophan and lysin (Wilson, 1921), yet both pellagra and ergotism have been attributed to latent or superimposed infection by McCollum, Crookshank and others, with the dietetic deficiency as a predisposing factor. The principal gain has been to emphasize the importance of the protective balanced diet of milk, eggs, fresh fruits, citrus, and leafy vegetables recommended by McCollum, McCarrison, and others. The inhibitory effect of starvation and over-feeding upon the gonads and sexual capacity was investigated by H. Stieve (1922–6[2]).

Recent advances in knowledge of the **metabolism of proteins** are associated with the work of Emil Fischer on the hydrolysis of their amino-acid constituents (1899–1906), Schröder (1882–5), Van Slyke and Myer (1913) on conversion of proteids into urea by NH_2 uptake (de-amination) in the liver or the tissues (Folin and Denis, 1912) and their "specific dynamic action" as energizers and heat-producers (Rubner, 1902). The limited power of the liver to reproduce amino-acids from ingested hydroxy-acids was shown by Embden and Smitz (1910–12), Knoop and Kertess (1911). In 1902 Otto Loewi showed that intact proteins in the food are not requisite for protein synthesis (growth), which disposes of the Voit-Pflüger controversy as to their supposed conversion into protoplasm. **Nitrogen metabolism,** as an expression of wear and tear in the tissues (nitrogen-increase) from muscular work, implies increase of uric acid (Hamill and Schryer, 1906), purins (M'Leod, 1899, Burian, 1905) and creatin (Brown and Cathcart, 1909–21), but this obtains only on excessive exertion, as shown by the urine of Marathon runners (Higgins and Benedict, 1911). In **carbohydrate metabolism** the work of Emil Fischer on the purins (1882–1906) and sugars (1884–1919) again looms large. The changes of substance involved in the ultimate production of CO_2 and water from sugar were

---

[1] For the dual nature of vitamin B, its heat-labile (antineuritic) and heat-stable (antipellagric) components, see S. L. Smith: Science, N. Y., 1918, n. s., lxvii, 494–496.

[2] H. Stieve: Die Unfruchtbarkeit als Folge unnatürlicher Lebensweise, München, 1926.

elucidated by Gustav Embden (1912–13), H. D. Dakin (1913) and their co-workers, and by Laquer and Myer (1923). The rôle of carbohydrates as protein-sparers and sources of muscular energy was shown even in starvation by Cathcart (1909). The discovery of insulin by Banting and Best (1922) threw new light on metabolism in diabetes. The undecipherable nature of pentose is indicated by some nine different views as to the nature of the pentose in the urine by fifteen observers. Metabolism of fat (synthesis from carbohydrates and storage) was investigated by Lebedev (1882) and Ida Smedley (1912–13); the rôle of lipoids in the cell membrane by E. Overton (1899), J. Loeb (1909), and Loewe (1912); hydrolysis of ingested fat in the stomach by Volhard (1900) and Willstätter (1924); catabolism of fats by Knoóp (1905), Embden (1906–8), Dakin (1908–23), and Leathes (1923–25); fat synthesis from proteins by Weinland (1908), Atkinson, Rappaport, and Lusk (1922). The known physiological fats were classified as lipids by Bloor (1925). The reversibility of lipase was demonstrated by Joseph H. Kastle and Arthur S. Loevenhart (1900) and confirmed by Armstrong and Gosney (1914–15). Nucleic acid metabolism was investigated by Levene (1912–25) and Jones (1923–25); purin metabolism by Hunter and Givens (1914), S. R. Benedict (Dalmatian coach-dog, 1916), Ackroyd and Hopkins (1916), Rose and Cox (1924–26). The apparatus for gasometry of the blood in common use are those of J. S. Haldane (1892–1918), with the gas-bag of C. J. Douglas (1911) and the portable respiration calorimeters of F. G. Benedict (1918) and others. The colorimetric methods of blood analysis were devised by Otto Folin and Wu (1919–22). Blood-sugar is estimated by Calvert's method (1924), blood-cholesterol by that of Myers and Wardell (1918), blood-urea by the non-colorimetric methods of Van Slyke and Cullen (1914) and Maclean (1921), who also devised similar ways of estimating blood-sugar (1919) and non-protein nitrogen (1921). Residual nitrogen was estimated by Bang (1915) and others; calcium-content (serum) by Kramer and Tisdall (1921–23) and the phosphate-content by Wesselow (1924) and others. Analysis of proteins by acid hydrolysis is effected by the methods of Emil Fischer (esterification, 1899–1906), Foreman (lime-alcohol, 1914; lead-salt method, 1919), Dakin (butyl alcohol extraction, 1918), Kingston and Schryver (carbamate method, 1924). Analysis by estimation of nitrogen partition was perfected by Donald Van Slyke (1911). The calorimetric tests for proteins were devised by Millon (1849), Ehrlich (diazo-reaction, 1883), Molisch (α-naphthol test, 1886–7), Salkowski (xanthoproteic test, 1888), Schiff (biuret test, 1896), Hopkins and Cole (glyoxylic reaction, 1901), Voisenet (HCl-NO₂ reaction, 1905), Rosenheim (formaldehyde test, 1906), Ruhemann (ninhydrin test, 1910) and Romieu (phosphoric acid reaction, 1925). Amino-nitrogen is estimated by the methods and apparatus of Donald Van Slyke (1911–15); amino-acids by the methods of Benedict (1909), Denis (1910), Van Slyke (1911), Folin and co-workers (1912–22).

The new science of endocrinology, although rooted in the prehistoric past, is virtually a creation of the 20th century.

In 1902, Sir William Maddock Bayliss (1860–1924) and Ernest H. Starling announced to the Royal Society that the secretion of pancreatic juice which is caused by introduction of acid into the duodenum is not a local reflex, but is produced by a substance (secretin) thrown out from the intestinal mucous membrane under the influence of the acid and carried thence by the blood-stream to the glands, as shown by experiment. Pavloff subsequently discovered enterokinase (1899) and Bayliss and Starling developed their theory of the chemical control of the body by means of "hormones" or chemical messengers, which pass from the organs and glands by the blood-channels to other parts of the body. This theory had already been adumbrated by Bordeu, was inherent in Darwin's "pangenesis," and seems admirably adapted to explain the many clinical phenomena produced by disturbances of the ductless glands, and the general theory of treatment by animal extracts. In 1903, Charles E. de M. Sajous (1852–   ), of Philadelphia, published a system of medicine based upon the internal secretions, in which the suprarenal, pituitary, and thyroid bodies are held to control the immunizing mechanism of the body. The old notion of "diathetic diseases" is now yielding to the concept of altered metabolism, much of which may be bound up with some *bouleversement* of hormonic equilibrium or some disturbance of function in the ductless glands. Operative surgery has played the most important part in working out the physiology and pathology of these glands, a branch of internal medicine which has, indeed, been almost entirely developed by scientific experimentation.

The starting-point of the doctrine of internal secretions was Claude Bernard's work on the glycogenic function (1848–57) and Addison's account of disease of the suprarenal capsules (1849–55). The former was thrown into striking relief through von Mering and Minkowski's experimental production of diabetes by excision of the pancreas (1889) and the later studies of E. L. Opie (1901), Ssoboleff (1902), and W. G. MacCallum (1909), showing that the presumable sources of this pancreatic glycosuria is in the islands of Langerhans. Addison's description of the suprarenal syndrome led Brown-Séquard to excise the adrenals in 1856, reproducing fatal symptoms resembling Addison's disease, and his result was repeatedly confirmed by Tizzoni (1886–89), Abelous and Langlois (1891–93), Schäfer, and others. In 1894–95, Oliver and Schäfer found that injection of the watery extract of the suprarenal gland into the blood produced marked slowing of the heart and rise of blood-pressure. The active principle was obtained in crystalline form by Jokichi Takamine in 1901. The description of hyperthyroidism or exophthalmic goiter by Parry (1786), Graves (1835), and Basedow (1840), and of hypothyroidism or myxedema by Curling (1850), Gull (1875) and Ord (1877) emphasized the mysterious importance of the thyroid gland, which was excised with fatal results (in the dog) by the Geneva physiologist, Moritz Schiff, in 1856. In 1882, Reverdin of Geneva produced experimental myxedema by total or partial thyroidectomy and, in 1883, Theodor Kocher of Bern reported that 30 out of 100 thyroidectomies were followed by a "cachexia strumipriva." In 1884, Schiff produced 60 cases of fatal excision in dogs, and pointed out that the animals could be saved by a previous graft of part of the glands, which led Murray (1891) and Howitz (1892) to the treatment of myxedema with thyroid extract, with very successful results. Horsley's observations on monkeys and the collective investigations of Sir Felix Semon showed that cretinism, myxedema, and cachexia thyreo-strumipriva are one and the same. The part played by the internal secretion was first pointed out by Schiff, and the isolation of iodothyrin by Baumann, in 1896, indicated its relation to iodine metabolism. In 1905, Erwin Payr transplanted a bit of thyroid from a woman to the spleen of her myxedematous daughter, with successful result. Thyroxin, isolated by E. C. Kendall (1914), is a stirring activator of metabolism and probably the hormone of the gland. It was formulated as $C_{11}H_{19}O_3NI_3$ by Kendall and Osterberg (1919). The synthetic product (Harington, 1925) has no effect on basal metabolism. The parathyroid glands were described by Ivar Sandström in 1880 and, in 1891, Eugène Gley showed that negative thyroidectomies in certain animals would be rendered speedily fatal if the four parathyroids were also removed. This was confirmed by Vassale and Generali (1896). Transplantation of the parathyroids was then essayed by von Eiselsberg (1892), Leischner (1907), and W. S. Halsted (1909), and it was shown that tetany will be produced if a transplanted gland is removed and *per contra* that the tetanic spasms will disappear after injecting the saline extract of the gland or after parathyroid feeding or transplantation. Halsted, in 1906, treated tetany successfully by administration of the parathyroids of beeves. In 1908, W. G. MacCallum and C. Voegtlin showed that exhibition of calcium salts will remove tetany, even in man, which seems to connect the parathyroids with calcium metabolism. A parathyroid hormone was isolated by I. B. Collip in 1926. The function of the thymus gland was first investigated by Friedleben (1858), but the effects of its excision or of the injection of its extracts are still obscure. Felix Platter (1614) and Kopp (1830) described early cases of thymus death in infants. The status lymphaticus was first sketched out by Richard Bright (1838) and more fully described by Paltauf (1889). Henderson got retarded atrophy of the gland on castration (1904), and Paton found that thymectomy increases the growth of the testes. The first experiment in physiological surgery upon human beings was made by the gynecologist, Robert Battey, who excised the normal healthy ovaries for the relief of neurotic and non-menstruating women (1872). The rationale of this operation, in relation to a supposed internal secretion from a specialized set of ovarian cells, has since been justified in many remarkable ways, particularly in osteomalacia and by the experiments of Starling and Lane-Claypon, which show that section of the mammary nerves or of the spinal cord in rabbits does not produce the inhibitory effect of Battey's operation upon pregnancy or lactation. The relation of the Leydig cells in the testis to internal secretion is *sub judice*, the most significant experiments so far being those of Brown-Séquard (1898–91) and Poehl (1896–7) upon the injection of testicular extracts. In the last thirty years, attention has centered upon the pituitary body. Fatal excisions of the gland in animals had been made by Marinesco (1892), Vassale and Secchi (1894), and others, but Nicholas Paulesco of Bucharest was the first to point out that removal of the anterior lobe is fatal and removal of the posterior lobe negative (1908). Meanwhile Mohr had described obesity with pituitary tumor (1840), Pierre Marie had shown the relation of the pituitary to acromegaly (macrosomia) and gigantism (1886), Fröhlich described pituitary tumor with obesity and sexual infantilism (1901), and Harvey Cushing and his associates at the Johns Hopkins Hospital actually produced an experimental pathologic reversion to the Fröhlich syndrome by partial excision of the anterior lobe in adult dogs (1908). Simmonds described pituitary dwarfism (anterior lobe deficiency 1914–18), Hutchinson and Gilford, progeria (1904), and H. M. Evans showed the effect of anterior lobe extract upon interruption or prevention of the œstrus. Cushing has shown that the anterior lobe secretion influences normal growth and sexual development, while the posterior lobe has to do with metabolism of carbohydrates and fats, the high tolerance of sugars in posterior lobe insufficiency yielding to treatment with pituitary extract. Cushing and his pupils have also shown the relation of the hypophysis to diabetes insipidus (1912) and hibernation (1913). Cushing visualizes the pituitary as conductor of the endocrine orchestra and notes that the Röntgen ray and the rat have done most for it. That the internal secretions control the configuration of the body and are the activators of emotion is emphasized in the writings of W. B. Cannon (1914–16), G. W. Crile (1915), L. F. Barker, and others.

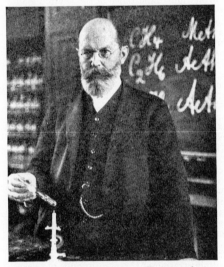

Popular treatises, professing to diagnose character in prominent persons from endocrine data, after the manner of phrenologists or of fortune-tellers' books, have tended to damage the theory latterly.

The doctrine of the correlation of the different internal secretions has been especially emphasized by the Viennese clinicians, Hans Eppinger, W. Falta, and C. Rüdinger (1908–9). Eppinger and Leo Hess[1] have also applied the ideas of Gaskell, Langley, and Sherrington as to the opposing functions of the two "autonomics" of the sympathetic system in the elucidation of the complex mechanism of physiological equilibrium and of visceral neurology (1910). They postulate two opposing diathetic conditions, vagotonus and sympathicotonus, described in 1892 by S. Solis Cohen as "vaso-motor ataxia," the semeiology of which can be thrown into relief by certain pharmacodynamic tests. These have been likened to "tuning keys by means of which we can operate upon the complicated stringed instrument of the body, and voluntarily make one string tighter to increase its vibrations, or another looser to dampen its function."[2] Eppinger and Hess also assume that the pancreas secretes a hormone, "autonomin," which antagonizes adrenalin, the hormone governing the sympathetic autonomic. While much of this is in dispute, it seems probable that the chemical hormones act *via* the blood upon the central nervous system, while the two opposing autonomics of the sympathetic system control the ductless glands and the visceral organs made up of smooth (involuntary) muscle.

Emil Fischer (1852–1919). (From a photograph in the Surgeon-General's Library.)

The most eminent physiological chemist of recent times was **Emil Fischer** (1852–1919), of Euskirchen, Rhenish Prussia, who was successively professor of chemistry at Munich (1879), Erlangen (1882), Würzburg (1885), and Berlin (1892).

Fischer discovered, isolated and formulated a host of new substances, such as phenylhydrazin (1875), which Abderhalden calls "the pathfinder of carbohydrate

---

[1] Eppinger and Hess: Die Vagotonie, Berlin, 1910.

[2] Januschke: Cited by L. F. Barker.

chemistry," the aliphatic hydrazins (1875–77), mannose, isomaltose, and the synthetic drugs veronal (1902), proponal (1905), saiodin (1905), and elarson (1913). He made vast researches in the synthesis of the purin compounds, including caffein, xanthin, theobromine (1879–1906); and developed a "family tree" of gout, demonstrating the purin nucleus as a sort of germ-plasm common to all the metabolic products of the disease. He synthetized and supplied structural formulæ for most of the sugar groups (1883–1919), including the six hexoses derived from mannitol, a hexose from formaldehyde, and fourteen out of the sixteen possible isomeric aldohexoses predicted by van't Hoff and Le Bel; and, in his studies of the polypeptides (1899–1906[1]), he linked together great chains of amino-acid substances (eventually 18 in all), to form these compounds, which are essential parts of the different protein molecules.

Fischer devised quantitative methods for isolating amino-acids, and demonstrated an amido (NH_2) nucleus common to all the proteins. His investigations of the enzymes (1884–1919) show that they are specific in action (1894–5), affecting only certain chemical substances, to which, as he puts it, they are related as a key to a lock or a glove to a hand, an analogy which Ehrlich cleverly applied in his side-chain theory. A brilliant stroke of genius was Fischer's deliberate attempt to produce a reliable hypnotic, ending in the synthesis of veronal (1904[2]). His last researches covered the depsides and tannin substances. During the war, he displayed phenomenal energy in furthering the manufacture of synthetic substitutes for nitrogenous products, animal fats and food-

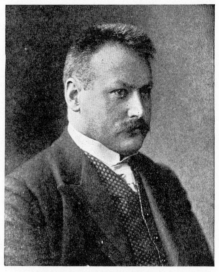

Emil Abderhalden (1877–   ).

stuffs. No chemist of modern times better deserved the honor of the Nobel prize, which he received in 1902.

Emil **Abderhalden** (1877–   ), of St. Gall, Switzerland, a pupil of Bunge and Emil Fischer and professor of physiology at Berne (1908) and Halle (1911), is the author of a bibliography of alcoholism (1897) and a text-book of physiological chemistry (1908). He edited a Handbook of Biochemic Technic (1909–10[3]), to which he added many new procedures, another great Handbook of Methods in Biological Investigation (1921–27[4]), of which 24 volumes have been published, a

---

[1] Fischer: Untersuchungen über Aminosäuren, Polypeptide und Proteine, Berlin, 1906.   [2] Fischer: Therap. d. Gegenwart, Berl., 1904, xlv, 145.

[3] Abderhalden: Handbuch der biochemischen Arbeitsmethoden, 4 v., Berlin and Vienna, 1910.

[4] Abderhalden: Handbuch der biologischen Arbeitsmethoden 24 v., Berlin and Vienna, 1921–27.

Biochemical Dictionary (1911), a book on nutrition (1917) and a text-book of physiology (1924). He has made a vast number of investigations of metabolism and food-stuffs, adopting Carl Ludwig's method of publishing his researches in collaboration with his many pupils. His special fields are the integration and disintegration of albuminoids and nucleic acids in the animal body, the protective ferments (1909–12), the metabolism of the cell (1911), the synthesis of its *Bausteine* (1912), and the synthesis of artificial food-stuffs, as tried out experimentally upon animals. In 1916 (with Fodor), he surpassed Emil Fischer by building up a polypeptide containing 19 amino-acids. He holds that the individual cells of animal and vegetable foods are made up of a number of chemical or phasic units which, in digestion and metabolism, are split up and transformed into other substances, to be assimilated by the body cells, according to their needs. In studying the protective ferments of the animal body Abderhalden evolved a biochemical test for pregnancy and other conditions by a ferment reaction (1912[1]). His contributions to the technic and methodology of biochemistry are of vast extent.

Among the outstanding biochemists and metabolists of recent times are: In Germany, Gustav **Embden** (1874–   ), of Hamburg, known for his work on the metabolism of fats (1906–8) and carbohydrates (1910–13), amino-acid synthesis in the liver (1910), lactic acid formation (1912) and lactacidogen (1914); Otto **Meyerhof** (1884–   ), of Hannover (chemistry of cell and muscle, 1912–24); Rudolf **Hoeber** (1873–   ), of Stettin (physical chemistry of cell and tissues, 1909–22); Otto **Warburg** (1883–   ), of Freiburg (cell and tissue respiration, 1908–24; charcoal model 1921–3; anaërobic metabolism in cancer, 1923–24); Richard **Willstätter** (1872–   ), of Carlsruhe (chlorophyll, 1913; enzymes, 1918–24); Adolf **Windaus** (1876–   ), of Göttingen (constitution of cholesterol, 1904–23); Nathanael **Pringsheim** (chlorophyll 1874–9); in England, Sir Gowland **Hopkins** (glutathione, 1921); Henry Edward **Armstrong** (enzymes, 1910–14); and, in America, Henry Drysdale **Dakin** (1880–   ), of London (carbohydrate metabolism, 1912; antiseptics, 1917; oxidations and reductions, 1922); Francis Gano **Benedict** (1870–   ), of Milwaukee (metabolism during inanition [1907], work [1909–13], rest [1910], fasting [1915], walking [1915], in diabetes [1910–12] and in infancy [1915]); Otto **Folin** (1867), of Atheda, Sweden, professor of biological chemistry at Harvard (1907), author of the well-known method of estimating creatin and creatinin in the urine (1904), the tests for amino-acids (1912–22), residual urinary nitrogen (1912–13), and blood analysis (1919–22); Donald B. **Van Slyke** (1883–   ), of Pike, New York (estimation of amino-acids, 1908–12; amino-acid and protein metabolism, 1912–16; acidosis, 1917–28; blood-gases and electrolytes, 1922–8; nephritis, 1921–8; gasometry, 1924–8); Graham **Lusk** (1866–   ), of Bridgeport, Conn. (D: n ratio, 1898; amino-acids, 1910;

---

[1] Abderhalden: Ztschr. f. physiol. Chem., Strassb., 1912, lxxvii, 249; lxxxi, 90.

nutrition, 1912–28); Thomas Burr **Osborne** (1859), of New Haven, Connecticut, and Lafayette Benedict **Mendel** (1872–   ), of Delhi, New York (synthetic food and vitamines, 1911–15); Phoebus Aaron **Levene** (1869–   ), of New York (nucleic acid metabolism, 1912–25; phosphatides, 1914–22; glycoproteids, 1914–21; nucleoproteins, 1925); Elmer Verner **McCollum** (1879–   ), of Fort Scott, Kansas (bone growth, nutrition requirements, 1911–25); Henry Clapp **Sherman** (1875–   ), of Ash Grove, Virginia (food chemistry and vitamines, 1918–24); John Raymond **Murlin** (1861–   ), of Ohio (infant metabolism, 1910–23); Eugene Floyd **Dubois** (1882–   ), of New York (metabolism in disease, 1915–27).

The leading spirit of recent **pathology** is Ludwig **Aschoff** (1866–   ), of Berlin, professor at Freiburg (1912), who, through his masters, Orth and Recklinghausen, stems directly from Virchow, and through his own pupils, Tawara, Kiyono, Suzuki, Ogata, Kawamura, has carried the Virchow tradition into Japan. A great systematist and philosopher, Aschoff strove to bring order and system into the bewildering complex of pathological reasoning, and through his work on pyelonephritis (1893) the different modalities of appendicitis (1908), thrombosis (1912), atherosclerosis (1908–14), phthisis (1922), his own treatises (1900–1909), and his other monographs on ovulation and menstruation, cholesterin gallstones, gastric ulcer, goiter, and fatty degeneration, has done much to stimulate thought and open out new views. His synthesis of the reticulo-endothelial system (1913–24) resembles Waldeyer's summation of the neuron theory (1891) in its orderly tendency, as also his classification of disease-reactions, viz., functional (recreative reaction), deficiency (regenerative reaction), destructive (reparatory reaction), infective (defensive reaction, *i. e.*, inflammation). He set the pace and posed the problems for German pathological work on war material, of which he has left enduring monuments in the eighth volume of the German Medical History of the War (1921), and the gigantic exhibitions of war specimens in the Kaiser Wilhelms Institut and his own Institute at Freiburg. The contributions of his school to Ziegler's *Beiträge* (1906–28) cover all aspects of pathology.

Among the outstanding pathologists of the newer trend are: Felix **Marchand** (1846–1928), of Leipzig, memorable for his work on inflammation and healing of wounds (1890–1921) and clasmatocytes (1901); Paul **Grawitz** (1850–   ), professor at Greifswald (aberrant hypernephroma, 1883–4; infantile jaundice, 1883; subcutaneous inflammation, 1887; suppuration, 1887–9; slumber cells, 1891–2); Hans **Chiari** (1851–1916), of Vienna (postmortem technic, 1894; history of pathology, 1903); Pio **Foà** (1848–1923), the leading pathologist of Italy, and Nicolaus Philip **Tendeloo** (   ), of Celebes (pulmonary diseases, 1902; tuberculosis (1905–23); James **Ewing** (1866–   ), of Pittsburgh (clinical pathology of blood, 1900–13; neoplastic diseases, 1919); Frank Burr **Mallory** (1862), of Cleveland, Ohio (endothelial leukocytes, 1898–26; histopathology, 1914); Eugene Lindsay **Opie** (1873–   ), of Staunton, Virginia (pancreatic diabetes, 1899–1902; influenza, pneumonia, 1917–19); Aldred Scott **Warthin** (1866–   ), of Greensburg, Indiana (pathology of hemolymph glands, hematopoietic system, syphilis, mustard gas poisoning); Edward B. **Krumbhaar** (1882–   ), of Philadelphia (heart-block, 1910–17; leucopenia in mustard gas poisoning, 1919; reticulosis, 1922; hemolytopoietic system, 1923; neutrophilic leukocytosis, 1924); Milton Charles **Winternitz** (1885–   ), of Baltimore, professor of pathology at Yale (influenza, 1919; war-gas poisoning, 1919); William George **MacCallum** (1874), of Dunnville, Ontario (tetany, 1908; pancreatic diabetes, 1909; pneumonia, 1918); Simeon Burt **Wolbach** (1880–   ) of Grand Island, Nebraska (Rocky Mountain fever, typhus fever, influenza); Horst **Oertel** (1873–   ), Oscar **Klotz** (1878–   ), of Preston, Ontario (arteriosclerosis, 1912; yellow fever, 1928); Dorothy Reed (Hodgkin's disease, 1902), and Maude E. Abbott (malformations of heart, 1908–27). The World War found the medical personnel of armies deficient in pathologists. The foundation of such newer periodicals as the Bologna *Archivio* (1922), the Paris *Annales* (1924), the Copenhagen *Acta* (1924), *Krankheits-Forschung* (Tendeloo, Leipzig, 1925), the *American Journal of Pathology* (F. B. Mallory, 1925), and the Chicago *Archives* (Ludwig Hektoen, 1926) illustrates the recent trend toward organization and system. The collection and preparations of pathological specimens from the World War in the Army Medical Museum (Washington) is due to the steadfast efforts of Louis B. Wilson and the officers subsequently detailed to this work, viz., Majors George R. Callender and James F. Coupal. This renaissance of pathology is in striking contrast with its deplorable status during the World War, when few surgeons competent to conduct a postmortem section could be found.

Of late years there has been an amazing increase in the literature of **psychology,** normal, morbid and comparative, including such related subjects as pedagogics, psycho-analysis, psychotherapy, epistemology, the scientific aspects of evidence and the relation of everyday thinking to border-line insanity. Psychology, defined by Jastrow as "a Colonial outpost of philosophy or, later, a protectorate of physiology" in its early phases, has steadily advanced through the physiological and psychophysical stages, to the comparative status, and is now an analogue of the general physiology of Claude Bernard. Psychophysics or quantitative psychology, as illustrated in the achievement of Wundt, Lotze, Fechner, and Herbart, and of McKeen Cattell in America, tended to "conceive sensations and stimuli as abstract or even instrumental realities like grammes or candle-powers or watts or ohms," and fell short of the profitable approach to the living organism, which must necessarily be qualitative or genetic (Jastrow[1]). Comparative psychology turns mainly upon Loeb's theory of tropisms in the lower forms (or the views of those who, like H. S. Jennings, oppose it) and the study of "behavior" in the higher animals (Watson). The mental development of the newborn infant has been specially studied by Kussmaul and Preyer. Pedagogics and juvenile psychology have been treated by Binet, Claparède, Stanley Hall, Séguin, Maria Montessori, and others. Among the leaders in morbid psychology is Pierre **Janet** (1859–   ), professor at the Collège de France, who developed the theory of psychologic automatism (1889), the relations between neuroses and fixed ideas (1898[2]) described psychasthenia (1903), and made extensive investigations of the mental status of hysteric patients (1903–8), emphasizing, in particular, the sexual factor in hysteria, but with the sound view that the sexual inadequacy of the neurotic is a symptom and not a cause, and that much alleged morbid heredity is the effect of bad domestic environment, the selfish hypocrisy of parents and suchlike. In 1905–8, Alfred **Binet** (1857–1911) and Th. **Simon** intro-

---

[1] J. Jastrow: Psychol. Rev., Princeton, 1927, xxxiv, 169–195.

[2] Janet: Année psychol., Paris, 1905–08, *passim.*

duced a series of graded tests for mental retardation by which it is possible to localize the developmental status of a patient's mind in relation to his age and the growth of his body (mental age), thus enabling school-teachers or school inspectors to segregate defective or "unusual" children. Another characteristic development is the exhaustive or intensive study of sexual psychology, with which modern writers, from scientific students like Krafft-Ebing and Havelock Ellis, down to insane men of letters like Nietzsche and Weininger, have been vastly preoccupied. The atmosphere of the present time, its art, poetry, fiction, and drama, is saturated with sexualism. Poets like Goethe, Swinburne, and Walt Whitman did much to dispel the ancient theological nightmare of the sinfulness of normal sexuality in men and women, and were forerunners of the scientific view that the instinct is an all-important part in normal human development, and has to be either recognized or reckoned with. Schopenhauer wrote on the subject with bitter and unsparing realism, and latterly women of such high repute as Rahel Varnhagen, Ellen Key, and Helen Putnam have considered the matter from a higher viewpoint, on account of its importance in connection with such problems as the proper hygiene and well-being of growing children, the growth of prostitution and commercialized vice, the social enslavement of women in crowded communities, and other degradations of a purely industrial age. In Germany, several periodicals are devoted to the sexual instinct alone, and the problem of biological teaching of school-children in these matters is under consideration. On the pathological side, there is the question of sexual perversion and the crimes resulting from it, for which, in young, healthy frontier communities like the United States no special provisions had been necessary in criminal procedure until the crowded conditions of modern cities brought the unsavory subject to the surface.[1] Recent thinking has been revolutionized by the revelation of the part played by suppressed or repressed sexuality in the development of neurotic conditions, the special achievement of Sigmund **Freud** (1856–   ), of Freiberg in Moravia, a pupil of Charcot, and professor of neurology at Vienna. Charcot, as we have seen, threw the sexual theory of hysteria into disrepute. Janet, from 1889 on, emphasized its emotional causation. Breuer and Freud introduced the cathartic treatment (questioning under hypnosis). Freud, in particular, interpreted the mechanism of hysteria as the resultant of a psychic traumatism or nervous shock, of sexual nature in the first instance, leading to morbid brooding and a kind of mental involution. Freudians hold the sexual factor to be existent in normal people, but

---

[1] J. L. Caspar, in his Practical Handbook of Legal Medicine (1856), regarded these crimes as among the "strange bubbles which sometimes rise from the low life of towns." Their modern study is due to Krafft-Ebing (1886) and to Leopold von Meerscheidt-Hüllesem, chief of police at Berlin, who showed the necessity of the segregation and surveillance, under humane restrictions, of perverted individuals in large cities, if only on account of blackmail and the homicidal tendencies which these characters are known to develop.

the way in which the individual reacts to the experience localizes the neurotic. The basic idea of Freud's subjective or dispositional psychology is that a large number of even ordinary mental processes come from hidden sources, unknown to the individual, whose tendency to fabricate reasons to justify the unsuspected reality is "rationalization" (Jones, 1908). Freud has also developed the theory of the psychic significance of dreams (*Traumdeutung*) and witticisms as unintentional determinisms, infantile amnesia, auto-erotism (Ellis), unconscious memories, absent-minded actions, anxiety-neuroses, also various aspects of

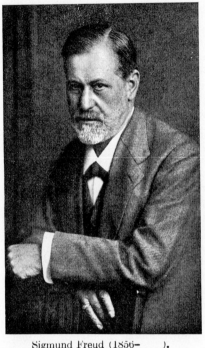

the "psychopathology of everyday life." He believes that there is a rigid determinism of psychical effects and that many complex mental processes never attain to consciousness and can be elicited only by a long process of "psychoanalysis," in developing which he was assisted by his pupil, C. G. Jung. Freud's first successful case, that of the patient "Dora," was of this kind. The correctness of his reasoning seems borne out by the successful treatment of hysteria through the disburdening of the mind or other appropriate psychotherapy. In his view, the basis of all sexual neuroses is the child's unconscious attachment to its parents, sometimes with hostility to the parent of the same sex. This "Œdipus complex" White regards as the "family romance,"[1] symbolizing the struggle of the individual to attain to self-confidence

Sigmund Freud (1856–   ).

and self-reliance by breaking away from dependence upon his parents. It is thus regarded as a measure of the degree of infantilism in the neurotic. Freud's reasoning about the effect of the mind upon the body (psychogenesis), the ambivalence of emotions (Bleuler), the mental levels of the conscious, the subconscious and its censor (Hughlings Jackson), the opposition between day-dreaming (wish-fulfilment) and reality, transferences, fixations, repressions, sublimations and regressions, has exerted a profound, and, in its popular aspects, a very dubious effect upon modern thought. The real interest of Freud is his profound insight into the workings of primitive mentality, or what Jelliffe calls "paleopsychology" (the historic past of the individual

---

[1] W. A. White: Mechanisms of Character Formation, New York, 1916, 145–176.

psyche). His school has occasioned abuses in medical practice and he himself has sometimes lapsed into extravagances of rationalization, which Jastrow wittily describes as giving "rich reasons for poor motives." In psychoanalysis, Freud has invented an instrument which can be exceedingly dangerous in intemperate, incompetent or unscrupulous hands. In America, his ideas have been followed by J. J. Putnam, A. A. Brill, William A. White, and others, and such variants as Bleuler's theory of normal "autistic thinking" go to show the very thin partitions which sometimes divide sanity from insanity.

Among Freud's pupils, all of whom branched out for themselves, was Alfred **Adler** (1870-   ), of Vienna, who stresses organic inferiority, sexual or other, as a prominent cause of neuroses (the inferiority complex, 1907). In this class of neurotics (Goethe's *incompletæ*), the sexual or other inadequacy is set off by a constant subconscious effort to assert and attain superiority (Nietzsche's "will to power"), the neurosis rooting in a constant overtaxing of bodily resources to compensate for the patent or latent inferiority. The strong deliberately choose plainness and simplicity. The neurotic, victimized by the "as if" tendency of Vahinger, acts on the assumption that he is strong, projects his own faults on to others, affects disdain, is fertile in reasons for failure, and combines a general faultfinding spirit with a self-imposed nimbus. This sound thesis Adler develops with great brilliancy, but lacks the lucid literary manner of Freud. Allied to this phase of constitutional psychology is Kretschmer's analysis of the manic-depressive and præcox (split personality) psychoses (1921). Janet's view of sexual inadequacy as a symptom rather than a cause of neuroses, is stressed in the writings of Wilhelm Stekel (1868-   ), of Vienna, which include an exhaustive analysis of the causes of impotence (1923) and an array of case histories which would have astounded Brantôme. Both Adler and Stekel favor Janet's view that much of alleged morbid heredity is chargeable to unfavorable domestic environment, harsh parentage, family slavery, and so on. The effect of the modern wave of sexual emancipation has been to capitalize and commercialize the ideas of the Freudian school, with occasional untoward results in fiction, on the stage and in actuality.

In striking contrast with the psychogenic philosophy is the behaviorist (comparative) psychology, an analogue of general physiology, which makes a clean sweep of "mind" and its attributes as a mere concept *in vacuo*, interprets mentality in terms of reaction to environment, indeed maintains that from amœba to man, the whole organism participates in thinking. **Behaviorism** was already implicit in the writings of William James, Stanley Hall, and others, but was specially developed by John Broadus **Watson** (1878-   ). It derives immediately from the work of Pavloff and his school on conditional reflexes in animals, which Watson applied to the nursery (1916). In Watson's treatises of 1914 and 1919, the centric idea of reaction to stimulus is developed with a scientific exactitude which has won the approval of all and sundry. Where behaviorism fails is in the determined effort to apply the rationale of the conditioned salivary reflex to the higher reaches of consciousness and deliberate thought. What was applicable to the lower stages of behavior becomes, in the words of Jastrow, "an acrobatic or verbalistic treatment, an ignoring of the realities, a juggling with formulæ, such as stimulus and response, denatured of the very quality that gives them significance," in brief, "the grin without the cat"; or "throwing out the baby with the bath." With reference to the two main trends which have dominated recent thought, Jastrow indulges the witticism that "psychology first lost its soul, and then its mind," but has now experienced "a change of heart and a change of mind." To see subconsciousness as virtually a sexual phenomenon, "a something not ourselves that makes for unrighteousness," is utterly to discourage the finer feelings and *nuances* of character. On the other hand, to envisage the human as a reliable reflex hound, registering salivary and movie emotions, is apt to make him seem, like Wilkie Collins' muscular Christians, "too unhealthily conscious of his unconscious healthiness," *i. e.*, a dreadful bore. Here K. S. Lashley's important experiments on learning processes in rats (1912–26), as interpreted by Herrick (1926[1]), may give us pause. Behaviorism has been most successful as comparative psychology, in elucidating the reflex life of animals, the infant, the anthropoid and the *primitif*. It is plain that in the higher animals, a function of the cerebrum (fore-brain) is to sublimate the instincts and affectivities radiating from the brain-stem and midbrain, that disorders of hunger (obesity), thirst (diabetes), sleep (insomnia) and sexual feeling (Fröhlich syndrome) are disturbances of inter-brain (infundibular) functions, wherefore instinctive actions and sensing of personality have little to do with intelligence and intellect. A set-off to Freudian and behavioristic reasoning is the *Gestalt* psychology of Kurt Koffka (1886–   ) and Wolfgang Köhler, which insists upon the psychic relativity of the laboratory animal, and the importance of the setting or background (*Gestalt*) as a configuration or constellation of factors, without which an object or happening has no significance whatever.

Parasitology and Chemotherapy.—In the last decade of the 19th century, as a result of the many improvements in microscopic and bacteriological technic, physicians began to study the animal and vegetable, and particularly the protozoan parasites as causes of disease, but the greatest triumphs in this field belong to the 20th century.

In the earlier period, Agostino Bassi had found the pathogenic organism (*Botrytis Bassiana*) of silkworm disease, or muscardine (1837), Schönlein, the achorion of favus (1839), Donné, the Trichomonas vaginalis (1837), Johannes Müller, the psorosperms (1841), David Grüby, the *Trypanosoma sanguinis* in frogs (1843), Davaine, the *Cercomonas hominis* (1857), Malmstem, the *Balantidium coli* (1857), Lambl, the *Giardia intestinalis* (1859) which Leeuwenhoek viewed *sans le savoir* in 1681. Küchenmeister discovered that parasites change their hosts (metaxenia) in 1851–53. Leuckart extended the general law of intermediary hosts to the Arthropoda and under his

---

[1] C. J. Herrick: Brains of Rats and Men, Chicago, 1926.

direction Fedschenko determined the life-history of Filaria medinensis in Cyclops (1869). This led to the studies of Patrick Manson on the development of Filaria bancrofti in mosquitoes (1879), Smith and Kilborne on ticks and Texas fever (1888), Bruce on the tsetse fly and nagana (1894), Ronald Ross on malaria and mosquitoes (1889–98), Finlay (1881), Walter Reed and his associates (1900) on yellow fever and Stegomyia. The first group of parasitic diseases to be investigated was that of the **protozoan dysenteries**, the pathogens of which had been seen by Lambl (1860), by Lewis (1870), and by Loesch (1875), who made drawings of both the innocuous and pathogenic forms, with the latter of which he was able to infect dogs. The greatest single monograph on dysentery is that of J. J. Woodward (1879), who saw the Loesch ameba, but did not sense its significance. Koch (1883) and Kartulis (1886–91) in Egypt, found amebæ to be invariably present in dysenteric postmortems, even of liver abscess, and differentiated between endemic dysentery due to amebæ, and epidemic dysentery due to bacteria. Osler confirmed this at the Johns Hopkins Hospital (1890). The term "amebic dysentery" was introduced by W. T. Councilman and H. A. Lafleur at the Johns Hopkins Hospital (1891), two types of parasites being recognized, the harmless *Amœba coli*, and the pathogenic *Amœba dysenteriæ*. These views were confirmed by Casagrandi and Barbagallo (1897), and particularly by Fritz Schaudinn, who styled the harmless form *Entamœba coli* and the pathogenic form *Entamœba histolytica* (1903). These species were first confirmed by Craig, who afterward found Viereck's pathogenic *Entamœba tetragena* in the Philippines and discovered a new species of diarrheal parasite, *Craigia (Paramœba) hominis* (1906), which Calkins regards as a new genus. Errors made by Schaudinn in the life-history of the pathogenic ameba were corrected when E. L. Walker and A. W. Sellards (1911–13) showed that *E. histolytica* and *E. tetragena* are identical, and that ingestion of cysts is necessary for infestation. Other pathogenic species of amebæ have been described by various observers, and diarrheal and dysenteric infections have also been found to be associated with Laverania, Leishmania, Balantidium coli, and the above-mentioned flagellate forms, Cercomonas, Trichomonas, and Lamblia. Meanwhile the question of bacillary dysentery had been settled by the discovery of bacilli by Shiga in Japan (1898), Kruse in Germany (1900), Flexner (1900), Strong and Musgrave at Manila (1900), and the Y-bacillus of Hiss and Russell (1903) in America. It is now known that most of tropical dysentery is bacillary. The *Endamœba buccalis*, described by Prowazek (1904), has been identified as an organism associated with pyorrhea alveolaris.

The symptoms of **hook-worm infection** were vaguely outlined in the Egyptian papyri, and for centuries the disease was variously known as Egyptian or tropical chlorosis, miner's or bricklayer's anemia, and St. Gothard tunnel disease. The parasite was described as Anchylostoma duodenale by Angelo Dubini (1843), and its causal relation to the disease was pointed out by Wilhelm Griesinger (1866). In 1900, Captain Bailey K. Ashford, U. S. Army, discovered the great prevalence of the disease in Porto Rico, and it was soon found to be very common among the rural population of the Southern States (U. S.) by Charles Wardell Stiles (1867–   ), of Spring Valley, New York, who discovered that the parasite of the American infections is a new species which he called Uncinaria americana (1902) and later Necator americanus. Stiles, who had already made his reputation in parasitology by his work on revision of species and nomenclature and his contributions to descriptive zoölogy, has since devoted himself, as professor of zoölogy in the U. S. Public Health and Marine-Hospital Service, to the task of exterminating the disease in the South, in connection with the Rockefeller Commission (now the International Health Board) established for this purpose in October, 1909. Under the administration of Wickliffe Rose, this Board soon succeeded in engaging the newspapers, boards of health, schools, and medical organizations of the South to coöperate in starting outdoor clinics, so that the local authorities are now able to take care of themselves by "intensive community health-work," and the Rockefeller Board has extended its activities to other fields. In three years (1910–12), no less than 393,566 persons were treated for hook-worm at these open-air clinics in the Southern States. In 1898, Arthur Looss (1861–1923) made the important discovery that the hookworm larva can penetrate the skin, reaching the intestines by a devious route, and this fact has enabled Stiles and Ashford to devise effective means of prophylaxis among rural populations. In Ashford's campaign against the disease in Porto Rico (1903–04), some 300,000 out of a population of a million have been treated, with a reduction of 90 per cent. in the mortality from anemia. **Pellagra,** which has latterly been identified in America, has been closely studied by Lombroso, Théophile Roussel, Sambon and others in Europe, and by James W. Babcock, Claude H. Lavinder,

45

Joseph Goldberger and his associates in the U. S. Public Service. Variously attributed to a parasite transmitted by the Simulium fly, or to food poisoning from photodynamic substances, it is now classed, with ergotism, beriberi, scurvy and rickets, among the deficiency diseases (avitaminoses), of Casimir Funk (1913[1]). Joseph Goldberger and his associates have demonstrated its experimental production in patients subsisting upon a faulty diet characterized by deficiency of a specific vitamine (1925) with alleviation and prevention by proper diet (1915–20), and production of the condition in the dog and the rat by experimental feeding (1926–7).

In 1911, Laveran's malarial parasite was obtained in pure cultures *in vitro* by Charles C. Bass, of New Orleans. Howard Taylor Ricketts (1870–1910), of Findlay, Ohio, a pupil of Hektoen, discovered that the Rocky Mountain spotted fever is transmitted by the wood-tick (*Dermacentor occidentalis*) in 1907, and (with R. M. Wilder) that Mexican typhus (*tabardillo*) is transmitted by the body-louse (*Pediculus vestimenti*) in 1910. This had already been demonstrated for European typhus by Charles Nicolle (1909), and in the same year, John F. Anderson and Joseph Goldberger, of the U. S. Public Health Service, had produced successful inoculations of typhus from man to monkey. The disease discovered by Nathan E. Brill in New York in 1910 was shown by Goldberger and Anderson to be a mild form of typhus.

The **trypanosomes** discovered by David Grüby (1809–98) in the frog (1843) and by Lewis in the rat (1878) were non-pathogenic, but a new interest in these organisms was awakened when Griffith Evans (1880) discovered in India that surra, a disease of horses, mules, camels and cattle, is caused by a variety which was afterward named by Steel and Crookshank, Trypanosoma evansi (1885–86). It is of record that the African traveler, David Livingstone, gave an accurate account of the tsetse fly disease in his *Missionary Travels* (1858, 94–97[2]). In 1894, Sir David Bruce (1855–   ) found that the tsetse fly disease or nagana of Zululand is due to the Trypanosoma brucei (Plimmer and Bradford, 1899), which he proved experimentally to be conveyed from the blood of big game animals to cattle and horses by this fly (*Glossina morsitans*). In the same year (1894) Rouget discovered T. equiperdum (Doflein, 1901) as the cause of dourine or *mal du coït* in horses; in 1901 Elmassian found T. equinum (Vosges, 1902) as the cause of *mal de caderas* in South American dogs and horses; Theiler (1902) found T. theileri (Bruce, 1902) in the bovine gall-sickness or *galziekte* of South Africa and T. dimorphon (Laveran and Mesnil, 1904) was found to be the cause of another animal disease in equatorial Africa by Dutton and Todd (1904). The most important find, however, was that of T. *gambiense* in the blood of man by J. Everett Dutton (1901), which was afterward seen by Aldo Castellani in the cerebrospinal fluid and blood of five cases of African sleeping sickness (1903). It was then shown by Bruce and Nabarro, of the Royal Society Commission, that the tsetse fly is the vector of the disease, and that Gambia fever, the disease first seen by Dutton and Todd in 1902, and sleeping sickness are two stages of the same infection. A Brazilian variety of human trypanosomiasis, due to T. cruzi and transmitted by a bug (*Conorhinus sanguisuga*), was described by Carlo Chagas (1909). The words "amebiasis" and "trypanosomiasis" were coined by W. E. Musgrave. Another remarkable organism was found in 1900 by Sir William Boog Leishman (1865–1926), in a postmortem film from a case of fever at Dum Dum, near Calcutta, and afterward described by him (May, 1903) as possibly a trypanosome. In July, 1903, Major C. Donovan found the same bodies in blood taken in life from splenic punctures. In July, 1904, Leonard Rogers announced the development of these parasites into flagellates and, in 1906–07, Walter Scott Patton described their development into flagellates in the bedbug. All these discoveries have associated the Leishman-Donovan bodies with the tropical splenomegaly, dumdum fever or kala-azar. In 1903, James Homer Wright found similar parasites (Leishmania tropica) in Oriental endemic ulcers, and Charles Nicolle found Leishmania infantum in infantile kala-azar (1908). In 1888, Victor Babes (1854–1926), a Roumanian physician, discovered a small protozoön in the blood of sheep suffering from an epizoötic disease called *carceag*, and the genus was called in his honor Babesia by Starcovici (1893), the term Piroplasma having been proposed by Patton (1895). A similar parasite was claimed by Babes as the cause of hemoglobinuric fever of European cattle, and in the same year Theobald Smith (1859–   ) found the organism, Pyrosoma bigeminum, in Texas fever, which, with F. L. Kilborne, he demonstrated to be transmitted by the tick. This was the first demonstration, after

---

[1] C. Funk: Die Vitamine, Wiesbaden, 1914.

[2] See E. W. Gudger: Boston Med. & Surg. Jour., 1919, clxxx, 523–527.

Manson's, of the transmission of infection by a blood-sucking insect. After this time, knowledge of the different piroplasmoses or babesioses grew apace, the best known being the canine form (Piroplasma or Babesia canis, Piana and Galli Valerio, 1895), the life cycle of which has been carefully traced by G. H. F. Nuttall and Graham Smith. The so-called Piroplasma hominis, assumed to be the cause of spotted fever of the Rocky Mountains, was shown by Craig to be an artefact in the erythrocytes (1904). In 1903, cell inclusions, staining deeply with methylene-blue-eosin, were found in the central nervous system in hydrophobia by Adelchi Negri (1876–1912) and a culture of these was made by Hideyo Noguchi in 1913. Cytoryctes variolæ, a protozoön found in the skin lesions of smallpox, was described by Giuseppe Guarnieri (1894) and its life-history was traced by Gary N. Calkins (1904), while similar bodies were found in variola by W. T. Councilman and others (1903) and by Mallory in scarlatina (1904). Histoplasma capsulatum found in a tropical splenomegaly on the Isthmus of Panama by Samuel Taylor Darling (1872–1925) in 1906 is said to be an yeast. The spirochete or spirillum of relapsing fever, discovered by one of Virchow's assistants, Otto Obermeier (1843–73), in 1873, was to open out the most important phase of parasitic diseases yet known, viz., the conquest of syphilis by Schaudinn, Wassermann and Ehrlich. In 1904, the spirochete of African relapsing fever (tick fever) was discovered independently by Nabarro, Ross and Milne in Uganda and by Dutton and Todd in the Congo and was called Spirochæte duttoni, in honor of Dutton, who died from the disease after he had proved its transmission by a tick (*Ornithodorus moubata*). The spirochete of the American variety of relapsing fever was discovered by Frederick G. Novy (1907). In 1903 Marchoux and Salimbeni proved that a Brazilian spirochætosis of domestic fowls is transmitted by the the tick *Argas persicus*.

Parasitology thus owes much of its present status to **medical etomology,** which is now taught at Harvard and Cornell Universities. The Army Medical School (Washington), and has been specially developed by Leland O. Howard (1898–1917), G. H. Nuttall (1899), Ronald Ross 1901), R. W. Doane (1910) A. W. Alcock (1911), W. S. Patton and F. W. Cragg (1913), W. A. Riley and O. A. Johannsen (1915). W. B. Herms (1915), A. E. Shipley (1917), A. C. Chandler (1918), W. D. Pierce (1921), and H. T. Fernald (1921).

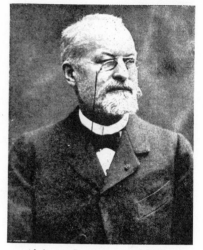

Alphonse Laveran (1845–1922).

Alphonse **Laveran** (1845–1922), of Paris, a Strassburg graduate of 1867 and Nobel prizeman of 1907, discovered the parasites of malarial fever (November 6, 1880) while an army surgeon in Algeria, and described them in all their various aspects (1881). He published no fewer than four separate treatises on paludism (1884, 1891, 1892, 1898), also *Trypanosomes et trypanosomiuses* (1904) and treatises on military medicine (1875) and military hygiene (1896).

Sir Ronald **Ross** (1857–   ), of the Indian Medical Service (1881–99), located the anopheles mosquito as the vector of malarial fever, discovered the Laveran plasmodia in the stomach wall of *Anopheles* which had fed upon the blood of malarial patients (1897), proved that the spores of the parasites are concentrated in the salivary gland of the insect (1898), and devised the culicidal methods (1902) which he employed with success in mosquito reduction in Sierra Leone. Lagos, the Gold Coast and Ismailia (1899–1902). For this work, which led to effective prevention of malarial fever all over the world, Ross received the Nobel prize in 1902. In mathematics, he has applied the theory of probabilities to the statistical prognosis of epidemics (*"a priori* pathometry,"* 1916). His plays, poems, and autobiography (1923) are the productions of a highly original mind.

Important advances in **protozoölogy** were made by Fritz **Schaudinn** (1871–1906), the son of an East Prussian innkeeper, who took his doctor's degree in zoölogy in Berlin in 1894, and, after some studies of the Foraminifera, devoted the rest of his life to the Protozoa.

As a descriptive zoölogist, he isolated many new species, but his first important contribution to medicine was the differentiation between the harmless Entamœba

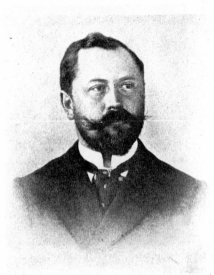

Fritz Schaudinn (1871–1906).

coli and the pathogenic Entamœba histolytica (1903). In addition to his work on amebic dysentery, which he carried out experimentally upon animals, Schaudinn confirmed the work of Ross and Grassi upon the malarial parasite, identifying Plasmodium vivax (Grassi and Feletti) as the cause of tertian fever (1902) and also confirmed Looss's demonstration of hook-worm infection through the skin (1904).

In May, 1905, working with Erich Hoffmann, Schaudinn crowned his life-work by the discovery of the Spirochæta pallida of syphilis.[1] Then, in a valuable paper of his own (October, 1905[2]), he described the morphology of the spirochetes, that of syphilis justifying the establishment of a new genus, Spironema or Treponema. Schaudinn's discovery of this almost invisible parasite was due to his incomparable skill in technic and staining methods. The causal relation was rapidly established by thousands of confirmatory observations made by enthusiastic microscopists all over the world. Schaudinn was Privatdocent at Berlin (1898) and became director of protozoölogy in the *Kaiserliches Gesundheitsamt* (1904) and the *Institut für Schiffs- und Trophenhygiene* at Hamburg (1906). In 1903 he founded the *Archiv für Protistenkunde*, the literary organ of protozoölogy, which he had found in the descriptive stage and left an experimental science.

The first steps in the conquest of syphilis had thus been made by professional zoölogists, Metchnikoff and Schaudinn. The next advances were made by an investigator who, although educated as a

---

[1] Arb. a. d. k. Gesundheitsamte, Berl., 1905, xxii, 527–534.

[2] Deutsche med. Wochenschr., Leipz. & Berl., 1905, xxxi, 1665–1667.

physician, really worked out his results as a chemist and pharmacologist.

Paul **Ehrlich** (1854–1915), of Strehlen, Silesia, a clinical assistant of Frerichs (1878–85) and Gerhardt (1885–89), and professor (1890) at Berlin, where he became an assistant in Koch's Institute, was entrusted (1896) with the directorship of the newly founded *Institut für Serumforschung* at Steglitz, which was transferred, under his direction, to the *Institut für experimentelle Therapie* at Frankfort on the Main (1899).

At Breslau, Ehrlich was but an indifferent student, occupying his time mainly with experiments on dye-stuffs and tissue staining, but the results of his labors soon appeared in his improved methods of drying and fixing blood-smears by heat, his triacid stain, his discovery of the mast cells and his detection of their granulations by basic aniline staining (1877), his division of the white blood-corpuscles into neutrophilic, basophilic and oxyphilic, his fuchsin stain for tubercle bacilli, based upon the discovery that they are acidfast (1882), his diazo-reaction of the urine, used in the diagnosis of typhoid fever (1882[1]), his sulpho-diazo-benzol test for bilirubin (1883[2]) and his method of intravital staining (1886[3]), in all of which he has been a great pioneer in merging descriptive cellular pathology into experimental intracellular chemistry. His studies on the blood are summarized in his treatise on anemia (with A. Lazarus, 1898). He was the pioneer of *Farbenanalyse* or the microchemical action of the tissues to dye-stuffs (1885–91). This is particularly true of his study of the oxygen requirements of the organism (1885), in which he applies the idea of a selective affinity between chemical substances and body tissues to protoplasmic chemistry and first outlines his "side-chain theory." This theory was suggested by August Kekulé's hypothesis of the closed benzene ring (1865), in which the six carbon atoms of this compound (C_6H_6) are assumed to form a stable hex-

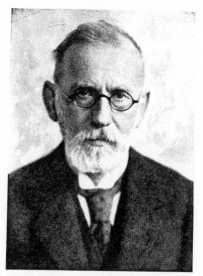

Paul Ehrlich (1854–1915).

agonal nucleus among themselves, while their fourth affinities are linked with unstable "side-chains" of easily replaceable hydrogen. Hoppe-Seyler had assumed that the emission and absorption of light in chlorophyll are accomplished not by the entire molecule itself, but by certain specialized groups of peripheral atoms. In like manner, Ehrlich assumed that the living protoplasmic molecule consists of a stable nucleus and unstable peripheral side-chains or chemo-receptors, which enable it to combine chemically with food substances and neutralize toxins or other poisons by throwing out detached side-chains into the blood. In spite of the enormous amount of criticism heaped upon this theory and its author, it may safely be affirmed that, as based upon a fundamental postulate in organic chemistry, it proved to be a valuable "heuristic principle" in developing the science of immunity and serum reactions. Thus, August **von Wassermann** (1866–1925) did not hesitate to affirm that without it he could never have hit upon the special and reliable hemolytic diagnosis of syphilis with which his name is associated and which was discovered one year

---

[1] Ehrlich: Ztschr. f. klin. Med., Berl., 1822, v, 285–288. Charité Ann., 1881, Berl., 1883, viii, 140–166.

[2] Centralbl. f. d. med. Wissensch., Berl., 1883, iv, 721.

[3] Deutsche med. Wchnschr., Leip. u. Berl., 1886, xii, 49–52.

after Schaudinn had found the parasite of the disease (1906[1]). The original Wassermann reaction has been much followed by such ingenious modifications and checks as the flocculation reactions of Meinicke (1911), Vernes (1917–19), Sachs-Georgi (1918) and Dold (1921), the sigma reaction of Dreyer and Ward (1921) and the simple, direct and sensitive test of R. L. Kahn (1921–26[2]), the effect of which is readily visible without the intervention of a special hemolytic indicator and bids fair to become a permanent aid in diagnosis. From the discoveries of Schaudinn and Wassermann, it became known that such immunes as come under Colles' and Profeta's law have the syphilitic spirochetes in their blood, whence Ehrlich reasoned that protozoan diseases cannot be treated by special antitoxins, but must be handled by drugs which can at once sterilize the patient's body of the parasites without injuring the body tissues. In attempting to treat trypanosomiasis in mice with certain specific dyes, he found that if the doses were too small to completely sterilize the animal of the parasite, a race of trypanosomes could be bred which proved permanently "fast" or resistant to the effects of the drug. This power of parasites to immunize themselves and their descendants against the action of drugs was the *Leitmotif* of the long series of "trial and error" experiments to find a *therapia sterilisans* against syphilis, and it proved to be the weak point in their final result, "606," or salvarsan. Salvarsan, which was first tried out by Ehrlich's Japanese assistant, S. Hata (1910), and has since been tested in thousands of cases, is, in itself, as reliable a specific as quinine in malarial infection, and is, moreover, a valuable prophylactic, in that it rapidly cleans up the ugly luetic sores and eruptions and sterilizes the blood, thus minimizing the possibility of infecting others. But the fact that it does not appear to reach some of the spirochetes, which, like the gonococcus, hide in other tissues, is responsible for disconcerting relapses, while "606" itself sometimes causes severe collateral effects upon the eye or the nervous system. The merits of "neo-salvarsan" ("914" in Ehrlich's experimental series) were greater, but it is hardly likely that any drug will prove a complete sterilizer under the above conditions. Salvarsan is, however, an ideal *therapia sterilisans* in the case of Treponema pertenue, the parasite of yaws. Ehrlich was the founder of hematology. He classified the leucocytes according to the presence or absence of granules, differentiated the leukemias, described polychromatophilia, distinguished between normoblasts and megaloblasts, lymphoid and myeloid tissues, showed that leucocytosis is a function of bone-marrow, studied aplastic anemia and laid the foundation for the study of the specific reactions of cells to various infections and stimuli. Of the other features of Ehrlich's scientific work, his introduction of such remedies as methylene-blue for quartan fever, trypan red for bovine piroplasmosis, arsenophenylglycin for the trypanosomiases; his proof that animals can be quantitatively immunized against vegetable poisons like abrin and ricin; his improvement of Behring's diphtheria antitoxin and his establishment of an international standard of purity for the same; his demonstration that cancer can be changed into sarcoma in animals by successive inoculations, and that the growth of cancer depends upon the presence of certain food substances in the body and that immunity from cancer depends upon their absence (atrepsy); his vast researches in the whole field of serology and immunity can only be mentioned.

In his skill in improvising hypotheses to meet the opponents of his theories, Ehrlich resembled Galen. In his predilection for quaint and archaic Latin phrases, he was like Paracelsus. But he did the most effective work since Pasteur and Koch in the science of infectious diseases, and added new territory to the domain of experimental pharmacology and therapeutics by his genius for research and his wonderful industry.

The trend of recent medicine from the bacterial theory of disease toward the biochemical is strongly marked in Ehrlich's work. The fallibility of the many tests for differentiating the pseudo-typhoid, pseudo-tubercle, pseudo-tetanus, and pseudo-diphtheritic bacilli, the variability in pathogenic status of fixed laboratory strains of definite

[1] Wassermann: Deutsche med. Wchnschr., Leipz. u. Berl., 1906, xxxii, 745.
[2] R. L. Kahn: Serum Diagnosis of Syphilis by Precipitation, Baltimore, 1925.

bacilli, the uncertain behavior of the typhoid bacillus as to fermentation on a sugar slope (Twort, 1907), the puzzling mutations and pleomorphisms, such as Neisser (1906), Jacobson (1910) and Penfold (1911) produced in the typhoid and coli germs, the apparent changes of one bacillus into another, the effect of meteorological conditions on inulin fermentation, the strange vagaries of agglutination and of Wassermann tests, all show the inadequacy of our present knowledge.

Jules **Bordet,** Director of the Institut Pasteur de Brabant (Brussels), who won the Nobel prize (1919), has been a great pioneer in the theory of serology and immunity reactions, for the phenomena of which he gives a simple and purely physical explanation. He discovered bacterial hemolysis (1898[1]), and, with Octave Gengou, fixation of the complement (1900–01[2]), and the specific bacillus of whooping-cough (1906[3]), the causal relation of which was demonstrated, according to Koch's postulates, by F. B. Mallory and others (1913[4]). As compared with Ehrlich's complex terminology, Bordet's theory of serum reactions is simplicity itself. He assumes that the toxin is neutralized by an antitoxin through absorption, comparable with that shown by a fabric in taking up dyes. Complete neutralization would be like complete saturation of the fabric with the dye-stuff, but if the toxin be added in divided doses, the last portion of the toxin could

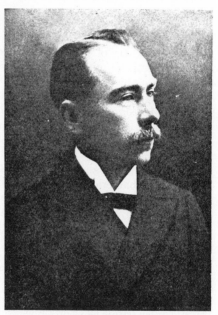

Jules Bordet.

not be absorbed, because its first portions have become supersaturated with antitoxins and can take up no more of them. Similarly, he assumes a *substance sensibilisatrice* in antitoxic sera which sensitizes the red blood-corpuscles or bacteria to the action of the alexins, as a mordant does for a dye-stuff. The disputes between Bordet and Ehrlich turn upon the simple fact that the former explains what he has seen in terms of physics, the latter in terms of structural chemistry.

---

[1] Ann. de l'Inst. Pasteur, Paris, 1898, xii, 688: 1899, xiii, 273.

[2] *Ibid.*, 1900, xiv, 257: 1901, xv, 289: 1902, xvi, 734. Deviation of the complement was discovered by A. Neisser and F. Wechsberg (München. med. Wochenschr., 1901, xlviii, 697–700).

[3] Ann. de l'Inst. Pasteur, Paris, 1906, xx, 731, 1 pl.: 1907, xxi, 720.

[4] Mallory, Horner and Henderson: Jour. Med. Research, Bost., 1913, xxvii, 391–397, 2 pl.

Among the advances in **serology** of striking interest are Quincke's lumbar puncture (1909) in cytodiagnosis, the discovery of agglutination by Bordet (1895) and Gruber (1896) and its application to the diagnosis of typhoid fever by Widal and Sicard (1896); the diagnostic use of tuberculin by the conjunctival reactions of Albert Calmette (1907) and Alfred Wolff-Eisner (1907), and the cutaneous reactions of Clemens von Pirquet (1907) and Ernst Moro (1908); Sir Almroth Wright's preventive inoculation against typhoid fever by dead cultures of the bacillus, with the opsonic index as a guide (1900); cobra venom reaction in insanity (Much-Holtzmann, 1909); Bela Schick's reaction for susceptibility to diphtheria antitoxin (1910–11); Emil Abderhalden's enzyme reaction in the diagnosis of pregnancy (1912). Many new modes of treatment with bacteria or bacterial products abound, such as Besredka's sensitized vaccines, Carl Spengler's employment of the bovine type of tubercle bacillus, and the use of bacilli attenuated in the cold-blooded animals against tuberculosis (Klebs, Friedmann), all of which have been on trial.

In the face of the bewildering array of laboratory findings which Rudolf Hoeber has assembled in his impressive monograph on the physical chemistry of the cell (1902), we really know very little of intracellular chemistry and metabolism. Nothing daunted, professional bacteriologists have taken comfort in the fact that bacteria, like certain major diseases, have existed and maintained their salient characteristics from remote periods of time, when the great dinosaurs and reptiles of the Mesozoic Era were infected with very modern specific infections and prehistoric man himself was assailed by arthritis deformans and tubercle. **Bacteriology** is now a highly organized science of immense practical efficiency, and two of its phases, environmental bacteriology and personal bacteriology, are basic in sanitation. Another phase, the taxonomic, has been a word of ambition among recent workers, who have clearly sensed the necessity of a complete revision of existing schemes of classification (**determinative bacteriology**).

Following the well-known morphological arrangement of Cohn (1875), the most prominent schemes of classification were those of W. Zopf (1883–5), Flügge (1886), Hueppe (1886), Migula (1890–1900), Lehmann and Neumann (1896), Erwin Smith (1905), Buchanan (1916–18), Breed and Conn (1919). In all these, the genus Coccaceæ, introduced by Zopf, played an important rôle. In 1917 and 1920, C.-E.-A. Winslow and other committeemen of the Society of American Bacteriologists issued two exhaustive reports on classification, culminating in a Manual of Determinative Bacteriology by David H. Bergey and others (1923), similar in scope to those of F. D. Chester (1901) and R. E. Buchanan (1925). This arrangement, introducing *Clostridium, Salmonella, Pasteurella, Neisseria* and other generic types, has proven of great value in identification and grouping. A remarkable simplification is the recent inclusion of *Bacillus abortus* (Bang, 1897), *Micrococcus melitensis* (Bruce, 1907), and possibly *B. tularense* (McCoy and Chapin, 1912) under the genus Brucella (Meyer and Shaw, 1920). The trend is illustrated in the paratyphoid enteritidis (Salmonella) group, which includes the pathogens of hog cholera (Salmon & Smith, 1886), paracolon infection (Gibert, 1895), paratyphoid infection (Achard & Bensaude, 1896, Schottmüller, 1900–1901, Uhlenhuth, 1909), meat poisoning (B. enteritidis, Gärtner, 1889), food poisoning (B. aertrycke, De Nobele, 1898), psittacosis (Nocard, 1893), equine abortion (Kilborne & Smith, 1893), "scours" (Thomassen, 1897) and rat plague (Danysz, 1900). During the second half of the 20th century **plant pathology** had been mainly phytopathology. The brilliant work of the Tulasne brothers on the Uredo and Ustilago smuts (1847–53), the famine resulting from the potato blight of 1844–45, and the determination of its cause by Anton de Bary (1861), the treatises of de Bary (1853), Julius Kühn (1858) and Ernst Hallier (1868) on vegetable pathology, the saving of the vineyards of France and the potato crops of America by the copper fungicide (Bordeaux mixture) devised by Alexis Millardet (1882–3), all stressed the overwhelming economic importance of the pathogenic fungi. On July 1, 1885, a section of mycology was established in the U. S. Department of Agriculture. To

Erwin F. **Smith** (1854–1927), of Gilbert's Mills, New York, who came to this bureau in 1886, we owe the conclusive demonstration of the existence of bacterial diseases in plants, first noticed by T. J. Burill in apple and pear blight (1878–84), and by Wakker in hyacinths (1883–89). Smith began his studies on bacterial wilt in cucumbers in 1893, demonstrated the bacterial origin of crown gall (1907–11), showed the resemblance of this vegetable tumor to cancer (1912–17) and culminated his life-work in three monumental volumes on *Bacteria in Relation to Plant Diseases* (1905–14), published by the Carnegie Institution of Washington. Smith, one of our most eminent men of science, was a poet and a scholar, whose benignant personality comprised all the known attributes of the "Beloved Physician." Meanwhile, through the interesting investigations of Ashford on tropical sprue (1908–14) and of Castellani on pathogenic moulds (1905–27), **medical mycology** is beginning to take its place in the science of **communicable diseases** which has been vastly forwarded by recent knowledge of diseases of animals and plants. Thus Bacillus coli (Escherich, 1886) produces lesions in animals similar to those of B. typhosus, and, as shown by Welch (1891), Levy (1891) and others, is responsible for the same immense variety of local diseases in man as the typhoid and paratyphoid bacilli. The Pasteurella group (Hueppe, 1886) is responsible for hemorrhagic septicemia in fowls (Perronciti, 1879; Pasteur, 1880), rabbits (Davaine, 1872; Koch, 1878), cattle (Kitt, 1885), swine (Loeffler & Schütz, 1886), and bubonic plague bacillus (Kitasato & Yersin, 1894). Scarlatina has been interpreted as a streptococcic infection of the throat by George F. and Gladys H. **Dick** (1923), who have produced a viable test for susceptibility by intracutaneous injection of the toxin in susceptibles (1924), immunization by inoculation of increasing skin test doses of the toxin (1924) and an antitoxic serum which can be used for prophylaxis or treatment (1924–25). The mycobacteria include the pathogens of tuberculosis in man (Koch, 1884), birds (Straus & Gamaléia, 1891), cattle (Smith, 1895–6) and cold-blooded animals (Klebs, 1900; Rupprecht, 1904; Weber & Taute, 1905); the bacilli of leprosy (Neisser, 1879; Hansen, 1880), rat leprosy (Stefansky, 1903), bovine paratuberculosis (Johne's bacillus, 1895) and many bacilli found in butter, hay and plant dust. To the Clostridia belong Pasteur's *Vibrion septique* (1861), the first pathogenic anaërobe to be described and now recognized as the causative agent of malignant edema (*C. septicum*), the organism ascribed to the same condition by Koch (1881), the bacillus (*C. chauvei*) of symptomatic anthrax (Arloing, 1887), the tetanus bacillus (Nicolaier, 1885), the Welch bacillus (*B. aërogenes*, 1892), the Bacillus botulinus (van Ermengem, 1897) and many organisms found in European War wounds by Adamson and others. The Hemophilus group includes the influenza bacillus (Pfeiffer 1892–93), the Hemophilus hemolyticus (Pritchett & Stillman, 1919), the bacillus of whooping-cough (Bordet & Gengou, 1906), the Koch-Weeks bacillus (1887), and the pathogen of septicemic cerebrospinal meningitis in rabbits (Cohen, 1909). The typing of pneumococci by Dochez, Gillespie, and Avery (1913–16) has thrown much light upon their relative virulence, and apart from the accepted pathogenic strains in bacillary dysentery there are many related pseudo-dysenteric types. Thus, bacteriological diagnosis tends to ultra-refinement.

The effects of **mixed infection** or bacterial symbiosis were investigated by Pavlovsky (1887), Emmerich (1887–99) and others, who showed that various bacteria heighten resistance to anthrax infection, while Roux and Yersin (1888–90), Monti (1889), Fessler (1891) and Pane (1894) showed increase of virulence in bacterial association. Mixed infections were classified by Wassermann and Keysser (1912). The **bactericidal action of the blood** was noted by John Hunter and demonstrated by Fodor (1887), Nuttall (1888), Buchner (alexins, 1890–95), von Behring and Nissen (1890). Pfeiffer discovered **bacteriolysis** of cholera bacilli in the peritoneal cavity (1895) and the theory of **bacteriolytic** and **hemolytic sera** was greatly extended by Bordet (sensibilizing substances 1898–9), Ehrlich and Morgenroth (amboceptors, antibodies, 1898–9). The stimulins of Metchnikoff were investigated by Denys and Leclef (1895), Wright and Douglas (opsonins, 1903–4), Neufeld and Rimpau (bacteriotropins, 1904–5). **Antitoxins** were discovered by von Behring and Kitasato (1890). **Toxin-antitoxin mixtures** were investigated in diphtheria by Ehrlich and Knorr (1895–7) and by Bordet (1899). Bacterial **agglutinins** were discovered by Gruber and Durham (1896), applied to typhoid diagnosis by Widal (1896) and shown to be absorbed from sera by bacteria (Castellani, 1902). **Precipitins** were discovered by R. Kraus (1898), applied to diagnosis by Ascoli (1911), employed to differentiate animal proteins by Wassermann and Schütz (1901–2), in medicolegal tests for human blood by Uhlenhuth (1900) and in differentiating animal species by Nuttall (1904). **Anaphylaxis,** known to Jenner and Magendie, was investigated by Richet

(1902–9), Theobald Smith (1903), Rosenau and Anderson (1906–7) and Otto (1906–7); **sensitization to foreign proteins** by Hericourt and Richet (1898), von Pirquet and Schick (**allergy,** 1903); **serum sickness** by Pirquet (1905); the **Arthus phenomenon** in secondary injections of horse-serum by M. Arthus (1903–6); **antianaphylaxis** or desensitization by Besredka and Steinhardt (1907), Anderson and Frost (1910); **protective ferments** by Abderhalden (1912); **anaphylatoxins** by Vaughan and Wheeler (1907), Doerr and Russ (1909), E. Friedberger (1910); Novy and de Kruif (1917); hay-fever by Dunbar (1893) and Wolff-Eisner (1906); **food idiosyncrasies** by Cooke and Van der Veer (1916), Wells and Osborne (1911), and Schloss (1920). Preventive vaccination with dead cultures was demonstrated by Brieger, Kitasato and Wassermann (1892) and Pfeiffer (1896). The theory of **local immunity** in the cells and tissues, without the intervention of antibodies was developed by Alexander **Besredka** (1925), who introduced sensitized vaccines (1913) and preventive inoculation against phthisis by B. C. G. or avirulent bovine bacillus vaccines (Bacillus-Calmette-Guérin, 1921–7).

Transmissible lysis of bacteria was discovered by F. W. Twort (1915) and F. d'Herelle (**bacteriophagy,** 1917) and investigated further by Bordet and Cinca (1920–21), Hans Zinsser (1922), Weiss and Arnold (1924) and others. D'Herelle postulates a self-reproducing bacteriophage (1918), Twort a pre-cellular (pre-bacterial) ultrascopic, filter passing virus. It is probable, however, that most viruses of this type are microörganisms as yet invisible. With reference to the statement of Doerr that filterability has no scientific meaning in relation to these "viruses," the important experiments of Stuart Mudd on electric polarisation of bacteria (1921–22) and of S. P. Kramer on bacterial filters (1926–27) open out new and hitherto unimaginable lines of approach and attack. The starting point of the doctrine of **filterable viruses** was the discovery of Loeffler and Frosch that the inoculable virus of foot-and-mouth disease will pass through the finest filters (1898), which had already been shown for the mosaic disease of tobacco by Ivanovski (1892) and Beijerinck (1893), with eventual cultivation of the virus by Olitsky (1925). The work of Mudd and Kramer has necessitated revision of previous notions of filterability, while that of Twort and d'Herelle envisages filterable viruses as ultrascopic organisms or states of substance.

It is a remarkable fact that many of the indeterminate diseases allocated to ultrascopic viruses are associated variously with cell inclusions of the type observed by Guarnieri (1892) or Negri (1903), bacterioid dots or chlamydozoa (Prowazek, 1907–8), Strongyloplasmata (Lipschütz, 1913) or the bacteria-like Rickettsia (1906–11), as indicated by the following tabulation[1]:

Vaccinia: From cowpox, (Jenner, 1796); from smallpox (Fischer, 1890; Voigt, 1905). Virus (Freyer, 1896–9; Negri, 1905).
Rabies: Virus (Pasteur, 1881; DiVesteat & Zagari, 1889). Cell inclusions (Negri, 1903–10). Black bodies (Koch & Riesling, 1910; Noguchi, 1913).
Bovine Pleuropneumonia: Virus (Pasteur, 1883; Nocard, 1898). Microörganisms (Bordet, 1910).
Yellow Fever: Bacillus X (Sternberg, 1888; Sanarelli, 1897). Virus (Walter Reed, 1901). *Leptospira icteroides* (Noguchi, 1919).
Smallpox: Cell inclusions (L. Pfeiffer, 1891; G. Guarnieri, 1892). Virus (Casagrandi, 1908).
Inundation Fever (Tsutsugamushi): Virus (Kitasato, 1893). Insect transmission (Miyajima & Asakawa, 1904). Cell inclusions (Kitashima & Miyajima, 1911–18). Virulent coccoid bodies (Ishiwara & Ogata, 1923). *Rickettsia Nipponica* (1923).
Verruca vulgaris (Warts): Virus (Jadassohn, 1895; Ciuffo, 1907).
Cattle-plague (*Rinderpest*): Virus (Koch, 1897; A. Theiler, 1897).
Foot-and-mouth Disease: Virus (Löffler & Frosch, 1897–8), Von Betigh bodies in lymph (1911).
South African Horse-sickness (*Pferdesterbe*): Virus (Macfadyen, 1900). Insect transmission (Theiler, 1903). Chlamydozoa (Kuhn, 1911).

---

[1] Prepared mainly from the chapter on micro-organisms of undetermined character in W. W. Ford's Text-book of Bacteriology, Philadelphia, 1927, 1003–1052.

Trachoma: Virus (Greef, 1900–8); Chlamydozoa (Halberstädter & Prowazek, 1907). Immunization (Nicolle, 1911–13).
Fowl-pest (*Hühnerpest*): Virus (Centanni & Savonuzzi, 1901; Marchoux, 1908). Chlamydozoa (Prowazek, 1908).
Canine Pseudorabies: Virus (Aujeszky, 1902; Schmiedhöffer, 1910).
Heartwater: Insect transmission (Lounsbury, 1902; Theiler & Robertson, 1903). Virus (Theiler, 1903; Edington, 1904). *Rickettsia ruminantium* (E. V. Cowdry, 1925).
Rocky Mountain Spotted Fever: Tick transmission (Wilson & Chowning, 1902). Rickettsia bodies (Ricketts, 1906–11; Wolbach, 1919–23).
Fowl-pox (Epithelioma contagiosa): Virus (Marx & Sticker, 1902–03). Chlamydozoa (Borrel, 1904; Prowazek & Lipschütz, 1908). Immunization (Manteufel 1910).
Sheep-pox (*Clavelée*): Virus and Chlamydozoa (Borrel, 1903).
Hog Cholera (*Schweinepest*): Virus (De Schweinitz, Dorset, Bolton, McBride, 1903–4). Cell inclusions (Uhlehnath & Boïng, 1910). Immunization (Preisz, 1898).
Equine Swamp Fever (Pernicious Anemia): Virus (Carrée & Vallée, 1904).
Canine Distemper (*Hundestaupe*): Virus (Carrée, 1905). Cell inclusions (Standfuss & Lentz, 1909).
Molluscum Contagiosum: Virus (Juliusberg, 1905). *Strongyloplasma hominis* (Lipschütz, 1913).
Dengue: Mosquito transmission (Graham, 1903; Cleland & Bradley, 1917–18; Siler, 1925). Virus (Ashburn & Craig, 1907). Chlamydozoa (Harris & Duval, 1924).
Mumps: Virus from saliva (Granata, 1908; Martha Wollstein, 1918).
Infectious Avian Leukemia (Moore): Virus (Ellermann & Bang, 1908–9). Cell inclusions (Hirschfeld & Jacobi, 1909).
Pappataci (Three-day) Fever: Virus (Doerr & Russ, 1908–11; Birt, 1908–10). Phlebotomus transmission (Doerr).
Tabardillo (Mexican typhus): Virus (Anderson & Goldberger, 1909–10).
Equine Cerebrospinal Meningitis (Borna's Disease): Cell inclusions (Joest, 1909–11).
Alastrim (Benign Smallpox): Cell inclusions (Carini, 1910). Virus (Aragao, 1911; MacCallum & Moody 1921).
Poliomyelitis: Virus (Flexner & Lewis, 1910; Landsteiner & Levaditi, 1910). Globoid bodies (Flexner, 1910–17).
Typhus Fever: Louse transmission (Nicolle, 1910–12; Ricketts & Wilder, 1910). Cell inclusions (Prowazek, 1916). Rickettsia Prowazeki (Rickets, 1910; Prowazek, 1913–15).
Avian Diphtheria: Virus Uhlenhuth (1910). Microörganisms (Bordet & Fally, 1910).
Measles: Virus (Hektoen, 1905–19; Nicolle, 1911–21). Transmission (Goldberger & Anderson, 1911). Bacteria (Ruth Tunnicliff diplococcus, 1917; Caronia, 1921–23). Convalescent Serum (Degkwitz, 1922–7). Cell inclusions (Döhle, 1911–12).
Pink-eye (*Pferdestaupe*): Virus (Bemelmans, 1913). Contagion (Clark, 1894).
Trench or Volhynian (Five day) Fever (Graham & Herringham, 1915; His & Werner, 1916): Virus (McNee & Renshaw, 1916). Louse transmission (Strong *et al.*, 1918). *Rickettsia quintana* (Töpfer, 1916).
Australian Encephalomyelitis: Virus (Cleland & Campbell, 1919).
Encephalitis lethargica: Virus (Loewe, Hirschfeld & Strauss, 1919). Coccoid bodies (Loewe & Strauss, 1920). Intranuclear bodies (Levaditi *et al.*, 1922).
Herpes: Virus (Grüter, 1919; Lowenstein, 1919; Goodposture & Teague, 1923).
Ovine Stomatitis (*Chancre du mouton*): Virus (Aynaud, 1923).
Varicella: Viruses (Rivers & Tillett, 1924). Cell inclusions (Tyzzer, 1905).

It is plain from the above that many communicable diseases are as yet undecipherable.

Tropical medicine, vaguely rooted in antiquity, came into being largely through the exploration of the globe by navigators and the settlements made in tropical and torrid regions by Spain, England, Holland, France and Germany. It owes its scientific status to the development of bacteriology, parasitology, protozoölogy, medical entomology and medical mycology. It had its authentic start with the organization of the Indian Medical Service of the British Army (1764), and some of the best work done in the early period clusters around the names of Lind, Wade, Russell, Fayrer, MacNamara, Malcolmson, Corbyn, Waring, Vandyke, Carter, Sir Leonard Rogers, and Sir Ronald Ross. Many valuable observations are to be found in the writings of Sir Richard Burton, but the real prime mover was Sir Patrick Manson. As the problem of colonial expansion became of moment in the 20th century, it was natural that there should be a large outcropping of worthwhile periodicals, and that institutes of tropical medicine should be established in the centers of shipping and commerce, notably London (1899), Liverpool (1899), Hamburg (1900), Brussels (1906), and San Juan, Porto Rico (1917), which will be a clearing-house and seed-plant for developments in the Antilles, Central and South America. The sense of the International Congress at Singapore (1924) was that each important tropical area has its own particular climate, ecology and diseases. Castellani says that it is not wise for a physician to attempt practice in the tropics without some "basic course of instruction in one of these schools."

The beginnings were the observations on parasites in Egyptian papyri and Babylonian baked bricks, the clinical data on leprosy, malaria, plague and diphtheria (*ulcera Syriaca*) in Hippocrates, Aretæus, the Bible and the Talmud, the Hindu notations on mosquitoes (malaria), rats (plague), diabetes and dysentery, the account of snake-bite in Lucan's *Pharsalia*, and the stressing of the icteric and diabetic diatheses in Arabic pathology. The introduction of cinchona bark (1638–70) was the *point d'appui* of the clinical studies of Sydenham, Morton, Lancisi and Torti on malarial fever. Laveran's discovery of the malarial parasite (1880) is signalized by Castellani as the *impetum faciens* of the brilliant achievements of Manson (filariasis), Ross (malaria), Dutton (trypanosomiasis), Bruce (tsetse fly nagana, Malta fever), Ashford (hook-worm, sprue), Stiles and Looss (hook-worm) and Schaudinn (dysentery, syphilis) in tropical parasitology. The service of the U. S. Army Medical Department in the Philippines (1900) and Antilles (1900) was distinguished by a rapid output of effective work, culminating in the sanitation of the Panama Canal Zone. Equally significant was the work of Parkes (London, 1851), Pruner Bey (Cairo, 1851), Koch (Cholera Commission, 1883), Pettenkofer (Munich, 1892–4), Koch (Hamburg, 1892) and the international conferences held after the opening of the Suez Canal (1869) with reference to warding off cholera and plague. Medical officers of the French Army and Navy did valuable work on malaria, Cochin China diarrhœa and other phases. In Japan, Ogata first differentiated infantile beriberi (1888), from the adult type, but the autonomy of the infantile variety was definitely established, clinically and pathologically, by José Albert (Manila) in 1908. In the Dutch East Indies, Christian Eijkman (1858–   ) was remarkable for his investigations on beriberi (1897–1906). Among the Germans, Theodor Bilharz (*Schistosoma hæmatobium*, 1852), Erwin Baelz (1845–1913) and H. B. Scheube (1851–   ), who did much to advance parasitology in Japan, B. A. E. Nocht (1857–1927), director of the Hamburg Institute of Naval and Tropical Medicine, Albert Plehn, investigator in Cameroon and author of a treatise on tropical hygiene (1906), Arthur Looss (hook-worm infestation, 1898) and L. Külz, who wrote on hygiene and diseases of tropical natives (1911–19), are outstanding. In Italy, the names of Baccelli, Golgi, Marchiafava, Celli, Grassi, Bignami are associated with malarial fever, and Aldo Castellani with the parasites of sleeping sickness (1903) and yaws (1905) and the best historical treatise on tropical medicine (1910). The relative immunity of most tropical natives to parasitic and surgical infections, comparable with the immunity of the carabao to surra, has been stressed by Walter Mendelson (1923–7).

Sir Patrick **Manson** (1844–1922), of Aberdeen, Scotland, and a medical graduate of its university (1866), entered the Chinese Imperial

Maritime Customs Service under Sir Robert Hart, and, landing on the beach of Formosa on a dark night in June (1866), embarked upon an energetic career in tropical surgery, in which he learned Chinese, invented a trocar for liver abscess, made postmortems in cemeteries, and saw all manner of tropical diseases, which he reported in the *Customs Gazette* (1871–83).

In 1872, he described tinea nigra, the fungus of which is Foxia Mansoni (Castellani, 1905) and gave the first correct description of tinea imbricata and its fungus (Trichophyton Mansoni). In 1877, he found filaria in elephantiasis and in 1878 discovered the transmission of *Filaria bancrofti* by the Culex mosquito. In 1880, simultaneously with Baelz, he found Paragonimus Westermanni in human sputum. He was the first after Hillary (1766) to give a correct description of tropical sprue (1880), the puzzling Cochin China diarrhea of the French naval surgeons (1864–80). He discovered *Sparganum mansoni* (1883), *Filaria hominis* (1891), the larval stage of *Filaria loa* (1891), its rôle in Calabar swelling (1893) and the eggs of *Schistosomum mansoni* (1903). He was the first to maintain that blackwater (hemoglobinuric) fever is distinct from malaria (1893) saw *Trypanosoma gambiense* before Ford (1900), described epidemic gangrenous rectitis (1907) and the double continued fever of the tropics (1907), performed the classical experiment of transmitting tertian malarial fever by an anopheline upon his own son, and was the inspirer and mentor of Ronald Ross. His Manual of 1898 sums up his vast experience in the semeiology of tropical diseases.

After a sojourn in England, Manson returned to Hong Kong (1886) and started a school of tropical medicine. In 1890, he left China, commenced practice in Cavendish Square, and, in 1898, started the London School of Tropical Medicine in a small house near the Albert Docks. It was funded by Lord Milner, moved to Endsleigh Gardens and is now endowed by the Rockefeller Institute (1927). Manson was knighted in 1903, and was well described by Blanchard as "the father of tropical medicine."

Great practical advances in the science of infectious diseases have been made in recent times through the coöperation of **army medical officers.**

The work of Alphonse Laveran on malarial fever, of Ferdinand Widal on typhoid fever, of Friedrich Löffler and Emil Behring on diphtheria, of Colonel Sir Ronald Ross on malarial fever, of Surgeon-General Sir David Bruce on Malta fever and sleeping sickness, of Colonel Sir William Boog Leishman (1865–1926), Major Donovan and Colonel Sir Leonard Rogers on kala-azar, will compare favorably with what John Hunter or Helmholtz accomplished during their period of military service.

One of the last and best of the noble line of the Indian Medical Service is Lieut.-Col. Robert **McCarrison** (1878–   ), who entered the service in 1901, and has been on almost continual duty in India to date, latterly at the Pasteur Institute at Coonoor. In 1906, he described the three-day fever endemic in Upper India since 1895, which is probably identical with Dalmatian pappataci fever. He is further distinguished by his investigations of the infectious endemic goiter of Kashmir (1913), the thyroid gland (1917), beriberi and other deficiency diseases (1921–4), particularly the remarkable degenerative changes in the viscera and general lowering of digestive capacity produced by vitamin B- or C-deficiency anterior to beriberi or scurvy. This is one

of the most significant contributions to the rôle of nutrition in preventive medicine. In the United States Army, the labors of such men
as William Beaumont, Jonathan **Letterman** (1824–72), who revived
Larrey's methods of rapid evacuation of the wounded and reorganized
the whole administration of medical service in the field, William A.
Hammond, creator of the Army Medical Museum, Joseph Janvier
Woodward (1833–84), pioneer in photo-micrography, Alfred A. Woodhull (1837–   ), who introduced the Indian method of giving massive
doses of ipecac in dysentery,[1] Billings, Otis, Smart and Huntington
have set an example which has been followed by a number of able
officers in recent times. A great pioneer in the study of bacteriology
in America was Surgeon-General George M. **Sternberg** (1838–1915),

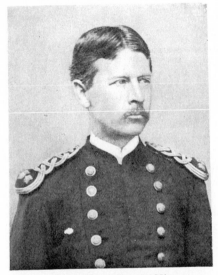

who isolated the diplococcus of
pneumonia simultaneously with
Pasteur (1880[2]), published valuable treatises on bacteriology
(1892) and disinfection (1900),
and through the localization of
"Bacillus X" in yellow fever as a
negative find, cleared the ground
for later investigators. During
his administration, Major Walter
Reed (1851–1902), of Virginia,
who had studied under Welch at
Johns Hopkins and had done good
work on the pathology of typhoid
fever in his laboratory (1895), was
detailed as the head of a Board,
including James Carroll, Aristide
Agramonte and Jesse W. Lazear,
to study yellow fever in Cuba, then
occupied by the American Army

Walter Reed (1851–1902).

(1900). Carlos Finlay (1833–
1915) had already advanced the theory that the disease is transmitted by
the Stegomyia mosquito (1881), but when the Army Board went to
Cuba, the Bacillus icteroides of Sanarelli held the field. In 1900,
Henry R. Carter (U. S. Public Health Service) had shown that a lapse
of twelve to fifteen days is necessary before a case of yellow fever becomes dangerous to others. Reed and his associates soon disposed of
Sanarelli's bacillus (identical with the Bacillus X of Sternberg) and
proceeded at once to attack the problem of transmission by mosquitoes.
During the course of their experiments,[3] twenty-two cases of yellow fever
were produced experimentally, fourteen by infected mosquito-bites, six

[1] Woodhull: Studies, chiefly clinical, in the non-emetic use of ipecacuanha,
Philadelphia, 1876.
[2] Sternberg: Rep. Nat. Bd. Health, 1881, Washington, 1882, iii, 87–92.
[3] Reed (*et al.*), Philadelphia Med. Jour., 1900, vi, 790–796.

by the injection of blood, and two by the injection of filtered blood-serum, thus proving the existence of a filterable virus (1901[1]), confirmed by Rosenau at Vera Cruz (1903), while seven enlisted men disposed of the fomites theory of transmission by sleeping in infected bedding. Carroll was the first to submit to mosquito inoculation and came through an attack of yellow fever successfully. Lazear died from the effects of an accidental mosquito-bite. Thus it was proven, according to the most rigorous conventions of formal logic, that the cause of yellow fever is either an ultra-microscopic organism or a filterable virus which is transmitted to man by a particular species of mosquito, the *Aëdes* (*Stegomyia*) *ægypti*. With reference to the conditions under which the experiment was performed, particularly the period of development in the body of the mosquito, the demonstration of the Army Board is one of the most brilliant and conclusive in the history of science. Its economic importance is indicated by the immense saving of life and money through the eradication of yellow fever in the United States and the West Indies, if not throughout the entire world. The New Orleans epidemic of 1905 was promptly checked by the U. S. Public Health Service and yellow fever was eradicated from Mexico by Licéaga and from Rio by Oswaldo Cruz. In February, 1901, shortly after Reed had proved his case, Major William C. **Gorgas** (1854–1920), of Mobile, Alabama, as chief sanitary officer of Havana, Cuba, began to screen yellow fever patients and destroy mosquitos, and, in three months, Havana was freed from the disease for the first time in 150 years. In connection with the work on the Panama Canal, Gorgas freed that part of the Isthmus not only from yellow fever, but from all dangerous infections, and through this great triumph in sanitation, Panama, formerly a notorious plague spot of disease, the "White Man's Grave," as it was called, is now one of the healthiest communities in existence. In 1913–14, General Gorgas, at the invitation of the Chamber of Mines of Johannesburg. South Africa, investigated the causes of the high death-rate from pneumonia among the native miners of the Rand, and devoted the summer and autumn of 1916 to a survey of the endemic foci of yellow fever in South America for the Rockefeller Foundation, upon which work he was engaged at the time of his death. The investigations of typhoid fever incidence in camp during the Spanish-American War (1898), by Walter Reed, Victor C. Vaughan and Edward O. Shakespeare demonstrated the transmission of the disease by flies.

During the American occupation of Porto Rico, the island population was vaccinated and freed from smallpox under Colonel John Van R. Hoff, and shortly afterward Colonel Bailey K. Ashford discovered hook-worm infection in the island (1900[2]) and eradicated the disease, found sprue in Porto Rico (1908), identified *Monilia psilosis* as its exciting cause (1914) and founded the Institute of Tropical Medicine at San Juan (1917) which has recently acquired a sumptuous habitat (1926). Colonel Charles F. Craig (1872–   ) demonstrated the existence of

---

[1] Tr. Ass. Am. Phys., Phila., 1901, xvi, 45–72.

[2] Ashford: New York Med. Jour., 1900, lxxi, 552–556.

malaria carriers (1902–05[1]); showed that the so called Piroplasma hominis of Rocky Mountain spotted fever is really an artefact in the erythrocytes (1904); and, in the Philippines, showed with Colonel Percy M. Ashburn that the cause of dengue is a filterable virus (1907[2]). Craig is also the author of extensive monographs on the malarial fevers (1901, 1909), the parasitic amebæ in man (1911) and of recent work on the hemolysins, cytolysins and complement-fixing substances of Entamœba histolytica (1927). Captain Henry J. Nichols (1877–1927) collaborated with Ehrlich in his initial work on salvarsan (1910) and has since investigated the experimental production of yaws (1910–11). Under the administration of Surgeon-General George H. Torney, Major Frederick F. Russell, in 1909, began the huge experiment of vaccinating the United States Army against typhoid fever, after the methods advocated by André Chantemesse (1851–1919) and F. Widal in France (1888), Pfeiffer and Kolle in Germany (1896), and Wright and Semple in England (1896). From a morbidity of 173 (16 fatal) cases of typhoid in 1909, Russell was able to bring his statistics down to 9 cases of the disease with one fatality in 1912, while at present the army is absolutely free from typhoid. The mobilization of United States troops on the Mexican border in 1912[3] gave Major Russell an opportunity such as never came even to Jenner or Pasteur, viz., that of testing his vaccine at a huge outdoor clinic consisting of some 20,000 men. The absolute success of his experiment is now a matter of history. Colonel Edward B. Vedder (1878–   ), of New York City, has made important studies in beriberi as a deficiency disease, summed up in his treatise of 1913, and was the first to determine the specific amebicidal action of emetine in the treatment of amebic dysentery (1910–11[4]). In 1911, Captains Ernest R. Gentry and Thomas L. Ferenbaugh discovered that Malta fever is endemic in Southwestern Texas, and transmitted by the goats of the goat-ranches. In 1916, Major George B. Foster made an important investigation of the causation of common colds by a filterable virus. In 1925, Colonel Joseph F. Siler and Majors Milton W. Hall and Arthur P. Hitchens demonstrated (in 47 cases) the transmission of dengue by Aëdes ægypti, thus nullifying the long accepted belief that Culex fatigans is the vector (Graham, 1903), verifying the preliminary observation of Cleland and Bradley (1917) and demonstrating the exact mechanism of transmission (identical with that of yellow fever). Lieut. Col. Charles E. Woodruff (1860–1915) investigated the deleterious effects of tropical light upon the blonde northern races (1905) and wrote interesting volumes on Expansion of Races (1909) and Medical Ethnology (1915). Colonel George Ensign Bushnell (1853–1924) was one of the leading American students of tuberculosis, particularly of its effects upon troops in the World War and upon natives of the tropics. He showed that endemic tropical tuberculosis either destroys the weak in infancy or immunizes the strong by virtual preventive inoculation, whence the devastating effects of the disease in non-immunized areas. In his Mütter lecture (1902) Colonel Louis A. La Garde (1849–1920) demonstrated that sterile gunshot wounds are non-existent, because the microörganisms in powder or projectiles are not destroyed by the heat of firing, but conveyed directly into the wound. He wrote a standard treatise on gunshot injuries (1914). The manuals of military hygiene by Colonel Valery Harvard (1909) and x-ray technic by Captain Arthur C. Christie (1913) are in the same class. Col. Edward L. Munson, once editor of the Military Surgeon, is the author of important works on military hygiene (1901), sanitary tactics, the military shoe (1912) and the Management of Men (1921). All these works, with the various manuals of military medicine by Charles S. Tripler (1858), Alfred A. Woodhull (1898), Paul F. Straub (1910), Charles F. Mason (1912), and others, have added much to the lustre of the U. S. Army Medical Corps at home and abroad.

Intimately connected with the history of communicable diseases is the illustrious bead-roll of its medical martyrs. With Servetus and Semmelweis, who died for their opinions, should be classed such names as Daniel A. Carrion (verrugas), Jesse W. Lazear (yellow fever), Alexander

---

[1] Craig: Ann. Med., Phila., 1905, 982; 1029.

[2] Craig and Ashburn: Philippine Jour. Sc., Manila, 1907, B. ii, 93–146.

[3] Russell: Harvey Lecture, 1913.

[4] Vedder: Bull. Manila Med. Soc., 1911, iii, 48–53. Jour. Trop. Med., Lond., 1911, xiv, 149–152.

Yersin and Hermann Franz Müller (bubonic plague), Tito Carbone (Malta fever), Allen MacFadyen (typhoid and Malta fever), J. Everett Dutton (African relapsing fever), Howard Taylor Ricketts (tabardillo), A. W. Bacot (typhus fever), Thomas B. McClintick (Rocky Mountain fever), William Ironside Bruce (aplastic anemia), Pirie (kala-azar), Gaspar Vianna (postmortem sepsis), Adrian Stokes and Noguchi (yellow fever), all of whom lost their lives in investigating the diseases with which their names are associated. Another group includes Bergonié, Spence, Blackall, Hall-Edwards, Albers-Schönberg, Leonard, Caldwell, Dodd, Kassabian, and other victims of x-ray injuries. Among those who have run definite risks by experimenting upon themselves are John Hunter, Hammond, Carroll, Halsted, Henry Head and L. F. Barker.

Recent **surgery** undoubtedly owes most to Wilhelm Konrad **Röntgen** (1845–1922), of Lennep (Rhineland), who became professor of physics at Strassburg (1876), Giessen (1879), Würzburg (1888), and Munich (1899). Child of a German farmer and a Dutch mother, Röntgen was educated at Utrecht, but being a dreamer, hating routine and standardization, he was but an indifferent student until he came under the influence of Clausius, the teacher of Willard Gibbs (at Zurich), and later an assistant of Kundt, whom he accompanied to Würzburg. In 1895, while experimenting with a Crookes tube, with reference to Hittorf (cathode) and

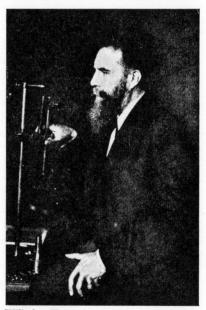

Wilhelm Konrad Röntgen (1845–1922).

Lenard rays, Röntgen got strange accidental shadows of solid objects, and by making his tube light-proof, a greenish fluorescent light could be thrown upon a platinobarium screen 9 feet away, a new kind of radiation. These rays passed through most substances, the soft parts of the body in particular, so that the bones of his hand, as being denser, were boldly revealed upon a photographic plate. Upon communicating his discovery to the Würzburg Society on December 28, 1895, Röntgen modestly called the new rays x-rays, but upon motion of Kölliker, who predicted their usefulness in medicine and surgery, they were named Röntgen rays. In spite of the award of the Nobel prize (1901) and the world-wide fame which was his, Röntgen, a simple, honest, truth-loving nature, began to hate publicity when his discovery was imputed to his assistant. Wounded by the vituperation, he sank more and more into himself and was accessible only to students

46

and to visitors of character, breeding and ability. Saddened by the war, of which he predicted the outcome, he retired from his chair, and, wife and friends gone, he died on February 10, 1922, a lonely, isolated man, neglected by the younger generation. Like Faraday, he was no mathematician, but a wonderful stimulator of capable youth, "a mid-wife of mind," and one of the noblest and greatest men of his generation.

The applications of **Röntgenology** to surgery and medicine were developed with amazing rapidity and in less than twenty years the new science was on a firmer footing than most. **Röntgenography** was immediately applied by the surgeon to the diagnosis and location of fractures, dislocations, foreign bodies, and embedded projectiles, by the dentist to the teeth, by the physiologist to the elucidation of function, by the medico-legal expert to the detection of concealed objects and the diagnosis of death (Vaillant, 1907). An early pioneer was W. B. Cannon, who elucidated the movements of the stomach (1898) and intestines (1902) in animals by using bismuth paste, which was carried over to surgery by E. Beck (1906). Further improvements in technique led to such novelties as pneumoperitoneum (Weber, 1915), ventriculography (Dandy, 1918) and cholecystography (Graham and Cole, 1923–24). Röntgentherapy started with the discovery of the possibility of epilation in nævus pilosus and hypertrichosis by Leopold Freund of Vienna (1896) and the next five years were devoted to empirical therapy of cutaneous lesions, notably lupus (Schiff and Kümmell, 1897; Pusey, 1900), psoriasis (Ziemssen, 1898), favus (Freund, 1898), eczema (Hahn, 1898), superficial epithelioma (Stenbeck and Sjögren, 1899–1900) and alopecia (Kienböck, 1900). The new period was ushered in by G. **Holzknecht** and **Kienböck,** who introduced scientific dosage (1900–2); **Albers-Schönberg** who invented the compression diaphragm (1902–3), which intensified the object by cutting out secondary rays, showed the injurious effect of the rays upon internal organs, notably azospermia (1903) and devised the leaden chamber for the protection of operators from sterility (Philipp, 1905); and by **Perthes,** who introduced **deep therapy** (1903). Senn applied the x-rays to the treatment of leukemia (1902–3) and Heineke noted their selective effect upon lymphatic organs (1903–4). Tubes of calcium glass (Grunmach, 1905) and of lead glass (Wichmann, 1905) added to the comfort of the eyes and the safety of the operator, while the sulphur-zinc screen of Danneberg (1906) made for more distinct pictures. The observations on the effects of irradiation upon the growth of young animals (Perthes, 1903) in suppressing sweat (Buschke and Schmidt, 1905), on the leucocytes (Aubertin and Beaujard, 1904), the testicle (Bergonié and Tribondeau, 1904), the ovary (Halberstaedter, 1905), the eye (Birch Hirschfeld, 1907) and in the production of cholin in the blood (Benjamin, 1907) opened out new viewpoints. Meanwhile congresses of Röntgenology had been held at Paris (1900), Berne (1902), and Milan (1904) and a Röntgen Society was founded in Berlin (1905). The pioneer work of Kienböck, Holzknecht, Albers-Schönberg and Perthes was continued in France by Beclère (Paris), Bergonié (Bordeaux), Leduc (Nancy) and Bordier (Lyons), in England by Hall Edwards, Morton, and Sequeira, in America by Pusey, Senn, Coley, Williams, Baetjer, Beck, and Stelwagon. In 1904, Foveau de Courmelles began to treat uterine myomata by x-rays and during 1906–10 much was done by Holzknecht, Wetterer, Albers-Schönberg, and others in irradiation for uterine tumors and hemorrhage, while following Beclère's work on deep therapy in tuberculous lymphoma (1905), Holzknecht, Kienböck, Wetterer, Freund, Barjon, Beclère, and Rudis-Jicinsky did much for the treatment of surgical tuberculosis (bones and joints). The introduction of such new devices as the **Coolidge tube** (1913[1]) and the **Potter-Bucky diaphragm** (1913–24[2]) mark the beginning of a new period. Finsen's treatment of smallpox pustules by exclusion of ultraviolet light (1893) and of lupus by its concentration (1895), the invention of the mercury vapor lamps of Leo Arons (1896), Peter Cooper Hewitt (quartz lamp, 1901), and Kromayer (1904), the discovery of **radium** by the **Curies** (1898), the applications of **radium therapy** to lupus (Danlos and Block, 1901) and malignant tumors (Danysz, 1903), of **ultraviolet light** (1903) and Alpine sunlight (1910) to tuberculosis by Rollier, and to rickets by Kurt **Huldschinsky** (1918), along with the introduction of **diathermy** by Franz **Nagelschmidt** (1894) have extended the possibilities of phototherapy and

1 W. D. Coolidge: Am. J. Roentgenol., Detroit, 1913–14, n. s., i, 115–124.
2 G. Bucky: Arch. Roentgenol., Lond., 1913–14, xviii, 6–9.

radiotherapy to all manner of diseases and surgical conditions. **Cancer,** in particular, still remains very much of a surgeon's problem and has shown an alarming increase of late years. Apart from the occasional successes of radium-therapy in superficial epithelioma and other local malignancies, the best results have so far been obtained with the knife. On the pathogenetic side, the first successful transplants in rodents were made by Arthur Hanau (1889), who committed suicide on account of the neglect his work encountered. It was confirmed and followed up by Moran (1894), Leo Loeb (1901) and Jensen (1902–3), who carried sarcoma through some 40 generations of mice. During 1910–15, the initial observation of Pott on soot cancer in chimney sweeps (1775) was extended to tobacco smoking, betel nut chewing, biliary calculus, nematoda (Borrel, 1910), Kangri burns (Neve, 1910), tar (Bayon, 1912), culminating in the brilliant work of Fibiger on nematode irritation in mice, which was accomplished under overwhelming difficulties (1914). All this tended to confirm the initial observation of Virchow that the exciting cause of malignancy is local irritation. The remarkable experiments of Peyton Rous on the transference of sarcoma in Plymouth Rock chickens by transplants or inoculation with a cell-free filtrate (1911–14) were continued by Carrel and Burrows (1911), A. Fischer Drew, and others of the Rockefeller Institute, who improved the nutritive media. In 1926, Gye and Bernard announced that the Rous sarcoma virus is made of two negative components, one obtained from a cell-free filtrate killed with chloroform, the other from a "primary culture" kept at standstill until its potency is *nil*, and that these combined will produce a positive result on inoculation. The inert component is supposed to contain the basic virus common to all malignant tumors, the chloroformed filtrate contains the specific nutritive substance (trephone) characteristic of particular types of tumor. The most striking and significant experimentation was that of **Maude Slye** (Chicago) who by selective breeding of mice showed that resistance to malignancy is a Mendelian dominant, susceptibility a recessive, which can either of them be bred into or out of susceptible or resistant generations according to the laws of genetics (1913–28). Thus cancer may be a superimposed or acquired diathesis which can be stimulated to malignant activity by local irritation, even from microorganisms or parasites. Murphy regards resistance as a lymphocytosis which can be accelerated by gentle Röntgen irradiation and destroyed by strong x-ray stimulation. In the treatment of malignant tumors, radiotherapy goes hand in hand with surgical intervention, supplementing it in the early stages, supplanting it in the later. In sarcoma, the x-ray seems preferable to a mutilating operation.

Thus the possibilities of irradiation, of serum-, vaccine- and protein-therapy, of iodine in goiter and of irradiated cod-liver oil and foods in rickets, of alcohol injections in neuralgia, of artificial hyperemia and transfusion, prelude the "biological period," in which the surgeon becomes more and more of an internist, and surgery itself more conservative. The note of **preventive surgery** was sounded in Volkmann's treatment of tuberculosis of the bones and joints by iodine, cod-liver oil and diet. Bier now rejects all joint operations except amputation. In many conditions, the surgeon is now *messerscheu.* Apart from Röntgenology, recent surgery owes much to improvements in **anesthesia.**

Following the suicide of Horace Wells (1848), nitrous oxide anesthesia was discarded, but was revived by its original discoverer G. Q. Colton (1862) and, in 1868, was used in combination with oxygen by Edmund Andrews, of Chicago, to forestall asphyxia. Up to 1900, chloroform was the preferred anesthetic in the Western states, but the NO_2-O (gas oxygen) mixture was revived by Goldmann (1900), Halsted and Crile, who, by 1901, had employed it in 575 major operations, forestalling shock by a preliminary injection of scopolamine and morphine (**anoci-association**). The two gases were used in sequence by J. T. Gwathmey (1914) and the mixture played a great part in the surgery of the Western Front (1914–18). Meanwhile, following the introduction of cocaine by Anrep (1879–84) and Koller (1884), **Halsted** developed all its possibilities in **conduction anesthesia** (nerve-blocking) after hazardous experimentation upon himself (1885), while Corning (1885), Matas (1899) and Bier (1899) employed it by the spinal route. The **infiltration anesthesia** of C. L. **Schleich** (1894–5) was already known to Halsted, who even got results with plain water. Conduction anesthesia was put into general practice by **Crile** (1897–1900) and **Cushing** (1900). Novocaine (Einhorn, 1905) was employed by Balfour (1913) in nerve-blocking and is now the accepted anesthetic in surgery and dentistry, e. g., in craniotomy (Cushing). The open drop method in administering ether was introduced by Prince (1893) to replace the Morton flask and Clover cone (rebreathing) and occasioned longstanding controversy. In 1913, **Gwathmey** proposed rectal injection of ether and oil preceded by morphine and MgSO₄ injections to replace inhalation anesthesia and (with Karsner, 1917) oral administration of this mixture in painful dressings. Gwathmey further improved this method (**synergistic anesthesia**) in 1922. In aid of abolishing shock, Crile employs diathermy to the liver, digitalis to the heart, hypodermoclysis of water and oxygen, transfusion, insulin (diabetes), ammonia and novasurol (cardiac edema). In chest surgery, Gwathmey employs oxygen and a volatile narcotic to avoid pneumothorax in high-pressure anesthesia (Tiegel's principle).

Among the many neurological operations introduced in the 20th century are intracranial trigeminal neurotomy (1901) and hypoglossolaryngeal anastomosis (1924) by C. H. Frazier, anterolateral cordotomy for neuralgia (Spiller and Frazer, 1911), periarterial sympathectomy (Leriche, 1917–22), cervical sympathectomy for Raynaud's disease (Adson and Brown, 1925), the experiments of Royle and Hunter on sympathetic ramisection for spasticity (1924). In visceral surgery, we may note valvular cecostomy (Gibson, 1900), appendicostomy (Weir, 1902), gastroduodenostomy (Finney, 1902), gastro-enterostomy for peptic ulcer (W. J. Mayo, Moynihan), and omentopexy (Ransohoff, 1912); in thoracic surgery, pleural discission (Ransohoff, 1906), pleurectomy (W. L. Keller, 1922), the remarkable success of Rehn (1896–1927), and Tuffier (1920) in suturing the heart and the operation of E. C. Cutter for mitral stenosis (1926); in genito-urinary surgery, the operations for excision of the prostate by Sir P. J. Freyer (1901) and H. H. Young (1903).

Friedrich **Trendelenburg** (1844–1924), of Berlin, a pupil of Langenbeck, is memorable for his graduating dissertation on ancient Indian surgery (1866), his work on stricture of the trachea (tampon-cannula, 1869), his introduction of gastrostomy in esophageal stricture (1877) and for his high pelvic posture in operating on the viscera (1881). He was the first to suture the patella in Germany (1878) and, in 1908, essayed the feat of operating for embolism of the pulmonary artery, which he lived to see repeated with success by his pupil Kirschner (1924). He was a founder (1872) and historian (1923) of the German Surgical Society and left a charming autobiography (1924).

The acknowledged leader of recent German surgery is August **Bier** (1861–   ), who succeeded von Bergmann at Berlin (1907), introduced intraspinal anesthesia with cocaine (1899), a new method of treating amputation stumps (1900), and active and passive hyperemia as an adjuvant in surgical therapy (1903[1]), in which he was preceded by Hugh Owen Thomas (1876–86). Latterly, Bier has stood out sturdily for conservative methods, particularly in the surgery of the joints. His defence of Hahnemann (1925) is really a brief for *milde Macht* in therapeutics. His recent survey of the medical doctrines of the past (1927[2]) places him among the ablest philosophical historians of our profession. In cocaine anesthesia by the spinal route, Bier was preceded by James Leonard Corning[3] (1855–1923), of New York City, in 1885, and by Rudolph Matas (1899). Infiltration anesthesia (1894) was introduced

---

[1] Bier: Hyperämie als Heilmittel, Leipzig, 1903.

[2] Bier: Gedanken eines Arztes über Medizin. München. med. Wochenschr., 1926–28, *passim*.

[3] Corning: New York Med. Jour., 1885, xlii, 483: xlii, 317.

by Carl Ludwig Schleich (1859–1922), who left an engaging auto-biography (1926).

Ernst Ferdinand **Sauerbruch** (1875–   ), of Barmen, Rhenish Prussia, professor at Marburg (1907), while working in Mikulicz's clinic at Breslau, greatly advanced the possibilities of intrathoracic surgery by his invention of the pneumatic chamber at reduced atmospheric (negative) pressure for the prevention of pneumothorax (1903–04). The idea of using differential pressure was first conceived by Quénu and Tuffier in 1896. Sauerbruch also devised the positive pressure cabinet in which a patient breathes compressed air, while the pleural cavity is opened at ordinary atmospheric pressure. The earlier cabinets were clumsy and had many inconveniences, but, with the modern improvements of Sauerbruch and Willy Meyer (cabinet for differential positive and negative pressure), great advances in the surgery of the esophagus and the chest have been made. Forced respiration in poisoning was first used by George Edward Fell, of Buffalo, N. Y., on July 23, 1887,[1] and this led to positive pressure by means of intubation (the Fell-O'Dwyer method), which was also recommended by Rudolph Matas in 1899. In 1909,[2] Samuel James Meltzer and John Auer, of the Rockefeller Institute, greatly simplified matters by the method of intratracheal insufflation of air through a tube passed into the trachea, producing "continuous respiration without respiratory movements." Maintenance of respiration in a strapped animal by means of a bellows had been demonstrated by Vesalius and Robert Hooke, but the ingenious Meltzer-Auer experiment made the procedure viable and was a true advance in physiological surgery.

Prominent German surgeons of today are Hans **Kehr** (1862–1916), author of authoritative treatises on gall-stone surgery (1896–1901); Emil Werner **Körte** (1853–   ), of Berlin, who has excelled in pancreatic (1898–1903) and visceral surgery; Edwin **Payr** (1871–   ), of Innsbruck, director of the University Clinic at Leipzig, who has worked in intestinal suturing and thyroid transplantation (1906); Erich **Lexer** (1867), of Würzburg, professor and director of the Surgical Clinic at Jena, who investigated the microörganisms of acute osteo-myelitis (1897), and made a great reputation in the war by his effective work on plastic surgery, particularly of the bones and joints.[3] Victor **Schmieden** (1874–   ), of Berlin, director of the Frankfort Clinic, wrote a book on military surgery (with Borchard, 1920) and has done remarkable work on the suprarenal gland, the pericardium and other organs. Apart from his surgical skill, Heinrich Ernst **Albers-Schönberg** (1865–1921), of Hamburg, a medical graduate of Leipzig (1891), was

---

[1] Fell: Tr. Internat. Med. Cong., Wash., 1887, i, 237. Buffalo Med. & Surg. Jour., 1887–88, xxvii, 145–157.

[2] Meltzer and Auer: Jour. Exper. Med., N. Y., 1909, xi, 622–625.

[3] For which see, H. G. Beyer: Johns Hopkins Hosp. Bull., Balt., 1916, xxvi, 267–270.

the leader of Röntgenology in Germany. In 1897, he started a private Röntgenological institute, founded the leading periodical of the science (*Fortschritte*, 1897) and, in 1919, was appointed to the first chair of the subject (University of Hamburg). In 1903, he published a textbook, discovered the deleterious effect of x-rays on the gonads, and invented a compression diaphragm. He described total marmorization of the bones (1904), and died a martyr to x-ray cancer (1921), which had set in about 1908. Georg **Perthes** (1869–1927), successor of Bruns at Tübingen (1910), described the osteochondritic deformity of the hip (1910–20), noted by A. T. Legg in 1909, and was the originator of deep Röntgen-therapy (1903) and a prime-mover of the treatment of cancer by irradiation.

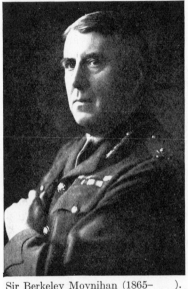

Sir Berkeley Moynihan (1865–   ).

Much effective work in visceral surgery has been done by Eugène Doyen (Paris), César Roux (Lausanne), Werner Körte (Berlin), A. W. Mayo-Robson (London), Sir Berkeley Moynihan (Leeds), John B. Murphy (Chicago), Charles H. Mayo and William J. Mayo (Rochester, Minnesota), and John M. T. Finney (Baltimore); in the surgery of the head by von Bergmann, MacEwen, W. W. Keen, H. Schloffer, Harvey Cushing; in the surgery of the vascular system by Erwin Payr (Leipzig), W. T. Halsted, J. B. Murphy, Alexis Carrel; in osteoplastic and orthopedic surgery by Albert Hoffa, Erich Lexer, E. Lorenz, J. B. Murphy, John B. Roberts, and the remarkable group of New England orthopedists, viz., Edward H. Bradford, Robert W. Lovett, and James W. Sever, who introduced the treatment of scoliosis by plaster jackets applied in suspension, Edville G. Abbott (Portland, Maine), who introduced the treatment of lateral curvature by application of jackets in flexion (1911), Robert B. Osgood, who, simultaneously with C. Schlatter, described adolescent apophysitis of the tibia (1903) and studied poliomyelitis carriers (1913), Charles F. Painter, who excised the innominate bone (1908), Joel Ernest Goldthwait, of Marblehead, Massachusetts, who has done much to simplify the complicated subject of "rheumatic disorders" by his classification of arthritis into the villous, infectious, atrophic and hypertrophic varieties (1904), and Ernest A. Codman, who described subacromial bursitis as a common cause of shoulder disability (1906–11), the pathology and treatment of which were further elucidated by Walter M. Brickner, of New York (1915). In the treatment of Pott's disease, fractures and deformities by bonegrafts, Fred H. Albee (1876–   ), of New York, has achieved a well-deserved reputation (1911–15[1]). The Italian method of cineplastic treatment of amputation stumps was introduced by G. Vanghetti (1906).

Of English surgeons who have rendered distinguished service during the European War, Sir Berkeley **Moynihan** (1865–   ), of Malta, made valuable contributions on retro-peritoneal hernia (1899), gallstones (1904), abdominal operations (1905), surgery of the spleen and

---

[1] F. H. Albee: Bone-graft Surgery, Philadelphia, 1915.

pancreas (1908), duodenal ulcer (1910), gunshot wounds (1917), and an interesting volume of essays (*Pathology of the Living*, 1910). He collaborated with A. W. M. Robson in his treatises on diseases of the stomach (1901) and pancreas (1902), and with Sir George Henry **Makins** (1853–   ), in his book on surgery of the stomach and intestines (1912). Makins' *Surgical Experiences in South Africa* (1901) is a clinical study of the effects of small-calibre bullets. He also wrote the Bradshaw lecture on gunshot wounds of arteries (1914) and a treatise on gunshot injuries of the blood-vessels (1919). Sir Anthony Alfred **Bowlby** (1855–   ) is author of treatises on *Surgical Pathology and Morbid Anatomy* (1887) and *Injuries and Diseases of Nerves* (1889). Sir Robert **Jones** (1855–

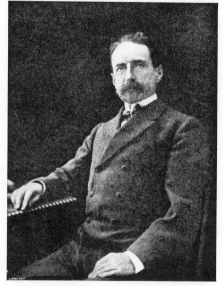

), of Rhyl, Wales, the guiding spirit of the British and American orthopedic services during the war, is the author of a book on injuries of the joints (1915), *Notes on Military Orthopedics* (1917) and *Orthopedic Surgery* (with R. W. Lovett, 1923). Alfred Herbert **Tubby** (1862–   ), consulting surgeon of the British Mediterranean (1915) and Egyptian Expeditionary Forces (1916–19), has written treatises on *Deformities* (1896), and (with Jones) on the modern surgery of paralyses (1903). Sir William Arbuthnot **Lane** (1856–   ), of Fort George, Scotland, noted for his work on the treatment of fractures by plates and screws

Théodore Tuffier (1857–   ).

(1892–1905) and on treatment of chronic intestinal stasis (Lane's kink) by short-circuiting the intestine (1903), wrote a manual of operative surgery (1886) and played an important part in the administration of surgical service during the war.

As in 18th century Paris, Tuffier, Terrillon, Chassaignac, Faure, Jaboulay, Hartmann, Pozzi, Delbet, Quénu, Doyen, Kirmisson, Morestin, Albarran, Leriche, and Lecène have made many innovations in surgical procedure and have sometimes included gynecological work as part of their specialty.

Marin-Théodore **Tuffier** (1857–   ), of Bellême (Orne), a Paris medical graduate of 1885, who taught surgery at the Paris Faculty and experimental surgery at the Sorbonne, is the author of experimental studies on the surgery of the kidney (1889), and of monographs on the surgical treatment of phthisis (1897–1909), subarachnoid cocaine anesthesia (1901), the semeiology of the blood in surgery (1905), and the surgery of the stomach (1907). He popularized spinal anesthesia in France, was a pioneer in pyelography and ovarian transplantation, and during the war collaborated with P.-E.-J. Simonin (1864–1926), in standardizing wound treatment and other administrative phases of military surgery along the whole French line. Like Menetrier and Ledoux-Lebard, he is an accomplished connoisseur and collector of *objets d'art.* Hippolyte **Morestin** (1869–1919), a Paris graduate of 1894, was a dexterous operator in all branches of general surgery, particularly in such difficult feats as his methods in sliding hernia (1900), spino-facial anastomosis (1901), resection of the wrist (1902) and the inter-ilio-abdominal amputation (1903). He made many con-

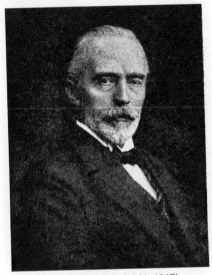

Theodor Kocher (1841–1917).

tributions to anatomy, wrote a treatise on diseases of the joints, and, after 1904, devoted himself almost exclusively to plastic and maxillofacial surgery, of which he was one of the most brilliant exponents during the war. Of recent French surgeons, René **Leriche** (1879–   ), who introduced periarterial sympathectomy (1917–22), has written on fractures (1916–17) and diseases of the bones (1926), and Paul **Lecène** on general pathology (1909) and the history of surgery (1923).

The last few years are remarkable for a revival of Hunterian or **physiological surgery.** Just as Marion Sims and Billroth, in their specialties, advanced the clinical pathology of visceral diseases, so we find Kocher, Horsley, von Eiselsberg, Halsted, Crile, Cushing. Carrel, Murphy, not only thinking physiologically in their work, but making many new departures by means of experimentation on animals. John Hunter, Merrem and Sir Astley Cooper did this, as also Jameson and Gross in America, but until latterly the method had been almost non-existent.

By common consent, the leader of this group was Theodor **Kocher** (1841–1917), of Bern, Switzerland, who was a pupil of Langenbeck and Billroth, and held the chair of surgery in his native town until his death (1872–1917).

Kocher was remarkable for his method of reducing dislocations of the shoulder-joint (1870[1]), for his contributions on hernia, osteomyelitis, his operations for ar-

---

[1] Kocher: Berl. klin. Wochenschr., 1870, vii, 101–105.

tificial anus, his hydrodynamic theory of the effect of gunshot wounds, and especially for his work on the thyroid gland. He was the first to excise the thyroid for goiter (1878[1]), and performed this difficult operation over 2000 times with only $4\frac{1}{2}$ per cent. mortality. In 1883,[2] he published his description of "cachexia strumipriva," which he had found as a sequel in 30 out of his first 100 thyroidectomies, and which, in connection with the pioneer experiments of Moritz Schiff on dogs (1859) and the work of the Reverdins and Horsley, inaugurated the physiology and physiological surgery of the ductless glands. Kocher also applied experimental surgery to the physiology of the brain and spinal cord. In 1912 he conceived the idea of injecting sterilized coagulene (derived by Fonio from the blood-platelets) to accelerate coagulation in internal hemorrhage.

Kocher was a slow, careful, precise and absolutely skilful operator, a typical scientific surgeon, who obtained the completest clinical history of his patients before beginning, and with whom success was an almost foregone conclusion. He maintained an absolutely aseptic field of operation and was a master of minute dissecting. His text-book of operative surgery (1894) is an index of his great learning. In appendicitis *à chaux* and *à froid* he was excelled by his pupil César Roux (1857–   ), whose post-haste, sleight-of-hand methods, sometimes to the exclusion of anesthesia and antisepsis, were more like the sensational, cinematographic operating of Doyen (Paris) than the painstaking, conscientious ways of Lister, Halsted, and Kocher himself. In general, the less showy the operating, the better the patient's chances.[3]

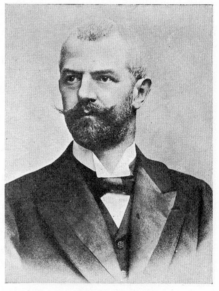

Anton von Eiselsberg (1860–   ).

The leading surgeon of Austria is Anton **von Eiselsberg** (1860–   ), of Steinhaus, Austria, professor of surgery at Utrecht (1893), Königsberg (1896) and Vienna (1901), and a pupil of Billroth. He was one

[1] Cor.-Bl. f. Schweiz. Aerzte, Basel, 1878, viii, 702–705.

[2] Arch. f. klin. Chir., Berl., 1883, xxix, 254–337.

[3] As Professor Harvey Cushing says, in his telling address before the International Medical Congress (London, 1913): "The accurate and detailed methods, in the use of which Kocher and Halsted were for so long the notable examples, have spread into all clinics—at least into those clinics where you or I would wish to entrust ourselves for operation. Observers no longer expect to be thrilled in an operating room; the spectacular public performances of the past, no longer condoned, are replaced by the quiet, rather tedious procedures which few beyond the operator, his assistants, and the immediate bystander can profitably see. The patient on the table, like the passenger in a car, runs greater risks if he have a loquacious driver, or one who takes close corners, exceeds the speed limit, or rides to admiration," Brit. Med. Jour., London, 1913, ii, 294.

of the first to notice the appearance of tetany after goiter operations (1890), and, in 1892, he produced tetany experimentally by excising a cat's thyroid which he had successfully transplanted into the abdominal parietes.[1] He has also studied the metastases of thyroid cancer, was a prominent worker in pituitary surgery, and did effective work during the World War.

William Stewart **Halsted** (1852–1922), of New York, was professor of surgery in the Johns Hopkins University (1889–1922). In 1884, he first performed refusion or centripetal transfusion of a patient's own blood, after defibrination, in CO-poisoning. He was a pioneer in conduction and infiltration anesthesia by cocaine (1885); was the first to ligate the subclavian artery in the first portion with success (1891[2]);

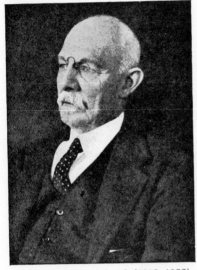

William Stewart Halsted (1852–1922).

devised the well-known supraclavicular operation for cancer of the breast (1889[3]), and, simultaneously with Edoardo Bassini (1814–1924), the modern operation for hernia (1889[4]), which, in its later phase (1893), diverges widely from Bassini's in technic. In 1916 he first excised Vater's ampulla for cancer. He did much work in experimental surgery, particularly in circular (1887) and bulkhead suturing of the intestines (1910), occlusion of the aorta and larger arteries by means of a metal band as a substitute for ligation (1909[5]), and in auto- and iso-transplantations of the parathyroid glands (1909[6]), which, in connection with H. Leischner's classical paper of 1907, have had much to do with establishing the functional status of these organs. In aid of a strictly aseptic technic he introduced gutta-percha tissue in drainage (1880–81), rubber gloves (1890), silver foil dressing (1896), transfixion of bleeding tissues and vessels by fine needles and finest silk. Quietly and unobtrusively, Halsted taught the delicate art of the perfect healing of wounds, which was never and nowhere more beautifully demonstrated than at his clinic.

George Washington **Crile** (1864–   ), of Chile, Ohio, professor of

[1] Von Eiselsberg: Wien. klin. Wochenschr., 1892, v, 81–85.

[2] Halsted: Johns Hopkins Hosp. Bull., Balt., 1892, iii, 93.

[3] Johns Hopkins Hosp. Rep., Balt., 1890–91, ii, 277–280; Tr. Am. Surg. Assoc., Phila., 1898, xvi, 144–181, 5 pl.

[4] Johns Hopkins Hosp. Bull., Balt., 1889–90, i, 12; 1893, iv, 17, 3 pl.

[5] J. Exper. Med., N. Y., 1909, xi, 373–391, 3 pl.

[6] Ibid., 175–199, 2 pl.: 1912, xv, 205–215, 2 pl.

clinical surgery in the Western Reserve University since 1890, is the author of highly original experimental researches on surgical shock (1899), blood-pressure in surgery (1903), hemorrhage and transfusion (1909), which procedure he has carried almost to perfection by his skill and technic. He has introduced various new operations for cancer of the lip, uterine prolapse, etc., and was the first after Halsted to perform a major operation with intraneural injections of cocaine as an anesthetic (1887). He has worked with particular ability in minute "block dissections" of the lymphatics in cancer. His operations on the head and neck for this condition (1908) are comparable with the Halsted breast excision or the Wertheim-Clark operation for uterine cancer. His theory of "anoci-association," the blocking of shock in operations by the combination of general and local anesthesia (morphia and scopolamine followed by nitrous oxid and novocaine), with less than 1 per cent. mortality, is his most important contribution to surgery. He has later evolved a bipolar theory of the electric nature of living processes (1926), in which the acid nucleus of the cell is the positive component, the cytoplasm the negative agent of oxidation, with the cell-membrane as condenser and the brain and liver as positive and negative poles respectively.

Harvey **Cushing** (1869–   ), of Cleveland, Ohio, professor of surgery at the Johns Hopkins (1902–11) and Harvard Universities (1912), stands *facile princeps* in neurological surgery, particularly in surgery of the head and the pituitary body.

He has done original work in experimental physiology, pathology and surgery, such as experimental production of gall-stones (1899), experimental production of valvular heart lesions in the dog, with successful operative treatment of the same (1908), successful treatment of facial paralysis in man by anastomosis of the spinal accessory and facial nerves (1903); he has introduced such new procedures as anesthetic nerve-blocking (1898), lumbar drainage in hydrocephalus, cross-bow incision in opening the base of the brain, and has done more than any other surgeon to demonstrate the possibility of operative relief for intracranial conditions notably in decompression for intracranial hemorrhages in the newborn (1905) and inaccessible tumors (1905), the surgery of the pituitary body (1909–12) and of tumors of the eighth nerve (1917). Cushing described the longitudinal sinus disease (1917), has done much for the pathology of the cerebello-pontine syndrome (1917), and the meningiomata (Cavendish Lecture, 1922) and (with Percival Bailey) has made a histological classification of the cerebellar gliomata (1926), correlating the clinical signs with the kind of tumor.

In his work on the pituitary body, Cushing has thrown much light on its physiological functions by the experimental production of sexual infantilism in animals, by the study of pituitary metabolism in disease, pregnancy, hibernation and other conditions, and by the general consideration of its disorders as "dyspituitarism." His monograph on this subject (1912[1]) contains his mode of operating and is an exhaustive study of the condition as approached from the physiological, pathological, clinical and surgical sides. His writings are informed with unique knowledge of the history of surgery and his *Life of Sir William Osler* (1925) is one of the best and most successful of medical biographies.

---

[1] Cushing: The Pituitary Body and its Disorders, Philadelphia, 1912.

Of recent American neurological surgeons, Charles Harrison **Frazier** (1870–   ), of Germantown, Pennsylvania, is the *opérateur par excellence* in trigeminal neuralgia, for which he has employed Spiller's idea of subtotal section of the posterior roots in such wise as to avoid motor disturbances and keratitis, with brilliant success in 396 cases (1901–26), as also in Spiller's device of chordotomy for unendurable pain (1899), with avoidance of injury to the pyramidal tract.   Charles A. **Elsberg** (1871–   ), of New York, has specialized in surgery of the spinal cord, of which he has written a well-known treatise (1925), and Walter E. **Dandy** (1888–   ), of Baltimore, is notable for his work on the experimental production on hydrocephalus (with Blackfan, 1911–14), its operative treatment (1921), the method of ventriculography (1918) and ventricular estimation (1923) and an operation for cerebellopontine tumors (1925).

Great advances in **vascular surgery** have been made by the experimental method, with the aid of the aseptic absorbable ligature.

Indeed, the first case of a successful venous suture was the celebrated "Eck fistula" (1877), which has since been applied by Pavloff and others in experiments requiring the physiological exclusion of the liver.   In 1881, Vincenz Czerny tried to suture an eroded jugular vein, with fatal results, but Schede succeeded in suturing the femoral vein, and, by 1892, had 30 successful cases.   In 1890, Jassinovski made 26 experimental arterial sutures upon animals, all lateral, and was followed by Dörfler (1890), who, like Murphy and Silberberg before him, employed a suture passing through all three arterial coats.   By proceeding aseptically, he avoided thrombosis, and, in 1891, Durant applied the method with success in two cases of arterial suture in man.   These were all lateral sutures.   The first end-to-end suture of veins was attempted with success upon a dog by Hirsch in 1881, and, in 1898, Jaboulay and Briau successfully applied their U-suture to the severed carotid artery of a donkey, to be followed with equal success upon animals by Salomoni and Tomaselli.   The first successful circular suturing of blood-vessels in man was done by

John Benjamin **Murphy** (1857–1916), of Appleton, Wisconsin, professor of surgery in the Northwestern University, Chicago (1895–1916), who was unquestionably the most effective teacher of his subject in the West.   After many experimental end-to-end resections of wounded arteries and veins, he successfully united a femoral artery, severed by a gunshot wound, in 1896.[1]

Murphy had already done epoch-making work in the production of "cholecysto-intestinal, gastro-intestinal, entero-intestinal anastomosis and approximation without sutures" by means of a special button (1892[2]), which was preceded by the decalcified bone-plates of Nicholas Senn, potato and turnip plates, etc.   Meanwhile, Robert Abbe (1851–1928), of New York, had introduced catgut rings for intestinal suturing (1892[3]), and had attempted prosthetic union of blood-vessels by means of a fine glass tube (1894), which was improved upon by Erwin Payr's device of absorbable magnesium cylinders (1900).   In 1897[4] Murphy introduced end-to-end suture of blood-vessels by means of invagination, the intima being brought into apposition with the adventitia, but, although there was no hemorrhage, the circulation was restored in only 4 cases out of 13, on account of the narrowing of the lumen of the

---

[1] Murphy: Med. Record, N. Y., 1897, li, 73–88.

[2] Murphy: *Ibid.*, 1892, xlii, 665–676.

[3] Abbe: Med. Record, N. Y., 1892, xli, 365–370.

[4] Murphy: *Ibid.*, 1897, li, 73–88.

vessels, with consequent thrombosis. This was finally obviated by the triangular suture of Carrel (1900). Before this innovation, Höpfner and others had transplanted pieces of artery or vein by means of Payr's magnesium rings, and Ullmann had tried to transplant a kidney in the dog in 1902. All these experiments fell through, however, on account of septic complications, and even Carrel succeeded only by dint of the most refined asepsis.

Murphy developed anastomosis of the intestines by invagination and had remarkable results with bone-grafts, which, curiously, do not succeed, as a rule, unless the sliver of tissue used is autogenous—from the patient himself. The graft will, in time, reproduce the exact contour of the defective bone, in accordance with Driesch's morphological law of the "totipotency of protoplasm."

Rudolph **Matas** (1860–   ), of New Orleans, has greatly improved the operation for the radical cure of aneurysm by his procedure of aneurysmorrhaphy (1902[1]), *i. e.*, intra-saccular suturing or closing the mouths of the vessels entering into the aneurysm, and was one of the earliest to work in nerve-blocking (1898–9), spinal anesthesia (1899), and laryngeal intubation (1902).

Alexis **Carrel** (1873–   ), of Sainte-Foy-les-Lyon, France, a graduate of the University of Lyons (1900), who came to America in 1905 and is now a member of the Rockefeller Institute, has revolutionized the surgery of the vascular system and made great advances in physiology and physiological surgery, for which he became a Nobel prizeman in 1912. In 1902, he published his first paper on vascular anastomoses and visceral transplantation,[2] in which he showed that perfect end-to-end anastomosis of blood-vessels can be secured by inserting in the opposing ends a triple-threaded suture, which, when drawn tightly, converts the round lumen of the vessel into an equilateral triangle, thus securing closest apposition, without leakage, preserving the continuity of the lumen, and so avoiding thrombosis. Before Carrel's time, a wounded artery was treated only by ligation in continuity. From end-to-end anastomosis of arteries he advanced, by means of specially invented needles and rigid asepsis, to the substitution of a lost piece of an artery by pieces of artery or vein, and thence to the transplantation of organs from animal to animal. Thus, he has transplanted a kidney, with its vascular supply, from cat to cat, secretion of urine beginning before the end of the operation, and this feat not only proved successful in man, but has been extended to other viscera also. Transplantations in mass of blood-vessels, organs, viscera, and limbs have been also successful.[3]

Carrel's investigations of the latent life of arteries (1910[4]) led to the preservation of portions of blood-vessels in cold storage for days or weeks before using them in transplantation. Latterly, he has applied the principle of R. G. Harrison's experiment on extravital cultivation of nerve-cells (1907–14) to the extravital cultivation

---

[1] Matas: Tr. Am. Surg. Assoc., Phila., 1902, xx, 396–434, 16 pl.

[2] Carrel: Lyon méd., 1902, xcviii, 859–864.

[3] Jour. Am. Med. Assoc., Chicago, 1908, li, 1662–1667.

[4] Jour. Exper. Med., N. Y., 1910, xii, 460–486.

and rejuvenation of tissues (1911[1]), culminating in his remarkable experiment of keeping the excised viscera of an animal alive and functionating physiologically *in vitro* (1912[2]). He has also succeeded in activating and accelerating the growth of connective tissue by dressings of thyroidal, splenic, embryonic, and other animal extracts (1913). He has isolated tissue cells in pure cultures and developed technical methods by which these strains can be kept indefinitely in an active condition outside the body.

During the World War, Carrel did work of lasting value in the treatment of wound infection with the Dakin solution and on the rate of healing of wounds. In 1919, he began to develop methods for the physiological study of tissues *in vitro*, in which each cell-type is identified, not only by its morphological characteristics, but by its specific physiological properties, a dynamic transformation of classical cytology, which includes his recent studies on the leucocytic trephones (1923), explantation, growth-activation or inhibition of malignant tumors.[3]

Internal medicine, in its recent phases, harks back to the two main trends of Greek medicine, the Coan and the Cnidian: on the one hand, the time-honored Hippocratic reliance on the natural powers of the mind and the five senses in diagnosis (without which the physician is nothing), revision of semeiology (Mackenzie), simple lines of therapy, merging, on the extreme left, into such extravagances of general (humoral) pathology as the doctrine that there is only one disease, the rest turning upon imbalance of protective substances in the blood plasma (syzygiology); on the other hand, an almost bewildering array of laboratory tests, instrumentation, specialism, etiological theorizing, improvisation of sera and vaccines or vagaries of protein or protean therapy, which tend to merge bedside medicine into the ancillary devices it utilizes, to enslave the mind of the physician by making him dependent upon artificial aids and, *in extremis*, to turn the patient himself into a laboratory animal. Between the two lies the Golden Mean, the *via media* followed by all practitioners of sound sense, ripe judgment and varied experience. It has been well said that no sane man today could read all the current literature on any medical specialty and retain his reason. The actual advances made are those which have stood the acid tests of experience and practical application.

In **diagnosis**, apart from the biochemical methods and blood tests of Folin, Van Slyke, and others, the methods of estimating the sedimentation rate of erythrocytes devised by Fahraeus (1918–21), Linzemeier (1920), Westergren (1921), Katz (1922), Zeckwer and Goodell (1925) are of little positive value and most of the functional tests are prognostic. The tests for **renal function** comprise all phases of urinalysis, including total nitrogen (Kjeldahl, 1913), residual (non-protein) nitrogen (Morris, 1911; Folin and Dennis, 1912–13; McLean, 1914–16); provocative polyuria (Albarran, 1905; Straus-Grunwald, 1905), total urea (Marshall, 1913–14), provocative urea elimination (F. C. MacLean, 1915), renal test-meals (Mosenthal, 1915), methylene-blue (Achard and Castaigne, 1897), indigo-carmine (Volcker and Joseph, 1903), phenolsulphonephthalein (Rowntree and Geraghty, 1910–12), benzoic acid

---

[1] Carrel: Jour. Am. Med. Assoc., Chicago, 1911, lvii, 1611.

[2] Jour. Exper. Med., N. Y., 1913, xviii, 155–161.

[3] For an exhaustive bibliography and history of explantation, see A. Krontowski: Ergebn. d. Physiol., München, 1928, xxvi, 370–500.

(Kingsbury and Swanson, 1921), blood-cholesterol (Epstein, 1917) and blood-chlorides (de Wesselow, 1923). Cryoscopy (Korányi, 1894) and the Ambard coefficient (1910) are now little used by comparison with these tests which afford indices of the functional capacity of the kidney in renal and cardiac disease, pregnancy, and surgical conditions, analogous to the information given by the indicator diagram on a steam-engine. In diabetes and the glycosurias, the tests of Benedict for urinary sugar (1908), of Frommer (1905) and Rothera (1908) for acetone bodies, of Van Slyke for total acetone bodies (1917), of Sørensen (pH 1909), Sellard (1917), Van Slyke (1918), for acidosis and ketosis, with those of Haldane and Priestley (1905) and Fredericia (1914) for alveolar CO_2-tension are commonly employed, while insulin (Banting and Best, 1922), as being the main coefficient in sugar metabolism, has thrown much light upon carbohydrate tolerance. The tests of **pancreatic function** include those of Loewi (1908), Wohlgemüth (urinary diastase, 1908–10) and Cammidge (1912). **Hepatic function** is estimated by such tests as those of Ehrlich (1886–1901), Schlesinger (1903), Fouchet (1917) and Van den Bergh (1918) for bile-pigments (urine and blood), levulose-tolerance (Strauss, 1901), indican (Strauss, 1902), galactose (Bauer, 1906), coagulation time (Wright and Colebrook, 1921), fibrinogen content (Whipple and Horwitz, 1911), fibrinolysis time (Goodpasture, 1914), blood lipase (Lowenhart, 1902; Whipple, 1913); hemoclasia or leucocytosis after meals (Widal, 1920–21); the phenoltetrachlorphthalein test for global eliminative capacity (Rowntree, Hurwitz, and Bloomfield, 1913) and duodenal drainage of bile by the method of Meltzer (1917) and Lyon 1919).[1]

In Graves' disease, the aceto-nitril test (Reid Hunt, 1919), the eye signs with the rest of Barker's eight symptoms, the adrenalin mydriasis test (Loewi, 1907), the adrenalin tests of Emil Goetsch (1918, 1920) and the Read formula for basal metabolism (1922) are of moment; in suprarenal disease, adrenalin glycosuria (Blum, 1901), adrenalin mydriasis (Meltzer, 1904; Ehrmann, 1905), and the supra-renal white line of Émile Sergent (1903); in pituitary disease, the x-ray picture, ocular changes, sugar tolerance, basal metabolism, blood-pressure, glycosuria, and the thermic reaction (Cushing, 1918); in cardiac insufficiency, the blood-pressure tests of Graupner (1902–6) and Schott (1912), the staircase test (Selig, 1905). In the cardiac arrhythmias, polygraphy (Mackenzie-Lewis, 1892), electrocardiography (Einthoven, 1903) and determination of systolic and diastolic pressures with the sphygmomanometers of Riva Rocci (1896) and Erlanger (1902), the oscillometer of Pachon (1909) by the methods of Marey (1876), Strasburger (1904), Korotkoff (1905) or Ehret (1909), following the rule of Rolleston (1923) for age, are well known; as also the cutaneous protein reactions of Dunbar (1903), Chandler Walker (1918) and Coke (1923) for hay-fever and asthma, and the susceptibility tests of Bela Schick (1913), George and Gladys Dick (1924), for diphtheria and scarlatina. Apart from the functional tests, the blood (neutrophile) picture of Joseph Arneth (1904), the differential leucocytometer of Schilling (1911), blood grouping by hemo-agglutination (Landsteiner, 1899–1901), and its applications to the differentiation of race (Manoiloff, 1922–25), and the jurisprudence of paternity (Ottenberg, 1921) are notable, as also the concepts sickle-cell anemia (Herrick, 1910), goat's milk anemia (von Jaksch, Hayem, 1889; Glanzmann, 1916) and agranulocytosis (Werner Schutz, 1922), thrombo-angiitis obliterans (Leo Buerger, 1908), the remarkable work of Emanuel Libman and his pupils on various types of endocarditis (1910–23) and the description of cyanotic sclerosis of the pulmonary artery, with polycythemia (*cardiacos negros*) by Abel Ayerza (1901) illustrate some of the recent advances made in the field of the blood and the circulation. Glandular fever (Filatoff-Pfeiffer, 1889) is now interpreted as an infectious mononucleosis.

In **gastro-enterology,** much is due to Röntgenography, to the Coolidge tube (1913), to W. B. Cannon who introduced the bismuth meal in animals (1897–8), to Holzknecht, Haudek and Groedel, who popularized the use of the fluorescent screen and made the first effective serial plates of the stomach in man (1909–12), to A. F. Hurst who made x-ray studies of defecation and constipation (1908), to Biggert, who studied the stomach and bowel with bismuth meal and bismuth enema, to Weber, who introduced pneumoperitoneum (1913), and to E. A. **Graham** and W. H. **Cole,** who devised Röntgenography of the gall-bladder (1923–4). The important studies of Cannon and Washburn on hunger contractions in connection with gastric pain (1912), of Anton J. Carlson (1875–   ) on the nature of hunger-contractions

---

[1] For functional tests, see the Manual of W. M. Barton (Boston, 1917).

(1913), of Mann and Whipple on exclusion of the liver and extra-hepatic secretion of bile, of Boyden, Mann and Higgins on the mechanism of evacuation of the gall-bladder (1924–6), the discovery of the sphincter of the common bile-duct (Oddi, 1887) by Simon P. Gage (1879) and the introduction of non-surgical drainage of the gall-bladder by S. G. Meltzer (1917) and Lyon (1919) are among the brilliant achievements of recent Americans, which include the studies of C. Eggleston and A. C. Hatcher on the action of emetics and the mechanism of vomiting (1912–25), of J. T. Case on intestinal stasis (1914–15), of W. C. Alvarez on the mechanism of gastro-intestinal peristalsis (1914–27) and of A. C. Ivy on the physiology of gastric secretion (1920–25). In 1905, W. J. Mayo showed that duodenal ulcer is ten times more frequent than gastric ulcer, the significance of the pyloric vein in differential diagnosis and (with Moynihan) perfected the technic of its treatment by gastro-enterostomy (1906). Duodenal intubation with the small tube is associated with the name of Einhorn, fractional intubation of the stomach (soft tube) with that of Rehfuss (1914). The principal dietetic schemes for gastric ulcer are those of Leube (1897), Lenhartz (1904), Lambert (1908) and Sippy (1915). The story of recent developments in gastro-enterology has been effectively conveyed by Walter C. Alvarez.[1]

Tests of **gastric function** include the test-meals of Ewald (1890) and Rehfuss (1914), x-ray examination (Cannon, 1898), and detection of blood in the fæces. The pharmacologic tests for vagotonia and sympathicotonia (Eppinger and Hess, 1910) are still *sub judice.*

In **neurology,** many new tests for neurosyphilis by examination of the cerebro-spinal fluid have been introduced, notably the butyric acid test (Noguchi, 1909), the colloidal gold reaction (Lange, 1912), the estimates of globulin increase of Nonne and Apelt (1907–8) and Pandy (1910) and of protein content (Mestrezat, 1912; Loche-longue-Levinson, 1919). The simplified complement-fixation test of R. L. Kahn (1924) supplements the Wassermann reaction (1906) and, on account of its extreme simplicity, bids fair to supplant it in America. The psycho-galvanic reflex was first described by I. R. Tarchanoff (1890) and applied to clinical phenomena through the apparatus devised by him. In respect of semeiology, the data from gunshot wounds in the World War brought out many new phases, notably those on peripheral nerve lesions (Tinel, Athanassio-Benisty), chronic progressive cerebellar tremor (Holmes, 1914); the longitudinal sinus disease (Cushing, 1917); the syndromes of the foramen, lacerum posterius (Vernet, 1916), cerebellar irritation (Goldstein and Reichmann, 1916–17), and retroparotid space (Villaret, 1918), while the thalamus opticus syndrome of Déjerine (1903) and Roussy (1906) was further elucidated by Henry Head and Gordon Holmes (1918). Déjerine summarized the clinical phenomena of spinal radiculitis (1905) and the spinal arthropathies (with Cellier, 1920); described olivo-ponto-cerebellar atrophy (Déjerine-Thomas, 1900), the tabetic muscular atrophies (Déjerine-Sottas, 1906) and the parietal lobe syndrome (1914). Through the work of Déjerine and Tilney, the syndromes of Jackson (1886), Avellis (1891), Schmidt (1892), Bonnier (1902), Babinski-Nageotte (1902), Cestan-Chenois (1903) and Tapia (1905–6) are now allocated to lesions of the medulla, those of Gubler-Weber (1855–63), Millard-Gubler (1855–58), Foville (1858), Benedikt (1872), and Varet (1905) to lesions of the pons. To the basal ganglia are assigned syndromes of the thalamus opticus (Déjerine-Roussy, 1903–6) and corpora striata (C. & O. Vogt, 1921), including paralysis agitans and Parkinsonism (1817), muscular dystonia (Oppenheim, 1900), and degeneration of the lenticular nucleus (Kinnier-Wilson, 1913); to the cerebellum the asynergia (1899) and adiadokokinesis (1902) of Babinski, the combined cerebro-cerebellar degeneration of Holmes (1907) and the cerebello-pontine angle tumors developed by Stewart and Holmes (1904), Starr (1910), Cushing (1918), and others. Gradenigo's syndrome (1904) is otitic abducens (sixth nerve) paralysis. The myatonic type of muscular atrophy (myatonia congenita) was described by Oppenheim (1900), the distal types by Gowers (1902) and Spiller (1906) the ascending and descending forms of unilateral sclerosis by Mills and Spiller (1900–1906). Unconsciousness of illness or physical discomfort, noticed by Knapp with reference to foreign bodies in the eye (1882), was first studied by Anton (1899), and latterly in hemiplegia by Poetzl (1924) and Sapiro (1925). The many ways of producing experimental epilepsy, from the cerebral anemia of Kellie and Astley Cooper (1824) to pulmonary hyperventilation (O. Foerster, 1925) have gone far to reduce it from the status of a disease to that of a symptom.

---

[1] Alvarez: The Mechanics of the Digestive Tract, New York, 1928.

Two main currents of recent **therapeutics** are purposeful dietetics (nutritional therapy) and protein therapy.

The work of the metabolists, Eijkmann (1897), Henriques and Hansen (1905), Hopkins (1906–12), Funk (1911), McCollum, Davis *et al.* (1911–18), Osborne and Mendel (1912–15), Goldberger (1915–20), McCarrison (1921–7) on the deficiency diseases has shown conclusively that a monotone diet, lacking in the proper accessory food factors (vitamins) will produce grave pathological effects in the viscera, the nervous system, the sexual apparatus, and other parts of the body which may get beyond control if allowed to go too far.

Dietetics, one of the basic principles of Hippocratic therapy, has, therefore, come into its own again. In the artificial life of city people, the adjustments of the body to food are as delicate and dubious as those in the newborn infant.

Forced fasting and "girth control" in persons otherwise "plump and pleasing" tend to toxic urine, constipation, and worse things. McCarrison has recently produced goiter and vesical calculus by an experimental diet in rats (1927). Carlson's fasting Italian (Zetti) got naught but constipation and leukemia. Horace Fletcher really cultivated constipation and suffered from chronic toxemia and decayed teeth, while his son-in-law died of colonic stasis and malnutrition. William James said of Fletcherism: "It nearly killed me." The Russian famine brought on amenorrhea, sexual impotence and exposure to unusual diseases through lowered resistance. Natural savage man has 3 to 4 stools *per diem*, while the highly concentrated meat and cereal diet of Americans makes for stasis, acidosis and high blood-pressure, as shown in Chinese put upon this diet. The conclusions of McCarrison, McCollum, and others are that an ideal normal diet would consist of whole wheat, milk, and milk products, uncooked vegetables, sprouted legumes, fresh meats and fruit, with specific avoidance of white bread, tea, sugar, boiled vegetables, margarine, tinned meats and jams, which injure the system through the boric and sulphurous acids and formaldehyde employed as preservatives. The peculiar diets of tropical, arctic, and other natives are probably natural adjustments of individual metabolism to environment. There is truth in the homely German proverb: *Man ist was er isst (homo est quod est).*

Salient among the recent triumphs of **nutritional therapy** is the prevention and arrest of **goiter** by overcoming iodin deficiency.

In 1909–13, David **Marine** and C. H. Lenhart demonstrated the effects of iodine on goiter in brook-trout and other animals, and following the discovery of **thyroxin** in the thyroid gland by E. C. **Kendall** (1914), reduced the incidence of goiter in over 2000 schoolgirls of the goiter belt (Akron, Ohio) by exhibition of small doses of sodium iodide (1917–20). Similar results were then obtained in the Swiss Cantons by R. Klinger (1918–22), with a reduction from 87.6 per cent. (1919) to 13.1 per cent. (1922) in St. Gall. The use of butter-fat against xerophthalmia, keratomalacia, and night-blindness (Osborne and Mendel, 1913), of unhusked rice against adult beriberi (1897) and of tiqui tiqui extract against infantile beriberi (1912), of cod-liver oil (E. Mellanby, 1919) and foods irradiated with ultraviolet light (Steenbock and Black, 1924) against rickets, the uselessness of cooked vegetables and fruits against scurvy (E. M. Delf, 1921) are among the advances in **vitamin therapy.** In 1925, G. H. Whipple and F. S. Robscheit-Robbins showed the beneficial effect of raw beef liver upon blood regeneration in anemia, which was then applied to the treatment of **pernicious anemia** in practice by G. R. Minot and W. P. Murphy (1926).

The rationale of **protein therapy** is, roughly speaking, "a hair of the dog that bit you," or one disease cures another; but its scientific *locus standi* is Weigert's law, viz., that a local injury or necrosis will usually start reparative processes in excess of requirements (1871–3), or

47

as Pflüger expressed it in 1877: "Injury is the incentive to removal of injury." It includes anything from acupuncture, the seton, the moxa, bloodletting, emesis, or blistering up to the treatment of neurosyphilis by superinfection with malaria. The theory of the subject grew up around the treatment of bacterial infections with specific sera and vaccines, which were soon found to have a non-specific therapeutic effect in other diseases.

In 1905, Winter showed that a stopped heart can be resuscitated by adrenalin injections and in 1906, Rudolph Schmitt began to treat various diseases with parenteral injections of milk. The beneficial effect of malarial infection in epilepsy was known to Hippocrates and no less than 164 cases of its curative effects in paresis and insanity were recorded by earlier writers.[1] In 1887, Julius **Wagner von Jauregg** (1857–), of Vienna, postulated the general theory of the influence of febrile diseases upon psychoses and after some twenty years of observation of the beneficial effect of such diseases upon paresis, began to inoculate paretic soldiers with malaria in 1917. In spite of some fatalities, his success was so striking that he received the Nobel prize in 1927. Meanwhile, Felix Plaut got similar results with relapsing fever (1919). Kunde, Hall, and Gerty have treated paresis by foreign proteins without the use of the living plasmodium (1926). Gordonoff (1925) showed that a drop of chlorophyll will revive a heart at standstill. Wildegans got hæmolytic effects from injection of foreign blood-corpuscles (1926), and Dold an anaphylactic protein reaction from injection of non-toxic autogenous blood-serum when previously shaken. Along such lines, Bier has attempted to explain the rationale of Hahnemann's triturations, succussions and potencies. The general consensus of opinion is that protein therapy is more commonly successful, not in general but in local infections, such as the arthritides, gonorrhea, asthma, neurosyphilis, cutaneous and ocular diseases. The reactions are different in different animals, and as toxic doses are fatal, and the threshold dose varies in different individuals, the method is fraught with danger, e. g., in the use of krysolgan and sanocrysin in phthisis. Protein therapy and stimulotherapy appear to obey the Arndt-Schulz law (1885–7), viz., that weak stimuli accelerate vital activities, strong stimuli inhibit them, maximal stimuli abolish or destroy them.

Among the novelties of recent therapeutics are cisterna puncture (Ayer, 1919–20); the experiments of L. H. Weed, McKibben, Foley, and others on the effects of injection or ingestion of hypertonic salt-solutions in lowering brain bulk and intracranial tension (1919–20); the treatment of impoverished nutrition in infants by insulin fattening (McKim Marriott, 1924) and adults (Falta, 1925); the extensive use of all modes of irradiation, of detoxicated drugs, toxins and venoms, and of old remedies, such as the heliotherapy of Cælius Aurelianus, lead in cancer (Blair Bell, 1922) or urea as a diuretic (Klemperer, 1895). The journals swarm with new remedies of specific or synthetic type, the most remarkable, if not reliable, being insulin (Banting and Best, 1922); ephedrine (Nagai, 1887); krysolgan (A. Feldt, 1917), sanocrysin (Holger Møllgaard, 1924), plasmochin (Elberfeld group, 1925), ergosterin (György, et al., 1927) or the general use of iodine as antiseptic (Pregl's solution, 1921).

Obstetrics has only just entered the preventive phase, but **antenatal care** (puericulture) is now a matter of world-wide interest. Much was due, in the first instance, to the writings of John William **Ballantyne** (1861–1923) on Diseases of the Fœtus (1892–5), Antenatal Pathology and Hygiene (1902–4), and latterly to the reports of E. L. **Holland**

---

[1] A. Maisani: Med. Prat., Napoli, 1927, xii, 284.

(1922) and **Janet Campbell** (1924) on maternal and fetal mortality. Schemes for ante-natal care comprise complete examination of the expectant mother with reference to the dangers of faulty obstetrics and puerperal diseases to mother and child, improved training for students and midwives and general education of the public as to standards of efficiency to be maintained. Among the most striking manifestoes are the colored posters of the Department of Maternal and Infant Welfare of the Central Soviet Government, designed to warn and counsel expectant mothers in a population of over a hundred million illiterate people. Some 80,000 of these posters were distributed in 1924.

The recognition of autogenous puerperal sepsis and its prevention by aseptic and mild antiseptic measures is of recent date. Fleming claims that strong antiseptics destroy the bactericidal power of leucocytes (1917). By far the most striking advance in preventive obstetrics is the expectant treatment of eclampsia by means of quietude, isolation in a dark room, and exhibition of sedatives and purgatives, which was introduced by Vassili Vassilievich **Stroganoff** (1857–   ) in 1897,[1] with such recent modifications as the additional use of magnesium sulphate (E. M. Lazard, 1897) or its intramuscular injection (Lee Dorset). The technic of pedalic version has been improved by Irving W. Potter (1918–22). The low (cervical) Cesarean section originated by H. Sellheim (1908–10) has been perfected and popularized by J. B. DeLee (1916–19) and A. C. Beck (1920). New forceps for particular manœuvres have been devised by Christian Kjelland (1915), Barton (1925) and Piper. The high fetal and neonatal mortality due to intracranial hemorrhage from lacerations of the tentorium cerebri and falx cerebelli has been demonstrated by E. L. Holland (1922) and others, and the dangers of rapid compression of the fetal head in breech extraction and forceps delivery recognized. The advantages and dangers of the use of pituitrin in lingering labor (Blair Bell, 1906–25) are matters of discussion. In anesthesia, there is the same casuistry with reference to the numerous methods available, notably morphine and scopolamine hypodermically (Steinbüchel, 1902) or per rectum (Krönig and Gauss, 1913), nitrous oxide, ethylene (Luckhardt, 1922) or the synergistic method of Gwathmey (1923), in which intramuscular injections of morphine and magnesium sulphate are combined with rectal injection of quinine, alcohol, and ether in olive oil. X-rays were first used in obstetric diagnosis by Davis and Varnier (1896) and latterly (*via* pneumoperitoneum) by R. Peterson (1922).

In **gynecology** the most notable advance has been the establishment of the true nature of ovarian endometriomata (chocolate cysts) by J. A. Sampson (1922[2]), and the assimilation of these tumors, along with the uterine adenomyomata of Recklinghausen (1896) and Cullen (1906) to the aberrant neoplasms of Grawitz type. They were classified as solenomata by F. Jayle (1926) and the histology of ovarian endometrioma was worked out by Bailey (1924). On the therapeutic side, the most telling advance is the diagnosis and treatment of sterility from occlusion of the Fallopian tubes by insufflation of the tubes with gas, devised by I. C. **Rubin** (1920[3]) of New York. Ernst Wertheim's radical operation for cervical cancer (1906), Tuffier's work on ovarian grafting (1907–21), the work of Fothergill (1915–16) and Ward on the radical cure of prolapse and the general therapeutic application of radiant energy and diathermy (Nagelschmidt, 1908; Cumberbatch, 1921) have their place in the historic sequence. In connection with recent work on irradiation of the ovary, Klein found the stimulating effect of the ovarian hormones to be no more than that of a simple hyperemia (1927). An exhaustive encyclopedia of gynecology is that of Josef Halban and Ludwig Seitz (1924–7[4]).

The Nobel prize in medicine for 1911 was awarded to Allvar **Gullstrand** (1862–   ), of Landskrona, Sweden, professor of **ophthalmology**

[1] V. V. Stroganoff: Vrach, St. Petersb., 1900, xxi, 1137–1140.

[2] J. A. Sampson: Arch. Surg., Chicago, 1921, iii, 245–323.

[3] I. C. Rubin: Jour. Am. Med. Assoc., Chicago, 1920, lxxiv, 1017: lxxv, 661.

[4] Halban & Seitz: Biologie und Pathologie des Weibes. 10 v., Berlin, 1924–7.

in the University of Upsala (1894), for his mathematical investigations of dioptrics or the science of the refraction of light through the transparent media of the living eye. As Willard Gibbs founded the chemical theory of heterogenous substances, so Gullstrand has founded the dioptrics of heterogeneous media.

Formerly, the image in the eye was regarded as a schematic, "co-linear," or point-for-point arrangement, like that studied on the lenses of optical instruments. The course of the rays in astigmatism, for instance, was represented by the diagrammatic Sturm's conoid. Gullstrand took up the study of the ocular image from the viewpoint of reality, clearly differentiating its actual formation from its optical projection. He showed that the assemblage of rays in Sturm's conoid has not the slightest resemblance to the actual condition in astigmatism. By applying the methods of mathematical physics, especially those of Sir William Rowan Hamilton (1828), he treated the problem as one concerning a set of widely diffused bundles of rays, refracted through a system of continually curving planes, and showed that, during accommodation, the index of refraction of the lens is augmented by an actual change in its structure. His principal works on this theme are his study of astigmatism (1891), his General Theory of Monochromatic Aberrations (1900[1]), and his essays on dioptrics of the crystalline lens (1908) and the real optic image (1906). In 1889, he introduced a practical method of estimating corneal astigmatism by a single observation, an advantage possessed by a single instrument, the Sutcliffe ophthalmometer. In 1892, he introduced a photographic method of locating a paralyzed ocular muscle. He also introduced a micrometric method of estimating the photographed corneal reflex, as giving the most exact knowledge of the form of the normal and diseased cornea. His work in this field is not unlike Burdon-Sanderson's photographic determinations of reaction time in muscle. In 1907, he showed that the yellow color of

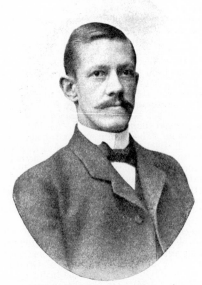

Allvar Gullstrand (1862–   ).

the macula in the retina is a cadaveric phenomenon, not existing in life; and, as above stated, he discovered the intracapsular mechanism of accommodation.[2] He also devised the reflexless stationary ophthalmoscope (1912), which excludes all light not belonging to the ophthalmoscopic image, and is thus free from all reflections from the mirror or the eye itself, giving a better image, better stereoscopic effect, and a wider field of vision. He has invented corrective glasses with aspherical lenses for those operated on for cataract, which give cleaner cut and more luminous images, with wider range of vision, than spherical lenses with the same focal distance; and latterly the slit-lamp (1902) which permits of microscopic study of the living eye.

Two prominent innovations in **eye surgery** of recent times have been made by officers of the Indian Medical Service. The operation of extraction of cataract within the capsule was introduced by Lieut.-

---

[1] Gullstrand: Allgemeine Theorie der monochromatischen Aberrationen, Upsala, 1900.

[2] Arch. f. Ophth., Berl., 1912, lxxii, 169–190.

Colonel **Henry Smith** in 1900,[1] and his success with it has been remarkable. As a benefactor of humankind, he is known all over northern India, where the reflection of the pitiless sunlight from the dusty plains tells with terrific force upon the eyes of the natives. His clinics at Jullundur and Amritsar, in the Punjab, are frequented not only by stream of blind people, coming by every mode of travel, but by ophthalmic surgeons, even from the western United States, who travel across the world to learn his methods. He teaches by making the pupil perform the operation before him. He averages about 3000 extractions a year, and, by 1910, he had 24,000 to his credit, of which 20,000 were done by the intracapsular method. Another new operation, that of sclerocorneal trephining for glaucoma, was in-troduced by Major Robert Henry **Elliot,** I. M. S., in August, 1909.[2] The operation of von Graefe had held the field for half a century, Lagrange and Herbert had em-phasized the value of sclerectomy, and even corneal trephining had been essayed by Argyll Robert-son, Blanco, Fröhlich, and Free-land Fergus, but Elliot has made the operation his own by many improvements and has made it viable. Latterly, diathermy and protein-therapy have proved ef-fective weapons in the manage-ment of diseases of the eye.

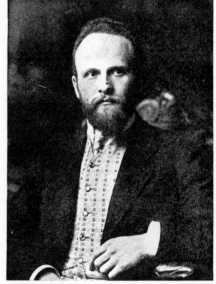

Robert Bárány (1876–). (From a photograph in the Surgeon-General's Library.)

In the field of **otology** Robert **Bárány** (1876–), of Vienna, Privatdocent at the University, has done much to clear up the hazy subject of aural vertigo, or Ménière's disease, especially in differentiating it from allied or adjacent lesions in the cerebellum, from epilepsy, or from ordinary nystagmus (1906[3]).

Labyrinthine vertigo or "vestibular nystagmus" is interpreted by Bárány as a disturbance of function of the vestibular nerve or the organs to which it is distributed, and he has traced its origin to a large number of different causes with which it might be confused. He has introduced a number of ingenious differential tests, such as production of nystagmus by irrigation of the external meatus with cold or warm water (caloric test) or by having a patient try to point at an object with his eyes shut after having previously touched it (static test), and he has been able to prove his case by successful operations on the cerebellum or the internal ear. He has also devised a "noise machine" for testing paracusis Willisii, and other diagnostic novelties.

[1] H. Smith: Indian Med. Gaz., Calcutta, 1900, xxxv, 240; 1901, xxxvi, 220· 1905, xl, 327.

[2] Elliot: Ophthalmoscope, Lond., 1909, vii, 804–808.

[3] Bárány: Arch. f. Ohrenh., Leipz., 1906, lxviii, 1–30, and later publications.

Recent advances in **oto-rhino-laryngology** have been mainly along lines of improved instrumentation, such as the use of the electric audiometer in testing for deafness, indeed, the use of mechanical and biochemical aids as surrogates for the evidence gained by the senses has extended to nearly all branches of practical medicine.

This is notable even in **toxicology** and medical jurisprudence, *e. g.*, in such devices as Thorpe's electrolytic modification of the Marsh-Berzelius test for arsenic, the use of functional liver tests in hepatic poisoning by 606 or 914, the Stas-Otto-Dragendorff method for alkaloidal poisoning (used in the Crippen case), the spectroscopic method of Hartridge (1912) for estimation of minute traces of carbon monoxide in the blood, the Uhlenhuth-Nuttall (precipitin) test for blood-stains (1902–5), the negation of paternity by blood-grouping (1921), and the identification of the pistol in homicide by rifling and marks on the bullet.

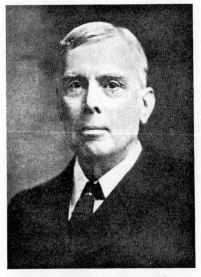

Charles Creighton (1847–1927).

The rise of modern **epidemiology** is associated with William Farr's article on vital statistics (1837) and his subsequent letters on causes of death in England (1839–70), which stimulated activity in the Statistical Society of London (founded 1834) and led to the foundation of the Epidemiological Society (August, 1850), by Babington, Brodie, Simon, Southwood Smith, Murchison and other leading spirits of the time.

The modern English school stems from Charles **Creighton** (1847–1927), a medical graduate of Aberdeen (1878) and London (1881), who translated Hirsch's great work on medical geography for the Sydenham Society (1883–6). His *History of Epidemics in Britain* (1891–94) is now admitted to be a classic of unimpeachable accuracy, but he was amateurish and outmoded in pathology, a believer in dyscrasias, miasms and effluvia, and his unfortunate brief against vaccination (1889), with his subsequent attack on Jenner (1889), rendered him anathema in British opinion, isolated him as a recusant, and delivered him into the hands of the anti-vaccinationists. No one excelled Creighton in his power to get at the real meaning of the older writers, but he was constitutionally incapable of doing justice to the present and maintained, with dogged tenacity, that whatever is generally accepted is necessarily false. This paradoxical twist in his mentality exposed him to a lifetime of ostracism and poverty, which he bore with manful indifference, despising the pseudohistorians who evaluate the ancients not in relation to their time, but only in so far as they square with recent viewpoints. He died a lonely, forsaken man, and has only just come into his own as the founder of modern British epidemiology.

Of the newer men who have come under Creighton's influence, Major **Greenwood** (1880–   ), professor of epidemiology in the University of London (1926), has made valuable studies of Sydenham (1919) and Galen (1921) as epidemiologists, industrial hygiene (1921), and vital statistics; Sir William Heaton **Hamer** has investigated English epidemiology (1906), typhoid carriers (1911), cerebrospinal fever (1917), and influenza (1927). Francis Graham **Crookshank** (1873–   ), of Wimbledon (Surrey), has edited a valuable historical study of influenza (1926) and represents the extreme left of the Baillou-Sydenham school of remote cosmic and telluric factors in causation (epidemic constitutions). John **Brownlee** (1868–1927) stems more directly from Farr. He turned out a large amount of very unequal work, his best findings being those on the periodicity of measles and other diseases (1914–24). He devised "periodograms" and upheld Farr's law that the death-rate varies directly with density of population (1861–70), which Yule found to "fit the figures (ideal facts), but not the (real) facts." Of the mathematicians who have cultivated the advanced methods of Pearson, George Udney **Yule** (1871–   ), lecturer on statistics at Cambridge, has advanced the soundest views in his *Introduction to the Theory of Statistics* (1911); Sir Ronald **Ross** (1857–   ) has obtained epidemic curves corresponding with the normal bell-shaped Farr-Pearson curve, showing the proportion of the total population affected in a given time and variants showing the effect of natality, immigration, emigration, and other external factors upon an epidemic and its subsidence from exhaustion of susceptible material (1916). In America, Raymond **Pearl** has analyzed the effects of density of population in lowering the birth-rate (1920–27), and has obtained a logistic curve of population-growth (1926). At the Rockefeller Institute, under direction of Simon **Flexner,** the methods of Danysz (1900), Bainbridge (1909) and Topley (1918–20) in **experimental epidemiology** were carried out on a grand scale in villages of mice by H. L. Amoss, L. T. Webster and others (1918–24). The effects of introduction of new susceptible material upon the epidemic curves (exaltation of virulence) and their subsidence (acquired immunity following extinction of susceptible material) were studied and it was shown that epidemics arise from increased dosage of bacteria, which is again accelerated or diminished by factors determining susceptibility or resistance in the population.[1] The ablest historian of epidemiology in recent times is Georg **Sticker** (1860–   ), of Cologne, who has dealt with the space-time phases in his exhaustive clinical monographs on whooping cough (1896), hay-fever (1896), plague (1908–10), influenza (1911), cholera (1912), dengue (1914), colds (1915), leprosy (1924), tropical fevers (1925), and his scholarly surveys of the general history of epidemic diseases.

Of the brilliant group of Italian clinicians and epidemiologists, Angelo **Dubini** first described the European hook-worm disease (1843) and electric chorea (1846); Salvatore **Tommasi** (1813–88), of Turin, professor of clinical medicine at Pavia (1861) and Naples (1865), and the ablest Italian clinician of his time, reformed Italian medicine by making a clean sweep of the school theories of Rasori in North Italy, Maurizio Bufalini (1787–1875) in Central Italy, and the diathetic school of Southern Italy, in favor of a physiological interpretation of pathology; the versatile and highly cultured veteran Guido **Baccelli** (1832–1916), of Rome, evoked the incomparable Renaissance glory of Italy in medicine and became widely known by his account of aphonic pectoriloquy in pleural effusion (Baccelli's sign, 1875), by his methods of treating aortic aneurysm by the introduction of a coil of metal in the walls (1876) and the injection treatment of malaria with quinine (1890), syphilis with corrosive sublimate (1894), and tetanus with carbolic acid (1905). At Naples, Arnaldo **Cantani** (1837–93) founded the first

---

[1] L. T. Webster: Bull. New York Acad. Med., 1928, 2. s., iv, 20–26.

bacteriological laboratory in Italy (1885) and was remarkable for his work on disorders of metabolism (1873; 1883), enteroclysis (1878–9) and progressive cutaneous atrophy (1881); Mariano **Semmola** (1831–96) wrote an important work on albuminuria and nephritis (1850); Antonio **Cardarelli** (1821–1916) was memorable for his tracheal sign in aortic aneurysm; and Gaetano **Rummo** (1852–1917) for his work on cardioptosis and as founder of *Riforma medica* (1885).   At Padua, Achille **De Giovani** (1837–1916) was a pioneer in the application of anthropometry to the clinical study of the constitution.   At Pavia, Carlo **Forlanini** originated artificial pneumothorax.   At Genoa, Enrico **De Renzi** (1839–1921) was director of the medical clinic and did good work on diabetes and tuberculosis.   At Bologna, Angelo **Murri** (1841–) investigated temperature and fever (1873–4) and bigeminal pulse (1887).   At Catania, Salvatore **Tommaselli** (1830–1902) studied quinine intoxication in malaria (Tommaselli's syndrome).   Camillo **Golgi** (1843–1926), the eminent histologist, Corrado **Tommasi-Crudeli** (1834–1900), of Rome, a pupil of Virchow, Ettore **Marchiafava** (1847–1916), the leading pathologist of Italy, Angelo **Celli** (1858–1914), Battista **Grassi** (1855–1925), Amico **Bignami** and Vittorio **Ascoli,** Baccelli's successor at Rome, all made their mark by effective work on malarial fever.   Pietro **Grocco** (1856–1916), of Pavia, described paravertebral dulness on the opposite side in pleural effusion (Grocco's triangle, 1902). Guido **Banti** (1852–1925) described splenomegalic anemia (1898). Adelchi **Negri** (1876–1912) discovered the Negri bodies in hydrophobia (1903–4). Aldo **Castellani,** a medical graduate of Florence (1899) [1876–   ], now professor of tropical medicine in Tulane University, New Orleans, found Dutton's Trypanosoma gambiense in the cerebro-spinal fluid of sleeping sickness patients (1903), and the spirochæte of yaws (1905), was a pioneer in investigating the bronchomycoses which simulate phthisis (1905–27), the tonsillomycoses (1926), the mycotic forms of pruritus of the anus and vulva (1927), infestation of the scalp with Trichophyton Louisianicum (1927) and (with A. J. Chalmers) wrote the best modern book on tropical medicine (1910); Angelo **Maffucci** (1845–1903) and Edoardo **Maragliano** (1849–   ), of Genoa, are memorable for their work in tuberculosis; Giuseppe **Sanarelli** for investigations of yellow fever; Giuseppe **Guarnieri** (1856–1918) for his work on the supposed parasites of variola and vaccinia (1894); as neurologists Andrea **Verga** (1811–95), Augusto **Tamburini** (1848–1919), Enrico **Morselli** (1852–   ) and Leonardo **Bianchi;** as pathologists Pio **Foà** (1848–1922) and Benedetto **Morpurgo;** in endocrinology, Giulio Vassale and Niccolò Pende.

Here may be signalized two recent phases of 20th century medicine, namely, the **rise of medicine in Latin America and Japan.**

Although up to recent years, the Latin-American countries have been intellectually provinces of Spain, with some impetus from French and German influences here and there, the medicine of Latin America bids fair to surpass that of Spain. With all reverence for the name of Ramón y Cajal, one of the greatest histologists of all time, his strenuous efforts for university autonomy in medical teaching availed little. In spite of the work of Juan Ferran of Barcelona on vaccination against cholera and tuberculosis (1885–1919), Barraquer (progressive lipodystrophy, 1906; cataract extraction, 1917), Tolosa Latour, Gomez Ocãna, Salvador Cardenal (1853–1927), the leading surgeon or the journalist reformer, Rodriguez Mendez, Spanish medicine[1] has been dominated by what the Spaniards themselves call "caciquism" (nepotism). Medical practice is poorly paid and the doctors are driven to the bread-basket view of life. In the western hemisphere, Mexico had the first hospital (1524), the first chair of medicine (1578–80), the first medical books to be printed (1570, 1578) and the first medical periodical (1772). Some 315 medical books were published between 1570 and 1833 (León). Eminent in Mexican medicine are the names of Eduardo Licéaga (1836–1920), the surgeons Rafael Lavista, Luis Muñoz, the obstetricians Juan Maria Rodriguez, and Juan Duque de Estrada, the statistician Antonia Peñafiel and the eminent medical historian and anthropologist, Nicolas León. In Cuba, Carlos Juan Finlay (1833–1915) first stated the theory of mosquito-borne yellow fever (1881), and excellent work has since been done by Juan Guiteras (1853–1925), Aristides Agramonte (yellow fever) and Juan Santos Fernandez (1847–1922) (ophthalmology). Brazil numbers such remarkable physicians as Gaspar Vianna, who introduced antimony tartrate injections in kala-azar, Torres Homem, Miguel Conto, Francisco de Castro, Rocha Faria, Oscar Clark, José de Mendonca, Emilio Ribas, Cruz, and Chagas. Parasitology received a great impetus at the hands of Oswaldo Gonçalvez **Cruz** (1872–1917), who became director of public health at Rio in 1903, and through his energetic and drastic reforms was ultimately accepted as sanitary dictator of Brazil. In 1901, he founded the Institute at Maguinhos to which the citizens of Rio gave his name in 1908. Here Carlos **Chagas** discovered the Trypanosoma Cruzi and described the infective thyroiditis produced by it (1909), and Cruz discovered the anopheline sub-species Chagasia and a species of Psorophora. From this Institute have emanated innumerable investigations of the novel insects, parasites and venomous reptiles with which Brazil abounds, usually published in the transactions of the Institute or in the columns of the *Brazil Medico*. The Instituto Butantan (Sao Paulo), founded by Vital Brazil (1899[2]), was one of the earliest distributing stations for large-scale production of sera against snake-poisoning and was an incentive to the foundation of an Antivenin Institute at San Antonio (Texas), directed by Col. M. L. Crimmins, U. S. Army (retired). The leading sanitarians of Argentina were Carlos Malbrãn, who founded the first chair of bacteriology in Buenos Aires, and his successor, José Penna (died 1919), who founded a chair of clinical epidemiology (1884), completed the National Bacteriological Institute (1916) and described the sequelæ of spider bite (1894). Excellent beginnings in scientific medicine have been made in Buenos Aires, Caracas, Lima, and other South American cities.[3] In the Philippines the names of the martyr-patriot José Rizal (1862–96), José Albert (infantile beri beri, 1908–24), T. H. Pardo de Tavera (Filippino materia medica, 1892), C. Manalang (hookworm), Fernando Calderon (medical education), and Vicente Jesus (public hygiene) are worthy of note.

Modern Japan has now 50,000 doctors, 21 medical schools, over 100 government and prefecture hospitals, about 1000 private hospitals, about 8000 isolation hospitals, 10 leper hospitals, one insane hospital, 8 research institutes and nearly 50 medical journals, of varying merit. Medical education and investigation have thriven largely under German influence. Anatomy was established in Japan by Kazuyoshi Taguchi, physiology by Kenji Ozawa, biochemistry by Muneo Kumagawa (1839–1902) and Torasaburo Araki, pathology by Moriharu Miura, bacteriology by Shibasaburo Kitasato and Masaki Ogata. Kitasato is the

---

[1] For an account of recent improvements in public hygiene, see Arthur Seligmann, Leipzig, diss., 1925.

[2] Vital Brazil: A defensa contra o ophidismo, São Paulo, 1911. The Instituto Soro-Therapeutico de Butantan is now directed by Dr. Afranio do Amaral.

[3] For a full account of recent medical developments and institutions in Latin America, see F. H. Martin: South America, New York, 1927.

founder of the Governmental (1892) and the Kitasato Institutes (1914) for Infectious Diseases in Tokyo.

The bacillus of dysentery was discovered by Kiyoshi Shiga (1897). In parasitology, introduced by Isao Ijima, Japan has already achieved a most brilliant record, particularly in the science of the trematode worms. In 1904, Fujiro Katsurada and Akira Fujinami discovered Schistosomum Japonicum and described schistosomiasis, the intermediate host having been discovered by Keinosuke Mujairi and Minoru Suzuki. Metagonimus Yokogawai and its second intermediate host were, both of them, discovered by Sadamu Yokogawa in 1913, and the first intermediate host by M. Muto (1916). Ryukichi Inada and Yutaka Ido discovered the spirochete of infectious jaundice (Weil's disease) and developed a successful serum-therapy for the infection in 1914–15. The parasite of rat-bite fever (Spirochæta muris) was discovered by Kenzo Futaki and Kikutaro Ishiwara (1915). The second intermediate host of Clonorchis sinensis was discovered by Harujiro Kobayashi (1911–14); the intermediate host of Paragonimus Westermanii (Ringer, 1879) by Koan Nakagawa (1914–15). The migratory course of human ascaris was demonstrated by Sadao Yoshida, and the experimental production of cancer from continuous stimulus by Katasusaburo Yamagawa and Koichi Ichikawa (1915). In 1920, Hideyo Noguchi discovered the parasite of yellow fever (*Leptospira icteroides*) at Guayaquil and died a martyr to the disease in Africa (1928).

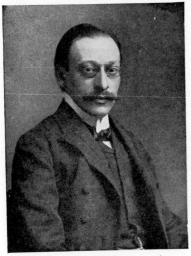

Max Neuburger (1868–   ).

The last ten or twenty years have witnessed an unusual growth of interest in the **history of medicine.** Apart from the great Leipzig plant, the subject is now taught in most of the German universities (Sigerist). In Vienna, the veteran Max **Neuburger** (1868–   ), author of valuable histories of the physiology of the nervous system in the 17th to 18th centuries (1897), the mechanism of specific nutrition (1900), antitoxic therapy (1900), German neuropathology (1912), Austrian and Viennese medicine (1918–22), medicine in Josephus (1919), the healing power of nature (1926), and a superlative history of medicine (1906–11), began to teach the subject as privatdocent forty years ago (1898) and succeeded to Puschmann's chair (1904), with an Institute and museum in the old Josephinum.

The subject is now taught at Jena by Theodor **Meyer-Steineg** (1873–   ), author of studies of Thessalos of Tralles (1910), Galenic physiology (1912–13), Roman military hospitals (1912) and an illustrated survey of medical history (with Sudhoff, 1920); at Freiburg, by Paul **Diepgen** (1878), of Aix, author of studies of Arnold of Villanova (1909–22), a medical chronology (with Aschoff, 1920) and histories of medicine (1913–24), and of German medicine (1923); at Düsseldorf by Wilhelm **Haberling** (1871), of Liegnitz, notable for the best recent studies of the history of military medicine (1910–18); at Wurtzburg, Georg **Sticker** (1860–   ), of Cologne, the historian of epidemiology (1896–1924); at Rostock by Walter **von Brunn** (1876–   ), of Göttingen, author of studies of the Hanseatic barber-surgeons' guilds (1921), modern German medical periodicals (1925), Caspar Stromayr (1925) and a history of surgery (1925); at Bonn by Karl Schmiz (1877–   ), historian of the

Bonn Medical Faculty (1920); at Frankfurt by Richard Koch (1882–); at Berlin by Max **Wellmann** (1863–) of Stettin, editor of Dioscorides (1906–14), Philumenos (1908) and an expert in classical philology; at Leipzig by Henry E. **Sigerist** (1891–), who succeeded to Sudhoff's chair and the editorship of his *Archiv* in 1925. At the University of London, Charles **Singer** (1876–), author of many valuable studies, has lectured on the history of medicine and science since 1921. At Edinburgh, John Dixon **Comrie** (1875), author of a history of Scottish medicine (1927), has lectured to students since 1913. At Strassburg, Ernest **Wickersheimer** (1880–), of Bar-le-Duc (Meuse), as librarian of the Sorbonne (1909), the Academy of Medicine (1910–19) and of the University Library at Strassburg (1919), has devoted his life mainly to research work, notably of French medicine of the Renaissance period (1905), French medical periodicals (1908), the history of the Paris Medical Faculty during 1359–1516 (1915), and many aspects of French medicine up to the 18th century. In the same trend are Erich Ebstein (1880–) of Göttingen, who, at Leipzig, has made remarkable studies of the history of diseases, therapeutic methods and of secular literature; Max Meyerhof (Arabic ophthalmology); Franz Hübotter (Chinese medicine); Ernst Seidel (Arabic, Armenian, and Persian medicine); Conrad Brunner (Swiss medicine); Édouard Jeanselme (Byzantine medicine); Pierre-Eugène Menetrier (French medicine); J. W. S. Johnsson (Danish medicine); and in classical philology, Max Wellmann, Diels, Rose, Ilberg, Ulrich von Wilamovitz-Moellendorf, Jones, Withington and Heidel, who have worthily sustained the tradition established early in the 19th century by Adamantios Coray (1748–1833).

In the United States, chairs have been held by Cordell (Baltimore), Packard (Philadelphia) and others, and intramural teaching of an informal kind was introduced at the Johns Hopkins Hospital by Osler and Welch, at Harvard by Streeter, and at the Mayo Clinic. The pioneer in post-graduate teaching was William Snow **Miller** (1858–), of Stirling, Massachusetts, who, in connection with his chair of anatomy at the University of Wisconsin, has conducted an extramural *seminar* at

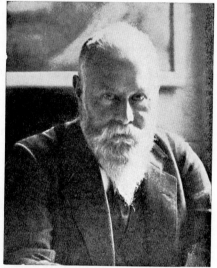

Karl Sudhoff (1853–). (From a portrait in the Surgeon-General's Library.)

Madison since 1909, with an output of some 50 papers since 1911. An offshoot exists at the University of Oregon (1927) and there are many promising beginnings all over the Northwest and the Pacific Coast. In 1926, William H. **Welch** was appointed professor of history of medicine in the Johns Hopkins University, with a prospective Institute and Library, which will undoubtedly become a center for post-graduate instruction in methods of research work and a seed-plant of medical culture.

The most important advance of recent years was the foundation of the *Institut für Geschichte der Medizin* at Leipzig, in 1905, under the direction of Karl Sudhoff, for whom a special chair of the subject was created in the University (1905). This Institute and its publications are supported by a special endowment of 500,000 marks left for this purpose by the widow of the late Professor Theodor Puschmann, and in accepting the directorship Professor Sudhoff stipulated that a separate home for the new specialty should be erected. Karl **Sudhoff** (1853–), of Frankfort on the Main, who had practised medicine for many years before this event, and is entirely self-taught in medical history, began his studies with his important investigations of Paracelsus (including a thorough study of the Paracelsus manuscripts), started in 1876, and published 1887–99, which are still authoritative. He has written exhaustive and scholarly monographs on the iatro-mathematicians of the 15th and 16th centuries (1902), manuscript and other 15th century medical illustrations (1907), the early history of anatomical illustration (1908), German medical incunabula (1908), the Greek papyri of the Alexandrian Period (1909), ancient balneology (1910), and the early history of syphilis (1912). In addition to these researches, all of the highest order, Sudhoff has published a host of minor investigations of value, particularly in the *Archiv für Geschichte der Medizin*, which he founded in 1908. He has made many of the rarer medical texts accessible to German readers through his *Klassiker der Medizin*, a series of inexpensive reprints which, in style and *format*, are like Ostwald's well-known editions of scientific classics. His method of investigation was a new departure. With the financial resources at his command, he has traveled far and wide in search of rare or un-printed medical manuscripts and illustrations in the European libraries, private and public, and, by photographing these and collating them, he has been able to apply the inductive method with signal ability in bringing out many new facts, settling disputed points, and exploding much of the traditional *Papierwissenschaft* which has been slavishly accepted to date. Thus he has shown, by collation of unprinted manu-scripts, that up to Vesalius, the textual illustration of anatomy was for centuries based upon servile tradition and almost devoid of any signs of original observation. No one has written more effectively upon anatomical illustration since Choulant. Sudhoff has also devel-oped the whole science of the *Lasstafelkunst*, against which Paracelsus brayed with such obscene vigor in his *Liber Paragranum* (1859), and, during this research, he discovered the first medical publication to be set in type, Gutenberg's purgation calendar of 1457, in the Bibliothèque nationale in Paris. His philological researches on the Alexandrian papyri (1909) throw much light on the status of Egyptian medicine in this period, and his later investigations of the early history of syphilis (1912–26), which we have already described, furnishes a formidable argu-ment against the theory of the American origin of the disease. His path-breaking study of medieval surgery (1914) was completed in 1918. He had revised Pagel's *Einführung* (1915), in addition to a beautifully illustrated survey of medical history of his own (with Meyer-Steineg, 1922), has published a history of dentistry (1921), an anthology of pediatric incunabula (1925), books on Cos and Cnidos (1926), pre-historic German medicine (1928), and has collaborated with Arnold Klebs in a study of the existing incunabula on plague (1926). He has also added much to our knowledge of the advancement of state medicine during the Middle Ages. His original investigations and re-productions of the medieval writings on leprosy, plague and syphilis, including the preventive ordinances, go far beyond the labors of Haeser in this field. To look through his wonderful catalogue of the Dresden Historical Exhibit (1911) is to realize how little one knows about the history of hygiene. His vast reading gives him an insight into medieval medicine, such as is possessed by no other living man, and his conversation alone is said to be an inspiration to his pupils. Sudhoff believes that classical philologists who have exhausted the possibilities of the secular literature of Greece and Rome, should try their teeth on the older medical writings and help to elucidate them. His exhaustive study of the German medical incunabula (1908) supplements and completes the work of Choulant, and was a forerunner of the movement, started in Berlin (1904), to get up an international catalogue of all the incunabula in public and private libraries, in order to decide the many unsettled points as to time, place of publication and authorship.

With the work of this distinguished scholar, our sketch of recent medicine may fitly close.

CULTURAL AND SOCIAL ASPECTS OF MODERN MEDICINE

READERS of Lecky's "History of European Morals" will recall the impressive pages in which he discusses the effects of the modern spirit of industrialism upon ethical relations, even upon sexual morality. Two types of character, he says, are apt to be produced—the thrifty and cautious, which has "all that cast of virtues which is designated by the term 'respectability' "; and the speculative, enterprising type, which is "restless, fiery, and uncertain, very liable to fall into great and conspicuous vices, impatient of routine, but by no means unfavorable to strong feelings, to great generosity or resolution." The first type is prevalent in poor, isolated communities, the second among the busy marts of commerce. These phases of the great industrial movement of modern life have not been without their effect upon medical practice. During the 19th century, we see the physician becoming more and more impersonal, more of a business man and not so much influenced by the social and ethical obligations which were certainly a characteristic of the 18th century physician. The "family doctor" of the past has well-nigh disappeared, except in small communities, and, in the modern period, we find the city physicians, under stress of competition, driven to unusual protective devices to hold their own. The reasons for this are not far to seek. They have been set forth at sufficient length in Mr. Bernard Shaw's clever but superficial tirades on the commercialization of the medical profession. Otto Juettner, in his interesting life of Daniel Drake, tells of a certain gruff physician in the Western Reserve in the early thirties who, when summoned to see any patient of whose financial status he was ignorant, always demanded, on entering the room: "Who pays this bill?" This is a crude instance, yet compare it with what Abraham Flexner says about the careers of the two Hunters, Matthew Baillie, Bright, Addison, and Hodgkin:

"These men all ran substantially the same course. As unknown youths they became assistants in the dead-house or the out-patient department of the hospital. This was their opportunity; obscurity was their protection. They spent years in working out, on both pathological and clinical sides, the important problems with which their names are severally associated. When, at the close of a decade, they had achieved scientific eminence, they were whirled off into busy practices. The rest of their active lives they spent as prosperous consultants, visiting the hospital and teaching in its medical school, of course, but without the leisure, environment, or stimulus requisite to further scientific pursuit. The hospital as an institution was indifferent; other inducement there was none. Fifteen or twenty unproductive years followed. Thus men blossomed early, but they left no seed; they had no scientific heirs; they established no line."[1]

While John Hunter left many remarkable pupils, and Addison and Hodgkin were anything but "prosperous consultants," it is not unlikely

---

[1] A. Flexner: Medical Education in Europe, New York, 1912, 13.

that a good consulting practice, a comfortable berth in Harley Street, has been a prominent ambition of the London practitioner in the later period. Even in Germany, Flexner is disposed to admit "a growing suspicion that the idealism of the clinical professors is yielding to the temptation, perhaps the need, of increased income. . . . The scale of living has been altered by industrial prosperity; new ideals, material in character, are creeping in." From the days of John Hunter's unwilling quest after "that damned guinea" to the disputes of our own time about "fee-splitting," contract practice, lodge doctors, *Kranken-kassen*, patent medicines, unqualified practitioners and socialization of medicine, the necessity of struggling for a competence, instead of having it assured by family practice, as in the 18th century, has wrought a change in the modern physician. The ideal is scientific and impersonal, to be as efficient as an engineer and to look and act like one.

In spite of themselves, men are influenced by the social conditions which impinge upon them. It is a noticeable fact that the pictures of Americans of the Civil War generation have a more sincere and ideal look than those of the present time. The modern type everywhere is one of clean-cut business efficiency. In the advancement of science this has been an immeasurable gain. Modern science has done away with the idea of personal infallibility, has centered itself upon results and has a fine probity of its own. "The scientific gentleman," said Billings, "is the blue-ribbon of our day." It is to the credit of modern medicine that, in spite of intense competition, thousands of physicians have continued to practise their profession along the old honorable lines, giving largely and nobly of their time to the poor, although, in the crowded streets of finance, a man whose heart is better than his head is a fool by definition. The most enlightened physicians of today are advancing preventive medicine, which tends to do away with a great deal of medical practice. "Certainly men who regularly render a large part of their services gratuitously and are constantly striving to eradicate their own means of livelihood cannot be convicted of being altogether mercenary."[1]

As Harvey Cushing quaintly puts it: "Dr. Pound of Cure Lane is being superseded by his young disciple, Dr. Ounce of Prevention Street."[2]

The increased cost of living, the automobile, expensive office appointments and instruments, foreign study and travel, make heavy inroads on the modern physician's income, and, hence, have almost tripled the rate of **medical fees.** In other words, the purchasing power of money is steadily declining. According to the laws of economics, the greater the supply of gold, the more it becomes a commodity and the fewer the things it will buy. It is easier to get money nowadays than unadulterated food and raiment or unscamped labor, and, as

---

[1] J. B. Nichols: "Medical Sectarianism," Wash. Med. Ann., 1913, xii, 12.
[2] Cushing: Brit. Med. Journal, Lond., 1913, ii, 291.

labor-saving inventions destroy leisure, time becomes more valuable than money.

At the end of the 18th century (1798), the professional charges of "practitioners of physic and surgery in the State of New York"[1] were $1 for an ordinary visit or $1.25, with a single dose of medicine, 12 cents each for pills and powders, $5 for a consultation ("verbal advice") or a night visit, $1 to $2 for bloodletting, $4 for cupping, $100 each for amputating a joint, excising an eye, operating for aneurysm, while operating for hernia, stone, or cataract cost $125; an ordinary labor case was $15 to $25; a difficult one, $25 to $40. S. C. Busey, commencing practice in Washington, D. C., in 1849, got $1 a visit, and "many times the bill was settled with a fraction, and often a small fraction, of that amount."[2] At present, the average bill for a city visit in Washington is $3 to $5, and with $5, $30 and $100 as a minimum in consultations, obstetrical and surgical cases respectively. In larger cities, the minimum fee for a visit may be as high as $25 with some practitioners. In England, the average consultation fee was a guinea up to 1870, after which it became customary to ask two guineas for the first visit and one guinea afterward. If travel were required, the charge was an additional guinea a mile, until about 1845, when railway locomotion reduced this to two guineas per three miles (Power). In the country districts, or among the poor, visits may be variously ten shillings, five shillings, eighteen pence, or sixpence. The country doctor usually charged for the medicines he prepared and supplied rather than the advice rendered, e. g., bleeding 1s. 6d., bolus 1s. 6d., draught and pill 1s. 9 d., iter (journey to house) 1s. 6d. The Poor Law appointment in 1845 was usually £20 per annum for each parish, 10s. extra for a midwifery case, with an additional 2s. 6d. if the patient lived three miles away (Power[3]). The socialization of medicine by **panel practice** has imposed much extra work at small compensation upon English physicians, as it doubled the labors of those not on military duty in the recent war.

In France, during the Napoleonic wars, a cabinet consultation or a city visit was 10 sous (1805–39); by 1850 it was 1 franc. Bloodletting was 1 livre; an accouchement, 12 livres. In Prussia (1906), physicians and patients made whatever bargain they chose: 2 to 20 marks for an office visit, 1 to 10 marks for a subsequent visit or a consultation, 4 to 10 marks for a confinement, with half as much again for twins, 3 to 15 marks for removing a tonsil, 10 to 30 marks for setting a fracture. In 1892, over half the physicians of Berlin were making less than 3000 marks annually; about one-tenth were making over 10,000. In 1908, the salary of a professor ordinarius was 4800 marks, with increases of 400 marks every four years, up to a limit of 7200 marks at the end of twenty-four years' service. Outside Berlin, it began with 4200 and ends with 6600 marks. A salaried extraordinarius got 2600 marks to start with, 4800 marks as the limit. In Austria, the extraordinarius started with 3200 kronen and reached 4000 kronen in a decade. Flexner says that a prominent German professor disclosed the sources of his income as "$300 as hospital physician, paid by the city; $2000 as professor, paid by the state; $5000 in student fees. He also does some consultant practice in the afternoon."[4] The lowering and fluctuation of monetary values during the World War was such that it is impossible to estimate the effect upon medical fees in limited space.

Modern art, like that of the 17th century, has represented medical subjects in varied and manifold ways. One prominent characteristic of modernity, "the strange disease of modern life," is to seek what is odd and new, and, in art, to find inspiration in ugliness. Goya's canvasses in the Prado, for instance, and particularly his etchings, are triumphs of the *macabre*. His figurations of teratology, idiocy, insanity, death by violence, and general bloodshed show the curious interest in the horrible, the solemn delight in death which the Goncourts thought essen-

---

[1] J. J. Walsh: "Physicians' Fees down the Ages," Internat. Clin., Phila., 1910, 20 s., iv, 259–275.

[2] Samuel C. Busey: Personal Reminiscences, Washington, 1895, 63.

[3] D. A. Power: Janus, Amst., 1909, xiv, 292–293.

[4] Flexner: *Op. cit.*, pp. 148, 293–299.

tially Spanish: "*Le génie de l'horreur, c'est le génie de l'Espagne.*" The Musée Wiertz in Brussels affords another example of this tendency. Infanticide, suicide, premature burial, and eroticism are the special themes of this artist. Charcot gives an interesting group of blind men by the Japanese artist Hokusai. The impressionist Degas, working with the precision of a Dutch interior painter, has excelled in rendering the artificial movement of the ballerina. His nudes are as ugly as those of Rembrandt. A more recent development is the *scabreux*, which has been exhaustively treated by modern cartoonists and caricaturists, like Gavarni, and in the canvasses of the German Secessionists, some of whom have represented childbirth, for instance, with appalling frankness. Every recent *Salon des réfusés* at Paris has had something of this kind. Along more conventional lines there have been plenty of paintings representing doctors at the bedside or surgeons operating in clinic; and of pictures of the old-fashioned literary type, which tell a story, such as Wilhelm von Kaulbach's *Narrenhaus* (1837), E. Hamman's Vesalius; Germain Colot cutting for stone in the presence of Louis XI (1414), by Rivoulon; Paré operating on the outskirts of a besieged town by L. Matout; the *Pestifères de Jaffe* of Antoine-Jean Gros; Géricault's *Femme Paralytique* (1820); *La Mort de Bichat* by Louis Hersent; Robert Henry's *Pinel à la Salpêtrière;* Feyen-Perrin's *Leçon de Velpeau;* or Péan demonstrating hemostasis by forcipressure (L. Gervex). Others, such as Andrea Cefaly's dentist (1875), Geoffroy's sick boy taking castor oil, Gibelin's society dame undergoing venesection, Laurent Gsell's picture of Pasteur inoculating against hydrophobia, Edelfelt's "Pasteur in his laboratory," Camille Bellanger's art-students dissecting at the École pratique, A. Brouillet's picture of Charcot demonstrating a hysterical case at the Salpêtrière, or Julian Story's laboratory at St. Lazare, show the tendency toward realistic or photographic representation. Carolus Duran, Sargent, Cecilia Beaux, and others have made many esteemed oil portraits of recent physicians. Many modern medical men have illustrated their own works, in particular the Bells, Bright, Hodgkin, Henle, His, Leidy, and Lister. Auvert, Cruveilhier, Bright, Lebert, Hope and Carswell left great polychrome atlases of disease. The young Pasteur made unique pastels of his parents and others. Paul Richer made a beautiful drawing of Charcot, and Charcot himself was a talented draftsman and decorator of porcelain. His pencil followed the lead of the comic and the fantastic, and his caricatures of the Paris Faculty, as friends in council (*L'Aréopage*) and in Indian file (*en queue*), are delicious. Sir Seymour Haden, the surgeon, was one of the most accomplished of modern etchers. The exhibits of artistic productions by physicians at the New York Academy of Medicine (1927), and in Toronto (1927), were distinct revelations as to the number of medical men who are now following the graphic and plastic arts without ostentation. In sculpture, we have Alfred Boucher's bas relief of Tobias restoring his father to sight (Musée de Troyes), Falguière's full-length statue of Charcot

48

(Salpêtrière, 1898), Paul Richer's statue of Pasteur at Chartres, and the more conventional figures of English and American physicians in various localities. Rodin has made a large number of curious shorthand notations of human anatomy, as preparatory to his peculiar mode of treating marble. Of the many recent monuments to Servetus, we may mention the figure on the funeral pyre in the Place de Montrouge (Paris) by Jean Baffier, the contemplative Servetus, in doctor's cap and gown, in the vestibule of the Museo Velasquez at Madrid, the statue of the martyr in prison by Roche (Annemasse), the Rodinesque nude by Joseph Bernard at Vienne (Isère), the gowned seated figure on the portico of the edifice of the Faculty of Medicine at Zaragoza, and the expiatory plinth of rough-hewn granite at Geneva. Servetus has also been commemorated in a play by the Spanish dramatist and physician, José Echegaray (*La muerte en los labios*[1]).

As modern physicians have been abundantly caricatured in the graphic arts, so the business-like tendencies of the profession in our own time have afforded liberal opportunities for literary satire. Baas has hit off the early 19th century doctors of this type as characterized "by the fashionable cut of their clothing, their universal greetings and rapid gait, their imperturbable amiability, and the thermometer, stethoscope, percussion hammer, etc., peeping out of their coat pockets."[2] All this implies a somewhat sweeping survey of a whole period, but we find similar traits of smartness in such characters as Dickens' Dr. Slammer in *Pickwick* or Dr. Jobling in *Martin Chuzzlewit*, and Charles Reade's Dr. Aberford in *Christie Johnstone*. Thackeray's Dr. Firmin and Wilkie Collins's Dr. Downward represent types of a craftier and more dubious kind. The best imaginative portrait of the high-bred physician of intellectual type is that of Lydgate, in George Eliot's *Middlemarch*, a novel which, on the whole, affords the most effective side-light on English medicine in the late Georgian and early Victorian periods. The keenest edge of the author's satire is reached in the medical gossip of the gentlewomen in the tenth chapter. Mrs. Cadwallader likens Casaubon, the fossil bridegroom of the beautiful Dorothea, to a dose of medicine, "nasty to take and sure to disagree"; and Lady Chettam, in discussing Lydgate's superior family connections, observes:

"One does not expect it in a practitioner of that kind. For my own part, I like a medical man more on a footing with my servants; they are often all the cleverer. I assure you I found poor Hicks' judgment unfailing; I never knew him wrong. He was coarse and butcherlike, but he knew my constitution."

The same note is sounded in Major Pendennis' horror lest a lady marry her uncle's doctor, which would seem a far cry from the present esteem in which physicians are held. Henry James' *Washington Square* (1880) opens with an amusing assurance of their superior status in the

---

[1] Osler mentions another: "The Reformer of Geneva" (privately printed, 1897) by Professor Shields (Princeton).

[2] Baas: *Op. cit.*, p. 770.

United States. Balzac immortalized the French country doctor.[1] No less than Dupuytren was the original of his Desplein, and Bouillaud was his Horace Bianchon.[2] Flaubert's Homais is a satirical study of the provincial French apothecary. Samuel Warren, Charles Lever, O. W. Holmes, Weir Mitchell, Mrs. Reinhardt have all delineated the physician from different angles. Mitchell has made a clever study of a quack.[3] The medical students of Dickens, Albert Smith, and others are sufficiently well known. Turgenieff's Bazaroff,[4] the agnostic, anarchistic student of Eastern European type, is a genuine creation.

Latterly, the *docteur doctorant* is seldom absent from fiction and the drama, which are often preoccupied with some phase of pathology, from Ibsen's *Ghosts* and Tolstoi's *Ivan Ilyich* to the recent avalanche of biographies, novels and plays engendered by Freudian doctrine. Satire at the expense of medicine was resumed in Samuel Butler's *Erewhon* (1872), and continued by Bernard Shaw (*The Doctor's Dilemma*), Octave Mirbeau (*L'épidémie*), Hermann Hesse (*Kurgast*), Michel Corday (*Les embrasés*), André Couvreur (*Caresco*), H. E. Wells (*Tono Bungay*), Thomas Mann (*Zauberburg*), Sinclair Lewis (*Arrowsmith*) and particularly in the farce of *Knock* (1926) by Jules Romains (Louis Farigoule), which illustrates the potency of herd instincts and crowd psychology in the encouragement of quackery. Dostoievsky, James Joyce, and many others have illuminated sundry aspects of morbid and sexual psychology, even as Balzac, in the Esther-Vautrin series, grappled with the sexual genesis of crime. As medicine and hygiene are concerned with nearly every phase of human activity, there is hardly any literary work of consequence which does not deal incidentally with some phase of medicine. The great Library of the Paris Medical Faculty contains, in fact, full sets of the greater writers of France, for this reason.

From the novels of Smollett and the plays of Schiller to the *Causeries du Lundi*, the dramas of Echegaray and Arthur Schnitzler or the poems of Sherrington and Henry Head, the literary productions of medical men make an imposing list. Dana, Cushing, and John Fallon have made remarkable collections of medical poets. Among the physicians who were amateurs of music are Felix Plater, Athanasius Kircher, Caspar Bartholinus, Boerhaave, Auenbrugger, Arbuthnot, Withering, Helmholtz, Carl Ludwig, T. W. Engelmann, Henle, Max Schultze, Sir Richard Owen, Sir Robert Christison, Billroth, Naunyn, Kahlbaum, Wilhelm Ebstein, Julius Jacobson, Ludimar Hermann, Duke Karl Theodor of Bavaria, Alfred de Bary, Borodin, Jacques Loeb, Herter, Gerster, and Hemmeter.

The conditions of **medical education** in modern times may be briefly stated as follows: The teaching of medicine as a science, as something of larger scope than its practice, began with the foundation of laboratories and with the gradual assemblage of specialties as units in university instruction. From Boerhaave's time on, great teachers

---

[1] Balzac: Le médecin de campagne (1833).

[2] A. Lutaud: Bull. Soc. franç. d. hist. de méd., Paris, 1920, xiv, 373: 1925, xix, 145.

[3] Weir Mitchell: The Autobiography of a Quack, New York, 1900.

[4] Turgenieff: Fathers and Sons (1862).

have always had a limited number of brilliant pupils, who had it in themselves to be w,hat they were, but the average medical student did not begin to come into contact with the actual working facts and experiences necessary for his "education," until he was given an opportunity to test and try things for himself, and this was only possible, even in anatomy, when practical work was substituted for routine didactic lecturing, often based upon fantastic theories emanating from the teacher's brain. German university teaching was for a long time didactic, but with the foundation of such laboratories as Purkinje's at Breslau (1824), Liebig's at Giessen (1825), or Virchow's at Berlin (1856), there was a new departure; and, although it took a long time for the new movement to get under way, yet, after the advent of Virchow and his contemporaries, the modern world was going to school to Germany in the sciences upon which medicine is based, while England and France excelled mainly in the organization of hospital and clinical teaching. As late as 1842, Helmholtz, graduating as an army surgeon, discussed, among other theses, a surgical operation which, like Haller in the past, he had never seen or tried. While German medicine was in the throes of "Nature Philosophy," Laennec and Louis, Bright and Addison, Graves and Stokes, Dupuytren and Astley Cooper, were turning out crowds of competent clinicians and surgeons. German medical education is based upon the sound assumption that all the specialties, even dentistry or obstetrics, are so many phases of physics and chemistry, and there is hardly one of her eminent teachers who has not done original work in some fundamental branch of medicine at the beginning of his career. In the United States, conditions were entirely different. In colonial times, the medical student, however poorly educated, had, at least, the advantage of being under a preceptor, and thus coming into actual contact with some details of medical practice. But in the stress and competition of a growing democracy, this custom was soon discontinued, and while one or two medical schools maintained a certain level of excellence, a vast number of inferior schools were permitted to spring up which had no reason for existence beyond the primitive necessity of having doctors "before there was any way of educating them" (Flexner). In the first half of the century, ambitious and enterprising American students, who had the means, were going to Paris to study under Louis, or to Astley Cooper in London; in the later period, they were swarming to Virchow in Berlin, to Charcot in Paris, or to Billroth in Vienna. It was only toward the end of the 19th century, under the direction of Eliot at Harvard, Billings, Welch, and Osler at the Johns Hopkins, and Pepper in Philadelphia, that medical teaching began to be true university teaching, in the sense of training a student to make use of his own mind as a substitute for blind acceptance of dogma. In the early period, scores of able American physicians, it is true, came out of inferior schools and learned their medicine by practising it, but what they accomplished was due to themselves and not to the conditions from which they sprang.

On the continent, clinical medicine was ably taught by Corvisart, Laennec, Louis and Trousseau in Paris, Schönlein and Frerichs in Berlin, Skoda and Oppolzer in Vienna. At this time, "snap diagnoses," like sleight-of-hand surgery, were the fashion. Corvisart once remarked that the subject of an oil painting must have been a victim of heart disease, and it proved to be so. Hebra and Joseph Bell could detect the occupations as well as the diseases of their patients. Frerichs was so infatuated with this cult that he never admitted a diagnosis to be wrong. Yet the most exact methods known were employed in the clinics. Corvisart was the reviver of percussion. The stethoscope, in Laennec's hands, was the means of developing the science of diseases of the chest. Louis and the Irish clinicians introduced pulse timing by the watch. Piorry invented the pleximeter. Wunderlich put clinical thermometry upon a scientific basis. The stethoscope was first mentioned in the Harvard Catalogue in 1868–69, the microscope in 1869–70. Thermometers began to make their appearance in English hospitals about 1866–67, and came into general use about 1868–70. They were about 10 inches long, so large, in fact, that it took at least five minutes for them to register the axillary temperature, and so clumsy that, as Brunton relates, they were carried under the arm, "as one might carry a gun."[1] Their reduction in size, indeed the invention of the pocket thermometer, was due to Sir Clifford Allbutt (1868). Neither Keen nor Tyson saw a clinical thermometer or a hypodermic syringe during 1862–65. Billings, however, in taking care of the wounded from the seven days before Richmond (1862), had provided himself with both.[2]

In 1840, Schönlein introduced the novelty of lecturing in German at the Charité, while Geheimrat Wolff, his Berlin rival, conducted in opposition a "lateinische Klinik," where there was neither percussion nor auscultation, and this pedantry was not suspended until shortly before Schönlein's retirement in 1857. Schönlein's clinics, as described by Naunyn,[3] were of the highest scientific order. Upon entering the ward, the short, fat Schönlein would sink into a comfortable armchair beside the patient's bed, while his assistant read the case-history with the necessary details of auscultation and percussion and all the chemical and microscopical findings. He would then rise and examine the patient, and, dropping into his chair again, proceed to develop his diagnosis upon pathological grounds, and then discuss the case from the point of view of etiology and therapy. If a patient died, there was an autopsy with an "epicrisis" in which possible errors in diagnosis were discussed. After Schönlein came Frerichs (1859), who kept up

---

[1] Sir Lauder Brunton: Lancet, London, 1916, i, 317. See, also, the interesting history of clinical thermometry by G. Sims Woodhead and P. C. Varrier-Jones in Lancet, Lond., 1916, i, 173; 281; 338; 450; 495.

[2] J. S. Billings: Tr. Coll. Phys., Phila., 1905, 115–116. Clinical thermometry was popularized in the United States by Édouard Séguin's books of 1873 and 1876.

[3] B. Naunyn: Die Berliner Schule vor 50 Jahren (Samml. klin. Vortr., No. 478), Leipz., 1908, 210, 211.

the same traditions. He would examine new cases directly upon entering, and, if he found that his assistants had thoroughly studied them, the histories would be read, with all the accessory data of examination of urine, excreta, sputum, larynx, even the fundus of the eye; while microscopic slides would be demonstrated and pictures (often from his private collection) handed about among the students. He never nagged or bullied his assistants, treating them, Naunyn says, as if they were essential organs of his own body. His recapitulation of the case, with diagnosis, sometimes theatrical, was esteemed a masterpiece. It rested upon a rigorous scientific basis, yet, in closing with his subject, Frerichs favored the minute bedside casuistry of the English; and the patient, if not removed in time, sometimes heard a bad prognosis. Therapy was carefully considered by Frerichs and prescriptions forthcoming, as part of the subject, although, Naunyn thinks, the results did not greatly concern him. Upon the recovery or death of the patient, Frerichs gave a vivid and instructive epicrisis and, at the end of each semester came the "general epicrisis" in which all the cases gone over were carefully reviewed.[1] Upon such teaching as this was based the German development of internal medicine as a science, even down to the great clinics of Naunyn or Friedrich Müller. Traube, who became clinical director of the other wing of the Charité in 1853, was also esteemed for his exact diagnoses.[2] He was more conscientious and sincere in bedside examination, more interested in his patients than Frerichs, and was consequently better liked in private practice; but, according to Naunyn, he knew little chemistry, was an almost servile follower of Virchow in pathology, and, in his efforts to make clinical medicine subservient to physiology, sometimes lapsed into wire-drawn subtleties and superfine distinctions. Virchow favored Traube and hated Frerichs, so that the relations of these two were never cordial. Naunyn relates[3] that it was a common circumstance for the two great clinicians to stalk by at the head of their classes in the Charité without taking the slightest notice of each other, and their pupils were tacitly forbidden to associate in public. Meanwhile Virchow was the bright particular star of the Berlin School, a political revolutionary in his youth, an intellectual tyrant in old age. His public lectures, at which he was often late for political reasons, were diffuse, tedious, and difficult to follow, on account of his lengthy, often involved, sentences, but he was a brilliant master at the postmortem table and merciless in examining students.[4] To the north of the old Charité stands the new Charité, an ugly, gloomy building with grated windows containing

---

[1] Naunyn: *Op. cit.*, 212, 215–218.

[2] For example, that of aortic aneurysm by laryngoscopic detection of paralysis of the left vocal cord (Deutsche Klinik, Berl., 1860, xii, 395: 1861, xiii, 263). Osler relates that on one occasion, when a postmortem did not confirm his views, Traube simply said, "*Wir haben nicht richtig gedacht!*"

[3] Naunyn: *Op. cit.*, 219.

[4] His occasional bitterness Naunyn attributes to the hardships of his early youth.

the insane, the syphilitic, and a "combined station," the patients of which were sick convicts taken from the prisons. Of this "combined station" Virchow was physician-in-chief, and here, most assiduous in his duties, he actually posed as a "clinician."[1] At Vienna, Skoda was all for auscultation, Rokitansky all for postmortems, and Oppolzer was the best all-round teacher. Of the later Berlin group, it was said: "Gerhardt makes a diagnosis usually, Senator often, Leyden never" (Jacobi). Leyden, when his clinical assistant reported *"unreine Herztöne,"* said: "Very well, then, wash them" (A. C. Klebs). In England, Addison was easily the greatest clinical lecturer of his time, handsome, brilliant, and eloquent, but feared by his students on account of his cold, arbitrary manners and his martial outside. The genial, even-tempered Bright ran him an easy second, and although not so imposing in the lecture room, did more scientific work in the end and had a much larger practice. With Bright, Addison, and Hodgkin, pathology and clinical medicine went hand in hand. After them came Gull, Wilks, and Fagge, all effective teachers. In France, Trousseau was the most vivid and picturesque lecturer of the period, setting the pace for Dieulafoy, Marie, and other teachers of the courteous, quick-minded French type. Charcot's public clinics were unique of their kind, and designed to meet the needs of the great throngs who followed them. In order to throw his teaching into stronger relief, he demonstrated his cases in a miniature theater, the stage of which was furnished with footlights and all the scenic accessories of illumination from different angles. The patients stood before the footlights or in the limelight, if necessary, while Charcot, from the side of the stage, elucidated their cases in a slow, distinct manner. His voice being low, and his audiences the largest of any clinic in Europe, he deliberately dramatized and visualized the essential features of a case by mimicking the various gaits, tremors, tics, spasms, and constrained postures himself. When the patient was dismissed, the pathological lesion would immediately be thrown upon a screen at the back of the stage. Charcot's screen effects have now given place to the epidiascope and the cinematograph, which has been utilized by some modern surgeons as the only way of making a large concourse of students see the details of an operation.[2]

In the earlier American schools, clinical teaching was largely didactic. Most of the schools lacked true clinical facilities, and hospital work was usually accessible only to those who obtained positions as internes

---

[1] "Die Assistenzärzte jener Abteilung, erzählten oft, wie regelmässig und ausführlich er dort die Visite mache, und wie gern er den Arzt spiele," Naunyn, *op. cit.*, 215, 222. This may have been part of Virchow's ironical program in reference to Frerichs. M. Regensburger relates that he once saw Frerichs harpoon the biceps of a living patient to secure a preparation of trichina. Four days later the patient died of pyemia. The case was posted by Virchow, who began the necropsy by mimicking the solemn pontifical manner of Frerichs: "Gentlemen, another sacrifice to our science!" (California State Jour. Med., San Francisco, 1914, xii, 179).

[2] Naunyn, for instance, has likened Langenbeck's clinic in Berlin to an arena in which one saw Langenbeck himself, a number of backs, and great streams of blood, a common enough experience in the larger surgical centers.

or externes. These deficiencies were set off, in the later period, by the post-graduate school, in which the teaching was entirely practical, and which Flexner has satirically dubbed "an undergraduate repair shop."[1] Private preceptors and quiz-masters were employed by those who could afford it during their medical courses. A good example is to be had in Busey's account of the private teaching of George B. Wood, of Philadelphia, about the middle of the 19th century. Wood, a grave, dignified Quaker who had a private botanic garden, spent $20,000 on diagrams and models, and gave over $60,000 in endowments to the University of Pennsylvania and the College of Physicians of Philadelphia. He met his students nightly at his private house, around a table lighted by silver candelabra, and here he would examine them, line by line, precept by precept, through the two volumes of his book on practice of medicine.[2] This method was fairly typical of American teaching in the period. Its defects were that it was a mere pedagogic rubbing in of what had already been heard in routine lectures, with hardly any practical clinical experiences whatever. W. W. Keen says that the Philadelphia clinics, "until Da Costa, in the session of 1866–67, took hold of them, were about as inane and useless as one could imagine."[3] Bedside teaching in pediatrics, and indeed, in internal medicine also, was employed by Jacobi in New York in 1862–4. What clinical teaching should be is sensed in Flexner's spirited account of Friedrich Müller's clinic at Munich:

"A path is opened in order to wheel the patient in. The professor reads the history, displays on the blackboard the temperature chart, then, in quick, clear fashion, explores the patient, pointing out what he finds, discoursing on its significance, suggesting alternative explanations, until he settles down on the most probable diagnosis. This furnishes the topic for development and further illustration. The etiology, the pathology, the therapeutics, of the condition are set forth with wonderful vigor and lucidity. . . . A master mind at work is exhibited daily to two hundred students or more."[4]

Teaching of this type depends upon the man, and, other things being equal, has existed in the past here and there. The means of its more general extension in the present were afforded by the liberality of monarchical governments in Europe and of millionaires in America.

As far as original research is concerned, brilliant investigators have seldom failed of obtaining laboratories or institutes in the end, as witness the cases of Purkinje at Breslau (1824), Liebig at Giessen (1825), Buchheim at Dorpat (1849), Virchow at Berlin (1856), Bowditch at Harvard (1871), Schmiedeberg at Strassburg (1872), Pettenkofer at Munich (1879), Liebreich at Berlin (1883), Welch at Baltimore (1884), Pasteur at Paris (1888), Pavloff at Petrograd (1890), Koch at Berlin (1891), Kitasato at Tokyo (1892), Mosso at Turin (1894), and Ehrlich at Frankfort (1896), the Imperial Institute for Experimental Medicine at Petrograd (1890), the Lister Institute for Preventive Medicine at London (1891), the Institute Oswaldo Cruz at Rio de Janeiro (1901), or such American institutions as the laboratories established in Philadelphia by William Pepper (1895), the Wistar Institute of Anatomy and Biology at Philadelphia (1892), the Rockefeller Institute in New York (1901), the John

---

[1] Flexner: Medical Education in the United States, New York, 1910, 174.

[2] Busey: *Op. cit.*, 31–37, 45–46.   [3] W. W. Keen: Jeffersonian, Phila., 1912, xiv, 3.

[4] Flexner: Medical Education in Europe, p. 170.

McCormick Institute for Infectious Diseases in Chicago (1902), the Henry Phipps Institute for Tuberculosis in Philadelphia (1903), The Carnegie Institution of Washington (1903), the Rudolf Spreckels Laboratory (1910), the Henry Phipps Psychiatric Clinic of Baltimore (1913), the Otho S. A. Sprague Institute (1911). Nearly every university, medical school, hospital, or health department in the country has now a pathological laboratory. Cleveland (Ohio) has recently acquired a Pathological Institute of modern type.

The **nuclei of medical education** in the United States and Canada have invariably been associated with some eminent name or names.

With the foundation of the Medical Faculty of the University of Pennsylvania (1765) are associated Morgan, Shippen and Rush; with that of King's College, New York (1768), John Jones and Samuel Bard; with that of Harvard (1783), John Warren and Benjamin Waterhouse; with that of Dartmouth (1797), Nathan Smith; with the College of Physicians and Surgeons, New York (1810), Samuel Bard, David Hosack, Valentine Mott, Wright Post, Samuel Latham Mitchill and John W. Francis; with the Medical Department of Yale (1810), Nathan Smith, Jonathan Knight and Benjamin Silliman; with that of Transylvania University, Lexington, Ky. (1817), Benjamin W. Dudley and Daniel Drake; with that of the Medical College of Ohio, Cincinnati (1819), Daniel Drake; with that of Bowdoin College, Brunswick, Me. (1820), Nathan Smith; with the Medical College of South Carolina, Charleston (1824), Samuel Henry Dickson; with the Jefferson Medical College, Philadelphia (1825), George McClellan, John Eberle and Nathan R. Smith; with the Rush Medical College, Chicago (1837), Daniel Brainerd. A remarkable center of medical education in its day was the College of Physicians and Surgeons of the Western District of the State of New York, founded June 12, 1812, and located at Fairfield, N. Y. In its palmy days, this was the second largest medical school in the country, with a roster of 217 students in 1834, and a total record of 3123 students and 589 graduates. Its faculty included such men as Lyman Spalding, T. Romeyn Beck, Reuben D. Mussey, and Frank H. Hamilton.[1] Upon its extinction in 1840, its effects were divided between the medical schools of Albany and Geneva, N. Y., the latter of which (opened February 10, 1835) became, in 1872, the present Medical Department of Syracuse University, associated with the names of H. D. Didama, Willard Parker and Alonzo Clark.

The Medical Faculty of McGill University, Montreal (1829), sprang from a course of teaching at the Montreal General Hospital (1820), which originated as a small house in Craig Street (1819), acquired for the sick by the Female Benevolent Society, organized to relieve the suffering poor of Montreal during the severe Canadian winter of 1817. The Faculty acquired its splendid new buildings in 1901.[2]

In 1869, according to the Bureau of Education, there were 72 medical colleges in the United States, of which 59 were regular, 7 homeopathic, 5 eclectic and one botanic (Tyson). In 1859 the Chicago Medical College introduced the novelty of a three years' graded course of study, but the requirements were not rigidly adhered to. The first real reform in American medical education was made, in 1871, by President Charles W. Eliot, of Harvard, who raised the entrance requirements of the Harvard Medical School, lengthened its curriculum to three years, and graded it, providing at the same time better facilities for clinical and laboratory instructions. In 1880, the three years' course, of nine months each, was extended to four years; in 1892–93 it was made obligatory; and an academic degree was required for admission in 1901. The three years' graded course was introduced in

---

[1] N. S. Davis: Contributions to the History of Medical Education (etc.), Washington, 1877.

[2] Maude E. Abbott: An Historical Sketch of the Medical Faculty of McGill University, Montreal, 1902.

the medical departments of the Universities of Pennsylvania and Syracuse in 1877, to be followed by Ann Arbor (1880) and others. In 1893, the Johns Hopkins Medical School, organized by President Daniel C. Gilman, John S. Billings, Henry Newell Martin, and William H. Welch, was opened, and with it came the opportunity for teaching scientific medicine by modern methods. Billing's original recommendations for the Johns Hopkins Hospital (1875[1]) included:

Not only the care of the sick poor, but the graded accommodation of pay and private patients in rooms or suites of rooms, proper education of physicians and nurses, and, above all, the promotion of "discoveries in the science and art of medicine, and to make these known for the general good." He insisted that the out-patient department should be connected with the building set apart for the instruction of students, and separated from the administration buildings; that clinical instruction should be mostly given in the wards and out-patient department, and not in an amphitheater, except in the surgical unit; that medical cases should not be brought from beds to an amphitheater; that there should be two pharmacies and a training-school for nurses; and that a perfect system of records, financial, historical, and clinical, should be kept. With Osler as physician-in-chief, Welch, Halsted, and Kelly in the chairs of pathology, surgery, and gynecology, a brilliant and efficient medical faculty was soon developed, with actual work in wards, clinics, dispensaries, laboratories, and dead-house as the basis of teaching. A bachelor's degree is required for admission, the students serve as clinical clerks and surgical dressers, after the Scotch and English fashion; the laboratories and clinics coöperate as hospital units, as in Germany. Billings lectured on medical history before the hospital was opened; the subject was furthered by Osler's evenings with his students at his home and by the meetings of the Hospital Historical Club. Osler required his students to read and report on the foreign medical journals, and otherwise develop the art of self-direction. The example of Johns Hopkins soon set the pace for Boston, Philadelphia, New Haven, Ann Arbor, Chicago, and elsewhere. The New York Polyclinic, our first institution for post graduate instruction was founded by John A. Wyeth (1881) and opened in 1882. At the University of Pennsylvania, a fourth-year course of entirely practical work was introduced in 1892–93, laboratories of hygiene (1892) and clinical medicine (1895) were added through William Pepper's efforts, and, in 1903, the Phipps Institute for Tuberculosis was added as a clinical plant. On September 25, 1906, the Harvard Medical School acquired a magnificent set of new buildings. Such American schools as the Jefferson (Philadelphia), the University of Michigan (Ann Arbor), the Rush and Northwestern (Chicago), the University of Minnesota (St. Paul), have now very good laboratory and clinical facilities, and there is much prospect of improvement in the South. The Medical Department at Washington University (St. Louis) has recently acquired a handsome endowment and buildings. Minneapolis is equally well off in this respect. The two leading Canadian schools, McGill (Montreal) and the University of Toronto, are organized on the English plan and are of a high grade of excellence. In the teaching and practice of surgery, the **Mayo Clinic,** at Rochester, Minnesota, has become a Mecca for post-graduate instruction, at the same time, the most highly organized exemplar of group medicine in existence. It had its start in Saint Mary's Hospital, erected by the Convent of the Sisters of Saint Francis (Rochester, 1889) for Dr. William Wardell Mayo (1819–1911), whose sons developed the plant to its present high efficiency.[2] It now controls 5 buildings, with 5 attached to the Kahler Corporation, in all 1345 active and 440 convalescent beds, handles about 65,000 patients annually, with an average floating population of about 2300, a permanent staff of 155 members, a non-permanent staff of 285, 1000 nurses, and 1100 extra personnel. Scientific work is done in all branches of medicine and recorded in a periodical, and incoming surgeons are salaried and retained, after a year's trial, by fitness alone.

In 1909–11, Abraham Flexner, at the instance of the Carnegie Foundation for the Advancement of Teaching, made two close and

---

[1] Hospital Plans, five essays, New York, 1875, 3–11, *passim.*

[2] Sketch of the History of the Mayo Clinic, Philadelphia, 1926.

comprehensive studies of the status of medical education at home and abroad,[1] and his strictures on American conditions excited a storm of comment and criticism, although Flexner's descriptions of what he saw are truthful and sincere, and therefore authoritative. Many inferior medical schools, brought face to face with the fact that "An unpleasant truth is better than a pleasant falsehood," doubtless resented an invitation to go out of business if they could not improve themselves. That there have been too many American medical schools— 39 in Illinois, 14 in Chicago, 42 in Missouri, with 12 survivors, 43 in New York, with 11 survivors, 27 in Indiana, with 2 survivors, 20 in Pennsylvania, with 8 survivors, 18 in Tennessee, with 9 survivors, 20 in Cincinnati, 11 in Louisville—was an inevitable resultant of conditions of growth in a democracy, as also the amazing overplus in the number of physicians—one doctor on the average for every 691 persons in the entire United States, 1 : 460 in New York, 1 : 580 in Chicago, 1 : 365 in Washington, D. C., as against 1 : 1940 in the whole German Empire; 1 :2120 in Austria, and 1 :2834 in France (1913). The surface explanation is simple. There are more people in the world, consequently more physicians. American conditions indicated a definite lack of restrictive requirements. Billings, in his survey of American medicine in 1876, accepted these conditions philosophically for two important reasons, viz., that a young man who has spent so many years "in the study of medicine as it ought to be studied, that is to say, in preparing himself to study and investigate for the rest of his life, will not settle in certain districts," and that to set a definite standard for medical matriculation, graduation, and registration would be hazardous in a country of such wide extent, since, to be uniform, it must necessarily be made a low one.[2] Moreover, the financial and other resources for improving medical education on a grand scale were not at that time forthcoming in this country. The present ideal is summed up in Weir Mitchell's aphorism that "the rate of advance in medicine is to be tested by what the country doctor is," in other words, the people of the United States should see to it that they have the same highly trained physicians that every peasant can have in Germany. Of his early student days in the Western Reserve (1857–60), Billings wrote: "They taught us medicine as you teach boys to swim, by throwing them into the water"; and, in 1878, he believed that it would be long before the annual number of medical graduates at the Johns Hopkins exceeded 25. Yet, in the third year, there were 32, and today many are settling in the smaller localities of the South and elsewhere, showing that advantages for income and investigation have materially improved since the Centennial year. The future of American medical education is, like all other higher developments, simply in the hands of the only aristocracy we strive for—the aristocracy of an enlightened public opinion. One ideal of our coun-

---

[1] Flexner: Medical Education in the United States and Canada, New York, 1910. Medical Education in Europe, New York, 1912.

[2] J. S. Billings, Am. Jour. Med. Sc., Phila., 1876, n. s., lxxii, 480.

try, what Emerson called its "mysterious destiny," has been the old ideal of the democratic New England community—the "conversion of raw material into efficiency," and its results and failures can be properly judged only by this standard. During the World War and after, there has been a great dearth of physicians in all civil and rural communities. In Massachusetts, 73 towns were without any registered physician (1920[1]), in Vermont 102 (1923), in Montana "several large counties" (1923), and worse conditions obtain in other parts of the country, where the deficiency has to be supplied by Public Health Nurses. Raymond Pearl[2] finds that these difficulties are fundamentally economic, and physicians, like other sensible people today, "do business where business is good and avoid places where business is bad." The difficulties encountered in providing adequate medical assistance for vast tracts of territory were well illustrated in pre-war Russia, where all accredited physicians had to be university medical graduates. The deficiency was supplied by the institution of "civil Feldscherism," which came into being with the emancipation of the serfs (February 19, 1861), and was a subject of heated dispute. The military Feldschers were originally those pupils of Peter the Great's medical school at Moscow, who had suffered a *capitis diminutio* for insubordination or inefficiency and were abased to the level of playing regimental barber or nurse to the barrack hospital. The civil Feldscher has been defined as the "leib-medik of the moujik," in other words, a half-fledged, half-educated medical assistant, deputized by government to take care of the vast numbers of peasants, of whom the *mirs* or village communities of pre-war Russia were largely made up.[3] The village doctor received the peasant at stated intervals, the Feldscher looked after him the rest of the time, while "flying corps" of oculists and other specialists were occasionally sent across the Caucasus into Siberia or wherever needed. The Feldscher, like the public health nurse, was thus a sort of *pis aller*, and the reason for his existence was a tacit agreement that it is better to have a half-doctor than no doctor at all.

The tendencies of German, French, and English medical teaching have been determined by the racial and national characteristics of these peoples, which are as definite as the physical configuration or the chemical composition of their bodies. The Anglo-Saxon has the supreme virtue of "saving common sense," with its corollaries of sobriety and decency, but is deficient in imaginative sympathy, and fumbles with things he does not understand. The French, in the view of Stuart Mill, tend to "thought without knowledge," may even simulate thought, prefer form to substance, and abide in stereotypy and established bureaucratic routine. Germanic erudition tends to "knowledge without thought," values substance more than form, is easily gulled by

---

[1] Boston Med. & Surg. Jour., 1920, clxxxii, 327.

[2] Pearl: Jour. Am. Med. Assoc., Chicago, 1925, lxxxiv, 1024–1028.

[3] Lancet, Lond., 1897, ii, 359–361.

pedantry, hollow bombast, dull or blatant pomposity, bull-dozing (*imponiren*) and the specious trappings of titular position and authority. The composite American, while simple, plain, sensible and practical at his best, is prone to hasty generalization, snap judgments, the posting of Arcadian ideals, "the passion for the beneficent edict," whence an illimitable capacity for self-deception with regard to values settled ages ago. The tendencies of German medicine spring from the fact that it began as a branch of philosophy in the medieval universities, and not, like the French and the English, around and about hospitals (Flexner[1]). Hence, German university teaching has ever followed the ideal of academic freedom. Education being, as Flexner says, a game in which the student must make the first move, he is left to think and act for himself, and if he becomes a poll-parrot, it is his own fault. German professors and students alike migrate from town to town, as in the Middle Ages, and university appointments are not local, but based solely upon fitness and ability. The medical Faculty of Berlin is made up of outsiders. When the student has passed his university and state examinations, he may practise or, if he has distinguished himself by original research, become a Privatdocent, with the *venia legendi* or right to teach on his own account, from which status he may, if he builds up his reputation, rise through the various grades of professorship. Conditions like these make for original research and, given the university origins of German medicine, it seems natural that the very idea of scientific laboratories, of hygienic or psychiatric institutes, should have originated in Germany. Add to this the sharply drawn distinctions between *Wehrstand*, *Lehrstand*, and *Nährstand*, and the singular fitness of the race for classifying and coördinating knowledge. The faults of the German system are mainly along practical lines and are summed up in the phrase "survival of the fittest." The nurses, as in France, are of poor quality, but there is no dearth of clinical material, only difficulty in making it available for large bodies of students, who are usually taught, not in the wards, but in the amphitheater. "The dullest rustic," says Flexner, "has long since grasped the idea that the professor is chosen for his skill and learning." The hospitals are full of patients, but to get in close touch with them, one must be either a *Hospitant* (Famulus) or a *Praktikant*, and the former has the advantage. The *Hospitant* can follow his chiefs through the wards and examine patients, but otherwise, as a professor's fag, engaged in recording cases, examining urine, preparing slides, and other things which Sir Clifford Allbutt designates as "merely clerks' work," his opportunities are not overwhelmingly sought for by German students. The *Praktikant* is "a non-resident interne of vague status,"[2] abruptly chosen from his class and pitchforked into the clinical arena, where, as a raw student, his ignorance is thrown into the lime-

---

[1] A. Flexner: Medical Education, New York, 1925, 19–58, *passim*.
[2] Flexner: *Ibid.*, 163.

light, and his chief has little time to correct his fumbling. He must sink or swim on his own merits, and his inexperience sets off the brilliant summaries of the chief, much as pretty women enhance the impression of their beauty by association with ugly women. The German professor, a high priest of his science and its teaching, his brain stored with classified knowledge, is liable to acquire a heaviness of mind which may degenerate into top-heaviness. His autocratic position may sometimes be manifested as a "stiff *Vornehmheit*," an unpleasantly impersonal manner toward pupils or patients,[1] which is in odd contrast with the easy informality of the best modern English, French, and American traditions. The advantages of modern French and English clinical teaching are precisely in the latter direction. The relations between teacher and pupil, professor and patient, are less official and formal, and the ideal is, in Huxley's phrase, to make the greatest possible number fit to survive. Parisian patients are even said to contribute much to the success of clinical instruction by their quick, intelligent replies.[2] In Paris, the hospitals, being public charities, are thrown open to students everywhere, and the whole aim of French teaching is bedside instruction. Ward teaching is cleverly exploited by means of *stagiaires* or student assistants, of whom each professor has to train a large number, and to whom two or three beas each are allotted for self-instruction. Stagiaires, externes and internes, are quizzed, in succession, by a running fire of questions from the chief, as he considers each case, and, so informal is procedure that it is no discourtesy for even an outsider to ask pertinent questions.[3] The student is put into the hospital wards directly upon matriculation and continues clinical work in the different specialties until he graduates, when he must write and publish a thesis. It is then open to him to compete for the position of *agrégé* or assistant professor by means of the *concours* or public examination. *Agrégés* are now chosen from lists of eligibles who have passed the examinations, but the system is exposed to the evils of favoritism, and often excludes the right man; the position is not as valuable as a hospital appointment (Flexner). The French graduating theses differ from the German or Russian in that, as a rule, they are exceedingly clever and well-written *résumés* of what is known rather than records of original work. They are invaluable for reference. As with the French, the strong point of English medical teaching is clinical instruction. Emerson said of the English that "theirs is a logic that brings salt to soup, hammer to nail, oar to boat," and, neces-

---

[1] This may be regarded as of little moment, since the general testimony is in accordance with Flexner's view that, all things considered, patients and pupils are very fairly treated in Germany.

[2] Flexner: *Op. cit.* (1912), 229–230.

[3] Flexner: *Op. cit.* (1912), 229–230. On November 21, 1822, the Paris Medical Faculty was suppressed by royal mandate on account of a noisy political *chahut* among the students, who stampeded an oration of Desgenettes; to be resumed in March, 1823, with an entirely new faculty. P. Menetrier: Bull. Soc. franç. d'hist. de méd., Paris, 1922, xii, 440–445.

sarily, the physician to the bedside. The English hospitals are not, as with the Germans and French, governmental institutions or public charities, but are supported by voluntary contributions, and, with the exception of Oxford, where medical teaching is academic, and Cambridge, where it is confined to the fundamental sciences, the English type of instruction is that of the hospital medical school. Here, the student is given the same clinical advantages as obtain in Paris, the nursing system is the finest in the world, but the institutions not being connected with universities, little opportunity for post-graduate or other instruction for outsiders has been afforded until recently.[1] Of the English clinical teacher, Flexner says, "No matter who or how many attend his lectures, his pupils are specifically those with whom he talks at the bedside." These make their rounds daily with the house physician, rendering complete case histories with microscopic findings. All are put through their paces twice weekly, in a rigorous but urbane, informal spirit, by the senior physician. The same thing obtains at the final examination, which is a severely practical grilling, although the bearing of the examiners is said to be "informal, sympathetic, and easy, even to the point of joining in tea with the onlookers who happen to be present when that national function becomes due."[2]

In modern teaching of the fundamental sciences, the principal drawback has been the didactic or expository lecture. In anatomy, this vogue was started by the 18th century men, the so-called "surgeon-anatomists," and particularly by the Monros at Edinburgh, of whom the "evergreen *tertius*," up to 1846, "unconcernedly at noon ate cranberry tarts in the midst of grinning students at a small pastry cook's, and with digestion unimpaired the next hour read his grandfather's essays on hydrophobia as part of an anatomical course."[3] Honest John Bell, tilting vainly against these ineptitudes of "the windy and wordy school," pointed out that "in Dr. Monro's class, unless there be a fortunate succession of bloody murders, not three subjects are dissected in the year," while "nerves and arteries which the surgeon has to dissect at the peril of his patient's life" were demonstrated an a subject fished up from the bottom of a tub of spirits and exhibited at a distance of a hundred feet.[4] Robert Knox describes the anatomical teaching in London during 1810–25 as the crudest conceivable: "There were in the metropolis but two great schools. In one of these the course began with hernia and the fasciæ and ended with hernia and the fasciæ. The lecturer read the descriptions of the muscles from Fyfe's wretched work. At the other a man of high genius (Abernethy), affecting to despise descriptive anatomy, which his natural indolence and the spirit of his age and country prevented him mastering, talked of the abdominal muscles as so many steaks, which he buffoon-like tossed over each other, when dissected, counting them as steak first, steak second, steak third, muscles and tendons which the first of descriptive anatomists have failed clearly to describe."[5] But even after Bichat, Bell and Knox, and the Warburton act of 1832, anatomy was still treated as the handmaid of surgery (or of the fine arts) until the modern Germans—Henle, Gegenbaur, Waldeyer—correlated it with histology, morphology, and embryology. The dingy, ill-lighted malodorous dissecting room, where, as Flexner says, "eight or ten inexpert boys hack away at a cadaver until it is reduced to shreds," still survives in some localities in the United States.

---

[1] Flexner, in his superlative book on "Medical Education," accounts for these developments.

[2] Flexner: *Op. cit.* (1912), 188–205, 282.

[3] Lonsdale: Cited by Stirling (Some Apostles of Physiology, London, 1902, 119).

[4] John Bell: Letters on Professional Character and Manners, Edinburgh, 1810, cited by Flexner.

[5] R. Knox: Lancet, Lond., 1854, ii, 393.

The anatomical laboratory or institute, such as the Clover-Leaf Hall at Munich, with 500 students dissecting at once under the eye of the professor, or Mall's series of separate rooms at the Johns Hopkins, or Harvard, with its extensive cold-storage plants, is an innovation of recent date. Dearth of material and too many students are the great handicaps, and, even in Germany, Flexner argues, the most scientific lecturing will never compensate for insufficient experience in dissecting. In England, where the utilitarian view has prevailed, it is significant that there have been no great anatomists since the time of Sir Charles Bell. Horner, Holmes, Harrison Allen, Leidy and Dwight were able teachers in America, but the modern scientific methods were introduced by Minot at Harvard and by Mall at the Johns Hopkins. Mall isolated his students in separate rooms and did away entirely with descriptive lectures.[1] Edmond Souchon (1842–1924) who did much for anatomical teaching at New Orleans, founded a unique museum for didactic purposes at Tulane University. France has had no physiologists of the first rank since Claude Bernard, unless we regard Pasteur as an example. In England, Foster at Cambridge and Burdon Sanderson at Oxford, both pupils of Sharpey, set the pace in physiological teaching. In America advanced instruction began when Bowditch opened the first physiological laboratory at Harvard in 1871 and Huxley brought Newell Martin to the Johns Hopkins (1876). The traditions were ably kept up by Porter in Boston, Howell in Baltimore, and others. German physiological teaching, the highest development of the century, grew out of the great laboratories of Johannes Müller at Berlin, Ludwig at Leipzig and Voit at Munich, but, even in Germany, it is urged that there is too much elaborated lecturing and too little laboratory work (Flexner). The laboratory founded at Turin under S. Berruti in 1851 was a center of great activity under Jacob Moleschott (1861–79) and Angelo Mosso (1888–93). In 1894, Mosso acquired a handsome new building. Hydrophysiology received a great impetus at the Naples Zoölogical Station, founded by Anton Dohrn in 1871. In pathology, all Europe sat at the feet of Virchow and his pupils, of whom Cohnheim was the teacher of Welch, who with Prudden, brought experimental pathology and bacteriology to America. Welch established a research laboratory at the Johns Hopkins in 1884. The first university chair of pathology was that held by Lobstein at Strassburg (1819), while in Vienna, Biermayer was made professor extraordinarius (1821), to be followed by Johannes Wagner (1830) and Rokitansky (professor ordinarius 1844). Meanwhile, Cruveilhier had been appointed to the first chair in the Paris Faculty (1836) and Virchow became professor ordinarius at Würzburg (1849) and Berlin (1856). The French indifference to pathology is shown by the fact that two neurologists, Charcot and Marie, held the chair for years, the former succeeding Vulpian in 1872. Marie was appointed to Victor Cornil's chair, "very much," as Osler puts it, "as if Allan Starr or Dana were selected as successor to Prudden." Bacteriology has been best taught in France at the Pasteur Institute and its branches; in Germany, at the institutes of Koch, Ehrlich, von Behring and others; in Belgium, by Bordet; in America, by Welch, Simon Flexner, Vaughan, Novy, Abbott, Ernst and others. "Bacteriology," says Flexner, "transformed hygiene from an empirical art into an experimental science," and the teaching of the two has gone hand in hand since the foundation of Koch's Institute. Experimental pharmacology was first taught by Magendie in France and by Buchheim, Traube, and Schmiedeberg in Germany. Brunton, Ringer, Langley and Cushny in London, Fraser in Edinburgh, respresent the height of English teaching. H. C. Wood founded clinical pharmacology in America and taught therapeutics by means of charades. Cushny at Ann Arbor, and Abel at the Johns Hopkins introduced the modern German methods. The medicinal plant-garden of the College of Pharmacy of the University of Minnesota (Minneapolis) was started in 1910–11, and was followed by similar gardens at the Universities of Wisconsin (Madison), Michigan (Ann Arbor), Nebraska (Lincoln) and Washington (Seattle). In 1781, John Hunter found himself unable to answer a simple, important question put to him by a judge in a poisoning case. Impressed by this and other shortcomings of medical evidence in criminal trials, Andrew Duncan, Sr., memorialized the patrons of the University of Edinburgh and even approached the Crown authorities in aid of founding a chair of forensic medicine. Through his repeated efforts, the Edinburgh chair, the first in Great Britain, was instituted by the Crown in 1806. Germany had preceded this record by some fifty years. Louis gave

---

[1] For a full account of the status of anatomy and its teaching in America, see C. R. Bardeen, Bull. Univ. Wisconsin, Madison, 1905 (No. 115), scient. ser. iii, No. 4, 85–208.

voluntary lectures in Paris before the Revolution, and a chair was subsequently founded at the École de santé (1794). Stringham began to give voluntary lectures at the College of Physicians and Surgeons of New York and was appointed professor in 1813. Romeyn Beck acquired a chair in the Western Medical College in 1815. The example was followed by other schools. By 1832–33 every medical school in Great Britain had lectures on forensic medicine. Attendance was irregular. Christison's class in 1822 consisted mainly of law students. Edinburgh made it a compulsory subject in 1833, and separate examinations were required by London University in 1863. None are required in Germany and Austria.[1] Legal medicine is now best taught at Vienna, where all judicial autopsies, coroner's cases, and anything medical connected with court-room procedure, are under control of the university professor; in Paris and Lyons, in connection with the admirable service of the Prefecture of Police; and at Edinburgh, where the professor is also police surgeon. It is ably argued by Flexner that the most scientific lecturing in all the subjects mentioned will be imperfectly assimilated if the student has not received proper preliminary instruction in physics, chemistry, and general biology. In clinical medicine, not even the splendid lectures of a Charcot or a Friedrich Müller can take the place of bedside teaching, which it is one of the chief merits of English medicine to have consistently followed.

Schools of tropical medicine were established at London (1899), Liverpool (1899), Hamburg (1900), and Brussels (1906), an Imperial Bacteriological Laboratory at Muktesar (1895), a Plague Research Laboratory at Bombay (1896), Pasteur Institute Laboratories at Kasauli (1900) and Guindy, Madras (1905), also a Sleeping Sickness Bureau (1908) and an Indian Research Fund (1911).

In 1916, a School of Hygiene and Public Health was established (by endowment of the Rockefeller Foundation) at the Johns Hopkins University, under the directorship of William H. Welch (1916–26) and William H. Howell (1926). It coöperates with the schools of medicine and engineering.

America, beginning with Elizabeth Blackwell's graduation in 1849, was the pioneer in **medical education for women.** In the United States and Canada, women can now study medicine anywhere on the same terms as men.

The Woman's Medical College of Pennsylvania (Philadelphia) was organized in 1850, and the Woman's Medical College of Baltimore in 1882. The earliest lady graduates after Elizabeth Blackwell were Sarah Adamson Dolly (1849), Emma Blackwell (1850), Ann Preston (1850), Marie Zakrzewska (1850) and Mary Putnam Jacobi (1870). The English Medical Register of 1858 contains the name of a single lady graduate of Geneva, and a second was examined and qualified in 1865. The first Swiss lady graduate was Marie Heim-Vögtlin (1845–1916). In 1874, the London School of Medicine for Women was opened with fourteen students; and, in 1896, they acquired the privilege of resident posts at the Royal Free Hospital. In the same year, the Royal College of Physicians in Ireland and the London University admitted them to the privilege of examination. No other London hospital schools are open to women, but the universities of Durham, Manchester, Liverpool, Birmingham, Leeds, and Bristol are co-educational. At Glasgow, Aberdeen, Dundee, and St. Andrew's they are given every facility, but there has been much opposition in Edinburgh. On the continent, the Swiss universities took the lead in 1876, the German states followed, one by one, Prussia being the last to throw open the right of university instruction and graduation to women in 1908. Dorothea Christiana Erxleven was the first woman to receive a medical degree in Germany (Halle, 1754). In Holland, Aletta Jacobs was the first women to study medicine. She passed her state examination in 1878. A medical degree was given to Catherine van Tussenbroek in the same year. Paris, Vienna, Rome, Brussels, Upsala, and Copenhagen are now all co-educational. The faculties of Paris and Bern are the most frequented. Crowds of enthusiastic young Russian Jewesses flock to the latter, and turn out huge annual batches of inaugural dissertations. The number of women graduates who get into practice is said to be relatively small, probably by reason of marriage.

---

[1] H. Littlejohn: Tr. Med.-Leg. Soc., Lond., 1914–15, xii, 3–6.

Of the many admirable **hospitals** constructed in the modern period, the pavilion system attained a high plane of development in the Johns Hopkins Hospital, planned by J. S. Billings and opened in 1889, and the Hamburg-Eppendorf pavilion, opened in the same year. In hygienic advantages and economy of administration, these structures marked a great advance upon the huge, many-storied buildings (block hospitals) of the past. The Peter Bent Brigham Hospital at Boston (1913), also originally planned by Billings, follows the same idea. With the opening of the Rudolf Virchow Hospital at Berlin (1906) a new idea was introduced, that of a community of separate pavilions as detached hospital units, and upon this plan are based such hospitals as the new Allgemeines Krankenhaus at Vienna, the Toronto General Hospital, the Barnes Hospital (St. Louis), and the Cincinnati General Hospital. Latterly, the tendency, even in Germany, has been away from extreme decentralization and toward a compromise between the pavilion and block systems, the advantage being greater economy in space, excavation, piping and plumbing, also economy and centralization of administration. Examples are to be found in the New Cook County Hospital (Chicago), the Henry Phipps Psychiatric and Brady Urologic Clinics (Baltimore) and the new buildings of Bellevue (New York). In noting the more recent move away from hospitals of the dispersed unit type toward concentrated buildings of the skyscraper type, Goldwater points out that they are an inevitable feature of our overcrowded larger cities and that whatever errors in planning and construction they (or any other hospitals) may have are a necessary outcome of the conditions, financial or local, under which they were produced. The last fifty years have been called the "dark age in hospital planning." Due to the high cost of hospital construction and dearth of available ground to build upon, the ideal has become that of the hotel or office building and the economic slogan of building committees—"deal with public charity as a private business," is bad for administration and social service. The wards tend to become smaller and darker as to cubic air-space and light, the hermetic corridors are non-ventilated, as also the nurses' station, or the laundry and x-ray room in the cellar, while the anesthesia and recovery rooms are as "gloomy inside as the fourth circle in Dante's Inferno" (Goldwater). The tendency to shoot up into the air, as in the Allegheny General Hospital (Pittsburgh) or the structures of the New York Medical Center (1928) is inevitable in our overcrowded American cities.[1] In 1927, there were 6946 hospitals (859,445 beds) in the United States, or 50 more (22,869 beds) than in 1926; 248 (20,894 beds) in the United States Possessions, and 458 (62,500 beds) in Canada.

The first **children's hospitals** to be established in this country were the Child's Hospital and Nursery in New York (1854) and the Children's Hospital of Philadelphia (1855).

Some 37 **institutions for the blind** were established in Great Britain between

---

[1] S. S. Goldwater: Mod. Hospital, Chicago, 1927, xxviii, 49–52.

1791 and 1897. The Berners Street workshop, started by Miss Gilbert, the blind daughter of the Bishop of Chichester, set a model which has been widely copied. Following the example of France and England, asylums for the blind were established at Vienna (1804) by W. Klein, Berlin (1806), Amsterdam, Prague and Dresden in 1808, and there are now more than 150 on the continent, mostly governmental. The first American school for the blind was the Perkins Institution, founded at Boston by John D. Fisher in 1829, under state aid. Here Samuel G. Howe, who also founded the first American school for the feeble-minded (1848) became director (1831) and educated Laura Bridgman. Institutions for the blind were established in New York (1831), Philadelphia (1833), Columbus, Ohio (1837), Staunton, Virginia (1839), and now every state in the Union makes provision for this purpose. **Schools for the deaf** were established at Edinburgh (1810), Glasgow (1819), and elsewhere. There are now over 99 in Germany, 95 in Great Britain, 71 in France, 47 in Italy, 38 in Austro-Hungary, 34 in Russia, and 126 in the United States. The American movement began with the investigations of Thomas Hopkins Gallaudet in Europe (1815), and the foundation of the Connecticut Asylum (1816). The Columbia Institution (Washington, D. C.) was founded by Congress in 1857, under the direction of Edward M. Gallaudet. The *American Annals of the Deaf and Dumb* (1847) was started by Edward Allan Fay, author of *Marriages of the Deaf in America* (1898), and the histories of the American schools (1893). The Volta Bureau (Washington, D. C.) was founded in 1890 by Alexander Graham Bell.

The introduction of outdoor life and **open-air sanitaria for phthisical patients** is a feature of modern medicine. Open-air treatment existed in Scotland about 1747 and a seaside hospital for scrofula was opened at Margate in 1791. George **Bodington** (1799–1882), of Sutton Colfield, England, in his *Essay on the Treatment of Pulmonary Consumption* (1840) anticipated many modern views as to the advantages of cold dry air for "healing and closing of cavities and ulcers of the lungs," as also of exercise in the open and abundant nutrition; but his theory was so roughly handled by the medical critics of his day that he was discouraged from carrying it into practice to any extent. The first sanitarium for phthisical patients was established at Görbersdorf, in the Waldenburg Mountains, by Hermann **Brehmer** (1826–99), in 1859. It still exists, and its success has led to the foundation of many similar institutions in mountain and winter resorts, notably those of Carl **Spengler** at Davos and Edward Livingstone **Trudeau** (1848–1915) at Saranac Lake in the Adirondacks. In 1876, Peter **Dettweiler** (1837–1904) founded the sanitarium at Falkenstein in the Taunus, introducing the reclining chair for rest cure in the open air, portable receptacles for sputa, and other novelties. By 1886, England had 19 hospitals for consumptives. The sanitarium movement in Germany was especially fostered by Ernst **von Leyden** and there are now thousands of such institutions all over the world. Apart from mountain and winter resorts, like Asheville or Sankt Moritz, the climatic treatment includes the arid and semi-tropical, like Arizona or Yalta (Crimea), and the maritime, like the Riviera and Algiers. The seashore sanitaria also include those for scrofula, with which the coast-lines of countries like Italy and Norway are dotted.

The first International Congress for tuberculosis was held July 25–31, 1888, at Paris, and, after the sixth (1901), an International Association was formed, which hold annual "conferences" in different cities (1902–13, resumed 1921), to prepare for triennial international congresses. Of these, three were held before the war at Paris

(1905), Washington (1908), and Rome (1911). A French society of similar title exists in Paris, and publishes a *Revue*. Since the gift of the Phipps Institute in 1903, the subject has awakened keen interest in America, especially through the labors of Trudeau, Vincent Y. Bowditch, L. F. Flick, Arnold Klebs, S. Adolphus Knopf, Henry Barton Jacobs, George Ensign Bushnell (1853–1924), Frank Billings, Edward R. Baldwin, Lawrason Brown, Theodore Bernard Sachs (1868–1916), and others.

The **nursing** of the sick at the hands of trained, well-bred women is an institution of modern times. The period from the latter part of the 17th century up to the middle of the 19th was the "dark age" of sick nursing, in which the status and competence of female attendants had sunk as low as the hospitals in which they served. Outside the Roman Catholic orders, in which discipline and decency still prevailed, this was almost universally the case. The pudgy, slatternly, dowdy-looking female, of drunken and dubious habits, was the type, from the old colored prints to the time of Sairey Gamp. In 1857, the servant nurses in the larger London hospitals were referred to in the *Times* as follows:

"Lectured by Committees, preached at by chaplains, scowled on by treasurers and stewards, scolded by matrons, sworn at by surgeons, bullied by dressers, grumbled at and abused by patients, insulted if old and ill-favored, talked flippantly to, if middle-aged and good-humoured, tempted and seduced if young and well-looking —they are what any woman might be under the same circumstances."[1]

The idea of training nurses to attend the sick in a special school for the purpose originated with Theodor **Fliedner** (1800–64), pastor at Kaiserswerth on the Rhine, and his wife Friederike, who, in 1833, turned the garden-house of their pastorate into an asylum for discharged female prisoners, and in October, 1836, founded the first school for deaconesses (*Diaconissenanstalt*), which became the model for similar institutions in Germany and elsewhere. To the Fliedners came, in 1840, Elizabeth Fry, famous for her extension of John Howard's work in sanitating prisons, and later **Florence Nightingale** (1823–1910), an English lady, born at Florence, Italy, who devoted her whole life to sick nursing and, indeed, made it the model institution which it is in English-speaking countries today. When the Crimean War broke out in March, 1854, Miss Nightingale, at the instance of Lord Sidney Herbert, then Secretary of War, went out with a body of nurses to take charge of the barrack hospital at Scutari, where her ministrations and reforms soon became a matter of history. In the face of the indifference of public officials and the opposition of narrow bureaucrats, she received the loyal support of Lord Raglan and the hardworking army surgeons, and, within ten days, was feeding nearly 1000 men from her diet kitchen. In three months, she was providing 10,000 men with clothes and other necessities from her own supplies. The effect of her unexampled success was such that after her return to England a sum of £50,000—the Nightingale Fund—was raised to establish a school for

---

[1] London Times, April 15, 1857. Cited by Nutting and Dock, History of Nursing, New York, 1907, i, 505.

nurses at St. Thomas' Hospital, which was opened on June 15, 1860, with fifteen probationers, who were scientifically trained as "new style nurses." These soon filled up vacancies in the larger hospitals, which brought about a wholesale regeneration of English nursing. Nightingale nurses were sought for everywhere. On the panels of the diplomas of the British College of Nurses are inscribed, along with Fry and Nightingale, the names of such famous English nurses as Ethel Fenwick, Rebecca Strong, Margaret Huxley, Agnes Jones, Margaret Breay and Isla Stuart.

The adoption of the Geneva Convention (1864) created the necessity for better nursing on the continent: and, in America, the movement was especially furthered by Elizabeth Blackwell and Marie Zakrzewska, who founded the first training-school for nurses in the United States (1873). Elizabeth Blackwell (1821–1910), of Bristol, England, the first lady medical graduate in England (1849), Clara Barton (1821–1912), of Oxford, Massachusetts, and Louisa Lee Schuyler (1837–1926), who founded the Bellevue School for Nurses (1873) were instrumental in organizing sick nursing and medical aid during the Civil War. The Connecticut Training School for Nurses, now part of Yale University, was founded by Francis Bacon (1832–1921) and others (October 1, 1873). During the Spanish-American War, army nursing was organized by Anita Newcomb McGee; and during the European War by Dora E. Thompson, Jane B. Delano (1862–1919) and Julia Stimpson. By the Act of March 3, 1919, Congress attached nursing services to five branches of the Government, viz., the Army, Navy, Public Health Service, Veteran's Bureau, and Indian Bureau. In 1873, three training-schools were established at the Bellevue, New Haven, and Massachusetts General Hospitals, and the Johns Hopkins Training-School for Nurses was superintended by Miss M. Adelaide Nutting, who, with Miss Lavinia L. Dock, wrote a *History of Nursing* (1907).

Miss Nightingale's *Notes on Hospitals* (1859) and *Notes on Nursing* (1860) are true medical classics, distinguished by the rarest common sense and simplicity of statement. She defined nursing as "helping the patient to live," introduced the modern standards of training and *esprit de corps*, and early grasped the idea that diseases are not "separate entities, which must exist, like cats and dogs," but altered conditions, qualitative disturbances of normal physiological processes, through which the patient is passing. While she did not know the bacterial theory of infectious diseases, she realized that absolute cleanliness, fresh air, pure water, light and efficient drainage are the surest means of preventing them.

Since the time of Pinel and Reil, Tuke and Conolly, the proper study and **care of the insane** has been an object of ambition, often dimly realized. When Esquirol succeeded Pinel at the Salpêtrière, in 1810, he made great reforms in housing and regimen, traveled all over France to carry out Pinel's ideas, founded ten new asylums and was the first to lecture on psychiatry (1817). Gardner Hill introduced the idea of "no restraint" at Lincoln Asylum, England (1836) and, in 1839, in the face of bitter opposition, John Conolly discarded all mechanical restraints at the Hanwell Asylum. The abuses attending the commitment and care of the insane in private asylums were vigorously attacked by Charles Reade in *Hard Cash* (1863).

Early American institutions were the State Hospital at Williamsburg, Va. (1773), the Bloomingdale Asylum, New York (1809), now at White Plains (1821), the Friends Asylum, at Frankford, outside Philadelphia (1817), the McLean Hospital, Boston (1818), the Hospitals at Columbia, South Carolina (1828), and Worcester, Mass. (1833), the Hartford and Brattleboro Retreats (1836–38), and the New Jersey State Asylum at Trenton (1848). The last was established through the propagandism of Miss Dorothea Lynde Dix, of Maine, whose work in ameliorating the condition of the insane in America, and even in Great Britain, is similar to John Howard's prison and hospital reforms. She is said to have been instrumental in founding no less than 32 asylums. With the opening of the Utica State Hospital in 1843, began what Hurd calls "the era of awakening,"[1] and by 1850 the movement for State provision for the insane was well on its way. The State asylums at Willard (1869) and Binghamton, New York (1881), were founded to set off the barbarities in the treatment of the chronic insane in county asylums. The largest American hospitals are those at Binghamton and Washington, D. C. Pliny Earle, in 1867, emphasized the importance of suitable employment for the insane. In 1885, Daniel Hack Tuke made a sweeping attack on American and Canadian asylums, and in 1894,[2] Weir Mitchell pointed out the deficiencies in the proper care and treatment of the insane, discussed the general "woodenness" of boards, the evils of political control, and indicated the absolute lack of any scientific study of insanity in American hospitals. The latter idea originated with the Germans. The very first article which Griesinger penned for his *Archiv* (1868[3]) proposed a reorganization of the German hospitals and outlined the idea of a psychiatric clinic, where the patients should be studied and treated, as in hospital, before commitment or discharge. In Berlin, Ideler had demonstrated cases at the Charité in 1832, to be followed by Griesinger (1866), Westphal (1869), and Jolly (1890). Psychiatric clinics were opened at Strassburg (1872), Basel (1876), Breslau (1877), Bonn (1882), Freiburg (1887), Halle (1891), and elsewhere, the movement culminating in the fine institution opened by Kraepelin at Munich November 7, 1904. On April 16, 1913, the Psychiatric Clinic, donated to the Johns Hopkins University by Henry Phipps, and modeled along the German lines, was opened at Baltimore under the direction of Professor Adolf Meyer. Kraepelin's new Institute was opened on June 13 1928.

The first attempt at the **training of idiots** was made by the celebrated otologist J.-M. G. Itard in 1800 upon a wild boy found in a forest in central France, and known as the "savage of Aveyron." Subsequent efforts made by Ferret at Bicêtre (1828) and Falret at the Salpêtrière (1831) proved futile. Success was at length attained by Edouard Séguin, a pupil of Itard and Esquirol, during 1837–48. He was made instructor at Bicêtre (1842) and in 1844, the Academy of Sciences reported favorably upon his ideas. Returning to America, he established schools in several states, after which his methods, summarized in his treatise on idiocy (1846), were taken up all over the country. Subsequent work by Guggenbühl on cretins (1842), by Saegert in Berlin (1842) and elsewhere, was equally successful, and later the subject became a matter of legislation.

In the development of national and international regulation of **public hygiene,** necessity has been the mother of invention. There was nothing spontaneous about the movement. It was simply forced upon the attention of legislators by the modern outbreaks of epidemic disease and by the evils resulting from poverty, shiftlessness, overcrowding, industrial conditions and migration of people from place to place. Its developments have been slow. The first big scare came from the invasion of Asiatic cholera (1826–37), which had been endemic in India for centuries, was pandemic in Asia during 1816–30, had spread over Russia by 1830, skirted Northeastern Germany in 1831, reaching England in June of the same year, and Calais, March, 1832, and invaded America *via* Quebec and New York. Heinrich Heine has left a graphic and memorable account of its outbreak in Paris. On March

---

[1] H. M. Hurd: The Institutional Care of the Insane, Baltimore, 1916.

[2] Mitchell: Proc. Am. Med.-Psychol. Ass., 1894, Utica, N. Y., 1895, i, 101–121.

[3] W. Griesinger: Arch. f. Psychiat., Berl., 1868–69, i, 8–43.

29th, the night of *mi-carême*, a masked ball was in progress, the *chahut* in full swing. Suddenly, the gayest of the harlequins collapsed, cold in the limbs, and, underneath his mask, "violet-blue" in the face. Laughter died out, dancing ceased, and in a short while carriage-loads of people were hurried from the *redoute* to the Hôtel Dieu to die, and, to prevent a panic among the patients, were thrust into rude graves in their dominoes. Soon the public halls were filled with dead bodies, sewed in sacks for want of coffins. Long lines of hearses stood *en queue* outside Père Lachaise. Everybody wore flannel bandages. The rich gathered up their belongings and fled the town. Over 120,000 passports were issued at the Hôtel de Ville. A *guillotine ambulante* was stalking abroad, and its effect upon the excitable Parisians reduplicated the scenes of the Revolution or of the plague at Milan. With signal intelligence, Heine puts his finger upon the chief obstacle which public health movements have ever encountered, viz., the dread of disturbing private business. In this case, an *émeute*, with barricades, was stirred up among the rag-pickers, who resented the removal from the streets of the piles of offal from which they derived their livelihood. The suspicion of secret poisoning was raised, as a counter-theory to that of infection, the cry *"à la lanterne"* was heard, and six persons were murdered and naked corpses dragged through the streets, under this belief. Finally the public press quieted the panic, and the *Commission sanitaire* was able to accomplish something.[1] On September 1 and 2, 1858, the Quarantine Station on Staten Island, New York, was attacked and destroyed by deliberate action of citizens, who had been tormented for fifty years with devastating yellow fever epidemics, attributed to its lax administration and this "act of salutary and well-intentioned violence" was sustained by the local court.[2] Similar panics, such as the shot-gun quarantines at the South during yellow fever, with the lugubrious "Bring out your dead!" emphasized the necessity of enlightened organized control of public health.

Cholera was again pandemic in 1840–50, 1852–60, 1863–73, and at later intervals in Europe. It is still wide-spread in the Far East. **Influenza** was epidemic at intervals during 1800–81 and pandemic in 1830–33, 1836–37, 1847–48, 1889–90 and 1918–19. Visitations of 1800–1803 were of cerebral or nervous type. The Parisian invasion of 1829 was preceded by acrodynia (1827–29); while epidemics of 1836–37 and 1841–45 (gastro-intestinal modality) were accompanied by infantile poliomyelitis, and by such modes of myoclonic encephalitis as Dubini's electric chorea (1846). The great wave of 1847–48 was mainly catarrhal, the lesser waves (1851–57) nervous; that of 1866–67 was followed by poliomyelitis in Norway (Ruhräh); that of 1873–75 was preceded by poliomyelitis in Philadelphia (1871–74) and followed by the first epidemic of poliomyelitis in France (1875); that of 1889–90 was preceded by poliomyelitis in Sweden (Medin, 1887), and followed by the nona of Lombardy and Hungary, identified by Netter (1918) with the lethargic encephalitis, and preceding the great pandemic of 1918–19 (Economo, 1917). The epidemic of 1918–19 was probably transmitted from China (March, 1918) by Indo-Chinese troops landing in France (Zinsser) and was notable for rheumatic or dengue-like manifestations followed by fatal pneumonias and empyemas, frontal and maxillary sinus infections and en-

---

[1] Heine: Französische Zustände, letter of April 9, 1832 (Sämmtliche Werke, Cotta ed., Leipzig, xi, 88–102).

[2] F. H. Garrison: Bull. New York Acad. Med., 1926, 2. s., ii, 1–5.

cephalitis. Nervous manifestations were early noted by Zeviani (1800–1803), Peyton Blakiston (1837), Graves (1837), Broussais (1837) and Dunglison (1848), while Peacock stressed the pulmonary and gastro-intestinal modalities (1848). But for a century, the main trend of opinion was in favor of the classical catarrhal fever standardized by Saillant (1780) and clinically delimited in 1896[1] by Otto Leichtenstern (1845–1900). The recent view of influenza as a disease of protean modalities is largely the work of the English school of epidemiologists. **Cerebrospinal fever** appeared periodically at the intervals 1805–30, 1837–50, 1854–74 and 1875 to the present time; yellow fever in the Southern States in 1853, 1867, 1873, 1878, and 1897–99. **Typhus fever** was rife during the Napoleonic wars and smote Ireland severely in 1817, 1819, and 1846. Typhoid, scarlatina, measles, and other infections appeared at intervals. Bubonic **plague** was spread from Hong Kong all over the world from 1894 on, and without modern sanitation, the pandemic would probably have attained to medieval proportions. Politics came near wrecking the situation in San Francisco in 1907–8, and it was only through the Marine Hospital Service experts, who diagnosed the disease and destroyed the rodent carriers, that the city, perhaps the country, was saved. This was the first time that a city was made rat-proof. The epidemic character of poliomyelitis was first noted by Medin in Sweden (1887), and its incidence in the Scandinavian countries, Austria, and the United States (1907–10) has been severe. Its pathology was ably investigated by Simon Flexner, who isolated a germ in 1913.

In 1762, a sanitary council had been established in every Prussian province, but it was not until the second pandemic of cholera (1840–59) that France and England began to wake up to the task of organizing public health. In 1840, a national organization of *Conseils d'hygiène* for the cities, with special committees for the provinces, was formed in France, the essence of which still survives. The English code of sanitary legislation, in some respects, the best and most progressive in the modern world, had its origins in the definite and determined reaction which set in, early in the 19th century, against the pernicious *laissez faire, laisser aller* doctrines of Adam Smith, Malthus, James Mill, and other professors of the "dismal science." About 1765, such inventions as the spinning jenny created a large industrial class, recruited from the rural districts of England, Scotland, and Ireland. Following the French Revolution and furthered by the developments of mechanic arts and machinery, a huge manufacturing class arose, with an industrial proletariat as its vassals. This, with steam transportation, caused rapid urbanization, so that by 1851, about half, and by 1911, three-fourths of the population of England and Wales were huddled in towns, and thus exposed to the evils of overcrowding, poverty and bad sanitation. In relation to famine and epidemic diseases, Edmund Burke (1795), advocated masterly inactivity, *i. e.*, "a wise and salutary neglect" on the part of government (Creighton). The Cobden-Manchester school of manufacturers, so despised by Carlyle, maintained that the public and the government have no right to interfere with business enterprises, and were even supported by Nassau, sr., and John Bright. Even Humboldt and Stuart Mill maintained that the state should not concern itself with public health and social welfare, except in so far as these are jeopardized by individual action. In consequence, poverty, prostitution, disease and mortality rates increased apace. Children, indentured as apprentices, were practically

---

[1] O. Leichtenstern: Influenza und Dengue, Wien, 1896.

sold into slavery and subjected to shocking cruelty by the hard-fisted taskmasters who exploited them. The foundation of Methodism at Oxford by John and Charles Wesley (1729), John Howard's prison reforms, the efforts of Tuke, Pinel and Reil for humane treatment of the insane, the Abolition Act of 1807, and Romilly's efforts to humanize the penal code (1808), all tended to the development of altruistic sentiment (Morris). Through the humanitarian efforts of such able writers as Charles Dickens, Charles Reade, Mrs. Gaskell (Mary Barton), William Carleton (Irish novels), Thomas Carlyle, Goethe (Mignon) and Victor Hugo (Cosette), it began presently to be perceived that the real wealth of a nation is its population, as Johann Peter Frank had originally maintained; and that the food-fallacy in Malthus lay in the fact that production of food itself depends upon the number, ability and industry of the people producing it, upon material production (including machinery and labor-saving devices), and upon adequate means of transportation, without which, as in the recent war, whole communities may starve with superabundant food near at hand. So potent was Chadwick's propagandism for public health that it became a watchword in the speeches of Beaconsfield, who cleverly substituted *sanitas* for the *vanitas vanitatum* of Ecclesiastes.[1] As Newsholme observes, philanthropy was the motor power in initiating sanitary reform, but the driving power came from the great expense of sanitary Poor-Law administration and actual fear of the ever-recurring epidemics of communicable diseases.[2] The present motto of the Royal Society of Medicine affirms the ancient conviction of Herophilus that life without robust health is useless and valueless: *Non est vivere sed valere vita.*[3]

Early English legislation, such as the Peel Act of 1802, to preserve the "health and morals" of cotton-spinners and factory hands, was directed mainly toward the hygiene of occupations, particularly child labor. The Factory Act of 1833 restricted hours of labor in children and introduced professional inspectors of factories; the Poor-Law Amendment Act, of 1834, placed local relief of poverty under centralized government control, grouped parishes into "unions" for this purpose, and interdicted outdoor relief to able-bodied men. In 1848, Parliament passed the Public Health Act, based upon the startling returns of the Health of Towns Commission (1844) and constituting a General Board of Health, with sanitary inspectors to report upon the health of cities. This was followed by a long line of progressive **legislation**, including the Common Lodging Houses Acts (1851, 1853), the Nuisances Removal Act (1855), the Burial Act (1855), the act of 1858 transferring the powers of the General Board of Health to the Privy Council, the organization of the Local Government Board (1870), the Public Health Act of 1875, the Infectious Diseases (Notification) Acts of 1889 and 1899, the Infectious Diseases (Prevention) Act (1890), the Contagious Diseases (Animals) Act (1891), the Public Health (London) Act (1891), the Isolation Hospitals Act (1893), the Local Government Act of 1894, the Public Health (Ports) Act (1896), the Vaccination Acts of 1898 and 1907, the Rivers Pollution Prevention Act (1898), the Provision of Meals Act for school children's lunches

---

[1] Speech at Aylesbury (1864). At Manchester (April 3, 1872), he said: "After all, the first consideration of a Ministry should be the health of the people."

[2] Sir A. Newsholme: Public Health and Insurance, Baltimore, 1920, i, 70. Sir M. Morris: The Story of English Public Health, London, 1919.

[3] Stendhal's slap at the "strictly business" tendency of Americans of his period (*Et propter vitam vivendi perdere causas*) is apposite here, with reference to the lag in public sanitation before the time of Lemuel Shattuck (1850).

(1902), the Notification of Births Act (1907), the Housing and Town-Planning Act (1909), the National Insurance Act (1911) and the Notification of Births (Extension) Act (1915). The investigations and reforms instituted by Lord Ashley (1833) in regard to child labor, culminating in his famous reports on mines and collieries (1842–43), led to a succession of acts (1844–1912) which have raised the age limit of employment to twelve years. Children were forbidden to work in white lead in 1878, the factory acts of 1864, 1867, 1870 and 1878 were extended to workshops in 1891, a Coal Mines Regulation Act was passed in 1896, Workmen's Compensation Acts in 1897 and 1906, and, in 1901, medical officers of health were required to keep registers of workshops and report upon them annually. Medical inspection and treatment of school children were delegated to the Board of Education in 1907. The delegation of the treatment of disease in paupers to the Poor Law authorities, of disease prevention to the Local Government Board (1871) and of medical inspection of school children to the Board of Education (1907) was contrary to the fundamental principles of sound administration, since it decentralized authority, assigning duties of identical order to different organizations, on the *ad hoc* principle, with consequent overlapping of functions, group competition and obliteration of the true objects of community service and team-work. This was further intensified in the National Insurance Act of 1911, which through a tax levied upon working people, employers and the state, guarantees weekly sickness and maternity benefits, sanatorium treatment in tuberculosis and attendance by a contract physician (panel practice) to about one-third the total population, with no provision for nursing, surgery, hospitalization, special treatment or medical aid other than of ordinary character; although complete medical and sanitary service would have been available to the total population if placed under one central body. On July 1, 1919, the Local Government Board was abolished and sanitary administration was centralized in the Ministry of Health, with Sir Christopher Addison (1869–) as the first minister. He was succeeded by Sir George Newman (1870–). Child labor laws were enacted in Massachusetts (1836, 1842), Connecticut (1842), Maine (1847), Pennsylvania (1848), but there was no industrial dust legislation until the Massachusetts act of 1877 and no provisions for factory inspection prior to those of Massachusetts in 1888. The best pioneer work was done by the U. S. Department of Labor and much was accomplished through the labors of George M. Kober, W. Gilman Thompson, John B. Andrews, Alice Hamilton, J. W. Schereschewsky, S. S. Goldwater, and others. Industrial museums of safety have been established at Berlin (1904), Vienna (1909), New York (1911), and twelve other cities. A traveling exhibit of this kind was set up in Washington in 1915–16. The first clinic for occupational diseases was opened at Milan on March 20, 1910. Another was established at New York by S. S. Goldwater in 1915. Research Institutes for industrial hygiene have been opened at Frankfort on the Main (1910), Pittsburgh, Pa. (1915), and other cities. The *loi Roussel* of December 23, 1874 (France), for the protection of friendless children, was a great advance in humanitarian legislation. In the reforms of prisons, insane asylums and dangerous trades, the effect of the writings of Charles Dickens and Charles Reade should not be forgotten. The speech delivered by Dickens at the anniversary festival of the Hospital for Sick Children, London, on February 9, 1858, is radiant with the genius of humanity, one of the strongest pleas ever made in behalf of social medicine by a man of letters.

The mechanism of **infant welfare** activities, vaguely foreshadowed by Soranus of Ephesus, Aulus Gallius, Oribasius, St. Vincent de Paul and other humanitarians, originated in France, in the foundation of crèches, or day nurseries for the infants of working mothers, by Firmin Marbeau (November 11, 1844), in the two laws for the protection of infants and children (1874, 1889), through the influence of Théophile Roussel (1816–1903), and in the remarkable methods instituted at Villiers-le-Duc by **Morel de Villiers** (1854–63) and his son (1884–1903), in consequence of which the infant mortality of this hamlet was reduced to a stable zero during 1893–1903. These methods were taken up by Benjamin **Broadbent**, major of Huddersfield (England) and applied with success, since 1902, by its medical officer of health, S. G. H. **Moore.** Through the pioneer work of the borough of Huddersfield, the Notification of Births Act was passed (1907). Infant mortality work was then taken up by English public health officials, notably A. K. Chalmers at Glasgow (1906) and J. F. J. Sykes at St. Pancras, culminating in the four epochal reports of Sir Arthur **Newsholme** to the Local Government Board (1910–16), which are the basic texts of infant welfare work. Newsholme maintains that infant mortality is of multiplex causation, to be met by multiple infant welfare activities. To these, the leading pediatrists of England and other countries have devoted their best efforts. In 1912, the Children's Bureau was established at Washington by the government, under the direction of Miss Julia C. Lathrop. Infant welfare activities in America have been largely furthered by women, notably Dr. S. Josephine Baker (New York), Mrs. Mary Lowell Putnam (Boston), Miss Ellen C. Babbitt (New York) and Dr. Helen MacMurchy (Toronto). In England, Dr. Janet Lane-Claypon has done splendid and efficient work for this cause.

The ghastly details of intra-mural burial, the overcrowding of church-yards with successive layers of dead bodies, were referred to in *Hamlet, Tom Jones,* Dickens' *Bleak House* and Swinburne's *Bothwell* (Act II, sc. 2). The development of extra-mural cemeteries was due to the propagandism of Sir Edward Chadwick, whose reports (1843–55) led to the Burial Act (1855), abolishing inhumation within the limits of cities. Pietro Capparoni describes a similar Napoleonic ordinance of 1809.[1] England has now a very efficient corps of medical officers of health, a body which is almost extinct in France. Every German university has now a hygienic institute, and the Germans *physikus* is at once a public health official and an expert in legal medicine. In Russia, public sanitation was virtually non-existent until the advent of Ivan Ivanovich **Molleson** (1842–1920), who, after some experience with village practice, started the first permanent Sanitary Commission at Perm (1871) and became its first public health officer. Having thus secured governmental backing of the cause of public health, he thereafter led a peripatetic life devoted to extension of the hygienic idea at Novgorod (1872), Perm (1873–81), Astrachan (1881), Iroit (1882), Perm (1888), Saratov (1889), Tambov (1896), Kaluga (1906) and Voronezh (1911–20). He was unquestionably the originator of public health officers in Russia. In the United States there were no advances in public hygiene beyond a few stray smallpox regulations, until after the second cholera pandemic, when a sanitary survey of Massachusetts was made in 1849 by the Massachusetts Sanitary Commission, of which **Lemuel Shattuck** (1793–1859) was the prime-mover. The famous report of the Commission (1850) stressed the enormous amount of ill health and physical debility in American cities consequent upon insanitary conditions and the need for local investigation and control of such defects; but it was not until 1869 that the Massachusetts State Board of Health, the first permanent organization of its kind was established. A temporary acting State Board of Health for Louisiana had been established at New Orleans in 1855, and followed by Massachusetts (1869), District of Columbia (1870), California (1871), Virginia (1871), Minnesota (1872), Louisiana (1873), Michigan (1873[2]), Alabama (1875), Georgia (1875), Maryland (1875), Colorado (1876), and Wisconsin (1876). The metropolitan Board of Health of New York City was authorized only after considerable legislative opposition (1866). In 1901, only ten states had a satisfactory system of vital statistics (Kober). The American Public Health Association was organized in 1872. Quarantine regulations against yellow fever were established in Philadelphia in 1856 and later, but owing to the jealous insistence of the seaboard cities upon the right to operate their own stations and enforce their own laws, there was no uniform system of regulation until February 15, 1893, when Congress passed an act establishing a national quarantine system and vesting its powers in the Marine Hospital (Public Health) Service. The cholera epidemic of 1872–73 led to the appointment of a Cholera Commission, and the yellow fever epidemic of 1878 to the creation by Congress of a National Board of Health (March, 1878), which died out from lack of appropriations. Its place has been taken, since 1883 by the U. S. Marine Hospital Service, which was created originally for the medical care of merchant seamen (1798), eventually took over quarantine functions in ports without state or municipal quarantine control, and is now the U. S. Public Health Service. This service has a good Hygienic Laboratory and its experts have done much admirable work, particularly in the establishment of the disease **tularemia** which was first observed in squirrels by G. W. McCoy (1911), who with C. W. Chapin discovered the pathogenic agent (*Bacterium tularense*, 1912) which was isolated in man by Wherry and Lamb (1914). The disease was identified as such and named by Edward Francis (1919–21), who demonstrated its transmission to man by the deer-fly and by all manner of insects and rodents. It was independently observed in Japan by H. Ohara (1925), who inoculated his own wife. In such matters as the supervision of milk supply, child hygiene, and the close and ac-

---

[1] Capparoni : Riv. di storia crit. d. sc. med., Rome, 1915, vi, 586.

[2] For an interesting account of the constructive work of Henry B. Baker in the Michigan State Board, see Jour. Mich. State Med. Soc., Grand Rapids, 1916, xv, 424–427.

curate registration of disease—the sanitary surveys for diagnosing the condition of a sick community which Paul M. Kellogg has likened to "blue-prints"—the best recent work has been done by the State Boards of Massachusetts, Michigan (H. B. Baker), Pennsylvania (Samuel Gibson Dixon, 1852–1918), Illinois (John A. Rauch), Maryland (John S. Fulton), in connection with the municipal government of Washington, D. C. (G. M. Kober, W. C. Woodward), by the Department of Health of New York City, the excellent status of which is due to the altruistic labors of Stephen Smith (1823–1922), Hermann Michael Biggs (1859–1923), William H. Park, S. S. Goldwater, and others. The latter is now of special importance in relation to the great overplus of foreign population in the Borough of Manhattan. Hygienic improvements in nearly all countries and cities have produced a very striking diminution in the death-rate and a corresponding increase in the mean duration of life. The great **sewage** system of Chicago, viz., the Illinois and Michigan (1836–48), the New Drainage Canal (1892–1900), which reversed the flow of the Chicago River away from Lake Michigan, and the Illinois and Mississippi (Hennepin) Canal (1892–1907), with their extensions, viz., the North Shore Channel (1908–10), the Lake Front Sewer (1913–16), the Evanston Front Sewer (1916–20), the Calumet Sag Channel (1916–22), and the six great divisions of the Sanitary District (for sewage treatment), has had a striking effect upon the reduction of the total death-rate and typhoid mortality.[1] The celebrated Paris sewers were installed by M.-F.-E. Belgrand in 1854–56, with sewage-farm at Gennevilliers (1869–72), those of Hamburg in 1842, to be followed by Frankfort (1867), Danzig (1869), Berlin, built by James Hobrecht, (1873–83[2]), with farm at Osdorf, and Munich, activated by Pettenkofer (1868–92[3]). Sewer canals existed in Vienna from 1338, but the present network of canalisation was begun in 1830 and continued at intervals down to 1920. The pneumatic systems of Charles Liernur (1867), employed at Delft and Amsterdam, and of Isaac Shone (1878) are virtually systems of drainage by pumping for smaller cities. In England, where sewage is commonly discharged into the sea, filtration beds were first employed at Wimbledon in 1876. Prior to 1847, the sewers of London were merely drains for storm-water, and the discharge of sewage into them was not permitted before that time. The present system was begun in 1849, continued by the Metropolitan Board of Works (1856–88), according to plans of Sir James Bazalguette (1859–75) and completed by the London County Council, in all 288 miles. The labors of Edward Frankland (1825–99) and the experts of the Rivers Pollution Commission established the principle of sewage purification by means of intermittent filtration through different soils (1868–74). This was vastly improved by H. F. Mills, T. M. Drown, and William T. Sedgwick (1855–1921) at the Lawrence Experiment Station of the Massachusetts State Board of Health (1887). Fermentation of stored sewage in a closed tank was developed from the *fosses fixées* of Mouras (1860), by Scott-Moncrieff (1891), Talbot at Urbana, Illinois (1894), and Donald Cameron at Exeter, England (1895), who named the process. Passage through coke and stone in closed iron cylinders (contact system) was devised by W. J. Dibdin, chemist of the London County Council. Trickling filtration was introduced by Lowcock at Malvern, England (1892), and by Colonel G. E. Waring at Newport (1894[4]). The improvements in sewage disposal, activated by Pettenkofer in Munich and Virchow in Berlin, or the bacterial system of purification, introduced in England by William J. Dibdin (1896), have had great effect upon the mortality of typhoid fever and other water-borne diseases, as also the purification of the **water-supply** by sand filtration. This was introduced by the Chelsea Company in London in 1829, but did not reach perfection until recent times. In 1837, it was said that, in contradistinction to foreign cities, London swallowed its filth but seldom smelt it. The London Supply consists of a consolidation (storage and interconnection) of the Chelsea (1721), Lambeth (1783), Vauxhall (1805), West Middlesex (1806), Kent (1810), Grand Junction (1811) and Southwark Water Works, effected by the Metropolis Water Act (1902), which authorized the Metropolitan Water Board to acomplish this end (June 24, 1904). The supply is derived mainly from the Thames and Lea Rivers. The Liverpool Supply (1880–9) is derived from the Vyrnwy Lake, the largest reservoir in Europe. The New York City Supply comes from the Old Croton Aqueduct (1837–43), the Bronx River Conduit (1880–85), the New Croton Aqueduct (1884–93) and the New Aqueduct from the Catskills (1905–

---

[1] R. W. Putnam: Mil. Surgeon, Wash., 1926, lviii, 243–258.

[2] J. Hobrecht: Die Canalisation von Berlin. Berlin, 1884.

[3] M. Niedermayer: Arch. f. Hyg., München, 1893, xvii, 677–703.

[4] C.-E. A. Winslow: Technol. Quart., Boston, 1905, xvii, 318–332.

9), including a filtration plant at Scarsdale and the Ashokan, Kensico, Hill View and Jerome Park Reservoirs.[1] The investigation of lead-poisoning at Claremont, the English estate of Louis Philippe, by his physician, Gueneau de Mussy (1848–49), showed some of the dangers of piping, but that water is a vehicle of infection was not recognized until well after the London cholera epidemic of 1854, in which John Snow traced the infection to a pump in Broad Street. Although Snow's views were opposed by Farr and Sir J. Simon (1855), removal of the pump-handle stopped the epidemic. In the cholera epidemic of 1866, it was shown that the infection came from unfiltered water, furnished by one of the Metropolitan Water Companies, which had been ordered filtered by the act of 1852 (15. and 16. Victoria, cap. 84). The writings of William Budd (1871–73) fortified the theory of water-borne cholera and typhoid by establishing the fact that infection comes from the dejecta of the patients. The typhoid epidemic at Lausen, Switzerland (1872), which came from water passing through a hill, upset belief in the water theory, and real progress came only with bacteriology. The "drinking-water theory" finally gained ascendancy over the pythogenic or filth theory (Murchison), and the "ground-water" theory (Pettenkofer) through the Lowell and Lawrence epidemic of 1890, investigated by W. T. Sedgwick, and the fact that Hamburg, with unfiltered water, suffered severely from cholera in 1892, while the adjoining city of Altona enjoyed almost complete immunity through filtration. Sedgwick established the important principle that "quiet water, not running water, purifies itself." The filter at Lawrence, Mass. (1894), was "the first in America to stand between a water both highly polluted and highly infected and a large industrial population."[2] The Belmont filtration plant of Philadelphia (1893) and the Washington plant (1905) have been most effective in checking typhoid. In Germany, the great filtration plants of Berlin and Hamburg, the work of W. P. Dunbar at the Hamburg Testing Station, and the ingenious "Imhoff System" (1909–10) of sewage purification devised by Carl Imhoff (1876–   ), employed in the Emscher Thal, are worthy of special note. Prussia has probably the best system of preventing the **adulteration of food and drugs** punishing such offenses, not by fines, but by actual imprisonment. Bismarck declared the adulterers of food to be, next to the anarchists, the greatest enemies of the German people. The society against food adulteration, founded in Hamburg in 1878, became eventually the *Verein für öffentliche Gesundheitspflege*. The *Kaiserliches Gesundheitsamt* (founded 1876) drafted a law in 1878, patterned after the English law of August 11, 1875, and it was passed on May 14, 1879, and followed by a long line of similar enactments, the most important being the ordinance of February 22, 1894, for certifying food-chemists and protecting manufacturers against the false indictments of the incompetent *Winkelchemiker*. There was no pure food legislation in the United States until 1881, when laws were passed simultaneously by New York, New Jersey, and Michigan, and no adequate national legislation until the passage of the Food and Drugs Act of June 30, 1906 (abolished June 30, 1927) and the Meat Inspection Act of 1906, which still seems upon a somewhat unsatisfactory basis.

The movement for "Birth Control," a commonplace right of continental European women, although interdicted by our federal and State laws, has been advocated, mainly by William J. Robinson and others. As stated by Dr. A. Jacobi, before the New York Academy of Medicine (May 26, 1915), the object of this idea is primarily eugenic, to improve the quality of the human stock by the limitation of reckless begetting, by the deliberate regulation of the number and time of arrival of children, and by enlarging the responsibility of paternity.

In the distant past, a few severe and even cruel laws were enacted and enforced to protect society from the criminal. The tendency of recent times has been the proliferation of complex codes of petty statutes, many of them vastly curtailing the private rights of the individual, with the superadded paradox of leaving society at the mercy of the criminal, since almost any law can be evaded by sharp practice and chicanery. The great danger of the hour is legal and

---

[1] A. D. Flinn: Century Mag., N. Y., Sept., 1909.

[2] See W. T. Sedgwick: Jour. New Engl. Water Works Ass., Bost., 1900–1901, xv, 315; 1916, xxx, 183.

medical Bolshevism, which springs from the basest of human passions, namely, a mean envy of the private personal rights, possessions and privileges of others. As was shown in the French Revolution, crowd psychology, the spirit of the mob is fatal to medicine. The object of scientific teaching is to level the people up to its standards. It cannot be levelled down to popular standards. While much has been learned, especially from army experience in the recent war, as to the value of centralization and organization in group medicine, such schemes as compelling the people to "sell themselves" health insurance (admittedly a failure in England) are subversive of the true aims of medical science, since they are exposed to the *caveat emptor* fallacy on either side and many thus lead to abuses of privilege by malingerers. With arrangements of this kind, legitimate medicine has nothing whatever to do.

Sectarianism and **quackery** have flourished apace in modern life, often under strange guises. According to Flexner, "the homeopath is the only sectarian found at all in Great Britain or on the Continent," because a qualified physician, no matter what he may call himself, must pass the necessary examinations in order to practice. The proportion of homeopaths was 211 : 30,558 in Germany in 1909, and 193 : 31,154 in Great Britain in 1907. In America, under existing conditions, every species of medical sect—osteopathy, chiropraxis, Christian Science, eclecticism, botanic medicine, etc.—has been permitted to flourish. In 1902, there were 126 non-sectarian, 22 homeopathic, 9 eclectic, and 2 physiomedical schools in the United States, as against 74 non-sectarian, 2 homeopathic, and 3 eclectic in 1927. There are no sectarian institutions in Canada. In respect of fiduciary allegiance to Hahnemann's original doctrines, the modern homeopath is often like a skeptical or backsliding clergyman. Scientific medicine is neither homeopathic nor allopathic. Upon the subject of treatment, which is often very much in the air, hinges the whole matter of tolerance of sectarianism and quackery. In the past, as we have seen, many important features of medical treatment were actually introduced by laymen. Therapeutics, in fact, began with herb-doctoring. It is the purely experimental status of actual therapeutics which opens a loophole for the modern quack. "The very candor of scientific medicine gives him his chance, for, just where the scientific physician admits his inadequacy, the charlatan is most positive" (Flexner). The tendency to consult quacks is analogous to the physician's liability to be deluded by wild-cat investments. "Some of the most responsible doctors," says Robert Morris, "will always be in the hands of financial fakers, and some of the most responsible business men will always be in the hands of medical fakers." In the early part of the 19th century, John St. John Long, a handsome imposter, who traded upon his influence over women without meeting their advances, had enormous success in England, and even Napoleon consulted the pythoness Lenormand. Under the law of 1815 (55 George III, cap. 194), an English apothecary was still entitled to diagnose and prescribe, and the Society of Apothecaries was authorized to license him for registration in the Medical Register; but, in 1886, the old-time strife was settled by requiring that the governing bodies in medicine, surgery, and pharmacy should grant no certificate or license unless the candidate should qualify by examination in all three branches. On June 21, 1869, Germany made the serious mistake of passing a statute abolishing the obligations of physicians to attend urgent calls and to treat the poor *gratis*, which incidentally let down the bars to all unlicensed practitioners who might profess merely to treat disease.[1] The effect of this "*Kurierfreiheit*," a reflex of the democratic idealism of Virchow, was a tremendous outpouring of nature-healers, faith-healers, Baunscheidtists, exorcists, masseurs and masseuses, and devotees of vegetarianism, Kneippism, *Nacktkultur*, blue and green electricity, and occultism of all kinds.

Police returns show as many as 1013 registered quacks in Berlin (1903), as against 28 in 1879, and 1349 quacks out of 3584 physicians in 1909. There were 4104 registered quacks in Prussia in 1902, 5148 in 1903, and, in 1905, there were 6137, and 2112 in Saxony. In Great Britain, qualified physicians have been listed in the Medical Register since the Medical Act of 1858, but there is no police registration of quacks. As in Germany and the United States, they may use the mails and advertise *ad libitum*. "The newspapers, the billboards, and the 'bus give the charlatan easy and continuous access" (Flexner). There were 31,592 licenses for the sale and manufacture of proprietary remedies in 1894–95 at five shillings each, and 40,734 in 1904–05. The blue book report issued by the Privy Council Office in 1910 shows that herbalists, bone-setters, nature-healers, abortionists, venereal and consumption specialists, hernia and cancer quacks abound. As in Germany, they are punished when caught in heinous malpractice or murder, but they are usually too shrewd to be caught.[2] The British Medical Journal devoted a whole number to the exposure of quackery in 1911. In France, there are better laws, but they are not rigidly enforced.

America has been a paradise for quacks, from the time of Perkins down to the electronic reactions of Abrams and the cults pilloried by Morris Fishbein. Nowhere have patent medicine vendors made so much money. "What need of Aladdin's lamp when we can build a palace with a patent pill" was one of Lowell's witticisms, and it illustrates the easy-going, humorous, American tolerance of humbuggery and fraud. The complex scheme of medical laws in our several states is inferior to the old English system, which had a few liberal laws, seldom changed through the centuries, but susceptible of an elastic interpretation where the merits of the case required it. As under our divorce laws, a divorced or separated couple may change their marital status as they cross successive state lines, so a border physician in Indiana was non-suited for his fee for the after-treatment of an amputation over

---

[1] See, in addition to Flexner's observations, H. Magnus: Die Kurierfreiheit, Breslau, 1905.

[2] The case against the "healers" of the novelist Harold Frederic, whose death at the hands of these "Christian Scientists," in 1898, was, as Bernard Shaw puts it, "a sort of sealing with his blood of the contemptuous disbelief in and dislike of doctors he had bitterly expressed in his books," was reluctantly dismissed by Justice Hawkins at the Central Police Court, London, on the ground of insufficient evidence as to Frederic's own part in the transaction.

the state line, although the operation itself was excused as within the legal exception of an emergency; while a confidential communication made in New Jersey by a Colorado patient was held not to be privileged when the Jersey physician gave testimony in a Colorado court.[1] People tend to become lawless through a multiplicity of useless laws, an odd contrast to the simple common law book of Switzerland, which any peasant can understand and use. The difficulties with a multiplex system of laws are sensed in Lord Beaconsfield's aphorism that where the social order is very strong (in rural communities) it can put up with weak government; where the social order is weak (in large cities) it requires strong government. The whole theory of interpretation of existing law is contained in Bismarck's view that there are times (e. g., in peace) when government must be liberal, and times (e. g., in war) when it must be despotic. "Everything changes, nothing is constant here below." As it is, quacks have commonly thriven best in our liberal and thickly settled states and cities and not at all in the agricultural districts of the South, where doctors are few and society is very strong. So long as therapeutics is what it is, quackery is almost beyond the reach of legislation,[2] and, as in France, rigid legislation might turn out to be a farce. The newspapers, reaping the harvests they do from advertising quackery, are indifferent, although the location, citation, and exposure of quacks and quack medicines have latterly afforded rare sport for keen-sighted journalists who are something more than pressmen. The only serious attempts to take up the cudgels on behalf of the public are those made by the British Medical Association and the American Medical Association.

The **British Medical Association** was organized on July 19, 1832, in the board room of the Worcester Infirmary, at the instance of the late Sir Charles Hastings, who was then physician to the Infirmary. Since its foundation, meetings have been held in different cities of Great Britain each year, and the Association now has many home and colonial branches. Its published transactions, 1832–53, and the *Provincial Medical and Surgical Journal* (1840–53), succeeded by the *Association Medical Journal* (1853–57), were also its organs until the *British Medical Journal* was founded in 1857. As representing the united profession of Great Britain, the Association has played an important part in the development of English medicine in the modern period, particularly in medical reform, looking after parliamentary bills relating to public health legislation and poor laws, and in the exposure and censure of quackery, patent nostrums, and other frauds. In 1909, it published *Secret Remedies*, a convenient directory of current nostrums.

In 1847, the **American Medical Association** was organized, owing its inception to a national convention of delegates from medical societies and colleges called by the Medical Society of New York State, largely through the efforts of Nathan Smith Davis, to improve the then disgraceful status of medical education in the United States. During the first fifty years of its existence, its activities were confined to discussion rather than accomplishment, and its membership was limited to specially elected delegates. Since its reorganization at St. Paul, in 1901, membership in the Association has been based upon membership in the state medical societies, which are again based upon membership in the county societies. Both state and national

---

[1] See, on this head, the able legal study of C. A. Boston in Med. Times, N. Y., 1916, xliv, i, 113; 153.

[2] The advertising and sale of secret unofficial remedies was interdicted in France by the laws of 1803 and 1805, which have usually been ignored. (G. Bourgeau: Paris diss. No. 83, 1916, p. 37.)

organizations have a specially elected House of Delegates to transact business, which welds the whole profession of the country into an efficient organized body, capable of accomplishing things. Under the earlier dispensation, the aims of the Association were restricted mainly to the narrower problems of medical ethics; its present purpose is largely the direction of public opinion in regard to public hygiene and medical education. In spite of much opposition, the Association, in the last twelve years of its existence, has accomplished many important things, first and foremost, in checking, through its Council on Pharmacy and Chemistry, the exploitation of the medical profession by patent medicine makers and the swindling of the people by quacks and quackery. Special records of "New and Non-Official Remedies," proprietary medicines, diploma-mills and other frauds being kept and published for public use. It has vastly improved the status of the state medical societies as to increase in membership and efficiency, so that where formerly the state societies published meager volumes of "transactions" at rare intervals, there were, by 1910, some twenty-two state society journals, a great improvement in the centralization of periodical literature. The Council on Medical Education (1904), has, through its propaganda in the last 25 years, done much to decrease the number of low grade medical schools and consequently of incompetent or unscrupulous physicians. It has also done much to secure four-year courses and "full time" professors for the more scientific disciplines. According to data recently supplied by the Association, there have been some 335 medical colleges, with 118 other institutions of dubious character, in the United States during the period 1765–1913, of which there were 6 in existence in 1810, 160 in 1904, 95 in 1816–17, and 88 in 1920; of the latter 75 were non-sectarian, 5 homeopathic, 1 eclectic, and 3 nondescript. Since 1904, 94 medical schools have ceased to exist, 53 by merger, 41 by extinction. During 1912–13, some 14 medical colleges were closed, and 2 in 1916–17. In 1927, there were 19,662 medical students, as against 11,826 in 1880, 28,142 in 1904 and 12,137 in 1919; and 4035 medical graduates for the year 1927 as against 3241 in 1880, 5747 in 1904 and 2656 in 1919. These decreases indicate, of course, the prospect of a corresponding average improvement in quality. There are "fewer but better colleges," 57 of which met the improved requirements for admission of the Association of American Medical Colleges on January 1, 1912, and 71 in 1927, during which year there were 80 medical colleges in the United States and 9 in Canada.[1] The present proportion of physicians to the total population of the United States is 149,521 : 118,628,000, or one physician to every 793 persons. In proportion to the actual population, South Dakota had the fewest physicians in 1920 (1 : 1160) and the District of Columbia the most (1 : 365), exclusive of some 500 government physicians who did not practice (otherwise 1 : 259). During 1913–27, the population has increased by 23,925,500, while there are 124 fewer doctors. Thirteen State licensing boards have recently insisted on higher preliminary requirements. Finally, through its Council on Health and Public Instruction, the Association has now public speakers in practically every state of the Union, who instruct the people directly in regard to infectious diseases. The *Journal of the American Medical Association*, founded in 1883, was edited by Nathan Smith Davis (1883–88), latterly by George H. Simmons (1899–1924) and Morris Fishbein (1924). Apart from its own Journal, the Association now controls eight periodicals and publishes a useful Directory of physicians in the United States and Canada.

There is no modern science or group of sciences which has so many current **periodicals** as medicine. In striking contrast with the 18th century, which had but few medical periodicals, our own time, particularly our own country, has literally swarmed with medical journals, many of which are, as the Germans say, *Eintagsfliegen*—of ephemeral duration. Each one has, or has had, its use in some particular locality or as subserving the interests of some theory or sect, some "ism" or "pathy." There are too many medical periodicals in the modern world. Mr. Charles Perry Fisher estimated some 1654 current up to January, 1913.[2] Of these, 630 were American, 461 German,

---

[1] Jour. Amer. Med. Assoc., Chicago, 1920, lxxv, 379–415: 1927, lxxxix, 601–610, *passim*.   [2] Bull. Med. Library Assoc., Balt., 1913, n. s., ii, 22.

268 French, 152 British, 75 Italian, 29 Spanish. In the Surgeon-General's Library there were some 1895 on hand in 1916–17, 1240 in 1920–21, 1925 in 1927. In the first series (1880–95) of the Index Catalogue 4920 medical periodicals were indexed; at the end of the fiscal year, June 30, 1916, the total number indexed (1880–1916) was 8289. The great number of medical periodicals, as of medical societies, in the United States is due, not to social or scientific conditions, but, as in Russia, to the extent of national territory and to the expansion of cities.[1] All countries have periodicals which are obviously "home-grown" and intended for home consumption. As a rule, the journals of the larger cities—Boston, New York, Philadelphia, Chicago, New Orleans, and others—are of better quality and of more metropolitan character than those of the several States, but some of the latter have attained a much higher standard by the centralization of State medical societies, through which the State medical journal is also the organ of the State medical society. Through the major part of the 19th century American medical journalism, of the provincial type, was so "inebriated with the exuberance of its own verbosity," so high-strung in faction-breeding, so shrill with the feline amenities of controversy that Billings characterized it in an "untranslatable French criticism": *Il y a trop de tintamarre là dedans, trop de brouillamini.* Carlyle's "cackle as of Babel" conveys the exact sense of this French pronouncement. The writers of the period, in the words of Dr. Holmes, "chewed the juice out of all the superlatives of the language in Fourth of July orations," as witness such spread-eagle titles as the *Granite State Medical Revolutionist and Hygienic Advertiser*, the *Georgia Blister and Critic*, the *Poughkeepsie Thomsonian*, the *Puget Sound Sanitarian and Prohibitionist*, the *Quarterly Review of Narcotic Inebriety*, the *Divine Science of Health*, the *Southern Homeopathic Pellet*, the *Indiana Scalpel*, the *Uric Acid Monthly*, and the *Dental Jairus*. The tide was turned by the caustic critique of Billings in the Centennial year (1876[2]), which, along with the subsequent *Index Medicus* (1879) and *Index Catalogue* (1880), did much to elevate the status of American medical literature.

Following the Medical Repository (1797–1824) came, in order of time, the Philadelphia Medical Museum (1804–11), the Philadelphia Medical and Physical Journal (1804–09), the Medical and Agricultural Register (Boston, 1806–07), the Baltimore Medical and Physical Recorder (1808–09), the American Medical and Philosophical Register (1810–14), the New England Journal of Medicine and Surgery (Boston, 1812–28), the American Medical Recorder (Philadelphia, 1818–29), and the Philadelphia Journal of the Medical and Physical Sciences, founded in 1820 by Nathaniel Chapman. In 1827, Chapman started a new series of the last journal under the title "American Journal of the Medical Sciences," which, under

---

[1] In 1881, Dr. James R. Chadwick, late librarian of the Boston Medical Library, said: "In England, it is possible for those who are specially interested in gynecology and obstetrics to attend the meetings of the Obstetrical Society of London, as actually happens, whereas in America the distances to be traversed are so great as to render this impossible." (Boston Med. and Surg. Journal, 1881, cv, 245). At the present time there are national American societies for all the specialties, which meet annually.

[2] J. S. Billings in: A Century of American Medicine, Philadelphia, 1876, 328–343.

the subsequent editorship of Isaac Hays, I. Minis Hays and others, has been, for a long period, the best of the American monthly medical periodicals. Among the best of the medical weeklies have been the Boston Medical and Surgical Journal (1828), which has been edited by such men as John Collins Warren, Francis Minot, George B. Shattuck (1845–1923) and others, and has just celebrated its centenary (1928); the Medical News (Philadelphia, 1843–1905), founded by I. Minis Hays; The New York Medical Journal (1865–1925), which, of late years, has been edited with great ability by the late Frank P. Foster (1841–1911) and laterly by Charles E. de M. Sajous, Claude Lamont Wheeler (1864–1916) and Smith Ely Jelliffe; the Medical Record (1866–1925), edited by George F. Shrady, and, latterly, by Thomas L. Stedman. The Philadelphia Medical Journal (1898–1903) and American Medicine (Philadelphia, 1901) were originally edited by George M. Gould. Among the best periodicals devoted to special subjects are The American Journal of Obstetrics (New York, 1868–1917), founded by Emil Noeggerath and Abraham Jacobi; The Annals of Surgery (1885–), edited by Lewis Stephen Pilcher (1845–); The American Journal of Physiology (Boston, 1898); The Archives of Ophthalmology and Otology (New York, 1869), founded by Herman Knapp; The Journal of Experimental Medicine (New York, 1896), founded by William H. Welch; the American Journal of Anatomy (Baltimore, 1901); the Journal of Medical Research (Boston, 1901–24), continued as the American Journal of Pathology (1925), edited by Frank B. Mallory; The Journal of Infectious Diseases (Chicago, 1904), founded by Ludvig Hektoen; The Journal of Biological Chemistry (New York, 1905), founded by Christian A. Herter; The Journal of Morphology (Boston, 1887), founded by the late Charles O. Whitman, the Journal of Experimental Zoölogy (Baltimore, 1904), edited by Ross Granville Harrison; Surgery, Gynecology, and Obstetrics (Chicago, 1905), founded and edited by Franklin H. Martin; the Journal of Laboratory and Clinical Medicine (St. Louis, 1916), founded by Victor C. Vaughan, and the Journal of Bacteriology (Baltimore, 1916).

The better sort of medical periodicals may be roughly divided into three classes: those devoted exclusively to purely scientific and experimental researches; those devoted to the specialties; and those which include, along with clinical and surgical cases, papers, original or sophomorical, upon set subjects, reports of progress, abstracts, reviews, translations, historical tidbits, facetiæ, and medical gossip. In periodicals of the first class, Germany takes the lead in number. In respect of quality, the transactions of such learned bodies as the Royal Society of London, the scientific academies of France, Prussia, Saxony, Bavaria, Austria, Italy, or the Société de biologie of Paris, stand first, as regards occasional contributions to fundamental physiological science. Then come the publications of university laboratories and clinics, of medical societies, institutes, and other foundations, in relation to which the titles Acta, Annalen, Arbeiten, Archiv, Beiträge, Berichte, Centralblatt, Folia, Jahrbuch, Mitteilungen, Monatsschrift, Sammlung, Verhandlungen, Veröffentlichungen, Vierteljahresschrift, or Zeitschrift usually connote something of positive value, while Blätter, Correspondenzblatt, Calender, Organ, Repertorium, Wochenschrift, or Zeitung have a more dubious implication. Of annual publications, Ergebnisse contain valuable résumés of current scientific work; Jahresberichte, the equivalents of our year-books, are useful for bibliographical reference or statistical compilation. As a rule, the periodicals devoted to anatomy, physiology, bacteriology, psychology, anthropology, surgery, or the different medical specialties are good of their kind in any country. The veterinary journals are sometimes of better quality than the dental. Homeopathic journals are almost uniformly poor, and journals devoted to osteopathy, anti-vivisection, and other fads have no scientific value whatever. Of the general medical periodicals of the third class, the *Wochenschriften* of the larger Germanic cities—Berlin, Munich, Vienna—the *British Medical Journal, The Lancet,* and the journals of the larger cities of Great Britain—Edinburgh, Glasgow, Dublin, Bristol—are all of the best quality. The corresponding publications in the Latin, Scandinavian, and Slavic countries are of unequal value. Aside from decadent literature, almost anything printed in France is well written, and the witty *feuilletons* in the Parisian medical journals are no exception to the rule. Some, like the *Chronique médical,* are *capables de tout* in this respect. Many of the French and Italian weeklies are printed on large, inconvenient sheets like newspapers, which suggests the advantages of Ostwald's idea of a definite *Weltformat,* a uniform size and shape for all scientific books and periodicals. An undesirable feature of the smaller-size Latin periodicals is the actual advertisement of nostrums within the text, or the binding of such advertisements between the leaves of the journal. Italy is almost unique in glorifying the names of great and small reputations eponymically by bestowing them upon medical periodicals,[1] *e. g.,* in the case of *Cesalpino, Cirillo, Ercolani, Fracastori, Galvani, Guglielmo da Saliceto, Ingrassia, Malpighi, Morgagni, Orosi, Pisani, Ramazzini, Selmi, Spallanzani, Tommasi, Valsalva, Zacchia.*

The tendency toward extreme specialization is indicated in such titles as *Arbeiterschutz* (1925,) *Brain* (1879), *Cancer* (1923), *Encéphale* (1906), *Endocrinology* (1917), *Eos* (1905), *Epilepsia* (1909), *Genetica* (1919), *Hæmatologica* (1920), *Heart* (1909), *Imago* (1912), *Lepra* (1909), *Mental Hygiene* (1917), *Mutterschutz* (1905), *Nevraxe* (1909), *Nippiologia* (1915), *Seuchenbekämpfung* (1924), *Tuberculosis* (1902), *Tumori* (1911), *Vita sexualis* (1896), while the historical spirit is patent in *Æsculape* 1923), *Caducée* (1901), *Chiron* (1805), *Hippocrates* (1898), *Isis* (1913) and *Janus* (1896). In 1927, some 36 journals were devoted to biology (general physiology), 14 to cancer, 6 to endocrinology, 8 to genetics, 14 to history of medicine, 10 to industrial hygiene, 19 to pathology, 40 to psychology and psycho-analysis (5), 15 to psychiatry, 26 to radiology, 7 to social hygiene, 17 to tropical medicine, and 33 to tuberculosis (on file in the S. G. O. Library).

Most of the Spanish medical journals are inferior even to those of South America in quality. The beautiful language of Spain is a social rather than a scientific medium, and much of her medical literature is taken up with rhetoric and *problemas para solucionar.* Printed with aniline inks upon inferior paper, most of our valued medical productions will have crumbled or their contents faded away in a century or more, and criticism of medical periodicals seems idle or ungracious. The slightest of them may subserve a useful purpose in setting some anxious inquirer upon the path of study or of original investigation. Walsh, in his studies of medieval medicine, has emphasized the fact that the human mind soon tires of difficult or insoluble problems and may drop a subject for centuries. To insure continuity of interest there must be constant rejuvenation and restimulation, and

---

[1] The Dutch journals "Pieter Camper," and "Boerhaave" are other examples. Most of these eponymic titles ended with the war.

in no phase of modern activity is it so imperative that the scientific spirit should burn and shine like a sacred fire, as in the field of medicine. The highest function of the medical journalist today is to introduce new currents of scientific ideas and to keep them in circulation. The public would be much better protected from quacks if our newspapers drew their information from reliable representatives of the medical press,[1] instead of from reporters, untrained in science and with a mania for advertising the sensational.

One of the most striking features of modern medicine was the tendency toward **internationalism,** even on the field of battle. In 1862, Henri Dunant (1828–1910), a Swiss philanthropist, published his "Souvenir de Solferino," and this account of the barbarities of warfare led to the International Conference of the Red Cross Societies at Geneva in 1863, and to the signing, on August 22, 1864, of the Geneva Convention, in which fourteen different States pledged themselves to regard the sick and wounded, as also the army medical and nursing staffs, as neutrals on the battlefield. This movement was warmly supported by Queen Augusta of Prussia and the Grand Duchess Maria Pavlovna of Russia, and today its intention is carried out over all the civilized world.

In 1867, the first international medical congress was opened at Paris, at the instance of Henri Guitrac, to be followed by those at Florence (1869), Vienna (1873), Brussels (1875), Geneva (1877), Amsterdam (1879), London (1881), Copenhagen (1884), Washington (1887), Berlin (1890), Rome (1894), Moscow (1897), Paris (1900), Madrid (1903), Lisbon (1906), Budapest (1909), and London (1913). It had already been preceded by international congresses on statistics (Brussels, 1851), hygiene and demography (Brussels, 1852), ophthalmology (Brussels, 1857), veterinary medicine (Hamburg, 1863), anthropology (Spezia, 1865), and pharmacy (Brunswick, 1865), and was followed by a series on otology (New York, 1876), laryngology (Milan, 1880), criminal anthropology (Rome, 1885), tuberculosis (Paris, 1888), dermatology (Paris, 1889), physiology (Basel, 1889), psychology (Paris, 1890), gynecology and obstetrics (Brussels, 1892), alcoholism (Brussels, 1894), tuberculosis (Paris, 1895), leprosy (Berlin, 1897), dentistry (1900), surgery (Brussels, 1902), care of the insane (Antwerp, 1902), unification of heroic remedies (Brussels, 1902), milk (Brussels, 1903), habitations (Paris, 1904), school hygiene (Nuremberg, 1904), physiotherapy (Liège, 1905), cancer (Heidelberg, 1906), pellagra (Turin, 1906), occupational diseases (Milan, 1906), sleeping sickness (1907), epilepsy (Budapest, 1909), tropical medicine (Manila, 1910), comparative pathology (Paris, 1912), eugenics (London, 1912), and history of medicine (Antwerp, 1920). These are only a few of such international gatherings, which include almost every specialty.

Another sign of the international spirit is the award of the **Nobel prizes** for medicine to von Behring (1901), Ronald Ross (1902), Finsen (1903), Pavloff (1904), Koch (1905), Golgi and Ramón y Cajal (1906), Laveran (1907), Metchnikoff and Ehrlich (1908), Kocher (1909), Kossel (1910), Gullstrand (1911), Carrel (1912), Richet (1913), Bárány (1914), Bordet (1919), August Krogh (1920[2]), A. V. Hill and Otto Meyerhof (1922), Banting and MacLeod (1923), Einthoven (1924–5), Johannes Fibiger (1926), Julius Wagner von Jauregg (1927) as also to Roentgen (1901), Becquerel and the Curies (1903) in physics, Emil Fischer (1902), Pregl (1923) and Zsigmondy (1925), in chemistry and Henri Dunant for promotion of peace (1901).

[1] This is now the case with the leading New York newspapers. For the harm done by the press in misleading statements and flamboyant advertising of proprietary remedies and quack procedures, see the Paris thesis of Dr. Georges Bourgeau: Les erreurs et les dangers de la grande presse en matière médicale, 1916, No. 83.

[2] No awards of the Nobel prize in medicine were made during 1915–18, 1921, and 1924.

MEDICINE IN THE WORLD WAR AND AFTER

The war of 1914–18, which Sudermann ultimately defined as "the most gigantic imbecility since the Crusades," meant, as we now see it, the débâcle of the 19th century civilization. In Spengler's view, it was a historic change of phase (with "strong contrapuntal accents") fore-ordained hundreds of years ago. Viewed from a closer angle we can trace each move, checkmate, gambit and counter-gambit leading up to the disaster in the remarkable chronology of events which Wilfrid Scawen Blunt appended to his Diaries of 1888–1914,[1] and there can be no doubt that the issue was not primarily an expression of racial antagonism, but "a clash of imperialist interests, primarily economical, brought about by financiers, diplomats, and soldiers, who, for short-sighted ends, played upon mob psychology" (Norman Thomas). But whether a biological process, a coil of fate or a smoke-screen for graft and profiteering, it remained, in its consequences, a black tragedy for European humanity. In the words of Hrdlicka, "they have suffered much."

Viewed after the lapse of a decade, the medical innovations and inventions of the war period seem clever, respectable, but not particularly brilliant. The administrative achievement was, however, truly remarkable.

The opening of the war revealed Germany in a state of perfect military preparedness, England and France in a state of partial preparedness, and our own country in the gerundive state of being about to be prepared. Yet, twenty months after our entry into the war (April 6, 1917), the armistice was signed (November 11, 1918).

To raise medical personnel, England had to draw some 11,000 civilian practitioners; in France, the whole medical profession was mobilized; and in our Army, expanded twenty-fold over the army of 1916, no less than 29,602 physicians were in uniform as reserve officers, in fact, the élite of our American profession flocked to the colors. Under the administration of the late General William C. Gorgas, the Surgeon-General's Office was expanded to gigantic proportions, commensurate with our far-flung array of 32 training camps, each a community of 30,000–40,000 soldiers. On the Western front, medical administration was an affair of providing for the supplies, sanitation, hospitalization, medical and surgical services of immense training areas, hospital areas, lines of communication and miles of trenches, while the open fighting at the end of the war brought up a new problem, the complex sanitation of vast moving armies. The chief surgeons of the American Expeditionary Forces during the fighting period were Colonel A. E. Bradley and Generals Merritte W. Ireland and Walter D. McCaw. The medical establishment of the British Army was administered by General Sir Alfred Keogh and later General Sir John Goodwin, that of the French Army by P.-E.-J. Simonin (1864–1920), Tuffier and Justin Godart. The Surgeon-General of the German Army during the war period was Lieut. Gen. Otto von Schjerning (1853–1921).

For medicine, the greatest triumph of the war was in the direct application of the science of infectious diseases to military sanitation, the group sanitation, in fact, of armies of millions. Apart from the statistics of the German Army in 1870–71, and of the Japanese Army in 1904–5, this was the first war of magnitude in history in which the mortality from battle casualties exceeded that from communicable diseases. In the European War, the official German losses were 1,531,048 killed, 4,211,569 wounded, 155,013 died from disease, 991,340 missing, with 762,796 deaths

---

[1] W. S. Blunt: My Diaries, New York, 1922, ii, 460–476. The interest of Blunt is that, while flagrantly disloyal to country, his judgments of men and things were usually right and true, confirming the view of Turgenieff that a man of the world, of a particular class and type. is most apt to be *"bon juge en pareille matière."* The touchstone of the 19th century civilization is in the noble sentence of Max von Pettenkofer: "The belief in something higher than ourselves, in an intangible, unattainable ideal, is the source of all human culture and of all progress" (1869).

in the civilian population from food shortage (total 6,888,770). In our Civil War, there were 44,238 killed in action, 246,712 wounded, 31,978 (10.48 per 1000) died from wounds, 186,216 (61.04 per 1000) died from disease. In the World War, 34,249 of our forces were killed in action, 224,089 wounded were admitted to hospital, of whom 13,691 (4.5 per 1000) died, and 50,714 (16.67 per 1000) died from disease. Thus there were four times as many deaths from disease in the Civil War as in the World War, while our recent death-rate from wounds in hospital was reduced one-half. In other words, the next greatest medical achievement in the World War was the conquest of wound infection. Trench warfare in soil contaminated by decades of cultivation made every soldier a potential bacillus carrier. On the battle front sepsis was inevitable, the aseptic ritual impossible, and the revival of Listerism (treatment of infected wounds by antisepsis) was a foregone conclusion. Passing through the experimental phase of dressing with colored antiseptic pastes, salt pack and hypertonic solution (Wright), there was at length evolved the physico-chemical principle of wound irrigation by a solution of a gas in a liquid (Carrel-Dakin), and later, the mechanical principle of *débridement* or wound excision with *épluchage* and primary suture (Gray, 1915; Lemaître, 1917–18[1]) which was known to Desault (1790) and Larrey (1812[2]). H. D. Dakin's device of setting free chlorine gas from sodium hypochlorite or dichloramine-T constitutes the most refined antisepsis. The excision of all devitalized wound tissues prior to suture is an aseptic principle of the first order, of capital importance in industrial or future war surgery. These were the only innovations made in Western front surgery, which was, however, remarkable for the use of Röntgenography on a grand scale and ingenuity in maxillo-facial surgery and the treatment of gunshot fractures.[3]

In internal medicine, some new and strange pathologic concepts came into play, such as the longitudinal sinus disease, Volhynian (five-day) fever, trench-foot, trench-nephritis, spirochætal jaundice, the toxic jaundices from picric acid, trinitrotoluene and tetrachlorethane poisoning, the effects of gassing, gas gangrene, and other complications of wound infection the disorders of peripheral nerves and the effects of gunshot wounds upon the nervous system, particularly from shell shock and wind contusion, gas gangrene from the bacillus Welchii, and other complications of wound infection.

The mental tests of Binet and others were introduced into our recruiting system for the first time by Robert M. Yerkes (1917), and revealed the large percentage of twelve-year-old minds in our recent population. Psychology and neuro-psychiatry did much for mobilization by weeding out mental defectives, always bad risks for armies. The motley complex of neurotic phenomena going under the name of "shell-shock," much of which occurred in the safe zones behind the battlefront, illustrated the transformation of mental emotion into physical commotion, and was carefully studied by F. W. Mott, T. W. Salmon and others. Great impetus was given to the study of wound shock by the investigations of W. T. Porter, Cannon, Crile and Turck (cytost). The effects of gunshot wounds on peripheral nerves were intensively studied by Marie, Jules Tinel (1916[4]), Mme. Athanassio-Benisty (1916–17) and others, including the Peripheral Nerve Committee of our Medical Corps.

Of communicable diseases, measles, mumps and meningitis smote our camps heavily during 1917–18, due to the fact that country boys, being seldom exposed, are non-immune; and the great epidemic of Spanish influenza (1918–19), with its complicating pneumonias and empyemas, was more fatal everywhere than the war itself. That measles is a respiratory affection, transmitted *via* the air-passages, was emphasized by E. L. Munson in the Texan epidemic of 1917, and from that time on interest became concentrated on the sputum-borne infections (including measles, meningitis, scarlatina) as the outstanding problem of preventive medicine. Contact infection by hand and breath became of cardinal importance, since the first principles of public hygiene were obliterated in the slave-ship overcrowding of public vehicles and places, consequent upon war conditions everywhere.

The net result of war experience was the novel hygienic principle that the infected or exposed individual is more dangerous to society

---

[1] H. W. M. Gray: Brit. Med. Jour., Lond., 1915, ii, 317.

[2] Larrey: Mémoires de chirurgie militaire, Paris, 1912, i, 50; 307.

[3] M. W. Ireland: Jour. Am. Med. Assoc., Chicago, 1921, lxxvi, 763–769.

[4] J. Tinel: Les blessures des nerfs, Paris, 1916.

than the disease itself. Community welfare now demands not only isolation of carriers, contacts and suspects, but also education of the individual to realize that, as long as he is a disease carrier, he must voluntarily protect the community from himself.

That trench fever (P. U. O.) is a louse-borne infection was realized by the British Commission under Gen. Sir David Bruce and finally demonstrated by the American Commission under R. P. Strong. The relation of pediculosis to typhus (noted by Tobias Cober in 1606) became of moment on the Eastern front, particularly in Servia, where many American physicians succumbed to the disease. In the trenches every soldier became lousy and "Fighting the Cootie," by the various methods of delousing, taxed the ingenuity of all military sanitarians. Spirochetal jaundice (Weil's disease) was investigated by R. Inada and Y. Ito (1914 –15), Adrian Stokes and others; effort syndrome (D. A. H.) by Thomas Lewis. Trench-foot (*Gamaschenkrankheit*) was resolved by Osler into the equation: Cold bite + muscle inertia = trench-foot. Volhynian fever was first described by H. Werner (1916). Under the leadership of General Sir Robert Jones, H. Morestin and others, orthopedic or reconstructional surgery of mangled bones and limbs was materially advanced in England. In the treatment of gunshot fractures, the use of continuous extension by the Hodgen splint and Balkan frame greatly accelerated the evacuation of the wounded and their prompt return to duty. In Belgium, C. Willems substituted the principle of early active mobilization of joint lesions for the old orthopedic teaching. Remarkable was the work of Alexis Carrel at Compiegne on wound treatment, of Crile, Gwathmey, Karsner, and Marshall on gas-oxygen anesthesia, of H. D. Gillies (Sidcup), Delageniere (Le Mans), H. Morestin (Val de Grâce), A. C. Valadier (Boulogne), Derwent Wood (London) and of Hayes, Hutchinson, Blair and other Americans at Neuilly on maxillo-facial surgery, of J. A. Blake (Neuilly), M. Sinclair (Wimereux), H. D. Souttar (Netley), R. Leriche (Lyons) and of Gosset, J. P. Goldthwaite, H. Osgood, N. Allison and W. L. Keller on fractures and splints, of Pedro Chutro (Paris), on fractures and bone-sinuses, of H. Cushing (Boulogne) on brain surgery, of Morestin, Chutro and Gosset on cranioplasty by cartilaginous grafts, of Stassen (Port Villez) on amputation, of Tuffier (Paris) on reamputation, of Vanghetti on cineplastic amputation, and of Arbuthnot Lane, Calot, Tuffier, Morestin, P. Bastianelli and E. Lexer (Hamburg) on general plastic and orthopedic surgery. Reconstruction and reëducation of the disabled, planned in Germany ten years before the war, has been carried forward everywhere on a grand scale, and vocational rehabilitation, adumbrated by Juan Luis Vives (1531), became a matter of national administration.

The physiological requirements of aviators and the pathology, prevention and treatment of war-gassing were entirely new subjects, in the development of which American medical officers played an important part. Notable contributions to the pathology of war-gas poisoning were the studies of Sir Leonard Hill (1915–20), E. B. Krumbhaar (1918–19), A. S. Warthin (1919), M. V. Winternitz (1920), F. P. Underhill (1920) and H. L. Gilchrist (1922).

Through infant welfare activities, in the very midst of the war, the infant death-rate was, in 1916, brought down to 91 per 1000 in England, and 97 in Scotland, in both cases the lowest on record. In Germany, although 40 per cent. fewer babies were born in 1916 than in 1913, the infant death-rate of 164 in 1914 was well kept down thereafter. In France, due to the increased employment of women in munition factories, there was a steady rise in infant mortality after 1915, reaching 126 in 1917. As the war-time birth-rate was 50 per cent. less than normal and 40 per cent. less than the annual death-rate, France was facing national extinction and the employment of nursing mothers as munition workers was strongly opposed by the Academy of Medicine. Much was accomplished by infant welfare units (400 strong) sent overseas by the Red Cross, under direction of William Palmer Lucas and operating over the whole area of France.

Improved sanitation was a coefficient in the prevention of typhoidal infections by trivalent vaccines, in the tetravaccines employed against typhoid, the two paratyphoids, and cholera. Remarkable success attended the treatment of burns by the paraffin-resin solution (ambrine) of Barthe de Sandifort (keritherapy[1]); the purification of army water-supplies; the localization of projectiles in the body by the

---

[1] Barthe: Jour. de méd. int., Par., 1913, xvii, 211–214.

Hirtz compass, the electrovibrator of Bergonié, and by the wholesale exploitation of Röntgenology; the application of wonderful prosthetic devices improvised to serve as artificial hands and limbs; and in the training of the badly mangled defectives, of the blind and deaf and of cardiac, pulmonary, and neurotic defectives for future efficiency in life.

The effects of the World War upon the civilian population of Europe were serious and lasted over a full decade. The people were keyed up to extreme phases of high nervous tension through the tremendous issues at stake, as evidenced by the great increase in heart disease, neurotic conditions, general mortality and the consequences of exaggerated sexuality or of atrophy of the gonads from starvation, fear and mental worry. In Germany, Friedrich Müller tells us, gout disappeared entirely with deficiency of meat, but the indigestible warbread, compounded of bran, turnips, potatoes and whole wheat, along with the subsequent reduction in diet to 1100–960 (officially 1350) calories, produced not only loss of weight, but muscular atrophy, loss of strength, and eventually hunger edema. There was general lowering of body temperature, pulse-rate, systolic blood-pressure and basal metabolism, with consequent lowering of bodily resistance and increased mortality among the aged, the infantile, the poor, the insane, the tubercular (50 to 90 per cent.), the pneumonic and of patients undergoing surgical operations. The starved could no longer keep their bodies warm, children ceased to play, infantile rickets increased eightfold, and a new kind of babies (*Kriegsneugeborene*) came into being, underdeveloped at birth, with symptoms of constant restlessness and automatic grasping movements. The German collapse in 1918 was, in part, due to starvation in the zone of the interior, which brought on revolution and its consequences. As time wore on, the illustrated and comic journals abounded in pictures of gaunt-faced men and extremely attenuated women, very different from the jolly, well-nourished Germans of old. In Vienna, Constantinople and the larger cities, the enriched profiteers fed well while the poor starved. The gentle, the refined, the learned were driven into menial employments and prostitution. In aid of the starving infants of Vienna, von Pirquet introduced feeding by "nems" (energy in 1 c.c. of milk), estimated by a height: weight ratio in place of calories (1917), and latterly "pelidisi" feeding. In the middle of the war, France faced depopulation through the general adult mortality and the employment of nursing mothers in the munition factories. Women became too indifferent or too excited to nurse their children. That the abnormal restlessness of recent people, at work or at play, is a neurotic phenomenon, engendered in part by wartime or post-bellum excitement, is self-evident, for similar manifestations were observable in the French Revolution or after the Napoleonic Wars. In Russia, the extreme phases of hypertension and apathy were exhibited on a gigantic scale.[1]

---

[1] W. H. Gantt: Brit. Med. Jour., Lond., 1924, i, 1055: ii, 336; 553: 1926, ii, 303; 747; 757; 802: 1927, ii, 739.

During the war period (1914–17), the two revolutions (1917), the resumption of war (1918–19), and the famine (1919–23), Russia suffered more from starvation, civil disorder, physical and mental suffering than all the other nations combined, exhibiting a higher mortality from disease than she had sustained from the World War and the subsequent bloodshed. During the famine period, 10,000,000 died of starvation alone, while the rest of Europe experienced a general decline in the death-rate after 1918. In 1919–20, the ration was 272–611 calories, which was raised to 1500 in 1921, while some 11,000,000 were fed by the American and British Relief Commissions. The mortality from hunger edema and hunger cachexia was 50 per cent. The starved ate berries, roots and leaves, fought over the carcasses of dead animals, and even came to cannibalism, which was witnessed by Gantt and the American relief officers. The mental effect was a singular apathy, inability to concentrate, weakened will power, impaired memory, loss of affection, compassion, and the desire to be clean. In the larger cities, learned professors shovelled snow and stood in the bread line while the less-favored tried to be put in jail to be rationed. Coincident with the second revolution and the famine was a gigantic incidence of communicable diseases. Typhus and relapsing fever were rare before 1914, but after the war (1914–17) affected 35,000,000. Cholera ran from 205,000 cases (1921) to 9 in 1925, and was exceeded only by the great Russian epidemic of 1892, which was also coincident with famine. Smallpox mounted to 166,000 cases in 1919. Malarial fever, always rampant in Russia, affected 3,170,547 people in 1914 and by 1922 had spread all over Russia, even to Archangel, the shores of the Arctic and the Caucasus (6500 feet above sea level). In 1923, there were 6,000,000 registered cases, probably a third of the actual number. The Anopheles now infests the huts of the peasants in winter time, and many infants are infected. Through scarcity of quinine, the mortality reached 40 per cent. in some areas. Cold, dampness, and lack of clothing were responsible for 30–50 per cent. mortality from measles during 1919–20, and scarlatina increased apace in 1922. Tuberculosis increased in all the combatant nations during and after the war, to be followed eventually by a lower death-rate from the killing off of chronics and susceptibles. In Leningrad, the rate fell from 50.7 (1920) to 29.8 (1927). Syphilis increased all over the civilized world in consequence of the war, as much as 20 per cent. in Germany (1923) and 80–95 per cent. in Russia during the same period (1922–23). There was no decrease in general paralysis in Russia, in spite of the omnipresence of malaria. The spread of venereal diseases was greatest among the young and was due to ignorance, illiteracy overcrowding, lack of drugs, and pansexuality. There was little among the educated classes, most of whom fled the country. Starvation, mental distraction, and fear produced impotence and amenorrhea, in the intelligent. Friedrich Müller states that both inanition and obesity (overfeeding) tend to produce atrophy of the gonads (sterility and impotence), as borne out by Stieve's experiments on animals (1922–6). Pavloff believes that the conditions which have undermined Russian society are due to the throwing down of all moral restraints, in other words, the psychotic effects of extreme sexual license and of the Freudian repressions are identical in the long run. In the neurotic, *les extrêmes se touchent*. The changes in the type and incidence of disease were extraordinary. Obesity, alcoholism, scurvy, diabetes, gout, drug habit, and gastritis, appendicitis, biliary disorders, and constipation disappeared, for excellent reasons. Pneumonia, typhoid fever, cancer, endocrine disorders and epilepsy remained stationary. There was marked increase of acute enteritis, peptic ulcer, visceral ptoses, noma, pyorrhea, flatulence and meteorism; of functional neuroses, and psychoses and neurasthenia, particularly in women and children; of circulatory disorders, particularly arteriosclerosis, hypertension, angina pectoris, and other cardiac disorders, which doubled in 1914–17, while anemia and dyspnea were almost universal and nephritis remained stationary. Tubal pregnancy, puerperal fever, and abortion have increased since 1918–19, but eclampsia remained stationary, with low mortality, in consequence of the effective Stroganoff treatment. Dirt, squalor, uncleanliness, lack of disinfectants and lowered bodily resistance brought about an enormous increase of surgical infections, dry gangrene, bed-sores, purulent tendovaginitis, varix, thrombophlebitis, and lymphangitis and operative wounds took months to heal. The rough, irritating food increased peptic ulcer six-fold (1920–22); gangrene necessitated many amputations, and the increase in gastric cancer stimulated new operative procedures. The general physical habitus became smaller and thinner, the features narrower, and sharper, and there was great increase in stillbirths and monsters. The way to reconstruction through the period following the organization of the Soviet government was long and tedious. The customs, institutions and economic organization of the old régime were entirely obliterated. Communism was applied to every person,

child or thing. There were practically no funds, food or fuel, no definite organization of agriculture or commerce. Trading was abolished and penalized and the
"N. E. P." ("New Economic Policy") of the Soviet (1921) activated little beyond
meagre rationing and running the hospitals. There was a distinct lack of drugs and
of doctors (1 : 5800), of whom one-third perished in the famine. Of medical schools,
there were three in Leningrad, two in Moscow, one each in Kiev, Odessa, Kazan,
Saratov, Kharkov (1805), Ekaterinoslav (1915), Perm (1917), Krasnodar (1924)
and the transferred faculties of Warsaw and Dorpat (Jurjev) at Rostov and Voronezh and no graduates during 1915–17. In 1922, 58 were graduated from the old
Military-Medical Academy and 136 out of 2481 students at the Leningrad Medical
Institute (founded 1917). One-tenth of Russian physicians in this period were women.
All grades and titles were abolished, the equivalent of an M. D. degree being a certificate of qualification granted on presentation of a thesis. Existing professors, necessarily Soviet-appointed, were retained unless counter-revolutionary. Before 1914
the maximum salary was about $300 monthly. During 1917–21, only rations were
given. In 1921, the N. E. P. allotted $5 monthly, which has since been raised to
$17.50 with a ration of 1500 calories (Pavloff's present compensation).

The social extravagances of Russian communism—religion as "a
popular opiate," free legalized abortion, automatic dissolution of marriage and, in consequence, great armies of deserted, homeless children
at large—have obtained before in history and will doubtless right themselves as the economic status of the people improves. Panmixia means
promiscuous population of the world from unfit material which Nature,
in turn, pitilessly destroys; and where marriage ceases to be, in the
words of the Roman law, "a partnership for things human and divine,"
with particular reference to the rearing of children, society is governed
from below, which, as Bismarck said, "cannot be," no more than
thinkers and scientists can be evolved *per saltum* out of social orders
"unused to thinking" (Robinson). The truth is that the main issues
of the period were economic rather than moral or intellectual, a necessary consequence of the wartime starvation. The dreams of the liberals
went down in ashes and tears,[1] and the peoples of Russia, Italy, Spain,
Poland, Hungary became virtual prisoners of war, under military
regimen, sometimes despotic, while the higher aims and aspirations of
the individual were scrapped for the bare necessities of food, raiment,
shelter and sexual gratification. The impact of the war was little felt
in America, but some of the end-results were similar, set off by the
general prosperity of the people, and have been well described by
recent novelists. Some European observers[2] have seen the amusing fashions of recent vintage, *e. g.*, extremist emancipation of women's heads
and legs, the assimilation of the elderly to the gracile, boyish flapper type,
Reformkleider resembling bags or sacks, the desire to be thin and to
appear young, exhibitionism (*Nackt-und Freiluftkultur*) and suchlike, as
neurotic consequences of the high tension of the war period, as with the
incroyables and *merveilleuses* of the French Revolution. The theater became a *tout à l'égout* and the murders, as Wells observes, are now "mostly
sexual." Followers of Spengler maintain that the present civilization
will run down and wear out in some 400 years. But, as Emerson observed, the *Zeitgeist* "is a nimble swimmer and snaps his fingers in the

---

[1] Survey, N. Y., Feb. 1, 1926 *passim*.   [2] Ramón y Cajal: Charlas de café, Madrid,1920.

face of laws." European humanity has weathered such things before and may outface and outpace the most dismal Jeremiads. The period is one of endless mechanical inventions which save labor but destroy leisure, in which the masculine rôle superimposed upon women in war was carried over into peace time, a period of Ångström units, synthetic clothes, shoes, foods, drugs and biological products, of micro-music, television, medical and hygienic *Rundfunksprachen*, medical consultations by wireless at sea, aëro-transportation, health insurance, illegitimate parents, paternity tests, artificial rejuvenation, mercerized silk, paper socks, shirts, and napkins and other advantages of the levelling effects of machinery. As we enter the machine age, the salient fact about medicine is the trend toward **socialization.** For the general practitioner, this means simply that, in consequence of the dearth of physicians in smaller communities and the high cost of hospitalization, he must live up to newer responsibilities, while public health nurses and social welfare workers, like the Feldshers of pre-war Russia, take over the care of doctorless areas. Sir Andrew McPhail very dourly and doughtily upholds the older traditions of Victorian England and Scotland.[1] But few people in modern life can save money, even for doctor's bills, hence become easy victims of cultists and quacks. It is argued that if the family doctor is now called upon to practice preventive medicine, in the sense of examining and instructing his clientèle with reference to avoiding diseases, he will lose none of his ancient glory or his income. The danger is, however, not so much with the true bedside physician, who is born, not made, but from the inevitable tussle between abuse of privilege, on one side, and inadequate or indifferent medical service on the other. It is fallacious to suppose that general medicine has kept pace with actual knowledge of communicable diseases, most of which are now preventable. The family doctor has been stripped of his personal infallibility, his likeness to a priest or a family solicitor, and is so busy that he is apathetic or indifferent to the burning questions of the hour. One of these is the delegation of medical and hygienic problems to laymen, uninstructed in either medicine or science, with the inevitable increase of meaningless paper work by complex "administration" and red-tape, which, it is said, has driven the best medical officers out of the health bureaus into the field and opens out the perspective of isolation or emergency hospitals with "a clerk-in-charge."

Moore, in his recent survey of American conditions,[2] says that at present some 1,019,500 persons are engaged in wholetime medical and hygienic activities in the United States, that disabling diseases cost two billion, decreased efficiency in industry two billion, hospitals five billion, drugs 700 million dollars annually, that we were fifty years behind Europe in securing adequate compensation laws to injured workmen (1910–20), and that medicine has not kept pace with recent social change and advancements in science, due to dearth of funds, personnel, physicians and hospitals, inability of many people to pay for medical treatment, inadequate incomes and hospital facilities and consequent indifference on the part of physicians. In consequence, 70 per cent. of hospital service is state supported, public, and pay clinics are increas-

[1] Macphail: Brit. Med. Jour., Lond., 1927, II, 373–380.

[2] H. H. Moore: American Medicine and the People's Health, New York, 1927.

ingly consulted, large industrial plants are supplying better medical service to their wage-earners than can be had in private life, most universities afford medical service with physical examinations, but health insurance, while compulsory in most European countries, is apparently too paternalistic for American wage-earners. There are apparently too many physicians in the cities, some of which are too healthy to support doctors, while there is distinct shortage in rural, isolated, and inaccessible areas. To offset this difficulty in rural New York, a bill providing for health centers (hospitalization and medical service) was drafted by Hermann M. Biggs (1920), and passed in modified form in 1923. Such centers now exist in East Harlem (1923), Boston (1924–27), Troy (1925), Oakland, Philadelphia, Cleveland and elsewhere. The medical center for New York City will comprise a 20-story State Building, the Columbia, Presbyterian, Sloan Maternity and Babies Hospitals, the Vanderbilt Clinic, and a Neurological Institute. It will be the salient experiment in social medicine. Laboratory service is now afforded by all the states of the Union. At the head stands the Hygienic Laboratory of the U. S. Public Health Service, with its effective output of scientific work and valuable publications. In 1925, some 618 private diagnostic laboratories reported to the American Medical Association. Of these 125 provided treatment. In 1924, twenty states were manufacturing and distributing biological products. The Children's Bureau (1912) of the Department of Labor administers the provisions of the Maternity and Infancy (Sheppard-Towner) Act (1921), the merits of which are still *subjudice*. The Chamberlain-Kahn Act for combating venereal diseases (1919) was utilized in gradually decreasing allotments out of $1,000,000 appropriation annually during 1919–27, after which no further appropriations were made. On June 30, 1927, the Bureau of Chemistry (Department of Agriculture) was abolished, and with it the administration of the Pure Food and Drugs Act (1906).

In England, recent legislation on infant and maternity welfare, *e. g.*, the Puerperal Fever and Puerperal Pyrexia Regulations (1926), the Ophthalmia Neonatorum Regulations (1926), the Midwives and Maternity Homes Act (1926), the Adoption of Children Act (1926), the Additional Rules of the Central Midwives Board (1927), and similar glosses superimposed upon the Maternity and Child Welfare Act of 1918, is described as "almost bewildering" in variety and extent. The Housing (Rural Workers) Act (1927) is an experiment, viable up to 1931.

Thus, there is not only lag and maladjustment of administrative machinery, but with a people so spontaneous as Americans, it may be scrapped or changed overnight if found too costly, or to conflict with social, political or personal moments of energy or inertia. The objections of conservative practitioners to socialized or standardized medicine are that the people have already been cozened, stultified, nagged and enslaved by a complex network of superimposed laws and regulations, which are not true codified expressions of total public sentiment, but defeat their own object by encouraging evasion, chicanery, hypocrisy, vice, vulgarity and corruption of the young; that to apply this principle to the practice of medicine is to degrade the physician to the level of a unionized vassal, destroy his individuality, encourage insolence of office and supercilious bureaucracy, with mere conventional handling or neglect of patients; in brief, to expose the science and art of medicine to the coxcombry of impertinent supervision by lay-meddlers of Citizen Fixit type. These are, indeed, grave objections, yet medicine owes much to discoveries of the non-medical, as also to the great manufacturing and power-producing plants of recent times; and doubtless the difficulty will be resolved by intelligent participation and coöperation of the doctor himself, who, it is argued, "is so wrapped up in practice that he does not know what is happening to him." In Germany, as far back as 1901, the difficulties with the *Kurierfreiheit* law (1869), compulsory panel practice, health insurance (1887), and the many physicians' strikes in the German cities, led to the organization of a protective league of physicians against the encroachments of state-management of medicine (*Hartmann-Bund*), organized by Hermann Hartmann (1863–1923), which issues a periodical (*Aerztliche Mitteilungen*, 1901–28) and has acquired a home of its own (1926). Yet since the war German medicine has moved rapidly in the direction of socialization, particularly in recent laws concerning the practice of medicine (Bavaria, 1927), the legalization of abortion (May 14, 1927), the emancipation of the prostitute from the controlled (1918) to the *vogelfrei* status (1927) and the public stations dispensing free advice and examination to couples contemplating matrimony or for the treatment of venereal disease. The intense interest of the people in social medicine came to a focus in the recent hygienic exposition (*Gesolei*) at Düsseldorf (1926), an essential folk-exhibition organized by Arthur Schlossmann, with the coöperation of local societies and many commercial plants, mobilizing the resources of the modern poster, diorama, film, dummy figure, model and transparent image in a most graphic and effective way. The Cattaraugus Health Demonstration (1927) is an American experiment in the same trend.[1] The opposition between mechanized medicine (*Kaninchenmedizin*) and orthodox bedside practice has been ably discussed by Bier, Sauerbruch, Much and other leading spirits, particularly Erwin Liek,[2] who files a strong brief for the ethical aspect of Hippocratic medicine, with its implication that, at the bedside, science is not an end, but a means to an end; as against machine-diagnosis, perfunctory paper-work (panel practice) on 90 to 100 people *per diem*, with consequent envisaging of the patient as a mere routine *numero*, or otherwise as an interesting case or *Versuchsthier*. In the view of Sauerbruch, a theorist is not a practitioner, while Trendelenburg argues that the difficulty is not between physician and medical (laboratory) man, but between good and bad doctors. The mere sacro-sanctity of the doctor *quâ* physician is thus disappearing. The profession will become more and more self-critical as to the inclusion of incompetent or unscrupulous representatives, without recourse to de Kruif's expedient of "anti-physician." Fishbein[3] points out that the fallacy in "selling medicine to the public" is that the people are already oversold as to luxuries, cannot pay for necessities, and so fall into exploitation by quacks. Sauerbruch argues that intuition, apart from talent for observation, must be inborn in the true Asclepiad and opposes Sigerist's view that any given medical student is plastic material, awaiting only a moulder or carver. To have no specific talent for bedside practice is, however, not necessarily to be a *raté* and Cushing has taken an able lead in encouraging some of his students to take up medical journalism, editorial duties and other lines.

---

[1] See Sir Arthur Newsholme: The New York Health Demonstrations, New York, 1927.

[2] E. Liek: Der Arzt und seine Sendung, München, 1926.

[3] M. Fishbein: Socialized medicine, Nation, N. Y., 1928, cxxvi, 484–486.

Panel practice leads to careless prescribing from a merely perfunctory routine attitude toward patients, and it is argued that unless sanitary and social welfare arrangements are simple and well considered enough to be automatic, they are a public nuisance. With the exception of work emanating from Pavloff's Reflex Tower at Leningrad, nearly all the Russian medical journals are preoccupied with socialized medicine. The famine, and the consequent ravages of disease, necessitated a giant organization, the watchwords of which are the deification of science, religion as a popular opiate, good opera, and health for the masses.

Connected with the Peoples' Commissariat of Public Health (1918) are the Soviet Central Scientific Institute of Public Health (1919), comprising Institutes of Protozoan Diseases (1918), of communicable diseases (1918), for control of sera and vaccines (1919), of physiological nutrition (1919), of hygiene (1919), of biochemistry (1921), of microbiology (1921), of experimental biology (1921), and of tuberculosis (1922). There are hospital provisions for up to 250,000 beds, but only one physician per 20,000 people in areas of 50 square kilometers, which are usually doctored by Feldshers. The Röntgen Institute at Leningrad (under Professor Nemeneff) the largest in Europe, handles a tremendous clientèle and turns out 40,000 x-ray plates daily. There is a Health Resort Clinic, where the indications for balneological treatment are taught and whence patients are sent to mineral stations, usually at state or industrial expense. In like manner, the National Public Health Department of Moscow is fused with seven other institutions devoted to bacteriology, protozoology, chemistry, pharmacology, serum-control, and a Biophysical Institute, under Professor Lazareff. An Ethnopark displays figures of all the Russian races in groups. There are separate institutes for physical culture and industrial diseases, 25 stationary and 80 mobilized exhibits of various kinds, 26 dispensaries for ambulatory cases, handling 1000 patients each *per diem*, a large Venereal Dispensary, 25 Diet Kitchens for Diabetics and Dyspeptics, and night asylums (sanatoria) for vagrants. Of 33,000 physicians, some 29,500 are virtual chattels of the state, at salaries of $20—$65 monthly, most of the doctors being "country-shy" on account of the dreary isolation of the rural districts and the vast distances to be travelled in practice. The medical faculties have been increased from 7 to 24, but the students come from the peasantry and the industrial proletariate since the migration of the intelligentsia and have no preliminary training whatever. In the five-year courses, the first three years are devoted to the basic disciplines, with laboratory work. The last two to clinical work, but an additional year in hospital is planned. Time is wasted on social hygiene and the political theory of Soviet organization. State examinations were minimized in wartime and abolished after the Revolution. All titles being abolished, graduates receive certificates of qualification and a diploma licensing to practice. Lenin's Central Committee for Improvement of the Condition of Teachers and Scholars (*Zekubu*) rations, pensions, and finds places for thousands, and has a magnificent marble casino.

The most effective of the Soviet methods of exploiting public, rural and personal hygiene is by way of brilliant polychrome posters, which, after the fashion of Indian picture-writing or the tavern sign, warn the illiterate peasantry as to the dangers of quackery, venereal diseases, industrial accidents, abortion, and sepsis. The main argument objected against Leninized medicine, with its countless institutes, laboratories and folk-exhibits, its ways of handling abortion, marriage, venereal disease and tuberculosis, is that it is overcentralized. All sanitary arrangements are directed by one popular ministry, under Dr. Semaschko. But it is in Russia that the great future problems of social medicine will be tried out on a grand scale.

The status of **medical education** since the war has been carefully studied by **Abraham Flexner** (1925[1]).

At the start, he stresses the increasing trend toward elimination of superstition and speculation, the stationary, uncritical status of empirical medicine and the necessity of viewing clinical observation and laboratory experimentation as coequal, if medical education is to retain a scientific quality. Medical problems, as Gay observes, arise at the bedside and are answered largely in the laboratory, but scientific method must not operate in a vacuum and the defects of English, French, German, and American medical education spring from their origins, viz., clinically, around hospitals, from the incorporation of medicine in the medieval university curriculum as a branch of philosophy (*Physica*) and in the case of American medicine, empirically and caravan-wise, out of post-colonial pioneering. There are thus three kinds of medical schools, the clinical (English and French), university (German), and the proprietary (early American). In consequence, English students were followers of some clinical master. French students were hampered by the bureaucratic barrier of *agrégation*, the *concours* and lack of laboratory facilities. German medicine was obfuscated by philosophising until the advent of university clinics and laboratories, was temporarily demoralized by the crass materialism of the pre-war period and now lacks funds for progressive work. American medical education was shiftless, heterogenous, multifarious (over 500 schools) and is still affected by sectarianism, competition along futile lines, politics and the narrowing effects of favoritism and inbreeding, which Flexner illustrates by the fact that in North European medicine there is no such favored being as a Berlin, Leyden, or Stockholm "man."

American clinical instruction was below the University grade, but following the arguments of Mall and Barker, the full-time idea was introduced at the Hospital of the Rockefeller Institute (1909), whole-time chairs in medicine, surgery, pediatrics, obstetrics, and psychiatry were established at the Johns Hopkins Medical School (1913), and there are now more than 30 full-time clinical chairs in the United States, Canada, and England. In preliminary medical education, Latin is requisite in German, French, and Danish schools, not so in Holland, Sweden, Russia, England and the United States, where actual training of the mind has become very superficial and uneven since the war. American medical students have, further, no training in foreign languages and little proficiency in the use of English. French medical training puts the raw student into the clinic directly upon matriculation and keeps him at it for five years along with other studies, a process which is wasted upon students with no particular aptitude for bedside practice. English medical schools have latterly adopted the "block" system, whereby the student cannot take up anatomy and physiology without preliminary grounding in chemistry and physics, nor pass on to clinical work without absolving the basic disciplines. This plan is followed, with some modifications, in Germany, Austria, Holland, Belgium, Switzerland, and Denmark. In Sweden, the basic disciplines, laboratory branches, and clinics are sharply separated and taken each at a time, the courses lasting from six to twelve years.

In Denmark, a very clever modification of the French system seems effective, namely attendance of clinics by first-year students, which is not resumed until two years later. German clinical instruction still fails through the predominance of demonstrative exposition over actual participation. In America, success will turn largely upon the acquisition of university hospitals by medical faculties which is now in progress. Laboratory training has naturally fallen off in war-worn Europe, through lack of funds, and hardly anywhere has the practical exercise won entirely over the didactic lecture and the demonstrative exposition. American medical education is marred by over-organization, or what Flexner calls the "passion for attending to details in mechanical and standardized fashion," but is very unequal, ranging from best to worst, and attempts to do too much for the student who discovers that "medicine is difficult to learn and impossible to teach." In consequence of the higher cost of living, the amounts devoted to medical education in the budgets of various American universities have increased anywhere from 100 to 900 per cent. since the war, and have been tripled in England and Canada; but, on the continent, salaries and budgets have decreased (in Germany) or have been merely scaled to cover the decreased purchasing power of money (in France). The price of laboratories has increased 40–50 per cent. in Germany and 70 per cent. in England.

---

[1] A. Flexner: Medical Education, New York, 1925.

It is thus due to lack of funds and facilities for experimentation that we find continental Europeans turning to such comparatively sterile fields as the constitution, characterology, eidetics, racial hygiene, the vagaries of psycho-analysis or pedagogics and the maunderings of **"medical philosophy,"** which, far from helping toward "the logical clarification of thoughts," seems as confusing and unrewarding as in the days of Hegel and Schelling. It is, however, an expression of the difficulty voiced by W. J. Mayo, that the profession has on hand, at present, too much knowledge, cannot keep pace with it, and needs to have it organized. Among those who continue to darken counsel by words without wisdom are the fabricators of medical theories, most of them as old as the hills, the adjudicators between vitalism and materialism (both meaningless terms), those who maintain the Columbian origin of syphilis and the votaries of cultism, from the pretended diagnosis of diseases by the iris (*Augendiagnose*) to the amazing examples of non-medical follies ridiculed by Fishbein. In striking contrast is the splendid practical assistance rendered to medicine and hygiene by the great industrial and manufacturing plants, notably those of Henry S. Wellcome (London), Bayer (Elberfeld), Schering, Zeiss, Edison, Eastman, Pullman, the United States Radium Corporation, the United Fruit Company (tropical medicine), and the medical publishers. A salient feature of the recent brilliant output of experimental medicine is the rapid development of a large number of talented **women as investigators,** *e. g.*, among Americans, following Mary Putnam Jacobi, who won a Paris Faculty medal for her thesis on acid and neutral fats (1870), the late Mme. Déjerine (neurology), Maude Slye (cancer), Florence Sabin (hematology), Alice Hamilton (industrial medicine), Gladys Dick (scarlatina), Dorothy Reed (Hodgkin's disease), Ruth Tunnicliff (measles, meningitis), Margaret Lewis (mitochondria), Alice C. Evans (Brucella), Anna Williams (diphtheria), Martha Wollstein (serology), Louise Pearce (experimental medicine), Lydia and Louise Rabinovich (bacteriology; resuscitation), Clara Jacobson (trophic nerves), Mary Swartz Rose (food chemistry), Lydia De Witt (pathology), Amy Daniels (nutrition), Katharine M. Howell (serology), Nina Simmonds (biochemistry), Josephine B. Neal (meningitis, encephalitis), Miss N. M. Stevens (embryology); in England, Janet Lane-Claypon (ovarian hormones), Ida Smedley (fat-metabolism), Harriette Chick (proteins), and in Canada, Maude Abbott (congenital malformations of heart). Among those who have been promotors of infant welfare are Mary Lowell Putnam (Boston), Jane Addams (Chicago), Julia C. Lathrop (Washington), S. Josephine Baker (New York), Ellen C. Babbitt (New York), Lillian Welsh (Baltimore), Janet Lane-Claypon (London), Janet Campbell (Liverpool), and Helen MacMurchy (Toronto).

A matter of concern to **preventive medicine** is the remarkable increase in mortality from heart disease, pneumonia, nephritis, cancer, and tuberculosis.

51

Recent statistics from the Department of Commerce show that of 1,285,927 deaths occurring in about 90 per cent. of our population during 1926 (as against 1,219,019 for the total 1925 registration), 209,370 were from heart disease as against 191,226 in 1925, 107,797 from pneumonia, 103,332 from nephritis, 99,833 from cancer and 91,568 from tuberculosis. The increase in cardiac disease is in part attributable to the high tension at which recent people live or are required to live, that in pneumonia to exposure and scanty attire in our changeable climate, that in nephritis to nation-wide consumption of poisonous alcoholic brews and decoctions, that in cancer to the fact that, since normal expectation of life has increased from thirty-five (1825) to fifty-five years (1925), more people survive to the age of cancer-incidence.

Concern about **cancer** has led to the formation of many societies, institutes and periodicals devoted to the subject. National conferences, such as that held at Lake Mohonk (1926), illuminate the difficulties implicit in the idea of preventing a disease which appears to be the effect of irritation of any kind superimposed upon a diathesis in which the Mendelian dominant (resistance) has been overcome by the recessive (susceptibility) through accidental or transmitted mutation (Maude Slye). Control of **tuberculosis** is largely a matter of increase of material prosperity, better food, more creature comforts, and is credited with forwarding early diagnosis, the open-air life, public health nursing, coördinated study of major diseases the world over, sanitary and life-extension surveys and other phases of concerted attack by all manner of specialists (Welch). The problem of the respiratory affections is still in the "sparingly soluble" state. In consequence of better material conditions and better knowledge of nutritional requirements, **infant mortality** has been reduced 50 per cent. since 1908, and is now less a matter of diarrhea and enteritis than of premature births from faulty ante-natal hygiene and obstetrics. The problem of **birth-control,** a guaranteed right of European women, turns upon two words in Section 211 of the Penal Code, a result of the Comstock Bill, passed on February 11, 1873, against the express warning of Senator Conkling that it might not express the codified will of the people.[1] Still's recent work on "place in family as a cause of disease" (1927[2]) verifies Karl Pearson's findings as to the handicaps of the first born. A first pregnancy is a risk to the child, but congenital defects or lowered resistance to disease are not repeated in families, whence the right of women to "space their babies" or to see that they come into the world (if at all) under the best hygienic and economic conditions. Weir Mitchell said that the treatment of neurasthenia and neuroses should begin in the preceding generation. The dreadful hardships and exposure to disease of our pioneers in the backwoods, which Hektoen has so effectively described,[3] are partly responsible for "worn-out stock," a fact which led Oliver Wendell Holmes to his famous paradox: Whether the American Continent is capable of sustaining life? This paradox of poor health, fragile physique, and general debility in a rich, fertile country was, in fact, the

[1] Mary Ware Dennett: Birth Control Laws, New York, 1926.

[2] G. F. Still: Lancet, London, 1927, ii, 795; 853.

[3] K. Gjerset and L. Hektoen: Norwegian-Am. Histor. Assoc. Stud. & Rec., Minneapolis, 1926, i, 1–59.

theme stressed by Lemuel Shattuck in his famous report of 1850. The newer generation starts under sanitary conditions more favorable for improved vigor.

Some lift to the cause of **international hygiene** was attained at the International Convention of Health of the League of Nations at Geneva (May, 1926), at which disinfestation against typhus on the Russian frontier, smallpox quarantine (vaccination) in Greece, regulation of Danube traffic, the establishment of a headquarters for Eastern sanitation at Singapore, station-grown cinchona, telegraphic notification of oncoming epidemics, mapping of national disease-incidence, opium conferences and the establishment of a great clearing-house of sanitary information at Geneva were considered. The close studies of the incidence of cholera in the Punjab by Sir Leonard Rogers (1927–8[1]) and of bubonic plague in the same area by Lieut. Col. W. H. C. Forster (1927) are in the same trend. Rogers recommends preventive inoculation of all pilgrims leaving Punjab districts for fairs and Forster holds that vaccination against plague, which is only voluntary at the peak of an epidemic, should be planned and executed four months ahead, since the peak (March–May) is dependent upon flea-reproduction, which again turns upon humidity and is negligible in dry seasons. In Egypt, the gigantic quarantine station at El Tor sets an effective cordon for thousands of pilgrims, continuing the work in which Clot-Bey, Pruner-Bey and Ruffer were so efficient. For ages, Asia has been the matrix of the major epidemics and China has endemic areas of all manner of diseases. The sanitation of these vast areas, if attainable, is one of the big problems of the future.

Since the war, there has been a growing sentiment in favor of Kant's ideal of universal peace, set off by endemic outbursts of warfare at intervals all over the globe. The conclusion is obvious; indeed, Ramón y Cajal affirms that since civilized man required millions of years to attain to his present estate, it will take an equal period of time for the finer anatomy of the brain to become specialized up to the pacificist ideal. As with individuals, wars are "wished" upon peaceful, friendly (and therefore defenceless) nations, never upon those keen and able to defend themselves. Yet wars never settled anything and, like revolutions, are merely agencies for transformations of energy and transfers of power. The recent war effected the transvaluations predicted by Nietzsche, the "changing morality" of "sinners purged of conscience and made happy in their sinning . . . the strong made to exult, the weak robbed of their old sad romance."[2] Several English novelists have recently glorified murder, and our latter-day huzzies despatch their lords like the ladies in Brantôme—*en le tuant virilement de ses propres mains*. The salient note is that of Mencken's "beauty-hating races," and of the traits signalized by anthropologists as the immemorial hall-marks of the peasant—"envy, malice and greed." Triumph of peasant *mes-*

---

[1] Rogers: Indian Med. Research Mem.; Calcutta, 1928, No. 9.   [2] H. L. Mencken.

quinerie means necessarily ridicule of *noblesse oblige* and of the ancient
ideals of the past.[1] The decline of a civilization is like Pitt-Rivers'
account of the extinction of the Polynesian population[2] by the disappearance of their ancestral traditions, with consequent ascendancy of
purely animal instincts. Hundreds of young people, unequal to the
conflict between early training, older ideals and the newer conditions,
have gone down in suicide and worse things, and, as stated, many
recent neurotic and cardiac manifestations of disease are attributable
to the same cause. Poor Otto Weininger's mad ravings against the
"coitus-cult" are set off by the *vantardise* of the senile and the neurotic.
Much of the recent American furore about the natural function of sex
was a kind of compensatory hypertrophy against prohibition, a *naïf*
discovery of "Little Jack Horner" type. As the lady in Elmer Davies'
novel observes: "Everybody talks sex now but some people are still a
little afraid of it. A formula for being sexual and moral at the same
time would sell like anti-fat tablets." Apart from venery, the problem
of the venereal diseases turns, as Crookshank has so ably shown,[3] upon
the simple fact that the sentiment of honor, never very plentiful anywhere, becomes a vanishing fraction in a democratic society. As
medical officers of armies know, physicians could stop venereal disease
if all persons were activated by personal honor. These are some of the
problems which confront socialized medicine.

   The medicine of the future is beset by the pitfalls of mass-production, commercialism, newspaper exploitation, the soullessness of corporations, the deification of corporations, the conflict between group-
medicine and specialization, the natural lawlessness engendered by
complex regulations and regimentation, the periodic flights into mysticism to which the human mind is liable and the human tendency of
patients to flock to quacks and cultists when orthodox medicine, and
above all, its many specialists, fail to help or to heal. But the signs
of change are everywhere apparent. Billroth maintained that internal
medicine must become more surgical. The surgeon of today is becoming more and more of an internist. Some, indeed, affirm that
medicine is destined to be dissipated into mere phasic aspects of
chemistry, physics, microbiology or the other disciplines upon which
it rests. Rather is recent scientific medicine like the newer music (of
tones instead of familiar notes), a matter of vibrations discernible only
to the "inner ear," and which await synthesis and orchestration into
the majestic symphony which may very well be for the people of the
future. With fine insight, Hans Much has declared the spirit of bedside medicine (the "Art" of Hippocrates) to be, first of all, ethical:
Ueber Hippocrates sprechen heisst über das Wesen der Medizin sprechen.
He who does not feel this truth is not to be envied, for whatever else
he may be, he is assuredly no physician, has no perception of the long

---

[1] Der Bauer ist ein Schelm und wenn er schläft des Mittags. German proverb.

[2] G. H. L. Pitt-Rivers: The Clash of Culture, London, 1927.

[3] F. G. Crookshank: Brit. Jour. Vener. Dis., Lond., 1926, ii, 36–50.

foreground in which medicine was "the foster mother of all the sciences," as it has latterly become the most potent agent of civilization the world has known. It is in this spirit that a great physician once said that love of his profession had elevated and sustained him, when all else had turned to dust and ashes—

> "With wide embracing love
> Thy spirit animates eternal years,
> Pervades and broods above,
> Changes, sustains, dissolves, creates and rears."

It is true that some physicians are vain, self-seeking, of the prima donna type, and there be others of the medieval category of *die Heil-ärzte welche heilen nicht, Heilärtze welche krank Machen*. Since the war, crime has not been entirely unknown in the medical profession. In an entirely honorable spirit, the German medical periodicals have recently posted instances of physicians who practised thuggee and dacoity methods upon their patients and the doctor as "rough-neck" has appeared upon the American stage, a far cry from the big, humanitarian spirit of such recent men as Charcot, Pasteur, Lister, Osler, Metchnikoff, Ehrlich, who may be said to have envisaged the entire human race as their virtual patients. The ethical spirit is, therefore, the Palladium, the soul of medicine, the *consecratio medici*—

> "And when it fails, fight as we will, we die;
> And while it lasts, we cannot wholly end."

It is with this thought in mind that Sudhoff has said: "Medicine is a sacred calling and he who makes it ridiculous is guilty of sacrilege." Implicit in the original definition of things sacred (*sacra*) is the ancient idea that a curse as well as a blessing attaches to them. The physician has shed the assumption of sacerdotal or pontifical infallibility which obscured his vision in the past; but his feeling for the ethical requirements of his profession should be, as Sudhoff says, a sacred thing.[1]

In the face of much irresponsible writing about the "science of medicine" and its probable future, it is well to consider the serious commentary of Wunderlich[2] seventy years ago (1858), which could not be improved upon today:

"The medicine of our era has no use for pathologic dogmas, realizing, as it does, that nothing can be known of organic changes if the nature of the changes themselves is not understood. It accepts neither an exclusively humoral nor an exclusively solidist pathology, since fluids and solids are both parts of the organism. It declines to draw analogies from chemical hypotheses unless the combinations and dissolutions of substance can be followed up and elucidated in the sick patient. It cherishes no fancy that the limits of visibility can unveil the secret of life, but it regards no

---

[1] See, on this head, the "sittliche Förderung" of W. Gmelin in: Arch. f. Rassen.- u. Gesellschaftsbiol., München, 1927–28, xx, 28–51.

[2] C. A. Wunderlich: Geschichte der Medizin, Stuttgart, 1859, 364–366. Translated by Dr. Albert Allemann.

fact as worthless, whether attaching to gross anatomy or to the minutest particles of the body. It sees the human patient as an organism which cannot be too thoroughly studied, and in so far as it aims to be the science of disease, no more and no less, present-day medicine may be called physiological.

"If our science admits of no domination by its basic or subordinate branches, with even greater energy does it resent outside interference. For it has ceased to discuss problems which, whatever their general importance, bear no relation to its own field of observation. Transcendental problems lie beyond its scope and for them it has neither a reply nor a solution. Toward such, it has the right to maintain a strict, if respectful, neutrality. No one, more than the physician, is convinced that the needs of the human mind are beyond all knowledge of nature; no one is more penetrated with the duty of respecting peace of mind and happiness in the possession of ideal things as sacred. Those who, neglecting this fact, have penetrated into fields foreign to natural science, cease thereby to be natural scientists. Natural science must content itself with as much of truth as is contained in natural phenomena, and that part is not small. . . . But no one today is so vain as to regard himself as infallible. And modern science, which can never be too rigorous in method and acid tests, is tolerant of concrete conclusions, if based upon sound principles and demonstrable fact. There is, therefore, no longer any dogmatic or doctrinal method of healing, but anything is admissible or justifiable if based upon methodically ascertained facts or, failing these, upon conscientious consideration of reality. . . It is true that in recent times, a dilettante interest in nature has become fashionable and so much has the reading of scientific articles in periodicals and attendance upon popular lectures become a self-imposed cult that it would seem, at first sight, as if the physician's duties had been lightened thereby. With the best intentions, many physicians have even attempted to educate the people as to the achievements as well as the aims of science. But let us at least have no illusions as to lay views of natural science, particularly with reference to the findings of medicine. In an age of table-tipping and ghostly communications, no one can regard public opinion as ripe enough to pass upon natural phenomena. . . . If the physician should sometimes suffer from injustice and misunderstanding, should his honest work be now and then ignored or even sneered at, he must bear in mind that in the majestic eye of Nature, the individual is nothing. And however depressed he may feel when intriguers and mountebanks blow about their ephemeral successes, he may be sure that these upstarts will be overtaken, in the end, by the Erinnyes of conscience. For natural science is a proud, silently advancing power, of whose might the spheres most threatened by it have hardly a notion. Just its singularity and its grandeur is that it showers its gifts upon friends and foes and scoffers alike, that it conquers and maintains its dominion by its blessings, as it noiselessly subdues and dissolves unreason.

"What then is the future, the distant aim of medicine? Its bases, as far as valid, are imperishable. But it is the characteristic of natural science that it is illimitable, enlarges its spheres of investigation as it advances. What will be its future problems? No one can tell. But so much is certain: the future work of medicine lies neither in exclusively physical nor chemical investigation, nor in the shaping of neuropathology nor in hematology, nor cytology, nor in super-subtle diagnosis, nor in the rehabilitation or rediscovery of therapeutic principles. The future aim of medicine is that of any other science and identical with that of medicine at all times: It is the task of seeking and finding the truth, whatever and wherever it is and by whatsoever ways it may be found."

To the younger generation this old-fashioned pronouncement, like Beethoven's music, now "a voice from another world," may seem academic, outmoded, *geheimrätlich*. But it affords an excellent corrective for our natural human tendency to form hasty, shallow and superficial judgments from a mere folding spy-glass view of the complex conditions around and about us, namely, the passing of the older order of things, the advent of a newer world, as yet "powerless to be born," of which Anatole France observed: *L'avenir est caché même à ceux qui le font.* We see the grave, serious Wunderlich, imbued with the ancient Hippocratic tradition, pursuing these reveries, in the quiet habit of his life; but what he really says is: "Wherever the art of medicine is loved, there also is love for humanity."[1] The aim of modern medicine, coördinate with the advancement of all the sciences, is the prediction and control of phenomena, the prevention as well as the cure of disease. Preventive and social medicine can and should have no fairer ideal than that of the beautiful sentence of Minot: "We have enthroned science in the imagination, but we have crowned her with modesty, for she is at once the reality of human power and the personification of human fallibility."

---

[1] Hippocrates: Precepts, vi (Littré, ix, 258).

APPENDICES

I. CHRONOLOGY OF MEDICINE AND PUBLIC HYGIENE

B. C.

7000–2000. Neolithic Age in Europe (Osborn).

5000–4500. Dawn of Sumerian, Egyptian and Minoan cultures.

3400–2500. Old Kingdom: Egypt (Breasted).

2980.　Im-hotep.

2900–2625. Age of the Pyramid builders (Breasted).

2697.　Huang-ti.

2500.　Surgical operations depicted upon tomb of Pharaohs at Saqquarah.

2445–1731. Middle Kingdom: Egypt (Breasted).

2250.　**Code Hammurabi** (Babylon).

2000–1000. Bronze Age in Europe (Osborn).

1580–1200. New Empire: Egypt (Breasted).

1500.　**Ebers Papyrus.**

1300.　Berlin Papyrus.

1000–500. Earlier Iron Age (Halstatt culture) in Europe.

950.　Homer.

800.　Period of Brahminic medicine.

776.　First Olympiad.

753.　Founding of Rome.

639–544. Thales of Miletus.

600.　Massage and acupuncture practised by the Japanese.

　Lex regia (post-mortem Cæsarean section).

590.　Tarquinius Priscus begins canalisation of Rome (Cloaca Maxima).

585.　Eclipse of sun as predicted by Thales (May 28).

580–489. **Pythagoras.**

532.　Eupalinus of Megara tunnels water-supply of Samos from Leucothean Spring.

522.　Democedes founds a medical school at Athens.

504–443. **Empedocles.**

500.　Later Iron Age (La Tène culture).

500–428. Anaxagoras.

494.　Ædiles (sanitary police) in Rome.

490.　Battle of Marathon.

480.　Thermopylæ and Salamis.

461–430. Age of Pericles.

460–370. **Hippocrates.**

449.　Roman Law of the Twelve Tables.

435–432. Meton reforms calendar (365 days).

431–404. Peloponnesian War.

430–425. **Plague of Athens.**

429–347. Plato.

400.　Thucydides describes plague at Athens.

384–322. **Aristotle.**

370–286. **Theophrastus of Eresos.**

370.　Herbal of Diocles of Carystos.

338–323. Alexander the Great.

331.　Foundation of Alexandria.

323–30. Ptolemies.

312.　Censorship of Appius Claudius; **first Roman aqueduct** (*Aqua Appia*) constructed (11 miles).

310–250. **Erasistratus.**

300.　**Alexandrian School.** Euclid.

272–269. Aqueduct of 43 miles (*Anio Vetus*) constructed under Manius Curius Dentatus.

280.　**Herophilus.**

212.　Archimedes killed at capture of Syracuse.

180.　Aqueduct to Pergamon constructed under Eumenes II.

146.　Siege of Corinth.

144–140. Marcian Aqueduct (*Aqua Marcia*) constructed (61.75 miles) under Quintus Marcius Rex.

125.	Aqua Tepula (11 miles) completed under censorship of Cæpio and Longinus.
124.	**Asclepiades of Prusa (Bithynia) born.**
120–63.	Mithridates.
100.	**Central heating in Rome.**
99–55.	Lucretius: *De rerum natura.*
81–58.	Apollonius of Kitium.
80.	Mithridates, King of Pontus, experiments with poisons.
59.	Julius Caesar orders publication of *Acta diurna.*
50.	Themison.
45.	Sosigenes introduces Julian Calendar (365¼ days).
33.	Aqua Julia (15½ miles), Aqua Virgo (14 miles) constructed under Marcus Vipsanius Agrippa.
31 B. C.–14 A. D.	Augustus Cæsar; Augustan Aqueduct (*Aqua Alsietina*) constructed.
30 B. C.–476 A. D.	Roman period in Egypt.
24.	Prevalence of heat-stroke ends Arabian campaign of Aelius Gellius (Dio Cassius, LIII, 29).
18.	Vipsanius Agrippa constructs Aqueduct of Nîmes (Pont du Gard).

A. D.

14–37.	Tiberius. Celsus.
21.	Roman baths (*thermæ*) opened by Vipsanius Agrippa.
23–79.	Pliny the Elder.
38–52.	Aqua Claudia (46 miles) and Anio Novus (58 miles) begun under Caligula and completed under Claudius.
45.	Scribonius Largus.
50.	Athenæus of Attila (founder of Pneumatic School) devises method of filtering water.
54–68.	Nero. Dioscorides.
79.	Plague following eruption of Vesuvius.
97.	Sextus Julius Frontius publishes book on Roman water-supply (*De aquis urbis Romæ*)
98–117.	Trajan. **Rufus of Ephesus.**
97.	Sextus Julius Frontius appointed water inspector (*Curator aquarum*) in Rome.
109.	Aqua Trajana (36½ miles) completed under Trajan.
117–138.	Hadrian. **Aretæus. Soranus of Ephesus.**
	Aretæus describes leprosy, tetanus, diabetes and diphtheria (*ulcera Syriaca*)
125.	Plague of Orosius.
131–201.	**Galen.**
146.	Destruction of Corinth.
150.	Ptolemy (geocentric astronomy).
164–180.	Plague of Antoninus.
220.	Archagathus practices in Rome.
226.	Alexander Severus constructs Aqua Alexandrina (14 miles).
251–266.	Plague of Cyprian.
302.	Eusebius, Bishop of Cæsarea, describes Syrian epidemic of **smallpox.**
303.	Martyrdom of Saints Cosmas and Damian.
325–403.	**Oribasius.**
335.	Constantine closes the Asclepieia and other pagan temples.
369.	**Hospital of St. Basil** erected at Cæsarea by Justinian.
375.	Plague Hospital at Edessa.
395–1453.	Byzantine Empire.
400.	**Fabiola founds first nosocomium in Western Europe.**
476.	Fall of Western Roman Empire.
480–524.	Boëthius.
480–544.	St. Benedict of Nursia.
490–575.	Cassiodorus.
493–526.	Reign of Theodoric the Great.
500.	Theodoric builds aqueduct for Spoleto (Umbria).
507–711.	Visigoths in Spain.
525–605.	**Alexander of Tralles.**
527–565.	Justinian I. **Aëtius of Amida.**
528.	**Monte Cassino founded** (by Benedict of Nursia).
538–593.	Gregory of Tours.
542.	Nosocomia founded at Lyons by Childebert I and at Arles by Cæsarius
543.	Plague of Justinian.
568–774.	Establishment of Lombards in Italy.
569.	Tabari describes appearance of smallpox at the siege of Mecca.
570.	Marius, Bishop of Avenches, employs the term "variola."
571–632.	Mohammed.

580.	Hospital at Merida founded by Bishop Masona.
	Epidemic quinsy (*esquinancie*) mentioned in Chronicle of St. Denis.
581.	Gregory of Tours describes smallpox epidemic at Tours.
583.	Council of Lyons interdicts migration of lepers.
590.	Epidemic of St. Anthony's fire (ergotism) in France.
600.	Aaron describes smallpox in his *Pandectæ*.
610.	Hospital of St. John the Almsgiver at Ephesus.
622.	Mohammed's Hegira.
625–690.	Paul of Ægina.
639–968.	Mohammedan period in Egypt (Eastern Caliphate).
644.	Edict of Rotharus, King of Lombardy, for segregation of lepers.
651.	Hôtel-Dieu founded by Saint Landry, Bishop of Paris (first mentioned 829).
675.	Monastic records of smallpox in Ireland.
732.	Battle of Poitiers.
	Museum "Shoso-in" founded at Nara (Japan).
738.	School of Montpellier founded.
749–1258.	Eastern Caliphate.
768–814.	Charlemagne.
776–856.	Hrabanus Maurus.
786–802.	Reign of Harun al-Rashid.
793.	Famine and high mortality in England (Anglo-Saxon Chronicle).
794.	St. Albans Hospital (England).
799.	Coronation of Charlemagne.
809–873.	Joannitius.
820–1517.	Rise of Venetian Republic.
825.	Xenodochium at Mont St. Cenis.
827.	Walafrid Strabo composes his *Hortulus* (poem on the medicinal plants in the cloister garden at Reichenau).
829.	Hôtel-Dieu (Paris) first mentioned.
830.	Monastic infirmary at St. Gall.
830–920.	Isaac Judæus.
848–856.	School of Salerno first heard of.
856.	Epidemic angina at Rome (Baronius).
857–884.	Bertharius, Abbot of Monte Cassino.
860–932.	Rhazes (smallpox and measles).
871–901.	Alfred the Great.
897–899.	Three years' mortality of men and cattle in England (Danish Invasion).
898.	Soror founds Hospital of Santa Maria della Scala at Siena.
962.	Hospice St. Bernard.
968.	St. Conrad's Hospital at Constance (Switzerland) founded.
969–1171.	Fatimite Caliphate (Egypt).
980–1036.	Avicenna.
1004.	Epidemic suffocative angina at Rome (Baronius).
1020–1087.	Constantinus Africanus.
1021.	Dancing mania.
1039.	Fatal angina (*cynanche*) in Eastern Empire (Cedrenus).
1046.	Pestilence and murrain in England (Anglo-Saxon Chronicle).
1048–1049.	High mortality of men and cattle in England (Anglo-Saxon Chronicle).
1050.	Albucasis.
1066.	Battle of Hastings.
1073–1080.	Gregory VII.
1080.	Hospital for Lepers at Harbledown, England, near Canterbury (rebuilt 1276).
1084.	St. John's Hospital, Canterbury (now almshouse).
1086.	English Domesday Book (social-economic survey) completed.
1087.	Anglo-Saxon Chronicle notes correlation between famine and fever (1086–7).
1096–1272.	Crusades.
1099.	Order of St. John of Jerusalem founded.
1099–1179.	St. Hildegard.
1100–1180.	Rise of Salernitan School (High Salerno).
1103–1105.	Pestilence and murrain in England (Anglo-Saxon Chronicle).
1110–1113.	University of Paris founded (Papal license, 1215).
1112.	"Destructive pestilence" in England (Anglo-Saxon Chronicle).
1114–1187.	Gerard of Cremona.
1116.	Thibaut d'Estampes called to Oxford (assembly of students).
1125.	"Most dire famine, pestilence and murrain in all England" (Anglo-Saxon Chronicle).

1126–1198.	**Averroës. Avenzoar.**
1131.	Council of Rheims forbids clerics to practise medicine.
1132.	Holy Cross Hospital founded at Winchester.
1135–1204.	**Moses Maimonides.**
1136.	Leper Hospital at Ilford, England.
1137.	**St. Bartholomew's Hospital** (London) founded by Rahere.
1138–1254.	Hohenstaufen Emperors.
1139.	Lateran Council interdicts surgery among the higher clergy.
1140.	**Nicolaus Salernitanus** (*Antidotarium*).
	Mercurials recommended in *Circa instans* of Matthæus Platearius.
	King Roger II of Sicily restricts medical practice to licentiates.
1145.	William VIII of Montpellier founds Hospital of the Holy Ghost (Montpellier).
	Seiken publishes book on Japanese materia medica.
1158.	**University of Bologna** founded.
1161.	Jewish physicians burned at Prague on charge of "poisoning wells."
	Order of Henry II (England) regulating public stews.
1162–1202.	City of Arles (France) issues medical ordinances.
1162–1546.	Parliamentary recognition of public stews (London).
1163.	Council of Tours ("Ecclesia abhorret a sanguine").
1167–68.	Migration of students from Paris to **Oxford** to form a "studium generale."
1170.	**Ruggiero Frugardi** of Salerno completes *Practica Chirurgiæ*.
1171–1252.	Abbasid (Ayyubid) Empire (Egypt).
1172.	Dysentery among troops of Henry II in Ireland.
1180.	**University of Montpellier** founded (reorganized 1289).
1181.	William VIII, Count of Montpellier, declares Montpellier a free school of medicine.
1187.	Saladin takes Jerusalem.
1191.	**Teutonic Order** authorized by Clement III.
1193–1280.	**Albertus Magnus.**
1193–7.	Great general famine and pestilence in England. .
1196.	Account of famine fever by William of Newburgh.
1197.	St. Mary's Spital in London.
1198.	**Hospital movement** inaugurated by **Innocent III.**
1200.	School of Arts and Medicine at Perugia (*studium generale*, 1308).
1201.	**Oxford** first called a **University.**
	Unprecedented plague and murrain in England.
1201–1277.	**Saliceto.**
1204.	Innocent III opens **Santo Spirito in Sassia Hospital** (Rome).
1209.	Migration of students from Oxford to **Cambridge.**
1210.	**Collège de St. Côme** founded at Paris by Jean Pitard.
	Franciscan Order recognized by Innocent III.
1211.	Innocent III recognizes **University of Paris.**
1214.	Ugo Borgognoni made city physician of Bologna at a fixed salary.
1214–94.	**Roger Bacon.**
1215.	Magna Charta.
	St. Thomas's Hospital founded by Peter, Bishop of Winchester (rebuilt 1693).
1220.	Montpellier statute organizing Universitas medicorum with right of students to choose preceptor (August 17).
1222.	**University of Padua** started by migration of students from Bologna (Library, 1629).
1223.	**Cambridge** first called a **University.**
1223–1226.	Louis VIII. 2000 lazar houses in France.
1223–1303.	Taddeo Alderotti.
1224.	Frederick II issues law regulating the study of medicine.
	Frederick II founds University of Naples.
1226.	St. Mary Magdalene, Glastonbury, rebuilt.
1227–1274.	Thomas Aquinas.
1228.	University of Vercelli founded (abolished, 1372).
	500 students at Padua.
1229.	University of Toulouse started.
1229–34.	University of Naples abolished.
1230.	Examination of candidates by two masters for right to practice at Montpellier.
1230–40.	**Roland of Parma** edits Roger's *Practica Chirurgiæ* (1170).
1231.	**Salerno** constituted a **medical school** by Frederick II.
	Gregory IX issues bull *Parens scientiarum* authorizing faculties to govern universities.
1233.	Apothecary shop at Wetzlar.
	Gregory IX charters University of Toulouse (1229) as a "studium generale."

1234.   Frederick II revives University of Naples (without medical faculty).

1235–1311. **Arnold of Villanova.**

1235–1315. Raymond Lully.

1236.   Water piped to London from Paddington.

1237–60. Decline of University of Padua (tyranny of Ezzelin).

1240.   Montpellier statute specifying six months practice outside city as essential for license (January 14).

        Law of Frederick II favoring dissection and regulating surgery and pharmacy.

1242.   Roger Bacon refers to gunpowder.

1243.   University of Salamanca founded by Ferdinand III of Castile (April 6).

1244–5. **University of Oxford** chartered by Henry III.

1245.   Savoy Hospital, London (rebuilt 1509).

1246–8. **University of Siena** started (*studium generale*, 1275; charter 1357).

1247.   **Hospital of St. Mary of Bethlehem** founded as a priory by Simon Fitzmary.

        Pestilence and famine in England (Matthew Paris).

        Council of LeMans prohibits surgery to monks.

1248.   University of Piacenza founded by Papal charter (reconstituted, 1398).

1249.   University College (Oxford) founded by William of Durham.

1250.   Matthew Paris calls inmates of leper-houses, *miselli* (measles).

        Joinville describes **scurvy** in troops of Louis IX at siege of Cairo.

1250–1320. **Peter of Abano.**

1252.   Conrad II moves University of Naples to Salerno.

        Bruno of Longoburg completes his *Chirurgia magna.*

1252–1517. Mameluke dynasties (Egypt).

1253.   University College, Oxford, founded.

1254.   Alphonso X (the Wise) authorizes *studium generale* at Seville (December 28).

1256.   Enfranchisement of serfs at Bologna.

1257.   **Sorbonne** founded at Paris.

1257–9. Famine fever in Britain (Matthew Paris).

1259.   King Manfred revives University of Naples.

1260.   University (studium) started at Valladolid.

1260–1320. **Henri de Mondeville.**

1263.   Balliol College (Oxford) founded.

1264.   Merton College (Oxford) founded.

1265.   English House of Commons organized.

1265–1308. Duns Scotus.

1265–1321. Dante.

1266.   End of Western Caliphate.

        University of Perugia founded.

        Charles I reorganizes University of Naples (October 24).

        Theodoric completes surgical treatise (aseptic treatment of wounds).

1267.   Council of Venice forbids Jews to practice medicine among Christians.

        St. Edmund Hall (Oxford) founded.

1270–80. **Spectacles** introduced by Venetian (Murano) glassmakers.

1272.   Law school at Parma (University, 1422).

1275.   **Saliceto** completes his *Cyrurgia* (June 7–8).

1281.   Guildhall order forbidding swine in the streets of London.

1282.   Sicilian Vespers.

1282–1549. Charnel-house (ossuary) for dead in St. Paul's church-yard (London).

1283.   Lepers excluded from Berwick on Tweed.

1284.   Peterhouse College (Cambridge) founded.

1285.   Conduit for London water-supply constructed at West Cheap.

        Postmortem of case of pest at Cremona (Chronicle of Salimbene of Parma, 1288).

1285–1307. Bernard de Gordon teaches at Montpellier.

1287.   **Plica Polonica** in Poland after Mongol invasion.

1289.   Pope Nicholas IV charters University of Montpellier (1181) as a *studium generale* (October 26).

1290.   Pope Nicholas IV charters University of Lisbon.

1295–96. **Lanfranc** completes his *Chirurgia magna.*

1296.   Epidemics of flux in England.

1300.   University of Lerida founded by James II of Spain.

        Boniface VIII issues bull *De sepulturis.*

1300–68. **Guy de Chauliac.**

1301.   Abdul Hamid II founds Public Library (Oumoumiye) at Stamboul (Constantinople).

1302.   Creation of the States General in France.

1302.	Bartolomeo de Varignana performs first judicial postmortem (Bologna).
1303.	Boniface VIII charters Universities of Rome (June 6) and Avignon.
1304.	Fernando IV of Castile endows University (studium) at Valladolid (May 24).
	Henri de Mondeville teaches anatomy at Montpellier.
1305.	Clement V charters Universities of Orleans and Angers.
	City Hospital of Siena established.
1306–16.	Henri de Mondeville writes his surgical treatise.
1308.	Clement V charters University of Perugia as studium generale (September 8).
	Clement V permits removal of University of Lisbon to Coimbra.
1309.	Papal See removed to Avignon.
	King Diniz of Portugal charters University of Coimbra (February 15).
1311.	Guildhall order forbidding flaying of dead horses in London.
1312.	University of Palermo started (charter, 1806).
1314.	Exeter College (Oxford) founded.
	Mondeville employs miniature paintings in his anatomy.
1315–16.	Famine and throat infection (pestis gutturosa) in Britain (Trokelowe's Annals).
1316.	City surgeon at Lübeck at 16 marks ($4) per annum.
	Mondino's Anothomia completed.
1317.	John XXII issues bull Spondent pariter against abuses of alchemy.
1318.	University of Treviso chartered by Frederick the Fair.
1319.	First criminal prosecution for body-snatching.
1320–21.	University started at Florence (charter, 1349).
1321.	John XXII issues bull establishing medical school at Perugia.
1322.	Famine and mortality in army of Edward II in Scotland.
1326.	John XXII issues bull Super illius specula against practice of magic.
	Oriel College (Oxford) founded.
1328.	City Physician at Strassburg.
1330.	Introduction of gunpowder in warfare.
1331.	First mention of firearms by Muratori.
1332.	John XXII charters University of Cahors as a studium generale.
1333.	Public medico-botanical garden at Venice.
1336–1453.	Hundred Years' War.
1338.	Exodus of students from Bologna to Pisa.
1339.	Benedict XII charters University of Grenoble as a studium generale.
1340.	Alphonso IV moves University of Coimbra back to Lisbon.
	14,000 students at Oxford.
1341.	Gentile da Foligno gives public dissection at Padua.
1343.	Clement VI charters University of Pisa as "studium generale" (September 3).
	Report on faulty sanitation (nuisances) in London White Book (Liber albus).
1345.	First apothecary shop in London.
	Illustrated anatomical treatise of Guido de Vigevano.
1345–50.	Schools of arts, law and medicine at Valencia.
1346.	Clement VI charters University of Valladolid (1304) as a "studium generale" (July 30 Library, 1484).
	Ordinance of Edward III driving lepers from London.
	Cannon used at battle of Crécy.
1347.	Pembroke Hall (Cambridge) founded.
	Pope Clement IV charters University of Prague (January 26).
1348.	Board of Health and quarantine (quaranta giorni) established at Venice.
	Gonville and Caius College (University of Cambridge) founded.
	Emperor Karl IV charters University of Prague (April 7) as a "studium generale."
1348–50.	Black Death (magna mortalitas).
	Guy de Chauliac succors plague-stricken at Avignon.
1349.	Clement VI charters University of Florence (1320) as "studium generale" (May 31).
	Act prohibiting alms to sturdy and valiant beggars (England).
1350.	Trinity Hall (Cambridge) founded.
1352.	Report on extra-mural nuisances, London (26. Edward III).
1354.	Pedro IV founds University of Huesca.
1354–5.	Alphonso IV moves University at Lisbon back to Coimbra.
1355.	Charles IV charters University of Arezzo (1215) as "studium generale."
1357.	Charles IV charters University of Siena (1246) as a "studium generale."
	Royal order against throwing of filth into Thames (London).
1360.	Innocent VI recognizes University of Bologna as a "studium generale."
1361.	Charles IV charters University of Pavia (April 13).
1361–91.	Lesser epidemic waves of Black Death in Great Britain.

1363.	Guy de Chauliac completes his surgery.
1364.	Casimir the Great charters University of Cracow as a "studium generale" (May 12. Library, 1517).
1364.	University of Pisa (1343) rechartered by Urban V (November 10).
1365.	Duke Rudolph IV founds University of Vienna (March 12. Library, 1775). University of Orange founded by Charles IV.
1367.	University of Fünfkirchen founded by King Louis of Hungary.
1370.	John of Arderne writes surgical treatises.
1371.	Seven professors in medical faculty at Bologna. Royal order forbidding slaughtering of animals in London and suburbs.
1373–5.	Boccaccio lectures at Florence.
1374.	City ordinance of Reggio against the plague. Dancing mania at Aix, Cologne, and Metz. Venice excludes plague-ridden ships from harbor.
1376.	Board of medical examiners in London.
1376–7.	Return of Popes to Rome. Ragusa exacts thirty (*Trentina*), later forty days' quarantine (*Quarantina*).
1377.	University of Coimbra moved back to Lisbon.
1379.	Clement VII charters Universities of Erfurt and Perpignan.
1383.	First quarantine of Marseilles harbor.
1385.	Urban VI charters University of Heidelberg as a "studium generale" (October 23; opened October 28, 1386).
1388.	Urban VI charters University of Cologne as a "studium generale." First English Sanitary Act (17. Richard II). Salaried city veterinarian at Ulm.
1389.	Urban VI recharters University of Erfurt (1379). Boniface IX authorizes University of Pavia (1361).
1391.	Boniface IX charters University of Ferrara as a *studium generale* (March 4). University of Lerida permitted to dissect a body every three years.
1398.	University of Pavia moved to Piacenza.
1399.	Beginning of *Acta Facultatis Medicæ Viennensis* (May 6).
1402.	Boniface IX charters University of Würzburg (December 10) (reorganized 1582).
1403.	Quarantine lazaretto at Venice.
1404.	University of Turin founded by House of Savoy (revived, 1713; 1720). University of Pavia (Piacenza) closed. First public dissection at Vienna (February 12).
1406.	Emperor Wenzel makes surgery respectable in Germany. University of Pisa closed.
1409.	Alexander V charters University of Leipzig as a "studium generale" (September 9) (Library, 1543). Alexander V authorizes studium generale at Aix in Provence. Insane asylum at Seville.
1410.	Insane asylum at Padua.
1411.	University of St. Andrews founded by Bishop Henry Wardlaw.
1412.	Filippo Maria Visconti revives University of Pavia. Dancing mania at Strassburg (Chapel of St. Vitus, Zabern).
1414.	Jail fever (64 deaths) in Newgate and Ludgate Prisons (Stow's Chronicle).
1415.	Ordinance (3. Henry V) against extra-mural nuisances (London).
1419.	Pope Martin V charters University of Rostock (February 13).
1422.	University of Parma founded (Library, 1781). University founded at Dôle (France).
1425.	Insane asylum at Saragossa.
1426.	University of Louvain founded.
1429–31.	Syphilis mentioned in Italian (Uffizi) and Swiss archives.
1431.	Charles VII founds University of Poitiers (chartered by Eugenius IV).
1432.	Henry VI of England founds University of Caën (Calvados).
1437.	Eugenius IV charters University of Caën (1432). City Library at Ulm.
1439.	Johannes von Gmünd prints first calendar (in block-type).
1440–50.	Invention of printing.
1441.	Eugenius IV founds University of Bordeaux as a *studium generale*.
1444.	Eugenius IV charters University of Catania, Sicily (April 18).
1450.	Niklaus Krebs of Cues (Cardinal Cusanus) suggests timing the pulse (1440), and weighing blood and urine. Vatican Library (Rome) founded.

1450.   Nicholas V founds University of Barcelona.
            University of Treves founded (academic sessions, 1473).
1451.   Bernardo di Rapallo devises perineal operation for stone.
            Nicholas V founds University of Glasgow as a studium generale (reorganized, 1577).
1452.   **Barber surgeons of Hamburg** (*Meister Bartscheerer*) incorporated.
            Ratisbon ordinance for midwives (*Regensburger Hebammenbuch*).
1452–1519. **Leonardo da Vinci.**
1453.   Fall of Constantinople (end of Byzantine Empire).
1454.   **Gutenburg Bible** printed.
            Calixtus III charters University of Freiburg (Bull of April 20, 1455).
1456.   **University of Greifswald** chartered by Calixtus III (May 29).
            Ospedale maggiore (Milan) founded.
1457.   Gutenberg **Purgation-Calendar** printed (**first medical publication**).
            Peter Schöffer prints Psalter with improved types.
            University of Freiburg founded by Albrecht VI (opened April 26, 1460).
1459.   Pius II charters Universities of Ingolstadt (April 7) and Basel (November 12).
1460.   **University of Basel** opened (April 4).
            Heinrich von Pfolspeundt writes treatise on surgery.
            Savonarola notes effect of contracted pelvis in labor (Aranzio, 1587).
1462.   Sack of Mainz by Adolph of Nassau drives German printers over Europe.
            Bloodletting-Calendar printed at Mainz.
1463.   Pius II charters University of Nantes.
            Syphilis (*le gros mal*) mentioned in open court at Dijon (July 25).
1465.   Paul II charters Universities at Bourges and Budapest.
1467.   Subiaco Cicero printed.
            Gerson's tracts on self-abuse printed.
1468.   Biblioteca Marciana founded at Venice.
1469.   Pliny's Natural History printed.
1469–71.   **Ferrari da Grado's** *Practica* printed.
1470.   Medical treatises by **Valescus de Taranta** and **Matthæus Sylvaticus** printed.
            Bismuth known in Germany (Chronicle of Petrus Albinus, 1590).
            Johann Hartlieb's palmistry printed.
1471.   Jenson prints treatises by **Mesue** and **Nicolaus Salernitanus** (*Antidotarium*).
1472.   Duke Ludwig of Bavaria opens University of Ingolstadt.
            Hochenburg *Regimen sanitatis* (German text) printed.
            Bagellardo's treatise on **pediatrics** printed.
1473.   University of Florence (studium generale) moved to Pisa (November 1).
            Simone de Cordo's *Synonyma* printed (**first medical dictionary**).
            Ulrich Ellenbog publishes tract on poisonous gases and fumes.
1473–1543. Copernicus (heliocentric astronomy).
1474.   University of Zaragoza founded.
1474–5.   Caxton prints in England.
1475.   Sixtus IV charters **University of Copenhagen** (June 19) (reorganized, 1537).
1475–1564. Michael Angelo.
1476.   **Saliceto's "Cyrurgia"** printed.
            Saliceto describes renal dropsy.
            Sixtus IV charters University of Mainz.
            Ulrich Hahn (Rome) invents printing of music.
1477.   **Universities of Tübingen and Upsala** founded.
1478.   **First edition of Celsus** printed at Florence.
            Mondino's *Anothomia* printed at Leipzig.
            Spanish Inquisition.
1478–9.   Epidemic of plague in London.
1479.   **First edition of Avicenna** printed.
1480.   Latin text of **Regimen Sanitatis** printed.
            Herbarium of pseudo-Apuleius printed at Rome.
            Matthias Corvinus introduces morocco bindings.
1484.   Innocent VIII authorizes **burning of witches** in bull *Summis desiderantes*.
1484–5.   Peter Schöffer (Mainz) prints herbal (*Hortus Sanitatis*).
1485.   Sweating-sickness appears in England.
1486.   First Latin edition of Rhazes printed.
            English epidemic of **sweating-sickness.**
            Statute (3. Henry VII [1488–9], Cap. 3) regulating slaughter-houses.
1489.   168 bath-houses at Ulm.
            "Malleus malleficarum" (Witches' Codex) of Jacob Sprenger printed.

1490. University of Heidelberg moves to Speyer on account of plague.

1490–1553. **Rabelais.**

1491. Jacob Meidenbach's **Hortus sanitatis** printed.

    Ketham's *Fasciculus Medicinæ* published.

1492. Discovery of America.

    John of Gaddesden's *Rosa anglica* printed.

    Nicholas Leonicenus corrects botanical errors in Pliny.

    Hartmann Schedel describes diphtheria epidemic at Nuremberg.

1493. Smallpox in Germany.

1493–1551. **Paracelsus.**

1494. **University of Aberdeen** founded as a studium generale.

    Scillacio traces **syphilis** to the South of France.

1495. Maximilian I mentions syphilis in **Edict against Blasphemers.**

    English statute (2. Henry VII, cap. 19) against contagion by fomites (bedding).

1496. Albert Dürer's drawing of a syphilitic printed.

    Bathing in common prohibited at Nuremberg.

    Charles VIII creates four salaried medical chairs at Montpelher; renewed by Louis XII.

1496–1500. Spread of syphilis in Europe.

1497. Aldine edition of Theophrastus printed.

    Vasco da Gama doubles the Cape (November 22).

    Scurvy on Vasco da Gama's voyage.

1498. Florentine *Ricettario* (**first official pharmacopœia).**

    First notices of syphilis in Scotland and England.

1499. University of Alcala founded.

    Johann **Peyligk** publishes anatomical drawings.

1499–1500. Plague in England.

1500. Jacob Nufer performs **first Cæsarean section** on living subject.

    Berengario da Carpi treats syphilis with mercurial inunctions.

1500–1501. Alexander VI charters University of Valencia.

1501. **Magnus Hundt's** *Anthropologium* published.

    Studium generale at Santiago.

    Morbus Hungaricus pandemic in Europe.

    African negroes first brought to West Indies.

1502. Maximilian I constitutes **University of Wittenberg** (July 6) as a "studium **generale'**

    (reorganized as University of Halle, 1693; Library, 1696).

1504. Julius II authorizes Universities of Santiago (December 17).

1505. **Royal College of Surgeons of Edinburgh** chartered.

    Julius II charters University of Seville (1254).

    Peter Hele (Nuremberg) adds hands to clock.

1506. University of Frankfort on the Oder founded by bull of Julius II.

    Bankside stews in Southwark (London) suppressed.

1507. **Benivieni's** collection of **post-mortem sections** printed.

1508. **Guaiac** wood brought from America.

    Sweating-sickness in England.

    Symphorien Champier publishes history of medicine.

    Jerome of Brunswick's Book on Wound-Surgery published.

    Plague in England.

1509–1547. Reign of Henry VIII.

1510. Peter Hele (Henlein) of Nuremberg makes **pocket watches.**

    Pandemic influenza in Europe.

1510–90. **Ambroïse Paré.**

1513. **Eucharius Röslin's** *Rosegarten* printed.

1513–15. Plague in England.

1514. **Gunshot wounds** first described in Vigo's "Practica."

    Peter Martyr notes smallpox (*variolæ*) in England.

    Brissot opposes derivative blood-letting.

1514–15. Acts of Henry VIII for repopulation of the Isle of Wight.

1514–64. **Vesalius.**

1517. **Fugitive anatomical plates** published by Johann Schott of Mainz.

    Gersdorff's Field-Book of Wound-Surgery published.

    Malignant sore throat (diphtheria) in Amsterdam and the Rhineland.

    Sweating-sickness in England.

    Montpellier statute authorizing students to accompany doctors in private practice.

    Sir Thomas More's *Utopia.*

    Library (Bibljoteka Jagiellonska) at Cracow.

1517–1521. Reformation.
1517–1524. **Linacre** publishes **translations of Galen.**
1517–1928. Ottoman Empire (Egypt).
1518.   **Royal College of Physicians** (England) founded (September 23).
        Bibliothèque Nationale (Paris) founded.
        Nuremberg ordinance regulating sale of food.
1519.   **Friesen's** *Spiegl der Artzny* and *Synonima* published.
1519–1522. Magellan circumnavigates the globe.
1519–1556. Charles V, King of Spain and Emperor of Germany.
1520.   Scurvy on Magellan's voyage.
1521.   **Black Assizes** of Cambridge (**jail fever**).
1521–1523. **Berengario da Carpi** publishes anatomical treatises.
1524.   Linacre foundation of medical lectures at Oxford and Cambridge.
        Cortes erects **first hospital in city of Mexico.**
        Lucas van Leyden's portrait of Ferdinand I of Spain (adenoid face).
1525.   **First Latin translation of Hippocrates** published at Rome.
1526.   Clement VII charters University of Santiago.
        Gymnasium Ægidianum founded at Nuremberg (moved to Altdorf, 1575; University
          1578)
        First (Aldine) Greek text of Hippocrates published at Venice.
        Paracelsus founds **chemotherapy.**
1526–94.   Palestrina.
1527.   Philip, Landgrave of Hesse, founds first Protestant **University at Marburg** (May 30).
        Sack of Rome by Charles V (decline of Italian humanism).
1528.   First Aldine edition of Paul of Ægina.
1529.   City Library at Hamburg founded.
        Sweating-sickness in England.
1529–30.   **Sweating-sickness** spreads over Europe.
1530.   Collège de France (Paris) founded (reconstituted, 1831).
        Fracastorius' poem on syphilis published.
        Otto Brunfels publishes his atlas of plants.
        Sarsaparilla introduced.
1530–31.   English act against vagabonds.
1530–37.   University of Copenhagen closed.
1531.   Clement VII founds University of Granada.
        Plague in England.
1532.   **Albert Dürer's** treatise on human symmetry published.
        Act of Parliament (23. Henry VIII, cap. 5) instituting Commissions of Sewers in England
        Rabelais publishes first Latin version of the aphorisms of Hippocrates.
        Parish bills of mortality in London.
1533.   Charles V issues **Constitutio Criminalis Carolina.**
        Buonafede holds **first chair of materia medica** at Padua.
1533–92.   Montaigne.
        Autopsy of double human monster in San Domingo (July 18).
1534.   Aldine edition of Aetius published.
        Jesuit order founded.
        Appearance of first Russian medical book: "The Benign Cool Vineyard."
1535.   **Mariano Santo di Barletta** gives first account of **median lithotomy.**
        Scurvy on Jacques Cartier's second expedition.
1535–6.   Plague in England.
1535–98.   Spread of epidemic pneumonia from Venice (beginning of general prevalence to date).
1536.   Ambroïse Paré makes first excision of elbow-joint.
        Escola medico-cirurgica founded at Lisbon (reorganized, 1826).
        Paracelsus' *Chirurgia Magna* published.
1536–9.   Dissolution of English monasteries by Act of Parliament.
1537.   University of Lisbon moved back to Coimbra (reorganized, 1772).
        Christian III revives University of Copenhagen (September 9).
        Vesalius graduates at Basel.
        Dryander's *Anatomia* published.
1538.   Vesalius publishes his *Tabulæ anatomicæ sex.*
        University of Santo Tomas (San Domingo) founded.
        Henry VIII orders recording of christenings, marriages and deaths in English parish
          registers.
1538–40.   Pandemic dysentery (Hirsch).
1539.   Cardan improves formulation of theory of probabilities.

1539.   Influenza in England and Europe.
1540.   Paul III founds University of Macerata (July 1).
        English barbers and surgeons united as **"Commonalty of the Barbers and Surgeons."**
        Statute of Henry VIII permitting four dissections annually.
        Valerius Cordus discovers **sulphuric ether.**
        Mattioli treats syphilis by internal use of mercury.
        Raynald translates Röslin as *The Byrth of Mankynde.*
        Sebastianus Austrius plagiarizes pediatric treatise of Cornelius Roelants.
1542.   **Leonhard Fuchs** attempts a rational botanical nomenclature (*Historia stirpium*).
1543.   Copernicus describes revolution of planets around the sun (1507).
        Vesalius publishes the **Fabrica** (June 1) and founds modern anatomy.
        University Library (Biblioteca Albertina) at Leipzig founded.
        Plague in England.
        Water-supply and sewage plant (with farm) at Bünzlau (Silesia).
        English apothecaries legalized by Act of Parliament.
        Henry VIII issues ordinance against plague.
1544.   Albert III founds **University of Königsberg** (August 17, Library, 1534).
        St. Bartholomew's Hospital refounded under superintendence of Thomas Vicary.
        Botanic Garden at University of Pisa.
1545.   **Paré** improves **amputation** and **treatment of gunshot wounds.**
        Giambattista da Monte gives **bedside instruction at Padua.**
        Botanic Garden at Padua.
1545–1563. Council of Trent.
1546.   Valerius Cordus publishes **first German pharmacopœia.**
        Ingrassias describes stapes.
        Jerome Bock's "Kräuterbuch" published.
        London stews suppressed.
        Georg Agricola describes **ventilation of mines** (*De re metallica*).
        Brassavola revives tracheotomy.
        Fracastorius publishes treatise on contagious diseases.
        Regius Professorship of Physic founded at Cambridge.
1547.   Canano notes valves in veins.
        Insane asylum established at St. Mary of Bethlehem ("**Bedlam**"), London.
        The Dominican Penot (Toulouse) lays down basic principles of **hydrotherapy** (*De aquæ
        naturalibus virtute*).
        Plague in England.
1548.   University of Messina founded (reorganized 1838).
1549.   **Anatomical theater at Padua.**
1550.   **Paré's** essay on **podalic version** published.
        Average expectation of life eight and one-half years (Chadwick).
        Bartolommeo Maggi proves that gunshot wounds are not poisonous.
        Conrad Gesner publishes *Historia animalium.*
        Hollerius prescribes spectacles for myopia.
1550–1600. Giordano Bruno: plurality of worlds; infinity of universe.
1551.   Anatomical theaters at Paris and Montpellier.
        University of Mexico founded.
        Pierre Belon shows homology between skeletons of birds and man.
        Last epidemic of sweating-sickness in England.
        Influenza (*coqueluche*) in France.
        City Library (Bibliotheca Vadiana) at St. Gall (Switzerland).
1552.   **Caius** publishes treatise on sweating-sickness.
        Matthæus Friedrich publishes **first tract on alcoholism.**
1553.   **Servetus** describes the pulmonary circulation.
        The collection *De Balneis* published.
        University of Lima founded.
1554.   **Johann Lange** describes **chlorosis** (*morbus virgineus*).
        Fernelius publishes treatise on **special pathology** in his *Medicina.*
        Cardan obtains **absolute alcohol.**
        Jacob Rueff's midwifery (*De conceptu*) published.
        Editio princeps of Aretæus printed at Paris.
1555.   Diet of Augsburg.
        Pierre Franco performs **suprapubic lithotomy.**
1556.   University of Sassari (Sardinia) founded (Library, 1550–62).
        Saxon National Library at Dresden founded.
        Studium generale at Sassari, Sardinia (*University*, 1634).

1556–1598. Philip II.
1557. Lommius publishes treatise on dietetic treatment of fevers.
1557–8. Epidemic influenza (Europe and England).
1558. Ferdinand I charters and opens University of Jena (February 2).
    Cornaro publishes treatise on **personal hygiene.**
    Nicolas Massa decompresses brain for traumatic aphasia.
1558–1603. Reign of Elizabeth.
1559. Caspar Stromayer's ophthalmic treatise (Sudhoff).
1560. Pius IV authorizes University of Douai (opened 1562).
    Maurolycus describes myopia, hypermetropia and the optics of the lens.
    Pierre Franco introduces high lithotomy.
    Monardes introduces balsam of Peru.
    Botanic Garden at Zürich.
1561. **Fallopius** publishes *Observationes anatomicæ* (Fallopian tubes).
    Paré founds **orthopedics.**
    Pierre Franco's treatise on **hernia** published.
    Adam Lonitzer introduces ergot.
    St. Thomas's Hospital (London) founded.
1561–1626. **Francis Bacon.**
1562. University of Lille founded (Library, 1883).
    Witchcraft made a capital offense in England.
    Czech translation of Mattioli's commentary on Dioscorides published at Prague.
    First Elizabethan Act (V, cap. 3) for relief of poverty.
1562–1568. Pandemic plague.
1562–1601. English Poor-Laws under Elizabeth.
1562–1629. Huguenot wars in France.
1563. Witchcraft a capital crime in Scotland.
    Collegio Borromeo (Pavia) founded.
    Plague in London.
    John Jones publishes *Dyall of Agues.*
1564. **Medical dictionaries** of Stephanus and Gorræus published.
    Eustachius discovers abducens nerve, thoracic duct, and suprarenal glands.
    Aranzi advances human embryology in *De humano fœtu.*
    Malignant angina (diphtheria) among children in the Rhineland (Wier).
1564–1616. Shakespeare.
1564–1642. Galileo.
1565. Statute of Elizabeth permitting dissection of executed criminals.
    Jean Nicot brings **tobacco** plant to France.
1566. Johann Sturm's "Akademie" opened at Strassburg.
1566–7. Plague among English troops in Ireland.
1567. **Ulisse Aldrovandi** establishes botanical garden in Bologna.
    Paracelsus' account of **miners' phthisis** published.
    Donati describes epidemic smallpox and measles at Mantua.
1568. **Constantino Varolio** describes the pons Varolii.
    Paré differentiates between syphilis and smallpox (greater and lesser pox).
    Mercator introduces projection maps.
    Duke of Alba introduces **musketry.**
    Portuguese introduce surgery in Japan.
1568–9. London and Westminster ordinances against plague.
    Severe plague epidemic in Edinburgh.
1570. **Felix Platter** urges psychic treatment of the insane.
    Plague on the Continent (Europe).
    Fabricius ab Aquapondente discovers function of valves of veins (published 1603).
1571. Battle of Lepanto.
    Francisco Bravo describes **tabardillo** (Mexican typhus).
    Laurentian Library (Biblioteca Medicea Laurenziana) founded at Florence.
    Barber-Surgeons Board (Stockholm) constituted.
1571–93. Cesalpino speculates on the circulation of the blood.
1571–1630. Johann **Kepler:** elliptical orbit of planets (1609–21).
1572. University founded at Pont-à-Mousson, Lorraine (December 5).
    Geronimo Mercuriali publishes his treatise on **skin diseases.**
    Lead poisoning (*colica Pictonum*) in Poitou.
    Society of Antiquaries of London founded.
1573. **Adam Lonitzer's** ordinance for midwives (Frankfort on the Main).
    Paré introduces version.

1574.   Gregory XIII charters University of Oviedo.
1574–1577. Pandemic plague.
1575.   **Universities of Leyden and Helmstädt** founded.
    Paré describes monoxide poisoning.
    Volcher **Coiter** establishes **comparative osteology.**
    Paré introduces massage and artificial eyes.
    Baillou describes laryngeal croup as a new disease (*morbus incognitus*).
1576.   Paracelsus publishes tract on mineral waters.
1577.   Botanic garden at Leyden.
    Black Assizes of Oxford (510 deaths from jail [typhus] fever).
1578.   **Guillaume de Baillou** describes **whooping-cough** (*quinta*).
    Chair of Medicine in University of Mexico.
    Rudolph II charters University of Altdorf (opened, 1580).
    King Stefan Bathory founds University of Wilna (Poland) (Library, 1570).
1578–83. Five-year bills of mortality in London (plague-period).
1578–1657. **William Harvey.**
1579.   William **Clowes** publishes **first English treatise on syphilis.**
    Botanic garden at Leipzig.
1579–1664. "City *Remembrancia*" on municipal hygiene (London).
1580.   Scurvy on Drake's voyage around the world.
    Prospero Alpino introduces **moxa** and coffee from the Orient.
1580–82. Influenza in Europe.
1580–84. Plague in London.
1581.   London ordinance against plague (Bills of Mortality).
    Rousset's treatise on **Cæsarean section** published.
1582.   **University of Edinburgh** chartered by James VI (Library, 1580).
    Augsburg Collegium medicum founded.
1582–1632. Measures against overcrowding and overbuilding in London.
1583.   **Georg Bartisch's** *Augendienst* published.
    Cesalpino classifies plants in his *De plantis.*
    Della Porta's *Phytognomonica* published.
1583–1618. Diphtheria (*garrotillo*) epidemic in Spain.
1584.   Sir Walter Raleigh brings **curare** from Guiana and introduces the potato.
    Schenck von Grafenburg experiments on artificial respiration in asphyxia.
1584–8. Plague in Scotland.
1585.   **Guillemeau's** treatise on diseases of the eye published.
    Pope Sixtus V restores Alexandrian Aqueduct at Rome as Aqua Felice.
    Elizabethan Act (27, cap. 20) authorizing convection of **water-supply** to Plymouth from Dartmoor (Drake's Water-Leet).
1585–6. Scurvy on Drake's voyage to Spanish Main.
1586.   University of Graz (Styria) chartered (October 22) and opened (April 14).
    Della Porta's *Physiognomia* published.
    Exeter Black Assizes (spread of jail-fever by prisoners).
1587.   Aranzio gives first description of deformed pelvis.
1588.   Defeat of Spanish Armada.
    Anatomical theater at Basel.
    Clusius plants potatoes in Vienna and Frankfort.
    Dr. Timothy Bright introduces shorthand (Ratcliffe, 1580).
    Maffei introduces tea.
1589.   Galileo demonstrates law of falling bodies.
1589–1611. Henri IV.
1590.   **Compound microscope** invented by Hans and Zacharias Janssen.
    José d'Acosta describes **mountain sickness.**
1591.   Trinity College (Dublin) founded (University 1593).
    Pandemic plague.
1592.   Georg Hoefnagel publishes microscopic observations of insects (50 plates).
    Botanic garden at Montpellier.
1592–3. Plague in London.
1593.   Marischal College (Aberdeen) founded by George Keith, Earl Marischal.
    Elizabethan Act (35, cap. 6) against overcrowding of London houses.
1595.   **Libavius** publishes *Alchymia* (**first treatise on chemistry**).
    Joseph du Chesne (Quercetanus) uses calomel.
    City of Passau issues ordinance for midwives.
    Mahuang (*Ephedra*) noted by Shi Cheng Li.
1596.   Peter Lowe publishes essay on the "Spanish Sickness" (syphilis).

1596.   Harington's *Metamorphosis of Ajax* published.
1596–7.   Dysentery noted in England.
1597.   **Tagliacozzi** publishes treatise on **plastic surgery.**
               Codronchi's treatise on medical jurisprudence published.
               Israel Spach's *Gynæcia* published.
               Influenza in Italy.
               James VI of Scotland publishes "Demonology."
               Botanic Garden at Paris (Jardin des Plantes, 1635).
1598.   Edict of Nantes.
               Medical Faculty added to University at Pont-à-Mousson, Lorraine (1572).
               Mercurio gives picture of the "Walcher position" in *La Comare.*
               Fedeli establishes necessity of post-mortem in jurisprudence of poisoning.
               Carlo Ruini publishes treatise on anatomy of the horse.
               Medical Department, University of Mexico, founded.
1599.   **Ulisse Aldrovandi's** *Historia animalium* published.
               Libavius isolates bismuth nitrate.
               Peter Lowe founds Royal Faculty of Physicians and Surgeons of Glasgow.
1599–1660.   Velasquez.
1600.   Queen Elizabeth charters **East India Company** (December 31).
               Fourth Elizabethan Poor-Law (43, cap. 2) authorizing apprenticeship of children.
               Gilbert's *De magnete* published.
               Fabry of Hilden removes foreign bodies from the cornea with magnet.
               University of Harderwijk founded.
               "Foglietti" (newspaper) published in Venice.
1601.   **James Lancaster** (Purchas' *Pilgrims*) mentions effect of lemon-juice against **scurvy** (voyage of 1600).
               University of Manila started.
1602.   Bodleian Library (Oxford) founded.
               Hamlet produced.
               Harvey graduates (M. D.) at Padua.
               Felix Platter publishes the first classification of diseases.
               First pharmacy in Russia.
               Fedeli publishes treatise on **medical jurisprudence.**
               Florian Matthis first performs **gastrotomy.**
1602–30.   Thomas Dekker's plague pamphlets.
1603.   Prince Cesi founds the **Accademia dei Lincei** at Rome (reorganized, 1847).
               Rise of London as a metropolis.
               University of Cagliari (Sardinia) founded.
               Clusius introduces gamboge (used as purge, 1610).
1604.   Johann **Kepler** demonstrates inversion of optic image on the retina.
1604–9.   Galileo elucidates law of falling bodies (1589).
1605.   Verhoeven publishes newspaper at Antwerp.
               Population of London, 224,275 (Creighton).
               Autopsies of victims of scurvy on Ste. Croix Island (Champlain's Voyages).
               Botanic garden at Giessen.
1605–13.   London Water Reservoirs from Ware to Clerkenwell.
1606–69.   Rembrandt.
1607.   Settlement of Jamestown, Virginia (May 13).
               Rudolph II charters **University of Giessen** (May 19) (Library, 1612).
1608.   Shakespeare outlines the semeiology of syphilis in *Timon of Athens.*
               Oswald Croll introduces many new preparations in *Basilica Chymica.*
               Thomas Coryate attempts to introduce table-forks in England (Italy, 1080).
1609.   United Netherlands.
               Henry Hudson anchors "Half Moon" in New York Bay.
               Galileo invents telescope.
               Kepler's *Astronomia Nova* published.
               Jalap brought from Mexico.
               Ambrosian Library at Milan founded.
               Louise Bourgeois publishes obstetric treatise.
1609–18.   Kepler states laws of planetary motion.
1610.   Galileo devises microscope.
               Trautmann performs Cæsarean section (April 21).
               Cristoforo Guarinoni describes gummata of the brain.
               Van Helmont defines gases and likens respiration to combustion.
               Minderer introduces ammonium acetate (spiritus Mindereri).

1610.	Leather book-bindings introduced in France.
	Rosicrucian Order founded.
1610–13.	Smallpox in Scotland and England.
1611.	Union of Brandenburg and Prussia.
	University of Santo Tomas (Manila) founded.
	Pope Paul V restores Aqueduct of Trajan at Rome.
	Villa Real, and others, describe epidemic diphtheria (*garrotillo*) in Spain.
1612–13.	Epidemic ague (influenza) in England.
1613.	Lord Mayor of London interdicts brewing of strong beer.
	University of Cordova (Argentine) founded.
	1400 students at Padua.
1614.	**University of Groningen** founded (August 23) (Library, 1615).
	Rodericus à Castro publishes treatise on medical jurisprudence.
1615.	*Frankfurter Postamtszeitung* (newspaper) published.
	Sir Hugh Myddelton improves **London water-supply** (New River).
	Bartolotti discovers milk-sugar.
	Christoph Scheiner introduces pin-hole test (optometry).
	Libavius publishes treatise on **transfusion** (*Chirurgia transfusoria*).
1615–16.	**Harvey** lectures on the **circulation of the blood.**
1616.	University of Paderborn founded.
	Cesare Magati treats wounds with plain water.
1617.	Briggs and Napier introduce logarithms.
	John Woodall, in his *Surgeon's Mate*, features value of **lemon-juice in scurvy.**
	Guild of Apothecaries of the City of London founded.
1618.	**First edition of London Pharmacopœia.**
	Annibal **Albertini** publishes treatise on **heart diseases.**
	Martin **Böhme** publishes veterinary treatise (*Ross-Artzeney*).
1618–42.	Diphtheria spreads from Spain to Italy.
1618–1648.	Thirty Years' War.
1619.	**Christoph Scheiner's** *Oculus* published.
1619–20.	London Company of Bakers punished for falsifying weight of bread (penny-loaves).
1620.	Landing of the Pilgrims at Plymouth, Massachusetts (December 21).
	Bacon's *Novum Organum* published.
	Botanic Garden at Strassburg.
	Raymund Minderer's *Medicina militaris* published.
	Van Helmont teaches survival of a chemical substance in its compounds (Conservation of Matter).
	Pharmaceutical Department (*Prikaz*) in Russia.
	Caspar Bauhin classifies plants.
	Van Helmont stresses chemical rôle of gastric juice and bile in digestion.
	Fabry of Hilden emphasizes rôle of head injuries in psychoses.
1621.	Universities of Strassburg and Rinteln founded by Emperor Ferdinand II.
	Zacchias publishes treatise on medical jurisprudence.
	Cornelius Drebbel improves the microscope.
	Botanic Garden at Oxford.
1622.	**Aselli** discovers the **mesenteric glands** and **lacteal vessels.**
	Richard Hawkins' account of scurvy on voyage of 1593 (use of lemon-juice) published.
	London Weekly News published.
	Drebbel invents submarine.
1622–1763.	**Molière.**
1623.	New Netherlands colonized by the Dutch.
	University of Alcala moved to Madrid.
	Medical Faculty added to University of Altdorf.
1623–5.	Purpuric fever in Britain.
1624.	Louis Savot improves fireplace (inside air and flue).
1625.	Botanic Garden at Altdorf.
	Jean Riolan stresses pigmentation of the skin as a criterion of race.
	High mortality from plague in London.
1626.	**Jardin des Plantes** at Paris (1597).
1628.	**Harvey** publishes *De Motu Cordis*.
1628–1885.	Smallpox endemic in London.
1629.	Botanic Garden at Jena.
	Severino makes first resection of the wrist.
	London Bills of Mortality begin to specify causes of death.
	Sennert describes sequels of alcoholism.

1629.	**Petroleum** described by the Franciscan friar De la Roche d'Allion.
1629–31.	Plague in London.
1630.	**Thuillier** *père* holds that *ignis sacer* (**ergotism**) is due to poisoning by corn smut.
	Samuel Hafenreffer advances dermatology in his *Nosodochium*.
1630–38.	Treatment of malarial fever with **cinchona bark** known in Peru (Countess of Chinchon).
1631.	**Théophraste Renaudot** edits *Gazette de France* (May 30).
	Adrian van Mynsicht introduces tartar emetic.
1632.	Gustavus Adolphus founds University of Dorpat.
	University of Amsterdam founded as "Athenæum illustre."
	Botanic Garden at Hampton Court.
1632–77.	Spinoza.
1633.	Stephen Bradwell publishes **first book on first-aid.**
	Domenico **Marchetti** operates for renal calculus.
1634.	Smallpox epidemic in London.
1635.	Richelieu founds the Académie française.
	University of Budapest founded at Tyrnau.
1636.	**Harvard College** founded by act of General Court of Massachusetts (October 28).
	University of Utrecht (1634) founded (Library, 1581).
	Assembly of Virginia passes act regulating physicians' fees.
	William Briggs describes papilla of optic nerve.
	Malachias Geiger (*Fontigraphia*) mentions cachexia from overdosage of **iodine in goitre.**
	Plague in London.
1636–77.	**Francis Glisson** becomes Regius Professor of Physic at Cambridge.
1637.	**Descartes** shows that accommodation depends upon change in form of lens.
	Descartes founds analytical geometry (*Géométrie*).
	Royal College of Physicians issues report upon public health.
1638.	Cornelius Drebbel improves the **thermometer.**
	University of Lima, Peru (1553), acquires Medical Faculty.
	Padre Acugna, a Portuguese monk, introduces oil of copaiva.
	Assembly of Maryland passes act regulating surgeons' fees.
1639.	**First printing press in North America** (Cambridge, Massachusetts).
	First hospital in Canada.
	Virginia Assembly passes law regulating medical practice (October 2).
1639–50.	**Juan del Vigo** introduces **cinchona** into Spain and Italy.
1640.	Queen Christina charters University of Åbo.
	Coup de barre (probably **yellow fever**) at Guadeloupe (Dutertre).
	Bay State Psalm Book published.
	Marcus Banzer introduces artificial tympanum (*De auditione læsa*).
	Van Helmont investigates combination of acids and alkalies (salts).
	Werner Rolfink revives **dissecting** (*rolfinken*) in Germany.
1640–1688.	The Great Elector.
1641.	Heavy smallpox incidence in London.
	Kircher publishes *Magnes*.
1642.	**Jacob Bontius** describes **beriberi.**
	Peter Barba publishes book on use of cinchona in malarial fever.
1642–1649.	Civil War in England.
1642–1727.	Newton.
1643.	Torricelli constructs **barometer.**
	Mazarin Library (Paris) founded.
	Sir Edward Greaves describes **typhus fever** as a "new disease" in England.
1644.	**Descartes** elucidates **reflex action.**
	Descartes' treatise on dioptrics published.
	Hôtel Dieu in Montreal.
1644.	Matthew Hopkins, the witch finder.
1645.	Battle of Naseby.
	Royal ("Invisible") **Society** founded in London.
	City Library (Breslau) founded.
1646.	**Sanctorius** describes new instruments in his commentary on Avicenna.
	Diemerbroek publishes monograph on plague.
	Severino employs freezing mixtures (snow and ice) in surgical anesthesia.
	Syphilis appears in Boston, Mass.
1647.	**Pecquet** discovers receptaculum chyli and the circulation of chyle.
	Wirsung discovers **pancreatic duct.**
	Massachusetts act against pollution of Boston Harbor.
	Brancacci Library (Naples) founded.

1647.	Giles **Firmin** lectures on anatomy in Massachusetts.
1647–8.	Dutertre describes first definite epidemic of **yellow fever** in West Indies.
1648.	Peace of Westphalia.
	University of Bamberg founded.
	Van Helmont's *Ortus medicinæ* published.
	Athanasius Kircher describes the ear trumpet.
	Glauber investigates mineral acids.
	Francesco Redi disproves theory of spontaneous generation.
	Quarantine statute enacted by General Court of Massachusetts Bay.
	Riolan classifies skin diseases.
1649.	Royal Academy of Medical Sciences at Palermo.
	Act regulating the practice of medicine in Massachusetts.
	Dysentery among Cromwell's troops in Ireland.
	Fatal smallpox epidemic in London.
1649–1660.	Commonwealth in England.
1650.	**Glisson** describes **rickets** in *De rachitide.*
	Franciscus Sylvius shows association of tubercles with pulmonary phthisis.
	Johann Sperling publishes *Zoologia Physica* (man's place in nature).
1651.	**Harvey's** treatise on **embryology** (*De generatione animaliun*) published.
	Highmore discovers the **maxillary sinus.**
	Rudbeck and Thomas **Bartholin** discover the **lymphatics of the intestines.**
	Isaac Minnius severs sterno-mastoid for torticollis.
1652.	Johann Hoppe describes miliary fever.
	Lorenz Bausch founds the Academia Naturæ Curiosorum.
1653–1659.	Protectorate in England.
1654.	Otto von Guericke of Magdeburg introduces the **air-pump** (1641).
	Glisson describes the **capsule of the liver** in *Anatomia hepatis.*
	Engel Apotheke at Darmstadt.
	Pascal advances theory of probabilities.
	University of Herborn founded.
1654–1715.	Reign of Louis XIV.
1655.	University of Duisburg founded.
	Scultetus publishes his "Armamentarium."
1655–6.	Fatal epidemic of dysentery and fever among Cromwell's troops in Jamaica.
1656.	**Wharton's** "Adenographia" published.
	Rolfink shows that **cataract** is clouding of the lens.
	Lazar houses abolished in France.
1657.	Accademia del Cimento founded at Florence.
	Botanic Garden at Upsala.
	Wolfgang **Hoefer** describes **cretinism** in *Hercules medicus.*
	Jan à Gehema urges that field chests of drugs be furnished armies by the state.
	Comenius publishes *Orbis pictus.*
1657–9.	Epidemic catarrhal fever (ague) in England.
1657–1669.	Pandemic malarial fever.
1658.	**Swammerdam** discovers **red blood-corpuscles.**
	Wepfer demonstrates hemorrhagic lesion of the brain in **apoplexy.**
	Muffet's *Theater of Insects* published.
	Athanasius Kircher attributes plague to a contagium animatum and finds bacteria in milk.
	Sir John Winter invents ventilating fireplace (outside air).
1658–1665.	Typhus and influenza in England (Willis).
1659.	**Malpighi** outlines lymphadenoma (**Hodgkin's disease**).
	Willis describes war-time typhus of 1643.
	Severe smallpox epidemic in London.
	Diphtheria at Roxbury, Massachusetts.
	Royal Library (Berlin) founded.
1660.	**Schneider** shows that nasal secretion does not come from pituitary body (Galen).
	Willis describes **puerperal fever.**
	Hermann **Conring** publishes statistical treatise (*Examen rerum publicarum*).
	Malpighi discovers capillary anastomosis.
1660–85.	Charles II.
1661.	University of Lemberg (Lwow) founded.
	Stensen discovers **duct of parotid gland.**
	Malpighi publishes first account of **capillary system** (*De pulmonibus*).
	Stenson discovers **parotid duct.**
	Robert Boyle defines chemical elements and isolates acetone.

1661. **Typhoid fever** epidemic in England described by Willis (*Pathologia cerebri*, 1667, ch. 8).
  Scarlatina appears in England.
  Biblioteca Alessandrina (University of Rome) founded.
  Charles II charters the Royal Society.
  St. Bartholomew's Hospital (London) founded.
  John Graunt founds **medical statistics.**
  Population of London 460,000 (John Graunt).
  Descartes publishes first **treatise on physiology** (*De homine*).
  Lorenzo **Bellini** discovers excretory ducts of kidneys.
  De Graaf shows that ova arise in the **ovary.**
  Meibom discovers Meibomian glands.

1663. **First hospital in American colonies** (Long Island, N. Y.).
  Medical Faculty (Collegium Medicum) in Stockholm.
  Hendrik van Roonhuyze publishes treatise on gynecology (operation for **vesico-vaginal fistula**).
  Sylvius treats of **digestion** as a fermentation.

1663–65. Plague in England.

1664. **Willis's** *Cerebri anatome* published (**classification of cerebral nerves**).
  Swammerdam discovers **valves of lymphatics.**
  Henshaw invents pneumatic cabinet (differential pressure).
  De Graaf examines **pancreatic juice.**
  Solleysel transmits **glanders** from horse to horse.
  De la Martinière describes gonorrheal rheumatism.

1664–5. Royal Society (London) publishes *Transactions.*

1665. Newton discovers binomial theorem (published 1669) and law of gravitation.
  Great Plague of London.
  William Boghurst differentiates plague from spotted (typhus) fever in *London's Dreadful Visitation* (bills of mortality).
  Duke Christian Albrecht of Holstein founds **University of Kiel** (October 5).
  Richard Lower performs transfusion of blood from dog to dog.
  Ruysch investigates blood-vessels by anatomical injection.
  Colbert founds **Académie des sciences** (Paris).
  Royal Library at Copenhagen founded.
  Hooke's *Micrographia* published (**description of plant-cells**).
  First number of **Journal des sçavans** published (January 5).

1666. **Great Fire of London.**
  University of Lund founded (December 19).
  Newton describes solar spectrum.
  Malpighi's treatise on the viscera published.
  Coroners appointed for each county of Maryland.

1666–1675. Smallpox in Europe.

1667. Royal College of Physicians of Ireland (Dublin) founded.
  Jean Denis (Paris) performs first **transfusion of blood** from lamb to man.
  Swammerdam describes **docimasia** of fetal lungs.
  Hooke shows true function of lungs by artificial respiration.
  Walter Needham shows that fetus is nourished by the placenta.
  Alexander VII founds Library and Botanic Garden (University of Rome).
  Act for rebuilding London after fire of 1666.
  End of plague in England (epidemic at Nottingham).

1667–9. Smallpox in England (Sydenham).

1668. **Mayow** finds "igneo-aërial spirit" (**oxygen**) essential for combustion and respiration.
  Engel Apotheke in Darmstadt (1654) becomes Merck's Fabrik.
  Mauriceau's obstetric treatise published.
  Yellow fever appears in New York.

1668–9. Fatal aphthous fever in Leyden and other Dutch towns.

1668–1672. Epidemic dysentery in England (described by Sydenham and Morton).
  University of Agram (Zagreb) founded (Library, 1606).

1669. **Richard Lower's** *Tractatus de corde* published.
  Stensen founds statigraphic geology (*De solido intra solidum*).
  Brand discovers phosphorus.
  Lower shows that venous blood takes up air in the lungs.

1669–72. Dysentery and infantile summer diarrhea in England (Sydenham and Willis).

1669–74. Leopold I founds University of Innsbruck (Tyrol) as Academia Leopoldina (charter April 7, 1677). (Library, 1746).

1670. Malpighi discovers **Malpighian bodies** in spleen and kidneys.

1670.	Swammerdam discovers muscle-tonus.
	Willis discovers sweet taste of **diabetic urine** (*De medicamentorum operationibus*).
	Kerckring describes valvulæ conniventes of small intestine.
	Zambeccari performs **nephrectomy** on dogs.
	Physic Garden (now Royal Botanic Garden) at Edinburgh.
	Parliamentary Act for enlarging streets of London.
	Arsenic poisoning at Paris (Ste. Croix and Brinvilliers).
1671.	**Redi's** treatise on the **generation of insects** published.
	Newton publishes *Methodus fluxionum* (differential calculus).
	Joh. von Muralt teaches anatomy in Zürich.
	"Buying the smallpox" a custom in Poland.
	University of Urbino opened as a "studium generale."
	Yellow fever at Barbados.
1672.	**Willis** describes dementia præcox and general paralysis in *De anima brutorum*.
	Newton announces theory of light and colors.
	Le Gras brings **ipecac** to Europe from America (Piso, 1648).
	De Graaf describes the **Graafian follicles** in the ovary.
1672–82.	System of water-piping for Versailles constructed from Ranneken's plans.
1673.	**Malpighi** describes development of the chick.
	Leeuwenhoek makes **microscopes.**
	Botanic Garden at Chelsea.
1674.	**Printing press at Boston,** Massachusetts.
	Velsch publishes monograph on Filaria medinensis.
	Willis describes whooping-cough (Baillou, 1578).
	Malebranche surmises existence of motor-nerves.
	Morel invents **tourniquet** for checking hemorrhage.
	Hammen, a pupil of Leeuwenhoek, discovers **spermatozoa.**
	Fatal smallpox epidemic in London.
1675.	Leeuwenhoek discovers **protozoa.**
	Malpighi's *Anatome plantarum* published.
	Influenza in England.
	Sydenham differentiates scarlatina from measles.
1676.	Richard **Wiseman** describes tuberculosis of joints (tumor albus).
	Isaac Barlow invents repeating watch.
1677.	Kaiserliche Leopoldinische Akademie der Naturforscher founded.
	Leeuwenhoek observes spermatozoa.
	Hooke notes **fungoid disease of plants.**
	Glisson's doctrine of **irritability of tissues** (1662) published.
	Peyer describes **lymphoid follicles** in small intestine.
	Smallpox in Boston (**Thacher's Brief Rule** published).
1677–9.	Smallpox epidemic in London.
1677–1681.	Pandemic malarial fever in Europe.
1678.	Duke Francis II of Este founds University of Modena (November 5).
	De Marchetti shows anastomosis of arterioles and veins by injection.
	Measures to prevent smallpox in Boston (May 6).
1678–9.	Epidemic catarrhal fever (ague).
1679.	**Rivinus** discovers **sublingual duct.**
	Leeuwenhoek discovers **striped muscle.**
	Nicolas de Blegny publishes the **first medical periodical** (*Nouvelles découvertes*).
	Bonet's *Sepulchretum* published.
	Influenza in England.
	Botanic Garden at Berlin.
	James **Yonge** describes **flap amputation.**
1680.	Denis Papin constructs a miniature steam engine.
	Leeuwenhoek discovers **yeast plant.**
	Caspar Bartholin discovers excretory duct of sublingual gland.
	De Marchetti performs nephrotomy for renal calculus.
	Plague hospital at Magdeburg.
1680–1681.	**Borelli's** *De motu animalium* published.
1680–88.	Stephan Blankaart publishes *Collectanea Medico-physica* (periodical) at Amsterdam.
1681.	Royal College of Physicians of Edinburgh founded.
	Heavy smallpox mortality in London.
	Printing press at Williamsburg, Virginia.
1681–2.	**First medical congress** held at Rome (Congresso medico romano).
1682.	**Brunner** describes **duodenal glands** (discovered 1672).

1682.   **Nehemiah Grew's** *Anatomy of Plants* published.
             Newton demonstrates law of gravitation (1665–6).
             Botanic Garden at Amsterdam.
1682–1725.   Peter the Great.
1683.   Duke Francis II of Este charters University of Modena (Library, 1772).
             Sydenham's treatise on gout published.
             Leeuwenhoek describes and figures **bacteria** (September 17).
             Edward **Tyson** investigates **intestinal worms.**
             Abbé de la Roque publishes *Le Journal de Médicine* (Paris).
             Duverney publishes first treatise on **otology.**
1683–1848.   Chemical laboratory at Oxford.
1684.   Bernier classifies races of mankind by color of the skin.
             Sir Robert Sibbald notes scarlatina as a new disease in Edinburgh.
             Royal Academy of Sciences at Modena founded.
             Medicina Curiosa, London (**first English medical journal**), published (June 17).
1685.   Revocation of the Edict of Nantes.
             Medical Faculty at the University of Edinburgh.
             Barber-Surgeons' school at Stockholm reorganized as Societas chirurgica.
             Printing press at Philadelphia.
             Bidloo's *Anatomia* published.
             Vieussens' *Nevrographia* published.
             Deventer investigates contracted pelvis in labor.
             Paul **Portal** publishes obstetric treatise.
             Prussian ordinance regulating medical fees.
1685–6.   Typhus fever in England (Sydenham).
1685–1750.   Johann Sebastian Bach.
1686.   **Sydenham** describes **chorea minor.**
             Leibnitz publishes treatise on integral calculus (*De geometria recondita*).
             Joh. von **Muralt** opens Collegium in Zürich with lectures in the vernacular (January 5).
             Malpighi publishes treatise on fungi (*De plantis qui in aliis vegetant*).
1687.   Newton's *Principia* completed and published.
             Newton demonstrates parallelegram of forces (Stevinus, 1586).
             Muralt publishes course of anatomical lectures (Zürich).
             Sir William Petty publishes *Essays in Political Arithmetic.*
1688.   Influenza epidemic in England.
1688–89.   Revolution in England.
1689.   **Richard Morton's** *Phthisiologia* published.
             Walter Harris publishes treatise on **diseases of children.**
             Leeuwenhoek discovers rods in retina, and finer anatomy of cornea.
             Dysentery and typhus fever at sieges of Londonderry and Dundalk (Ireland).
1690.   **Locke's** *Essay on the Human Understanding* published.
             Publick Occurrences (newspaper) published at Boston, Massachusetts.
             Justine Siegemundin publishes treatise on midwifery.
             Floyer counts the pulse by the watch.
1691.   University at Dôle (1422) moved to Besançon.
             Clopton **Havers** publishes *Osteologia nova* (Haversian canals).
             Autopsy of Governor Slaughter in New York.
             Yellow fever in Boston.
             Regia Accademia dei fisiocritici in Siena.
1692.   Salem Witchcraft.
             Ammann teaches **deaf-mutes.**
             Stahl advances doctrine of psychogenic disorders and psychotherapy.
1692–1890.   King's and Queen's College of Physicians in Ireland (Dublin).
1693.   College of William and Mary founded at Williamsburg, Virginia.
             University of Halle founded (Library, 1696).
             St. Thomas's Hospital (London) rebuilt.
             Printing press in New York.
             Quarantine against yellow fever in Boston Harbor.
             Molyneux describes influenza of 1693 in England.
             Baglivi describes **heat-stroke** in Rome.
             Acoluthus (Breslau) resects the lower jaw.
             Edmund **Halley** prepares **Breslau Table.**
1693–9.   "Seven ill years" (famine and fever) in England and Scotland.
1694.   Camerarius gives experimental proof of sexuality in plants.
             High fever mortality in London.

1694–5.   Loss of 600 sailors on "Tiger" from yellow fever off Barbados.

1694–1788. Voltaire.

1695.   Nehemiah Grew discovers magnesium sulphate in Epsom waters (**Epsom salts**).

1696.   Window-tax deprives habitations of light and air in England (7.-8. William and Mary, cap. 18).

1697.   Anatomical theater erected in Surgeons' Hall at Edinburgh.
        Pacchioni discovers glands in the dura mater.
        Biblioteca casanatense (Rome) founded.

1698.   **Stahl's** treatise on **diseases of the portal system** published.
        Statute of Monpellier requiring visits of students to hospital and city patients.

1699.   History and Memoirs of the French Academy of Sciences published.
        Tyson's *Orang Outang* published.
        Infectious diseases act in Massachusetts.

1700.   **Königliche Preussische Akademie der Wissenschaften** founded at **Berlin.**
        Ramazzini publishes treatise on **trade diseases.**
        Real Academia de medicina y cirurgia (Seville) founded.
        Lorenzo Terraneo investigates **gonorrhea.**
        Quarantine Act, Pennsylvania.

1701.   Frederick Elector of Brandenburg, crowned King of Prussia.
        Variolation (human inoculation) against smallpox practised in Constantinople.
        Yale College founded (New Haven).
        Smallpox prevention act (Massachusetts) authorizing impressment of houses for isolation of patients.
        Robert Houstoun taps ovarian cyst.

1701–13. War of the Spanish Succession.

1701–33. **Deventer's** *Novum lumen* published.

1701–86. Diphtheria endemic and epidemic in Spain.

1702.   **University of Breslau** founded by Leopold I (October 21).
        Stahl states phlogiston theory.
        Smallpox in Boston.

1702–14. Reign of Queen Anne.

1703.   Foundation of St. Petersburg.
        House of Lords authorizes apothecaries to prescribe as well as dispense drugs.
        Leeuwenhoek discovers parthenogenesis of plant lice.

1704.   Newton's treatise on Optics published.
        Valsalva publishes *De aure humana* ("Valsalva's method").
        John Freind lectures on chemistry (Oxford).
        Dr. Eysenbart practises as a mountebank in Germany.

1705.   Robert Elliot first professor of anatomy at Edinburgh.
        Brisseau and **Maître Jan** show that **cataract** is the clouded lens.

1706.   Academy of Sciences (Montpellier) founded.
        Marsili establishes **first laboratory of marine zoölogy** at Marseilles.
        Freind describes diseases of troops on Lord Peterborough's Spanish expedition.
        Moscow Court Hospital (*Hofspital*) founded.

1707.   Senckenburg Foundation for advancement of science.
        Edict of Louis XIV specifying free 10 o'clock clinic for poor in French medical schools.
        Dionis' *Cours d'opérations de chirurgie* published.
        Union of Scotland with England.
        Influenza pandemic in Europe.

1708–77. **Haller.**

1709.   Boerhaave describes heat-stroke as "insolation."

1709–10. Malignant fever in London.

1710.   **Charité** Hospital opened at **Berlin.**
        English quarantine act.
        Royal Scientific Society at Upsala founded.
        Morand and Le Dran perform first exarticulation of shoulder-joint.
        Sir David Hamilton describes "miliary fevers."
        Anel operates for aneurysm by ligating above the sac.
        Pourfoir du Petit founds doctrine of contralateral innervation.
        Thomas Newcomen invents fire engine.
        Santorini discovers muscle and cartilage in larynx.
        Severe smallpox epidemic in England.
        School of Physic at Trinity College, Dublin.
        Hospital at York (England).

1711.   John Shore invents **tuning fork.**

1711.   Lancisi founds **medical library** (Biblioteca Lancisiana) at Rome.
          Heister makes first post-mortem of **appendicitis.**
          Bernard de Mandeville describes the vapors (hysteria) and **spleen** (hypochondria).
1712.   Influenza epidemic.
          Engelbert Kämpfer describes Madura foot as "perical."
          Torti (Modena) uses cinchona bark in **pernicious malarial fever.**
1712–78. Rousseau.
1713.   St. Côme merged into **Académie de chirurgie** (Paris).
          Theatrum anatomicum founded in Berlin.
          Real Academia española (Madrid).
          Botanic Garden at St. Petersburg.
          Anel catheterizes lachrymal ducts.
          Nicolaus Gauger publishes memoir on heating (elliptical ventilating fireplace).
1714.   Accession of House of Hanover (England).
          G. D. Fahrenheit constructs 212 degree **thermometer.**
          Epidemics of typhus fever and smallpox in London.
          Leibnitz recommends pavilion system of hospital construction (barracks) to forestall
            infection.
1714–15. **Timoni** and **Pylarini** communicate Asiatic practice of **smallpox inoculation** to Royal
            Society.
1715.   J.-L. **Petit** differentiates between compression and concussion of the brain.
          Vieussens publishes treatise on heart dis?ases.
          J. T. Hensing discovers phosphorus in the brain.
1715–65. Material prosperity (decline of fevers) in England.
1716.   Surgeon General appointed in German Army at 900 marks per annum.
          Abraham de Moivre publishes *Doctrine of Chances.*
          New York City issues ordinance for midwives.
          Hospital at Salisbury (England).
1717.   Timoni has daughter inoculated against smallpox.
          Gauthier (naval surgeon) invents apparatus for distilling sea-water.
          Heister's Anatomical Compend displaces that of Philip Verheyen (1693).
          Hospital for infectious diseases in Boston.
1718.   Theatrum anatomicum in Vienna.
          Lady Mary Wortley Montagu has son inoculated for smallpox.
          Pierre Dionis describes tubal pregnancy.
          Heister's *Chirurgie* published.
          Hoffmann's anodyne.
          Edward **Strother** describes **puerperal fever.**
          Botanical Garden at Madrid.
1718–19. Typhus fever in England described by Clifton Wintringham.
1719.   Westminster Hospital (London) founded.
          Kaspar Neumann isolates **thymol.**
          M**ɔ**rgagni describes syphilis of brain, lungs, and viscera.
          Dysentery pandemic in Europe.
          Heavy smallpox mortality in London.
          Hospital at Cambridge, England.
          National Library at Turin founded.
          Epidemic of plague at Marseilles.
          Epidemic of influenza (*fierro chuto*) in Peru.
          Richard Mead publishes "Short Discourse" on plague.
          Act of Parliament (7. George I, Cap. 8) enforcing Mead's recommendations (repealed
            1721).
1720.   University of Turin reopened (new buildings).
1721.   General Holtzendorff creates "Collegium medico-chirurgicum" at Berlin.
          Palfyn exhibits **obstetric forceps** to French Academy of Surgery.
          Zabdiel Boylston inoculates for smallpox in Boston (June 26).
          University of Dijon (Côte d'Or) started (Papal bull, April 16, 1723).
          Apothecaries Company of London organized.
          Water supplied to London from Thames by Chelsea Water Company.
          School of Naval Medicine at Rochefort-sur-Mer (Library, 1793).
          Floyer's *Psychrolusia* published.
          Daniel Defoe writes *Journal of the Plague Year.*
1721–2.   Smallpox epidemic in Boston.
1722.   "Buying the smallpox" (inoculation scabs) current in Wales.
1723.   **Cheselden's** treatise on lithotomy published.

1723.	Montpellier statute authorizing students' clinic at Hôpital St. Éloi (February 6). University of Dijon (1721) authorized. Yellow fever reaches London (from Lisbon).
1724.	**Guyot** of Versailles attempts **catheterization of the Eustachian tubes.** Imperial Russian Academy of Sciences (St. Petersburg) founded (Library, 1714). John Maubray gives private instruction in obstetrics in England. A. **de Moivre** publishes *Annuities upon lives.*
1724–1804.	Kant.
1725.	Prussian edict regulating practice of medicine. **Guy's Hospital** (London) opened (January 6). Freind's History of Physick published. Universidad Central de Venezuela (Caracas) founded.
1726.	**Stephen Hales** makes first measurement of **blood-pressure.** Freind presents memorial of College of Physicians to Parliament on prevalence of alcoholism. Albinus, Winslow and Du Verney describe tendon-sheaths. H. F. Albertini correlates dyspnea with heart disease.
1727.	**Pourfour du Petit** investigates functions of **cervical sympathetic.** Cheselden performs lateral operation for stone. Benjamin Franklin founds American Philosophical Society (Philadelphia). Pope Benedict XIII founds University of Camerino (July 25).
1727–9.	Epidemic catarrhal fever (ague) in England.
1728.	**Fauchard** publishes *Le chirurgien dentiste.* Michael **Alberti** describes epidemic **whooping-cough.** **Cheselden** introduces iridiotomy for **artificial pupil** (1720).
1728–93.	**John Hunter.**
1729.	Influenza pandemic in Europe. Royal Infirmary (Edinburgh) opened. Dean Swift's *Modest Proposal* on famine and beggary in Ireland. Edward Strother describes epidemic fevers of 1726–9.
1730.	**Daviel** improves **cataract operation.** Black Assizes (jail-fever) at Taunton. James **Douglas** describes the **peritoneum.** Gaspar Casal describes **pellagra** as "mal de la rosa." Lambert resects lower jaw (Fauchard). **Réaumur** introduces 80 degree **thermometer.** Frobenius describes preparation of sulphuric ether. Royal Botanic Garden at Kew, near London.
1730–31.	Thomas Cadwalader teaches anatomy in Philadelphia.
1731.	Friedrich **Hoffmann** describes **chlorosis.** **Le Dran** improves **lithotomy.** J.-L. Petit investigates hemostasis in amputation. **Académie royale de chirurgie** (Paris) founded (December 18). **Philadelphia Hospital** founded. Royal Dublin Society (Ireland) founded.
1732.	Christian VI reorganizes University of Copenhagen (March 3). **Boerhaave's** *Elementa chemiæ* published. **Winslow's** *Exposition anatomique* published. Abraham Chovet publishes *Syllabus* for anatomical classes in Philadelphia. Influenza pandemic in Europe.
1732–7.	George II founds University of Göttingen (Lectures, 1734; Library, 1735–6).
1733.	**Library of the Paris Medical Faculty** founded. St. George's Hospital (London) founded. Cheselden's *Osteographia* published. George Cheyne describes "**Cheyne-Stokes respiration.**" Stephen Hales produces dropsy by injecting water into the veins. Zedler employs bismuth in salves. John Machin describes ichthyosis histrix in the Lambert family. Influenza epidemic in England. Real Academia Nacional de Medicina (Madrid) founded.
1734.	Joseph Rogers describes epidemic diseases of Cork, Ireland (1708–34). National Library at Naples founded. Friedrich Wilhelm I of Prussia issues **first regulations for field hospitals.**
1734–5.	J. F. Cassebohm investigates anatomy of the ear (*De aure humana*).
1734–6.	**Huxham** describes fevers of Devon and Cornwall.

1735.   Linnæus' *Systema naturæ* (classification of animals) published.
        Werlhof describes **purpura hæmorrhagica.**
        Medical Society in Boston founded.
        Huxham describes ship-fever (malignant typhus) on warships off Plymouth and Portsmouth.
        English laws against witchcraft repealed.
1735–6. William Douglas describes first appearance of scarlatina in New England.
1736.   Edinburgh Hospital founded.
        J.-L. **Petit opens mastoid** for abscess in middle ear.
        Haller investigates cardiac movements and function of **bile** in digestion of fats.
        École préparatoire de médecine at Rouen.
1736–40. Astruc publishes influential treatise on venereal diseases.
1737.   **University of Göttingen** (Georgia Augusta) formally opened (September 17).
        Influenza and equine epizoötic cough in England (Huxham).
        Royal Medical Society of Edinburgh founded.
        Radcliffe Library (Oxford) founded.
1738.   Haller called to Göttingen.
        Friedrich Hoffmann investigates fever.
        Lieberkühn invents reflector microscope.
        Heavy smallpox epidemic in Charleston, South Carolina.
        Daniel Bernouilli states the kinetic theory of gases.
1739.   Special **chair of midwifery** in the University of Edinburgh.
        Letherland notes scarlatinal sore throat in London.
        Percival Pott recommends external use of bismuth.
        F.-S. **Morand** makes first **excision of hip-joint.**
        Royal Swedish Academy of Science founded.
        Hospital at Aberdeen (Scotland).
1740.   University of Pennsylvania founded as "College of Philadelphia."
        Ship-fever of Cartagena expedition described by Smollett.
        Bishop Berkeley's *Querist* (1737–8) on food-economics and famine in Ireland.
        London Hospital founded.
        Friedrich Hoffmann describes **rubella.**
        Thomas Dover invents **"Dover's Powder."**
1740–41. Famine and typhus fever in Ireland.
1740–42. Smallpox epidemics in England and Scotland.
1740–48. War of Austrian Succession.
1740–86. Reign of Frederick the Great.
        Hot-air heating at Neues Palais (Potsdam).
1741.   Chair of clinical medicine at Edinburgh.
        Süssmilch's treatise on **vital statistics** published.
        John **Atkins** describes **sleeping sickness** in Guinea.
        Timoni's child dies of smallpox in spite of inoculation (1717).
        Archibald **Cleland** catheterizes Eustachian tube.
1741–2. Epidemic famine-fever in England.
1742.   **Celsius** invents 100 degree **thermometer.**
        Anatomical theater in Zürich opened.
        Linnæus describes **aphasia.**
        Pandemic influenza in Europe.
        Royal Danish Scientific Society founded (November 13).
1743.   **University of Erlangen** chartered (February 21) and opened (November 4) by **Karl VII.**
        Epidemic of "influenza" in Italy and England.
        Kirkpatrick introduces attenuated "arm to arm" inoculation against smallpox.
        University founded at Santiago (Chile).
        Red Cross arrangement at battle of Dettingen (June 27).
        Pringle (1750–52) describes dysentery and typhus among troops after Dettingen.
        Frederick the Great separates main hospitals from flying ambulances.
1743–58. Stephen **Hales** publishes treatises on ventilators.
1743–98. Inoculation against smallpox a lucrative practice in England.
1744.   **Trembley** investigates **regeneration** of tissues in hydrozoa.
        Euler creates calculus of variations.
        Alexander **Monro** publishes handbook of comparative anatomy.
        Academy of Sciences at Rouen.
1745.   Barbers separated from higher surgeons in England (Act of June 24).
        Middlesex Hospital (London) founded.
        Ambulatory clinic opened at Prague.

1745.	**Heberden's** *Antitheriaka* published (improvement of London Pharmacopœia).
	C. G. Kratzenstein employs **electrotherapy** in paralysis.
	William Cooke introduces **steam heating.**
1745-6.	Formidable epidemic of ship-fever (typhus) among English troops in Jacobite Rebellion.
1745-99.	Spread of diphtheria from Spain to the Continent, England and America.
1746.	College of New Jersey (Princeton University) founded.
	English window-tax of 1696 shifted to tenement houses (20. George II).
	Academy of Sciences (Amiens) organized.
	Sir Richard Manningham describes **typhoid fever** as febricula (Murchison).
	Haller investigates **mechanism of breathing** (*De respiratione*).
	London Lock Hospital founded.
	Antoine Deparcieux introduces idea of "mean expectation of life."
	Theden introduces compressive bandage in hemostasis (Esmarch, 1873).
	Total complement of d'Anville's fleet wiped out by fever and scurvy at Halifax.
	Middlesex County Hospital for smallpox opened in London.
1747.	**Haller's** *Primæ lineæ physiologiæ* published.
1748.	Collegium medico-chirurgicum at Dresden.
	Medical Faculty (Colegio de cirurgia) at Cadiz.
	Meckel describes **sphenopalatine ganglion.**
	John Starr describes malignant sore throat in Cornwall (England).
	Fothergill publishes account of **ulcerated sore throat.**
1749.	Medical Society in New York.
	British Lying-in Hospital (London) founded.
	Senac's treatise on the **heart** published.
	Lafosse investigates pathology of glanders.
	Meyer orders phthisical patients to mountains at Appenzell.
	Nathaniel Cotton describes scarlatina at St. Albans (England).
	Buffon's Natural History published.
1749-64.	Swedish vital statistics first locate prominent rôle of **whooping-cough** in infant mortality (43,393 deaths).
1749-1827.	Laplace.
1749-1832.	Goethe.
1750.	Griffith **Hughes** gives classic account of **yellow fever** of 1715 (Barbados).
	City of London Lying-in Hospital founded.
	Antonio Nuñez Ribero Sanchez introduces **corrosive sublimate** in syphilis.
	Black Assizes at Old Bailey (London); court-room epidemic of jail-fever.
	Russel describes Aleppo button (**endemic ulcer**).
	Zittmann's decoction.
	Thomas Walker first physician to settle in the West (United States).
	Musée de Luxembourg (Paris) established.
1751.	Haller founds Königliche Gesellschaft der Wissenschaften (Göttingen).
	Pennsylvania Hospital founded at Philadelphia.
	Albergo dei poveri (Milan) founded.
	Diphtheria appears in New York.
1751-5.	Fothergill reports monthly on putrid and miliary fevers in England.
1752.	**Haller** publishes memoir on **specific irritability of tissues.**
	Smellie's *Midwifery* published.
	Pringle's treatise on *Diseases of the Army* published.
	Réaumur experiments on **digestion** in birds.
	Huxham describes epidemic diseases of 1728-52 (Plymouth).
	Seraphim Hospital (Stockholm) opened for teaching purposes.
	Pennsylvania Hospital (Philadelphia) opened.
	Queen Charlotte's Lying-in Hospital at London founded.
	Medical Society founded in London.
	St. George's Hospital (London) founded.
	Heavy smallpox mortality in London.
1753.	**Daviel** publishes memoir on extraction of **cataract.**
	Lind's Treatise on Scurvy published.
	Levret's *Art des Accouchemens* published.
	Linnæus publishes classification of plants (*Species plantarum*).
	British Museum (London) founded (Library, 1753).
	Prussian Academy of Useful Sciences (Erfurt) founded.
	Cadwallader Colden describes "throat distemper" in New York.
1754.	**Van Swieten** organizes **clinical instruction** in Vienna.
	Watson describes scleroderma at Curzio's clinic.

1754.   Botanic Garden at Vienna.
           Kings College (Columbia University) founded at New York.
           Epidemic of throat distemper (diphtheria and scarlatina) in New England.
1754–7.   Black discovers CO_2.
1755.   Earthquake of Lisbon.
           University of Moscow founded by Czarina Elizabeth.
           Heavy epidemic of whooping-cough in Sweden.
           Zinn's atlas of the eye published.
1756.   Meath Hospital, Dublin, founded.
           Pfaff's treatise on dentistry published.
           Nicolas André describes infraorbital neuralgia.
           Royal Central Statistical Bureau (Stockholm) established (reorganized 1858).
1756–63.   Seven Years' War.
1757.   William Hunter describes arteriovenous aneurysm.
           Huxham describes malignant sore throat at Plymouth (1751–7).
           Lind's treatise on naval hygiene published.
1758.   Return of Halley's comet (end of comet theory of disease).
           De Haën employs thermometry in clinical work.
           Influenza epidemic in Scotland (Whytt).
           Lind joins Haslar Hospital.
           John Fordyce describes miliary (putrid) fever.
           Richard Brocklesby introduces ridge-ventilation in decentralized barrack hospitals
1758–62.   Epidemic dysentery in England.
1759.   Königliche Bayerische Akademie der Wissenschaften founded at Munich.
           Wolff's *Theoria generationis* published.
           Local epidemic influenza in Peru and Bolivia.
           Mestivier describes and operates for localized appendicitis.
           First public dissection in American Colonies by John Bard and Peter Middleton.
           John Bard operates for extra-uterine pregnancy.
           Physic Garden at Kew (England).
1760.   William Shippen, Jr., lectures on anatomy in Philadelphia.
           Royal Norse Scientific Society at Trondhjem.
           Thomas Goulard notes curative effect of lead in cancer.
           Cullen introduces Scotch douche.
           Act to regulate practice of medicine in New York City.
1760–76.   Benjamin Martin improves microscopes.
1761.   Morgagni's *De sedibus* published.
           Auenbrugger's *Inventum novum* published.
           Pope Clement XI gives MS. of Eustachius to Lancisi.
           École Nationale Vétérinaire (Lyons) founded.
1761–3.   Joseph Black differentiates between specific and latent heat.
1761–5.   Astruc publishes system of gynecology.
1762.   Plenciz states theory of contagium animatum.
           Roederer and Wagler describe typhoid fever at Göttingen.
           Influenza epidemic in Europe.
           John Clayton's *Flora Virginica* published.
           Shippen's private maternity hospital established at Philadelphia.
           Library of Pennsylvania Hospital founded (first in America).
           Bilguer resects wrist.
           Stoerk introduces aconite and other narcotics.
           Botanic Garden at Cambridge (England).
           Surgical clinic opened at Lisbon.
1762–96.   Reign of Catherine II of Russia.
1763.   Catherine II founds Secret Hospital for Venereal Diseases at St. Petersburg.
           Senckenburg Foundation at Frankfurt a. M.
           Botanic Garden at Madrid.
           Linnæus creates scientific nosology in *Genera morborum*.
1764.   Cotugno describes sciatica.
           Louis introduces digital compression for hemorrhage.
           School of Surgery founded in Barcelona.
           Botanic Garden at St. Vincent.
           First pavilion hospital at Plymouth.
           Vogel introduces the term "paranoia."
1764–6.   Sutton and assistants inoculate 19,792 persons with unripe smallpox virus (no deaths).
1765.   Medical Department of University of Pennsylvania founded.

1765. **Fontana** publishes memoir on viper poison.
Library of the Sorbonne (Paris) founded.
Francis Home describes false membrane in diphtheritic croup.
R. B. Hirsch names ganglion of sensory root of fifth nerve after **Gasser.**
Royal Veterinary High-School at Dresden planned (erected 1774).
James Watt invents steam-engine (Patents, 1769–84).
Catherine II founds the Hermitage at St. Petersburg (Public Museum, 1852).
1765–6. École Nationale Vétérinaire at Alfort.
1766. **Cavendish** discovers hydrogen.
Desault's bandage for fractures introduced.
Improvement of streets of London (Paving Act).
New Jersey State Medical Society founded.
1767. **Heberden** describes **varicella.**
Sir George **Baker** publishes essay on **lead colic** in Devonshire.
Charles **White** resects shoulder-joint.
Kay and Hargreaves invent spinning jenny (beginning of Industrial Revolution in England).
Library of Montpellier Medical Faculty started (gift of 1200 books).
Influenza pandemic in Europe.
Medical School, King's College, New York, founded.
Heberden describes London influenza of 1767.
1768. Louis XV moves University of Pont-à-Mousson to Nancy.
Wolff's memoir on embryology of the intestines published.
Robert **Whytt** describes **tuberculous meningitis.**
Heberden describes **angina pectoris.**
Gimbernat's ligament discovered.
Theatrum anatomicum at Frankfurt a. M.
Dr. Johnson discusses St. Kilda boat-cold (contagion of influenza).
Lind's treatise on **tropical medicine** published.
1769. Guy's Hospital (London) founded.
Dartmouth College (Hanover, New Hampshire) founded.
Cullen's *Synopsis nosologiæ* published.
Constitutio criminalis Theresiana (Law of **torture**).
Pott's treatise on **fractures and dislocations** published.
Watt's steam-engine (1765) patented.
Peter Middleton publishes first American book on history of medicine.
Medical Society of New York City, founded.
University of Malta (La Valletta) founded.
Palatine Library (Parma) founded.
1770. Maria Theresa reorganizes University of Pavia.
William Hunter founds **school of anatomy in Great Windmill Street.**
Rutty describes **relapsing fever.**
Cotugno demonstrates albumen in the urine.
School of Obstetrics (Scuola pareggiate) at Venice.
General Dispensary in Aldersgate Street (London).
John Rutty publishes continuous records of weather and diseases in Dublin during 1724–64.
Willan describes scarlatina in London.
William Hunter describes **retroversion of the uterus.**
Schilling describes yaws ("Indian pox").
Abbé de l'Épée invents sign language for **deaf-mutes.**
First medical degree in United States conferred upon Robert Tucker by King's College.
Pennsylvania quarantine act.
1770–71. Smallpox destroys three million people in East Indies.
1770–1827. Beethoven.
1771. Rev. Richard Price constructs first life-table for actuaries (Northampton Table).
Arkwright perfects spinning jenny.
Louis Vitet publishes *Médecine vétérinaire.*
George **Armstrong** describes **congenital pyloric stenosis.**
John Hunter's treatise on the **teeth** published.
1771–2. Diphtheria epidemic in New York.
1771–4. **Priestley** and **Scheele** isolate **oxygen** ("dephlogisticated air").
1772. University of Coimbra reorganized.
Beginnings of modern Japanese medicine.
Encyclopédie (Diderot and d'Alembert) completed.
Heavy smallpox mortality in London.

1772.   **Rutherford** discovers **nitrogen.**
         Priestley discovers nitrogen and **nitrous oxide.**
         Mercurio Volante (Mexico) published (October 17).
         New Jersey act to regulate the practice of medicine.
         Haygarth reports on public health and diseases of Chester (England).
         Royal Academy of Belgium (Brussels) founded.
1773.   Medical Society of London founded.
         James Sims publishes continuous records of epidemic diseases in Tyrone (1765–72).
         First insane asylum in U. S. at Williamsburg, Virginia.
         Fothergill describes **facial neuralgia.**
         Charles **White** urges asepsis to prevent **puerperal fever.**
         John Howard begins visitations of English prisons.
         Botanic Garden at Coimbra.
         James **Lind** shows possibility of delousing and prevention of **typhus** by baking clothes.
         Jesuit Order suppressed by Clement XIV.
         University of Münster (Westphalia) founded (reorganized 1818, 1902).
1773–74. Revolution in Russia.
1774.   **William Hunter's** *Anatomia uteri* published.
         Benjamin **Jesty** vaccinates against smallpox (Dorsetshire).
         Andersch discovers glossopharyngeal nerve.
         Haygarth describes typhus fever in Chester, England (1772–4).
         Priestley discovers **ammonia** and sulphur dioxide.
         Scheele discovers **chlorine.**
         John Howard testifies in House of Commons as to status of jails in England ("Winter's Journey").
         Acts of Parliament for sanitary improvement of prisons.
         Royal Czech Society of Sciences (Prague) founded (reorganized 1784, 1918).
         Royal Veterinary High-School (Dresden) opened.
         Priestley announces his discovery of "dephlogisticated air" (1774).
1775.   **Lavoisier** isolates and defines **oxygen.**
         Pole and Dobson find grape-sugar in the urine.
         Conradi isolates **cholesterin** in bile (Chevreuil, 1824).
         Pandemic influenza.
         Diphtheria epidemic in New England.
         John Morgan appointed Director General of American Army.
         Botanic Garden at Vienna.
1775–83. American Revolution.
1776.   Declaration of Independence.
         Marie Theresa establishes Academy of Sciences at Agram (Croatia).
         Cullen's "First Lines" published.
         Adam Smith publishes *Wealth of Nations.*
         Jasser operates successfully on the **mastoid.**
         Black Assize at Dublin (infection of court by a single prisoner).
         Scheele and Bergmann discover uric acid in vesical calculi.
         Fothergill describes tic douloureux.
         Plenck's classification of skin diseases published.
         Centenary of Royal Society (institution of Copley Medal for work in experimental science).
         Cruikshank discovers that severed nerves will grow together.
1776–1805. Scarlatina pandemic in both hemispheres.
1777.   **Lavoisier** describes exchange of gases **in respiration.**
         Sigault performs **symphysiotomy.**
         John Howard's investigations of **prisons** and hospitals published.
         Newcastle Dispensary, for smallpox inoculation, founded by John Clark (October 1).
         Bonnemain employs **warm-water heating** in greenhouses.
         Josef II founds Veterinary School at Vienna (July 23).
         William **Shippen** chosen Director General of American Army Medical Department.
         Lorry publishes *Doctrina de Morbus Cutaneis* (classification).
         Veterinary High School at Vienna.
1777–8. Levison describes scarlatina epidemic in London.
1777–89. John Clark reports on typhus and other diseases at Newcastle.
1777–97. First University of Bonn (Charter 1784; opened 1786).
1778.   Count Rumford investigates mechanical equivalent of heat.
         C. C. von **Siebold** performs **symphysiotomy** in Germany.
         Withering describes scarlatina epidemic in Birmingham.
         Veterinary High School at Hanover founded.

1778.	**William Brown** publishes first **American pharmacopœia** in Philadelphia.

1778.   **William Brown** publishes first **American pharmacopœia** in Philadelphia.
Lichtenberg differentiates between positive and negative electricity.
Royal Batavian Society of Arts and Sciences at Weltvreden, Java (oldest in Asia).

1779.   University of Palermo founded.
Academy of Sciences (Lisbon) founded.
J. P. **Frank** issues first system of **public hygiene** (vol. i, April 24).
Bylon of Java describes **dengue.**
Academia das Sciencias (Lisbon) founded.
Ingenhousz discovers process of respiration in plants.
Pott describes deformity and paralysis from spinal caries.
Notation of causes of death begun in English naval hospitals.
Mesmer's memoir on **animal magnetism** published.
Hôpital Necker (Paris) founded.

1779–80.   Heavy typhus fever epidemic in Channel fleet off Portsmouth (England).

1779–83.   Dysentery pandemic in Europe.

1780.   University of Oxford establishes chair of clinical medicine.
University of Münster inaugurated.
University of Naples reorganized.
Chabert's memoir on **animal anthrax** published.
Benjamin **Franklin** invents **bifocal lenses.**
Guyton de Morveau stresses danger of **industrial lead poisoning.**
Hôpital Cochin (Paris) founded.
Board of Health at Petersburg, Virginia.
Benjamin Moseley describes yellow fever in Jamaica.
Foreign Medical Review (London) founded.
American Academy of Arts and Sciences founded at Boston.

1780–85.   Epidemic catarrhal fever (influenza) in England.
Pandemic dysentery (Hirsch).

1781.   Cavendish effects synthesis and ascertains composition of water.
Lavoisier investigates **metabolism.**
Kant's "Critique of Pure Reason" published.
Massachusetts Medical Society founded.
Manchester Literary and Philosophical Society founded.

1782.   **Medical Department of Harvard University** founded.
Medico-chirurgical Institute in Zürich opened (April 28).
Senebier discovers effect of light on **chlorophyll.**
Heysham describes epidemic of typhus fever at Carlisle (1781).
Epidemic influenza in England and Scotland.
A. M. Lorgna founds Società italiana delle scienze (Rome).
University of Innsbruck reduced to a lyceum by Joseph II.

1783.   Austria separates surgeons from barbers.
Fox's East India Bill (impeachment of Warren Hastings, 1788).
Lambeth **Water Works** (London Supply) constructed.
Dispensary opened at Whitehaven (England).
Spallanzani investigates acidity of **gastric juice.**
Royal Society of Edinburgh founded (Transactions, 1788).
Hunterian Museum at Glasgow founded.
Marschall (Strassburg) excises a prolapsed cancerous uterus.
Probable cholera epidemic at Hurdwar festival (India).
Argand burner invented.

1783–85.   Minckelaers introduces **gas-lighting** in Louvain.
Cavendish establishes composition of air.
Lavoisier decomposes water and overthrows phlogiston theory.

1784.   **Allgemeines Krankenhaus** opened at **Vienna** (August 16).
Kings College (New York) rechartered as Columbia College.
Goethe and **Vicq d'Az**/**r** discover **intermaxillary bone.**
Cotugno discovers **cerebrospinal fluid.**
James Watt constructs steam radiator for his work-room.
Pellagra hospital in Lengano (Italy).
Royal College of Surgeons in Ireland founded.
Asiatic Society of Bengal (Calcutta) founded.
Catherine II founds Obukhovski Hospital at St. Petersburg.

1785.   **Josephinum** established at Vienna.
Cartwright invents power loom.
Fowler introduces potassium arsenate (**Fowler's solution**).

1785.   **John Hunter** discovers collateral circulation and introduces proximal ligation in **aneurysm**.
       Cod-liver oil first used by English physicians.
       Withering's treatise on the fox-glove (**digitalis**) published.
       Charles White describes phlegmasia alba dolens.
       Children exposed to smallpox in Chester (England) as a means of immunization (Haygarth).
       Sir Gilbert **Blane** publishes treatise on **naval medicine**.
       Hôpital Beaujon (Paris) founded.
       Royal Irish Academy (Dublin) founded.
       Chair of anatomy established in the University of Dublin.
       Watt patents device for smoke abatement.
       London Hospital Medical College.
       University of Georgia (U. S. A.) founded.
       Justus Perthes founds Geographische Anstalt (Gotha).

1786.   Josef II erects university buildings at Budapest.
       John Hunter publishes *Treatise on the Venereal Diseases*.
       Inoculation against smallpox begun at Newcastle Dispensary (founded 1777).
       Parry describes **exophthalmic goiter** (Basedow, 1840).
       Lettsom describes **drug habit** and alcoholism.
       A. F. Miller attempts classification of micro-organisms.
       Vicq d'Azyr publishes treatise on comparative anatomy.
       P.-F. **Moreau** excises **elbow-joint**.
       James Sims describes scarlatina epidemic in London (1786).
       Fourcroy and Thouret discover adipocere.
       Royal College of Physicians (London) publishes transactions.
       Josef II founds Royal Hungarian Veterinary High-school at Budapest (December 12).
       Botanic Garden at Calcutta.

1787.   **College of Physicians of Philadelphia** founded (Library, 1788).
       Western University of Pennsylvania (Pittsburgh) founded.
       Mascagni publishes atlas of the **lymphatics**.
       Paullitzky introduces **ergot** in obstetrics.
       Guild of Bathkeepers abolished in Würzburg.
       Lavoisier constructs a gasometer.

1788.   University of Louvain removed to Brussels.
       Lagrange publishes *Mécanique Analytique*.
       John Filson, a medical student, surveys Cincinnati (Ohio).
       Influenza pandemic in Europe.
       Malacarne investigates **cretinism**.

1789.   **John Hunter** describes **intussusception**.
       Matthew Baillie describes dermoid **ovarian cysts**.
       Linnæan Society of London founded.
       Edward Wigglesworth constructs **first American life-table**.
       Société de médecine de Lyon founded.
       University of Georgetown (D. C.) founded.
       Medical Society of Delaware founded.
       Medical Society of South Carolina founded.
       Botanic Garden at Sydney (Australia).

1789–99. French Revolution.

1790.   Royal Veterinary Schools established at Berlin (June 1) and Munich.
       Gen. Arthur St. Clair (M. D., Edinburgh) names Cincinnati (Ohio).
       William Murdock introduces **coal-gas lighting**.
       John Ferriar reports on diseases of Manchester.

1791.   **Soemmerring** publishes first volume of his **anatomy**.
       University of Innsbruck restored to rank by Leopold II.
       New Hampshire Medical Society founded.
       Medical Department, Columbia College (New York) reorganized.
       Royal Veterinary College (London) established.
       Dr. Guillotin invents the guillotine.
       Royal School of Veterinary Medicine at Milan opened (February 1).
       Royal Sea-Bathing Infirmary for scrofula at Margate.

1791–99. William **Baynham** of Virginia operates for **extra-uterine pregnancy**.

1792.   **Galvani's** essay on **animal electricity** published.
       Voltaic pile.
       J. P. Frank describes appendicitis as "peritonitis muscularis."
       Law abolishing medical schools in France (August 12).
       Establishment of French Republic (September 21).

1792.   Fodéré publishes treatise on goiter and cretinism.
         W. C. Wells establishes rationale of prismatic spectacles.
         Young elucidates **accommodation of the eye.**
         J. T. Lowitz discovers glucose.
         Sprengel's History of Medicine published.
         Larrey introduces flying ambulances.
         Connecticut Medical Society founded.
         Cotton gin (Eli Whitney).

1792–4.   First Russian medical periodical (*Vrachevnie Viedomosti*) published.

1792–1824. Porcelain hot-air stoves in vogue.

1793.   Matthew **Baillie's** *Morbid Anatomy* published.
         Abernethy introduces neurectomy.
         Benjamin Bell differentiates between gonorrhea and syphilis.
         Matthew Carey describes **yellow fever** epidemic in Philadelphia.
         Veterinary School at Madrid.

1793–94.   Reign of Terror in France.

1794.   Lavoisier beheaded (May 8).
         John Hunter publishes treatise on **blood, inflammation, and gunshot wounds.**
         John Hunter describes **transplantation** of animal tissues.
         Thomas Percival's code of medical ethics privately printed (published, 1803).
         Dalton describes **color-blindness** (October 31).
         Scarpa's *Tabulæ nevrologicæ* published.
         Board of Health at Philadelphia, Pennsylvania.
         Erasmus Darwin's *Zoönomia* (use and disuse, protective mimicry) published.
         Écoles de santé authorized in France (December 4).
         Gumpertz publishes Greek text of Asclepiades.
         University of Tennessee (Knoxville) founded.

1794–1815. University of Bonn closed.

1795.   Surgeon General Görcke founds Pepinière (Kaiser-Wilhelms-Akademie, 1895) at Berlin.
         Institut de France founded (August 22).
         Abernethian Society (London) founded.
         Hôpital St. Antoine (Paris) founded.

1795–6.   Société de médecine de Paris founded.

1795–1815. Reil edits *Archiv für Physiologie.*

1795–1836. Hufeland edits *Journal der praktischen Arzneikunde.*

1796.   **Jenner** vaccinates William Phipps (May 14).
         Abernethy first ligates external iliac artery.
         Wright Post successfully ligates femoral artery in America.
         Anderson College of Medicine (Glasgow) founded.
         Houses of Recovery (fever hospitals) opened at Manchester and Stockport (England).
         Blane standardizes rationing of lemon-juice against scurvy (Royal Navy).
         Hufeland publishes *Makrobiotik.*
         Count Rumford improves fireplaces.
         Biblioteca Nacional (Lisbon) founded.
         Board of Health at New York (City).
         Botanic Garden (Royal Dublin Society) at Glasnevin.
         Yellow fever in Boston.

1796–1800. Willan reports monthly on prevailing diseases of London.

1796–1815. Napoleonic Wars.

1797.   **Wollaston** discovers **uric acid in gouty** joints.
         Currie publishes reports on **hydrotherapy in typhoid fever.**
         John Rollo advocates meat diet in diabetes.
         Societas chirurgica (Stockholm) fused with Collegium medicum.
         Massachusetts Public Health Act, authorizing local boards of health.
         Société de médecine d'Angers founded.

1797–1805. Yellow fever prevalent in United States.

1797–1814. University of Louvain closed.

1797–1824. *Medical Repository* (New York) published.

1798.   **Jenner's** *Inquiry* published.
         Malthus' *Essay on Population* published.
         United States Marine Hospital Service established (Act of July 16).
         Imperial Medico-Military Academy founded at St. Petersburg.
         John Haslam describes **general paralysis** (Calmeil, 1826).
         Beddoes founds Pneumatic Institute at Clifton (oxygen-therapy).
         Paul Revere heads Board of Health at Boston, Massachusetts.

1798.   Société de médecine et de chirurgie (Bordeaux) founded.
             Medical School of Dartmouth College organized.
1798–9.   Dysentery and typhus fever among English troops in Ireland.
1798–1808.   **Willan's** treatise on **skin diseases** published.
1799.   De Carro introduces Jennerian **vaccination** on the continent (Vienna) and in Asia.
             Matthew **Baillie** describes **endocarditis.**
             Davy discovers anesthetic properties of **laughing gas** (NO_2).
             A. von Humboldt describes choke-damp and fire-damp (gas-mask and safety lamp).
             Fever Hospital at Waterford, Ireland.
             Medical and Chirurgical Faculty of Maryland (1789) incorporated (Library, 1830).
             Medical Library, Transylvania University (Lexington, Kentucky) founded.
             Act of Congress enjoining United States Federal Officers to coöperate in quarantine en-
               forcement.
1799–1800.   Robert **Willan** describes malignancy of typhus in London.
1799–1804.   Napoleon First Consul.
1799–1825.   Laplace publishes *Mécanique Céleste.*
1800.   "**Royal College of Surgeons in London**" chartered.
             University of Ingolstadt moved to Landshut.
             Bichat's *Traité des membranes* published.
             Order of Minister of Interior authorizing clinical instruction at Montpellier (April 29).
             Opening of Fever Hospital at Waterford (Ireland).
             Royal Institution of Great Britain founded.
             Library of Congress (Washington, D. C.) founded.
             Hedenus performs total **thyroidectomy** for goiter (October 8).
             Morveau (France) and Cruikshank (England) purify water by chlorination.
             Benjamin **Waterhouse** introduces Jennerian **vaccination** in New England.
             F. W. **Herschel** discovers **ultra-red rays** in spectrum.
             Cuvier's Comparative Anatomy published.
             Gillespie describes yellow fever on frigate *La Picque* (1795).
1801.   **Pinel** publishes psychiatric treatise.
             Thomas Young describes **astigmatism** and states undulatory theory of light.
             Astley Cooper perforates typanic membrane for obstruction of Eustachian tube.
             Osiander excises cervix uteri for cancer (May 5).
             Bichat's *Anatomie descriptive* published.
             India Office Library (London) founded.
             Willan reports on the diseases of London (1796–1800).
             Medical Society founded at Toulouse.
             J. W. **Ritter** discovers **ultra-violet rays** in spectrum.
1801–8.   Sir Humphry **Davy** invents **carbon** (electric) **arc light.**
1802.   **Heberden's** *Commentaries* published.
             United States Marine Hospitals at Norfolk (Virginia)and Boston (Massachusetts)..
             Samuel Brown vaccinates 500 people in Lexington, Kentucky.
             Conseil général de santé founded in France.
             Vaccination establishment (*Impfinstitut*) founded in Berlin (December 5).
             Bichat's *Anatomie générale* published.
             Royal Philosophical Society of Glasgow founded.
             London Fever Hospital established (Gray's Inn Lane).
             Gall speculates as to localization of cerebral functions (phrenology).
1803.   Odier employs bismuth internally.
             Société anatomique de Paris founded (December 3).
             Société de pharmacie de Paris founded.
             Influenza epidemic.
             Fort Dearborn (present Chicago), Illinois, built.
             Edict regulating medical instruction in France (June 8).
             Montpellier Medical Faculty reorganized (March 17).
             Thomas Percival publishes *Medical Ethics* (1794).
             Otto describes **hemophilia.**
             Schlesische Gesellschaft für vaterländische Kultur (Breslau) founded.
1803–8.   Lewis and Clark explore the Rocky Mountains and sources of the Mississippi.
1803–16.   Subsidence of malignant fevers in England (Creighton).
1804.   Universities of Kasan and Charkov founded by Alexander I.
             Beethoven completes *Eroica* Symphony (published 1806).
             Dalton states **atomic theory.**
             Scarpa describes **arteriosclerosis.**
             Laennec describes **peritonitis.**

1804.	Royal London Ophthalmic Hospital founded.
	House of Recovery (Fever) opened at Leeds.
	Deschamps publishes first treatise on diseases of the nose and sinuses.
1804–15.	Napoleon Emperor of the French.
1805.	Battle of Trafalgar.
	Troja (Naples) discards arm-to-arm vaccination for inoculation of cows from human subject (retrovaccination).
	Sertürner isolates **morphine.**
	Vieusseux describes **cerebrospinal meningitis** at Geneva.
	Vauxhall Company (London water-supply) established.
	Society of Physicians in Wilna (Poland).
	Royal Medical and Chirurgical Society (London) founded (chartered 1834).
1805–6.	Young and Laplace elucidate capillarity.
1805–26.	First Boston Medical Library.
1805–30.	Decline of malignant scarlatina in Great Britain.
1805–92.	Mehemet Ali dynasty (Egypt).
1806.	End of Holy Roman Empire.
	Fulton invents steamboat.
	Ferdinand III of Sicily charters University of Palermo (January 12).
	École préparatoire de médecine at Amiens.
	West London and East Middlesex water-supply companies established.
1807.	Compulsory vaccination introduced into Bavaria and Hesse.
	Act abolishing slave-trade (England).
	Swedish Medical Society (Svenska Läkaresällskapet) founded at Stockholm.
	École préparatoire de médecine at Angers.
	University Botanic Gardens at Dublin.
	College of Physicians and Surgeons (New York) founded.
	College of Medicine, University of Maryland (Baltimore) founded.
	Davy isolates Na, K, Ca, Mg, S and B.
1807–8.	James Clark reports on diseases at Nottingham.
	Heavy measles epidemic in England and Scotland.
1808.	Napoleon founds Université de France (law of May 10, 1806).
	Universities of Lyons (Rennes) and Clermont-Ferrand founded.
	Ralph **Cuming** performs **interscapular-thoracic amputation.**
	Physikalisch-medizinische Sozietät (Erlangen) founded by C. F. Harless (1773–1853).
	Medical Faculties at Bahia and Rio de Janeiro founded.
	Badham publishes treatise on **bronchitis.**
1808–19.	K. A. Rudolphi publishes system of helminthology.
1808–23.	Reforms in British penal code (Romilly, Mackintosh, Peel).
1809.	**University of Berlin** founded by Friedrich Wilhelm III of Prussia (August 16).
	Fusion of Universities of Erlangen and Altdorf.
	McDowell performs **ovariotomy** (December 13).
	Allan Burns describes **endocarditis.**
	Soemmerring invents electric telegraph.
	French Hospital founded at New York.
	Botanic Garden (Kruidtuin) at Antwerp.
	Lombard Institute of Sciences (Milan) founded.
	Yale Medical School founded.
	Kent Water Works (London Supply) established.
1810.	Hildenbrand publishes account of typhus and typhoid fever.
	Wells describes rheumatism of the heart.
	Bayle describes essential tubercle.
	Marzari attributes **pellagra** to corn.
	Nicolas Appert (France) patents process for **canning food.**
	Gas Company of London chartered by Parliament.
	Hufeland Gesellschaft (Berlin) founded.
	Wollaston discovers cystin in calculi.
	Davy analyzes corrosive sublimate.
1810–11.	University of Berlin opened.
1810–19.	**Gall** and **Spurzheim** publish treatise on the **nervous system.**
1810–23.	Chevreul investigates animal fats.
1811.	Frederik VI founds University of Christiania (Oslo) (September 2).
	Medico-Chirurgical Institute (Stockholm) founded for instruction of army and navy surgeons.
	Massachusetts General Hospital (Boston) established.

1811.	Napoleon abolishes University of Salerno (November 29).
	Sir Charles Bell discovers functions of spinal nerve-roots.
	Courtois discovers iodine in "varec" (ashes of sea-weed).
	F. L. Jahn popularizes gymnastics in Germany.
	Grand Junction Water Works (London Supply) established.
	Allen Burns describes chloroma.
	Keuffel discovers neurilemma.
	Notation of causes of death begun on British fleet.
1811–12.	J. G. Heine devises many new orthopedic apparatus.
1812.	University of Genoa founded.
	Parkinson describes perforative appendicitis.
	Legallois describes action of vagus on respiration.
	Academy of Natural Sciences founded at Philadelphia.
	Bellevue Hospital (New York) established.
1813.	Sutton differentiates delirium tremens from phrenitis.
	Langenbeck, sr., excises uterus for prolapse.
	Robert Watt publishes treatise on whooping-cough (chin-cough) and analyzes statistics of child-mortality.
	Ling introduces Swedish movements as therapy.
1813–15.	Orfila publishes treatise on toxicology.
1813–83.	Richard Wagner.
1814.	Royal Hospital for Diseases of the Chest (London) founded.
	Fraunhofer's lines in the solar spectrum discovered.
	Stephenson's first locomotive.
	London lighted with gas-lamps (April 1).
	State Library at St. Petersburg.
	London Medical Repository founded.
	Scott publishes *Waverley*.
1815.	German Confederation.
	Battle of Waterloo.
	Society of Apothecaries (England) licensed by Parliament.
	Medico-Chirurgical Society (Glasgow) founded.
	De Candolle shows discrepancy between morphologic relationship (serial homology) and physiologic species.
	University of Wittenberg removed to Halle.
	Davy invents safety lamp for coal-miners (fire-damp).
	Maelzel's metronome.
	Laennec discovers mediate auscultation (May 1).
	Guthrie amputates successfully at the hip-joint.
	Marcet discovers lipase (steapsine).
	Lisfranc performs exarticulation of tarso-metatarsal joint.
	Joshua Milne constructs Carlisle (mortality) table.
	Botanical Garden at Christiania (Oslo).
	Special chair of midwifery in Glasgow University.
1815–18.	Intermittent fever and typhus in Ireland.
1816.	Universities of Ghent, Liège, Louvain and Warsaw founded.
	Polish Academy of Sciences (Cracow) founded.
	Delpech performs subcutaneous tenotomy.
	Humboldt bases climatology upon isothermal lines.
	Guggemoos establishes School for Cretins at Salzburg.
	Laennec perfects stethoscope and publishes treatise on mediate auscultation.
	Medical Society at Hamburg founded.
	Lithium (Arfvedson) and selenium (Berzelius) discovered.
	Botanic Gardens at Sydney (New South Wales).
	Royal Ear Hospital (London) founded.
1817.	Universities of Ghent and Liège opened.
	Medico-Chirurgical Institute (Stockholm) becomes Caroline Institute.
	Franz I reorganizes University of Pavia.
	Medical Society of the District of Columbia (Washington) founded.
	Rhode Island Medical Society (Providence) founded.
	Medical Department, Transylvania University (Lexington, Kentucky) founded.
	Quine Medical Library, Chicago, founded.
	Pelletier isolates emetine.
	Parkinson describes paralysis agitans.
	Alibert describes scleroderma.

1817.	John **King** publishes book on **extra-uterine pregnancy.** Marcet discovers xanthin. Sir Astley **Cooper** ligates **abdominal aorta.**
1817–23.	Pandemic cholera.
1818.	Friedrich Wilhelm II of Prussia reorganizes **University of Bonn** (1777–79). University of St. Louis (Missouri) founded. **De Riemer** introduces **frozen sections.** **Valentine Mott** successfully ligates the innominate artery. Chevreul discovers butyric acid. J. F. **Meckel** systematizes human **abnormities.** **Orfila** stresses danger of **arsenic poisoning** from internal administration of bismuth. Proust discovers leucin. **Thénard** discovers **hydrogen peroxide.** **Caventou** and **Pelletier** isolate **strychnine.** Corvisart describes cardiac insufficiency (asystoly, Beau, 1856). Gall describes traumatic aphasia. Bateman reports on relapsing fever in London (1816–18). Prussian Pepinière (Berlin) becomes Friedrich Wilhelms Institut. Glasgow Cowpock Institution opened (August 28). Gesellschaft für Natur und Heilkunde in Dresden, founded.
1818–22.	Moreau de la Sarthe holds chair of medical history in Paris Faculty.
1819.	**University of St. Petersburg** founded by Alexander I. Bateman reports on diseases of London (Carey Street Dispensary, 1804–16). Library, Harvard Medical School (Boston), founded. **Caventou** and **Pelletier** isolate brucine, **veratrine,** and colchicin. Steamship crosses Atlantic Ocean. P. J. Roux performs staphylorrhaphy. **Lobstein** called to **first chair of pathology** (Strassburg). Medical College of Ohio founded. Hunterian Society (London) founded. Botanic Garden at Dresden.
1819–28.	John **Bostock** describes **hay-fever** as "summer catarrh."
1820.	**Académie de médecine** founded at Paris. C**o**indet uses i·dine in goiter (July 26). **Von Baer** publishes treatise on **embryology.** First U. S. Pharmacopœia published. Cincinnati Commercial Hospital founded. Philadelphia College of Apothecaries opened. United States Botanic Garden at Washington, D. C. **Caventou** and **Pelletier** isolate **quinine** and **cinchonin.**
1821.	**Itard's** treatise on **otology** published. Schilling demonstrates transmission of glanders to man. Cloquet publishes *Ophrésiologie* (nose and accessory sinuses). Anthony White resects the hip-joint. Charing Cross Hospital (London) founded. Academy of Medicine (Paris) institutes vaccine service. Leon Duvoir invents medium pressure (hot-water) heating. McGill College and University founded at Montreal. Philadelphia College of Pharmacy founded. Veterinary High Schools at Stuttgart and Stockholm. Royal Society of New South Wales (Sydney) founded. University at Buenos Aires founded. Société de médecine at Rouen. Central heating by natural gas at Fredonia, New York. Biermayer appointed to chair of pathology at Vienna. Illinois and Michigan Canal (Chicago sewage) authorized (begun 1836). Magendie founds *Journal de physiologie experimentale* (Paris).
1821–22.	Famine and fever in West Ireland.
1821–30.	Asiatic cholera described by Anglo-Indian surgeons.
1822.	**Magendie** demonstrates Bell's law of the s.inal **nerve-roots.** **James Jackson** describes **alcoholic neuritis.** Paris Medical Faculty suppressed (November 21). École préparatoire de médecine at Rouen. **Serul as** discovers **iodoform.** **Scherer** recommends **cod-liver oil.**

1822.	British Association for the Advancement of Science organized.
	Gesellschaft deutscher Naturforscher und Aerzte founded.
	Southwark Water Company (London Supply) established.
	Caroline Institute (Stockholm) becomes Caroline Medico-Chirurgical Institute (1571; 1751).
	Dieffenbach improves rhinoplasty and uranoplasty.
	F. Ollivier produces experimental hospital gangrene by auto-infection.
	J. N. Sauter performs hysterectomy (January 28).
	Fourier publishes treatise on heat.
	Medical Society of the County of Kings (Brooklyn) founded.
	Society of physicians at Riga.
1822–3.	Gaspard and Magendie produce experimental pyemia in animals.
1823.	Flourens demonstrates higher function of cerebrum (cerebration).
	George General Hospital (Hamburg) founded (October 20).
	Tiedemann and Gmelin investigate gastric and pancreatic juices.
	F. Wurzer investigates cod-liver oil (popular remedy since 1785).
	Purkinje investigates finger-prints.
	Chevreul publishes researches on animal fats.
	Chevallier brothers introduce achromatic microscope.
	Thomas Wakley founds the Lancet (London).
	Lembert performs enterorrhaphy.
	Paris Medical Faculty revived and reorganized.
	Società medico-chirurgica at Bologna.
	Royal (Dick) Veterinary College at Edinburgh founded.
	Cholera reaches Europe (Astrakhan).
1823–7.	G. B. Amici improves compound microscope.
1824.	Flourens publishes work on cerebral physiology.
	Chevreul investigates cholesterin (Conradi, 1775).
	Flourens experiments on the labyrinth.
	Prout investigates acidity of gastric juice.
	Graves reports on typhus fever in Galway (1821–22).
	Academy of Medicine (Cleveland, Ohio) founded.
	Franklin Institute (Philadelphia) founded.
	Accademia Medico-fisica founded at Florence.
	Sadi Carnot publishes Reflexions sur la puissance motrice du feu (second law of thermodynamics).
1825.	Purkinje discovers germinal vesicle in ovum.
	University of Virginia (Charlottesville) founded.
	Jefferson Medical College established at Philadelphia.
	G. B. Airy introduces spherical cylinders for astigmatism.
	James Copland uses potassium iodide in syphilis.
	Bouillaud describes and localizes aphasia.
	Nobili invents galvanometer.
	Faraday discovers benzol.
	Short introduces oleum tiglii from India.
	Andral and Louis describe tubercular peritonitis.
	Hungarian Academy of Sciences at Budapest founded.
	Chair of obstetrics revived at Montpellier (May 21).
	Fever hospital in New York City.
	National Veterinary School at Toulouse.
1825–6.	Richard Bright prepares colored plates of lesions of typhoid fever.
1825–7.	Dysentery and relapsing fever in England and Scotland.
1826.	University of Munich founded (by removal of University of Ingolstadt from Landshut).
	University of Abô (1640) moved to Helsingfors.
	École secondaire de médecine at Dijon.
	Regia Escola de cirurgia (Lisbon) founded.
	Laennec gives classical description of bronchitis and other thoracic diseases.
	Bretonneau describes diphtheritis.
	A. J. Balard discovers bromine and prepares potassium and sodium bromides.
	Becquerel invents differential galvanometer.
	Sir C. Bell states law of spinal nerve-roots (1811).
	Dutrochet stresses rôle of exosmosis and endosmosis in general physiology.
	Fresnel publishes memoir on the diffraction of light.
	Laennec maintains unity of scrofula and tuberculosis.
	Dupuytren describes congenital dislocation of the hip-joint.

1826.	**Calmeil** describes **general paralysis.**
	Botanic Garden at Brussels.
	University College (London) founded.
	Zoological Society of London founded.
	Guerney invents oxy-hydrogen (lime) light.
1826–8.	Relapsing fever in Ireland and Scotland.
	Piorry invents pleximeter.
	Ohm's law stated (*Die galvanische Kette*, 1828).
1826–31.	Rutgers Medical College of New Jersey.
1826–37.	Pandemic cholera.
1827.	Reichenbach isolates **creosote.**
	Von Baer discovers mammalian **ovum.**
	Richard **Bright** describes essential **nephritis.**
	Adams describes **heart-block.**
	Medical Gazette (London) founded.
	Amici and Cuthbert invent reflecting **microscope.**
	Isaac Hays founds *American Journal of the Medical Sciences* (Philadelphia).
	Daniel Drake founds *Western Journal of the Medical and Physical Sciences* (Cincinnati).
	Wöhler isolates alumin'um.
	Merck (Darmstadt) starts wholesale manufacture of **morphine.**
	John Walker (pharmacist) introduces **friction matches** at Stockton-on-Tees.
1827–8.	Epidemic of acrodynia.
1827–1912.	**Lord** Lister.
1827–9.	**Hodgkin** describes **aortic regurgitation.**
1828.	**Wöhler** effects **artificial synthesis of urea** from ammonium cyanate.
	Paris Bourse heated by high-pressure steam.
	Robert Brown describes Brownian movement.
	Medical Department, University of Georgia (Atlanta), founded.
	University College (London) opened (October 1).
	Sheffield School of Medicine (England).
	Boston Medical and Surgical Journal founded.
	Lancette française (*Gazette des hôpitaux*, Paris) founded.
	Glasgow Medical Journal founded.
	Medical Society of Leipzig founded.
1829.	Louis **Braille** introduces **printing for the blind.**
	Christison publishes *Treatise on Poisons.*
	Puchelt describes "perityphlitis."
	W. Wood describes **neuroma** (Odier, 1811).
	Benjamin **Babington** describes his "glottiscope."
	Andral describes sclerosis of the pulmonary artery.
	Gordon describes "hay asthma" (Bostock, 1819).
	Berzelius discovers **thorium.**
	Daguerre introduces **photography.**
	James Simpson constructs **first water-filter** (Chelsea Water Company, London).
1830.	J. J. Lister perfects achromatic microscope.
	Steinheim describes **tetany.**
	C. G. Ehrenberg discovers Bacterium termo.
	Kopp describes **thymus death.**
	Kaehler and Alms discover santonin.
	Reichenbach discovers paraffin.
	Priessnitz founds hydropathic establishment.
	Academia Nacional de Medicina (Rio de Janeiro) founded.
	Massachusetts anatomical law (disposition of unclaimed bodies).
	Malignant scarlatina reappears in Great Britain.
1830–31.	Cholera overruns Russia and invades Western Europe.
1830–48.	Reign of Louis Philippe.
1831.	Guthrie, Liebig and Soubeiran discover **chloroform.**
	Blaud's pills ($FeCO_3$).
	Liebig analyzes acetone (Boyle, 1661).
	William Henry sterilizes fomites of **scarlatina** patients with heat ($200°$ F.).
	Bouley describes intermittent lameness in horsès.
	Thackrah publishes book on trade diseases.
	Perkins introduces high-pressure (hot-water) heating.
	University Library (Berlin) founded.
	Harveian Society (London) founded.

1831. University of the City of New York founded.
       Medical Society at Bremen founded.
       University of Warsaw closed.
1832. **Universities of Zürich** and **Kiev** founded.
       British Medical Association founded.
       Hodgkin describes lymphadenoma (pseudoleukemia).
       Corrigan describes **aortic insufficiency.**
       Faraday describes galvanic and magnetic induction.
       Robiquet isolates codein.
       Chevreul isolates creatin.
       Anatomy Act passed in England.
       Boston Lying-in Hospital founded.
       Canadian Sanitary Commission organized.
       University of Wilna closed.
       Kay reports on sanitary status of cotton-spinners (Manchester, England).
       State School of Veterinary Medicine at Brussels.
       Liverpool Medical Institution founded.
       British quarantine against cholera.
1832–73. **Liebig** edits *Annalen der Chemie* (*Annalen der Pharmacie,* 1832–9).
1833. Johannes **Müller's** treatise on **physiology** published.
       Marshall **Hall** publishes memoir on **reflex action.**
       William **Beaumont** publishes experiments on **gastric digestion.**
       Biot and Persoz isolate diastase.
       Geiger and **Hesse** isolate **atropin** (Mein, 1831), hyoscyamin and aconitin.
       Quetelet introduces **anthropometry of children.**
       Carswell publishes Atlas of pathological anatomy.
       Ontario Act establishing Local Boards of Health.
       Zürich High-School (University) opened with Medical Faculty (April 29).
       Scientific Society (Isis) at Dresden.
       Gauss and Weber (Göttingen) introduce telegraphy.
       Medical Society (Aerztlicher Verein) at Munich.
       Lobstein describes osteopsathyrosis and arteriosclerosis.
       Pandemic influenza.
1834. Universities of Bern and Brussels founded.
       Royal Statistical Society of London founded.
       Faculté des Sciences (Lyons) founded.
       Medical Society of Ghent founded.
       Poor-Law Amendment Act (Great Britain).
       Westminster Hospital (London) founded.
       Runge isolates **carbolic acid.**
       Dumas obtains and names pure **chloroform.**
       Dumas and Péligot isolate methyl alcohol.
       Prout detects HCl in **gastric juice.**
       Tulane University of New Orleans founded.
1834–6. Dysentery pandemic in Central Europe.
1834–42. **Chadwick's** reports on health of English laboring classes (**Poor-Law reform**).
1834–45. *India Journal of Medical Science,* Calcutta (organ of Indian Medical Service).
1834–58. Johannes **Müller** edits *Archiv für Anatomie, Physiologie und wissenschaftliche Medicin.*
1835. **Louis** founds **medical statistics.**
       Cagniard de la Tour shows yeast to be a micro-organism.
       Berzelius defines catalysis.
       Malcolmson describes **beri-beri.**
       Owen discovers and describes **Trichina spiralis.**
       Cruveilhier describes disseminated sclerosis.
       Schwann discovers **pepsin.**
       L. G. de Koninck discovers phoridzin.
       Liebig isolates pure aldehyde.
       Medical Society of Lisbon founded.
       Finnish Medical Society (Finska Läkäresällskapet) at Helsingfors.
       Middlesex Hospital (London) founded.
       Musée Dupuytren (Paris) founded.
1835–7. University of Athens founded.
1835–9. Typhus fever epidemic in Scotland.
1836. University of London founded.
       Weber brothers investigate physiology of **locomotion.**

1836.
Quetelet founds social statistics (**demography**).
James **Marsh's** test for arsenic introduced.
Richard **Bright** describes acute yellow atrophy of the liver.
Cruveilhier demonstrates coagulation of blood in suppurative phlebitis (**pyemia**).
Sir Humphry **Davy** discovers **acetylene**.
Royal Pharmaceutic Institute (Stockholm) founded.
Cruveilhier occupies first chair of pathology in Paris Medical Faculty.
First dermatological clinic in United States (Broom Street Infirmary, New York).
Registration of Births and Deaths Act (England).
Child labor act (Massachusetts).

1836–41.
Boucher de Perthes investigates prehistoric man.

1836–48.
Illinois and Michigan Canal (**Chicago sewerage**) constructed (96 miles).

1837.
Gerhard differentiates between **typhus and typhoid fevers**.
Morse establishes telegraphic system.
Colles states law of maternal immunity in syphilis.
Bouillaud describes **endocarditis**.
Flourens discovers **respiratory center** in medulla (*nœud vitale*).
Jacob **Henle** describes epithelial tissues.
Schönlein describes peliosis rheumatica.
Bassi observes organisms of **silk-worm disease** (pebrine).
Magendie investigates **cerebrospinal fluid**.
Gustav **Magnus** demonstrates **respiratory function of blood**.
School of Medicine and Surgery (Kasr-el-Aini) at Cairo (Egypt).
Museum of Anthropology and Ethnology at St. Petersburg.
University of Michigan (Ann Arbor) founded.
Average expectation of life forty-five years (Chadwick).
Pharmaceutical Institute at Stockholm.
Rush Medical College (Chicago) chartered (opened 1843).
K. k. Gesellschaft der Aerzte founded at Vienna.

1837–8.
Southwood Smith reports on fevers at Nottingham.

1837–40.
Smallpox and typhus fever epidemic in England.

1837–43.
Old Croton Aqueduct (**New York City water supply**) constructed (41 miles).

1837–50.
Cerebrospinal meningitis spreads over Europe from Bayonne (France).

1838.
University of Messina founded.
Royal Venetian Institute of Science founded (April 15).
Medical College of Richmond (Virginia) founded.
Schleiden describes **plant cells**.
C. G. Ehrenberg publishes treatise on infusoria.
Malgaigne publishes treatise on **experimental surgery**.
Johannes **Müller's** treatise on **tumors** published.
Corrigan describes **pulmonary sclerosis**.
Mettauer successfully operates for **vesico-vaginal fistula**.
Southwood Smith reports on sickness and fever among London poor.
Botanic Garden at Kiev (Russia).
Royal Library (Brussels) founded.
Royal Orthopædic Hospital (London) founded.

1839.
Schwann publishes treatise on the **cell theory**.
Skoda's treatise on **percussion and auscultation** published.
Schönbein discovers ozone.
Schönlein discovers fungus of favus.
Rayer publishes treatise on renal diseases.
John Conolly introduces "no restraint" system in psychiatry.
Dieffenbach operates successfully for **strabismus**.
Arnott and Kay report on prevention of fever in London.
S. D. Gross lectures on pathology (Cincinnati).
University of Missouri (Columbia) founded.
First volume of **Littré's Hippocrates** published.
Wöhler isolates colloidal silver.
Royal Microscopical Society (London) founded.
American Statistical Association (Boston) founded.
First dental journal (New York).
Rowland Hill introduces **postage stamps**.

1839–79.
William Farr functions as statistical compiler in General Registrar's Office (London).

1840.
Jacob **Heine** describes infantile **poliomyelitis**.
Basedow describes **exophthalmic goiter**.

1840.   Henle publishes statement of germ theory of communicable diseases.
Clarke describes sleeping sickness in Sierra Leone.
Medical Department of Kemper College (St. Louis), first medical school west of the Mississippi.
Brompton Hospital for Consumption and Diseases of the Chest (London).
Free Vaccination Act (3.–4. Victoria, cap. 39), England.
École préparatoire de médecine at Tours.
G. J. Mulder founds chemistry of proteins.
Chapin A. Harris founds first dental school and society (Baltimore).

1840–49.   Pandemic cholera.

1841.   Henle's *Allgemeine Anatomie* published.
Medico-Psychological Association (London) founded.
Académie royale de médecine (Belgium) founded.
Dieffenbach treats stammering by section of the lingual muscles.
Kölliker describes development of spermatozoa.
Longet describes innervation of the larynx.
Longet allocates voluntary movements and sensation to the anterior and posterior columns of the cord.

1842.   J. R. Mayer states law of Conservation of Energy.
Rokitansky publishes treatise on pathology.
Long operates with ether anesthesia.
Wöhler effects synthesis of hippuric acid from benzoic acid.
Wöhler effects proteolysis.
Bérard differentiates between septicemia and pyemia.
Liebig publishes treatise on organic chemistry.
Dieffenbach publishes treatise on strabismus.
Bartolomeo Signorini excises lower jaw (September 27).
Anatomical Institute and New Canton Hospital (Zürich) opened.
Joussens (Brussels) introduces spot (colored pin) maps for localizing infectious diseases
School of Pharmacy (Pharmaceutical Society of Great Britain) in London.
Henle and Pfeufer found *Zeitschrift für rationelle Medicin* (Zürich).
Wunderlich founds *Archiv für physiologische Heilkunde* (Stuttgart).

1842–4.   Relapsing fever epidemic in Scotland.
1842–50.   Cerebrospinal meningitis in United States.
1843.   O. W. Holmes points out contagiousness of puerperal fever.
Dubini discovers ankylostoma duodenale.
Carl Ludwig investigates mechanism of urinary secretion.
Klencke inoculates rabbits with tuberculosis.
Charles Gerhardt obtains acetanilide.
Charles Robin discovers Oïdium albicans.
Küchler introduces test types.
Wheatstone bridge invented.
Simpson, Huguier and Kiwisch introduce uterine sound.
Farr publishes life-table.
Sydenham Society founded (London).
École préparatoire de médecine at Dijon.
Société de chirurgie (Paris) founded.

1843–55.   Chadwick reports on intramural burial in English towns.
1844.   Rokitansky demonstrates tubercular nature of Pott's disease.
A. J. Balard discovers amyl nitrite.
Grüby discovers Trichophytin tonsurans as cause of herpes tonsurans.
Metropolitan Health of Towns Association (London) founded.
Society for Improvement of the Condition of the Laboring Classes (London) founded.
New York Pathological Society founded (incorporated, 1886).
Société centrale de médecine veterinaire (Paris) founded.
Royal College of Veterinary Surgeons (London) founded.
Association of Obstetricians and Gynecologists (Berlin) founded.
Negri first obtains smallpox vaccine by inoculation from cow to cow.

1845.   Queen's College (Belfast) founded.
Virchow elucidates embolism as the cause of pyemia.
Virchow and Hughes Bennett describe leukemia.
Andrew Buchanan investigates coagulation of the blood.
Langenbeck detects actinomyces.
University of Honduras (Tegacigalpa) founded (opened 1847).
Accademia médico-quirúrgica española (Madrid) founded.

1845.   Veterinary Society in Berlin.

1845–61.   Rynd (Dublin) employs **hypodermic injections**.

1846.   **Weber brothers** discover **inhibitory effect of vagus nerve**.
      Morton introduces **ether anesthesia**.
      Marion Sims invents vaginal **speculum**.
      Claude **Bernard** discovers digestive function of **pancreas**.
      Stokes describes **heart-block**.
      Liebig discovers tyrosin.
      Elias Howe patents sewing machine.
      Royal Saxon Academy of Sciences (Leipzig) founded.
      Smithsonian Institution of Washington founded.
      American Medical Association organized (first meeting, Philadelphia, 1847).
      Pathological Society (London) founded.

1846–8.   Dysentery and typhus in Europe.
      Kölliker describes **smooth muscle**.

1846–9.   Great famine and fever period in Ireland.

1846–51.   Epidemic cerebrospinal meningitis in Sweden.

1847.   **Helmholtz** publishes treatise on **Conservation of Energy**.
      Virchow founds *Archiv für pathologische Anatomie* (Berlin).
      Joule determines mechanical equivalent of heat.
      Sir **J. Y. Simpson** introduces **chloroform anesthesia** in obstetrics.
      Semmelweis discovers pathogenesis of **puerperal fever**.
      Donders elucidates movements of the eyes.
      Carl **Ludwig** invents **kymograph**.
      Gerlach injects capillaries with **carmine stain**.
      K. B. Reichert obtains oxyhæmoglobin.
      James Young distils **petroleum**.
      Royal Academy of Sciences founded at Vienna.
      New York Academy of Medicine founded (incorporated 1851).
      Warren Anatomical Museum (Harvard University).
      O. W. Holmes appointed Parkman professor of anatomy at Harvard.

1847–9.   Dysentery pandemic in United States.
      University of Messina closed.

1848.   **Helmholtz** locates source of **animal heat** in the muscles.
      Claude **Bernard** discovers **glycogenic function** of the liver.
      Du Bois-Reymond publishes treatise on **animal electricity**.
      Fehling introduces test for sugar in urine.
      Société de biologie founded (Paris).
      University of Wisconsin (Madison) founded.
      American Association for the Advancement of Science founded.
      School of Veterinary Medicine at Cordova (Spain).
      English Public Health Act creating general and local boards of health **passed**.

1848–9.   Cholera reaches England and Scotland.

1848–51.   University of Pavia closed.

1848–52.   Second French Republic.

1848–54.   Indian Government constructs Ganges Canal and restores Delhi Canal.

1848–58.   General Board of Health (England).

1849.   **Addison** describes **pernicious anemia and suprarenal disease**.
      Claude **Bernard** produces **diabetes by puncture of the fourth ventricle**.
      Marion Sims operates for **vesico-vaginal fistula**.
      Virchow professor of pathology at Würzburg.
      J. K. Mitchell publishes treatise on cryptogamous origin of malarial fever.
      Sédillot performs **gastrostomy**.
      Millon introduces **reagent for proteins**.
      John **Snow** publishes views on **water-borne cholera**.
      James Thomson establishes absolute scale of temperature (**thermometry**).
      Hutchinson invents spirometer.
      Physico-Medical Society at Würzburg.
      Central Board of Health (Canada) organized.
      Royal Canadian Institute (Toronto) founded.

1850.   University of Pisa reopened.
      Helmholtz measures the **velocity of nerve current**.
      Clausius demonstrates and establishes second law of thermodynamics (Carnot, 1824).
      Waller states law of degeneration of spinal nerves.
      Rayer and **Davaine** discover anthrax bacillus (Pollender, 1849).

1850.	Thomas **Way** demonstrates **purification of sewage** by fertilization of soil.
	Vierordt introduces **sphygmograph.**
	Daniel **Drake** publishes treatise on **Diseases of the Mississippi Valley.**
	William Detmold (New York) opens abscess of the brain.
	Northwestern University (Chicago) founded.
	Report on sanitary condition of Massachusetts (**Lemuel Shattuck**).
	Steady decline of population in Ireland (end of famine and fever).
	Royal Scientific Society of Dutch East Indies (Weltvreden) founded.
	Chicago Medical Society organized (April 19).
	Metropolitan Interments Act (England).
	Women's Medical College of Pennsylvania (Philadelphia) founded.
	Epidemiological Society (London) founded.
1850–52.	**Chatin** employs **iodine for prophylaxis of goitre.**
1851.	University of Minnesota (Minneapolis) founded.
	Helmholtz invents **ophthalmoscope.**
	Claude Bernard explains vasomotor function of **sympathetic nerves.**
	Ludwig and **Rahn** investigate nerves of **salivary secretion.**
	Michaelis publishes *Das enge Becken.*
	Funke discovers hemoglobin.
	Falret describes **circular insanity.**
	Nélaton describes **pelvic hematocele.**
	University of Pavia reopened (November 5).
	Medical Faculty of **Georgetown University** (D. C.) founded.
	Wiener medicinische Wochenschrift founded.
1851–3.	**Pravaz** introduces **hypodermic syringe.**
1852.	**Kölliker's** treatise on histology published.
	Pirogoff employs **frozen sections** in his *Anatome topographica.*
	International Congress of Hygiene at Brussels.
	Obstetrical Society (London) founded.
	Farr reports on **cholera** epidemic of 1848–9.
	Griesinger shows **ankylostoma** to be the cause of Egyptian chlorosis.
	Babo demonstrates the rapid separation of blood-corpuscles from the serum by **centrifugation.**
	Horace Green excises growths from larynx *per os.*
	Magnus **Huss** defines **alcoholism.**
	Langenbeck introduces **subcutaneous osteotomy.**
	Remak shows that growth of tissues is due to cell-division.
	Société médico-psychologique (Paris) founded.
	Hospital for Sick Children at Great Ormond Street, London.
	School of Military Medicine at Val-de-Grâce (Paris).
	School for Javanese physicians at Weltvreden.
	Mercy Hospital (Chicago) chartered (June 21).
	Tufts College (Medford, Massachusetts) founded (Medical School, 1893).
	St. Mary's Hospital (London) founded.
	Veterinary School at Léon (Spain).
1852–3.	B.-A. **Morel** describes *démence précoce.*
1852–70.	Second Empire in France.
1853.	University of Melbourne founded.
	Washington University (St. Louis) founded.
	Marion Sims publishes treatise on **vesico-vaginal fistula.**
	Stanislao **Cannizarro** obtains alcohols from aldehydes.
	Budge establishes functional independence of spinal cord (localization of centers).
	Farr publishes second English life-table.
	Cohn establishes vegetable nature of **bacteria.**
	Virchow discovers **neuroglia.**
	Gilman Kimball excises uterus for fibromyoma.
1853–56.	Crimean War: Florence Nightingale.
1854.	**Hittorf** investigates **electrolysis** (ions).
	Sir W. R. Hamilton introduces quaternions.
	California Academy of Sciences (San Francisco) founded.
	Dysentery pandemic in Europe.
	Graefe elucidates glaucoma and its treatment by iridectomy.
	Universities of Marseilles, Clermont-Ferrand and Nancy founded.
	Ehrenberg publishes treatise on micro-organisms.
	Boston **Medical Library** founded.

1854.	Claude **Bernard** discovers function of **vasodilator nerves.**
	Graham investigates **osmosis.**
	Credé introduces method of removing **placenta** by external manipulation.
	Middeldorpf introduces **galvanocautery** in major surgery.
	Chlorine treatment of London sewage authorized (English Royal Commission),
	Beauperthuy states theory of mosquito transmission of yellow fever.
	Spanish law regulating public health.
	Aerztliches Intelligenz-Blatt (*Münchner medicinische Wochenschrift*, 1886) founded.
	Graefe founds *Archiv für Ophthalmologie* (Berlin).
1854–6.	**Belgrand** constructs **sewers of Paris.**
1854–60.	Cerebrospinal meningitis epidemic in Sweden and Germany.
1855.	**Manuel Garcia** introduces **laryngoscope.**
	Addison publishes memoir on **diseases of the suprarenal capsules.**
	Farr publishes classification of diseases.
	Burmeister classifies insects.
	Remak employs galvanic current in diagnosis and therapy.
	Marion Sims founds Hospital for Women's Diseases (New York City).
	Royal Academy of Sciences (Amsterdam) founded.
	Water filtration compulsory in London.
	Bessemer steel process and **Bunsen burner** invented.
	Paris Exposition.
1855–61.	**Sidney Herbert's** reforms in military sanitation.
1855–76.	**John Simon** serves as Central Medical Officer (London).
1856.	Sir W. H. **Perkin** (1838–1907) obtains **aniline dyes** (coal-tar products).
	Panum investigates chemical products of **putrefaction.**
	Brücke investigates speech (phonetics).
	Caspar's treatise on **medical jurisprudence** published.
1856–7.	Berlin water supply filtered.
1856–9.	Pandemic diphtheria.
1856–60.	General spread of diphtheria in Europe and America.
	Virchow becomes professor of pathology in Berlin.
	Jobst and Hesse discover **physostigmin.**
1857.	**Graefe** introduces operation for **strabismus.**
	E. B. **Elliot** prepares first Massachusetts Life-table.
	Typhoid fever traced to milk (Penryth, England).
	Petters discovers **acetone in urine** and expiration of diabetics.
	Bouchut performs **intubation** of the larynx.
	Universities of Chicago, Calcutta and Madras founded.
	Lucien **Corvisart** shows that pancreatic juice can digest proteins.
	Pathological Society of Philadelphia founded.
	National Sanitary Convention at Philadelphia.
1858.	**Virchow's** *Cellularpathologie* published.
	Claude **Bernard** discovers vaso-constrictor and vaso-dilator nerves.
	Marcet discovers lipolytic power of gastric juice.
	Niemann isolates **cocaine** in Wöhler's laboratory.
	Pettenkofer proves that solid walls are permeable to air.
	Kekulé shows **quadrivalence of carbon atom.**
	English Public Health and Local Government Acts (transfer of functions of General Board of Health to Privy Council and Home Secretary).
	Medical Act (England) ascertaining status of qualified and registered practitioners.
	Veterinary High-School at Copenhagen.
	National Sanitary Conference at Baltimore (Maryland).
	Royal Dental Hospital (London).
1858–67.	Pullman cars introduced.
1859.	**Darwin's** *Origin of Species* published.
	Wagner completes score of *Tristan* (produced 1865).
	Kirchhoff and **Bunsen** discover **spectrum analysis.**
	Graefe describes **retinal embolism.**
	Landry describes **acute ascending paralysis.**
	Pflüger publishes memoir on **electrotonus.**
	Petroleum used in oil-lamps (Pennsylvania).
	Florence Nightingale publishes *Notes on Nursing.*
	Farr publishes Healthy District Life Table.
	Sir J. **Bazalgette** plans canalization (sewage disposal) of **London** (executed 1859–75).
	Hermann **Brehmer** opens hospital for phthisis at Görbersdorf.

1859.　　Kolbe synthetizes salicylic acid.
　　　　　Botanic Garden at Singapore.
　　　　　National Sanitary Convention at New York (City).
　　　　　Laboratory of Marine Zoology and Physiology at Concarneau (Finistère).
1860.　　Pasteur demonstrates presence of bacteria in air.
　　　　　Lemaire points out antiseptic properties of **carbolic acid.**
　　　　　Czermak introduces **rhinoscopy.**
　　　　　Donders introduces cylindrical and prismatic **spectacles for astigmatism.**
　　　　　Zenker describes **trichinosis.**
　　　　　Bouchut publishes *Du nervosisme.*
　　　　　G. J. Symons publishes *British Rainfall* (Vol. I).
　　　　　Berliner medicinische Gesellschaft founded.
　　　　　Institute of Veterinary Medicine at Turin.
　　　　　Adulteration of Food Act (England).
　　　　　England and Massachusetts enact first laws against adulteration of milk.
　　　　　Parkes becomes professor of military hygiene at Army Medical School (Chatham).
　　　　　National Sanitary Convention at Baltimore.
　　　　　Duchenne describes **bulbar paralysis.**
　　　　　Schultze introduces method of resuscitating **asphyxiated infants.**
　　　　　University of California founded.
1860–92.　Canalization of **Munich** for sewage-disposal (Pettenkofer).
1861.　　Ernst **Brand** introduces **hydrotherapy** in typhoid fever.
　　　　　Pasteur discovers anaërobic bacteria.
　　　　　Pettenkofer and **Voit** construct **calorimeter** (basal metabolism).
　　　　　E. B. Wollcott (Milwaukee) first excises renal tumor.
　　　　　Thure Brandt introduces **massage in gynæcology.**
　　　　　Ménière describes labyrinthine vertigo.
　　　　　Max Schultze defines protoplasm and cell.
　　　　　Broca discovers **speech center** in the brain.
　　　　　Buckminster Brown establishes Samaritan Hospital (New York).
　　　　　Massachusetts Institute of Technology (Boston) founded.
　　　　　Society of Psychiatrists (St. Petersburg) organized.
1861–65.　Civil War in the United States.
　　　　　National Sanitary Commission (United States).
1862.　　University of Urbino opened (1671).
　　　　　Raynaud describes **symmetrical gangrene.**
　　　　　Phœbus summarizes knowledge of "early summer catarrh" (hay fever).
　　　　　Donders publishes studies on **astigmatism** and **presbiopia.**
　　　　　Spencer Wells operates for tubercular peritonitis.
　　　　　Krassovsky performs first ovariotomy in Russia.
　　　　　Victor von Bruns performs **first laryngeal operation with laryngoscope.**
　　　　　Florence Nightingale establishes training school for nurses at St. Thomas's Hospital.
　　　　　Winternitz and Oppolzer found first hydropathic establishment at Vienna.
　　　　　University of Warsaw reopened as a High School (closed 1869).
　　　　　Entomological Society (Iris) at Dresden.
1863.　　Helmholtz's *Tonempfindungen* published.
　　　　　Deiters discovers glia cells (astrocytes).
　　　　　Virchow investigates **tumors.**
　　　　　Davaine produces anthrax experimentally.
　　　　　William **Banting** publishes *Letter on Corpulence.*
　　　　　Kahlbaum classifies insanity and defines paraphrenia as age-linked insanity (**neophrenia,** hebephrenia, presbyophrenia).
　　　　　Setchenoff's work on cerebral reflexes published.
　　　　　Pasteur investigates **silkworm disease.**
　　　　　Army Medical School (England) transferred to Royal Victoria Hospital (Netley).
　　　　　Old Cook County Hospital (Chicago) started.
　　　　　American Veterinary Medical Association (Detroit) founded.
　　　　　Biological station at Areachon (Gironde).
　　　　　National Academy of Sciences (Washington) founded.
　　　　　University of Belgrade (Jugoslavia) founded.
1863–5.　Pandemic cholera.
1863–82.　Ismail Pasha (first Khedive of Egypt).
1864.　　**Donders** publishes treatise on anomalies of **accommodation and refraction.**
　　　　　Traube investigates pathology of **fever.**
　　　　　Hlasiwetz and Barth obtain **resorcin.**

1864. **Cohnheim** elucidates mechanism of **inflammation** (diapedesis of leucocytes).
Parkes' *Manual of Practical Hygiene* published.
Geneva Convention.
Le Verrier founds Association française pour l'avancement des sciences.
Weir Mitchell describes causalgia.
Gray Herbarium (Harvard University) founded (Cambridge, Massachusetts).
German Psychiatric Society (Berlin).
Chicago Medical College incorporated.
St. Louis College of Pharmacy founded.
University of Bucharest (Roumania) founded.
Berliner klinische Wochenschrift founded.
Max Schultze founds *Archiv für mikroskopische Anatomie* (Bonn)
Use of milk from diseased cows prohibited in Boston.
St. Luke's Hospital (Chicago) opened.
Council of Hygiene (New York City).

1865. **Gregor Mendel** publishes memoir on **plant hybridity.**
Zander introduces **mechanotherapy.**
University of Odessa founded.
Cornell University founded at Ithaca.
St. Louis Public Library founded.
Yellow fever and Russian cattle-plague in England.
Report of Citizen's Association on sanitary condition of New York City.
Billings founds **Army Medical Library (Surgeon General's Office,** Washington**).**
First Roumanian Medical Society at Galatz.
Rivers Pollution Commission (Great Britain).
Chicago Hospital for Women founded.

1865–6. Asiatic cholera in Europe.
Villemin demonstrates **transmissibility of tuberculosis** by inoculation (Klencke, 1843).

1866. Seven Weeks' (Austro-Prussian) War.
Voit establishes **first hygienic laboratory in Munich.**
Ludwig and **Cyon** investigate the **vasomotor nerves.**
Marion Sims publishes *Clinical Notes on Uterine Surgery.*
Graefe describes **sympathetic ophthalmia.**
Liébault publishes treatise on hypnotism.
A. J. Ångström introduces Ångström units.
P. H. Watson (Edinburgh) performs first excision of larynx.
Academy of National Sciences at Agram.
Society of Physicians at Cracow.
Purkinje founds Society of Czech Physicians at Prague.
Metropolitan Health Board (New York City) established (April 21).

1867. **Lister** introduces **antiseptic surgery.**
Helmholtz publishes treatise on **physiological optics.**
Kussmaul introduces **intubation of the stomach.**
Moritz **Traube** devises **semi-permeable membranes.**
English Sanitary Act.
Charles Liernur introduces pneumatic system of disposal of sewage.
Bobbs performs **cholecystotomy.**
Percy Frankland introduces combustion process for measuring organic matter **in water.**
A. W. von Hoffmann discovers **formaldehyde.**
First International Medical Congress at Paris.
Siemens brothers introduce dynamo.
Dominion of Canada established (July 1).
Opening of Suez Canal and of Pacific Railway.
First tunnels for Chicago water-supply completed.
Clinical Society (London) founded.
Canadian Medical Association organized.
W. H. Draper lectures on dermatology (College of Physicians, New York).
Metropolitan Poor Law Act (England).
Chicago Board of Health organized.
Tenement House Law (New York City).

1868. **University of Tokyo** (Tokyo Teikoku Daigaku) founded (Library, 1872).
Haeckel's *Natürliche Schöpfungsgeschichte* published.
Darwin publishes treatise on *Variation in Animals and Plants.*
Heidenhain investigates salivary secretion.
Meyer (Copenhagen) describes **adenoid vegetations.**

1868. Pelechin introduces antisepsis in Russia.
   Kahlbaum defines katatonia.
   Boettcher discovers spermine.
   Hering and **Breuer** discover **self-regulation of respiration** (rôle of vagus).
   Schwendener investigates **symbiosis** in lichens.
   James Lenox founds Presbyterian Hospital (New York).
   American Otological Society (Boston) founded.
   East London Nursing Society founded.
   Jewish Hospital (Chicago) founded.
   Society of Czechoslovakian Physicians (Prague).
   Société de médecine légale (Paris) founded.
   English Pharmacy Act against unlicensed sale of poisons.
   Pflüger founds *Archiv für die gesamte Physiologie* (Bonn).
1869. University of Warsaw founded (moved to Rostov, 1915).
   Esmarch introduces **first-aid bandage.**
   Brown-Séquard introduces doctrine of **internal secretions.**
   Wunderlich publishes treatise on **clinical thermometry.**
   Virchow urges medical inspection of schools.
   Goltz investigates nerve centers in the frog.
   Gustav Simon excises kidney.
   Oscar **Liebreich** demonstrates hypnotic effect of **chloral** hydrate.
   Bevan Lewis **investigates** localization of function in the brain (histological).
   J. P. Kirkwood publishes report on filtration of river waters.
   Mendeléjeff and Lothar Meyer discover periodicity of elements.
   American Journal of Obstetrics founded.
   Torture abolished in Canton of Zug (Switzerland).
   Faculté de Médecine (Nancy) founded.
   Ceylon Medical College (Colombo) founded.
   American Museum of Natural History (New York City) founded.
   Chicago Medical College becomes Medical Department of Northwestern University.
   American Medical Editors Association (New York) founded.
   Hospital at Osaka (Japan).
   Massachusetts State Board of Health created.
   Ontario (Canada) Act for Registration of Vital Statistics.
   Tenement House Law (New York State).
1869–70. Pius IX restores Marcian Aqueduct (Rome) as Aqua Pia.
1869–71. Royal Sanitary Commission (Great Britain).
1869–1919. Mercy Hospital (Chicago) enlarged.
1870. **Fritsch** and **Hitzig** investigate **localization of functions of brain.**
   Thomas performs vaginal ovariotomy.
   Saemisch describes serpiginous ulcer of the cornea.
   Linoleum invented.
   Beginnings of general **central-heating** in Germany.
   Daremberg appointed to chair of medical history in Paris Medical Faculty.
   Metropolitan Asylums Board (England).
   Board of Health, District of Columbia, organized.
   Women's Medical College (Chicago) organized (August 2) (closed, 1902).
   Universities of Syracuse (New York) and Cincinnati (Ohio) founded.
   Wisconsin Academy of Sciences founded.
   Metropolitan Fever Hospitals (London) established.
   Ural Scientific Society at Sverdlovsk.
   Anthropological Society of Vienna founded.
   Volkmann founds *Sammlung Klinischer Vorträge* (Leipzig).
1870–71. Franco-Prussian War (test of vaccination).
1870–74. Anton **Dohrn** establishes marine zoological laboratory at Naples.
1870–88. *Medical and Surgical History of the War of the Rebellion* published.
1871. Establishment of German Empire and French Republic.
   Darwin's *Descent of Man* published.
   Weigert stains bacteria with carmine.
   Hammarsten discovers rôle of **fibrinogen** in coagulation of blood.
   Hoppe-Seyler discovers **nuclein** in the blood-corpuscles.
   English Local Government Board created.
   Biological Station (University of Odessa) at Sebastopol (Crimea).
   Boards of Health in California and Virginia.
   Royal Anthropological Institute (London) founded.

1871.   Munich Society of Anthropology founded.
        Italian Society of Anthropology (Florence) founded.
        New York Orthopedic Hospital founded.
1871-2.   First American filter for water-supply at Poughkeepsie, New York.
1871-80. General and widespread adulteration of food in the United States.
1871-1919. Local Government Board (England).
1872.   University of Strassburg reopened.
        University of Klausenburg (Kolozsvar) founded.
        University of Adelaide (Australia) founded.
        Billroth resects the esophagus.
        H. C. Wood investigates heat-stroke.
        Abbé introduces oil immersion lenses.
        Merck introduces pyoctanin (methyl violet).
        Battey performs normal **ovariotomy.**
        Noeggerath describes effects of **latent gonorrhea** in women.
        Typhoid fever epidemic from polluted water at Lausen (Switzerland).
        Metropolis Water Act (piping of water to London).
        Milk stations established by Diet Kitchen Association (New York).
        American Public Health Association holds first meeting (September 12).
        Presbyterian Hospital (New York) opened.
        Lacaze-Duthiers founds Biological Station at Roscoff.
        Tokyo Library (Ugeno Park).
        Infant life protection act passed in England.
        German Surgical Association (Berlin) founded.
        Chicago Public Library founded.
        Sociedad Cientifica Argentina at Buenos Aires.
        Society of Chersonese Physicians at Cherson (Ukraine).
        Society of Physicians at Ekaterinoslav (Ukraine).
        Medical Society at Stuttgart.
1873.   Academy of Geneva (1559) becomes University.
        Obermeier discovers spirillum of **relapsing fever.**
        Nussbaum introduces nerve-stretching.
        Esmarch introduces hemostatic bandage.
        Gull describes **myxedema.**
        Billroth excises the larynx.
        Schwartze and Eysell devise mastoid operation.
        Cuignet introduces retinoscopy.
        Clerk Maxwell publishes treatise on electricity and magnetism.
        Lippmann's electrometer.
        Cantani describes lathyrism.
        Laryngological Society of New York organized.
        Revaccination compulsory in Germany.
        German Public Health Association (Berlin) founded.
        League of German Medical Societies (Berlin).
        Boards of Health in 134 American cities.
        Institute of Municipal and County Engineers (Great Britain).
1873-83. James **Hobrecht** constructs canalization system for **sewage of Berlin.**
1874.   Cholera conference in Vienna.
        International postal service.
        Fiedler stresses danger of morphine habit.
        Loi Roussel enacted for the protection of infants (France).
        Ehrlich introduces dried blood smears and improves stain methods.
        Kahlbaum publishes monograph on **katatonia.**
        Miescher investigates nucleoproteids.
        Willy **Kühne** discovers **trypsin.**
        Sappey investigates the lymphatic system.
        N. Pringsheim investigates chlorophyll.
        Fryer builds furnace incinerator for refuse at Nottingham (England).
        Imperial Hygienic Laboratory at Tokyo.
        Veterinary Institute at Kazan.
        Illinois law regulating food supply.
        Society of Croatian Physicians at Agram.
        Alfieri Institute of Social Sciences at Florence.
        Sir Josiah Mason founds University of Birmingham as Mason College.
1875.   Universities of Lemberg and Czernowitz founded.

1875.　　　École d'Anthropologie (Paris) founded.
　　　　　Faculté de Médecine et Pharmacie (Lille) founded.
　　　　　Landois discovers **hemolysis** from transfusion of alien blood.
　　　　　Sir Thomas **Barlow** describes **infantile scurvy.**
　　　　　Hardy and Gerard introduce **pilocarpin.**
　　　　　Kühne and Nencki discover indol.
　　　　　Lösch observes **parasitic amebæ** in dysentery.
　　　　　Weir Mitchell introduces **rest cure.**
　　　　　Corfield establishes **first public health laboratory in England.**
　　　　　Imperial Hygienic Laboratory (Osaka).
　　　　　Chesebrough obtains **vaseline.**
　　　　　Meat inspection compulsory in Germany.
　　　　　English Public Health Act.
　　　　　Paul **Börner** founds *Deutsche medicinische Wochenschrift* (Berlin).
　　　　　English Sale of Food and Drugs Act.
　　　　　Boston Medical Library founded (opened October 18).
1875–6.　　Cold-storage meat sent overseas.
1875–7.　　Pandemic cholera.
1875–82.　 Artisans' Dwellings Improvement Acts (England).
1875–1902. **Gegenbaur** edits *Morphologisches Jahrbuch.*
1876.　　　**Imperial Board of Health** founded at Berlin (April 30).
　　　　　Royal Sanitary Institute founded (London).
　　　　　Johns Hopkins University founded.
　　　　　Athenæum ilustre (1632) becomes University of Amsterdam.
　　　　　University of Bristol founded.
　　　　　Royal Academy of Medicine founded at Rome.
　　　　　Physiological Society of London founded.
　　　　　Centennial Exposition, Philadelphia (July 4).
　　　　　International Hygienic Congress at Brussels.
　　　　　Sayre introduces **gypsum corset for spinal deformities.**
　　　　　Kolbe isolates **salicylic acid.**
　　　　　Eulenburg publishes handbook of industrial hygiene.
　　　　　Lombroso publishes treatise on criminal man.
　　　　　Fechner investigates synæsthesia.
　　　　　Paquelin cautery introduced.
　　　　　Porro introduces **Cæsarean section** with excision of adnexa.
　　　　　Koch obtains pure cultures of **anthrax bacilli** on artificial media.
　　　　　Pictet invents artificial manufacture of ice.
　　　　　Max **Nitze** introduces **cystoscope.**
　　　　　Société française d'hygiène (Paris) founded.
　　　　　Library, Medico-Chirurgical Faculty of Maryland, opened.
　　　　　Museo Kircheriano (Rome) becomes Pigorini Museum of Prehistory and **Ethnography.**
　　　　　Public baths and portable bathtubs (England).
　　　　　Jablochkoff kaolin arc-lamp invented.
　　　　　Peter **Dettweiler** treats consumptives at Falkenstein (rest cure in open air).
　　　　　American Dermatological Association (Boston) founded.
　　　　　Bell telephone introduced.
　　　　　American Chemical Society (Washington, D. C.) founded.
　　　　　American Library Association (Chicago) founded.
1876–7.　　Raoult-Bunte burette for gas analysis.
1876–8.　　Friedrich Siemens establishes **crematory** (Gotha).
1876–84.　 Decline of cerebrospinal meningitis.
1876–1909. New Cook County Hospital (Chicago) begun and completed.
1877.　　　T. J. **Burrill** (Illinois) discovers **organism of pear-blight.**
　　　　　Pasteur discovers bacillus of malignant edema.
　　　　　Esmarch introduces **aseptic bandage.**
　　　　　Ernst **von Bergmann** introduces corrosive sublimate antisepsis.
　　　　　Bezold describes **mastoiditis.**
　　　　　Paget describes **osteitis deformans.**
　　　　　Pictet and Cailletet liquefy gases.
　　　　　Stricker treats articular rheumatism with salicylic acid.
　　　　　Winternitz publishes treatise on **hydrotherapy.**
　　　　　Faculté de Médecine (Lyons) founded.
1877–78.　 Russo-Turkish War.
　　　　　Bollinger and Israel describe **actinomycosis.**

1877–1907. Progressive factory legislation in Massachusetts.
1878. **Koch** discovers causes of **traumatic infections.**
    Von Basch measures blood-pressure with sphygmomanometer.
    W. A. Freund excises cancerous uterus.
    Marine Hospital Service (United States) takes over national quarantine.
    Downes and Blunt demonstrate bactericidal effects of light (Royal Society).
    Nägeli discovers that bacteria are not given off by moist surfaces.
    Massachusetts law authorizing inspection of plumbing.
    Foster founds *Journal of Physiology* (London).
    Edison invents platinum wire (incandescent) electric lamp.
    International Congress of Hygiene at Paris.
    Chicago Pathological Society founded.
1878–9. Welch, Prudden, Sternberg and Salmon introduce bacteriology in United States.
1879. **Neisser** discovers gonococcus.
    Hansen and Neisser discover **lepra bacillus.**
    Max Nitze introduces cystoscopy.
    Manson discovers transmission of filariasis by mosquitoes.
    Parkes Museum of Hygiene opened (University Hospital, London).
    Billings and Fletcher start *Index Medicus.*
    Bechem and Post employ low-pressure steam in central heating.
    Parliament sanctions Thirlmere Aqueduct (96 miles) for water-supply of Manchester.
    Factory and Workshops Act (England).
    Hygienic Institute (University of Munich) opened by Pettenkofer (authorized 1872).
    Anthropological Society of Washington (D. C.) founded.
    German food law passed (May 14).
1879–82. National Board of Health (United States).
1880. **Pasteur** discovers streptococcus, staphylococcus, and pneumococcus (Sternberg).
    Pasteur immunizes against chicken-cholera by attenuated cultures.
    Eberth isolates **typhoid bacillus.**
    Miquel devises exact methods for enumerating bacteria in water.
    Cold-storage meat successfully transported to Australia.
    Pasteur and **Sternberg** demonstrate carriage of **pneumonia bacillus** in healthy mouth.
    Sandström describes **parathyroid gland.**
    Mosetig Moorhof introduces iodine dressings in surgery.
    Balfour's *Embryology* published.
    Evans discovers trypanosome of Surra (T. Evansi).
    Merke (Berlin) investigates effect of steam upon pathogenic micro-organisms.
    Roeckner and Rothe devise method of purifying sewage by upward filtration.
    Von Jaksch defines physiological and pathological acetonuria.
    Billings publishes **Index Catalogue** (Vol. I).
    American Surgical Association founded.
    University of Tomsk (West Siberia) founded.
    Cambridge Medical Society (England).
    Government Calf Lymph Establishment at London.
    F. Rizzoli founds Orthopedic Institute at Rome.
    J. S. Billings constructs life-tables from data of United States Census.
    L. W. Meach compiles American Experience (Life) Table from data of 30 insurance companies.
    Ophthalmological Society (United Kingdom) founded.
    Parliament sanctions **Vyrnwy Aqueduct** (68 miles) for **water-supply of Liverpool.**
    London Association of Medical Women.
1880–1. **Laveran** discovers parasite of **malarial fever.**
1880–85. Bronx River Conduit (**New York City water-supply**) constructed.
1880–89. Hawksley and Deacon construct **Vyrnwy Water-works** (Liverpool supply).
1881. Billroth resects the pylorus for cancer, with success.
    Ogston discovers staphylococci in abscesses.
    Pasteur produces vaccine against anthrax.
    Food and Drug Law (New York State).
    Veterinary School at Lemberg (Galacia).
    Chicago Pathological Society (organized April 10, 1878).
    Vincenz Czerny introduces vaginal excision of uterine tumors.
    Hahn performs nephropexy.
    Wölfler introduces **gastro-enterostomy.**
    Medin discovers epidemic nature of **poliomyelitis.**
    Wundt investigates **reaction-time.**

1881.   **Soxhlet** estimates specific gravity of milk with lactodensimeter.
       Koch introduces gelatine-media (solid plate cultures) and steam sterilization.
       Grimaux obtains **codeine** from morphine.
       Government Animal Vaccination Establishment in Lambs' Conduit Street (London).
       Russian Surgical (Pirogoff) Society (St. Petersburg) organized.
       Société d'odontologie (Paris) founded.
       New York Polyclinic founded.
       College of Physicians and Surgeons (Chicago) incorporated (October 4; opened, 1882).
       Whooping-cough a leading cause of infant mortality in English vital statistics.
       Carlos Finlay surmises transmission of yellow fever by Stegomyia fasciata (August 14).
       Weiss (in Billroth's Clinic) describes post-operative tetany.
       Tyndall publishes *Essays on the Floating Matter of the Air.*
       University College of Liverpool founded.

1882.   **Koch** discovers **tubercle bacillus.**
       Gaskell investigates functions of vagus nerve.
       Löffler and Schütz isolate bacillus of glanders in pure culture.
       Bizzozero discovers **blood-platelets.**
       Horbaczewski synthetizes uric acid from glycocoll and urea.
       Walther Flemming investigates **cell division.**
       Bertillon introduces personal identification by anthropometry (Bertillonage).
       Max Sänger improves **Cæsarean section.**
       Liebreich introduces **lanolin.**
       Langenbuch excises the gall-bladder.
       Winiwarter performs cholecystenterostomy.
       First code for inspection of plumbing (Lawrence, Massachusetts).
       Holly introduces **central** (steam) **heating** at Lockport, New York.
       Lépine and Blanc describe pleuro-peritoneal tuberculosis.
       Grawitz describes **renal hypernephroma.**
       Public Health Act (Canada) passed.
       Provincial Board of Health (Ontario) organized.
       Royal Academy of Medicine in Ireland (Dublin) founded.
       New York Post-graduate Medical School and Hospital founded.
       Society for Psychic Research (London) founded.
       Michael Reese Hospital (Chicago) opened.
       Royal Society of Canada (Ottawa) founded.

1882–1904. Canizzaro and pupils investigate santonin group.
1882–1906. Emil Fischer investigates purin bodies.
1882–1913. Saccardo publishes *Sylloge Fungorum* (22 v.).

1883.   **Edwin Klebs** discovers **diphtheria bacillus.**
       Kjeldahl introduces method of estimating nitrogen.
       Golgi introduces **silver stain** for nerve-cells.
       Billroth and Senn anastomose ileum and colon.
       Pasteur vaccinates against anthrax.
       Metchnikoff states phagocytic theory of immunity.
       Unna introduces **ichthyol.**
       Koch discovers bacilli of cholera and infectious conjunctivitis.
       Lawson Tait operates for extra-uterine pregnancy.
       Adolf von Baeyer obtains formula of indigo.
       Fehleisen obtains pure cultures of streptococci in erysipelas.
       J. F. F. Hermans attributes faulty ventilating to humidity and overheating.
       Kühne and Chittenden demonstrate rôle of **trypsin** in digestion.
       Conner (Cincinnati) performs **gastrectomy.**
       A. F. A. King propounds theory of malarial transmission by **mosquitoes.**
       Parke's Museum (London) rebuilt.
       Pennsylvania Anatomical Law passed.
       Italian Society of Surgery (Rome) founded.
       Faculty of Medicine at Beirut (Syria).

1883–5.   Gustav Neuber (Kiel) introduces aseptic hospital.

1884.   **Nicolaier** discovers **tetanus bacillus.**
       Credé introduces silver nitrate instillations for infantile conjunctivitis.
       Lustgarten isolates smegma bacillus.
       Senn advances pancreatic surgery.
       Ludwig Knorr discovers **antipyrine.**
       Veit investigates tubal pregnancy.
       Riedel introduces salipyrin.

1884. Baumann discovers **sulphonal** (Kast, 1888).
Billroth excises pancreas for cancer.
Mikulicz operates for perforated typhoidal ulcer.
Gaffky obtains **pure culture of typhoid bacillus** (Eberth, 1880).
Loeffler obtains pure culture of diphtheria bacillus (Klebs, 1883).
Emmerich isolates **colon bacillus** (Escherich, 1886).
Hueppe investigates lactic acid bacilli in sour milk.
Chamberland invents porcelain bacterial filter.
Wilhelm Ebstein produces urinary calculi experimentally.
Bang and Stein cultivate bacilli of bovine tuberculosis.
Bernheim publishes treatise on suggestive-therapy.
Mergenthaler introduces linotyping.
Archæologic Museum at Epidaurus.
International Health Exhibit (London).
German workman's compensation law for industrial accidents.
United States Bureau of Labor established (June 27; in effect July 1, 1885).
Carl Koller employs **cocaine** in eye surgery.

1884–8. Hamburg-Eppendorf Hospital constructed.
1884–1919. Emil **Fischer** investigates carbohydrates and ferments.
1885. **O'Dwyer** improves **intubation of the larynx.**
Golgi discovers glia cells.
Yamanashi isolates **ephedrine** (Nagai, 1887).
Hermann Cohn introduces **examination of school-children** for visual acuity.
Bunge introduces hematogen.
Oscar Loewi discovers bactericidal property of formaldehyde (formalin).
Kossel isolates adenin.
Fraser introduces strophanthus.
H. Kümmell performs **choledochostomy.**
Bumm obtains pure cultures of gonococcus.
Hermann Rietschel appointed professor of heating (Technical High School, **Charlotten-**
burg).
Weismann publishes memoir on **continuity of the germ plasm.**
Ewald and **Boas** introduce test-breakfasts.
Halsted introduces **conduction anesthesia.**
Reilly (United States Army) constructs first **incinerator.**
Weigert introduces hematoxylin staining of nerve-fibers.
Princess Helena Pavlovna founds Clinical Institute (St. Petersburg).
Medical Society at Omsk (Siberia).
Medical Association of Montana (Billings) founded.
Institute of Military Hygiene at Madrid.
Trudeau Sanitarium at Saranac Lake, New York.

1885–6. Cholera survey in England.
1885–7. Auer von Welsbach patents and improves incandescent lamp mantle (Welsbach burner).
1885–93. New Croton Aqueduct (New York City water-supply) constructed (31 miles).
1886. **Nuttall** notes bactericidal power of blood-serum.
Von Bergmann introduces steam sterilization in surgery.
Filatow describes **glandular fever** and fourth disease.
Hirschsprung describes **megacolon.**
Escherich investigates bacteria of intestines in infants.
Fitz describes pathology of **appendicitis.**
Marie connects **acromegaly** with the pituitary body.
Weir Mitchell and Reichert investigate serpent venoms.
Marcel von Nencki introduces salol.
Soxhlet introduces **sterilized milk** for nutrition of infants.
Kopp, Cahn, and Hepp introduce acetanilide as **antifebrin** (Gerhardt, 1843).
Lehman investigates effect of industrial poisons.
Association of American Physicians (Boston) organized.
R. W. Felkin lectures on tropical medicine at Edinburgh.
New York Cancer Hospital founded.
Chicago Polyclinic opened (July 26).
Conseil de Santé (Quebec) organized.
Royal Institute of Public Health (London) founded.
Liverpool Biological Society founded.

1887. Clark University founded (Worcester, Mass.).
Bruce discovers coccus of **Malta fever.**

1887.   **Weichselbaum** discovers **meningococcus**.
     Salkowski discovers **phytosterin** (nucleus of vegetable fats).
     Wagner von Jauregg proposes treatment of infection by counter-infection.
     Fell introduces intratracheal anesthesia.
     Harvey Reed sutures pericardium.
     Sir John **Simon** publishes Public Health Reports.
     D'Arsonval introduces **high-frequency currents**.
     Howard **Kelly** performs **hysterorrhaphy**.
     Gowers and **Horsley** operate on the spinal cord.
     Gram introduces **diuretin**.
     Sewall immunizes pigeons against rattlesnake venom.
     Kast and Hinsberg introduce **phenacetin**.
     Sloane Maternity Hospital (New York) opened.
     Poor law medical officers abolished (England).
     American Orthopedic Association founded.
     Institute of Legal Medicine at Tokyo.
     Psychological Association (Berlin) founded.
     Newberry Library (Chicago) founded.
1887–9.   Hertz investigates electric waves.
1888.   Medical Department, University of Tomsk (1880), opened.
     Institut Pasteur founded.
     Roux and Yersin isolate toxin of diphtheria.
     Chantemesse and **Widal** introduce **vaccines against typhoid fever**.
     Weil describes **infectious jaundice** (Botkin, 1889).
     Victor Babes discovers piroplasm of carceag (Babesia).
     Ducrey isolates bacillus of chancroid.
     Nencki and Sieber isolate hematoporphyrin.
     Zuntz and Geppert construct respiration calorimeter.
     Celli demonstrates fly transmission of typhoid fever.
     Gee describes cœliac disease (intestinal infantilism, Herter, 1918).
     Parkes Museum merged into Sanitary Institute (Great Britain).
     Baumann and Kast introduce trional.
     Local Government Act (England).
     Bacteriological (public health) laboratory at Providence, Rhode Island.
     Experiment Station at Lawrence, Massachusetts.
     Public Health (Bacteriological) Laboratory at Rome (Italy).
     Alfieiri Institute of Social Sciences at Florence (1874).
     Marine Biological Laboratory at Woods Hole (Massachusetts).
     Société française d'ophthalmologie (Paris) founded.
     Museo pedagogico at Montevideo (Uruguay).
     École de service de santé militaire (Lyons) founded.
     American Association of Anatomists (Baltimore) organized.
     American Association of Railway Surgeons (Chicago) founded.
     Australasian Association for the Advancement of Science (Sydney) organized.
     Prehistoric Museum at Weimar.
1888–92. Dercum describes painful obesity.
1888–1906. Carlsberg Glyptothek (Copenhagen) constructed.
1889.   Johns Hopkins Hospital (Baltimore) and Hamburg-Eppendorf Hospital opened.
     University of Fribourg (Switzerland) opened (November 4).
     Hofmeister investigates proteins (crystallized egg-albumen).
     Buchner discovers **alexins**.
     Von Mering and **Minkowski** produce **experimental pancreatic diabetes**.
     Von Behring discovers **antitoxins**.
     Max **Einhorn** illuminates the stomach (gastrodiaphany).
     Von Jaksch describes **pseudoleukemic anemia**.
     Kitasato obtains pure cultures of tetanus bacillus.
     Pfeiffer describes glandular fever and discovers influenza bacillus.
     Pasteur, Chamberland, and Roux employ attenuated cultures in preventive inoculation.
     Salkowski investigates autodigestion of organs.
     Henry **Head** investigates mechanism of respiration.
     Conn (United States) investigates bacteriology of milk.
     Infant milk depots at Hamburg and New York (Henry Koplik).
     Roux and Yersin point out danger of diphtheria convalescents as carriers.
     Oscar **Lassar** introduces **public baths** (Berlin).
     University of Madras qualifies public health officers.
     Kocher performs hepaticostomy.

1889.   Vaughan and Novy teach bacteriology in Michigan.
        Von Bergmann publishes treatise on brain surgery.
        Queen Victoria's Jubilee Institute for Nurses chartered.
        Society of Scientists and Physicians at Tomsk (Siberia).
        Missouri Botanical Garden at St. Louis.
        Laboratory of Vegetable Biology at Fontainebleau.
1889–90.   Pandemic influenza.
1889–91.   **Brown-Séquard** establishes **organotherapy.**
1889–93.   Denver Aqueduct (16½ miles, from Platte River) constructed.
1890.   University of Lausanne founded (Académie, 1536).
        Imperial Institute of Experimental Medicine (St. Petersburg) founded.
        Koch introduces **tuberculin** and notes that tuberculous animals resist reinoculation.
        Behring treats **diphtheria** with **antitoxin.**
        Maffuci isolates avian tubercle bacillus (B. gallinaceus).
        Bowditch demonstrates **non-fatigability of nerve.**
        W. D. Miller elucidates bacteriology of dental caries.
        Pic standardizes treatment of tubercular peritonitis.
        Loeb develops theory of **tropisms.**
        Poehl isolates spermin from testis.
        Tarchanoff introduces **psychogalvanic reflex** in diagnosis.
        Emil Fischer investigates synthetic sugars.
        Schleich introduces **infiltration-anesthesia.**
        Head and Campbell investigate pathology of herpes zoster.
        S. M. Babcock develops method of estimating fats in milk.
        Czech Academy of Sciences and Arts at Prague founded.
        Institute Pasteur at Saigon (Cochin China).
        Biological Laboratory at Cold Spring Harbor (Long Island).
        Dermatological Society at Vienna founded.
        Botanical Garden at Tiflis (Siberia).
        Volta Bureau (Washington) founded by Alexander Graham Bell.
        German Pharmaceutical Society (Berlin) founded.
        State Institute for Experimental Medicine at St. Petersburg.
        Royal College of Physicians of Ireland (1667) revived.
        Écoles annexes de médecine navale at Brest, Rochefort, and Toulon.
        Archival Repository of Medical Literature at Berlin.
1890–93.   Behring and Kitasato develop antitoxin treatment of diphtheria.
        Pandemic influenza.
1890–1909.   Haberlandt investigates sensation in plants.
1891.   Institute for Infectious Diseases (Berlin) opened under Koch.
        Lister Institute for Preventive Medicine (London) opened.
        Waldeyer formulates the **Neuron Theory** (Ramón y Cajal, 1891).
        Quincke introduces **lumbar puncture.**
        Walter Snow urges recirculation of factory-air.
        Witzel performs gastrostomy (Kader, 1896).
        Halsted introduces rubber gloves in operative surgery.
        Michelson invents the interferometer.
        Bier introduces **artificial hyperemia.**
        Von Bergmann standardizes general aseptic ritual in surgery (Koch, 1881; G. Neuber, 1882–5).
        Peter Dettweiler builds first sanatorium for phthisical patients at Ruppertshain.
        Gabriel Lippmann introduces color photography.
        S. G. Hedin invents hematocrit.
        S. M. Copeman introduces glycerinated lymph for smallpox vaccination.
        Biological station at Glubokoe Lake (Russia).
        Institute de oftalmologia at Lisbon.
        Stanford University (California) founded.
        Association of American Medical Colleges (Chicago) founded.
        Department of Medicine, University of Texas (Galveston), founded.
1891–93.   S. P. Langley experiments with aëroplanes.
1891–1902.   **Manson** investigates **filariasis.**
1892.   State Hygienic Institute at Hamburg.
        Smith and Kilbourne demonstrate tick transmission of bovine piroplasmosis (Texas fever).
        Welch and Nuttall identify **gas bacillus** (Bacillus aërogenes).
        Halsted successfully ligates subclavian artery (first portion).
        Kossel and Neumann discover pentose in vegetable substances.

1892.   Ivanovski describes mosaic tobacco disease.
Calmette investigates serum therapy of cobra poisoning.
Francis Galton introduces identification by finger-prints (dactyloscopy).
Von Jaksch signalizes value of leucocytosis in diagnosis.
Salkowski and Jastrowitz describe pentosuria.
Sedgwick emphasizes necessity of fly-control in prevention of typhoid fever.
Bokay notes relation between varicella and herpes.
Frank Hartley resects Gasserian ganglion for trigeminal neuralgia.
Hans Buchner shows effect of sunlight on self-purification of streams.
Medical inspection of schools in New York City.
Laboratory of Hygiene (University of Pennsylvania) opened at Philadelphia.
Instituto Bacteriologico de Camara Pestana at Lisbon.
H. L. Coit organizes Medical Milk Commission (certified milk).
Royal Japanese Institute for Infectious Diseases at Chirokane (Tokyo).
American Psychological Association (New York) founded.
Wistar Institute of Anatomy and Biology (1808) incorporated (Philadelphia).
Public Health Act (Manitoba).
Cholera epidemic in Hamburg.
National Medical Society (Norsk Medcinske Selskab) at Christiania (Oslo).
Bibliographical Society (London) founded.
Biological station at Bergen (Norway).
Musée gréco-romaine at Alexandria (Egypt).

1892–1900. New Chicago Drainage Canal (28½ miles) constructed.
1892–1907. Illinois and Mississippi (Hennepin) Canal (Chicago sewerage) constructed (opened October 24, 1907).
1892–1913. Sherrington investigates reciprocal innervation of antagonistic muscles.
1892–1918. Haldane invents standard apparatus for estimating respiratory exchange (gasometry of the blood).

1893.   Finsen treats smallpox pustules by exclusion of ultra-violet light.
Gilbert discovers paracolon and paratyphoid bacilli.
G. R. Fowler performs pulmonary decortication.
Brunton and Cash investigate relation of pharmacological action to chemical structure.
Emil Fischer investigates the synthesis of glucosides.
Fedor Krause excises Gasserian ganglion for trigeminal neuralgia.
Anderson describes first mechanical water-filter.
First open (slow sand) filtration of water-supply at Lawrence, Massachusetts.
Hermann M. Biggs establishes Diagnostic Laboratory in New York City.
Nathan Straus establishes milk-stations in New York City (1893–1919).
Isolation Hospital Act (England).
Nurses' Settlement on East Side (New York City) founded by Lillian Wald and Miss Brewster.
Institut international de sociologie at Paris.
International Cholera Congress at Dresden.
Society of Anesthetists (London) founded.
Library, Medical Society of Denver, established.

1893–9.   Consolidation (storage and interconnection of conduits) of London water-supply.
1893–97. Erwin Smith investigates bacterial diseases of plants.
1893–1928. Freud describes sexual (anxiety) neuroses and develops psycho-analysis.

1894.   Kitasato and Yersin discover plague bacillus.
Kirstein devises direct laryngoscopy.
Yersin demonstrates identity of human and rat plague.
Dukes describes "fourth disease."
Paltauf (Vienna) takes over mass-production of diphtheria (antitoxic) serum.
Wölfler performs gastro-gastrostomy.
Bruce discovers trypanosome of nagana (T. Brucei).
Rouget discovers trypanosoma of dourine (T. equiperdum).
Banti describes splenic anemia.
Baumann discovers thyreoiodin.
Medical inspection of schools begun in United States.
Workmen's Compensation Act in Norway.
American Society of Heating and Ventilating Engineers founded.
New York Herald antitoxin fund turned over to Health Department.
Pasteur Institute in Tunis.
Cleveland (Ohio) Medical Library Association founded.
Local Government Act (England).

1894. International Loan Library for the Blind (*Deutsche Zentralbücherei*) at Leipzig.
Child Study Society (London) founded.
State Hydrophobia Vaccine Institute at Vienna.
Psychiatric Clinic at Rio de Janeiro.
Wellcome Physiological Research Laboratories (London) founded.
Institut Solvay (de physiologie) founded at Brussels.
Field Museum of Natural History (Chicago) founded.
University Biological Station at Dröbak, near Oslo (Norway).

1894–1925. J. N. Langley finances *Journal of Physiology* (founded 1878).

1895. Röntgen discovers **X-rays.**
Pfeiffer discovers **bacteriolysis** (Pfeiffer's phenomenon).
Finsen treats lupus by concentration of ultra-violet light.
Ronald Ross demonstrates development of malarial parasite in mosquito.
Calmette introduces serum against snake venoms.
Kocher investigates gunshot wounds from small-calibre bullets.
Zwaardemaker investigates smell and odors with olfactometer.
Wilhelm His reforms anatomical nomenclature.
Marconi introduces wireless telegraphy.
Cameron introduces septic tanks for purifying sewage sludge.
Herbert Haviland Field establishes Concilium Bibliographicum at Zürich.
Nobel Prize Foundation at Stockholm.
Proctor Marble Company (Vermont) employs nurses for sick employees.
Friedrich Wilhelms Institut (Berlin) becomes Kaiser-Wilhelms Akademie.
New York Public Library founded.
German Museum for Deaf-Mute Instruction at Leipzig.
Bureau of Laboratories (New York Health Department) established.
Imperial Institute of Veterinary Research at Muktesar (India).
Pasteur Institute for Indo-China at Uha-Trang (Annam).
State Serotherapeutic Institute at Vienna.
German Central Committee for Prevention of Tuberculosis at Berlin.
Pasteur Institute at Lille.
Institution of Sanitary Engineers (London) founded.
Instituto Medico at Sucre (Bolivia).
Universid Central (Quito, Ecuador) reorganized, with Medical Faculty.
École d'application des médecins et pharmaciens stagiaires (Toulon) founded (July 26).
Lane Medical Library (San Francisco) founded.

1895–1901. Jules and Augusta Dejerine publish treatise on anatomy of the nerve-centres.

1896. Max Gruber discovers **bacterial agglutination.**
Murphy performs successful circular anastomosis of blood-vessels.
Jaboulay performs sympathectomy for exophthalmic goitre.
Wright, Pfeiffer, and Kolle vaccinate against typhoid fever.
Widal and Sicard introduce **agglutination test** for typhoid fever.
Leo Arons (Berlin) invents mercury vapor lamp (elimination of red or orange rays).
Friedrich Bezold devises tuning-fork method of testing and training deaf-mutes.
Bourquelot and Bertrand discover tyrosinase.
W. J. Dibdin and Schweder invent method for **bacteriological purification of sewage.**
Casper employs ureteral cystoscopy and catherization in diagnosis of renal diseases.
Leopold Freund treats hypertrichosis with Röntgen rays.
Hammarsten discovers pentose in the pancreas.
Merling introduces **eucaine.**
Farina and Rehn operate on the heart.
Leichtenstern describes essential (three-day) influenza.
University of Lyons founded (July 10).
University of Caen (Calvados) revived.
First Congress of German Heating and Ventilating Engineers (Berlin).
Hermann Rietschel starts Testing Institute for heating and ventilating appliances at Charlottenburg (new buildings, 1906).
Stenbeck opens Röntgen Institute at Stockholm.
Welch founds *Journal of Experimental Medicine.*
Institute for Infectious Diseases at Bern (Switzerland).
Association française d'urologie (Paris) organized.
Institut Pasteur de la Loire-Inférieure (Nancy) founded (opened 1898).
Physicians' Temperance Society (Verein Abstinenter Aerzte) at Berlin.
Bacteriological Institute at Kiev (Ukraine).
Finsen's Phototherapeutic Institute (Medicinske Lysinstitut) at Copenhagen.

1896.   Bacteriological Laboratory at Bombay.
          National Union of Hungarian Physicians at Budapest.
          Botanical Garden at New York.
1896-8.   Schenck describes sporotrichosis.
1897.   **Shiga** discovers **dysentery bacillus.**
          Bordet discovers **bacterial hemolysis.**
          Emil Fischer synthesizes caffeine, theobromine, xanthin, guanin, and adenin.
          Flügge states theory of **droplet infection.**
          Jonnesco performs sympathectomy for glaucoma.
          Ogata finds plague bacilli in fleas of plague-ridden rats.
          Nuttall demonstrates fly-transmission of plague bacilli.
          Ehrlich states side-chain theory of immunity.
          E. Van Ermengem discovers Bacillus botulinus.
          E. Schiff and H. Kümmell treat lupus successfully with Röntgen rays.
          J. V. Laborde introduces **artificial respiration.**
          Horton Smith shows danger of chronic (urinary) **typhoid carriers.**
          Stroganoff introduces sedative (preventive) treatment of puerperal eclampsia.
          Nathan Brill describes mild endemic typhus in New York.
          Germano shows that dryness is fatal to bacteria.
          Apostoli introduces high-frequency electrotherapy (arsonvalisation) in gynecology.
          Kyoto Imperial University (Japan) founded.
          Röntgen Society (London) founded.
          Marine Biological Station at Westport (Scotland).
          Institut national d'hygiéne et de bacteriologie (Luxemburg) founded.
          G. C. Whipple establishes Mount Prospect Laboratory (Brooklyn Water Works).
          New York (State) adopts compulsory notification of tuberculosis (H. M. Biggs).
          Municipal Milk Station at Rochester, New York.
1897-8.   **MacCallum** demonstrates sexual conjugation of parasite of avian malaria.
1897-1902. **Cannon** investigates movements of stomach and intestines by Röntgenoscopy.
1897-1904. **Ramón y Cajal** publishes treatise on texture of the nervous system.
1898.   **P. and S. Curie** discover **radium.**
          Loeffler and **Frosch** investigate **filterable viruses.**
          Looss demonstrates **mechanism of hook-worm infection.**
          Theobald Smith isolates and cultivates **bovine tubercle bacilli.**
          Emil Fischer isolates the **purin nucleus** of uric acid transformation.
          Dreser introduces **heroin.**
          Simonds demonstrates transmission of bubonic plague by fleas.
          Bordet and Tsistovich demonstrate agglutinins, hemolysins and precipitins in blood-serum
             treated with alien blood-corpuscles.
          Killian introduces **direct bronchoscopy.**
          Vincent describes spirillo-bacillary angina.
          Tschirch explains chemical mechanism of common purgatives.
          L. O. Howard publishes Bulletin on mosquito-eradication.
          Arloing and Courmont introduce sero-agglutination of tubercle bacilli in diagnosis.
          Davis and Varnier employ X-rays in obstetric diagnosis.
          Affiliation of Rush Medical College with University of Chicago (January 5).
          Cornell University Medical College (New York City) founded.
          London College of Physiology founded.
          Faculty of Medicine at Porto Alegre (Brazil) organized.
          Philippine Health Service (Manila) organized (Board of Health, 1901).
          Bavarian Hydrologic Station at Munich.
          Prehistoric Museum at Ventimiglia (Italy).
          Institute for the Study of Malignant Disease (New York) founded.
          Mechanical water-filter installed at Elmira, New York.
          Experiments on chlorine purification of sewage at Hamburg.
          Samuel W. Abbott publishes second Massachusetts Life-table.
          State Sanitarium for Tuberculosis in Massachusetts.
          Marchoux founds Bacteriological Laboratory for East Africa at St. Louis (Senegal).
          German Pathological Society (Dresden) founded.
          Washington Academy of Sciences organized.
          Biological Experiment Station (Harvard University) at Cienfuegos, Cuba.
1898-1908. Zeppelin experiments with dirigible air-ships.
1898-1915. **Sherrington** investigates **decerebrate rigidity.**
          W. T. Porter finances *American Journal of Physiology.*
1898-1920. **Langley** investigates **autonomic system.**

1899.	**Reed, Carroll, Lazear,** and **Agramonte** demonstrate mosquito transmission of yellow fever.

Jacques Loeb produces chemical activation of sea-urchin egg.
Ramón y Cajal describes histology of cerebral cortex.
Weichselbaum and **Jaeger** isolate meningococcus.
Grassi and Bignami prove that Anopheles is sole transmitter of malaria.
Nuttall summarizes rôle of insects as vectors of communicable diseases.
Spiller introduces chordotomy for neuralgia.
Kossel states theory of protamin nucleus in protein transformations.
H. Dreser introduces aspirin.
Dewar liquefies air, oxygen, and hydrogen.
Beijerinck isolates filterable virus of mosaic tobacco disease.
Albert Hazen constructs slow sand water-filter for Albany, New York.
National University at Peking (China) founded.
London School of Hygiene and Tropical Medicine founded.
Liverpool School of Tropical Medicine founded.
Edinburgh School of Tropical Medicine founded.
Instituto Nacional de higiene de Alfonso XIII (Madrid) founded.
Medical Library Association (United States) founded.
Ehrlich's Institute for Experimental Medicine (Frankfurt) founded.
Children's Court at Chicago.
Moscow Odontological Society founded (disbanded 1919; revived 1922).
New York Zoological Park (Bronx) opened.
Societies of Neurology and of Pediatrics founded at Paris.
Royal Hygienic Institute at Posen.
Hackett Medical College (Canton, China) founded.
Cancer Commission of Harvard University founded.
American Anthropological Association (Washington, D. C.) founded.
Parliament authorizes Derwent Aqueduct (60 miles) for water-supply of Derby, Leicester, Sheffield, and Nottingham.
Vital Brazil founds Instituto Butantan (São Paulo, Brazil) for manufacture of serum against snake-venom.

1899–1900.	**Reed** completes demonstration of mosquito transmission of yellow fever.

Stenbeck treats cancer with Röntgen rays.

1899–1906.	**Emil Fischer** investigates amino-acid constituents of protein molecule.
1900.	**Gärtner** invents **tonometer** for measuring blood-pressure.

Bier introduces **spinal (cocaine) anesthesia** (Corning) into general surgery.
Widal and **Ravaut** introduce **cytodiagnosis.**
Gersung introduces prothetic (paraffin) injections.
Wertheim devises **radical operation for uterine cancer.**
Kastle and **Loevenhart** demonstrate **reversibility of enzymes** (lipase).
Sjögren and Stenbeck treat superficial epithelioma with X-rays.
A. Walkhoff shows destructive effect of radium on the tissues.
Willstätter and Bode produce synthetic cocaine.
Park recommends control of milk (New York City) by bacterial tests.
Woodhead disinfects water-supply of Maidstone (England) with chlorine after typhoid epidemic.
Danysz starts experimental epidemiology.
Mechanical water-filter installed at Lorraine (Ohio).
University of Odessa founded.
Hartmann-Bund (Verband der Aerzte Deutschlands) founded at Leipzig.
Institute for Medical Research at Kualu Lampur (Federated Malay States).
American Association of Pathologists and Bacteriologists (Boston) founded.
American Röntgen Ray Society founded.
Yale Botanical Garden at New Haven.
Institut général psychologique (Paris) founded.
College of Physicians and Surgeons (Chicago) becomes College of Medicine, University of Illinois (May 1).
German Central Cancer Committee (Berlin) founded.
Royal Hygienic Institute at Beuthen (Upper Silesia).
Volga Biological Station at Saratov (Russia).
Philippine Library and Museum (Manila) established.
Baylor University College of Medicine (Dallas, Texas) founded.

1900–1903.	**Leishman** and **Donovan** discover protozoön of **kala azar.**
1900–1904.	**Pschorr** and **Vongerichten** demonstrate phenanthren nucleus of morphine and codeine.
1900–1906.	**Mills** and **Spiller** describe unilateral type of spastic spinal paralysis.

55

1900–1922. Sixteen Indian cholera epidemics radiate from Kimbh Hardwar fair.

1901. De Vries states mutation theory.
Dutton and Ford discover trypanosome of sleeping sickness (Trypanosoma gambiense).
Bordet and Gengou demonstrate complement-fixation.
Aschkinazı and Caspari show that radium checks the growth of bacteria.
Dantes and Bloch treat lupus with radium.
Sjögren treats lupus with X-rays.
Landsteiner discovers blood-grouping (iso-agglutination).
Ayerza describes cyanotic sclerosis of pulmonary artery (cardios negros).
Emil Fischer devises ester method of isolating amino-acids.
Gowland Hopkins and Cole isolate tryptophan (Stadelmann, 1890).
Felix Marchand investigates wound-healing.
Takamine isolates adrenaline.
Pavloff isolates enterokinase.
Otto Cohnheim discovers erepsin.
Nencki and Marchlevski show relationship of hemoglobin and chlorophyll (hemopyrrol).
Uhlenhuth introduces precipitin test for blood-stains (Bordet, 1898).
Suddeck investigates ether intoxication.
Planck announces quanta theory of emission of radiant energy (verified by Einstein, 1905).
Temper and Pfützner construct central-heating plant at Dresden.
Elmassian discovers trypanosome of mal de caderas (T. Elmassiani).
Lister Institute of Preventive Medicine (London) founded.
Rockefeller Institute for Medical Research (New York) opened.
Instituto Oswaldo Cruz (Rio de Janeiro) opened.
Biometrika founded by Galton, Pearson, and Weldon.
Hygienic Laboratory, United States Public Health Service, opened.
State Institution for Investigation of Food Substances at Berlin.
German Orthopedic Society (Berlin) founded.
German Society for School-Hygiene (Berlin) founded.
German Society for History of Medicine and Science (Leipzig) founded.
State Serum Institute at Copenhagen.
Medico-Legal Society (London) founded.
Award of Nobel Prizes begun.
Museum of History of Medicine in Hôtel Dieu at Rouen.
Philippine Health Service (Manila) established (September 29).
Philippine Bureau of Science (Manila) established.
Nuttall founds Journal of Hygiene.

1901–5. Sanitary Institute (London) gives lectures to teachers on applied hygiene.

1901–26. Frazier introduces section of posterior (sensory) trigeminal roots for neuralgia.

1902. Carrel introduces new methods of vascular anastomosis and transplantation of tissues.
G. Kelling introduces exploration of peritoneal cavity by inflation.
Albers-Schönberg invents compression-diaphragm for Röntgenography.
Emil Fischer, Leuchs, and Weigert synthetize serin, glucosamin, and lysin.
R. Herzog discovers site of Asclepieion at Cos.
Holzknecht devises method of dosimetry for X-rays.
Robert Weir performs appendicostomy.
P. C. Hewitt perfects quartz mercury vapor lamp.
McClung isolates sex-chromosome.
Von Pirquet postulates formation of antibodies as termination of incubation period.
Ravenel isolates bovine tubercle bacillus from a tuberculous child.
Preston Kyes shows lecithin to be the complement of cobra-hemolysin.
Rutherford and Soddy demonstrate radio-activity of thorium and its emanation.
Schild introduces atoxyl.
H. von Tappeiner investigates photodynamic substances.
Steinbuchel introduces morphine-scopolamine anesthesia in obstetrics.
Finney performs gastro-duodenostomy.
Theiler discovers trypanosome of galziekte (T. Theileri).
J. R. Ewald investigates end organ of octavus (auditory) nerve.
John McCormick Institute for Infectious Diseases (Chicago) founded.
General Education Board (Rockefeller Foundation), New York.
Carnegie Institution of Washington founded.
Imperial Cancer Research Fund (England) founded.
Royal Army Medical College (London) founded.
Society of Bavarian Psychiatrists (Munich) founded.
Institute for Biological Experimentation at Vienna.

1902. Société française d'histoire de médecine (Paris) founded.
School of Tropical Medicine (Lisbon) founded.
Institut supérieur de vaccine (Vaccine Service of the Academy of Medicine) at Paris.
Society of German Food Chemists (Berlin) founded.
German Society for Prevention of Venereal Diseases (Berlin) founded.
National Serotherapeutic Institute at Vienna (new building, 1907).
American Anthropological Society (Andover, Massachusetts) organized.
Société de médecine physique (Antwerp) organized.
Metropolis Water Act (England).

1902–3. Jensen propagates cancer through several generations of mice.
1902–6. Bayliss and Starling investigate hormones.
1903. Metchnikoff inoculates higher apes with syphilis.
Von Pirquet and Schick identify serum-sickness with anaphylaxis.
Rollier treats surgical tuberculosis with ultraviolet light at Leysin.
Koch stresses danger of healthy typhoid carriers as agents of infection.
Emil Fischer and von Mehring introduce veronal.
Arthus produces local anaphylaxis.
Johannsen investigates pure line inheritance.
Danysz shows selective action of radium on malignant tumors.
Einthoven invents string galvanometer.
Albers-Schönberg notes sterilizing effect of X-rays on gonads.
Bruce demonstrates transmission of sleeping sickness by tsetse fly.
Benno Credé introduces collargol.
Dunbar discovers toxin and antitoxin (pollantin) of hay-fever.
Emil Fischer devises method of synthetizing polypeptides.
Josué produces experimental arteriosclerosis by adrenalin injections.
Mosetig-Moorhof devises method of plumbing bony cavities.
Posternac isolates phytin.
J. H. Wright discovers Leishmania bodies in endemic ulcers.
Riva Rocci invents sphygmomanometer.
Ramsay and Soddy demonstrate transmutation of radium into helium.
Schaudinn differentiates Entamœba histolytica from E. coli.
Siedentopf and Zsigmondy invent ultramicroscope.
Buchner and Meisenheimer discover enzymes of lactic acid and vinegar fermentation.
Almroth Wright and Douglass investigate opsonins.
Castellani discovers Trypanosoma Ugandæ.
Senn treats leukemia with Röntgen rays.
Dejerine describes thalamus opticus syndrome.
Janet describes psychasthenia.
Vaccination obligatory in Spain.
Henry Phipps Institute for Tuberculosis (Baltimore) opened.
American Society of Tropical Medicine (Philadelphia) founded.
Wellcome Tropical Research Laboratories at Khartoum (Soudan).
American Genetic Association (Washington) founded.
Medical Academy at Osaka (Japan) founded.
Société de médecine physique (Paris) founded.
Berlin Museum of Safety founded.
Germanic Museum (Munich) founded.
Permanent Exhibit for Industrial Welfare (Berlin) opened.
German Society for Prevention of Quackery (Berlin) founded.

1903–4. Frosch, Drigalski, and Dönitz establish theory of typhoid (bacillus) carriers.
1903–23. Bacteriological Institute at Zagreb (Jugoslavia).
1904. Atwater invents respiration calorimeter.
Sauerbruch introduces pneumatic cabinet for thoracic surgery.
Chittenden investigates minimum food requirements.
Max Cloetta introduces digalen.
Fourneau introduces stovaine (anesthesia).
Giemsa introduces modification of Romanovsky stain (1890) for protozoa (plasmodia and spirochætæ).
Schittenhelm isolates oxydase.
F. Stolz determines composition of adrenalin.
Weichardt investigates toxins of fatigue.
Arneth employs blood-picture in diagnosis.
Helene Stöcker founds *Die Neue Generation*.
Gradenigo describes sixth nerve syndrome.

1904.   Foveau de Courmelles treats uterine myomata by X-rays.
         University of Sofia (Bulgaria) founded (Medical Faculty, 1918).
         Deutsche physiologische Gesellschaft (Leipzig) founded.
         Physiological Society (Philadelphia) founded.
         Ethnological Society (London) founded.
         National Tuberculosis Association (New York) founded.
         Society for Experimental Psychology (Berlin) founded.
         Academia Nacional de Medicina (Caracas) founded.
         Tortugas Laboratory (Carnegie Biological Station) at Key West (Florida).
         Association international des médecins mécano-thérapeutes (Brussels) founded.
1905.   Schaudinn discovers parasite of syphilis (**Treponema pallidum**).
         Bordet and **Gengou** isolate **bacillus of whooping-cough.**
         Vassale employs parathyroid extract in tetany.
         Chaput employs stovaine in spinal anesthesia.
         König describes osteochondritis dissecans.
         Winter resuscitates the heart by adrenalin injections.
         Flügge and pupils show effects of **vitiated air** to be due to heat and humidity.
         Dutton and Koch demonstrate tick-transmission of African relapsing fever.
         Alfred Einhorn discovers **novocaine.**
         Ehrlich demonstrates change of experimental carcinoma transplants into **sarcoma.**
         Koch maintains that sleeping sickness is transmitted by several species of **Glossina.**
         Levaditi employs Ramón y Cajal's silver stain for spirochætes.
         Chapin abandons terminal disinfection at Providence (Rhode Island).
         Wright brothers make successful flight with aëroplane.
         Kaiserin Augusta-Victoria Haus (for combating infantile mortality) at Berlin.
         German Röntgen Society (Berlin) founded.
         Société de pathologie exotique (Paris) founded.
         King Edward VII College of Medicine (Singapore) founded.
         American Society for Psychical Research founded.
         Carnegie Laboratory for Plant Physiology at Tucson (Arizona).
         Institute of Ophthalmic Opticians at London.
         American Sociological Society (Chicago) founded.
         Vajirañana National Library of Siam at Bangkok.
1905–7. F. S. Lee investigates fatigue.
1906,   **Wassermann introduces serum diagnosis of syphilis.**
         Bárány develops theory of **vestibular nystagmus.**
         Einthoven obtains telecardiograms from the heart at a distance.
         Von Pirquet states doctrine of **allergy.**
         Ransohoff performs discission of the pleura.
         Voelcker and **von Lichtenberg** examine kidney with X-ray (**pyelography**).
         Parseval flies air-ship.
         E. Beck introduces bismuth paste in Röntgenography.
         MacDougal demonstrates heredity of experimentally acquired characteristics **in plants.**
         Neisser demonstrates susceptibility of lower apes to syphilis.
         Federal Food and Drugs Act (United States) passed (June 30; effective 1907).
         Provision of Children's Meals Act (England).
         Compulsory medical inspection of schools in Massachusetts.
         American Association for Labor Legislation founded (February 15).
         National Committee on Child Labor (United States) founded.
         Courses in public hygiene instituted at the University of Pennsylvania.
         Carnegie Nutrition Laboratory (Boston) opens.
         Institute for Experimental Cancer Research at Heidelberg.
         Institute for Experimental Pedagogics and Psychology at Leipzig.
         Chicago Tuberculosis Institute incorporated and opened.
         American Society of Biological Chemists (Ann Arbor) founded.
         Chemotherapeutic Institute (Georg Speyer Haus) at Frankfurt-on-the-Main.
         Institute for Applied Psychology at Berlin.
         State School of Tropical Medicine (Brussels) founded.
         Berlin Society for History of Medicine and Science founded.
         Pathological Society of Great Britain and Ireland (Cambridge) founded.
         Kaiserin Friedrich Haus (for Post-Graduate Medical Study) at Berlin.
         Entomological Society of America founded.
1906–13. **Willstätter** investigates **chlorophyll.**
1906–20. **Gowland Hopkins** investigates **accessory food-factors** (vitamins).
1906–25. Blair Bell introduces use of pituitrin as oxytocic in lingering labor.

1907. Von Pirquet introduces cutaneous reaction in tuberculosis.
Calmette and Wolff-Eisner introduce conjunctival reactions in tuberculosis.
Theobald Smith suggests use of toxin-antitoxin in diphtheria (Behring, 1912).
Emmerich and Löw obtain pyocyanase from Bacillus pyocyaneus.
Ricketts demonstrates tick-transmission of Rocky Mountain fever.
Emil Fischer obtains linkage of 18 amino-acids (protein molecule).
Ramsay obtains lithium by transmutation (irradiation) of copper.
Willstätter and Hocheder obtain phytol nucleus from chlorophyll molecule.
Adolf Schmidt employs functional test-meal in diagnosing intestinal disorders.
Zwirn performs keratoplasty in corneal opacity.
Fletcher and Hopkins demonstrate rôle of lactic-acid formation in normal muscle-contraction.
Benedict and Milner show that excess of CO_2 is harmless in a cool room.
Ramsay Hunt describes geniculate ganglion syndrome.
University of Saskatchewan (Saskatoon) founded (opened 1909).
Tokohu Imperial University at Sendai (Japan).
International Association of Medical Museums (Montreal) founded.
Royal Society of Tropical Medicine and Hygiene (London) founded.
Royal Medical and Chirurgical Society (1805) rechartered as Royal Society of Medicine (London).
Bureau international contre l'alcoolisme founded at Stockholm.
International Sleeping Sickness Congress at London.
Italian Society of Medical History (Florence) founded.
Notification of Births (Act) England.
Angelo Mosso founds Monte Rosa Institute (University of Turin) at Alagna Sefia.
Sudhoff founds *Archiv für Geschichte der Medizin* (Leipzig).

1907–8. Marage invents vocal siren (test for deafness) and photographs the voice.
1908. Leonard Finlay produces experimental rickets by deficient diet.
Bernstein investigates temperature-coefficients of muscular energy.
Buerger describes thrombo-angiitis obliterans.
Kamerlingh Onnes liquefies helium.
Willstätter and Benz show crystallized chlorophyll to be a magnesium product.
Gabriel Lippmann introduces relief-photography.
Zeppelin constructs improved air-ship.
Peking Union Medical College founded by Rockefeller Institute.
University of the Philippines (Manila) founded (College of Medicine, 1910).
Royal Army Medical College opened at Millbank.
Tropical Diseases Bureau (London) founded by Colonial Office.
Psycho-neurological Institute (St. Petersburg) founded.
Spanish Association for the Advancement of Sciences (Madrid) founded.
Institut für Radiumforschung at Vienna.
Clinic of Infantile Surgery at Montpellier.
Chicago adopts compulsory pasteurization of milk.
Bureau of Child Hygiene in New York City (Health Department).
American Public Health Association standardizes tests for milk.
Water-supply of Union Stock-yards (Chicago) disinfected by chlorine gas.
German Society for Racial Hygiene (Berlin) founded.
250 special hospitals for tuberculosis in United States.
International Moral Education Congress at London.
Denver (Colorado) Medical Society founded.
Biological Station at Kosina (Russia).

1908–9. Ante-natal hygiene started in New York and Boston.
1908–10. William Pasteur describes massive (post-operative) collapse of the lungs.
1909. Sørensen investigates hydrogen-ion concentration.
F. F. Russell vaccinates United States Army against typhoid fever.
Förster operates for locomotor ataxia.
Much introduces cobra-venom reaction for insanity.
Sherrington investigates proprioceptive reflexes.
Metropolitan Life Insurance Company (New York) introduces home-nursing for industrial policy-holders.
University of Neuchâtel founded (May 18).
Society of Medical History (Chicago) founded.
University College (National University of Ireland) at Dublin.
German Central Committee for Dentistry in School Children (Berlin) organized.
State Dental Institute at Christiania (Oslo) founded.

1909.	Society of Medical Missionaries (Leipzig) founded.
	German Medical School for Chinese at Woosung, Shanghai (now Fungchi Medical High School).
	Illinois Society for Mental Hygiene (Chicago) founded.
1909–13.	Marine and Lenhart standardize iodine treatment of goiter.
1909–25.	L. and M. Lapicque investigate chronaxia.
1910.	R. G. Harrison demonstrates outgrowth of nerve-fiber in extravital culture (1906–10).
	Flexner produces poliomyelitis experimentally.
	Vedder demonstrates amebicidal action of emetine.
	Rollier treats tuberculosis with ultraviolet light (heliotherapy) at Cergnat (École de Soleil).
	Chapin, Winslow, and Robinson emphasize danger of contact infection in communicable diseases.
	Martin Fischer explains edema as effect of acids on swelling of proteins.
	Hasselbalch devises formula for estimating hydrogen-ion concentration.
	Ehrlich and Hata introduce salvarsan (606).
	Adelaide Nutting establishes course of public-health nursing at Teachers College (Columbia University, New York).
	Nelson Morris Memorial Institute for Medical Research (Chicago) founded.
	Rockefeller Sanitary Commission for hookworm prevention (New York) organized.
	State Serum Institute (Copenhagen) founded.
	Laboratorie de police technique (Lyons) organized.
	Berlin Psychoanalytic Society founded.
	Veterinary High School (Lisbon) founded.
	Centenary of University of Berlin.
	National Committee for Preventing Blindness (United States) organized.
	Illinois State Commission on Industrial Diseases organized.
	Austrian Society for Investigation and Preventing of Cancer (Vienna) founded.
	Phonetic Laboratory at Hamburg.
	Association internationale des médecins scolaires founded.
	Clinic of Industrial Diseases (Milan) opened (March 20).
	Institut Pasteur at Algiers.
	Archæological Museum at Assuan (Egypt).
	Marine Laboratory (Pomona College) at Laguna Beach, California.
1910–11.	Medical Plant Garden (University of Minnesota) at Minneapolis.
1910–13.	Libman describes subacute bacterial endocarditis.
1910–19.	Dale, Laidlow, and Richards investigate histamin.
1910–24.	Carrel, Burrows (et al.) investigate tissue culture and transplantation.
1910–27.	A. V. Hill investigates thermodynamics of muscular contraction.
1911.	Carrel investigates extravital culture and rejuvenation of tissues.
	Cushing describes dyspituitarism.
	McCoy and Chapin isolate bacillus of tularemia.
	Naunyn describes infectious cholangitis.
	Peyton Rous transmits sarcoma via filterable virus.
	Gullstrand receives Nobel Prize for optical researches.
	Donnan introduces doctrine of equilibria about a semipermeable membrane impermeable to one ion only (Donnan equilibria).
	Abel isolates bufagin.
	Meinicke introduces flocculation test in syphilis.
	American Public Health Association publishes standard methods for examining milk.
	California establishes notification of veneral diseases (July 1).
	Universities of Oporto and Lisbon founded.
	Kyushu Imperial University at Fukuoka (Japan) founded.
	University of Iceland (Reykjavik) founded (June 11).
	Biochemical Society (London) founded.
	Otho S. A. Sprague Memorial Institute for Medical Research (Chicago) founded.
	National Council for Industrial Safety (United States) organized.
	International Society for Individual Psychology (Vienna) founded.
	Public Health Ministry (New Zealand) organized.
	Kaiser Wilhelm Society for Advancement of Science (Berlin) founded.
	Ontario Act regulating municipal milk supply.
	National Health Week (England).
	George Crocker Cancer Research Fund.
	Hygienic Exhibition at Dresden.
	Milk Institute at Wangen (Bavaria).
	Milk Institute at Fominskoe, Vologda (Russia).

1911–14.   Casimir **Funk** investigates **vitamines.**
1911–15.   **Van Slyke** devises methods of estimating amino-nitrogen and amino-acids.
1911–20.   American Museum of Safety at New York.
1911–27.   **Pavloff** investigates **conditional reflexes.**
1912.   **Bass** cultivates **malarial plasmodium** *in vitro.*
            Nicolle, Anderson, and **Goldberger** produce **experimental typhus** in monkey.
            Weber and **Lorey** effect X-ray examination of abdominal viscera (**pneumoperitoneum.**)
            Beurman and **Gougerot** describe **sporotrichosis.**
            Von Behring employs **toxin-antitoxin immunization** against diphtheria.
            Ransohoff performs omentopexy for gastric prolapse.
            Berlin Surgical Society founded.
            Naval Medical School (Royal Naval College) at Greenwich (England).
            South African Institute for Medical Research (Johannesburg) founded.
            National Organization for Public Health Nursing (United States) organized.
            German Hygienic Museum at Dresden (Exhibit of 1911).
            Division of Industrial Hygiene (United States Public Health Service) organized.
            German Society for Lighting Technics (Berlin) founded.
            Austrian Society for School Hygiene (Vienna) founded.
            Institute for Hygiene and Infectious Diseases at Saarbrücken (now Medical Bureau for
               the Saar Region).
            Ukrainian Medical Society at Lemberg (Lwow).
            "Ose" (Society for Jewish Hygiene) at St. Petersburg (transferred to Berlin, 1922).
            Lombard Medical Society (Società Lombarda) at Milan.
            Dr. F. G. Gade founds Pathological Institute at Bergen (Norway).
            Pathological Institute at Dortmund (Prussia).
1912–13.   **Gustav Embden** and co-workers investigate **carbohydrate metabolism.**
1912–14.   Institut du radium (Curie Foundation) erected at Paris.
1912–15.   Osborne and Mendel investigate effects of deficient diets.
1912–16.   **Cannon** investigates effect of adrenal secretion on emotions.
1912–22.   **Folin** and co-workers devise methods of estimating amino-acids.
1912–26.   Rudolf **Magnus** investigates **postural reflexes.**
1913.   **Abderhalden** introduces **ferment reactions.**
            Schick introduces **susceptibility test for diphtheria.**
            Krönig and **Gauss** introduce morphine-scopolamine anesthesia in obstetrics (**twilight
               sleep**).
            Barthe devises ambrine treatment for burns.
            Revival of doctrine of the constitution.
            Møllgaard introduces **sanocrysin.**
            Douglass, Haldane, Henderson, and Schneider investigate effect of acclimatization **to**
               high altitudes (Pike's Peak) on respiration.
            Dakin and **Dudley** investigate **intermediary metabolism** of carbohydrates and proteins.
            Kinnier Wilson describes degeneration of lenticular nucleus.
            Aschoff and **Landau** map out the reticulo-endothelial system.
            Holst and Frölich postulate vitamin C.
            Vianna employs antimony tartrate in Leishmaniasis.
            Coolidge tube introduced.
            Potter-Bucky diaphragm introduced.
            Bose investigates sensation in plants.
            Medical Research Committee (London) organized.
            International Medical Congress at London.
            Wellcome Medical and Medico-Historical Museums (London) founded.
            Rockefeller Foundation (New York) chartered.
            International Health Board (Rockefeller Foundation) organized.
            Institute for Cancer Research (New York) opened.
            Institute for Cancer Research at Hamburg.
            Eugenic Research Association (Cold Spring Harbor, Long Island) organized.
            Workmen's Compensation Acts effective in 41 countries.
            American Society of Experimental Pathology founded.
            United States Army Medical Research Board at Manila (reorganized, 1922).
            German Society for Applied Entomology (Munich) founded.
            Bibliographical Institute (Moscow) organized.
            Société lorraine de psychologie appliquée (Nancy) founded.
            Italian Association for Legal Medicine (Turin) founded.
            Cook County Psychopathic Hospital (Chicago) opened.
            New York State Commission on Ventilation organized.

1913.   Netherland Society for Prevention of Venereal Diseases (Amsterdam) founded.
             Mental Hygiene Committee (Baltimore) organized.
             Massachusetts Society for Mental Hygiene (Boston) organized.
             International Society for Investigation of Sex (Berlin) organized.
             Saxon Army Museum at Dresden.
             Botanic Garden at Cassel (Germany).
             National Botanic Gardens at Kirstenbosch (South Africa).
             Mycological Institute at Hamburg.
1913–15.   Sir Leonard Hill, Haldane, and others confirm Flügge's findings on effects of humid
             heat (1905).
1913–16.   Dochez, Gillespie, and Avery type the pneumococci.
             McCollum, Davis, and Kennedy allocate vitamines A and B.
1913–20.   **Bourquelot** investigates synthesis of glucosides.
1913–27.   **Maude Slye** experiments on hereditary susceptibility to and immunity from cancer.
1914.   Hungarian University at Pressburg founded.
             Royal Hungarian University at Debrecen founded.
             Dejerine describes parietal lobe syndrome (sensitive cortex).
             Margaret and Warren Lewis study mitochondria.
             Christiansen, Douglas, and Haldane investigate CO_2 carriage by the blood.
             Barcroft investigates effect of high altitudes at Cerro de Pasco.
             Prussian State University at Frankfurt-on-the-Main founded (June 10).
             St. Petersburg becomes Petrograd.
             China Medical Board (Rockefeller Foundation) organized.
             Kitasato Institute for Infectious Diseases (Tokyo) founded.
             Medical Research Council (London) organized (Medical Research Committee, 1913).
             National Institute for Medical Research (London) founded.
             Société de chimie biologique (Paris) founded.
             Pacific Association of Scientific Societies (Berkeley, California) organized.
             Government Institute for Physiotherapy (Moscow) founded.
             National Council for Combating Venereal Diseases (London) organized.
             American Social Hygiene Association (New York) organized.
             Graduate School of Tropical Medicine and Public Health (Manila) founded.
             Veterinary Institute at Christiania (Oslo).
             New School of Physiology at Cambridge (England) opened.
             Eugenics Education Society (Chicago) founded.
             City Institute of Obstetrics and Gynecology at Hamburg.
             Brady Urological Institute (Johns Hopkins University) at Baltimore.
1914–15.   Ido and Inada establish spirochætal origin of infectious jaundice.
1914–18.   World War.
1914–19.   **E. C. Kendall** discovers and investigates **thyroxin**.
1915.   **Carrel-Dakin treatment** of infected (gunshot) wounds.
             Delousing of troops organized.
             Preventive inoculation against tetanus in gunshot wounds.
             Organization of methods of **gas-defense**.
             Futaki and Ishiwara discover parasite of rat-bite fever.
             Simmonds describes pituitary dwarfism.
             Ramsay Hunt describes progressive cerebellar dyssynergy.
             Weber devises method of examining the abdominal viscera by Röntgenography (pneumo-
             peritoneum).
             Kjelland forceps introduced.
             Infant mortality rate (New York City) reduced from 27 (1885) to 9.4 per 1000.
             Mayo Foundation for Medical Education and Research (Rochester, Minnesota)
             organized.
             Institute of Medicine (Chicago) organized (April 22).
             S. S. Goldwater establishes occupation diseases clinic (New York City).
             New York City abandons terminal disinfection in favor of control of contacts and carriers.
             National Committee for Prevention of Blindness (United States) organized.
             Société française de pedagogie (Paris) founded.
             Milk and Dairies Act (England).
             American Association of Industrial Physicians and Surgeons founded.
1915–16.   Mott *et al.* investigate shell-shock.
1915–20.   **Goldberger** investigates pellagra.
1916.   Dakin introduces **dichloramin-T.**
             Werner describes **Volyhian fever.**
             Vanghetti introduces **cineplasty.**

1916. Bull introduces antitoxin for gas-gangrene.
Carlson investigates hunger.
Kasmelson treats purpura hemorrhagica by splenectomy.
Government exhibit of devices for industrial safety (National Museum, Washington).
Physiotherapeutic Institute (Petrograd) founded.
Experimental Institute for Nutritional Physiology (Moscow) founded.
American Radium Society (St. Louis) founded.
Higher Medical School for Women at Ekaterinoslav (Ukraine).
National Research Council (Washington, D. C.) organized.
Ekaterinoslav Medical Institute at Dripropetrovsk (Ukraine).
National Bacteriological Institute at Buenos Aires.

1916–7. University of Perm (Russia).

1917. Gray and Lemaître establish principle of **wound excision** (*débridement*) (Desault, 1790).
Von E.onomo describes **encephalitis lethargica**.
Mental tests employed in recruiting soldiers.
Willems standardizes early mobilization in wounds of joints.
Ruth Tunnicliff discovers diplococcus in measles.
Meltzer and Lyon introduce duodenal (non-surgical) drainage of gall-bladder.
Alice Evans establishes relation of Bacillus melitensis and B. abortus (**Brucella**).
Wagner von Jauregg treats **paresis** by superinfection with malarial fever.
Windau; extracts **cholesterin** (vitamin D) from cod-liver oil and formulates it.
Levaditi describes acute multiform erythema due to streptobacillus moniliformis.
University of Abô (1640) merged into separate Swedish and Finnish Universities.
Courses in public health started at Yale University.
School of Hygiene, Johns Hopkins University, established (instruction begun 1918).
Institute for Experimental Biology at Moscow (reorganized, 1920).
State Pharmaceutical Institute at Warsaw.
Municipal Contagious Diseases Hospital (Chicago) opened.
Institution for the Blind (Blindenstudienanstalt) at Marburg.
Netherlandish Society for Psychoanalysis (The Hague) founded.
Institut für Colloid-Forschung (Theodor Stern Haus) at Frankfurt-am-Main.
Bose Research Institute (Plant Physiology) at Calcutta.
Annals of Medical History (New York) started.

1917–18. State University at Samara.
American commission investigates trench-fever.
Heavy typhus epidemic in Mexico.

1918. State Universities I and II established at Moscow (Number I founded 1755).
State Universities established at Ekaterinoslav (Ukraine), Irkutsk (Siberia), Nijni Novgorod, Smolensk (Medical Faculty, 1920), Tiflis (Georgia) and Voronej.
Folk University at Taskent (Turkestan) founded.
Hokkaido Imperial University at Saparo (Japan) founded.
Medical Faculty, University of Pressburg, moved to Fünfkirchen (Pécs), Hungary.
Fahraeus introduces **erythrocyte-sedimentation** test.
Gordon Holmes investigates semeiology of gunshot injuries of cerebellum.
Dandy evolves method of Röntgenography of the brain by injection of air into the spinal cord (**ventriculography**).
Sachs-Georgi introduces flocculation test in syphilis.
Gilman Thompson (New York) organizes clinic for functional re-education of industrial and war cripples.
Chair of Industrial Hygiene established at Harvard University.
Kraepelin founds Psychiatric Institute (Deutsche Forschungsinstitut für Psychiatrie) at Munich.
Soviet Government founds First Tuberculosis Institute at Moscow.
Institute for Experimental Endocrinology at Moscow.
Industrial Fatigue Research Board (London) established.
Maternity Center Association for Prenatal Hygiene (New York City) founded.
Clinical Institute for Post-Graduate Medical Training at Kiev (Ukraine).
Medico-Biological Institute at Leningrad (now Röntgenological and Radiological Institute).
State Optical Institute at Leningrad.
Institute for Study of the Brain and Psychic Activity at Leningrad (Bechtereff director).
State Central Institute for Physical Education at Moscow.
State Institute for Microbiology and Epidemiology at Saratov.
State Radiologic Institute of Czechoslovakian Republic at Prague.
Central Epidemic Prevention Bureau in Temple of Heaven (Peking).

1918. Home for Investigation of Heating at Munich.
State Diagnostic and Serotherapeutic Institute at Ivanoice (Czechoslovakia).
British Orthopedic Association (London) founded.
Veterinary High-School at Brünn (Moravia).
Italian Society of Veterinary Medicine (Bologna) founded.
Odessa Pediatric Society founded.
Veterinary-Zoological Museum at Vitebsk.
Darwin Museum of Natural Science at Viatka.
Harkness Commonwealth Fund (New York) established.

1918–19. Spanish influenza pandemic.
Pan-Ukrainian Academy of Science (Kiev) founded.

1918–24. Flexner, Amoss, and Webster investigate experimental epidemiology.

1918–25. State Institution for Experimental Therapy and Control of Biological Products at Moscow.

1919. Universities established at Brünn (Masaryk University), Cologne, Hamburg (March 31),
Laibach (Llubjljana, Jugoslavia), Posen (Poland), and Riga (Latvia, September 28).
University of Jurjev (Dorpat, 1632) becomes University of Tartu (Esthonia).
Medical Faculty, University of Askrakhan (South Russian), organized.
University of Pressburg becomes University of Bratislava (Czechoslovakia).
University of Klausenburg becomes Roumanian University at Cluj (October 1).
University of Wilna (Poland) reopened.
British Ministry of Health established (July 1).
Mellanby produces **experimental rickets.**
Huldschinsky demonstrates **curative effect of sunlight** (quartz lamp) **on rickets.**
Swedish University at Abô (Tartu), Finland, opened (January 15).
Kolle and Ritz treat experimental (rabbit) syphilis with bismuth.
Dale and Laidlaw investigate histamin shock.
Weed and McKibben discover that intravenous injections of hypertonic solutions **lower**
brain-pressure.
E. Mellanby treats experimental rickets with cod-liver oil.
Mercurochrome introduced (Young, White, and Schwarz).
School of Hygiene and Public Health (Johns Hopkins University) opened at Baltimore.
Death-rate of New York City reduced from 28 (1869) to 12.93.
Sir James MacKenzie founds St. Andrews Institute for Clinical Research.
Württemburg State Bureau for Medical Investigation at Stuttgart.
Masaryk League against Tuberculosis (Prague) founded.
Czechoslovakian Congress for Tuberculosis organized (1923).
State Institute of Hygiene at Warsaw.
Boyce Thompson Institute for Plant Research at Yonkers, New York.
Institute for Theoretical and Applied Optics at Paris.
League of Red Cross Societies (Paris) founded.
Purkyne Neurological Society (Prague) founded.
Moscow Medical Institute founded.
Metchnikoff Institute for Infectious Diseases at Moscow.
State Institute for Social Hygiene at Moscow.
State Physico-Technical Röntgen Institute at Petrograd.
Chemico-Pharmaceutic Institute at Petrograd.
International Bureau of Labor at Geneva.
Psychiatric Clinic (Hamburg) opened.
Veterinary High-School (Petrograd) founded.
Société de pathologie végétale (Paris) founded.
Psychoanalytic Institute (Berlin) founded.
Institute for Sexual Science (Magnus Hirschfeld Stiftung) at Berlin.
Zoöpark at Moscow (Russian Acclimatization Society, 1864).

1919–20. Omsk Medical Institute (Siberia) founded.

1920. University of Warsaw (1869) becomes State University at Rostov-on-the-Don.
University of Odessa (1865) becomes Pedagogic High-School or "INO" (Institut Narodnoi
Osvity).
Medical Faculty, University of Odessa (1900) becomes State Medical Institute.
State University of the Soviet Republic of Armenia (Erwan) founded.
University of Kiev (1840) reorganized as Drahomanov Institute for Popular Culture.
Noguchi discovers **Leptospira** ictero-hæmorrhagiæ.
Widal defines **hemoclasia.**
Rubin insufflates Fallopian tubes in sterility.
J. B. Ayer introduces cisterna puncture (Wegeforth, Ayer, and Essick, 1919).
Sprunt and Evans envisage glandular fever as mononucleosis.

1920.
Meinicke introduces flocculation test.
Ravaut employs sodium thiosulphate in metallic poisoning (arsenic).
Association for Research in Nervous and Mental Diseases (New York) founded.
Union internationale contre la tuberculose (Paris) organized.
National Health Council (United States) organized.
National Child Health Council (United States) organized.
East German Academy of Social Hygiene (Breslau) founded.
West German Academy of Social Hygiene (Dresden) founded.
Society of Czechoslovakian Physicians (Pressburg) founded.
German Pharmacological Society (Cologne) founded.
Société internationale d'histoire de la médecine (Paris) founded.
Institut international d'anthropologie (Paris) founded.
Institute for Albumen Research (Hamburg) founded.
Russian Medical Society (Medizinskoe Obshestvo) in Berlin.
State Institute for Medical Sciences (Psycho-neurological Institute of 1908) at Leningrad.
State Scientific Public Health Institution at Moscow.
Sanitary-Hygienic Institute at Moscow.
State Bacteriological Institute "Immunity" (1912) at Moscow.
Institute for Tropical Diseases at Moscow.
State Psycho-Neurological Institute at Moscow.
State Institute of Physiatry and Orthopedics at Moscow.
Pasteur Museum at Strassburg.
Institute for History and Philosophy of Medicine (University of Cracow) founded.
Society for History and Literature of Veterinary Medicine (Berlin) founded.
Society of School and District Physicians (Magdeburg) founded.
Russian Eugenic Society (Moscow) founded.
Russian Protistological Society (Moscow) founded.
Chair of oto-rhino-laryngology established at Montpellier.
Institut Pasteur hellenique (Athens) opened.
State Institute of Dentistry (Warsaw) founded.
University Library, Odessa (1865), becomes Central Scientific Library.
Württemburg State Bureau for Veterinary Investigation at Stuttgart.
Odessa Surgical Society founded.
Accademia Leonardo da Vinci (Naples) founded.
Société française d'ethnographie (Paris) founded.
Institut vétérinaire exotique (Alfort) founded.
Haeckel Museum at Jena.
Bacteriological Laboratory at St. Louis becomes Biological (Pasteur) Institute at Dakar (Senegal).
Institute for Investigation of Industrial Diseases and Accidents at Dortmund (Prussia).

1921.
Septcentenary of University of Montpellier.
State University of White Russia (Minsk) founded.
Ukrainian University transferred from Vienna to Prague.
Medical Faculty, University of Charkov (1804), becomes Medical Institute.
University of Malta (1769) reorganized.
University of Kolozvár transferred to Szeged.
Rabindranath Tagore opens University at Santiniketan, Bengal.
Banting and Best isolate insulin.
Rio Hortega discovers microglia and oligodendroglia.
Langley publishes book on autonomic system.
Tonkah Kee founds University of Amoy (China).
A. F. Hess treats rickets by exposure to sunlight.
General use of iodine as an antiseptic (Pregl's solution).
Quarantine Station, New York City, turned over to United States Public Health Service (March 1).
New York Health Department operates 68 infant milk depots.
Industrial Health Service Bureau (Chicago) opened.
Harvard School of Public Health (Boston) founded.
Correspondence Committee on Social Insurance (International Bureau of Labor) at Geneva.
German National Station for Prevention of Alcoholism at Berlin.
State Hygienic Institute at Posen transferred to Landsberg (Prussia).
National Institute of Industrial Psychology at London.
Lichttechnisches Institut at Karlsruhe (Baden).

1921.	Institut Behring (for Experimental Therapy) at Marburg.
	Personnel Research Federation (New York City) organized.
	Institute of Microbiology at Saarbrücken (Saar District).
	Italian Society for Study of Sexual Questions at Rome.
	Pharmaceutic Institute at Charkov (Ukraine).
	Swiss Society of History of Medicine (Zürich) founded.
	Ukrainian State Psychoneurological Institute at Charkov.
	Biochemical Institute of the Commissariat of Public Health (Narkomzarav) at Moscow.
	Institute for Heating Technics at Moscow.
	Institute for Medico-Legal and Mental Tests at Moscow.
	Psychoanalytic Institute and Laboratory at Moscow.
	Sanitary Institute (1889) at Moscow.
	State Microbiological Institute at Moscow.
	State Venereological Institute at Moscow.
	Chemico-Pharmaceutic Institute at Odessa.
	Australian National Research Council (Sydney) organized.
	Eugenics Society (New Haven, Connecticut) founded.
	Society for Racial Hygiene (Kiel) founded.
	Royal Botanic Gardens at Peradeniya (Ceylon).
	Instituto experimental de veterinaria at Rio de Janeiro.
	Psycho-pedagogic Laboratory at Amsterdam.
	Gorgas Memorial Institute of Tropical and Preventive Medicine (Chicago) founded.
	Society of History of Science and Medicine (Munich) founded.
1921–3.	Otto **Warburg** devises charcoal model to illustrate cell-respiration.
	Gowland Hopkins isolates and investigates **glutathione.**
1921–5.	Bacteriological and Serum Institute for Anhalt Area at Dessau.
1921–6.	R. L. **Kahn** introduces serum test for syphilis.
1922.	Petrograd becomes Leningrad.
	Russian University in Prague founded.
	State University at Saratov founded.
	Medical Faculty, University of Astrakhan, becomes State Medical Lunacharski Institute.
	Finnish University at Tartu (Abô) opened (June 27).
	University at Kovno (Kaunas), Lithuania, founded.
	Blair Bell revives lead treatment for cancer.
	Schutz and Versé describe agranulocytosis.
	W. L. Keller improves operation of pleurectomy for empyema.
	H. Stieve investigates inhibitory effects of starvation and overfeeding upon sexual capacity.
	Sampson investigates ovarian endometrioma.
	Piper employs mercurochrome in puerperal sepsis.
	Correspondence Committee on Industrial Hygiene (International Bureau of Labor) at Geneva.
	German Society for Industrial Hygiene (Frankfurt-am-Main) founded.
	Liverpool Cancer Research.
	State Institute for Racial Biology at Upsala.
	Institute for History of Science at Heidelberg.
	Kolloid-Gesellschaft (Leipzig) founded.
	German Institute for Scientific Pedagogics at Münster.
	Institut für Jugendkunde at Magdeburg.
	State Institute for Post-graduate Medical Instruction (Clinical Institute, 1885) at Leningrad.
	State Radium Institute at Leningrad.
	House of the Learned (Dom Uchenych) at Moscow.
	State Institute for Skin and Venereal Diseases (Polyclinic, 1917) at Odessa.
	Biological Institute and Biostation (University of Perm) founded.
	Pan-Russian Pathological Society (Moscow) organized.
	Ose Society for Jewish Hygiene (Leningrad, 1912) moved to Berlin.
	Société de gastro-enterologie (Paris) founded.
	New England Heart Association (Boston) founded.
	Institut Pasteur at Brazaville (Congo).
	American Society of Clinical Pathologists (Denver, Colorado) founded.
	Animal Diseases Research Association of Scotland (Edinburgh) founded.
	Biological Institute at Guadalajara (Mexico).
1923.	Royal University of Milan founded (September 30).
	Health Organization of League of Nations at Geneva.

1923.   George and Gladys **Dick** discover hemolytic streptococcus of **scarlatina** and devise suscepti-
            bility test.
           Graham and **Cole** introduce **cholecystography** (examination of gall-bladder by X-rays).
           Luckhardt discovers anesthetic properties of acetylene gas.
           Gwathmey introduces **synergistic anesthesia.**
           Dandy evolves method of localizing brain tumors by ventricular estimation.
           Ross Institute and Hospital for Tropical Diseases (London) opened.
           International Education Board (Rockefeller Foundation) organized.
           Institute for Racial and Constitutional Anthropology at Vienna.
           Epidemiological Institute at Zagreb (Jugoslavia).
           State Scientific Institute for Maternity and Infant Welfare at Moscow.
           Scientific Institute for Microbiological Investigation at Moscow.
           Obuch Institute for Investigation of Industrial Diseases at Moscow.
           Cabinet for Study of Criminal Personality and Crime at Moscow.
           Pharmaceutic Institute at Oslo (Norway).
           Alfonso XIII Institute for Cancer Research at Madrid.
           Orthopedic Hospital and Institute at Madrid.
           Instituto Rubio (for training lay nurses) at Madrid.
           Swiss Institute for Physiology of High Altitudes and Tuberculosis at Davos.
           Cancer Institute at Buenos Aires (Argentina).
           Parapsychic Institute at Vienna.
           Maison des spirites at Paris.
           Viennese Society for Röntgenology founded.
           Czechoslovakian Biological Society (Brünn) founded.
           Eubiotic-Hygienic Society of Czechoslovakia (Pressburg) founded.
           Society of Russian Physicians in Czechoslovakia (Prague) founded.
           Society of Ukrainian Physicians in Czechoslovakia (Prague) founded.
           Latvian Scientific Society (Riga) founded.
           Society for Advancement of Applied Psychology (Berlin) organized.
           Prehistoric Museum at Eyzies-de-Tayac (Dordogne).
           Maudsley Hospital for nervous diseases (London) established.
1923–4.   Libman and Sacks describe atypical verrucous endocarditis.
1924.   **Calmette** vaccinates children against tuberculosis with **B. C. G.** (Bacillus Calmette-Guérin:
            non-virulent bovine culture).
           Gustav Magnus publishes monograph on postural reflexes.
           Steenbock and Black treat rickets by irradiating food with ultraviolet light.
           Marriott employs insulin-fattening for impoverished nutrition in infants.
           International Society of Medical Officers of Health (Geneva) organized.
           Italian League against Venereal Diseases (Rome) organized.
           Liga español contre el cancer (Madrid) organized.
           Russian Society of Endocrinology founded.
           Society for Prevention of Venereal Diseases (Pressburg, Czechoslovakia) founded.
           Polish Society for History and Philosophy of Medicine (Posen) founded (*Archiv*, 1925).
           Czechoslovakian Society of Röntgenologists and Radiologists (Prague) founded.
           Northwestern German Society of Internal Medicine (Rostock) founded.
           Society of Academic Teachers of Medical Röntgenology (Vienna) founded.
           Society of Psychiatrists (Leningrad) reorganized.
           Pedagogic Institute at Leipzig.
           Institute for Investigation of Psychology of Religions at Vienna.
           Institute for Social Medicine at Zagreb (Jugoslavia).
           Timiriaseff State Biological Institute at Moscow.
           State Institute for Scientific Pedagogics at Moscow.
           State Central Museum of Ethnology at Moscow.
           Institute for Comparative Culture at Oslo (Norway).
           American Society of Parasitologists (Baltimore) founded.
           Werner Siemens Institute for Röntgenology at Berlin.
           Incunabula Society (Wiegendruckgesellschaft) at Berlin.
           History of Science Society (United States) founded at Boston.
           American Society of Plant Physiologists (Chicago) founded.
           Medical Society (Denver, Colorado) founded.
1925.   Hebrew University of Jerusalem opened (April 1).
           University of Bari (Italy) opened.
           Hess, Weinstock, Steenbock, and Black demonstrate antirhachitic properties of **cholesterol**
            and phytostererol.
           O. Foerster investigates hyperventilation-epilepsy.

1925.   Whipple and Robschat-Robbins treat experimental anemia with raw liver.

International Health Board (New York) finances State Hygienic Institute of Czecho-slovakia (Prague).

Institute for Biological Research (Johns Hopkins University) at Baltimore.

Imperial German Academy of Natural Sciences (1652) at Halle.

Radiologic Institute (Foundation Bergonié) at Paris.

British Social Hygiene Council (London) organized (founded, 1914).

Sir Ronald Ross opens British Mosquito Control Institute at Hayling Island.

Fœderatio bio-climatica organized at Davos.

Society of Friends of History of Medicine (Lemberg) founded.

Confraternity for Psychology of Physical Exercise (Berlin) founded.

German Society for Disorders of the Voice and Speech (Berlin) founded.

Eastern Bureau (Health Section, League of Nations) at Singapore.

Hygienic Institute of Czechoslovakian Republic at Prague.

Ukrainian Biological Institute at Charkov.

International Union of Students (Geneva) organized.

Society of Physicians of Baltic Sea Bathing Resorts (Swinemünde) founded.

Museum of Gymnastics (Berlin).

Public Health Act (England).

Town-planning Act (England).

German Institute of Gynecology at Berlin.

1926.   **Minot and Murphy** introduce raw **liver diet in pernicious anemia.**

Vogel introduces ninhydrin (flocculation) test for pregnancy.

C. R. Harington effects synthesis of thyroxine.

Collip isolates **parathyroid hormone.**

Birkhaug investigates serology and serotherapy of erysipelas.

Ferry and Fisher investigate serology of measles.

Raymond Pearl obtains logistic curve for population growth.

W. H. Welch appointed professor of history of medicine in the Johns Hopkins University.

School of Hygiene, Johns Hopkins University (1916), officially opened.

School of Tropical Medicine (University of Porto Rico) opened at San Juan (October 1).

Society of British Neurological Surgeons (London) founded.

Benacheion Phythopathological Institute (Athens) opened.

Royal Veterinary Institute at Perugia.

Hygienic Exhibition (*Gesolei*) at Düsseldorf.

Hygienic Academy at Dresden.

Ukrainian Scientific Society in Berlin founded.

Scientific Institute for Investigation of Ukrainian Water-supply at Kiev.

University of Agra (United Provinces, India) founded.

Indo-Chinese School of Medicine and Pharmacy at Hanoi.

1927.   **Noguchi** shows causal relation of Bartonella bacilliformis to verruga and Oroya fever.

Ruth Tunnicliff introduces serum against measles.

Centenary of birth of Lord Lister (April 5).

Ronald Ross Gate of Commemoration unveiled at Calcutta (January 7).

Thomas Henry Simpson Memorial Institute for Medical Research (Ann Arbor) opened (February 16).

Dunn School of Pathology (Oxford) opened (March 11).

Institute of Optics (Paris) opened (March 17).

School of Hygiene (University of Toronto) opened (June 9).

Squier Neurological Clinic opened May 7th.

Pathological Laboratory and Research Institute (City of London Hospital for Diseases of Heart and Lungs) opened (July 19).

Museum of Gynecology at Berlin.

Ukrainian Organo-Therapeutic Institute at Charkov.

Ligue belge contre le rhumatisme (Antwerp) organized.

German Society for Prevention of Rheumatism (Berlin) founded.

Institute for Maternity and Infant-welfare at Kiev (Ukraine).

Psycho-Neurological Institute at Kiev.

Biological Society at Concepción (Chile) founded.

Centenary of *American Journal of Medical Sciences* (Philadelphia).

Legislation on abortion in Germany (May 14).

Bureau of Chemistry (United States Department of Agriculture) abolished (June 30); end of food inspection in United States.

German Food Law (October 1).

German law abolishing controlled prostitution (October 1).

1927.   Lindbergh crosses Atlantic in aëroplane.

United States Federal Caustic Poison Bill (Lye Bill) passed.

Brauer Institute (Hamburg) becomes Tuberculosis Institute.

1928.   Bicentenary of birth of John Hunter.

Tercentenary of publication of Harvey's *De Motu Cardis.*

Noguchi discovers pathogen of trachoma.

New Presbyterian Hospital (New York Medical Center) opened (March 17).

Squier Urological Clinic and Harkness Pavilion (New York Medical Center) opened (March 20).

Centenary of *Boston Medical and Surgical Journal, Glasgow Medical Journal,* and *Gazette des hôpitaux* (Paris).

Deutsche Forschungsanstalt für Psychiatrie (Munich) opened (June 13).

II. HINTS ON THE STUDY OF MEDICAL HISTORY

"Greater even than the greatest discovery is to keep open the way to future discoveries."—Abel (Mellon Lecture, 1915).

In the examination-papers of the U. S. Naval Academy, as they were publicly printed in the early eighties, one encountered a large number of questions like these:

Draw a map of Europe after the peace of Utrecht.

Show that the later Roman Republic was nominally a democracy but with aristocratic tendencies.

Ship lying head to wind, get underway under sail, and stand out on the port tack.

Make all preparations for a gale. Main tack and clew-garnet gone, what is to be done?

Show by a genealogical table, how Charles V obtained the different parts of his dominions, and draw a map of the same.

Design boilers to supply steam for an engine of 2000 I. H. P., etc.

In pedagogics of this kind, in which the Naval Academy was a pioneer, what a breezy, refreshing contrast to the kind of thing other students endured in the same period!

This method of teaching, the Socratic, which requires the student to use his own mind and do his own thinking, is now coming to be accepted everywhere as the best substitute for what Osborn describes as "the prevailing system of overfeeding, which stuffs, crams, pours in, spoon-feeds, and, as a sort of death-bed repentance, institutes creative work after graduation." The same authority instances "the famous method of teaching law re-discovered by the educational genius of Langdell," in which "the students do all the lecturing and discoursing, the professor lolls quietly in his chair and makes his comments."[1] At Weimar, as Amy Fay tells us, Liszt formed capable pianists by making his pupils do all the playing. "*Je ne suis pas un professeur du piano*," he would say, although he sometimes condescended to help them out with some difficult passage or some subtle nuance of expression. That is how Osler taught his students to think clinically, and the methods of teaching medicine by "case histories" introduced by Richard Cabot and others, are in the same trend. The extreme of spoon-feeding is Vivian Poore's "idiot savant," an asylum inmate, who could repeat most recondite passages learned by auditory memory, much as Blind Tom played the piano or as a type of Chinese servant, in preparing a pudding, is said to imitate every slightest gesture made beforehand by his mistress.[2]

One of the pioneers in teaching medical history by the newer methods was the late Dr. James Finlayson of Glasgow, who early saw that, for details and minutiæ, the printed volume is better than systematic lectures, and that medical libraries are really the laboratories in which the professor and his students must work. He sometimes amused himself by asking his hospital assistants "whether Galen wrote in Latin or Greek, and whether before or after the Christian era." Their wrong answers convinced him that the mere handling and inspection of some of Galen's works would have embedded the facts in their minds better than any spoken or written statement, and he accordingly gave demonstrations in the Library of the Faculty of Physicians and Surgeons, to which a small audience was invited. The same idea was utilized by Billings, Osler, Welch and others at the Johns Hopkins Hospital Historical Club, and its success is sufficiently evidenced in the work of some of the pupils. Finlayson's printed demonstrations of Hippocrates (1892), Galen (1892), Celsus (1892), Egyptian Medicine (1893), Herophilus and Erasistratus (1893) are perfect models of what such things should be—genial, simple and immensely interesting. The demonstrations by John S. Billings (Johns Hopkins Hosp. Bull., Balt., 1890, i, 29–31) and George Dock (Physician and Surgeon, Detroit, 1906, xxviii, 180–186) deserve study. The Syllabus and Specimen-extracts printed by Dr. John D. Comrie, lecturer on the history of medicine in the University of Edinburgh, utilize an idea of Wunderlich's in a very helpful and practical way.

Dr. C. N. B. Camac's "Epoch-making Contributions" (Philadelphia, 1909), from Lister, Harvey, Auenbrugger, Laennec, Jenner, *et al.*, is the best book of this kind for American students.

In the ordinary medical curriculum, the subject of medical history commonly goes a-begging, because set lectures have been found to be so inevitably dry and disappointing that students avoid them, even as pupils at musical conservatories are said to avoid the classes in harmony and counterpoint. It is a mistake to overburden the student with extra courses of lectures, given, say, in his graduating year, when such a course might defeat its own object by interfering with his work at the most important period of his student life; for his personal interest in medical history will naturally depend upon what he does with himself after graduation. Osler set off this difficulty by bringing historical topics directly into the clinics and by his evenings at home with his "boys." In any medical

---

[1] H. F. Osborn: Huxley and Education, New York, 1910, 25, 35.

[2] Poore: Treatise on Medical Jurisprudence, London, 1901, 403. Cited by George Pernet.

faculty of size, there will always be some member who takes a personal interest in encouraging and stimulating young men, after the example of Pasteur, Ludwig, Henle, Hyrtl, and of Welch, who, in his later period, has been content to live forward in the work of his pupils. Here, the field of medical history holds out perhaps the most attractive opportunity, and the following simple plan is suggested. Assuming that you have, like Osler, a personal interest in the welfare of students, ask any of your class who have the time or inclination, to look up a particular subject, such as Sydenham, or Laennec, or Virchow, or the history of our knowledge of the heart sounds, and report to you about it some evening, either at your home or elsewhere. At the meeting give each an opportunity for a five- or ten-minutes extempore talk on the given theme, and, as they speak, notice if they have really got at the inwardness of Sydenham, the significance of Laennec or the real facts about the heart sounds. Then amplify and correct by whatever you choose to say yourself, at the same time demonstrating books connected with the author or subject. In these days of large medical classes, compulsory attendance upon medico-historical demonstrations would require a good-sized room, preferably in a medical library, but a *laissez faire* policy will soon sift out your available material, and the smaller the gatherings, the better. Joseph Sylvester once lectured on the higher mathematics to an audience of one, Trousseau advised his students to get their bedside medicine in the little groups following the private clinics, and Finlayson made his medico-historical gatherings small enough to enable everyone present to take part. But whether your classes dwindle or no, apply the principle: *Repetitio mater studiorum.* See to it that the points you have attempted to bring out in your private evenings are brought out here and there in the different courses of lectures, by means of lantern slides and demonstrations of books, pictures, instruments or what not. As you proceed, different themes might be assigned to different students, sometimes their findings might be committed to writing, or a competition for an annual prize essay could be made possible by a small fund. The main object is to draw out the student's faculties and possibilities by making him do his own work entirely, and, in view of the gigantic proliferation of useless medical literature in our day, a great boon might be conferred upon the suffering medical humanity of the future by insisting that he be as brief as possible in writing or speaking. All of us are sinners in this respect. The ideal of each extempore talk or essay should be a *multum in parvo*, and to avoid *l'ennui de tout dire*. A humane habit of brevity will make the student a very acceptable contributor to medical gatherings and medical journals of the future. Try to make these evenings delightful ones for your students and they will keep your memory green when more cold-blooded teachers are forgotten. More than anything else will the student appreciate the fact that you are not there to hear yourself talk, but to help him to develop himself in writing and speaking. You teach boys to swim, as Billings said, by "throwing them into the

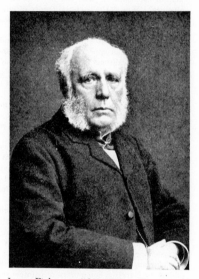

James Finlayson (1840–1906). (Courtesy of Sir William Osler.)

in water." The books, facts, and dates are as nothing comparison with the chance of giving the student an enlarged view of the *humaniora*, the nameless, unremembered things which help to make him a gentleman in his profession. Youth is, or ought to be, the period of generous self-surrender to ideals. Many fine traits, latent in young men, can be brought out by contact with a superior teacher. The general tendency of Osler's teaching, even in the clinic, has been admirably conveyed by Dr. Arnold Klebs:

"Never can one forget the scenes in the out-patient department, where he stood, surrounded by his boys, helping them as a friend in their struggles with some difficult case. He would go to one, put his arm around his shoulder, and then begin a friendly inquiry, interspersed with humorous remarks and allusions to the work done by special students on a given subject. Urging, encouraging, inspiring, so we saw him, exact always, dogmatic never, and when the humorous and friendly fire kindled in his eyes we could not help but love him and with him the task we had chosen as our life-work. Thus we imagine those *maîtres* of the old French school, a school no longer limited by national boundaries, one of those men who have trodden the paths through the wards of the Salpêtrière, the Charité and Lariboisière, tne Necker, the Hôtel Dieu, making apostles and missionaries in the great cause of scientific medicine."

The teacher who stands out best in the present writer's memory was a stalwart Viking from the state of Maine, who had his pupils assemble at his house of evenings to work over algebraic problems

In the center of the table, by the lamp, there was always a large pyramid of good-sized apples, which we boys were free to munch as we fiddled over our quadratic equations, while our teacher read his newspaper and his good wife pursued her knitting. Now and then, he would say, with a New England twinkle, "Be spry! be prompt! be brief!" as our fingers flew to get the solution. In his classroom, all the work was done by the students at the blackboard. There were no recitations, but, like Arthur Sherburne Hardy or Wentworth, our preceptor could always ascertain, by a few leading questions, whether his students understood algorithmics or not. In his rugged Northern way, he was like Liszt at Weimar.

As you proceed with your evenings, your own mind will suggest to you any number of topics for discussion: Why did English and continental physicians, for a long time, study the diseases of their cities in connection with the weather? "Epidemic constitutions," "Genius epidemicus." What are they? Why is meteorology important in medicine? How and why did physicians come to classify diseases like families of plants? What is a disease? Why is it not a "clinical entity"? What diseases were individualized by Hippocrates? Sydenham? Laennec? Contrast the first edition of Laennec's treatise on mediate auscultation with the second. When did Galen's influence disappear in internal medicine? Are we not still unconscious Galenists?

Why was epilepsy regarded as a contagious disease in the Middle Ages? Why was it called "morbus comitialis"? Why did the ancients call it the "sacred disease"? What famous men were epileptics? Why is the bacterial theory of infection giving place to the bio-chemical?

Why were medieval surgeons so cantankerous about their fees, and why did they shun major surgery?

Was syphilis really epidemic at Naples and elsewhere in 1494–95? What was Pasteur's explanation for the sudden appearance or disappearance of certain infectious diseases? What were Pettenkofer's initial conditions for the phenomenon of infection? How did sloven translating obstruct medical progress in the Middle Ages? How has the original meaning of the classics been obscured by overlaid material? Give the humorous side of certain medical controversies in the past. Why should we flit "when doctors disagree"?

What is the savage's concept of "making medicine"? Explain Huxley's statement that "medicine is the foster-mother of all the sciences." Why did medicine always lag behind the other sciences up to 1850? What did Sir Michael Foster mean when he said that "her children are always coming back to her"?

Medical history can be taught in this way either by the seminary plan of Finlayson, which has been so successfully employed by Professor W. S. Miller at the University of Wisconsin, or by the symposium or home plan of Osler, with inweaving of the subject in the clinics, laboratories and lecture rooms of the different medical disciplines and specialties. These methods have been used with success by George Dock (St. Louis), Harvey Cushing (Harvard), David Riesman (Philadelphia), and others.

Another pleasant way of studying the history of medicine is by means of the medical history club, which differs from the formal medico-historical society in that the papers read serve as an introduction to a congenial conversazione, with refreshments or otherwise. As the private musical club depends for its success upon the disinterested spirit of the refined amateur, so the law of the history club is that each member must shed all assumption or any trace of the professional jealousy which is common to physicians, musicians, politicians, and those possessed of histrionic or operatic talents. Stevenson said of the Barbizon community of painters that "formal manners being laid aside, essential courtesy was the more rigidly exacted; . . . to a touch of presumption or a word of hectoring these free Barbizonians were as sensitive as a tea party of maiden ladies." The medical history club will never thrive unless each individual member preserves the modest, consistent attitude of a learner. Michael Angelo's cartoon of Father Time in a go-cart, with the legend "Ancora imparo," might be its device, if such a club is to be a "going concern."

At the Johns Hopkins Hospital Historical Club, the usual plan is the reading of one or more formal papers followed by a general discussion. In these discussions, the luminous talks of Professor Welch have gone far to make the delicate appreciation of values in medical history a fine art. The program may be varied by the symposium idea or other features. At the Jenner evening at Harvard, Rosenau demonstrated actual vaccination and its effects upon a subsequent inoculation of smallpox. At the Washington evening on the Irish clinicians, Stokes, Graves, Corrigan and others were assigned to different men, while Stokes' life of George Petrie, Petrie's collection of Irish folk music and other curiosities were exhibited. At the Leidy evening, Dr. Joseph Leidy of Philadelphia exhibited many interesting relics of his illustrious uncle. Incidental music illustrating a period or a nation, such as Dvorak's terzetto in C for Bohemia, Purcell's Air from the Indian Queen for 17th century England, or something of Haydn or Schubert or Brahms for the Vienna school, might serve to break the monotony and add to the festal character of the evening.

Advanced instruction in medical history, that is, teaching the student how to utilize sources and conduct a medico-historical investigation, can only be given at an institute with the aid of a good medical library. At an institute, the student would be taught how to use the best reference books and bibliographical tools; how to detect and correct possible sources of error in medical writings and opinions, early and late; how to deal with medical manuscripts, the pathway to which lies through the earlier printed books; how to evolve new facts from the findings of erudition; and how to teach others to teach and to think historically. A medico-historical institute should therefore be not only a plant for research work but also a seed-plant of medical culture. This end would best be attained by the study of the general history of science in connection with the history of medicine. In 1906, Dr. Berthold Laufer filed an impressive plea for the study of the history of medicine and the natural sciences in this country.[1] The best account of institute teaching, including the best reference books, methods of research, exhibitions and museums, and the endowment of medico-historical research, is to be found in the valuable and exhaustive paper of Dr. Arnold Klebs (1914[2]) which all who are interested in the subject should read. Dr. George Sarton, of Harvard, a scholar learned in the mathematics and the history of culture, has endeavored to stimulate an interest in the establishment of an institute devoted to the history of the sciences and medicine, and it is to be hoped that his efforts may prove successful. Dr. Sarton is the founder and editor of "Isis," the first periodical to co-ordinate the results of historical research in all the sciences.

In pursuing medical history, whether as a private recreation or as a scientific discipline for the mind, the student may well consider the advice of the gifted mathematician N. H. Abel: Study the texts (*Si l'on veut faire des progrès dans le mathématiques, il faut étudier les maîtres et non pas les écoliers*). In other words, it is better to begin anywhere with some definite subject, such as Harvey or the history of fever, and study it exhaustively and well in the original texts, than to attempt to compass everything at once by superficial skimming. The subject of medical history is coextensive with the cultural history of the human race and no single mind can hope to absorb all of it. Here as elsewhere, "general knowledge means general ignorance" (Froude). Dr. John J. Abel is quite right when he says that "there should be in research work a cultural character, an artistic quality, elements that give to painting, music, and poetry their high place in the life of man." The real student of medical history will see his Hippocrates as he does his Homer, his Harvey as he does his Shakespeare, his Sydenham as he does his Milton. This is a large contract perhaps, but it is the royal road to learning anything well. Dr. Johnson said that if any man will read intelligently on any subject so many hours a day he will soon be learned. It is only in this way that the things we read become part and parcel of our mental being and "make incision in the memory." The best models in writing for the student are the charming essays of Osler, of which Sudhoff observed that they contain more of the true historical spirit than many a learned work of the professional historian. The reason is that Osler loved his old authors as he does his profession. If the student reads Greek or Latin, he will find much help in such admirable bilingual texts as Loeb's Classical Library for the ancient poets and authors, who abound in medico-historical details, Monro's Lucretius (1864), Alexander Lee's Celsus (1831), Littré's Hippocrates (1839–61), Daremberg's Oribasius (1851–76), Francis Adams' Aretæus (1856), Léon Meunier's Fracastorius (1893) and Sir Arthur Hort's Theophrastus (Loeb Classical Library, N. Y., 1916). For beginners, Sudhoff warmly recommends Theodor Beck's charming introduction to the Hippocratic canon by means of remarkably well-chosen excerpts (1907), a German bilingual which might well be translated for English and American students. Dr. C. N. B. Camac's "Counsels and Ideals" from the writings of William Osler (Boston, 1905), and the "Aphorisms and Reflections" of Huxley, selected by his wife (London, 1907), should be on every student's table. The historical publications of Burroughs, Wellcome & Company (London) are useful and accurate. But, as Carlyle says, "not many books are needful; an open, patient, valiant soul—that is the one thing needful." To this may be added a monition from Bernard Shaw: "Better keep yourself clean and bright; you are the window through which you must see the world."

[1] Laufer: Science, N. Y., 1907, n. s., xxv, 889–895.
[2] Klebs: Bull. Johns Hopkins Hosp., Baltimore, 1914, xxv, 1–10.

III. BIBLIOGRAPHIC NOTES FOR COLLATERAL READING

A. Histories of Medicine

Of the larger works, the *Grundriss* of Johann Hermann **Baas** (1838–1909), of Worms on the Rhine, translated into English by H. E. Handerson (New York, 1889), is still in many respects the most readable. The earlier works of Le Clerc (1696), Freind (1725–27), Schulze (1728), Haller (1751), Blumenbach (1786), and Kurt Sprengel (1792–1803), are mainly of antiquarian interest, while the histories of Hecker (1822–29), Bostock (1834), Puccinotti (1850–66), Meryon (1861), Daremberg (1870), and Bouchut (1873) are now of a vintage that could appeal only to the special "taster." Sprengel's work is unrivalled for its close rendering of the facts of ancient medicine and the unimpeachable accuracy of its footnotes. Heinrich **Haeser**'s great work (3d ed., 1875–82) is based upon original research and is remarkable for erudition but not always for accuracy. The third volume, on epidemic diseases, is invaluable. The merits of Baas's history are that he covers the whole ground in a thick, but not too long-winded, volume; that his statements of fact are all of them accurate as far as they go; that he gives a very thoroughgoing account of the different medical "theories," the condition of medicine and surgery in the different periods; and that he frequently carries his readers over many dull patches by his keen and frolicsome sense of humor. His faults are a certain diffuseness, the poor arrangement of his subject-matter, his long lists of relatively unimportant names, his failure to discriminate many things of scientific moment from things which are trivial, his whimsical tendency to wander away from his subject or to enlarge upon comic or erotic details and, finally, a curious lack of balance and proportion which, with all his glancing wit and humor, suggests, at times, an absolute contempt for the exigencies of literary style. He gives us many dates, but not always those we want, and like most medical historians Baas is at his weakest when he gets into the modern period. He cannot see the woods for the trees, dilates more upon theories than facts, is behind the times in his attitude toward the germ-theory, and has more to say about Broussais and Rasori than about Laennec or Louis, Charcot or Pasteur. Yet no modern historian has given a finer appreciation of the great English physicians, with whose practical aims he was evidently in cordial sympathy. Although a Rhinelander by birth, Baas represents the extreme North German or Protestant view of medical history. He is, everywhere, an essentially masculine-minded writer, hating all shams, humbuggery, frauds and superstitions. His footnotes and marginalia, like Gibbon's, suggest a certain sympathy with tabooed subjects. Nothing delights him more than to isolate some indecorous or inconsistent trait of character and brandish it aloft in what Swinburne calls "the broad light of German laughter."

Julius **Pagel**[1] published, in 1898, a one-volume history of medicine in the form of lectures. This is a very readable book, the work of a broad, good-natured, tolerant spirit, but sometimes inaccurate, and the bibliography is a hasty pudding. The new edition (1915), revised and partly re-written by Karl Sudhoff, has been purged of much inaccuracy, particularly in the earlier periods. In the latest revision (1922) it is practically a new book. The references are unique, such as only Sudhoff could furnish. In 1903–5, Pagel and Max Neuburger collaborated in bringing to editorial completion the *Handbuch der Geschichte der Medizin*, which was begun by Theodor Puschmann. This handbook, in three volumes, is the most reliable source of the larger reference works after Haeser. It is written upon the coöperative plan, and, in dealing with the modern period, the editors have resorted to the usual plan of allocating each specialty to a particular authority. As with many books written by different hands, these special monographs have, at times, a somewhat dry, perfunctory, and routine character. But the substantial merits of the Puschmann *Handbuch* as a reference work cannot be overestimated.

The best modern work is unquestionably the recent "History of Medicine" by Pagel's collaborator, Professor Max **Neuburger** (1868–   ), of Vienna, which is still coming out in parts and also in process of translation by Ernest Playfair (London, 1910–25). As an historian, Neuburger is eloquent, profound, absolutely sincere, and a good stylist. As a scholar, he is richer, deeper and more serious than Baas, and his accounts of folk medicine and of Greek and Arabian medicine are by far the better of the two. Yet he has no saving salt of humor and often exhibits the Germanic tendency to rhapsodize and to wander off into philosophic reverie. To present a philosophic synthesis of medical history is, in fact, the intention of his great work. He throws many new facts into the field, but does not always present them in a simple, direct manner. The second volume of Neuburger's treatise, covering medieval medicine, is a masterly synthesis, opening out many new viewpoints. The author's firm grasp of the complex details is everywhere manifest, but the reader is apt to lose himself at the first reading. The large first volume of the English translation is printed on light-weight cloth paper, a great comfort in

[1] A charming account of Pagel and his work by Drs. George Dock and M. G. Seelig of St. Louis is to be found in the Jour. Missouri State Med. Ass., St. Louis, 1910, ix, 366–369.

large-sized books. The substratum of erudition (footnotes and marginalia) has been largely omitted from the English version.

Of the smaller handbooks, Wunderlich's *Geschichte der Medizin* (1859) has never been translated and does not go beyond Schönlein's time. It is the work of a master clinician, and is interesting for its anthology of illustrative excerpts, including the different classifications of disease down to the time of Schönlein. The brief and little known sketches of William Farr (1839) and Edwin Klebs (1868) are highly original and suggestive. The *British Medical Almanack* of 1839 (pp. 113–178) contains the neat history up to Sydenham's time by the eminent English statist, William Farr. The preceding volumes of the journal (1836–38) contain his valuable medical chronologies. The *Medical History* of Edward T. Withington (London, 1894) is the work of a genuine scholar, written in an unusually engaging manner, with many valuable terminal notes and appendices. Unfortunately, it stops at the beginning of the 19th century, but it is based upon original research and there are few of the smaller sized books which convey so much accurate information. The *Epitome* of Roswell Park (1897) was preceded by the excellent history of Robley Dunglison (1872). Léon Meunier's *Histoire de la médecine* (Paris, 1911) has the merit of being very full on the modern period and is very readable, but not entirely accurate. The author often fubs us off with conversational counters and small talk. Five recent works of value may be signalized, viz., the compact history of Paul Diepgen (Sammlung Göschen, 1913–24). in primer-like, side-pocket form, is a remarkably terse, accurate, and reliable presentation, a little dry and rigorous in manner, but invaluable for the earlier periods, and the work of a master of the subject. The fourth volume (1924) is largely a history of modern German medicine. The Lowell Lectures of Sir William Osler (Yale Press, 1920) have all his accustomed charm of manner, with a number of unique illustrations and are especially to be recommended for beginners and cultivated lay readers. The "Survey" of Sudhoff and Meyer-Steineg (Jena, 1921), now in its third edition (1928), is an acknowledged masterpiece, and illustrated with the most instructive pictures which have ever been included in a work of this kind. The recent *Storia* (Milano, 1927) of the genial Arturo Castiglioni, author of *Il Volto d'Ippocrate* (1925) is a work of great merit, comprehensive, containing many unique illustrations, and is particularly valuable and reliable for Italian medicine. Charles Singer's *Short History* (1928) is the best primer on the subject in English.

B. Medical Biography

The earliest exhaustive collection is the *Dictionnaire historique de la médecine* (1755) of N.-F.-J. Eloy, which, in its later four-volume form (1778), is invaluable. Bayle and Thillaye's *Biographie médicale* (Paris, 1855) is a sort of medical "Who's Who" up to the middle of the 19th century, eminently useful as far as it goes. The seven volumes by A.-J.-L. Jourdain prefixed to the *Dictionnaire des sciences médicales* (Paris, Panckoucke, 1820–25) are indispensable, containing many valuable bibliographies. August Hirsch's *Biographisches Lexikon* (6 vols., Wien u. Leipzig, 1884–8), and Pagel's *Biographisches Lexikon* of 19th century physicians (Berlin u. Wien, 1901), are standard modern works, which may be supplemented by the many admirable biographies of English physicians in Leslie Stephen's *Dictionary of National Biography* (70 vols., London, 1885–1927), by the *Biographie francaise* (46 vols., Paris, 1852–77), the *Neuer Nekrolog der Deutschen* (1823–52), the *Biographisches Jahrbuch* (1896–1911), and other reference works listed in the extensive bibliography given by Hirsch. The sketches of great physicians in Meyer's *Geschichte der Botanik* (1854) are indispensable. The standard sources of American medical biography are those of James Thacher (1828) and Samuel D. Gross (1861), which are made up of extensive lives of a few men; Atkinson (1878), Stone (1894) and Watson (1896), which are good directories of contemporary names. Howard A. Kelly's Cyclopedia of American Medical Biography (Philadelphia, 1928) is the most recent work. For recent names, the various Who's Who's of different countries may be consulted, also Kürschner's *Deutscher Gelehrten-Kalender*, vols. 1–2, Berlin, 1925–6. For a complete bibliography of sources, see Bull. New York Acad. Med., 1928, 2, s., iv, 586–607 (F. H. Garrison). Of recent collections of biographical essays, those of G. T. Bettany (*Eminent Doctors*, 1885), Osler (*Alabama Student*, 1896), Sir B. W. Richardson (*Disciples of Æsculapius*, 1900), Victor Robinson (*Pathfinders*, 1912), G. Bilancioni (*Veteris vestigia flammæ*, 3v., Rome, 1922), A. Castiglioni (*Il Volto d'Ippocrate*, Milano, 1925), Pietro Capparoni (*Profili bio-bibliografici*, Rome, 1925), Sir George Newman (*Interpreters of Nature*, London, 1927), and J. C. Hemmeter (*Master Minds*, 1927) deserve especial mention.

For biographies of individuals, the following are either readable or otherwise valuable for reference or for a certain perspicuity.

Acland (Sir Henry W.): Memoir by J. B. Atlay, London, 1903.

Acosta (Cristobal): Life by J. Olmédilla y Puig, Madrid, 1899.

Adami: Brit. M. J., Lond., 1926, ii, 507–510.

Addison: Wilks & Bettany, History of Guy's Hospital, Lond., 1892, 221–234.—Guy's Hosp. Gaz., Lond., 1874, iii, 193; 201: 1901, xxii, 520, port., 1 pl.—Guy's Hosp. Rep., Lond., 1926, lxxvi, 253–279 (Sir W. Hale-White).

Albers-Schonberg: Fortschr. a. d. Geb. d. Röntgenstrahlen, Hamb., 1921, xxviii, 197–205 (R. Grashey).

Albertus Magnus: Janus, Bresl., 1846, i, 127–160 (L. Choulant).

Aldrich-Blake (Louisa): Life by Lord Riddell, London, 1926.

Alibert (J. L.): Achille Alfaric, Paris diss. No. 58, 1917.—Gaz. méd. de Paris, 1839, 2 s., vii, 193–198. Paris méd., suppl., 1914, 575–591 (L. Brodier).—Presse méd., Par.. 1923, xxxi, annexes, 1881–1884 (G. Thibierge).

Allbutt: Brit. M. J., Lond., 1925, i, 428; 485.—Lancet, Lond., 1925, i, 461–463.—Science, N. Y., 1925, lxi, 330–332 (F. H. Garrison).—Internat. Clin., Phila., 1926, 36 s., iii, 288–302 (Sir H. Rolleston).

Amatus Lusitanus: M. Lemos: Amato Lusitano, Oporto, 1907.—Ztschr. f. klin. Med., 1900, xli, 458; 1900–1901, xlii, 129 (Max Salomon).

Arbuthnot: Life by G. A. Aitken, Oxford, 1892.

Arderne (John): Sir D'Arcy Power's introduction to his treatises on fistula in ano (Early English Text Soc., No. 139, Lond., 1910), and *De arte phisicali* (London, 1922).

Aretæus: H. Locher: Aretæus, Zürich, 1857.—Francis Adams, Preface to "The Extant Works [etc.]," Lond., 1856, pp. v–xx.—München. med. Wchnschr., 1902, xlix, 1265–1267 (R. Kossmann).—Johns Hopkins Hosp. Bull., Balt., 1909, xx, 371–377 (E. F. Cordell).—Am. J. Clin. Med., Chicago, 1911, xvii, 1055–1058, *or* Pathfinders of Medicine, N. Y., 1912, 33–43 (V. Robinson).—Ztschr. f. d. ges. Neurol., Berl., 1923, lxxxvi, 227–246 (G. Ilberg).

Aristotle: T. L. Lones: Aristotle's Researches in Natural Science, Lond., 1912.—W. D'A. Thompson: On Aristotle as a Biologist, Oxford, 1913.—Arch. di storia d. sc., Roma, 1924, v. 5–11 (H. Balss).

von Arlt (C. F.): *Meine Erlebnisse*, Wiesbaden, 1887.

Arnold of Villanova: Arch. f. Gesch. d. Med., Leipz., 1909–16, *passim* (P. Diepgen).

Asclepiades: Biography by H. von Vilas, Wien, 1903.—N. Jahrb. f. d. klass. Altertum, Leipz., 1908, xxi, 684–703 (M. Wellmann).

Aselli: Arch. di storia d. sc., Roma, 1922, iii, 125–134 (V. Duccheschi).—Illustr. med. ital., Genoa, 1922, iv, 43–47 (A. Vedrani).

Atkinson (James): Ann. Med. Hist., N. Y., 1924, vi, 200–221 (J. Ruhräh).

Auenbrugger: Jahresb. d. Ver. d. Aerzte in Steiermark, Graz, 1866, ii, 19–52 (Clar).—Jahresb. d. Gesellsch. f. Nat.- u. Heilk. in Dresd., 1863, 59–72.—Tr. Cong. Am. Phys. & Surg., 1891, New Haven, 1892, ii, 180 (Weir Mitchell).—Walsh: Makers of Modern Medicine, N. Y., 1907, 55–85.

Aulus Gellius: Arch. di storia d. sc., Roma, 1925, vi, 1–17 (M. Neuburger).

Averroës: E. Renan: *Averroës et l'averroïsme*, Paris, 1852, 1865, 1869.

Avicenna: Paris thesis (No. 182) by J. Eddé, 1889.—*Also* (No. 261) by Mario Pariente, 1926.—Étude by Baron Carra de Vaux, in series "Les grands philosophes" (Paris, F. Alcan, 1900).—Johns Hopkins Hosp. Bull., Balt., 1908, xix, 157–160 (J. A. Chatard).—Arch. f. klin. Chir., Berl., 1884, xxx, 745–752 (H. Frölich).

Baccelli (Guido): Life by Gerrini (Turin, 1916) and A. Baccelli: *Mio padre* (Rome, 1924).

Bacon (Francis): Med. Life, N. Y., 1926, xxxiii, 149–169 (M. Neuburger).—The Nation, Lond., 1926, xxxix, 41–43 (C. Singer).—Bull. N. Y. Acad. Med., 1926, ii, 449–455 (F. H. Garrison).—Arch. f. Gesch. d. Med., Leipz., 1926, xviii, 113–129 (E. Wallach).

Bacon (Roger): *Essays* (ed. A. G. Little), Oxford, 1914, 337–372 (E. T. Withington); bibliography, 373–426 (A. G. Little).

von Baer: Selbstbiographie. 2. Aufl. Braunschweig, 1886.—Biographies by L. Stieda (1886), R. Stoelzle (1897), and W. Haacke (1905).—Allg. Wien. med. Ztg., 1877, xxii, 357: 369 (W. Waldeyer).—Ztschr. f. d. ges. Anat., 3 Abt., München and Berl., 1925, x, 508–512 (B. Ottow).

Baglivi: Ztschr. f. klin. Med., Berl., 1888–9, xv, 279; 475 (M. Salomon).—München. med. Wchnschr., 1907, liv, 1241, port. (K. Sudhoff).

Bard (John): Tr. Am. Ass. Obst. & Gynæc., 1918, N. Y., 1919, xxxi, 113–121 (G. K. Dickinson).

Bard (Samuel): Bull. New York Acad. Med., 1925, 2. s., i, 85–91 (F. H. Garrison).

Bartlett (Elisha): Boston M. & S. J., 1900, cxlii, 49–53 (Sir W. Osler).

Barton (Clara): Life by W. E. Barton, 2 v., Boston, 1922.

Battey (Robert): Diary; Therap. Gaz., Detroit, 1921, 3. s., xxxvii, 6 12–620 (H. A. Kelly).

Bayliss: Proc. Roy. Soc. Lond., 1926–7, S. B., xcix, pp. xxvii–xxxii, port. (J. Barcroft).—Ergebn. d. Physiol., München, 1926, xxv, pp. xx–xxiv (E. H. Starling).

Beaumont (William): Life and Letters by Jesse S. Myer (St. Louis, 1912). Also Physician & Surg. St. Louis, 1902, xxiv, 529–574 (Osler, Vaughan, *et al.*).

Beauperthuy: Arch. de parasitol., Par., 1919, xvi, 503–545 (R. Blanchard).—Ann. Med. Hist., N. Y., 1922, ɪv, 166–174 (C. A. Wood).

Béchamp: Ethel D. Hume, Béchamp or Pasteur? Chicago, 1923.

Bechtereff: Autobiography. Med. d. Gegenwart, Leipz., 1927, vi, 1–52.

von Behring (Emil): München. med. Wchnschr., 1917, lxiv, 1235–1239 (M. von Gruber).—Ztschr. f. Tuberc., Leipz., 1917, xxviii, 196–199 (H. Much).

Bell (John): Johns Hopkins Hosp. Bull., Balt., 1912, xxiii, 241–250 (E. R. Corson).

Bell (Sir Charles): Life by A. Pichot, Par., 1858, English transl., London, 1860.—Letters, London, 1870.—Johns Hopkins Hosp. Bull., Balt., 1910, xxi, 171–182 (E. R. Corson).—Brain, Lond., 1925, xlviii, 449–475 (H. C. Thomson).—Psychol. Rev., Princeton, N. J., 1926, xxxiii, 188–217 (L. Carmichael).

Benedetti (Alessandro): Atti. d. r. Ist. veneto di sc., 1916–17, lxxvi, 197–259 (R. Massalongo).

Benedikt (Moritz): *Aus meinem Leben*, Wien, 1906.

Benzi (Ugo): Riv. di storia crit. d. sc. med., Siena, 1921, xii, 75–95 (A. Castiglioni).

von Bergmann: *Kriegsbriefe* (A. Buchholtz) 2. Aufl., Leipz., 1911.—Deutsche Ztschr. f. Chir., Leipz. 1921, clxvi, 10–37 (R. Lampe).

Bergonié: Bull. Acad. de méd., Par., 1925, 3. s., xciii, 71–92 (E. Gley, *et al.*).

Bernard (Claude): Claude Bernard by Sir Michael Foster ("Masters of Medicine"), London, 1899. —Claude Bernard par Georges Barral ("Bibliothèque Gilon"), Paris, 1889. Also: Gaz. d'hôp. Paris, 1879, lii, 326; 333 (E. Renan).—Rev. philos., Par., 1919, lxxxvii, 72–101 (R. Lenoir).

Bernstein (Julius): Arch. f. d. ges. Physiol., 1919, clxxiv, 11–89 (A. von Tschermak).

Berthelot: Bull. Acad. de méd., Par., 1915, 3. s., lxxiv, 727–740 (G.-M. Debove).

Berzelius: Hygiea, Stockholm, 1924, lxxxvi, 857–871 (E. Nordenskiöld).

Bichat: Lancet, Lond., 1954, ii, 393–396 (R. Knox).—Bull. soc. franç. d'hist. de méd., Par., 1902, i 214; 261; 269; 277; 280; 285; 293; 309.—Interstate M. J., St. Louis, 1908, xv, 597; 667 (A. C. Eycleshymer).

Biggs (Hermann Michael): Health News, Albany, 1923, n. s., xviii, 159–184 (Nicoll, Parke *et al.*).

Bilharz: München. med. Wochenschr., 1925, lxxii, 480 (E. Ebstein).

Billings (John Shaw): Memoir by F. H. Garrison, New York, 1915.—Sketch by H. M. Lydenberg, Chicago, 1924.—Bull. N. Y. Public Library, 1913, xvii, 511–535 (S. Weir Mitchell, *et al.*).—Brit. M. J., Lond., 1913, i, 641–643 (Sir W. Osler, *et al.*).—Hospital, Lond., 1913, liii, 671–673 (Sir H. Burdett).—Nat. Acad. Sc. Biog. Mem., Wash., 1919, viii, 375–416 (S. Weir Mitchell & F. H. Garrison).

Billroth: Life by R. Gersuny, Wien, 1922.—Autobiography (Wien. med. Bl., 1894, xvii, 92–94) and his *Briefe* (7. Aufl., Hanover, 1906).—Arnold Huber, Zürich diss., 1923.—Berl. klin. Wchnschr., 1894, xxxi, 199–205 (J. Mikulicz); 205–207 (E. von Bergmann).—Deutsche Rundschau, Berl., 1893–4, xx, 274–277 (E. Hanslick).

Bird (Golding): Guy's Hosp. Rep., Lond., 1926, lxxvi, 1–20 (Sir W. Hale-White).

Black (Joseph): Life by Sir W. Ramsay, London, 1918.

Blanchard (Raphael): Science, N. Y., 1919, n. s., xlix, 391 (F. H. Garrison).—Bull. Acad. de méd. Par., 1924, 3. s., xcii, 850–861 (Doléris).—Bull. Soc. franç. d'hist. de méd., Par., 1924, xviii, 282–288 (Laignel-Lavastine).

Bloch (Ivan): Med. Life, N. Y., 1923, xxx, 57–70 (E. Ebstein).

Boerhaave: Life by W. Burton, London, 1746.—G. Neiret: Paris diss. No. 115, 1888.—Asclepiad, Lond., 1885, ii, 230–248, port. (Sir B. W. Richardson).—Janus, Leyden, 1918, xxiii, 195–369 (E. C. van Leersum, *et al.*).

du Bois Reymond (Emil): Life by H. Boruttau, Wien, 1922.—Deutsche med. Wchnschr., Leipz. u. Berl., 1897, xxiii, 17–19 (I. Munk).—Med. Chron., Manchester, 1896–7, n. s., vi, 241–250 (W. Stirling).—Nature, Lond., 1897, lv, 230 (J. Burdon Sanderson).

Borde (Andrew): Caledon. M. J., Glasgow, 1921, xi, 292; 300 (R. C. Buist).

Boughton (Gabriel): Lancet, Lond., 1927, i, 854 (G. C. Peachey).

Bouillaud: Bull. Soc. franç. d'hist. de méd., Par., 1925, xix, 145–158 (A. Lutaud).

Bourquelot (Émile): J. de pharm. et chim., Par., 1921, 7. s., xxiv, 403–464 (Bougault & Hérissey).— Rev. scient., Par., 1922, lx, 110–120 (J. Bougault).

Bowditch (Henry Ingersoll): Life and Letters by V. Y. Bowditch, 2 vols., Bost., 1902.

Bowditch (Henry Pickering): Mem. Nat. Acad. Sc., Wash., 1924, xvii, 183–196, port. (W. B. Cannon).

Bowman (Sir William): Ann. Med. Hist., N. Y., 1924, vi, 143–158 (B. Chance).

Brasdor (Pierre): Bull. Soc. franç. d'hist. de med., Par., 1922, xvi, 19–47 (Delaunay).

Bretonneau: Life and Letters by P. Triaire, 2 v. (Paris, 1892).—Proc. Roy. Soc. Med., Lond., 1924–5, xviii, Sect. Hist. Med., 1–12 (J. D. Rolleston).

Bright: Wilks & Bettany; History of Guy's Hospital, Lond., 1892, 212–221.—Johns Hopkins Hosp. Bull., Balt., 1912, xxiii, 173–186 (F. H. Garrison).—Guy's Hosp. Rep., Lond., 1921, lxxi, 1, 143; 1928, lxxxviii, 18 (Sir W. Hale-White).—*Ibid.*, Lond., 1927, lxxvii, 253–301 (W. S. Thayer).

Brinton (John H.): Personal Memoirs, New York, 1914.

Broadbent (Benjamin): Mother & Child, Balt., 1921, ii, 298–306.

Broadbent (Sir William): Life by Miss E. B. Broadbent, London, 1909.

Broca: Rev. d'anthrop., Par., 1880, 2. s., iii, 577–608, 1 phot. & bibliog. (S. Pozzi).—Bull. Soc. d'-anthrop. de Par., 1884, 3. s., vii, 921–956 (E. Dally).—J. Anthrop. Inst., Lond., 1880–81, x, 242–261, 1 phot. (E. W. Brabrook).—Saturday Lectures, Wash., 1882, 113–142 (R. Fletcher).—Bull. Acad. de méd., 1924, 3. s., xcii, 1347–1366 (C. Achard).

Brodie: Lives by H. W. Acland (Lond., 1864) and by Timothy Holmes ("Masters of Medicine"), Lond., 1897.—G. T. Bettany, Eminent Doctors, Lond., 1885, i, 286–303.

Brown (William): Mil. Surgeon, Wash., 1926, lix, 155 (Bessie W. Gahn).

Browne (Sir Thomas): Biography by Edmund Gosse, London and New York, 1905.—Brit. M. J., Lond., 1905, ii, 993–998 (Sir W. Osler).—Med. Library & Hist. J., Brooklyn, 1905, iii, 264–275 (C. Williams).—Macmillan's Mag., Lond., 1886, liv, 5–18 (Walter Pater).—Biometrika, Cambridge, 1922–3, xv, 1–76 (M. L. Tildesley).—Bibliography, Lancet, Lond., 1924, ii, 355 (H. P. Cholmeley).

Brunner (Joh. Conrad): Life by C. Kiepenheuer, Potsdam, 1927.—Samml. gemeinverst. Vortr., Hamb., 1888, n. F., 3. ser., No. 62 (C. Brunner).

Brunton (Sir T. L.): Brit. M. J., Lond., 1916, ii, 440; 478; 606.—Lancet, Lond., 1916, ii, 572–575.—Mil. Surgeon, Wash., 1917, xl, 369–377, port. (F. H. Garrison).

Budd (William): Bull. Johns Hopkins Hosp., Balt., 1916, xxvii, 208–215 (W. C. Rucker).

Buffon: Presse méd., Par., 1925, xxxiii, 361–363 (L. Roule).

Burdach: *Rückblick*, Leipzig, 1848.

Burdett (Sir Henry): Hospital, Lond., 1920–21, lxviii, 139–144.

Butts (Sir William): Ann. Med. Hist., N. Y., 1924, vi, 185–194 (T. N .Toomey).

Cadogan: Ann. Med. Hist., N. Y., 1925, vii, 15–92 (J. Ruhräh). Also Reprint.

Caelius Aurelianus: Janus, Haarlem, 1906, xi, 129; 208 (Meunier).

Caius (John): Memoir by John Venn, in Collective Works, ed. E. S. Roberts, Cambridge, 1912, 1–54.

Caldwell (Charles): Autobiography (Philadelphia, 1855).—Ann. Med. Hist., N. Y., 1921, iii, 156–178 (W. S. Middleton).

Cannizzaro (Stanislao): Arch. di storia di sc., Roma, 1926, vii, 67–79 (S. Baglioni), 80–82 (A. Mieli).

Cardan (Jerome): Lives by Henry Morley (2 vols., Lond., 1854) and by W. G. Waters, Lond., 1897.—Ann. Med. Hist., N. Y., 1921. iii, 122–135 (C. L. Dana).

Casserius: Life by G. Sterzi (Venice, 1910).

Celsus: Monograph by Carl Kissel (Giessen, 1844).—Max Wellmann: A. Cornelius Celsus (Berlin, 1913).—Fac. de méd. de Par. Confér. histor., 1866, 445–497 (P. Broca).—E. Littré, Médecine et Médecins, Par., 1872, 137–153.—Ann. Anat. & Surg., Brooklyn, 1882, v, 126; 177; 224; 280 (G. J. Fisher).—Glasgow M. J., 1892, xxxvii, 321–348 (J. Finlayson).—Handb. d. Gesch. d. Med., Jena, 1901–2, i, 415–443 (I. Bloch).—Neue Jahrb. f. d. klass. Altertum, Leipz., 1907, xix, 377–412 (J. Ilberg).—Classical Rev., Lond., 1908, xxii, 151–154 (Sir T. C. Allbutt).—Fortschr. d. med., Berl., 1909, xxvii, 1207; 1246.—Arch. f. Gesch. d. med., Leipz., 1924–5, xvi, 209–213 (M. Wellmann). For editions of Celsus, see Riv. di storia crit. d. sc. med., Siena, 1920, xi, 30; 34; 83; 144: 1922, xiii, 16 (D. Barduzzi).

Cesalpinus: Arch. f. d. ges. Physiol., Bonn, 1884, xxxv, 295–390 (H. Tollin).—Proc. Charaka Club, N. Y., 1910, iii, 150–156 (J. Collins).—Riv. di storia crit. d. sc. med. e nat., Faenza, 1912, iii, 73–92 (C. Cicone).—Cesalpino, Arezzo, 1916, xii, 237; 357; 413; 473: 1917, xiii, 73; 89; 153, 170; 222; 248; 263. 22 pl. (U. Viviani).

Chadwick (Sir Edwin): Lancet, Lond., 1924, i, 831; 882 (Sir W. J. Collins).

Champier (Symphorien): *Étude biographique* by P. Allut (Lyons, 1859).—F.-F.-A. Potton's *Études historiques*, Lyons, 1863.

Charcot: N. iconog. de la Salpêtrière, Par., 1893, vi, 241–250 (Gilles de la Tourette). Inauguration du monument: *Ibid.*, 1898, xi, 401–418, port. Charcot artiste, 489–516, 6 pl.—Arch. f. exper.

Path. u. Pharmakol., Leipzig., 1893-4, xxxiii, pp. i-x (B. Naunyn).—Deutsche Ztschr. f. Nervenh., Leipz., 1893, iv, pp. i-xv (W. Erb).—Sitzungsb. d. phys.-med. Soc. zu Erlangen (1894), 1895, Heft 26, 1-14 (A. von Strümpell).—Wien. med. Wchnschr., 1893, xliii, 1513-1520 (S. Freud).—Johns Hopkins Hosp. Bull., Balt., 1893, iv, 87 (Sir W. Osler).—Internat. Clin., Phila., 1894, 4. s., i, pp. xv-xxi, port. (M. A. Starr).—Ann. méd.-psychol., Par., 1925, lxxxiii, pt. 1, 385-392 (H. Colin); pt. 2, 54-86 (H. Courbon).—Rev. neurol., Par., 1925, xxxii, 731-745 (P. Marie); 746-756 (J. Babinski).—Internat. Clin., Phila., 1925, 35. s., iv, 244-272 (F. H. Garrison).

Chauveau (Auguste): Rev. gén. d. sc., Par., 1917, xxviii, 293-296 (J. P. Langlois).—Rec. de méd. vét., Par., 1917, xciii, 1; 101: 1918, xciv, 358.

Chevallier (J. B. A.): Deutsche Vrtljschr. f. öffentl. Gendhtspflg., Brnschwg., 1915, xlvii, 293-325 (M. J. Bauer).

Cheyne (George): Account of himself, London, 1743.

Chovet (Abraham): Anat. Rec., Phila., 1911, v, 147-172, 2 port. (W. S. Miller).—Ann. Med. Hist., N. Y., 1926, viii, 375-393 (W. S. Miller).

Christison (Sir Robert): Autobiography, 2 v., Edinb., 1885-6.

Clark (Alonzo): Bull. N. Y. Acad. Med., 1925, 2. s., i, 325-328 (F. H. Garrison).

Clift (William): Brit. M. J., Lond., 1923, ii, 1127-1132 (Sir A. Keith).

Codronchi: Riv. d. storia d. sc. med. e nat., Siena, 1923, xiv, 310-318 (G. Mazzini).

Cohn (Ferdinand): *Blätter der Erinnerung*, Breslau, 1901.

Cohn (Hermann): *Dreissig Jahre*, Breslau, 1897.

Cohnheim: Ges. Abhandl., Berl., 1885, pp. vii-li, port. (W. Kühne).—Arch. f. exper. Path. u. Pharmakol., Leipz., 1884, xviii, 3.-4. Hft., pp. i-x (E. Klebs).

Colles: Works (Sydenham Soc., Lond., 1881), i-xvi, port. (R. McDonnell).

Cooper (Sir Astley): Life by B. B. Cooper, 2 v., London, 1843.—Bradshaw Lecture by Sir W. Mac-Cormac, London, 1894.—Guy's Hosp. Rep., Lond., 1841, vi, 229-234.—Quarterly Rev., Lond., 1843, lxxi, 529-560.—G. T. Bettany, Eminent Doctors, Lond., 1885, i, 202-226.—Wilks & Bettany: History of Guy's Hospital, Lond., 1892, 317-329.—St. Barth. Hosp. Rep., Lond., 1922, lv, 9-36 (G. Keynes).

Cordus (Valerius): E. L. Greene: Landmarks of Botanical History, Wash., 1909, i, 270-314.—Zentralbl. f. Gynäk., Leipz., 1904, xxviii, 426-432 (K. Binz).—Isis, Brux., vii, 14-24 (C. D. Leake).

Cornil (Victor): Hyg. gén. et appliq., Par., 1908, iii, 257-259 (A. Chantemesse).—Presse méd., Par., 1908, xvi, 273-275 (M. Letulle).

Corrigan: Ann. Med. Hist., N. Y., 1925, vii, 354-361 (R. T. Williamson).

Corti (Alfonso): Anat. Anzeiger, Jena, 1914, xlvi, 368-382 (J. Schaffer).—Also [Abstr.] J. Am. Med. Assoc., Chicago, 1914, lxiii, 1676.—Arch. f. Gesch. d. Naturwissensch., 1914-15, v, 69-71 (G. Brückner).

Corvisart: Mém. Acad. de méd., Par., 1828, i, 107-133.—J. M. Lassus, Paris diss., 1927, No. 348.—Chron. méd., 1911, xviii, 350: 1921, xxviii, 75; 291.

Coste: Life by J. E. Lane: (Americana, 1928, xxii, No. 1), Mil. Surg., Wash., 1928, lxiii, 219-238.

Crateuas: Max Wellmann in Abhandl. d. k. Gesellsch. d. Wissensch., zu Göttingen, 1897, ii, 1-32 and Festgabe zu Fr. Süsemihl. Leipzig, 1898.

Creighton (Charles): Brit. M. J., Lond., 1927, ii, 240.—Lancet, Lond., 1927, ii, 250.—Aberdeen Univ. Rev., 1928, xv, 112-118 (W. Bulloch).—Bull. New York Acad. Med., 1928, 2. s., iv, 469-476 (F. H. Garrison).

Cruveilhier: Progres méd., Par., 1927, xlii, 357-364 (Ménétrier).

Cruz (Oswaldo): Brazil-med., Rio de Janeiro, 1897, xxxi, 51; 2751.—U. S. Nav. M. Bull., Wash., 1917, xi, 521-525 (W. C. Wells).

Cullen: Life by J. Thomson, 2 v., Edinb., 1859.—Asclepiad, Lond., 1890, vii, 148-177, 2 port. (Sir B. W. Richardson).—New York M. J., 1897, lxvi, 689-691 (F. Staples).—Edinb. M. J., 1925, n. s., xxxii, 17-30 (J. D. Comrie).

Currie (James): Memoir by W. W. Currie, Lond., 1831.—Ann. Med. History, N. Y., 1919-20, ii, 81 (Sir W. Osler).

Cushny: Brit. M. J., Lond., 1926, i, 455-457.—Med. Life, N. Y., 1926, xxx, 245-248 (J. D. Comrie).—Proc. Roy. Soc., Lond., 1926-7, S. B., c, pp. xix-xxvii, port. (H. H. Dale).—Science, N. Y., 1926, lxiii, 507-515 (J. J. Abel).

Cutbush (Edward): Ann. Med. Hist., N. Y., 1923, v, 337-386 (F. L. Pleadwell).

Czermak: Prag. med. Wochenschr., 1906, xxxi, 571-573 (R. von Jaksch).—Arch. f. Ophth., Leipz., 1906, lxv, pp. i-iv (E. Fuchs).

Darwin (Charles): Life and Letters by F. Darwin, 2 v., N. Y., 1898.—More Letters, 2 v., London, 1903.—Life by E. B. Poulton, London, 1896.—Gedenkschrift, Stuttgart, 1909.—Abernethian address by Sir T. L. Brunton, London, 1883.—Sketch by Karl Pearson, London, 1923.—Pamphlets by Grant Allen (New York, 1886) and A. E. Shipley (Cambridge, 1909).—British Museum (Natural History), Special guide No. 4. Memorials, London, 1910.—Proc. Roy. Soc., Lond., 1888, xliv, pp. i–xxxv (T. H. Huxley).—Deutsche Rundschau, Berl., 1888, lvii, 231–254 (T. W. Preyer).—Proc. Am. Phil. Soc., Phila., 1909, xlviii, pp. iii–lvii (Sir J. Bryce, et al.).—Pop. Sc. Monthly, N. Y., 1909, lxxiv, 315–343, 6 pl., 1 port. (H. F. Osborn).

Darwin (Erasmus): Science Progr., Lond., 1924, xviii, 447–453 (F. W. Shurlock).

Daviel: Marseille méd., 1925, lxii, 1358–1364 (Aubaret).

Dechambre (Amédée): Biography by L. Lereboullet, Paris, 1887.

Dee (John): Life by G. M. Hort, London, 1922.

Déjerine (Augusta): Encéphale, Par., 1928, xxiii, 75–88 (André-Thomas).—Rev. neurol., Par., 1927 xxxiv, pt. 2, 635–643 (G. Roussy).

Déjerine (Jules): Bull. Acad. de méd., Par., 1917, 3. s., lxxviii, 308–312.—Compt. rend. Soc. de biol., Par., 1917, lxxx, 416–420 (André-Thomas).—J. Nerv. & Ment. Dis., N. Y., 1917, xlvi, 239 (S. E. Jelliffe).

Delano (Jane): Pacific Coast J. Nurs., San Fran., 1919, xv, 266–268.

Desault: J. de méd. de Bordeaux, 1923, liii, 525–544 (P. Mauriac).

Descartes: R.-C.-C. Martin, Paris diss., 1924, No. 248.

Deventer: Janus, Amst., 1912, xvii, 425; 506 (B. J. Kouwer).—Geneesk. Gids's Gravenhage, 1924–5 ii, 438–443 (J. G. de Lint); 444–451 (P. C. T. van der Hoeven).

Diaz (Francisco): Dermat. Wchnschr., Leipz. & Hamb., 1925, lxxx, 516–519 (F. Lejeune).

Diderot: Würzb. Abhandl. a. d. gesamt Geb. d. Med., Leipz., 1925, xxii, 195–216 (E. van Jan).

Dieffenbach: H. Rohlfs: Gesch. f. deutsch. Med., Leipz., 1885, iv, 1–138.

Dietz (Johann): Autobiography, Munich, 1915. Translation: London, 1923.

Dieulafoy: Bull. et mém. Soc. méd. des hôp., Par., 1911, 3. s., xxxii, 755–769 (Siredey).

Dioscorides: E. L. Greene: Landmarks of Botanical History, Wash., 1909, i, 151–155.—Paris méd., 1919, xxviii, suppl., 336; 374 (L. Moulé).

Dodoens: D'Avorne: Éloge (Malines, 1850).—Janus, Leyden, 1917, xxii, 141–204 (E. C. van Leersum, et al.).—Nederl. Tijdschr. v. Geneesk., Amst., 1917, 2. R., liii, pt. 1, 2108–2139 (E. C. van Leersum, et al.).—Ber. d. deutsch., pharm. Gesellsch., Berl., 1918, xxviii, 51–53 (H. Schelenz).—Janus, Leyden, 1923, xxvii, 213–218 (F. W. T. Hunger).

Donders: Life by J. Moleschott, Giessen, 1888.—Sitzungsb. d. math.-phys. Cl. d. k. bayer. Akad. d. Wissensch., München, 1889, xix, 118–124 (C. von Voit).—Ann. d'ocul., Bruz., 1889, cii, 5–107, port. (J.-P. Nuel).—Arch. d'opht., Par., 1889, ix, 193–204 (E. Landolt).—Proc. Roy. Soc., Lond., 1890–91, xlix, pp. vii–xxiv, port. (W. B.).—Review of his work by Ernest Clark (London, 1914).

Douglas (William): Arch. Pediat., N. Y., 1922, xxxix, 593–600 (N. B. Foster).

Drake (Daniel): Memoirs by E. D. Mansfield, Cincinnati, 1851. Daniel Drake and his Followers, by Otto Juettner, Cincinnati, 1909. S. D. Gross, Lives (etc.), Phila., 1861, 614–662. Also: Jour. Am. Med. Ass., Chicago, 1895, xxv, 429–436 (W. Pepper). Also: Am. Jour. Med. Sc., Phila., 1876, n. s., lxxii, 451–452 (J. S. Billings).

Duchenne: C. Lasègue: Études méd., Par., 1884, i, 178–206.—Rev. internat. d'électrothér., Par., 1895–6, vi, 257–270 (Motet): 305–333, 1 pl., 2 port. (Inauguration du monument): 1899–1900, x, 69–90 (Brissaud).—Med. Rec., N. Y., 1908, lxxiii, 50–54 (J. Collins).—Presse méd., Par., 1925, xxxiii, 1601–1606 (G. Guillain).

Dudley (Benjamin W.): Med. Life, N. Y., 1926, xxx, 3–17 (A. H. Barkley).

Dupuytren: Vidal de Cassis: Essai historique (Paris, 1835).—H. Larrey: Discours (Paris, 1869).—Mém. Acad. de méd., Par., 1836, v, 51–82 (E. Pariset).—Monit. d. hôp., Par., 1856, iv, 145; 153; 161; 169 (Malgaigne).—Boston M. & S. J., 1916, clxxv, 489–494 (W. P. Coues).—Biog. Lexikon (Hirsch), Wien & Leipz., 1885, ii, 240–243 (Gurlt).—Bull. Soc. franç. d'hist. de méd. Par., 1920, xiv, 373–381 (A. Lutaud).

Durosiez: Feiga Helfenbein, Paris diss., 1922, No. 430.

Ehrlich (Paul): Festschrift, Jena, 1914.—Life by A. Lazarus, Wien, 1922.—Arch. f. Dermat. u. Syph., Wien & Leipz., 1915–16, cxxxi, 559–578, port. (A. Neisser).—Berl. klin. Wchnschr., 1914, li, 529–531 (Roux & Metchnikoff).—Deutsche med. Wchnschr., Leipz. u. Berl., 1915, xli, 1103; 1135 (A. von Wassermann).—Naturwissenschaften, Berl., 1914, ii, 243; 268: 1916, iv, 137; 149: 1919, vii, 165 (C. Oppenheimer, et al.).

Einthoven: Brit. M. J., Lond., 1927, ii, 664 (Sir T. Lewis).

Ellis (Havelock): Biographies by Isaac Goldberg, Boston, 1926, and H. Peterson, Boston, 1928.

Emmett (Thomas Addis): Reminiscences, N. Y., 1905.—Tr. Am. Gynec. Soc., Phila., 1919, xliv, 365–371, port. (J. R. Goffe).

Erasistratus: J. F. Hieronymus: Jena diss., 1790.—R. Fuchs: Erasistratea, Leipzig, 1892.—Glasgow M. J., 1893, 4. s., xxxix, 340–352 (J. Finlayson). Proc. Roy. Soc. Med., Lond., 1927, xx, Sect. Hist. Med., 21–28 (J. F. Dobson).

Erb: Deutsche Ztschr. f. Nervenh., Leipz., 1920–21, lxvii, pp. i–iv (M. Nonne); 1922, lxxiii, Heft 1–2, pp. i–xviii (F. Schultze).

Esmarch: H. Rohlfs: Gesch. d. deutsch. Med., Leipz., 1885, iv, 353–411.—München. med. Wchnschr., 1893, xl, 8 (A. Hoffa).—Berl. klin. Wchnschr., 1908, xlv, 578 (A. Brer).—Ztschr. f. Krankenpflg., Berl., 1903, xxv, 91; 1908, xxx, 65.—Med. Mag., Lond., 1893–4, ii, 9–21 (Zobeltitz).

Fabry of Hilden: Janus, Bresl., 1848, iii, 225–282 (Benedict).—Deutsches Arch. f. Gesch. d. Med., Leipz., 1883, vi, 1–25 (P. Müller).—Abhandl. z. Gesch. d. Med., Bresl., 1904, Heft xiii (R. J. Schaefer).—Janus, Amst., 1910, xv, 65–72, 1 port. (R. J. Schaefer).—München. med. Wchnschr., 1910, lvii, 1401–1403, port. (K. Sudhoff).—Johns Hopkins Hosp. Bull., Balt., 1905, xvi, 7–10 (W. B. Platt).

Farr (William): Johns Hopkins Univ. School. Hyg. De Lamar Sect., 1925–6, Balt., 1927, 203–220 (Sir A. Newsholme).

Fauchard: Paris méd., 1927, xvii, suppl., pp. i–viii (Boissier).

Favill (Henry Baird): Memorial volume, ed. J. Favill, Chicago, 1917.

Fayrer (Sir Joseph): Recollections of my Life, Edinb., 1900.

Fehling: Zentralbl. f. Gynäk., Leipz., 1925, xlix, 2866–2874 (P. Zweifel).

Fernel (Jean): P.-A. Capitaine: Paris diss., 1925, No. 96.—L. Figard: Un médecin philosophe, Paris, 1903,—Union méd., Par., 1864, 2. s., xxi, 497; 554 (A. Chéreau).—Deutsche Klinik, Berl., 1865, xvii, 2; 29; 41; 53 (R. Finckenstein).

Finlay (Carlos): Sanidad y Beneficencia, Habana, 1916, xv, 257: 1918, xx, 3–197 (E. Nuñez, et al.).—New Orl. M. & S. J., 1916, lxix, 55–60 (A. Agramonte).

Fischer (Emil): Life by Kurt Hoesch. Berlin, 1921.—Autobiography (*Aus meinem Leben*), Berlin, 1922.—Die Naturwissenschaften, Berl., 1919, vii, 841–882 (C. Harries, et al.).—München. med. Wochenschr., 1919, lxvi, 938–940 (E. Abderhalden).—Proc. Roy. Soc. Lond., 1921, S. A., xcviii, pp. 1–8 (M. O. F.).

Fitz (Reginald Heber): Boston M. & S. J., 1913, clxix, 893–903 (W. W. Keen, et al.).

Fletcher (Robert): Bristol M.-Chir. J., 1912, xxx, 289–294, port. (Sir W. Osler).—Index Med., Wash. 1912, x, No. 12 (F. H. Garrison).

Flint (Austin): Johns Hopkins Hosp., Balt., 1912, xxiii, 182–186 (H. R. M. Landis).

Flügge: Ztschr. f. Hyg., Berl., 1923, ci, 1. Heft.—Ztschr. f. Tuberk., Leipz., 1923–4, xxxix, 356–362 (B. Heymann).

Foà (Pio): Pathologica, Genova, 1924, xvi, 57–61 (A. Fabris).—Gior. di r. Accad. di med. di Torino, 1926, xxxii, 57–77 (F. Vanzetti).

Foster (Sir Michael): J. Physiol., Lond., 1906–7, xxxv, 233–246 (J. N. Langley).—Proc. Roy. Soc. Lond., 1908, s. B., lxxx, obit., pp. lxxi–lxxxi, port. (W. H. Gaskell).—Boston M. & S. J., 1907, clvi, 309–311 (W. T. Porter).—Publ. Med. Fac. Queen's Univ., Kingston, No. 7, 1913, 1–17 (J. G. Adami).—Maryland M. J., 1915, lviii, 105–118 (F. H. Garrison).

Fothergill: Memoirs by J. C. Lettsom, 4. ed., Lond., 1786.—Life by R. Hingston Fox (London, 1919).

Fournier (Alfred): Ann. de dermat. et syph., Par., 1914–15, 5. s., v, 513–528, port. (J. Darier).—Bull. Acad. de méd., Par., 1917, 3. s., lxxviii, 686–697 (G. M. Debove).

Fracastorius: Life by F. O. Mencken, Leipz., 1731.—A. Rittmann: Culturgesch. Abhandl., Brünn, 1869–70, 3. Heft.—Gior. ital. di mal. ven., Milano, 1885, xx, 1–11 (Gamberini).—Proc. Charaka Club, N. Y., 1906, ii, 5–20, 3 pl. (Sir W. Osler).—Science, N. Y., 1910, n. s., xxxi, 500; 857 (F. H. Garrison).—Ann. Med. History, N. Y., 1917–18, i, 1–34 (C. & D. Singer).

Francis (John W.): Bull. N. Y. Acad. Med., 1925, 2. s., i, 35–40 (F. H. Garrison).

Frank (J. P.): Autobiography, Vienna, 1802.—Biography by K. Doll, Karlsruhe, 1910, and the study of Frank's influence on social hygiene by K. E. F. Schmitz (Berlin, 1917).—H. Rohlfs: Gesch. d. deutsch. Med., Stuttg., 1880, ii, 127–211.—Med. Jahrb., Wien, 1886, n. F., i, 97–116 (H. von Bamberger).—Wien. klin. Wchnschr., 1909, xxii, 1341: 1913, xxvi, 627 (M. Neuburger).—Arch. di storia d. sc., Roma, 1923, iv, 326–330 (E. Ebstein).

Fraser (Sir T. R.): Brit. M. J., Lond., 1920, i, 100, port.—Lancet, Lond., 1920, i, 122.—Proc. Roy. Soc. Lond., 1920–21, xcii, s. B., pp. xi–xvii, port. (J. T. C.).

Frerichs: Arch. f. exper. Path. u. Pharmakol., Leipz., 1885, xix, pp. iii–viii (B. Naunyn).—Deutsche med. Wchnschr., Leipz. u. Berl., 1884, x, 257; 266; 279; 296: 1885, xi, 177 (E. Leyden).—Wien. med. Wchnschr., 1885, xxxv, 465; 497; 537 (E. Litten).

Freud: Life by Fritz Wittels, London, 1924. Autobiography in: Med. d. Gegenwart (Grote), Leipz., 1925, iv, 1–51, port.

Freund (Wilhelm Alexander): Memoirs (*Leben und Arbeit*), Berlin, 1913.—Zentralbl. f. Gynäk., Leipz., 1918, xliii, 73–82 (H. Bayer).

Friedenwald (Aaron): Life by Harry Friedenwald, Baltimore, 1906.

Fuchs (Ernst): Ztschr. f. Augenh., Berl., 1922, xlvii, 47–62.

Fuchs (Leonhard): Rep. Smithson. Inst., 1917, Wash., 1919, 635–647 (F. Neumann).

Gaddesden (John): Monograph by H. P. Cholmely. Oxford (Clarendon Press), 1912.

Galen: Sprengel: Beitr. z. Gesch. d. Med., Halle, 1794, i, 1. St., 117–195.—J. G. Ackermann in C. G. Kühn edition of Galen, v. 1, Leipzig, 1821.—Gaz. méd. de Par., 1847, 3. s., ii, 591; 603 (C. Daremberg).—*Ibid.*, 1858, 3. s., xiii, 43; 115; 171 (J.-E. Pétrequin).—Brit. M. J., Lond., 1892, i, 573; 730; 771 (J. Finlayson).—Middlesex Hosp. J., Lond., 1899, iii, 37–52 (Sir V. Horsley).—Naturwissenschaften, Berl., 1914, ii, 794–797 (K. Sudhoff).—For his practice, see: N. Jahrb. f. klass. Altertum, 1905, xv, 276–312 (J. Ilberg).—Also T. Meyer-Steineg: *Ein Tag im Leben des Galen*, Leipzig, 1913.—For Galenic physiology, see: Arch. f. Gesch. d. Med., Leipz., 1911–12, v, 172: 1912–13, vi, 417 (T. Meyer-Steineg).—M. Greenwood: Galen as an epidemiologist, Proc. Roy. Soc. Med., London, 1920–21, xiv, Sect. Hist. Med., 3–16.

Gall: Lives by B. Hollander (London, 1909) and A. Fronep (Leipzig, 1911).—Arch. f. Gesch. d. Med., Leipz., 1916–17, x, 3: 1918–19, xi, 93 (M. Neuburger).—Mitt. z. Gesch. d. Med., Leipz., 1917, xv, 435: 1919, xviii, 258 (M. Neuburger).

Galton (Sir Francis): Memories of my life, N. Y., 1909.—Life by Karl Pearson, 2 v., Cambridge, 1914–24.—Eugenics Rev., Lond., 1911–12, iii, 1–9 (M. C.).—Nature, Lond., 1910–11, lxxxv, 440–445.—Pop. Sc. Monthly, 1911, lxxix, 171–190 (J. A. Harris).

Galvani: J.-L. Alibert: Éloges historiques, Par., 1806, 187–338.—Arch. di storia d. sc., Roma, 1923, iv, 331–346 (G. Bilancioni).

Garcia (Manuel): Paris méd., 1925, lvii, 186–189 (Roshem).

Garth (Sir Samuel): Johns Hopkins Hosp. Bull., Balt., 1906, xvii, 1–17, port. (H. Cushing).

Gaskell (Walter Holbrook): Proc. Roy. Soc. Lond., 1914–15, s. B., lxxxvii, obit., pp. xxvii–xxxiii (J. N. Langley).—Science, N. Y., 1914, n. s., xl, 802–807 (F. H. Garrison and F. H. Pike).

Gaub: W. Dietze: Jena diss., 1927.

Gegenbaur (Carl): *Erlebtes und Erstrebtes*, Leipzig, 1901.—Jenaische Ztschr. f. Nature., Jena, 1925–6, lxii, 501–518, 3 port. (F. Maurer).

Gerster (Arpad G.): Recollections, N. Y., 1917.

Gesner (Conrad): Papers Bibliog. Soc. America, Chicago, 1916, x, 53–86 (J. E. Bay).

Gilbert (William): Jour. Roy. Nav. Med. Serv., 1916, ii, 495, 510 (C. Singer).

Gilles de Corbeil: Study by C. Vieillard, Paris, 1909.—Ann. Med. Hist., N. Y., 1925, vii, 362–378 (S. D'Irsay).

Glisson: Proc. Roy. Soc. Med., Lond., 1925–6, xix, Sect. Hist. Med., 111–122 (E. M. Little).

Golgi: Boll. d. Soc. med.-chir., Pavia, 1926, n. s., i, suppl., 1-48, port. (A. Perroncito).—Gior. d. r. Accad. di med. di Torino, 1927, 4. s., xxxiii, 31–52 (R. Morpurgo).—Ann. d'ig., Roma, 1926, xxxvi, 150–152 (G. Sanarelli).—Arch. Neurol. & Psychiat., Chicago, 1926, xv, 625–627 (H. R. Viets).

Goltz: Arch. f. d. ges. Physiol., Bonn, 1903, xciv, 1–64, port. (J. R. Ewald).

Gorgas: Life by Mrs. M. C. D. Gorgas and B. J. Hendrick, Garden City, N. Y., 1924.—Science, N. Y., 1920, n. s., lii, 53 (M. W. Ireland).—Am. J. Trop. Med., Balt., 1922, ii, 161–171 (J. F. Siler).

Gradenigo: Arch. ital. di otol., Torino, 1926, xxxviii, 111–117 (Bruzzi).

von Graefe (Albrecht): Life by E. Michaelis, Berlin, 1877.—C. Schweigger: *Rede*, Berlin, 1882.— J. Jacobson: *Verdienste* [etc.], Berlin, 1885.—Ber. ü. d. Versamml. d. ophth. Gesellsch., Stuttg., 1886, xxiv, 5–52 (Donders & Helmholtz).—Ann. d'ocul., Brux., 1872, lxvii, 5–56 (Warlomont).

von Graefe (Carl Ferdinand): H. Rohlfs: Gesch. d. deutsch. Med., Leipz., 1883, iii, 247–324.

Grassi (Benvenuto): Ann. di ottal., Roma, 1920, liii, 413–427 (G. Petella).

Grassi (Giovanni Battista): Naturwissenschaften, Berl., 1926, xiv, 225; 261 (C. Janicki).

Graves: Biography by W. Stokes in his "Studies in Physiology" (etc.), Lond., 1863, pp. i–lxxxiii. Also: Med. Times & Gaz., Lond., 1853, vi, 1–5 (W. Stokes).—Med. Hist. Meath Hosp., Dublin, 1888, 122–129, port.

Grawitz: Autobiography in: Med. d. Gegenwart (Grote), Leipz., 1923, ii, 23–75, port.

Gray (Henry): Am. J. M. Sc., Phila., 1908, n. s., cxxxvi, 429–435, port. (F. K. Boland).

Greenhill (William Alexander): Lancet, Lond., 1894, ii, 948.

Gross (S. D.): Autobiography, 2 v., Phila., 1887.—Tr. Am. Surg. Ass., Phila., 1897, xv, pp. xxxi–xlviii. —Am. J. M. Sc., Phila., 1884, n. s., lxxxviii, 293–308, port. (I. M. Hays).—Johns Hopkins Hosp. Bull., Balt., 1912, xxiii, 83–94 (C. W. G. Rohrer).

Grüby (David): Arch. de parasitol., Par., 1899, ii, 43–74, port. (R. Blanchard).—Dermat. Wochenschr., Leipz., 1926, lxxxiii, 512–516 (J. H. Rille).

Guérin (Alphonse): André Courbe, Paris diss., 1913, No. 45.

Gull (Sir William): Guy's Hosp. Rep., Lond., 1890, 3. s., xxxii, pp. xxv–xliii, port.—Wilks & Bettany. History of Guy's Hospital, Lond., 1892, 261–274.

Gurlt: Arch. f. klin. Chir., Berl., 1899, lviii, pp. i–vi (E. von Bergmann).

Guy de Chauliac: E. Nicaïse: Introduction to his edition of *La Grande Chirurgie*, Par., 1890, pp. lxxvii–cv (Bibliography of Guy), pp. cvi–cxci.—Confér. Inst. Fac. de méd. de Par., 1866, 173–208 (Follin).—Arch. f. Gesch. d. med., Leipz., 1919–20, xii, 8: 1921, xiii, 65 (W. von Brunn).

Guyon (Felix): Bull. et mém. Soc. de chir. de Par., 1923, xlix, 77–101 (J.-L. Faure).—J. d'urol., Par., 1920, ix, 323–333 (F. Legueu).

Haeckel: Autobiography (1852–6), Leipzig, 1921.—Life by W. Bölsche (English transl. by J. McCabe, Phila., 1906).—München med. Wochenschr., 1920, lxvii, 135 (R. Hertwig).—Monist, Chicago, 1920, xxx, 1–18 (R. C. Schiedt).

Hahnemann: Life by R. Haehl, 2 v., Leipzig, 1922.—Life by T. C. Bradford, Philadelphia, 1895.

Hales (Stephen): Gentleman's Mag., Lond., 1764, xxxiv, 273–278 (P. Collinson).—Dict. Nat. Biog., Lond., 1890, xxiv, 32–36 (Sir F. Darwin).—Johns Hopkins Hosp. Bull., Balt., 1904, xv, 185; 232 (P. M. Dawson).—Scient. Monthly, N. Y., 1916, iii, 439–454 (D. Fraser Harris).—Sir F. Darwin: Rustic Sounds, Lond., 1917, 115–139.

Hall (Marshall): Memoirs by Charlotte Hall, Lond., 1861.—Lancet, Lond., 1850, ii, 120–128, port.; 1857, ii, 172–175.—Dict. Nat. Biog., Lond., 1890, xxiv, 80–83 (G. T. Bettany).

Haller: Lives and Eulogies by J. G. Zimmermann (Zürich, 1755), E. G. Baldinger and C. G. Heyne (Göttingen, 1778), T. Henry (Warrington, 1783), R. C. Stiles (New York, 1867).—A. Lissauer (Berlin, 1873). See also Denkschrift, Bern, 1877. Hallers Wohnungen (etc.), by H. Kronecker, Bern, 1908, has many interesting illustrations.—Die Bildnisse (etc.), by Artur Weese, Bern, 1909, gives all extant portraits.—Especially interesting are "Haller Redivivus" by H. Kronecker (Mitth. d. naturf. Gesellsch. in Bern (1902), 1903, 203–226) and Harvey Cushing's paper in Am. Med., Phila., 1901, ii, 542; 580. See also Deutsche med. Wchnschr., Leipz. u. Berl., 1908, xxxiv, 1813–1815 (H. Kronecker).—München. med. Wchnschr., 1908, lv, 2142 (K. Sudhoff).—Johns Hopkins Hosp. Bull., Balt., 1908, xix, 65–73 (J. C. Hemmeter).—Bull. Soc. Med. History, Chicago, 1916, No. 4, 23–46 (C. B. Reed). For his literary life, see Ludwig Hirzel's introduction to Haller's *Gedichte*, Frauenfeld, 1882.

Halsted: Johns Hopkins Hosp. Bull., Balt., 1925, xxxvi, 2–59 (Matas, Welch, *et al.*).—Science, N. Y., 1922, n. s., lvi, 461–464 (H. Cushing).—Am. Mercury, N. Y., 1926, 396–401 (F. H. Garrison).

Harington (Sir John): Johns Hopkins Hosp. Bull., Balt., 1908, xix, 285–295 (J. G. Adami).

Harris (Walter): Ann. Med. History, N. Y., 1919–20, ii, 228–240 (J. Rührah).

Harvey (William): William Harvey by D'Arcy Power ("Masters of Medicine"), London, 1897.— Memorials of Harvey by J. H. Aveling, London, 1875.—Some Memoranda (etc.), by S. Weir Mitchell (Tr. Ass. Am. Phys., Phila., 1907, xxii, 737–763). Also, Reprint: New York, 1907.— Some recently discovered Letters (etc.), by S. Weir Mitchell, Philadelphia, 1912.—H. Milford: Portraits of Dr. William Harvey, Oxford Univ. Press, 1913.—Notice of an Unpublished Manuscript by G. E. Paget, London, 1801.—John Call Dalton's "Doctrines of the Circulation," Philadelphia, 1884, is the best history of the subject in English, and "Harvey's Views," etc., New York, 1915, by Dalton's pupil and successor, the late John G. Curtis, is another important contribution to American scholarship. The introduction to Charles Richet's text (Paris, 1879) is valuable. See, also, three addresses by T. H. Huxley in: Nature, London, 1878, xvii, 417; xviii, 146, and Pop. Sc. Monthly (Suppl.), New York, 1878, No. xi, 385–389. Also: Johns Hopkins Hosp. Bull., Baltimore, 1897, viii, 167–174 (W. K. Brooks). Also: St. Barth. Hosp. Rep., London, 1887, xxiii, 1–12 (W. Munk). Also: Lancet, London, 1878, ii, 776–778, 1 pl. (Sir B. W. Richardson). Also: Asclepiad, London, 1884, i, 39–44, 1 pl. (Sir B. W. Richardson).—Proc. Roy. Soc.

Med., Lond., 1916–17, x, Sect. Hist. Med., 33–59 (Sir D'A. Power).—Also: Harveian orations (listed in Index Catalogue, 1901, 2. s., vi, 780).—Bibliography by G. Keynes, Cambridge, 1928.

Hayem: Sang, Par., 1927, i, 59–68 (L. Rivet).

Heberden: Essay by A. C. Buller (London, 1879).—Pettigrew, Med. Portr. Gallery, Lond., 1840, iii, No. 7, 1–18, port.—Dict. Nat. Biog., Lond., 1891, xxv, 359 (J. F. Payne).—Ztschr. f. klin. Med., Berl., 1910, lxx, 352–357 (J. Pawinski).—St. Barth. Hosp. Rep., Lond., 1911, xlvi, 1–12 (Sir D. Duckworth).

Hebra: Allg. med. Centr.-Ztg., Berl., 1881, xvii, 1104–1198, *passim* (E. Schwimmer).—Pest. med.-chir. Presse, 1881, xvii, 812–888, *passim.*—Med. Rev. of Rev., N. Y., 1916, xxii, 719–724 (V. Robinson).—Wien. klin. Wchnschr., 1926, xxxix, 1353–1358 (L. Arzt).

Heim (Ernst Ludwig): Life by G. W. Kessler, 2 v., Leipz., 1835.—Rohlfs: Gesch. d. deutsch. Med., Stuttg., 1875, i, 480–519.

Heine: B. Bürger, Bonn diss., 1911.—Arch. f. klin. Chir., Berl., 1927–8, cxlix, 476–500 (H. Nahrath).

Heister: V. Fossel: Stud. z. Gesch. d. Med., Stuttg., 1909, 111–152.—Proc. Charaka Club, N. Y., 1906, ii, 131–141 (A. G. Gerster).

Helmholtz: Lives by L. Koenigsberger, 3 v., Brunswick, 1902 (English transl. by F. A. Welby, Oxford, 1906); and J. G. M'Kendrick, London, 1899. Bibliography by A. König, Leipzig, 1895. See also: Aerztl. Vereinsbl. f. Deutschl., Leipz., 1894, xxiii, 553–556 (C. Ludwig).—Arch. d'opht., Par., 1894, xiv, 721–842 (E. Landolt).—Rev. scient., Par., 1897, 4. s., viii; 321; 360 (E. du Bois Reymond).—Proc. Roy. Soc. Lond., 1896, lix, pp. xvii–xxx (A. W. R.).—J. Am. M. Ass., Chicago 1902, xxxviii, 549–926 (H. Friedenwald; H. Knapp, *et al.*).

van Helmont (J. B.): Studies by J. J. Loos (Heidelberg, 1807), D. H. Fraenkel (Leipzig, 1837), G. Rommelaere (Brussels, 1868).—Mém. d. concours . . . Acad. roy. de méd. de Belg., Brux., 1866, vi, 553–739 (J.-A. Mandon).—Bull. Acad. roy. de méd. de Belg., Brux., 1886, 2. s., ix, 985–1088 (Tallois).—J. hebd. de méd., Par., 1830, vi, 513–527 (E. Littré).—Med. Woche, Berl., 1903, 25; 33 (F. Strunz).

Hemmeter: Autobiography in: Med. d. Gegenwart, Leipz., 1924, iii, 1–62, port.

Henle: Life by F. R. Merkel, Braunschweig, 1909.—Life by Victor Robinson, New York, 1921.—See, also: Arch. f. mikr. Anat., Bonn, 1885–6, xxvi, pp. i–xxxii (W. Waldeyer).—Biol. Centralbl., Erlangen, 1885–6, v. 289–293 (W. Flemming).—Deutsche med. Wchnschr., Berl., 1885, xi, 463; 483 (K. Bardeleben).

Herophilus: K. F. H. Marx: Herophilus, Carlsruhe & Baden, 1838, Göttingen, 1842.—Rev. scient., Par., 1881, i, 12 (C. Daremberg).—Glasgow M. J., 1893, 4. s., xxxix, 321–340 (J. Finlayson).—Proc. Roy. Soc. Med., Lond., 1925, xviii, Sect. Hist. Med., 19–32 (J. F. Dobson).

Heubner: Autobiography, Med. d. Gegenwart (Grote), Leipz., 1925, iv, 93–124, port.—Klin. Wchn-schr., Berl., 1926, v, 2382–2384 (Finkelstein).

Hewson (William): Tr. Med. Soc., Lond., 1810, i, 51–63 (J. C. Lettsom).—Asclepiad, Lond., 1891, viii, 148–177 (Sir B. W. Richardson).—Dict. Nat. Biog., Lond., 1891, xxvii, 312 (J. F. Payne).

Heysham (John): Life by H. Lonsdale, London, 1870.

Hicks (Braxton): Select Essays (Sydenham Soc. Publ., vol. 173), Lond., 1901, 93–118, with bibliography (C. J. Cullingworth).

Hildegard (Saint): H. Fischer: *Die heilige Hildegarde,* Munich, 1927.

Hinton (James): Life by Mrs. Havelock Ellis (London, 1918).

Hippocrates: Introduction to Emile Littré's translation, v. 1, pp. 1–554, Par., 1839.—J. E. Pétrequin: *Chirurgie d' Hippocrate,* 2 v., Par., 1878.—J. Hornyánsky: Hippocrates, Budapest, 1910.—J. Hirschberg: *Vorlesungen,* Leipzig, 1922.—R. O. Moon: Hippocrates and his Successors, London, 1923.—H. Much: *Hippocrates der Grosse,* Stuttgart, 1926. Prolegomena by W. H. S. Jones and E. T. Withington in Loeb bilingual Hippocrates (4 v., London, 1923–8).—Brit. & For. Med.-Chir. Rev., Lond., 1866, xxxviii, 483–496 (Sir T. C. Allbutt).—Glasgow M. J., 1892, xxxvii, 253–271 (J. Finlayson).—Brit. M. J., Lond., 1906, i, 571–577 (R. Caton).—Harvard Stud. Class., Philol., Cambridge, 1914, xxv, 139–203 (W. A. Heidel).

Hirschberg (Julius): Klin. Monatsbl. f. Augenh., Stuttg., 1925, lxxiv, 497–501 (O. Fehr).—Arch. Ophth., N. Y., 1925, liv, 418–422 (H. Friedenwald).

His (Wilhelm): *Lebenserinnerungen,* Leipzig, 1903.—Am. J. Anat., Balt., 1904–5, iv, 139–161 (F. P. Mall).—Lancet, Lond., 1904, i, 1446–1449 (W. Stirling).—Deutsche med. Wchnschr., Leipz. u. Berl., 1904, xxx, 1438; 1469; 1509; (W. Waldeyer).—Verhandl. d. naturf. Gesellsch. in Basel, 1904, 434–464, port. (J. Kollmann).

Hodgkin (Thomas): Wilks & Bettany: Hist. Guy's Hosp., Lond., 1892, 380–386.—Guy's Hosp. Rep., Lond., 1878, 3. s., xxiii, 55–127 (Sir S. Wilks).—Guy's Hosp. Gaz., Lond., 1909, xxiii, 528; 1910, xxiv, 13 (Wilks).

Hoffmann (Heinrich): *Lebenserinnerungen*, Frankfurt, 1926.

Höfler (Max): München. med. Wochenschr., 1915, lxii, 79 (K. Sudhoff).

Holl (Moritz): Anat. Anz., Jena, 1922, lv, 12–29 (H. Rabl).

Holmes (O. W.): Lives by W. S. Kennedy (Bost., 1883), H. Lee (Bost., 1894) and J. T. Morse, Jr. (2 v., Boston, 1896).—Boston M. & S. J., 1894, cxxxi, 375–380, port.—Lancet, Lond., 1886, ii, 6–9 (Sir S. Wilks).—Brit. M. J., Lond., 1894, ii, 839–841 (Sir W. T. Gardner).—Johns Hopkins Hosp. Bull., Balt., 1894, v, 85–88 (Sir W. Osler).

Holt (Luther Emmett): Arch. Pediat., N. Y., 1924, xli, 1–4, port. (V. P. Gibney).—Science, N. Y., 1924, n. s., lix, 452 (T. M. Prudden).

Hooke (Robert): Dict. Nat. Biog., Lond., 1891, xxvi, 283–287 (Miss A. M. Clerke).—Am. Naturalist, Lancaster, Pa., 1919, liii, 247–264 (L. L. Woodruff).—Ann. Med. Hist., N. Y., 1927, ix, 227–243 (W. S. Middleton).

Hoppe-Seyler: Arch. f. path. Anat. (etc.), Berl., 1895, cxlii, 386–388 (R. Virchow).—Ztschr. f. physiol. Chem., Strassb., 1895, pp. i–lxii, port. (E. Baumann & A. Kossel).

Horner (J. F.): *Ein Lebensbild*, Frauenfeld, 1887.

Horsley (Sir Victor): Life by Stephen Paget (London, 1919).—Brit. M. J., Lond., 1916, ii, 162–167 port.—Lancet, Lond., 1916, ii, 200–203, port.

Howard (John): Lives by Aikin (1792), J. B. Brown (2. ed., 1823), T. Taylor (2. ed. 1836), Hepworth Dixon (2. ed., 1850).—Correspondence, edited by J. Field, London, 1855.—Also: Asclepiad, Lond. 1894, xi, 55–80 (Sir B. W. Richardson).

Howland (John): Bull. Johns Hopkins Hosp., Balt., 1927, xli, 311–321.

Huchard (Henri): Bull. Soc. méd. de l'Yonne, 1911, Auxerre, 1912, lii, 9–17 (L. Roché).

Hueppe: Autobiography in: Med. d. Gegenwart, Leipz., 1923, ii, 77–138, port.

Hufeland: Life by J. I. J. Sachs, Berl., 1832. Also Med. Alm., Berl., 1837, 39–54, port.—Berl. klin. Wochenschr., 1910, xlvii, 243–248 (D. von Hansemann).—München. med. Wochenschr., 1910, lvii, 250–252, port. (K. Sudhoff).

Hughlings-Jackson: Brit. M. J., Lond., 1911, ii, 950–954, port., 1551–1554 (Sir J. Hutchinson) 1912, i, 85 (C. A. Mercier).—Brain, Lond., 1903, xxvi, 305–366 (Sir W. Broadbent): 1915, xxviii, 1–190 (H. Head); 391–417 (J. Taylor).

Hunter (John): Stephen Paget: John Hunter ("Masters of Medicine"), London, 1897.—Memoirs (etc.) by J. Adams, London, 1917.—John Hunter and his Pupils by Samuel D. Gross, Philadelphia, 1881.—John Hunter and Odontology, by J. F. Colyer, London, 1913.—G. C. Peachy: Memoir of William and John Hunter, Plymouth, 1924.—Also Brit. Med. Jour., London, 1890, i, 738–740 (J. Finlayson); *Ibid.*, 1899, i, 389–395 (Sir W. MacCormac); *Ibid.*, 1886, i, 1093–1095 (Sir J. Paget); *Ibid.*, 1919, ii, 485–487 (Sir A. Keith).—J. Roy. Army Med. Corps, Lond., 1912, xix, 143–150 (H. A. L. Howell).—Osler Festschr., N. Y., 1919, i, 88–110 (Sir A. Keith). Also: Hunterian orations (listed in Index Catalogue, 1902, 2. s., vii, 483).

Hunter (William): William Hunter by R. Hingston Fox, London, 1901.

Huntington (George Sumner): Am. J. Anat., Phila., 1927, xxxix, 355–377.—Bull. N. Y. Acad. Med. 1928, 2. s., iv, 250–265.

Hutchinson (Jonathan): Brit. M. J., Lond., 1913, i, 1398; ii, 1632.—Lancet, Lond., 1913, i, 1832 ii, 430.—Ophth. Rev., Lond., 1913, xxxii, 225–230, port. (E. Nettleship).

Huxham: Dict. Nat. Biog., Lond., 1891, xxviii, 363 (N. Moore).—Johns Hopkins Hosp. Bull., 1906 xvii, 308–311 (W. G. Vogeler).

Huxley: Life and Letters by L. Huxley, 2 v., Lond., 1900.—Autobiographical sketch (Hosp. Gaz., Lond., 1891, xix, 312–314).—Proc. Roy. Soc., Lond., 1896, lix, pp. xlvi–lxvi, port. (Sir M. Foster).— Dict. Nat. Biog., Suppl., Lond., 1901, iii, 22–31 (W. F. R. Weldon).—Science, N. Y., 1896, n. s., iii, 147–154 (H. F. Osborn); 253–263 (T. Gill).—Rep. Smithson. Inst., 1898–1900, Wash., 1900, 701–728 (W. K. Brooks, *et al.*).—Nature, Lond., 1925, cxv, suppl. (Centenary), 697–752.—Bull. New York Acad. Med., 1925, 2. s., i, 399–404 (F. H. Garrison).

Hyrtl: Deutsche med. Wchnschr., Leipz. u. Berl., 1894, xx, 619 (K. von Bardeleben).—Wien. klin. Wchnschr., 1894, vii, 549; 556; 557.—Wien. med. Wchnschr., 1894, xliv, 1337; 1406.—Bull. Soc. Med. Hist., Chicago, 1923, iii, 96–108 (W. S. Miller).

In-hotep: Studies by Kurt Sethe, Leipzig, 1902; J. B. Hurry, Oxford, 1926, 2. ed., 1928.

Jackson (James): Memoir by J. J. Putnam, Boston & New York, 1905.—Boston M. & S. J., 1867–8, lxxvii, 106–109 (J. Bigelow & O. W. Holmes).

Jacobi (Abraham): Science, N. Y., 1919, n. s., l, 102–104 (F. H. Garrison).—Ann. Med. Hist., N. Y., 1919–20, ii, 194–205 (F. H. Garrison).—Med. Life, N. Y., 1928, xxxv, 213; 261 (V. Robinson).

Jacobi (Mary Putnam): A Pathfinder in Medicine, New York, 1925.

Janeway (E. G.): J. B. Clark: Personal Recollections, N. Y., 1917.—N. Y. M. J., 1912, xcv, 105–107 (Putnam).

Janeway (T. C.): Bull. Johns Hopkins Hosp., Balt., 1918, xxix, 142–148.—Science, N. Y., 1918, n. s., xlvii, 273–279 (L. F. Barker).

Jenner: Life by J. Baron, Lond., 1827–38.—Brit. M. J., Lond., 1894, i, 72; 1901, ii, 479; 1902, ii, 1; 1676.—J. Am. M. Ass., Chicago, 1896, xxvii, 312–317 (H. R. Storer).—New York M. J., 1902, lxxvi, 925; 978 (G. Dock).—Deutsche med. Wchnschr., 1896, xxii, 305–323 (Festnummer).— Scient. Monthly, N. Y., 1915–16, i, 66–85 (D. Fraser Harris).—Brit. M. J., Lond., 1923, i, 204–206 (Sir W. Hale-White).

Jex-Blake (Sophia): Life by Margaret G. Todd, London, 1918.—Woman's M. J., Cincin., 1920, xxvii, 179–185 (Helen MacMurchy).

Kelly (Howard): Johns Hopkins Hosp. Bull., Balt., 1919, xxx, 287–293 (T. S. Cullen); Bibliography, 293–302 (Minnie W. Blogg).

Kerner (Justinus): *Das Bilderbuch* (Stuttgart, 1886).

Klebs (Edwin): München. med. Wchnschr., 1914, lxi, 193; 251 (P. Ernst).—Lancet, Lond., 1913 ii, 1657 (F. H. Garrison).—Cor.-Bl. f. schweizer Aerzte, Basel, 1913, xliii, 1721–1729 (H. Strasser).

Knox (Robert): Life by H. Lonsdale, London, 1870.—Interstate M. J., St. Louis, 1915, xxii, 462–472 (A. C. Jacobson).

Koch: Biographies by W. Becker (Berlin, 1891), K. Wezel (Berlin, 1912), and M. Kirchner (Wien, 1924), Wien. klin. Wchnschr., 1903, xvi, 1377–1381 (R. Paltauf).—Deutsche med. Wchnschr., Leipz. u. Berl., 1910, xxxv, 2321: 1916, xlii, 653 (G. Gaffky).—J. de méd. de Brux., 1910, xv, 373–377 (J. Bordet).—Johns Hopkins Hosp. Bull., Balt., 1911, xxxiii, 415–425 (W. W. Ford); 425–428 (S. A. Knopf).—Parasitology, Lond., 1924–5, xvi, 214–238, 4 port. (G. H. F. Nuttall).

Kocher (Theodor): Cor.-Bl. f. Schweiz. Aertze, Basel, 1917, xlvii, 1217–1219.—München. med. Wochenschr., 1918, lxv, 78–80 (F. Sauerbruch).—U. S. Nav. M. Bull., Wash., 1918, xiii, 59–63 (A. C. Klebs).

Koeberlé (Eugène): Life by E. Pichevin, Strasbourg, 1914.—Rev. de gynéc., Par., 1915, xxiii, 311–342 (Gross).

Koenig (Franz): *Lebenserinnerungen* (Berlin, 1912).

Kölliker: *Erinnerungen*, Leipzig, 1899.—Ztschr. f. wissensch. Zoöl., Leipz., 1906, lxxxiv, pp. i–xxvi (Ehlers).—Anat. Anz., Jena, 1906, xxviii, 539–552 (W. Waldeyer).

Kossel: Ztschr. f. physiol. chem., 1927, clxix, 1–3.

Kraepelin: Allg. Ztschr. f. Psychiat., Berl. & Leipz., 1926–7, lxxxv, 443–458 (Weygandt).—Arch. f. d. ges. Psychol., Leipz., 1927, lviii, pp. i–xxxii, port. (W. Wirth).—Deutsche Ztschr. f. Nervenh. Leipz., 1927, xcvi, 1–7 (E. Trömner).—Med. Klin., Berl., 1926, xxii, 2018–2020 (Henneberg).

von Kries: Autobiography, Med. d. Gegenwart (Grote), 1925, iv, 125–187, port.

Krogh (August): Scient. Monthly, N. Y., 1921, xii, 381–383, port.

Kronecker (Hugo): Science, N. Y., 1914, n. s., xl, 441–444 (S. J. Meltzer).

Küchenmeister: Janus, Amst., 1900, v, 629–634 (J. C. Huber).

Kühne (Willy): Ztschr. f. Biol., München u. Leipz., 1900, n. F., xxii, pp. i–viii (C. von Voit).—Med. Chron., Manchester, 1901, 4. s., i, 401–415, port. (W. Stirling).

Kussmaul: *Jugenderinnerungen* (1899), 10. Aufl., Stuttg., 1919.—Life by T. H. Bast, New York, 1926. —München. med. Wchnschr., 1902, xlix, 281–286, port. (L. Edinger).—Therap. d. Gegenw., Berl., 1902, n. F., iv, 289–291 (B. Naunyn).—Deutsches Arch. f. klin. Med., Leipz., 1902, lxxiii, 1–89 (W. Fleiner).

Laboulbène: Life by L. Beurniar and P. Cambours, Dijon, 1901.

Laennec: Lives by A.-L.-J. Bayle (1826), H. Saintigon (1904), and Gerald Webb (1928).—Rouxeau (*Laennec avant, 1806*), Paris, 1912.—N. Orl. M. News & Hosp. Gaz., 1859–60, vi, 736–756 (A. Flint).—Conf. hist. Fac. de méd., Par., 1866, 61–107 (Chauffard).—Wash. M. Ann., 1910–11, ix, 250–260, 1 pl. (J. D. Morgan & D. S. Lamb).—Bull. Johns Hopkins Hosp., Balt., 1920, xxxi, 425–435 (W. S. Thayer).

Laguna (Andrés): Life by J. Olmedilla y Puig, Madrid, 1887.

Lamarck: Life by A. S. Packard, Lond., 1901.

Lancisi: A. Bacchini: *Il centenario lancisiano*, Roma, 1920.—Lancisi memorial number of Gior. di med. mil., Rome, 1920, lxviii, 541–642 (Marchiafava, *et al.*).—Internat. Clin., Phila., 1917, 27. s., ii, 292–308, 2 pl. (J. Foote).—Rassegna di clin. terap., Roma, 1920, xix, 97–119 (P. Capparoni).— Gior. di med. mil., Roma, 1920, lxviii, 543–636 (E. Marchiafava, *et al.*).

Lanfranc: J. Missouri M. Ass., St. Louis, 1910–11, vii, 402–408 (F. J. Lutz).

Langley: J. Physiol., Lond., 1926–7, lxi, 1–27, port. (Sir W. M. Fletcher).—Ergebn. d. Physiol., München, 1926, xxv, pp. xv–xix (R. du Bois-Reymond).

Larrey: Life by Paul Triaire, Tours, 1902.—John Hopkins Hosp. Bull., Balt., 1906, xvii, 195–215 (J. C. Da Costa).

Laveran: Bull. Soc. de path. exot., Par., 1922, xv, 373–378, port. (A. Calmette).—Ann. de l'Inst. Pasteur, Par., 1915, xxix, 405–414.—Proc. Roy. Soc., Lond., 1922, s. B., xciv, pp. xlix–liii, port. (Sir R. Ross).

Lavoisier: M. Berthelot: *La révolution chimique,* Paris, 1890.—John Hopkins Hosp. Bull., Balt., 1918, xxix, 254–264 (J. C. Hemmeter).—Scientia, Bologna, 1915, xvii, 321–327 (A. Mieli).

Leeuwenhoek: Asclepiad, Lond., 1885, ii, 319–346, port. (Sir B. W. Richardson).—J. Roy. Microsc. Soc., Lond., 1913, 121–135, port. (H. G. Plimmer).—Parasitology, Lond., 1923–4, xv, 308–319 (C. Dobell).

Leidy (Joseph): Proc. Acad. Nat. Sc., Phila., 1891, 342–388 (H. C. Chapman).—Pop. Sc. Monthly, N. Y., 1907, lxx, 311–314, port. (W. K. Brooks).—Science, N. Y., 1913, n. s., xxxvii, 809–814 (C. S. Minot); 1924, lix, 173–176 (H. F. Osborn).—Alumni Reg. Univ. Penn., Phila., 1919, xxi, 553–570 (F. H. Garrison).—J. Parasitol., Urbana, Ill., 1923–4, x, 1–21, 2 port. (H. B. Ward).

Leishman: J. Roy. Army Med. Corps, Lond., 1926, xlvii, 1–5, port.—J. Path. & Bact., Edinb., 1926, xxix, 515–528, port.

Leonardo da Vinci: See Index Catalogue, S. G. O., 1915, 2. s., xx, 256. Also: Bull. Med. Hist. Soc., Chicago, 1916, 66–83 (A. C. Klebs); Boston M. & S. J., 1916, clxxv, 1; 45 (A. C. Klebs).—Gior. di med. mil., Roma, 1919, lxvii, 1179–1281 (A. Angelucci, *et al.*).—Arch. di storia di sc., Roma, 1919, i, 157–174 (G. Bilancioni) [Bibliography], 177–185 (A. Mieli).

Lettsom: Life by T. J. Pettigrew, 3 vols., Lond., 1817.—Memoirs, Lond., 1817.—Dict. Nat. Biog., Lond., 1893, xxxiii, 134–136 (J. F. Payne).—Tr. M. Soc. Lond., 1917–18, xli, 1–61 (Sir St. C. Thompson).

Leyden: *Lebenserinnerungen,* Stuttg. u. Leipz., 1910.—Internat. Beitr. z. inn. Med., Berl., 1902, i, 1–12 port. (H. Nothnagel).—Mitt. a. d. Grenzgeb. d. Med. u. Chir., Jena, 1910, xxii, pp. i–iv (B. Naunyn).—Wien. klin. Wchnschr., 1910, xxiii, 1488–1490 (R. von Jaksch).

Liebig: Essay by T. L. W. von Bischoff, München, 1874.—Life by J. Volhard, 2 vols., Leipz., 1909.— Autobiography (Chem. News, Lond., 1891, lxiii, 265–276).—Faraday lecture by A. W. von Hofmann, Lond., 1876.—Allg. Wien. med. Ztg., 1899, xliv, 481; 494; 505; 514 (G. Klemperer).

Linacre: Sir W. Osler: Thomas Linacre, Cambridge, 1908.—Lancet, Lond,, 1928, i, 947–953 (Sir G. Newman).

Linnæus: Lives by Brightwell, London, 1858.—P. H. Malmston (Berlin, 1879).—T. M. Fries (London, 1923).—Album of Portraits by T. Tullberg., Stockh., 1907.—J. Am. M. Ass., Chicago, 1902, xxxix, 593–598 (L. Hektoen).—Janus, Amst., 1903, viii, 115–122 (W. Ebstein).—Med. Libr. & Histor. J., Brooklyn, 1904, ii, 173–184 (J. H. Hunt); 185–193 (A. Egdahl).—Proc. Wash. Acad. Sc., 1907, ix, 241–271 (E. L. Greene).

Lister (Lord): Life by Sir J. R. Godlee (London, 1917).—Collected Papers, Oxford, 1909, i, pp. i–xliv—G. T. Wrench (London, 1913). C. Dukes (London, 1924), and W. W. Cheyne (London, 1925).—J. R. Leeson: Lister as I know him, London, 1927.—Brit. M. J., Lond., 1912, i, 397–402.—Lancet, Lond., 1912, i, 465–472.—Clin. J., Lond., 1912–13, xli, 257–263 (Sir W. W. Cheyne). —Canad. J. M. & S., Toronto, 1912, xxx, 288–350 (Symposium).—Ann. Med. History, N. Y., 1919–20, ii, 93–108 (Sir St. C. Thomson).—Deutsche Ztschr. f. Chir., Leipz., 1912, cxx, 1–6 (E. Payr).—Brit. M. J., Lond., 1927, i, 656–658 (Sir B. Moynihan).—Bull. N. Y. Acad. Med., 1928, iv, 133–182 (A. Malloch et al.).

Littré: Notice by C.-A. Sainte-Beuve. Par., 1863. (Repr. from: Nouveaux lundis, v. 5, p. 200.) —Rev. d. deux mondes, Par., 1882, lii, 634–671 (C.-V. Daremberg).—Chron. méd., Par., 1895, i, 11–16, port. (Cabanès).—Bull. Acad. de méd., Par., 1919, 3. s., lxxxii, 433–458 (M. de Fleury): 1920, lxxxiii, 241–244 (Cabanès).—Isis, Brux., 1926, viii, 77–102, port. (L. Guinet).

Lobstein (Joh. Friedrich): Biography by E. Lobstein, Strassburg, 1878.

Locke (John): Janus, Amst., 1899, iv, 393; 457; 527; 579 (E. T. Withington).—Lancet, Lond., 1900, ii, 1115–1123 (Sir W. Osler).

Locy (William A.): Ann. Med. Hist., N. Y., 1925, vii, 190–192 (F. H. Garrison).

Loeb (Jacques): Sc. Progress, Lond., 1926, xx, 114–129 (T. B. Robertson).—J. Gen. Physiol., N. Y., 1925–6, viii, 654–664 (H. E. Armstrong).—Proc. Soc. Exper. Biol. & Med., N. Y., 1923–4, xxi, pp. i–xii (P. A. Levene et al.).—Naturwissenschaften, Berl., 1924, xii, 397–406 (C. Herbst).

Loeffler: Centralbl. f. Bakt., 1 Abt. Jena, 1915, lxxvi, 241–245 (Abel).—Deutsche med. Wochenschr., Leipz. & Berl., 1915, xli, 593–595 (G. Gaffky).—Parasitology, Lond., 1924–5, xvi, 241–238, port. (G. H. F. Nuttall).

Long (Crawford W.): U. S. 69. Congr. 1. Session, Senate Doc. No. 160, Washington, 1926.—Life by
F. L. Taylor, New York, 1928.—Johns Hopkins Hosp. Bull., Balt., 1897, viii, 174–184 (H. H.
Young).—Med. Press & Circ., Lond., 1916, ci, 36–38 (G. Foy).

Louis: Life by E.-J. Woillez, Par., 1873. Johns Hopkins Hosp. Bull., Balt., 1897, viii, 161–166 (Sir
W. Osler).—Colorado Med., Denver, 1926, xxiii, 269–275 (H. Sewall).

Lower (Richard): "Two Oxford Physiologists," by F. Gotch. Oxford, 1908.—Sir M. Foster. Lect.
Hist. Physiol., Cambridge, 1901, 181–185.

Ludwig (Carl): Memoir by J. von Kries. Freib. i. B. & Leipz., 1895.—Berl. klin. Wchnschr., 1895,
xxxv, 466 (H. Kronecker).—Med. Chron., Manchester, 1895–6, n. s., iii, 178–191 (W. Stirling).—
Proc. Roy. Soc. Lond., 1895–6, lix, pt. 2, pp. i–viii (Sir J. Burdon-Sanderson).—Science, N. Y.,
1916, n. s., xliv, 363–375 (W. P. Lombard).

MacCormac (Sir William): Autobiography. 2 v., London, 1884.

McDowell: Biographies by Mary Y. Ridenbaugh and A. Schachner (Philadelphia, 1922). New York,
1890.—Oration by S. D. Gross, Louisville, 1879.—Monatschr. f. Geburtsh. u. Gynäk., Berl.,
1909, xxx, 675–696 (A. Martin).

Mackenzie (Sir James): Brit. M. J., Lond., 1925, i, 242–244.—Lancet, Lond., 1925, i, 257–259.—
The Beloved Physician by R. McN. Wilson, London, 1926.

Macmichael (William): Life by F. R. Packard, The Gold-headed Cane, New York, 1915.—Dict. Nat.
Biog., Lond., 1893, xxxv, 229 (N. Moore).

Magendie: Leçon d'ouverture by Claude Bernard, Par., 1856. Éloge by P. Flourens, Par., 1858.
Also: Rep. Smithson. Inst. Wash., 1866, 91–125 (Flourens).—E. Littré: Médecine et médecins,
Par., 1872, 154–183.—Med. Libr. & Hist. J., Brooklyn, 1906, iv, 45; 198; 292; 364; 1907, v, 24,
2 port. (P. M. Dawson).—Bull. Soc. franç. d'hist. de méd., Par., 1926, xx, 251–258 (Ménétrier).

Maimonides (Moses): J. Pagel: Maimuni. Leipzig, 1908.—Studies by H. Kroner (Oberdorf-Bopfingen
1906–25).—Life by D. Yellin and I. Abrahams, Philadelphia, 1903.—Janus, Leyde, 1923, xxvii,
101; 286: 1924, xxvii, 61; 143; 193; 408; 455: 1925, xxix, 235 (H. Kroner).

Mall (Franklin Paine): Johns Hopkins Alumni Mag., Balt., 1917–18, vi, 261–263, port. (W. H.
Howell).—Bull. Johns Hopkins Hosp., Balt., 1918, xxix, 109–123.—Science, N. Y., 1918, n. s.,
xlvii, 249–254 (S. Flexner).

Malpighi: Lives by G. Atti (Bologna, 1847), E. Ferrario (Milan, 1860), U. Pizzoli (Milan, 1897),
M. Cardini (Rome, 1927).—Asclepiad, Lond., 1893, x, 385–406, port. (B. W. Richardson).—Sir M.
Foster, Lect. Hist. Physiol., Cambridge, 1901, 84–120.—Johns Hopkins Hosp. Bull., Balt., 1905,
xvii, 275–284 (W. G. MacCallum).—Ann. Med. Hist., N. Y., 1925, vii, 242–263 (J. M. Hayman).

Malthus: Life by J. Bonar, 2. ed., London, 1924.

Manson: Life by P. H. Manson-Bahr, London, 1927.

Marchand: Autobiography in: Med. d. Gegenwart, Leipz., 1923, 1–46.

Mareschal (Georges): Life by G. Mareschal de Bièvre, Paris, 1906.

Martin (Henry Newell): Proc. Roy. Soc. Lond., 1896, lx, pp. xx–xxiii (Sir M. Foster).

Martin (Sir James Ranald): Life by Sir J. Fayrer, Lond., 1897.

Matteuci (Carlo): Life by N. Bianchi, Torino, 1874.

Mattioli: Janus, Leyde, 1927, xxxi, 336–345 (H. Leclerc).

Mayow (John): "Two Oxford Physiologists" by F. Gotch. Oxford, 1908.—Sir M. Foster. Lect.
Hist. Physiol., Cambridge, 1901, 185–199.—Asclepiad, Lond., 1887, iv, 55–70, port. (B. W.
Richardson).—Dict. Nat. Biog., Lond., 1894, xxxvii, 175–177 (P. J. Hartog).

Mead: Memoirs by T. Lemon. Lond., 1755.—Gentlemen's Mag., Lond., 1754, xxiv, 510–515 (Matt-
ley).—W. McMichael and W. Munk: Gold-headed Cane. Lond., 1827, 56–118.—Asclepiad,
Lond., 1888, v, 49–79, port. (B. W. Richardson).—Dict. Nat. Biog., Lond., 1894, xxxvii, 181–186
(N. Moore).

Meltzer: Mem. Nat. Acad. Sc., Wash., 1926, xxi, 1–23, port. (W. H. Howell).

Mendel (Gregor): Life by H. Iltis, Berlin, 1924.—W. Bateson, Mendel's Principles of Heredity.
Cambridge, 1913, 327–334, 3 port.—J. J. Walsh, Catholic Churchmen in Science, Phila., 1906
195–221, port.

Mesmer: Erinnerungen by Justinus Kerner. Frankf. a. M., 1856.—F. Podmore: Mesmerism, Phila.,
1909. Life by R. Tischner, Munich, 1928. Brit. M. J., Lond., 1911, ii, 1555: 1921, i, 79; 133;
199; 249.

Metchnikoff (Elie): Life by Olga Metchnikoff, London, 1921.—A. Besredka: Histoire d'une idée,
Paris, 1921.—Ann. de l'Inst. Pasteur, Par., 1915, xxix, 357: 1916, xxx, 297.—Proc. Roy. Soc
Lond., 1917, lxxxix, pp. li–lix (Sir E. R. Lankester).

Mikulicz: Mitt. a. d. Grenzgeb. d. Med. u. Chir., Jena, 1907, Gedenkbd., 1–64, port. (W. Kausch).— München. med. Wchnschr., 1905, lii, 1297–1300, port. (Sauerbruch).—Wien. klin. Wchnschr., 1905, xviii, 671–674 (von Eiselsberg).

Minot (Charles Sedgwick): Anat. Rec., Phila., 1916, x, 133–155 [Bibliography], 156–164, port. (F. T. Lewis).—Proc. Am. Acad. Arts & Sc., Bost., 1918, liii, 841–847 (W. T. Councilman).

Mitchell (S. Weir): Memorial addresses, Phila., 1914.—Sketch by B. R. Tucker, Boston, 1914.— Brit. M. J., Lond., 1914, i, 119 (Sir W. Osler).—Nature, Lond., 1913–14, xcii, 534 (Sir L. Brunton). —Boston M. & S. J., 1914, clxx, 821–825 (J. J. Putnam).—J. Nerv. & Ment. Dis., N. Y., 1914, xli, 65–74 (C. K. Mills).

Monardes: Life by J. Olmedilla y Puig, Madrid, 1877.

Mondeville: J. L. Pagel, Leben, Lehre, und Leistungen (etc.), Berlin, 1892.—E. Nicaise's introduction to his translation of Mondeville, Paris, 1893, pp. v–lxxxii, with bibliography, pp. li–lxii.—Proc. Charaka Club, N. Y., 1910, iii, 70–98, port. (A. G. Gerster).

Montaigne: J. S. Taylor: Montaigne and Medicine, New York, 1922.

Moore (Sir Norman): Brit. M. J., Lond., 1922, ii, 1148; 1197.—St. Barth. Hosp. Rec., Lond., 1923, lvi, 95–104, port. (J. A. Ormerod).

Morestin (Hippolyte): Presse méd., Par., 1919, xxvii, annexes, 109 (J.-L. Faure).

Morgagni: F. Falk: Di pathologische Anatomie (etc.), Berlin, 1887.—Correspondence (*Carteggio inedito*), Bari, 1914.—Atti d. XI. Cong. med. internaz., 1894, Roma, 1895, i, 188–197 (R. Virchow). —Asclepiad, Lond., 1888, v, 147–173, port. (Sir B. W. Richardson).—J. J. Walsh, Makers of Modern Medicine, N. Y., 1907, 29–51.

Morgan (John): Journal of 1764, Phila., 1907.—Life by M. I. Wilbert, Phila., 1904.—Phila. J. M. & Phys. Sc., 1820, i, 439–442 (B. Rush).—Tr. Coll. Phys., Phila., 1887, centennial vol., 26–42 (W. S. W. Ruschenberger).

Morton (Richard): Med. Libr. & Hist. J., Brooklyn, 1904, ii, 1–7, port. (Sir W. Osler).

Mosso (Angelo): Arch. di fisiol., Firenze, 1910–11, ix, 121–130 (G. Funo & A. Herlitzka); [Bibliography], 131–136, port.—Lancet, Lond., 1910, ii, 1656.

Mott (Valentine): Memoir by S. D. Gross, Phila., 1868.—Bull. N. Y. Acad. Med., 1925, 2. s., i, 209–214 (F. H. Garrison).

Müller (Johannes): The recent biography by W. Haberling, Leipzig, 1924, is complete and authoritative.—Gedächtnisrede by R. Virchow, Berl., 1858 (Transl. in Edinb. M. J., 1858, iv, 452–527).— Abhandl. d. k. Akad. d. Wissensch. zu Berl. (1859), 1860, 25–191 (E. du Bois Reymond).—Johns Hopkins Hosp. Bull., Balt., 1896, vii, 16–18 (W. B. Platt).—Messenger, N. Y., 1903, 5. s., iii, 668–693 (J. J. Walsh).

Mumford (James Gregory): Boston M. & S. J., 1915, clxxii, 470–473 (R. C. Cabot).

Mundinus: Notizie by V. Joppi, Udine, 1873.—Ann. Anat. & Surg., Brooklyn, N. Y., 1882, xi, 35; 71 (G. J. Fisher).—Columbus M. J., 1896, xvii, 343–357 (J. E. Pilcher).—Med. Libr. & Hist. J., Brooklyn, N. Y., 1903, i, 1–8; 1906, iv, 311–331, 4 pl. (L. S. Pilcher).

von Muralt (Johann): Otto Obschlager: Zürich diss., 1926.

Murphy (John B.): Am. J. Obst., N. Y., 1917, lxxxv, 299–305, port. (C. W. Barrett).—Cleveland M. J., 1916, xv, 532 (G. W. Crile).—Med. Rec., N. Y., 1916, xl, 833 (G. E. Brewer).—Surg., Gynec., & Obst., N. Y., 1916, xxiii, 234 (W. J. Mayo).

Naunyn: *Erinnerungen*, München, 1925.—Med. Klin., Berl., 1925, xxi, 1866–1868 (Magnus Levy).— Deutsches Arch. f. klin. Med., Leipz., 1926, cl, 1–12 (F. Müller).

Neisser (Albert): Mitt. d. deutsch. Gesellsch. z. Bekämpf. d. Geschlechtskr., Leipz., 1916, xiv, 77–83 (A. Blaschko).—Ztschr. f. ärztl. Fortbild., Jena, 1916, xiii, 519; 545.

Nicaise: Éloge par P. Segond, Paris, 1903.

Nightingale (Florence): Life by Sir Edward Cook. 2 vols. Lond., 1913.—Nutting and Dock: History of Nursing, N. Y., 1912, 62–311.—L. Strachey: Eminent Victorians, London, 1918. 135–203.

Nocard: Bull. Soc. centr. de méd. vét., Par., 1924, lxxvii, 576–595 (Leclainche).

Noeggerath: Klin. Wchnschr., Berl., 1927, vii, 1926 (P. Diepgen).—München. med. Wochenschr., 1927, lxxiv, 1677 (Zinsser).—Ann. Med. Hist., N. Y., 1928, xi, 770–779 (H. S. Reichle).

Noguchi: Brit. M. J., Lond., 1928, i, 961.—J. A. M. A., Chicago, 1928, xc, 1727.

North (Elisha): Johns Hopkins Hosp. Bull., Balt., 1908, xix, 301–307 (W. R. Steiner).—Ann. Med. Hist., N. Y., 1924, vi, 245–257 (F. L. Pleadwell).

Nothnagel: Obituary by B. Naunyn, 1905. Biography by Max Neuburger, Vienna, 1922.—Wien. med. Wochenschr., 1910, lx, 2682–2688 (R. von Jaksch).

O'Dwyer (Joseph): Pediatrics, N. Y. & Lond., 1898, v, 95–97, port. (A. Jacobi).—J. J. Walsh: Makers of Modern Medicine, N. Y., 1907, 325–356.

Oken (Lorenz): Alexander Ecker: Lorenz Oken, Transl. by A. Fulk, London, 1883.

Oppolzer: Wien. klin. Wochenschr., 1908, xxi, 1109–1115 (M. Benedikt).—Mitt. z. Gesch. d. Med., Leipz., 1919, xviii, 170; 366 (E. Ebstein).

Orfila: Progrès méd., Par., 1927, xlii, 667–671 (Ménétrier).

Osler: Biography by Harvey Cushing; 2 v., Oxford Univ. Press, 1924.—Bull. No. IX, Internat. Assoc. Med. Mus. (edited by Maude Abbott), 2. ed. Montreal, 1927.—Brit. M. J., Lond., 1920, i, 21; 30; 64, port.—Nature, Lond., 1919–20, cv, 472 (Sir T. C. Allbutt).—Nation, N. Y., 1920, cx, 104–106 (W. S. Thayer).—Science, N. Y., 1920, n. s., li, 55–58 (F. H. Garrison).—Ann. Med. History, N. Y., 1919–20, ii, 157–187 (H. Cushing, et al.).—Therap. Gaz., Phila., 1920, 3. s., xxxvi, 160–164 (H. A. Hare).—Johns Hopkins Hosp. Bull., Balt., 1919, xxx, 195–218, 9 port. [Bibliography by Minnie Blogg, 219–233].—J. Canad. M. Ass., 1920.—München. med. Wochenschr., 1920, lxvii, 263 (F. Müller).—Bull. N. Y. Acad. Med., 1926, ii, 539–546 (F. H. Garrison).

Owen: Life by R. Owen. 2 v., Lond., 1895.—Proc. Roy. Soc. Lond., 1894, lv, suppl., pp. i–xiv (W. H. F.).—Johns Hopkins Hosp. Bull., Balt., 1911, xxii, 133–137 (C. W. G. Rohrer).

Pacini: Riv. d. storia d. sc. med. e nat., Siena, 1923, xiv, 182–212 (L. Castaldi).

Pagel (Julius): München. med. Wchnschr., 1912, lix, 425, port. (K. Sudhoff).—Klin.-therap. Wchnschr., Berl., 1912, xix, 205–208 (I. Bloch).—Arch. f. Gesch. d. Med., Leipz., 1912–13, vi, 71–79 (P. Richter).—J. Missouri M. Ass., St. Louis, 1913, ix, 366–369 (G. Dock).—Janus, Leyde, 1926, xxx, 179–191 (A. Pagel).

Pagenstecher: Lebenserennerungen, Leipzig, 1913.

Paget (Sir James): Memoirs and Letters by Stephen Paget, London, 1901.—Dict. Nat. Biog., Lond., 1901, suppl. iii, 240–242 (D'A. Power).—St. Barth. Hosp. J., Lond., 1901–2, ix, 17–21 (S. Paget).— Tr. Rhode Island M. Soc., 1902, Providence, 1903, vi, 504–525 (Helen C. Putnam).

Pappenheim (Arthur): Folia hæmatol., Leipz., 1916–17, xxi, pt. 1, 79–90 (T. Brugsch).

Paracelsus: Studies and biographies by: K. F. H. Marx (Göttingen, 1842), F. Mook (Würzb., 1876), J. Ferguson (Glasg., 1877–85), F. Hartmann (Lond., 1887), E. Schubert & K. Sudhoff (Frankf. a. M., 1887–9), K. Sudhoff (Versuch, Berl., 1894–9), F. Hartmann (Leipz., 1899), H. Magnus (Breslau, 1906), E. Schlegel (München, 1908), Anna M. Stoddart (Lond., 1911), and J. M. Stillman, Chicago, 1920. Also: Arch. f. d. ges. Med., Jena, 1841, i, 26–43 (H. Haeser).—Cor.-Bl. f. Schweiz. Aerzte, Basel, 1905, xxxi, 438–488 (M. Roth).—Zentralbl. f. Biblioth.-Wes., Leipz., 1893, x, 316; 385; xi, 169 (K. Sudhoff).—Isis, 1913–14, i, 62–94 (E. Radl).

Paré: Lives by J. F. Malgaigne (Œuvres complètes, Paris, 1840, i), Le Paulmier (Paris, 1884), S. Paget (London, 1897), F. R. Packard, New York, 1921. Also, Am. M.-Chir. Rev., Phila., 1869, v, 1059–1083 (S. D. Gross).

Parkes: J. Roy. Army Med. Corps, Lond., 1910, xiv, 227–231 (L. C. Parkes).

Parkinson: Johns Hopkins Hosp. Bull., Balt., 1912, xxiii, 33–45 (L. G. Rowntree).

Parry: Ann. Med. Hist., N. Y., 1925, vii, 205–215 (Sir H. Rolleston).

Pasteur: R. Vallery-Radot: La vie de Pasteur, Paris, 1900 (English transl., 2 v., Lond., 1911).— Lives by Mr. and Mrs. Percy Frankland (London, 1898), Stephen Paget (London, 1914), Émile Duclaux (English translation, Philadelphia, 1920), L. Descour (Paris, 1921, English translation, London, 1922), Louis Lumet (2. ed., Paris, 1923). Also: Rev. scient., Paris, 1895, 4. s., iv, 417–431 (Richet & Renan).—Berl. klin. Wchnschr., 1895, xxxii, 947 (R. Virchow).—Johns Hopkins Hosp. Bull., Balt., 1903, xiv, 325–334 (C. A. Herter).—Rev. de méd., Par., 1923, xl, 257; 330; 405 (C. Richet).

Patin (Guy): Lives by P. Pic, Paris, 1911; F. R. Packard, New York, 1925.

Pavloff: Boston M. & S. J., 1916, clxxiv, 799 (F. G. Benedict).—Brit. M. J., 1916, ii, 799 (W. M. Bayliss).—Med. Rev. of Rev., N. Y., 1916, xxii, 252–259 (V. Robinson).—Nature, Lond., 1916, xcvii, 9–11 (W. H. T.).—Bull. Battle Creek San. & Hosp. Clin., 1923–4, xix, 5–18.

Pavy (F. W.): Guy's Hosp. Rep., Lond., 1912, lxvi, 1–23 (F. Taylor).—Sc. Progress 20. Cent., Lond., 1912–13, vii, 13–47 (F. G. Hopkins).

Payne: Brit. M. J., Lond., 1910, ii, 1749–1754.

Payr: Autobiography in: Med. d. Gegenwart (Grote), Leipz., 1924, iii, 121–164, port.

Peachy (John): Janus, Leyden, 1918, xxiii, 121–158 (G. C. Peachey).

Pecquet: Jean Lucq. Paris diss., 1925, No. 22.—Bull. Soc. d. sc. méd. et biol. de Montpellier, 1921–2, iii, 32–60 (P. Gilis).

Pepper (William): Lives by F. N. Thorpe (Phila., 1904) and J. Tyson (Phila., 1901). Also Phila. M. J., 1899, iii, 607–611 (Sir W. Osler).

Percy: Life by C. Laurent, Versailles, 1827.

Perthes (Georg): Deutsche Ztschr. f. Chir., Leipz., 1927, cc, pp. xiii–xvi (F. Sauerbruch).

Peter of Abano: S. Ferreri: *Per la biografia*, Rome, 1918.—Ann. Med. Hist., N. Y., 1924, vi, 25, 53 (H. M. Brown).

Peters (Hermann): Ber. d. deutsch. pharm. Gesellsch., 1920, xxx, 333–339 (H. Schelenz).

Petersen (Jacob Julius): Janus, Haarlem, 1912, xvii, 357–362 (J. W. S. Johnsson).

Pettenkofer: Memoirs by C. von Voit (München, 1902), O. Neustätter (Wien, 1926), and E. E. Hume (New York, Hoeber, 1927).—Berl. klin. Wchnschr., 1901, xxxviii, 268; 301; 321 (M. Rubner).

Peyer (Joh. Conrad): Janus, Leyden, 1914, xix, 61–83 (R. Lang).

Pflüger: Memoir by M. Nussbaum. Bonn, 1909.—Arch. f. d. ges. Physiol., Bonn, 1910, cxxxii, 1–19 (E. von Cyon).

von Pfolspeundt (H.): Janus, Leyden, 1913, 109–119 (F. J. Lutz).

Pilcher (Louis Stephen): A Surgical Pilgrim's Progress, Philadelphia, 1925.

Pinel: R. Semelaigne: Paris diss., 1888, No. 166. Also his *Aliénistes et philanthropes*, Paris, 1912.— Mem. Acad. de méd., Par., 1828, i, 189–223 (E. Pariset); 224–231 (Esquirol).—Ann. méd.-psych., Par., 1885, 7. s., ii, 185–193 (A. Ritti): 1927, lxxxv, pt. 2, 30–89 (P. Courbon, *et al.*).—F. Tiffany: Philippe Pinel. [n. p., 1898].

Pirogoff: Autobiography (*Lebensfragen*), Stuttgart, J. G. Cotta, 1894.—Kazan. Med. Jour., 1911, xi, 171; 225; 299: 1912, xii, 53; 120; 196.—Med. & Surg., St. Louis, 1917, i, 5–13 (W. P. Coues).

Platter: *Selbstbiographie*, ed. by H. Boos, Leipzig, 1878.—*Tagebuchblätter*, ed. by H. Kohl, Leipzig, 1913.

Politzer: Monatschr. f. Ohrenh., Berl. & Wien, 1920, liv, 769–771 (V. Urbantschitsch).

Poncet (Antonin): Lyon chir., 1913, x, 329–336 (P. Leriche).

della Porta (G. B.): Am. Naturalist, Lancaster, Pa., 1918, lii, 455–461 (T. Holm).—L'Anomalo, Napoli, 1917, xiv, 161–224 (A. Zuccarelli, *et al.*).

Post (Wright): Memoir by Valentine Mott, N. Y., 1829.

Pott: Life by Sir J. Earle, prefacing Pott's "Chirurgical Works," London, 1790, i, pp. i–xlv.—Dict. Nat. Biog., Lond., 1896, xlvi, 207 (D'A. Power).—St. Barth. Hosp. Rep., Lond., 1894, xxx, 163–167 (Horder).—Boston M. & S. J., 1915, clxxii, 807–812 (R. W. Lovett).

Power (Henry): Autobiography. (Stratford-upon-Avon, 1912.)

Pozzi: Bull. Acad. de méd., Par., 1918, 3. s., lxxix, 448–452 (Hayem).

Pravaz: Paris méd., 1924, liv (annexes), 334–337.

Preuss (Julius): München. med. Wochenschr., 1914, lxi, 78 (Sudhoff).

Priessnitz: Biography by Philo vom Walde (Berlin, 1899).

Priestley (Joseph): Memoirs, Northumberland, 1806. Also: Pop. Sc. Monthly, N. Y., 1875, vi 90–107 (T. H. Huxley).

Pringle: Pettigrew: Med. Port. Gallery, Lond., 1840, ii, No. 14.—Dict. Nat. Biog., Lond., 1896, xlvi, 386 (J. F. Payne).

Prudden: Biographical Sketches, New Haven, 1927.

Purkinje: J. Am. M. Ass., Chicago, 1899, xxxii, 812–814 (R. Burton Opitz).—Arch. f. Krim.-Anthrop. u. Kriminalist., Leipz., 1906, xxii, 326–335 (G. Roscher).—Valuable analysis of his works by Th. Eiselt in: Vrtljschr. f. d. prakt. Heilk., Prag., 1859, lxiii, Beil., 1–20. Skandin. Arch. f. Physiol., Leipz., 1918, xxxvii, 1–116, 5 pl. (E. Thomsen).

Puschmann: München. med. Wochenschr., 1906, liii, 1–14 (Sudhoff).

Quatrefages: Bull. Soc. franç. d'hist. de méd., Par., 1926, xx, 309: 1927, xxi, 17; 201 (G. Herve & L. de Quatrefages).

Rabelais: F. Brémond: *Rabelais médecin*, Paris, 1879–88.—A. Heulhard: *Rabelais chirurgien*, Paris, 1885, and references in Index Catalogue.

Radcliffe: Life by J. B. Nias. Oxford, 1918.

Ramazzini: Franz Koelsch: Bernardino Ramazzini, Stuttgart, 1912. Also the Italian biographies of Maggiora (Modena, 1902–18), Piccinini (Milan, 1907), and Devoto (Genoa, 1923).

Ramón y Cajal: Autobiography (*Recuerdos de mi Vida.* 2 v., Madrid, 1901–17). Also (Abstract) in: Med. d. Gegenwart (Grote), Leipz., 1925, v, 131–176, port.—Arch. Neurol. & Psychiat., Chicago, 1926, xvi, 213–220 (W. Penfield).

Ranvier: Compt. rend. Soc. de biol., Par., 1922, lxxxvi, 1144–1152 (J. Nageotte).—Arch. d'anat. micr., Par., 1923, xix, No. 1, pp. i–lxxii (J. Jolly).

Rasori: Osp. maggiore, Milan, 1918, vi, 60–69 (C. Pasetti).

Récamier: P. Triaire: *Récamier et ses contemporains.* (Paris, 1899.)

Recklinghausen: Anat. Anz., Jena, 1910, xxxvii, 509–511 (Waldeyer).—Verhandl. d. deutsch. path. Gesellsch., Jena, 1912, xv, 478–488 (H. Chiari).—Proc. Am. Acad. Arts & Sc., Bost., 1918, liii, 872–875 (W. T. Councilman).

Redi: Life by Viviani (Arezzo, 1924).—Riv. di storia crit. di sc. med. e nat., Siena, 1922, xiii, 62–85 (G. M. Piccinini), 86–93 (A. Corsini): 1927, xviii, 167–193 (A. Ruzzauti).—Med. ital., Milano, 1925, vi, 251–261 (D. Barduzzi).—Scientia, Roma, 1927, xli, 25–34 (M. Cardini).—Ann. Med. Hist., N. Y., 1926, viii, 347–359 (R. Cole).

Reed (Walter): Biography by H. A. Kelly, Balt., 3. ed., 1923.—J. Hyg., Cambridge, 1903, iii, 292–296, port. (G. H. F. Nuttall).—Pop. Sc. Month., N. Y., 1904, lxv, 262–268 (W. D. McCaw).

Reil (Joh. Christian): Memoir by Heinrich Steffens, Halle, 1815.—*Gedenkrede* by Max Neuburger, Stuttgart, 1913.—*Gedächtnisrede* by R. C. A. C. Beneke, Halle a. S., 1913.—J. Nerv. & Ment. Dis., N. Y., 1916, xliii, 1–22 (W. A. White).

Remak (Robert): Berl. klin. Wchnschr., 1865, ii, 372.—Wien. med. Presse, 1865, xxxvii, 915 (M. Benedikt).

Renaudot (Théophraste): Life by G. Gilles de la Tourette. Par., 1884.—Gaz. d'hôp., Par., 1927, c, 605–609 (E. Forgue).—Albany M. Ann., 1907, xxviii, 599–623 (C. G. Cumston).

Retzius (Anders Adolf): Ann. Med. Hist., N. Y., 1924, vi, 16–24 (O. Larsell).

Retzius (Gustav Magnus): Anat. Anz., Jena, 1919–20, liii, 261–268 (Waldeyer-Hartz).—Nature, Lond., 1919–20, ciii, 448 (Sir A. Keith).—Scient. Month., 1920, x, 559–569 (O. Larsell).—Proc. Roy. Soc. Lond., 1920, xci, Obit. Notices, pp. xxxvi–xxxviii (E. A. Schäfer).

Rhazes: Proc. XVII Internat. Cong. Med., 1913, Lond., 1914, Sect. XXIII, 237–268 (G. S. A. Ranking).

Ricardus Anglicus: H. H. Beusing. Leipzig diss., 1922.—Dict. Nat. Biog., Lond., 1896, xlviii, 201 (C. L. Kingsford).—Janus, Leyde, 1924, xxviii, 397–403 (K. Sudhoff).

Richardson (Sir B. W.): *Vita medica,* New York, 1897.

Richet (Charles): Progrès méd., Par., 1926, xli, 792–803 (E. Gley); 803–806 (A. Philibert).

Richter (August Gottlieb): H. Rohlfs, Gesch. d. deutsch. Med., Leipz., 1883, iii, 33–172.

Ringer (Sidney): Proc. Roy. Soc. Lond., 1912, s. B., lxxxiv, pp. i–iii, port. (E. A. S.).—Biochem. J. Liverp., 1910–11, v, pp. i–xix (B. Moore).

Rivers (William H. R.): Brit. M. J., Lond., 1922, i, 936; 977.—Proc. Roy. Soc. Lond., 1923–4, s. B. xcv, pp. xliii–xlvii, port. (H. Head).

Robin (Charles): Bull. Soc. franç. d'hist. de méd., Par., 1925, xix, 8–15 (G. Variot).—Progrès méd., 1925, xl (suppl.), 65–67.

Rokitansky: Festreden, Wien. klin. Wchnschr., 1898, xi, 559–564.—Wien. med. Presse, 1874, xv, Fest-Nummer, 1–8 (J. Schnitzler); 1878, xix, 865–974 (Arneth); 1549–1554 (T. Meynert).—Prag. med. Wchnschr., 1878, iii, 309 (E. Klebs).—Allg. Wien. med. Ztg., 1879, xxiv, 141–143 (S. Stricker).

Röntgen: Strahlentherapie, Berl. & Wien, 1923, xv, 855–863 (W. Friedrich).—Wien. klin. Wochenschr., 1923, xxxvi, 432–435 (A. Eiselsberg).—Radiology, St. Paul, 1925, iv, 63; 139; 249 (I. S. Hirsch).

Roonhuyse: Nederl-Tijdschr. v. Geneesk., Haarlem, 1922, xvi, pt. 1, 856–874 (E. D. Baumann).

Rose (Valentin): Zentralbl. f. Bibliothekswesen, Leipz., 1917, xxxiv, 168–182 (E. Jacobs).

Röslin (Eucharius): Arch. f. Gesch. d. med., Leipz., 1907–8, i, 429–441 (K. Baas).

Ross (Sir Ronald): Memoirs, London, 1923.

Roux (César): Rev. méd. de la Suisse Rom., Genevè, 1927, xlvii, 121–145 (L. Perret).

Roux (Wilhelm): Autobiography in: Med. d. Gegenwart, Leipz., 1923, i, 141–206, port.—Anat. Anz., Jena, 1924–5, lix, 156–176 (D. Barfuth).

Ruffer (Sir M. A.): Ann. Med. History, N. Y., 1917–18, i, 218–220 (F. H. Garrison).

Rumford (Count): Bull. Soc. med. Hist., Chicago, 1913, i, 224–236 (H. M. Lyman).

Rush (Benjamin): Life by H. C. Goods, Berne, Indiana, 1918.—Recollections by J. C. Lettsom, Lond., 1915.—Reminiscences by T. D. Mitchell, Transylvania J. Med., Lexington, Ky., 1839, xii, 92–116.—S. D. Gross. Lives, etc., Phila., 1861, 17–85, port. (S. Jackson).—Asclepiad, Lond., 1885, ii, 38–57, port. (Sir B. W. Richardson).—J. Am. M. Ass., Chicago, 1889, xiii, 330–335 (H. R. Storer).—Med.-Leg. J., N. Y., 1886–7, iv, 238–273, port. (C. K. Mills).

Sahli: Autobiography. Med. d. Gegenwart (Grote), Leipz., 1925, v, 177–235, port.

Sainte-Beuve: Studies by F.-F.-E. Voizard, Paris, 1911, and G. Morin, Paris, 1928.—Gaz. hebd. d. sc. méd. de Bordeaux, 1919, xl, 342 (J. Sabrazès).—Presse méd., Par., 1919, xxvii, 961 (Laignel-Lavastine).

Salkowski: Biochem. Ztschr., Berl., 1923, cxxxviii, 1–4 (C. N.).

Sanctorius: Biography by A. Castiglioni (Bologna, 1920).—Resoc. r. Accad. med-chir. di Napoli (1889), 1890, xliii, 58–113 (M. del Gaizo).—Tr. Cong. Am. Phys. & Surg., 1891, N. Haven, 1892, ii, 188–198 (Weir Mitchell).—Illustr. med. ital., Genova, 1920, ii, 26–29 (A. Vedrani).—Riv. di storia d. sc. med. e nat., Siena, 1924, xv, 227–237 (D. Giordano & A. Castiglioni).

Sanderson (Sir John Burdon): Memoir by Lady Sanderson, Oxford, 1911.

Santorini: Atti r. Ist. veneto. di sc., 1915–16, lxxv, 1163–1188 (G. Cagnetto).

Saxtorph: Arch. mens. d'obst. et gynéc., Par., 1914, 192–232 (E. Ingerslev).

Scarpa: Discourse by S. Liberali, Treviso, 1834.—Mem. Acad. de méd., Par., 1838, vii, 1–28 (E. Pariset).—Asclepiad, Lond., 1886, iii, 128–148, port (Sir B. W. Richardson).

Schaudinn: Biography by Prowazek in his: Arbeiten, Hamb. & Leipz., 1911, pp. v–xii, port.

Schelenz (Hermann): Janus, Leyden, 1918, xxiii, 1–4, port. (J. W. S. Johnsson).—Ber. d. deutsch. pharm. Gesellsch., Berl., 1922, xxxii, 225–228 (G. Urdang).

Schiller: Index Catalogue, 2. s., xv, 201–202.

Schleich (Carl Ludwig): *Besonnte Vergangenheit*, Berlin, 1923.

Schmidt-Rimpler: Klin. Monatsbl. f. Augenh., Stuttg., 1916, xvi, 102–119 (T. Axenfeld).

Schmiedeberg: Arch. f. exper. Path. u. Pharmakol., Leipz., 1921, xc, pp. i–viii (Naunyn): 1922, xcii, pp. i–xvii (H. H. Meyer).

Schönlein: Gedächtnisrede by R. Virchow. Berl., 1865.—Berl. klin. Wchnschr., 1864, i, 276–279 (C. Griesinger).—Wien. med. Wchnschr., 1864, xiv, 107 (Frerichs).—Ztschr. f. klin. Med., Berl., 1910, lxxi, 471–477 (E. Ebstein).—Arch. f. Gesch. d. Med., Leipz., 1911–12, v, 449; 1915–16, ix, 209, 1 pl. (E. Ebstein).

Schultze (Max): Arch. f. mikr. Anat., Bonn, 1874, x, pp. i–xxiii, port. (G. Schwalbe).

Schulze (Joh. Heinrich): Life by J. M. Eder (Vienna, 1917).

Schwann: *Liber memorialis.* Düsseldorf, 1879.—Arch. f. mikr. Anat. Bonn, 1882–3, xxi, pp. i–xlix (J. Henle); 1909, lxxiv, 469–473, port. (O. Hertwig & W. Waldeyer).—Arch. f. path. Anat. (etc.), Berl., 1882, lxxxvii, 389–392 (R. Virchow).—Ztschr. f. physiol. Chem., Strassb., 1882, vi, 280–285 (A. Kossel).—Nature, Lond., 1881–2, xxv, 321–323 (Sir E. R. Lankester).—München. med. Wochenschr., 1910, lvii, 2703–2705 (K. Sudhoff).

Sedgwick (William Thompson): Biography by E. O. Jordan, G. C. Whipple, and C.-E.-A. Winslow, New Haven, Yale Press, 1924.

Semmelweis: Life by Sir J. W. Sinclair. Manchester, 1909.—Semmelweis Denkmal, Budapest, 1909.—Studies by A. Hegar (1882), J. Bruck (Wien. 1887), J. Grosse (Leipz. & Wien, 1898), F. Schürer von Waldheim (Wien & Leipzig, 1905) and Th. Malade (München, 1924).—Med. Rev. of Rev., N. Y., 1912, xviii, 232–246 (V. Robinson).—Ztschr. f. Geburtsh. u. Gynäk., Stuttg., 1924, lxxxviii, 314–334 (G. Sticker).—Ann. Med. Hist., N. Y., 1924, vi, 258–279 (P. M. Dawson).

Semon (Sir Felix): Autobiography, London, 1926.—P. McBride, Semon Lectures, London, 1913.

Senator: *Gedächtnisrede* by A. Goldscheider, Berl. klin. Wchnschr., 1911, xlviii, 1961–1968. Also: München. med. Wchnschr., 1911, lviii, 1733–1735 (A. Wolff-Eisner).

Sertürner: Biography by Franz Krömeke, Jena, 1925. Ber. d. deutsch. pharm. Gesellsch., 1917, xxvii, 500–507 (C. Stich): 1918, xxviii, 275–300 (H. Schelenz).

Servetus: Servetus and Calvin by Robert Willis, Lond., 1877.—Johns Hopkins Hosp. Bull., Balt., 1901, xxi, 1–11, 4 pl. (Sir W. Osler).—Janus, Leyde, 1915, xx, 331–360, 9 pl. (J. C. Hemmeter).—Osler Anniversary Volumes, N. Y., 1919, ii, 767–777 (L. L. Mackall).

Simpson (Sir James Y.): Lives by J. Duns (Edinb., 1873), Eva B. Simpson (Lond., 1896), and H. L. Gordon (Lond., 1897). Also Edinb. M. J., 1911, n. s., vi, Memorial No., 481–560, 9 pl.; vii, 12–17 (H. R. Storer); 505–512 (F. W. N. Haultain).

Sims (James Marion): "The Story of my Life" (N. Y., 1884).—"*Ueber Marion Sims*" by R. Olshausen (Berl., 1897).—Am. J. Obst., N. Y., 1884, xvii, 52–61, port. (P. F. Mundé).—Alabama M. & S. Age, Anniston, 1893–4, vi, 607–616 (T. A. Means).—Med. Rec., N. Y., 1894, xlvi, 705–708 (E. Souchon).—N. Orl. M. & S. J., 1895–6, n. s., xxiii, 455–460, 3 pl. (E. Souchon).—Ztschr. f. Geburtsh. u. Gynäk., Stuttg., 1913, lxxiii, 946–948 (A. Martin).

Skoda: Life by M. Sternberg, Wien, 1924.

Smellie: *William Smellie and his Contemporaries* by John Glaister, Glasgow, 1894. Memoir in: "Works" (New Sydenham Soc., 1876, vi) by A. H. McClintock.—St. Thomas's Hosp. Gaz., Lond., 1914, xxiv, 85–91 (J. S. Fairbairn).—Am. J. Obst., N. Y., 1919, lxxx, 150–160, port, 1 pl.

Smith (Nathan): Life and letters by Emily A. Smith, New Haven, 1914.

Smith (Stephen): Ann. Med. Hist., New York, 1917, i, 318–322 (F. H. Garrison).

Soemmerring: Life by W. Stricker (Frankf. a. M., 1862).—Ann. Med. Hist., N. Y., 1924, vi, 369–386, port. (T. H. Bast).

Soranus of Ephesus: Samml. klin. Vortr., Leipz., 1902, n. F., No. 335 (Gynäk. No. 121), 703–744 (J. Lachs).—Abhandl. d. K. sächs. Gesellsch. d. Wissensch., phil.-hist. Kl., Dresd., 1910, xxvii, No. 2 (J. Ilberg).—Proc. XVII Internat. Cong. Med., 1913, Lond., 1914, Sect. XXIII, 269–283 (A. H. F. Barbour).

Spalding (Lyman): Life by J. A. Spalding, Boston, 1916.

Spallanzani: J.-L. Alibert: Éloges historiques, Paris, 1806, 1–186.—J. Rosenwald. Paris diss., 1912, No. 59.—Sc. Progress, London, 1916, xl, 236–245 (B. Cummins).—Ann. Med. Hist., N. Y., 1924, vi, 177–186 (G. E. Burget).

Spens (Thomas): Edinb. M. J., 1914, n. s., xii, 51–55 (C. E. Lea).

Stahl: A. Lemoine: *Stahl et l'animisme* (Paris, 1858).—Arch. f. Gesch. d. Med., Leipz., 1926, xviii, 20–50 (R. Koch).

Starling: Brit. M. J., Lond., 1927, i, 900–906. Lancet, Lond., 1927, i, 1003.

Steinschneider (Moritz): Biog. Jahrb., 1907, Berl., 1909, xii, 171–175 (J. Pollak).—Bibliography by G. A. Kohut in: Steinschneider-Festschrift, Leipzig, 1896.

Stensen: Opera v. I (Copenhagen, 1909).—Sir M. Foster: Lect. Hist. Physiol., Cambridge, 1901, 106–110.—Med. Libr. & Hist. J., Brooklyn, 1904, ii, 166–182, port. (F. J. Lutz).—J. J. Walsh, Catholic Churchmen in Science, Phila., 1906, 137–166, port.—Johns Hopkins Hosp. Bull., Balt., 1914, xxv, 44–51 (W. S. Miller).

Sternberg (George M.): Biography by Martha L. Sternberg (Chicago, 1921).—Tr. Am. Soc. Trop. Med., N. Orl., 1916, x, 19–26 (E. L. Munson).—Bull. Johns Hopkins Hosp., Balt., 1921, xxxii, 1–5 (H. A. Kelly).

Stokes (Adrian): Guy's Hosp. Rep., Lond., 1928, lxxxviii, 1–17 (Sir W. Dunn).

Stokes (William): Life by Sir W. Stokes (Lond., 1897).—Dublin J. M. Sc., 1878, lxv, 186–200 (J. W. Moore).—Med. Hist. Meath Hosp., Dubl., 1888, 129–136, 1 pl.

Stoll: V. Fossel: Stud. z. Gesch. d. Med., Stuttg., 1909, 153–191.

Storer (Horatio R.): Boston M. & S. J., 1922, clxxxvii, 522: 1923, clxxxviii, 118.

Stromeyer: H. Rohlfs. Gesch. d. deutsch. Med., Leipz., 1885, iv, 139–260.—Wien. med. Wchnschr., 1876, xxxvi, 1064 (T. Billroth).

Strümpell: Autobiography, Leipzig, 1925.—E. Payr: *Gedächtnistede*, Leipzig, 1925.

Struensee: Bull. soc. franç. d'hist. de la med., Par., 1923, xvii, 232–237 (A. Lutaud).

Sudhoff: München. med. Wochenschr., 1923, lxx, 1414–1416 (P. Diepgen).—Bull. Soc. Med. Hist., Chicago, 1923, iii, 1–32 (F. H. Garrison); Bibliography, 33–50 (F. H. Garrison & A. N. Tasker).—Arch. di storia d. sc., Roma, 1924, v, 139–147 (H. E. Sigerist).

Süssmilch (J. P.): Publ. Am. Statist. Ass., Boston, 1900–1901, vii, 67–46 (F. S. Crum).

Swammerdam: Werk. v. h. Genootsch. t. Bevord. d. Nat.-Genees- en Heelk. te Amst., 1880, v, 1–64 (B. J. Stokvis).—Æsculape, Par., 1912, ii, 171–176 (H. Bouquet). See, also: novel "Swammerdam" by H. Klencke, 3 v. (Leipz., 1860).

van Swieten: Janus, Leyde, 1922, xxvi, 177–189 (V. Kreuzinger), Paris méd., 1922, xliv, annexe, 3–9 (A. Gilbert & P. Cornet).

Sydenham: Lives by J. F. Payne (Lond., 1900) and David Riesman (New York, 1926).—Tercentenary tribute by Sir G. Newman.—J. Brown: Horæ subsecivæ, Lond., 1858, 1–98.—K. Knav, Berlin diss., 1911.—Deutsche med. Wchnschr., Leipz., 1889, xv, 1068–1070 (Pagel).—Asclepiad, Lond., 1892, ix, 385–401, port., pl. (Sir B. W. Richardson).—Med. News, Phila., 1894, lxv, 234–236 (Sir H. Acland).—Janus, Amst., 1898, iii, 4–11 (J. F. Payne).—Bull. Acad. de méd., Par., 1924, 3. s., xci, 629–651.—Presse méd., Par., 1924, xxxii, 453–456 (A. Chauffard).—Klin. Wochenschr., Berl., 1924, iii, 1700–1703.—München. med. Wochenschr., 1924, lxxi, 1322–1324 (K. Sudhoff).—M. Greenwood on Sydenham as epidemiologist (Proc. Roy. Soc. Med., Lond., 1918–19, xii, Sect. Epidemiol., 55–76).

Sylvius (Franciscus): Sir M. Foster. Lect. Hist. Physiol., Cambridge, 1901, 145–173.—Johns Hopkins Hosp. Bull., Balt., 1909, xx, 329–339 (F. Baker).—Proc. Charaka Club, N. Y., 1910, iii, 14–28, 2 pl. (S. E. Jelliffe).

Syme: Memorials by R. Paterson, Edinb., 1874.

Tagliacozzi: Ann. Otol., Rhinol. & Laryngol., St. Louis, 1918, xxvii, 505–527 (M. and I. Frank).

Tait (Lawson): Life by W. J. S. McKay, London, 1922.—Brit. M. J., Lond., 1899, i, 1561–1564.—J. Am. M. Assoc., Chicago, 1899, xxxiii, 875–880 (C. A. L. Reed).—J. Obst. & Gynæc., Brit. Empire, Lond., 1921, n. s., xxviii, 117–123 (C. Martin).

Testut: Bull. Acad. de méd., Par., 1925, 3. s., xciii, 110–112.

Thackrah: J. Industrial Hyg., Boston, 1920, i, 578–581 (T. M. Legge).

Theophrastus of Eresos: E. L. Greene. Landmarks of Botanical History, Wash., 1909, i, 52–142.

Thiersch (Carl): Life by Justus Thiersch. Leipzig, 1922.

Thomas (Hugh Owen): Brit. M. J., Lond., 1896, ii, 71: 1917, ii, 175 (J. L. Thomas).—Orthop. Surg. (Jones), Lond., 1921, i, 3–23 (A. Keith).

Todd (Eli): Am. J. Insan., Balt., 1912–13, lxix, 761–785 (C. W. Page).

Toldt (Carl): *Autobiographie*, Berlin, 1922.

Tommasi: Bull. d. Mus. di zoöl., Torino, 1924, xxix, n. s., No. 15, 1–24 (G. Pierantoni).—Illustr. med. ital., Genova, 1921, iii, 114–117 (F. Del Greco).

Traube (Ludwig): Berl. klin. Wchnschr., 1876, xiii, 209 (R. Virchow).—Charité Ann., 1875, Berl., 1877, ii, 767–800, port. (E. Leyden).—Deutsche med. Wochenschr., Leipz. & Berl., 1918, xliv, 21–23 (W. Haberling).

Trendelenburg: Autobiography, Berlin, 1924.—Arch. f. klin. Chir., Berl., 1925, cxxxiv, pp. i–vi (W. Körte).—Deutsche med. Wochenschr., Leipz. & Berl., 1925, li, 279 (G. Perthes).

Tronchin: Life by H. Tronchin, Par., 1906.—Arch. f. Gesch. d. Med., Leipz., 1907–8, i, 81; 289 (A. Geyl).—Brit. M. J., Lond., 1913, ii, 133–136.—Paris méd., 1918, xxviii, suppl., 195–199.

Trotter (Thomas): J. Roy. Nav. M. Serv., Lond., 1919, v, 412–419 (Sir H. D. Rolleston).

Trousseau: P. Triaire: Bretonneau et ses correspondants, 2 v. (Paris, 1892).—Internat. Clin., Phila., 1916, 26. s., iii, 284–303 (F. H. Garrison).

Trudeau: Biography by S. Chalmers, Boston, 1916, Bull. Johns Hopkins Hosp., Balt., 1916, xxvii, 86–107 (W. B. James [et al.].—J. Am. M. Ass., Chicago, 1916, lxvi, 244–246 (S. A. Knopf).

Tschirch: *Erlebtes und Erstrebtes*, Bonn, 1921.

Tuke: R. Semelaigne: *Aliénistes et philanthropes*, Paris, 1912, 323–398.

Turner (Daniel): Ann. Med. Hist., N. Y., 1919, ii, 367–380 (J. E. Lane).

Turner (Sir William): Life by A. Logan Turner (Edinburgh, 1919).—Proc. Roy. Soc. Lond., 1916 lxxix, B. pp. xxxiv–xxxviii (M. A.).

Ughetti (G. B.): *Medici e clienti*, Palermo, 1898. *Viaggio*, Palermo, 1911.

Van Gehuchten: Bull. Acad. roy. de méd. de Belg., Brux., 1920, 4. s., xxx, 961–978 (Henrijean).

Vaughan (Victor C.): Autobiography, Indianapolis, 1926.

Venel: Zentralbl. f. chir. u. mech. Orthop., Berl., 1912, vi, 432–435 (M. Klemm).—Ztschr. f. Krüppelfürsorge, Hamb. & Leipz., 1914, vii, 216–224 (M. Kirmsse).

Vesalius: Études by A. Burggraeve, Ghent, 1841.—Lives by M. Roth (Berlin, 1892), J. M. Ball (St. Louis, 1910), J. Olmedilla y Puig (Madrid, 1913), and A. Corsini (Siena, 1916); also the Iconography of M. H. Spielmann (London, 1925).—Sir M. Foster: Lectures on the History of Physiology, Cambridge, 1901, 1–24.—Edinb. M. J., 1914, n. s., xiii, 324; 388, 1 pl. (G. M. Cullen).—Janus, Amst., 1914, xix, 397–523 (E. C. van Leersum, et al.).—*Ibid.*, 1915, xix, 435–507, 8 pl., 1 tab. (F. M. G. de Feyfer).—Nederl. Tijdschr. v. Geneesk., Amst., 1915, 2. R., li, pt. 1, 4–130 (E. C. van Leersum, et al.).—Med. Rec., N. Y., 1915, lxxvii, 245–247 (W. H. Welch, et al.).—Johns Hopkins Hosp. Bull., Balt., 1915, xxvi, 118–123 (W. H. Welch, et al.).—Bull. Soc. Med. Hist., Chicago, 1916, i, 47–65 (F. H. Garrison).—Arch. nederl. de physiol., La Haye, 1917, i, 129–147.—Verhandl. d. Gesellsch. deutsch. Naturf. u. Aerzte, Leipzig (1920), 1921, lxxxvi, 162–190.

Vicary (Thomas): Brit. J. Surg., Bristol, 1918, v, 359–362: 1920–21, viii, 240–258 (Sir D'A. Power).

Virchow: Biographies by W. Becher (Berl., 1891); C. Posner: 2. Aufl., Wien, 1921; K. Sudhoff: Leipzig, 1922—G. Braun: Zürich diss., 1925.—*Briefe* (Leipz., 1907).—*Gedächtnisrede* by W. Waldeyer (Abhandl. d. k. preuss. Akad. d. Wissensch., Berl., 1903, 1–52).—*Gedächtnis-Feier.* Verhandl. d. Berl. Gesellsch. f. Anthrop., 1902, 311–330, port.—Arch. f. path. Anat. (etc.), Berl., 1903, cxxi, 2–7 (F. von Recklinghausen).—Johns Hopkins Univ. Circ., Balt., 1891, xi, 17–19 (Sir W. Osler).—Phila. M. J., 1902, x, 360 (W. H. Welch).—Science, N. Y. & Lancaster, Pa., 1902, n. s., xv, 441–445 (F. Boas).—*Virchow-Bibliographie* (Berlin, 1901).—Virchow's Arch., Berl., 1921, ccxxxv, 1–30 (O. Lubarsch); 31–44 (J. Orth); 399–417 (E. Hesse); 418–443 (von Luschan).—Deutsche med. Wochenschr., Leipz. & Berl., 1921, xlvii, 1185–1188 (L. Aschoff); 1195 (G. Mamlock); 1192–1195 (R. Beneke).—Gustav Braun: Zürich diss., 1925.

Vitruvius: A. Söllner, Jena Med.-hist. Beitr., 1913, Heft 4.

Vulpian: Paris méd., 1912–13, xii (suppl.), 733–747 (J. Camus).—Bull. Acad. de méd., Par., 1927, xcvii, 724–738 (G. Hayem & E. Gley).—Rev. neurol., Par., 1927, l, 1087–1187.

Wakley (Thomas): Life by S. S. Sprigge, London, 1927.

Waldeyer-Hartz: *Lebenserinnerungen*, Bonn, 1921.—Anat. Anz., Jena, 1922–3, lvi, 1–53, port.

Warren (John Collins): Life by E. Warren, 2 vols., Bost., 1860.

Wassermann: Klin. Wochenschr., Berl., 1925, iv, 902 (H. Sachs).—Med. Klin., Berl., 1925, xxi, 491 (F. Kraus).

Weber (Sir Hermann): Autobiographical Reminiscences, London, 1919.

Weigert (Carl): Biography by R. Rieder, Berlin, 1906.—Ann. Med. Hist., N. Y., 1924, vi, 163–177 (H. Morrison).

Weismann (August): Science, N. Y., 1915, n. s., xli, 917–923 (E. G. Conklin).

Welch: Science, N. Y., 1920, n. s., lii, 417–433 (S. Flexner).—Bibliography by W. C. Burkett, Baltimore, 1917.

Wells (William Charles): Sketch by Elisha Bartlett (Louisville, 1849).—Ann. Ophth., St. Louis, 1909, xviii, 454–458.—Louisa S. Wells: Journal (New York Historical Society), 1906, 84–106.

Werlhof: Opera medica, Hannover, 1775, pars i, pp. i–xvii (J. E. Wichmann).—H. Rohlfs: Gesch. d. deutsch. Med., Stuttg., 1875, i, 32–81.

Wertheim: Wien. med. Wochenschr., 1920, lxx, 409–412 (J. Halban).

West (Samuel): Brit. M. J., 1908, i, 921–923.

Weyer (Johann): Biography by Carl Binz, 2. Aufl., Berlin, 1896.—Med. Mag., Lond., 1897, vi, 520; 609; 651; 769 (E. T. Withington).

White (Charles): Med. Libr. & Hist. J., Brooklyn, 1907, v, 1–18 (J. G. Adami).

White (J. William): Biography by Agnes Repplier, New York, 1919.

Whitman (Charles Otis): Am. Naturalist, Lancaster, Pa., 1917, li, 5–30 (C. B. Davenport).

Whytt (Robert): Tr. Roy. Soc. Edinb., 1861–2, xxiii, 99–131 (W. Seller).—Med. Libr. & Hist. J., Brooklyn, 1904, ii, 153–165, 1 pl. (J. Ruhräh).—Edinb. M. J., 1925, n. s., xxiii, 755–761 (J. D. Comrie).—Psychol. Rev., Lancaster, Pa., 1927, xxxiv, 287–304 (L. Carmichael).

Wickersheimer (Ernest): Bull. Soc. Med. Hist. Chicago, 1917–22, ii, 285–294 (F. H. Garrison).—Ann. Med. Hist., N. Y., 1922, iv, 389–394 (A. N. Tasker).

Wiedersheim (Robert): *Lebenserinnerungen*, Tübingen (1919).   Med. d. Gegenwart (Grote), Leipz., 1923, i, 207–227, port.

Wilks (Sir Samuel): Biographical Reminiscences (Lond., 1911).—Guy's Hosp. Gaz., Lond., 1911, xxv, 508–510, port.; Bibliography of his writings by William Wale: *Ibid.*, 512–520.—Brit. M. J., Lond., 1911, ii, 1384–1390, port.—Lancet, Lond., 1911, ii, 1441–1445, port.—Guy's Hosp. Rep. Lond., 1913, lxvii, 1–39 (W. H. White).

Willan (Robert): Arch. Dermat. and Syph., Chicago, 1926, n. s., xiii, 737–760 (J. E. Lane).

Willis (Thomas): Bull. Soc. Med. Hist., Chicago, 1923, iii, 215–232 (W. S. Miller).

Winslow: *L'Autobiographie*, Paris, 1912.

Winternitz (Wilhelm): München. med. Wochenschr., 1917, lxiv, 385 (J. Marcuse).—Wien. klin. Wochenschr., 1917, xxx, 347 (A. Strasser).

Wiseman (Richard): Life by Sir T. Longmore (Lond., 1891).—Sir B. W. Richardson, Disciples of Æsculapius, Lond., 1900, i, 158–175, port.—West. Lond. M. J., 1912, xvii, 203–205 (S. D. Clippingdale).

Withering: Life prefacing his "Miscellaneous Tracts," Lond., 1822, i, 1–206 [Bibliography], 207–209.—Proc. Roy. Soc. Med., Lond., 1915, viii, Sect. Hist. Med., 85–94 (A. R. Cushny).—Med. Press. & Circ., Lond., 1915, c, 39: 1917, ciii, 208 (G. Foy).

Wolff (Caspar Friedrich): Jenaische Ztschr. f. Med. u. Naturw., Jena, 1868, iv, 193–220 (A. Kirchhoff).—W. M. Wheeler: Woods Hole Biol. Lect., 1898, Bost., 1899, vi, 265–284.—[Sitzungsb. d. k. preuss. Akad. d. Wissensch., 1904 (W. Waldeyer).]

Wollaston: Sc. Progress, Lond., 1927, xxi, 81–95 (H. G. Wayling).

Wood (Horatio C.): Alumni Reg. Univ. Penn., Phila., 1906–7, xi, 196–200 (G. E. deSchweinitz.—Therap. Gaz., Phila., 1920, xliv, 322–324 (H. A. Hare).—Med. Rec., N. Y., 1920, xcviii, 393–396 (H. Beates, Jr.).—Tr. Coll. Phys., Phila., 1920, 3. s., xhi, 155–257 (G. E. deSchweinitz, *et al.*).

Wood (Leonard): Life by J. H. Sears, New York, 1919.

Woodward (Joseph Janvier): Nat. Acad. Sc. Biog. Mem., Wash., 1886, ii, 295–307 (J. S. Billings).—Mil. Surg., Wash., 1923, lii, 635–647 (J. C. Hemmeter).

Wunderlich: Arch. d. Heilk., Leipz., 1878, iv, 289–320 (O. Heubner); 321–329 (W. Roser).—Med. Klin., Berl., 1915, xi, 901–903 (A. Strümpell).

Wundt: Arch. f. d. ges. Psychol., Leipz., 1920, xl, Heft. 3–4, pp. i–xvi, 2 port (W. Wirth).—Ztschr. f. d. ges. Neurol., Berl., 1920, Orig., lxi, 351–362.—Am. J. Psychol., Worcester, 1921, xxxii, 161–178 (E. B. Titchener).—Psychol. Rev., Lancaster, Pa., 1921, xxviii, 153–188.

Young (John R.): Bull. Johns Hopkins Hosp., Balt., 1918, xxix, 186–191, 2 pl. (H. A. Kelly).

Young (Thomas): Lives by Gurney (Lond.. 1831) and Peacock (Lond., 1855).—Dict. Nat. Biog., Lond., 1900, lxiii, 393–399 (C. H. Lees).—Chicago Med. Recorder, 1913, xxxv, 129–136 (B. Holmes).—Am. J. Physiol. Optics, Southbridge, Mass., 1920, i, 9–14 (C. Sheard).

Yperman: Janus, Amst., 1913, xviii, 1; 197 (E. C. van Leersum).

Zacchias: V. Fossel: Stud. z. Gesch. d. Med., Stuttg., 1909, 46–110.

Zakrzewska (Marie): A Woman's Quest, New York, 1924.

Zander (J. G. W.): Allg. med. Centr.-ztg., 1922, xci, 1–3 (G. Schütz).

Zimmermann: Lives by Tissot (1797) and R. Ischer (1893).

Zuntz (Nathan): Berl. klin. Wochenschr., 1920, lvii, 433–435 (A. Loewy).—Arch. f. d. ges. Physiol., Berl., 1922, cxciv, 1–19 (A. Loewy).

C. Histories of Special Subjects

Alchemy: K. C. Schmieder: *Geschichte der Alchemie* (Halle, 1832).—E. Berthelot: *Les origines de l'alchimie* (Paris, 1885).

Alexandrian Medicine: K. Sudhoff: *Aerztliches aus griechischen Papyrus- Urkunden* (Leipzig, 1907).

American Medicine: James Thacher's sketch in his American Medical Biography, Bost., 1828, i, 9–85, which contains separate histories of medicine in the colonial states. Century (A) of American medicine (Phila., 1876), in particular the critical survey by J. S. Billings (pp. 290–366).—S. D. Gross: History of American Medical Literature (Phila., 1876).—J. M. Toner: Contributions (etc.) (Washington, 1874).—F. R. Packard: History of Medicine in the United States (Phila., 1901).—J. G. Mumford: A Narrative of Medicine in America (Phila., 1903).—University M. Mag., Phila., 1897–8, x, 136–140 (Sir W. Osler).—J. Am. M. Ass., Chicago, 1911, lviii, 437–441 (H. A. Kelly).—Med. Rec., N. Y., 1904, lxv, 361–367 (S. Smith); 1913, lxxxiv, 277–283 (T. Abbe).—Med. & Surg., St. Louis, 1917, i, 1068–1073 (C. Vabre).—Tr. Am. Surg. Ass., Phila., 1917, xxxv, 65–171 (E. Souchon).

Amulets and Talismans: S. Seligmann: *Die magischen Heil- und Schutzmittel*, Leipzig, 1927.—Elizabeth Villiers: *Amulette und Talismane*, München, 1927.

Anatomy: Ludwig Choulant's *Geschichte und Bibliographie der anatomischen Abbildung* (Leipzig, 1852), also translated, with additional matter by Mortimer Frank (Univ. Chicago Press, 1920); Hyrtl's studies of Arabic and Hebrew terms (1879), anatomical terminology (1880) and old German *termini technici* (1884); Robert von Töply's studies in mediæval anatomy (Leipzig, 1898), the *Histoire de l'anatomie plastique* of Mathias Duval and Édouard Cuyer (Paris, 1898), Ludwig Hopf on the early cultural phases (Abhandl. z. Gesch. d. Med., Breslau, 1904, Heft 9), and Karl Sudhoff on traditional (1907) and graphic phases of anatomy (1908) are the most remarkable works in this field. The anatomical illustration of the uterus alone is most exhaustively treated in F. La Torre's *L'utero attraverso i secoli* (Castello, 1917). The late Sir William Turner's history in the Encyclopædia Britannica (*sub voce* "Anatomy") and Frank Baker's article in Stedman's Reference Handbook (N. Y., 1913, i, 323–345) are the best monographs on the subject in English. Töply's monograph in the Puschmann Handbuch (1903, ii, 155–325) is a good routine and bibliographic account. Thomas Lauth's unfinished *Histoire de l'anatomie* (1815) is an earlier work. Anterior even to this is the *Historia anatomiæ* of Caspar Bauhinus (1597), which gives marginal bibliographical references to all the discoveries listed. A similar service is rendered by Sprengel (*passim*). I. H. Chievitz's *Anatomiens Historie*, in the Danish language (Copenhagen, 1904) has many interesting illustrations. In the atlas of J. G. de Lint (1925), the story is told in pictures—a new departure. W. W. Keen's Sketch of the Early History of Practical Anatomy (Philadelphia, 1874) is a valuable history of dissecting and injecting. For the history of anatomy in America, see Charles R. Bardeen (Bull. Univ. Wisconsin, Madison, 1905, No. 115, 85–208) and E. B. Krumbhaar (Ann. Med. Hist., N. Y., 1922, iv, 277–286). Of more recent works, Charles Singer's Evolution of Anatomy (New York, 1925), G. W. Corner's Anatomical Texts of the Earlier Middle Ages (Washington, Carnegie Inst., 1927), and E. Wickersheimer's edition of Mundinus and Vigevano (Paris, E. Droz, 1927) are worthy of especial note. For plastic (physiological) anatomy, see, F. H. Garrison: The Principles of Anatomic Illustration before Vesalius (New York, 1926) and the many recent German albums of *Plastik*. For Chinese anatomy: Anat. Rec., Phila., 1920–21, xx, 33–60 (E. V. Cowdry); 97–127 (E. T. Hsieh). For Oriental anatomy: Arch. f. Gesch. d. med., Leipz., 1919, xi, 177–182 (E. Hommel) and Mitt. d. anthrop.

Gesellsch. in Wien, 1926, lvi, 399–406 (L. Franz).   For early Italian anatomy: Illustr. med. ital., Genova, 1923, v, 3; 25; 101; 123 (G. Martinotti).   For *les gisants:* Bull. Soc. franç. d'hist. de méd., Par., 1926, xx, 85; 199 (Tricot-Royer).   For *écorchés:* Æsculape, Par., 1926, n. s., xvi, 1; 152 (H. Meige).   For fugitive sheets: Janus, Leyde, 1924, xxviii, 78–91, 7 pl. (J. G. de Lint) and Ann. Med. Hist., N. Y., 1925, vii, 1–5 (L. Crummer).   For cross-sectional anatomy, see, the introduction to the atlas of A. C. Eycleshymer & D. M. Schoemaker, N. Y., 1911, pp. ix–xvi. For terminology, see E. Brissaud: *Histoire des expressions populaires* (Paris, 1888); A. Bert & C. Pellanda: *La nomenclature anatomique et ses origines* (Paris, 1904); H. Triepel: *Die anatomischen Namen* (Wiesbaden, 1910), H. Holma's study of Assyro-Babylonian terms (Leipzig, 1911), F. Thöne's Kiel dissertation on Anglo-Saxon terms (1912), W. D. Baskett's thesis on Teutonic terms (Linguist. stud. Univ. Chicago, 1920, No. 5), and the above mentioned books of Hyrtl.

Anatomy (Comparative): J. Chaine: *Histoire d'anatomie comparative*, Bordeaux, 1925.

Anesthesia: Dublin J. M. Sc., 1875, lix, 32–38 (T. M. Madden).—*Ibid.*, 1888, lxxxvi, 284; 373; 485: 1889, lxxxvii, 116; 225; 305; 486 (G. Foy).—Deutsche Ztschr. f. Chir., Leipz., 1895–6, xlii, 517–596 (Th. Husemann).—Semi-centennial (The) of Anæsthesia (Bost., 1897).—Johns Hopkins Hosp. Bull., Balt., 1897, viii, 174–184 (H. H. Young).—J. T. Gwathmey: Anesthesia, N. Y., 1914, 1–29.—Scient. Monthly, N. Y., 1925, xx, 304–328 (C. D. Leake).—Marguerite Louise Baur: Zürich diss., 1927.

Anglo-Saxon Medicine: O. Cockayne: Leechdoms (etc.), (3 v., Lond., 1864–6).—J. F. Payne: English Medicine in the Anglo-Saxon Times (Oxford, 1904).—C. Singer: Early English Magic and Medicine, London, 1920.

Anthropology: A. C. Haddon: History of Anthropology, London and N. Y., 1910.

Arabian Medicine: F. Wüstenfeld: *Geschichte der arabischen Aerzte* (etc.) (Göttingen, 1840).—Djelal ed-din: *La médecine du prophète*, Trad. par N. Perron, Paris, 1869.—Lucien Leclerc's *Histoire de la médecine arabe* (2 vols., Paris, 1876).—Puschmann's Handbuch, Jena, 1902, i, 589–621 (Schrutz).—K. Opitz: *Die Medizin im Koran* (Stuttgart, 1906).—H. Kroner: *Zur Terminologie der arabischen Medizin*, Berlin, 1921.—E. G. Browne: Arabian Medicine, Cambridge, 1921.—D. Campbell: Arabian Medicine, 2 v., London, 1925.—M. W. Hilton-Simpson: Arab Medicine and Surgery, London, 1922.

Art (Medicine in): The subject was opened up by Virchow in Arch. f. path. Anat. (etc.), Berl., 1861, xxii, 190; 1862, xxiii, 194; and the material exhaustively listed by K. F. H. Marx (Abhandl. d. k. Gesellsch. d. Wissensch. zu Göttingen, 1861–2, x, 3–74; but was really the creation of Charcot and his pupils in the files of the *Nouvelle Iconographie de la Salpetrière*, Par., 1888–1913, *passim*. The two monographs of Charcot & P. Richer on the demoniac the deformed and the diseased in art (Paris, 1887–9); P. Richer's *L'art et la médecine* (Paris, 1902); Eugen Holländer's monographs on medicine in classical painting, caricature and plastic art (Stuttgart, 1903–12), Robert Müllerheim's *Die Wochenstube in der Kunst* (Stuttg., 1904), and F. Parkes Weber's Aspects of Death in Art (2. ed., Lond., 1914) are the best books on this subject.   Such essays as those of J. W. Churchman on Jan Steen and Velasquez (Johns Hopkins Hosp. Bull., Balt., 1907, xvii, 480; 1911, xxii, 383) and Mortimer Frank on Caricature in Medicine (Bull. Soc. Med. Hist., Chicago, 1911–15, i, 46–57), are well worth reading.

Assyro-Babylonian Medicine: F. von Oefele: *Keilschriftmedicin* (Abhandl 3. Gesch. d. med., Breslau, 1902, Heft 3).—F. Küchler: *Beiträge zur Kenntnis der assyrisch-babylonischen Medizin* (Leipzig, 1904).—Boissier: *Divination assyro-babylonienne*, Genève, 1905.—W. H. Ward: The Seal-cylinders of Western Asia (Washington, Carnegie Inst., 1910).—R. C. Thompson: Assyrian Medical Texts, London, 1923, and his The Assyrian Herbal, London, 1924.—Proc. Roy. Soc. Med., Sect. Hist. Med., London, 1914, vii, 109–176 (M. Jastrow).—Ann. Med. Hist., N. Y., 1917–18, i, 231–257 (M. Jastrow).—Arch. f. Gesch. d. med., Leipz., 1920–21, xiii, 1; 129: 1921–22, xiv, 26; 65 (E. Ebeling).

Astrology: C. A. Mercier: Astrology in Medicine, London, 1914.—F. Feerhow: *Die medizinische Astrologie*, Leipzig, 1914.—Siglo med., Madrid, 1871–5, xviii–xxii, *passim* (J. B. Ullersperger).—V. Fossel: Stud. z. Gesch. d. Med., Stuttg., 1909, 1–23.—New York Med. Monatschr., 1911, xxii, 31–35 (F. von Oefele).—Janus, Leyden, 1914, xix, 157–177 (E. Wickersheimer).

Austrian Medicine: M. Neuburger: *Die Entwicklung der Medizin in Oesterreich*, Vienna, 1918.—*Die alte medizinische Wien*, Wien, 1921.

Bacteriology: Friedrich Loeffler's *Vorlesungen* (1. Theil, Leipzig, 1887), incomplete, to be supplemented by Müller and Prausnitz (Puschmann's Handb., 1905, iii, 804–852) and Handb. d. path. Mikroörg., Jena, 1903, I, 1–28 (R. Abel).—S. Simon: Munich diss., 1907.—H. W. & H. J. Conn: Bacteriology, 2. ed., Baltimore, 1924, 13–66.—W. W. Ford: Text-book of Bacteriology, Phila., 1927, 18–31, and for history of individual micro-organisms, *passim*.

Balneology: E. Bäumer: Abhandl. z. Gesch. d. Med., Bresl., 1903, Heft vii.—J. Marcuse: *Bäder und Bäderwesen*, Stuttgart, 1903.—K. Sudhoff: *Aus dem antiken Badewesen*, 2 pts. (Berlin, 1910).

—A. Martin: *Deutsches Badewesen in vergangenen Tagen* (Jena, 1906).—P. Négrier: *Les bains à travers les âges*, Paris, 1925.—Also, Max Höfler's erudite study of the Sardinian baths in Ztschr. f. Balneol., Berl., 1918, xi, 51; 65; 77; 91. See, *also*, the bibliography in Index Cat., 1920, 3. s., ii, 331.

Bibliography (Medical): Haller's re-issue of the Boerhaave *Methodus Studii Medici* (2 vols., Amsterdam, 1751), and his bibliographies of botany (1771-2), anatomy (1774-7), surgery (1774-5) and practice of medicine (1776-8), make up the best of the 18th century contributions.—Carl Peter Callisen's *Medicinisches Schriftsteller-Lexicon* (33 vols., Copenhagen, 1830-45) is a sort of author Index-Catalogue of the latter half of the 18th and the first quarter of the 19th centuries. The earlier bibliographies of G. G. de Ploucquet (1808-9), Robert Watt (1824), James Atkinson (1834), and John Forbes (1835) are valuable. Ludwig Choulant's *Handbuch der Bücherkunde* (2. ed., Leipzig, 1840), and his *Bibliotheca medico-historica* (Leipzig, 1842), with Julius Rosenbaum's *Additamenta* (Halle, 1842-7), Haeser's *Bibliotheca epidemiographica* (Jena, 1843), with J. G. Thierfelder's "Additamenta" (Meissen, 1843; Greifswald, 1862), Rupprecht's *Bibliotheca medico-chirurgica* (Göttingen, 1847-92), W. Engelmann's *Bibliotheca medico-chirurgica* (Leipzig, 1848), Alphonse Sauly's *Bibliographie des sciences médicales* (Paris, 1874), and Lucien Hahn's *Essai de bibliographie médicale* (Paris, 1897) are invaluable works of their kind. Quérard's *La France littéraire* (12 vols., 1827-64) and Brunet's *Manuel du libraire* (8 vols., Paris, 1860-65, suppl., Paris, 1878-80) are especially good for French medicine. Spanish medicine has been exhaustively treated in the *Historia bibliografica* of Antonio Hernández Morejón (7 vols., Madrid, 1842-52) and the *Coleccion* of Miguel de la Plata y Marcos (Madrid, 1882).—National collections of the type of T. von Györy's *Bibliographia medica Hungariæ*, 1472-1899 (Budapest, 1900), L. Nielsen's *Dansk Bibliografi*, 1482-1550 (Copenhagen, 1919), J. Toriba Medina's *Biblioteca hispano-americana*, 1493-1810 (Santiago de Chile, 1898-1907) and the Mexican bibliographies of J. Garcia Icazbaleta (1886-1903), V. de Andrache (1900) and Nicolas León (1902-8) are now fairly plentiful. The most exhaustive modern bibliography of medicine is the Index Catalogue of the Library of the Surgeon-General's Office (37 vols., 1880-1928), supplemented by the monthly *Index Medicus* (1879-99; 1903-1926), the *Quarterly* Cumulative Index, Chicago, 1916-1926, and the Quarterly Cumulative Index Medicus, Chicago, 1926-8.—The hiatus caused by the suspension of publication of the *Index Medicus* was filled in part by the French *Bibliographia medica* (Paris, 1900-1902). For historic study of the fundamental texts, see the *Catalogue des sciences médicales* of the Bibliothèque impériale (3 vols., Paris, 1857-89), and the special bibliographies in the Index Catalogue, particularly its lists of historical texts (2. ser., xvii, pp. 89-178).

A valuable select bibliography of important scientific papers for the years 1800-1893 is the Royal Society's Catalogue (19 vols., London, 1867-1925), and for anatomy, physiology, bacteriology, chemistry, biology and anthropology, the International Catalogue of Scientific Literature, printed by the Royal Society (London, 1907-12). For parasitology, C. W. Stiles and A. Hassall's Index Catalogue of Medical Zoölogy (36 parts, Washington, 1902-12) is unique and invaluable. L. Pfeiffer's bibliography of smallpox and vaccination (Weimar, 1866), E. J. Warings's Bibliotheca Therapeutica (1878), H. C. Bolton's bibliography of chemistry (Washington, 1885-93), F. Schmid's bibliography of public hygiene (Berne, 1898-1906), Heinrich Laehr's bibliography of the literature of neurology (Berlin, 1900), H. de Rothschild's Bibliotheca lactaria (Paris, 1901), E. Roth's bibliography of nursing (Berlin, 1903), Gottlieb Port's index of dental literature (Heidelberg, 1904-14), and R. Ostertag on meat inspection (Stuttgart, 1905), Emil Abderhalden's bibliography of alcoholism (Berlin, 1904), John Ferguson's Bibliotheca Chemica (Glasgow, 1906), and the bibliographies of E. F. Cyriax on medical gymnastics (Worishöfen, 1909), W. Junks' Bibliographia botanica, Berlin, 1909, H. Gocht on Roentgen literature (Stuttgart, 1911-14), A. L. Caillet on psychic and occult sciences (Paris, 1912-13), Donald McMurtrie on crippled children (New York, 1913), the New York State Board of Charities on eugenics (Albany, 1913), A. C. Klebs on variolation (Baltimore, 1913), also F. Salveraggio on pellagra (Pavia, 1914), L. C. C. Krieger's Catalogue of the Mycological Library of Howard A. Kelly (Baltimore, 1924), H. Rost on suicide (Augsburg, 1927), and A. S. Lemon's *Bibliotheca Bacchica* (London, 1927) deserve mention.

For lists of periodicals see, the British Museum index, the abbreviations to the Royal Society's Catalogue of Scientific Papers (1867-1925), H. Scudder's catalogue of scientific serials (1633-1876) (Cambridge, 1879), the abbreviations to the Index Catalogue (1895, 1916), H. C. Bolton's catalogue of scientific and technical periodicals (1665-1895), 2. ed. (Wash., 1897), A. P. C. Griffin's Union List (Library of Congress, Washington, 1901), H. O. Severance's Guide (Ann Arbor, G. Wahr, 1914), the French *Annuaire des journaux périodiques* (Paris, 1881-1916), the catalogue of periodicals in the Royal Society of London (1912), the *Gesamt-Zeitschriften-Verzeichnis* of German libraries (Königl. Bibliothek, Berlin, 1914), the *Inventaire* of the Académie des sciences, covering scientific periodicals in Paris libraries (Paris, 1924-5) and the World-List of Scientific Periodicals, 2 v. (Oxford, 1925-7). For scientific societies, the section "Academies" of the British Museum Catalogue, the International Exchange Lists of the Smithsonian Institution and J. Müller's bibliography of German scientific societies (Berlin, 1883-7) are valuable.

Indispensable works for general reference in a library of large size are the Catalogues of the British Museum and of the Peabody Library of Baltimore, Maryland, Poggendorff's *Handwörterbuch der Geschichte der exakten Wissenschaften* (Leipzig, 1863–1926), Julius Petzholdt's *Bibliotheca bibliographica* (Leipzig, 1866), Lorenz's *Catalogue de la Librairie francaise* (Paris, 1867–1927), Heinsius' *Allgemeines Bücherlexicon* for the years 1700–1925 (36 vols., Leipzig, 1812–1927), Léon Vallée's *Bibliographie des bibliographies* (Paris, 1883), Henri Stein's *Manuel de bibliographie générale* (Paris, 1897) and A. Hortschansky's *Bibliographie des Bibliotheks- und Buchwesens* (Leipzig, 1905–13). For general use, Georg Schneider's *Handbuch der Bibliographie* (Leipzig, 1923) is unquestionably the best recent work. For the technique of bibliography, see the forms used by the Library of Congress, the Index Catalogue, the Dewey system and such essays as C. S. Minot: Woods Hole Biol. Lect., 1895, Boston, 1896, 149–168.

Anonymous and pseudonymous literature are well handled in Halkett & Laing's Dictionary (4 vols., Edinburgh, 1882–8), William Cushing's Initials & Pseudonyms (1. & 2. series), and anonyms (1890), Barbier's *Dictionarie des ouvrages anonymes et pseudonymes* (4 vols., Paris, 1822–7). To these may be added John Martin's Bibliography of privately printed books (2. ed., Lond., 1854), and the Bibliography of unfinished books in English by A. R. Corns and A. Sparke (Lond., 1915).

Biochemistry: F. Haurowitz: *Biochemie (seit, 1914)*, Dresden. Dorothy L. Jordan: Chemistry of the Proteins, London, 1926.

Biology (History of): J. A. Thomson: The Science of Life (Chicago & New York, 1899).—W. A. Locy: Biology and its Makers (New York, 1908).—G. B. Grassi: *I progressi della biologia* (Rome, 1911).—E. Rádl: *Geschichte der biologischen Theorien* (2. Aufl., Leipzig & Berlin, 1913).—C. Singer: Greek Biology and Greek Medicine, Oxford, 1922.—H. O. Taylor: Greek Biology and Medicine, Boston, 1922.—W. A. Locy: The Growth of Biology, New York, 1925.—E. Nordenskiöld: *Geschichte der Biologie*, Jena, 1926.

Birth-control: V. Robinson: Pioneers of Birth-control, N. Y., 1920.

Botanic Gardens: Ann. Missouri Botan. Garden, St. Louis, 1915, ii, 185–240 (A. W. Hill).

Botany: E. H. F. Meyer: *Geschichte der Botanik* (4 v., Königsberg, 1854).—J. von Sachs: *Geschichte der Botanik* (München, 1875).—G. Buschan: *Vorgeschichtliche Botanik* (Breslau, 1895).—J Wm. Harshberger: "The Botanists of Philadelphia" (Phila., 1899).—A. Hanson: *Die Entwicklung der Botanik* (Giessen, 1902).—E. L. Greene: "Landmarks of Botanical History" (Wash., 1909).—R. T. Günther's Oxford Gardens (Oxford, 1912), and Early British Botanists (Oxford, 1922); also: J. R. Green's History of Botany in the United Kingdom (London, 1914). See, also, Herbals. Also: J. Am. M. Ass., Chicago, 1911, lviii, 437–441 (H. A. Kelly).—Science, N. Y., 1914, n. s., xxxix, 299–319 (D. S. Johnson).

Byzantine Medicine: Glasgow M. J., 1913, lxxx, 321; 422 (Sir T. C. Allbutt).—H. Corlieu: *Les médecins grecs depuis la mort de Galien* (Paris, 1885).

Caduceus: Am. J. Archæol., Concord, N. H., 1916, xx, 175–211 (A. L. Frothingham).—Bull. M. Library Ass., Balt., 1919, ix, 13–16 (F. H. Garrison).

Canadian Medicine: W. Canniff: The Medical Profession in Upper Canada, 1783–1850, Toronto 1894.—J. J. Hagerty: Four Centuries of Medical History in Canada, 2 v., Toronto, 1928.

Cancer: J. E. Albert: *Das Carcinom* [etc.], Jena, 1887.—Jakob Wolff: *Die Lehre von der Krebskrankheit* (4 vols., Jena, 1907–28).—Ann. Med. Hist., N. Y., 1925, vii, 135–140 (E. B. Krumbhaar).—Bull. N. Y. Acad. Med., 1926, ii, 179–185 (F. H. Garrison).

Caricature (Medical): E. Hollander: *Karikatur und Satire in der Medizin*, 2. Aufl., Leipzig, 1925.—C. Veth: *De arts en de caricatur*, Amsterdam, 1926.—L. Nass: *Curiosités médico-artistiques*, 1.–3. series, Paris, (1907–14).—Bull. Soc. Med. Hist., Chicago, 1911–15, i, 46–57 (M. Frank).

Celtic Medicine: Proc. Am. Phil. Soc., Phila., 1887, xxiv, 136–166 (J. Mooney).

Chemistry: Histories by H. Kopp (Brnschwg., 1843–7, 1871–3), A. W. Hofmann (Berl., 1882), H. W. Picton (Lond., 1889), E. von Meyer (N. Y., 1891), W. Ostwald (Leipzig, 1908), A. Stange (Leipzig, 1908), M. M. P. Muir (N. Y., 1909), Sir E. Thorpe (2 v., Lond. & N. Y., 1909), J. C. Brown (Lond., 1913), T. E. Ekecrantz (Leipzig, 1913), T. M. Lowry (London, 1915), F. J. Moore (New York, 1918), and M. Delacre (Paris, 1920).—E. Berthelot: *La chimie au moyen âge* (Paris, 1896).—School Mines Quart., N. Y., 1905–6, xxvii, 87; 313; 388 (W. Ostwald).—Science, N. Y. & Lancaster, Pa., 1901, n. s., xiii, 803–809 (E. H. Keiser).—For American chemistry (1876–1926), see J. Am. Chem. Soc., Phila., 1926, xlviii (Jubilee Number), 1–254.

Chinese Medicine: M. Boym: *Clavis medica* (Frankfurt a. M., 1686).—A. Cleyer: *Specimen medicinæ sinicæ* (Frankfurt, 1682).—H. A. Giles: Chinese Biographical Dictionary (1897); History of Chinese Literature, 2. ed., 1910.—F. Hübotter: A Guide through Chinese Medical Writings, Kumamoto, 1924.—August Pfizmaier's translation of the pulse-lore of Chang Ke (1866), and his essays in Sitzungsb. d. phil.-hist. Cl. d. k. Akad. d. Wissensch., Wien, 1865–6, on Chinese pathology, semeiollogy and toxicology.—P. Dabry: *La médecine chez les Chinois* (Paris, 1863).—

J. Regnault: *Médecine et pharmacie chez les Chinois* (Paris, 1902).—Also: Janus, Amst., 1904, ix, 103; 159; 201; 257 (R. W. von Zaremba): Haarlem, 1908, xiii, 1; 121; 190; 268; 328 (Gruenhagen).— Arch. f. Gesch. d. Med., Leipz., 1913–14, vii, 115–128 (F. Hübotter).—Janus, Leyde, 1927, xxxi, 395– 412 (A. Fonahn).—U. S. Naval Med. Bull., Wash., 1927, xxv, 783–816 (J. L. McCartney).

Cholera: G. Sticker: Die Cholera (Giessen, 1912, 104–284).

Chronology (Medical): The tables prepared by Ludwig Choulant (1822), Casimir Broussais (1829), William Farr (1836–8), M. S. Krüger (1840), L. Aschoff (1898), and Julius Pagel (1908) are useful, as also the chronologies contained in the histories of Sprengel, E. Isensee, and E. Schwalbe.

Clinical Medicine: J. Peterson: *Hauptmomente in der älteren Geschichte der medicinischen Klinik* (Kopenhagen, 1890).—Knud Faber: Nosography, New York, 1923.

Contagion and Infection: Handb. d. pathog. Mikroörg. (Kolle & Wassermann), Jena, 1903, i, 223–306 (Wassermann).—G. Sticker: *Abhandlungen aus der Seuchengeschichte*, 2 v., Giessen, 1908–12.— Ann. Med. History, N. Y., 1917–18, i, 159–173 (A. C. Klebs).

Dante: De Renzi: *La medicina dei tempi di Dante*, Firenze, 1865.—L. Giuffrè: *Dante e le scienze mediche*, Bologna, 1925.—Arch. di storia d. sc., Roma, 1922, iii, 1–31 (E. Passera); 211–236 (A. Castiglioni); 237–243 (R. Sarra); 283–300 (G. Bilancioni); 1924, v, 101; 121 (A. Del Gaudio).— Riv. di antrop., Roma, 1924–5, xxvi, 3–17, 3 pl. (G. Sergi & F. Frassetto).

Deaf-mutism: Thomas Arnold: Education for Deaf-Mutes, Lond., 1888, 1–110.—Volta Rev., Wash. 1920, xxii, 391–421 (F. De Land).

Dengue: Monograph by G. Sticker (Wien, 1914).

Dentistry: Vincenzo Guerini's History of Dentistry (Philadelphia, 1909), and the discriminating review of Ashley Denham in Proc. Roy. Soc. Med., Lond., 1908–9, ii, Odont. Sect., 71–98. Also: Geist-Jacobi's *Geschichte der Zahnheilkunde* (Tübingen, 1896).—G. Cali's *L'odontoiatria attraverso i secoli*, Napoli, 1901.—C. R. E. Koch: History of Dental Surgery, 3 v., Fort Wayne, 1910; Dental Cosmos, Phila., 1920, lxii, 1–73.—A. G. Weber: *Bibliographiæ Stomatologicæ*, Havana, 1922.—C. Proskauer: *Culturgeschichte der Zahnheilkunde* (iconography), Berlin, 1926, and the exhaustive history of orthodontia by B. W. Weinberger (St. Louis, 1926).

Dermatology: Handb. d. Gesch. d. Med., Jena, 1905, iii, 393–463 (I. Bloch).—Lancet, Lond., 1911, i, 1555–1560 (J. H. Sequeira).—J. Am. M. Ass., Chicago, 1915, lxv, 469–474 (H. Fox).—Southern M. J., Birmingham, 1927, xx, 402–415 (J. M. King).—Arch. Dermat. & Syph., Chicago, 1924, ix, 675: 1928, xvii, 23 (H. Goodman).

Dietetics: H. Lichtenfelt: *Die Geschichte der Ernährung* (Berlin, 1913).—Festschr. z. 3. Sæcularfeier . . . d. med. Fac. Würzb., Leipz., 1882, ii, 17–41 (A. Stöhr).—Ztschr. f. diätet. u. phys. Therap., Leipz., 1898–9, 222–238 (J. Marcuse).—Pop. Sc. Month., N. Y., 1913, lxxxiii, 417–423 (J. B. Nichols).—Syst. Diet. (Sutherland), Lond., 1908, 25–67 (H. Campbell).

Diphtheria: J. Carlsen: *Bidrag*. Kjøbnhavn, 1890.—Bacteriology of Diphtheria (Nuttall & Smith), Cambridge, 1908, 1–52 (F. Loeffler).

Diseases (History of): C. G. Gruner: *Morborum antiquitates*, Breslau, 1774.—C. F. H. Marx: *Origines contagii*, Carlsruhe & Baden, 1827.—C. Pruys van der Hoeven: *De historia morborum*, Leyden, 1846.—Georg Kunkel: Munich diss., 1926.

Drugs: C. Pruys van der Hoeven: *De historia medicamentorum*, Leyden, 1847.—A. Schmidt: *Drogen und Drogenhandel im Altertum* (Leipzig, 1924).—F. A. Flückiger & D. Hanbury: *Pharmacographia*. (2. ed., London, 1879.)—A. Tschirch: *Pharmakognosie* (Leipzig, 1908–12).—Trousseau & Pidoux: *Traité de thérapeutique* (7. ed., Paris, 1868).—For history of vegetable drugs in U. S. P., see Bull. Lloyd Library, Cincinn., 1911, No. 18, 1–133 (J. U. Lloyd).

Dysentery: Arch. Path. & Lab. Med., Chicago, 1927, iii, 665–692 (G. R. Callender).

Education (Medical): T. Puschmann, *Geschichte des medizinischen Unterrichts* (etc.) (Leipzig, 1889).— N. I. Davis, "History of Medical Education" (etc.) (Chicago, 1851).—A. Flexner, "Reports to the Carnegie Foundation for the Advancement of Teaching" (Bull. No. 4, 6, N. Y., 1910–12).— Th. Billroth: The Medical Sciences in the German Universties (New York, 1924).—A. Flexner: Medical Education, New York, 1925. For the history of developments in different countries, see, Index Catalogue, 3. s., v, 128–138.

Egyptian Medicine: Papyros Ebers (ed. by G. Ebers). 2 v., Leipzig, 1875, later ed. W. Wrezinski, Leipzig, 1913, and transl. by H. Joachim (Berlin, G. Reimer, 1890).—Brugsch papyrus (Notice raisonnée (etc.), Leipzig, Hinrichs, 1863), also facsimile Brugsch major (Rec. de monum. egypt., Leipz., 1863, pt. 2, pp. lxxv–cvii).—Brugsch-minor (Abhandl. d. Berl. Akad. d. Wissensch., 1901).—The Hearst medical Papyrus, ed. by G. A. Reisner (Univ. Calif. Publ., v. 1).—The Petrie Papyri, ed. by T. L. Griffith (London, 1898).—K. Sudhoff, Aerztliches aus griechischen Papyrus-Urkunden, Leipzig, J. A. Barth, 1907.—Sir M. A. Ruffer: Studies in the Palæopathology of Ancient Egypt, London, 1921.—J. H. Breasted: The Edwin Smith Papyrus. New York Hist. Soc. Quart. Bull., 1922, vi, 1; 5. Also, Bull. Soc. Med. Hist., Chicago, 1923, iii, 58–78.—For

Hearst Papyrus: Proc. Roy. Soc. Lond., 1913–14, vi, Sect. Hist. Med., 97–102 (J. Offord).— Brit. M. J., Lond., 1926, i, 706 (E. M. Guest).—Prosper Alpinus, *De medicina Ægyptorum*, Venice, 1591.—Richard Millar, Disquisitions in the history of medicine, Edinburgh, 1811 (etc.).—Imhotep by J. B. Hurry, Oxford, 1928.—H. L. E. Lüring's Strassburg dissertation (Leipzig, 1888) is especially valuable as showing, by textual comparison, the indebtedness of the Greek and Roman writers to papyric medicine.—Medicine in Ancient Egypt by Bayard Holmes and P. G. Kitterman (Cincinnati, 1914) is very helpful.—For embalming, see, The Mummy by Sir E. A. Budge, Cambridge, 1925.—For an excellent résumé of Egyptian medicine, see Brit. M. J., Lond., 1893, i, 748; 1014; 1061 (J. Finlayson). Also: A. A. Nazmi, Montpellier diss., 1903.

Electrotherapy: H. A. Colwell: Essay on History of Electrotherapy, London, 1922.—Handb. d. physikal. Therap., Leipz., 1901, pt. 1, ii, 331–338 (Pagel).—Ann. d'électrobiol. (etc.), Par., 1904, vii, 129–146 (A. Tripier).—H. Chaufour: *Les origines du galvanisme*, Paris diss. No. 6, 1913.—Tr. XVII. Internat. Med. Cong., 1913, Lond., 1914, sect. XXIII, 347–350 (H. L. Jones). —St. Bartholomew's Hosp. J., Lond., 1913–14, xxi, 39; 61; 70; 90 (E. P. Cumberbatch).—Ztschr. f. phys. u. diätet, Heilmeth., Leipz., 1911, xv, 481 (F. Tichy).

Embryology: O. Hertwig: Lehrbuch (9. Aufl., Jena, 1910, 5–58).—Basel diss. by B. Bloch (1904).— W. A. Locy: "Biology and its Makers" (N. Y., 1908, 195–236).—St. Louis M. Rev., 1904, xlix, 273–281 (A. C. Eycleshymer).—Pop. Sc. Month., N. Y., 1906, lxix, 1–20 (C. S. Minot). Also Introduction to: "Manual" (etc.) by F. Keibel and F. P. Mall (Phila., 1910, v. 1).

Endocrinology: Lehrb. d. Organotherapie (Wagner-Jauregg & Bayer), Leipz., 1914, 1–26 (M. Höfler). —Endocrinology & Metabolism (Barker), N. Y., 1922, i, 45–78 (F. H. Garrison).

Endoscopy: Arch. f. Laryngol. u. Rhinol., Berl., 1915, xxix, 346–393 (G. Killian).

Epidemiology: Haeser: *Geschichte der Medizin*, 1882, iii, *passim.*—G. Sticker: *Abhandlungen* (etc.) (Giessen, 1908–12).—W. Ebstein: *Die Pest des Thukydides*, Stuttgart, 1899.—Handb. d. Gesch. d. Med., Jena, 1903, ii, 736–901 (V. Fossel).—Sudhoff-Festschrift (Essays [etc.]), Zürich, 1924, 3–62 (G. Sticker); 255–268 (F. H. Garrison).—Lancet, Lond., 1928, i, 1313: ii, 1.

Epigraphy (Medical): J. Arata: *L'arte medica nelle inscrizioni latine* (Genoa, 1902).—R. Blanchard: *Epigraphie médicale*, 2 v. (Paris, 1909–15).—Janus, Amst., 1909, xiv, 4; 111 (J. Oehler, with index of names).—See, also, the handbooks of Latin epigraphy by R. Cagnat (4. ed., Paris, 1914), J. C. Egbert (New York, 1896) and Sir J. E. Sandys (Cambridge, 1919).

Ethics (Medical): J. L. Pagel: *Medicinische Deontologie* (Berlin, 1897).—Grasset: *Principes fondamentaux de la déontologie médicale* (Paris, 1900).—C. D. Leake: *Percival's Medical Ethics*, Baltimore, 1927.—New York M. J., 1915, ci, 140; 205 (G. Wythe Cook).

Exercise (Physical): H. Mercuriali: *Artis gymnasticæ apud antiquos libri sex*, Venice, 1569.—F. E. Leonard: A Guide to the History of Physical Education (1923). 2. ed., Philadelphia, 1927.— E. A. Rice: Brief History of Physical Education, New York, 1926.

Fees (Medical): Internat. Clin., Phila., 1910, 20. s., iv, 259–275 (J. J. Walsh).—Johns Hopkins Hosp. Bull., Balt., 1898, ix, 183–186 (C. C. Bombaugh).—France méd., Par., 1906, liii, 300–304 (C. Vidal).—J. de sc. méd. de Lille, 1905, i, 543–548 (E. Leclair).—Janus, Amst., 1909, xiv, 287–293 (D'A. Power).—New York M. J. (etc.), 1912, xcvi, 370–373 (J. J. Walsh).—Caledon. M. J., Glasgow, 1914, x, 27–33.—Lancet, Lond., 1915, i, 1213.—Proc. Roy. Soc. Med., Lond., 1920, xiii, Sect. Hist. Med., 76–82 (D'A. Power).—Paris méd., 1924, iii (annexe), 124–127 (M. Boutard).

Folk-lore (Medical): W. G. Black: Folk-medicine (etc.) (Lond., 1883).—A. Bouchinet: *Des états primitifs de la médecine* (Paris thesis No. 194, 1891).—M. Bartels, *Die Medicin der Naturvölker* (Leipzig, 1893).—H. Magnus, *Die Volksmedizin* (Breslau, 1905).—O. von Hovorka & A. Kronfeld, *Vergleichende Volksmedizin* (etc.), 2 v., Stuttg., 1908–9.—Charlotte S. Burne: Handbook of Folklore, London, 1914.—D. Mackenzie: The Infancy of Medicine, London, 1927.—Boston M. & S. J., 1888, cxviii, 29; 57 (J. S. Billings).

Gastro-enterology: W. C. Alvarez: The Mechanics of the Digestive Tract, 2. ed., New York, 1928.

German Medicine: H. Rohlfs: *Geschichte der deutschen Medizin*, 4 v., Stuttgart, 1875–85.—A. Hirsch: *Geschichte der medicinischen Wissenschaften in Deutschland*, Berlin, 1893.—G. Sticker: *Die Entwickelung der ärztlichen Kunst in Deutschland*, Munich, 1927.

Graduation Ceremonies: Med. Libr. & Hist. J., Brooklyn, 1906, iv, 1–14 (W. W. Keen).

Greek Medicine: P. Girard: *L'Asclépieion d'Athènes* (Paris, 1882).—Alice Walton: The Cult of Asklepios, Boston, 1894.—M. Wellmann: *Die Fragmente der sikelischen Aerzte*, v. 1, Berlin, 1901. —W. R. Paton and L. Hicks: The Inscriptions of Cos, Oxford, 1891.—Also Handb. d. Gesch. d. Med., Jena, 1901, 153–402 (R. Fuchs). Also: C. V. Daremberg, *Etat de la médecine entre Homère et Hippocrate*, Par., 1867.—C. von Rittershain: *Der medicinische Wunderglaube* (Berlin, 1878).— A. Delfrasse & Henri Lechat: *Epidaure*, fol. Paris, 1895.—C. Moeller: *Die Medizin im Herodot*, Berlin, 1903.—M. Mollet: *La médecine chez les Grecs avant Hippocrate* (Paris, 1906).—O. Weinreich. *Antike Heilungswunder* (Giessen, 1909).—T. Gomperz: *Griechische Denker* (3. Aufl., Leipzig, 1911).

—Mary Hamilton: Incubation, Lond., 1906.—Jane E. Harrison: *Themis*, (Cambridge, 1912).— F. Kutsch. Giessen diss., 1913.—C. Singer: Greek Science and Modern Science (Oxford, 1920).— H. Diels: *Die Fragmente der Vorsokratiker*, 3 v., Berlin, 1922.—K. Sudhoff: *Kos und Knidos*, Munich, 1927.—H. E. Sigerist: *Antike Heilkunde (Tusculum Schriften*, No. 7, Munich, 1927).— Brit. & For. M.-Chir. Rev., Lond., 1886, xxxvii, 170; xxxviii, 483 (T. C. Allbutt).—J. de chir., Par., 1846, iv, 303; 332 (Malgaigne).—Brit. M. J., Lond., 1898, i, 1509; 1572 (R. Caton).—Boston M. & S. J., 1893, cxxviii, 129; 153 (Sir W. Osler).—For the MSS. of ancient Greek medical writers, see: H. Diels, *Die Handschriften der antiken Aerzte*, i-ii (Abhandl. d. k. preuss. Akad. d. Wissensch., Berl., 1905). See also: Homeric medicine.

Guilds (Medical): F. de Vigne, *Recherches historiques*, Gand, 1847.—*Mœurs et usages*, Gand, 1857.— Hoorebeke, *Description des méreaux*, Gand, 1877-9.—Rodocanachi: *Les corporations ouvrières à Rome*, Paris, 1894.—J. Colston: The Incorporated Trades of Edinburgh (1891).—E. Staley: The Guilds of Florence, London, 1906.—Renard: Guilds of the Middle Ages, London, 1919.— C. Welch: Coat Armor of the London Livery Companies, London, 1914.—J. Siebmacher: *Berufswappen*, Nürnberg, 1855, i, pt. 7, 44–48.

Gynecology: Franz von Winckel's *Ueberblick* in his Handb. d. Geburtsh. (Wiesbaden, 1903, i, 1. Teil, 1: 1904, ii, 1. Teil, 1; 1906, iii, 2. Teil, 1: 1907, iii, 3. Teil, 1) is the most exhaustive account of the whole subject. Kossmann (in the Puschmann Handbuch, 1905, iii, 953–980) gives a good short account. The essay by Handfield Jones at the beginning of Allbutt's System of Gynecology (1906) is an excellent free-hand discussion of the modern phases. The best account of American gynecology is the essay by Howard A. Kelly in the introduction to his Cyclopedia of American Medical Biography (Philadelphia, W. B. Saunders, 1912). Stewart McKay's History of Ancient Gynecology (1901).—F. Weindler's *Geschichte der gynäkologisch-anatomischen Abbildungen* (Dresden, 1908), A. Sachs on Biblical and Talmudic gynecology (Leipzig diss., 1909), F. Schauta's *Gynækologische Behandlung einst und jetzt* (Salzburg, 1910).—F. La Torre's *L'utero attraverso i secoli*, Castello, 1917.—W. Brütsch, Freiburg diss., 1922; Arch. f. Gesch. d. Med., Leipz., 1912–13, vi, 205–222 (C. Ferckel); 1915–16, viii, 297–349 (G. Bonelli); 1916–17, ix, 315: 1917–18, x, 124 (F. Reinhard); 1923, xv, 14–20 (G. Fischer), may be consulted; also: J. Lachs: Samml. klin. Vortr., n. F., Leipz., 1902, No. 335; 1904, No. 381 (Gyn. Nos. 121, 141).—Syst. Gynec. (Mann), Phila., 1887, i, 17–67 (E. W. Jenks).—Arch. f. Gynäk., Berl., 1923, cxx, 288–294 (I. Fischer) may also be consulted; also R. Kossmann: *Allgemeine Gynäkologie*, Berlin, 1903, 1–247.—*Biol. u. Path. des Weibes* (Halban & Seitz), Berl., 1924, i, 1–202 (I. Fischer).

Heart (Diseases of): G. A. Gibson: Diseases of the Heart, Edinburgh, 1898, *passim.*—R. O. Moon's "Growth" (etc.), Lond., 1927.—Janus, Bresl., 1847, ii, 53–124 (Landsberg).—Janus, Bresl., 1847, ii, 580; 1848, iii, 316 (P. J. Philipp). Also, Reprint (1856).

Heating, Lighting and Ventilation: J. P. Putnam: The Open Fireplace (1881), 2. ed., Boston, 1886.— O. Krell: *Altrömische Heizungen*, Munchen, 1901.—W. Hough: Bull. U. S. Nat. Mus., Wash., 1928, No. 141.—Gesundheits-Ingenieur, München, 1907, xxx, Festnummer, 10-25: 1914, xxxiv, 757–767 (H. Vetter).—Bull. New York Acad. Med., 1927, 2. s., iii, 57–67 (F. H. Garrison).

Heraldry (Medical): Antiquary, Lond., 1915, n. s., xi, 415; 455 (S. D. Clippingdale).—Chron. med., Par., 1918, xxv, 107–109 (Henry-André).

Herbals: A. Tschirch: *Handbuch der Pharmacognosie*, Leipz., 1910, 287–1072.—A. Arber: *Herbals* (Cambridge, 1912).—Eleanour S. Rohde: *The Old English Herbals* (London. 1922).—W. L. Schreiber: *Die Kräuterbucher des 15. und 16. Jahrhunderts*, München, 1924.—Sir E. A. Wallis Budge: The Divine Origin of the Craft of the Herbalist, London, 1928.—A. C. Klebs: Catalogue of *Early Herbals* (Lugano, 1925).—R. T. Gunther: *The Herbal of Apuleius Barbarus* (Oxford, Roxburgh Club, 1925).—C. Singer: The Herbal in Antiquity (Jour. Hellenic Studies, Lond., 1927, xlvii, 1–52, 10 col. pl.).—F. Hommel: Tschirch-Festschrift, Leipz., 1926, 72–79.—Käte Wengle: Zürich diss., 1926.

Hindu Medicine: F. Trendelenburg: *De veterum Indorum chirurgia* (Berlin, thesis, 1866).—A. F. R. Hoernle: The Bower Manuscript. Calcutta, 1893-8.—J. Jolly, Grundriss d. indo-arischen Philol. u. Alterthumsk., Strassburg, 1901, iii, Hft. 10.—P. Cordier, *Études sur la médecine hindoue* (Paris, 1894).—Jee, A Short History of Aryan Medical Science, London, 1896.—A. F. R. Hoernle: Studies in the Medicine of Ancient India, I. (Oxford, 1907).—Puschmann's Handbuch, Jena, 1901, i, 119–152 (I. Bloch).—Guy's Hosp. Gaz., Lond., 1889, n. s., iii, 117; 145; 157 (B. D. Basu).— Proc. Charaka Club, N. Y., 1902, i, 1–28 (B. Sachs).—G. Mukhopadhyaga: History of Indian Medicine, v. 1–2, Calcutta, 1923–6.

Histology: Univ. M. Mag., Phila., 1888–9, i, 82–87 (G. A. Piersol).

Homeric Medicine: J.-F. Malgaigne: *L'anatomie et la physiologie dans l' Homère*, Paris, 1842.—C. V. Daremberg: *La médecine dans Homère* (Paris, 1865).—H. Froelich: *Die Militärmedizin Homer's* (Stuttg., 1897).—O. Körner: *Ueber Wesen und Wert der homerischen Heilkunde* (Wiesbaden, 1904).—Paris thesis by A. Floquet (1912).—B. Coglievina: *Die homerische Medizin*

58

Graz, 1921. Also, O. Schmiedeberg on the drugs (Schrift. d. wissensch. Gesellsch. in Strassb., 1918, No. 36, 1–29) and L. Moulé on the hygiene (Bull. Soc. franç. d'hist. de méd., Par., 1923, xvii, 350–377).

Hospitals: Virchow: Virchow's Arch., Berl., 1860, xviii, 138; 273; xix, 43; 1861, xx, 166.—K. Sudhoff: *Aus der Geschichte des Krankenhauswesens,* Jena, 1913.—T. Meyer-Steineg: Jenaer med.-hist. Beitr., 1913, Hft. 9.—C. A. Mercier: Leper Houses and Mediæval Hospitals, London, 1915.— J. S. Taylor on the Hôtel Dieu (U. S. Naval Med. Bull., Wash., 1918, xii, 653–691, 2 pl.).— E. F. Stevens: The American Hospital, New York, 1918.—J. Drivon: Lyon méd., 1904, ciii; 545; 570; 630; 1924, cxxxiii, 160; 289 *passim.*

Hydrotherapy: M. J. Oertel, *Geschichte der Wasserheilkunde* (etc.) (Leipzig, 1835).—Handb. d. Gesch. d. Med., Jena, 1903, ii, 589–603 (von Oetele).—R. Metcalfe: The Rise and Progress of Hydrotherapy in England and Scotland, London, 1906.—V. van der Reis, Berlin diss., 1914.—Boston M. & S. J., 1906, cliv, 85–91 (J. H. Pratt).—Monatschr. f. phys. diätet. Heilmeth., München, 1909, i, 530–537 (F. Tichy).

Hygiene (Public): The subject has never been exhaustively treated. A glance at Professor Sudhoff's remarkable 593-page catalogue of the "Historische Abtheilung" of the Dresden Hygienic Exhibit (1911) will show its scope. Max Rubner's introduction to his "Handbuch der Hygiene" (vol. i, Leipzig, 1911) is a good historical sketch, as also Müller and Prausnitz in the Puschmann Handbuch (1905, iii, 783–852), and the historical review of W. H. Welch (New Haven, 1925).—A later study is that of A. Castiglioni in: Trattato d'igiene (Casagrandi), Torino, 1925. See, also: H. Hagen: *Antike Hygiene,* Hamburg, 1892.—J. Uffelmann: *Die öffentliche Hygiene in alten Rom.,* Berlin, 1881.—Max Rubner: *Zur Vorgeschichte der modernen Hygiene,* Berlin, 1895.—H. Delaunay: *L'hygiene publique à travers les âges,* Paris, 1906.—L. Kotelmann: *Gesundheitspflege im Mittelalter,* Hamburg, 1890.—Sir A. Newsholme's Public Health and Insurance, Baltimore, 1920, and his Evolution of Preventive Medicine, Baltimore, 1927.—A Half Century of Public Health, edited by Mazyck P. Ravenel for the American Public Health Association (New York, 1921) is a reliable account of recent American developments.—Sir John Simon's "English Sanitary Institutions" (1890), Sir Edwin Chadwick's "The Health of Nations" (1887), Sir M. Morris: The Story of British Public Health (London, 1919), "A History of Factory Legislation" by B. L. Hutchins and A. Harrison (1903), and "A Century of Public Hygiene in America" (1876) are good histories of legislative phases.—See, also: Ztschr. f. Med. Beamte, Berl., 1924, xxxvii, 350–373 (Wollenweber). For history of industrial hygiene under medieval trade-guilds, see Jour. Industr. Hyg., Boston, 1920, i, 475; 550; 578 (T. M. Legge). H. Kuttenkeuler (Die Naturwissenschaften, Berl., 1915, iii, 509; 521) gives a good history of German food chemistry and legislation. See, also: Hyg. Rundschau, Berl., 1917, xxvii, 609–613 (O. Spiegelberg).—For history of heating, ventilation, and lighting (with chronology): Bull. N. Y. Acad. Med., 1927, ii, 57–67 (F. H. Garrison).

Hypnotism: W. Preyer: *Die Entdeckung des Hypnotismus* (Berlin, 1881).—J. Bramwell: Hypnotism, 2. ed., London, 1906.—F. Podmore: Mesmerism and Christian Science (Phila., 1909). Also: Maryland M. J., 1910, liii, 81–97 (H. A. Kelly).

Iatromathematics: Karl Sudhoff: Abhandl. z. Gesch. d. Med., Breslau, 1902, Heft 2, and Jahresk. f. ärztl. Fortbild., München, 1919, 39–44.—Ann. Med. History, N. Y., 1917–18, i, 125–140 (E. C. Smith).

Incunabula (Study of the): R. A. Peddie's charming manual on Fifteenth-Century Books (London, 1913), and C. C. McCulloch: Bull. Med. Library Ass., Balt., 1915, v, 1–15. The earliest work was Michael Mattaire's *Annales typographici* (5 vols., Hague, Amsterdam & London, 1719–41), with supplement by Michael Denis (Vienna, 1789). G. W. Panzer's *Annales typographici* (11 vols., Nuremberg, 1793–1803) is the oldest chronological list by towns. Ludwig Hain's *Repertorium* (4 vols., Stuttgart, 1826–28), with Konrad Burger's *Register* (Leipzig, 1891), also the *Supplement* of Walter Arthur Copinger (3 vols., London, 1895–1902), Dietrich Reichling's *Appendices* (Munich, 1905–14), and Burger's *Supplement* (Leipzig, 1908) is the standard catalogue, which is further supplemented by Panzer's chronological *Annalen* of German incunabula (Nuremberg, 1788–1802), Choulant's *Handbuch der Bücherkunde* (Leipzig, 1828) and *Graphische Incunabeln* (Leipzig, 1858), J. W. Holtrop's list of incunabula at The Hague (1856), G. E. Klemming's *Sveriges bibliographi,* 1481–1600 (Upsala, 1889–92), the catalogue of M. Pellechet (v. 1–3, Paris, 1897–1909), P. Heitz's *Einblattdrucke* (Strassburg, 1906) and *Pestblätter* (with W. L. Schreiber, Strassburg, 1901), A. R. da Silva Carvalho's Oporto incunabula (1904), Konrad Haebler's Spanish incunabula (*Bibliografía Ibérica,* Leipzig, 1905), Konrad Burger's *Buchhändleranzeigen* (Leipzig, 1907), E. Voullième's catalogues of the Berlin (Leipzig, 1906–22) and Treves (Leipzig, 1910) incunabula and of German printers of the 15th century (1916), I. Collijn's lists of Upsala (1907) and Stockholm (1914–16) incunabula, Sudhoff's *Deutsche medizinische Inkunabeln* (Leipzig, 1908), R. G. C. Proctor's "Index" to the British Museum incunabula (London, 1898–1906), the British Museum Catalogue of XV Century Books (London, 1908–24), K. Burger's *Nummernkonkordanz* (Leipzig, 1908), Günther's *Wiegendrucke* of the Leipzig and Altenburg collections

(Leipzig, 1909), S. Sanpere y Miquel's Introduction to early Spanish printing and Catalan incunabula (Barcelona, 1909), the catalogues of illustrated incunabula by W. L. Schreiber (Leipzig, 1910–11), and L. S. Olschki (Florence, 1914), R. A. Peddie's *Conspectus incunabulorum* (Pt. 1, London, 1910), A. G. Roos (*Groningen incunabula*, 1912), Alblas and Van Someren (*Utrecht incunabula*, 1922), Castan (*Besançon incunabula*, 1923), A. W. Pollard and G. R. Redgrave's short catalogue of English Books printed in 1475–1640 (London, 1926), N. P. Kiseleff's lists of Russian incunabula (Moscow, 1912–13), G. P. Winship's Census of 15th Century Books owned in America (New York, 1919), A. C. Klebs and Sudhoff's *Pestschriften* (München, 1926), and the *Nachträge* to Hain (Leipzig, 1910), published by the Prussian Kommission für den Gesamtkatalog der Wiegendrucke, which has issued two volumes of a'*Gesamtkatalog* of all the incunabula in existence (Leipzig, 1925–6). Very important is its catalogue of single sheet incunables (*Einblattdrucke des XV. Jahrhunderts*, Halle a. S., 1914). For comparing and identifying the typography of the different imprints, Konrad Haebler's *Typenrepertorium* (4 vols., Halle, 1905–22) is indispensable and invaluable; also Konrad Burger's *Monumenta Germaniæ et Italiæ typographica* (Berlin, 1892–1916), G. Dunn's Photographs of Early Types (Wolley, 1899–1905), J. W. Holtrop's *Monuments typographiques des Pays Bas* (La Haye, 1868), O. Thierry-Poux's *Premiers monuments de l'imprimerie en France* (Paris, 1890), Gordon Duff's Early English Printing (London, 1896), Haebler's *Typographie iberique* (La Haye, 1901–2); for watermarks: C. M. Bricquet: *Les filigranes* (4 v., Leipzig, 1923); for engraver's marks: F. C. Nagler: *Die Monogrammisten*, 5 v., München, 1858–79 (Reprint, 1919). The above-mentioned manual of Peddie (1913) contains valuable bibliographies of initials, printers' marks, colophons, title-pages, signatures and watermarks, and a useful list of catalogues of collections by localities. For methods of cataloguing, see A. C. Klebs, Papers Bibliog. Soc. America, Chicago, 1916, x, 143–163.

Infection: *See* Contagion.

Influenza: G. Sticker: *Die Influenza*, Wien, 1911.—F. G. Crookshank (ed.): Influenza, London 1922.

Italian Medicine: The histories of S. DeRenzi (5 v.. *Napoli*, 1845–9), F. Puccinotti (3 v., Livorno' 1850–66), G. Bilancioni (Roma, 1920), D. Barduzzi (Torino, 1923), and A. Castiglioni (Milano 1927).

Japanese Medicine: Y. Fujikawa's *Geschichte der Medizin in Japan*, Tokyo, 1911.—Deutsches Arch. f. Gesch. d. Med., Leipz., 1878, i, 215–239 (A. Wernich).—K. Ogawa: History of Japanese Ophthalmology (Tokyo, 1904).

Jewish Medicine: T. Bartholinus: *De morbis biblicis*, Copenhagen, 1672.—E. Carmoly: *Histoire des médecins juifs*, Brussels, 1844.—R. Mead: *Medicina sacra* (London, 1749).—J. B. Friedreich: *Zur Bibel* (Nuremberg, 1848).—R. J. Wunderbar: *Biblisch-talmudische Medicin*. Riga & Leipzig, 1850–60.—J. Bergel: *Die Medicin der Talmudisten*, Leipzig, 1885.—A. Stern: *Medizin im Talmud*. Frankfurt a. M., 1909.—Max Grünwald: *Die Hygiene der Juden*, Dresden, 1911.—Julius Preuss, *Biblisch-talmudische Medizin*, Berlin, 1911.—A. Friedenwald: Jewish Physicians [etc.], Gratz. Coll. Pub., Phila., 1897, No. 1.—L. Venezianer: *Asaf Judæus*, 2. v. (Strassburg, 1916–17).— M. Neuburger: *Die Medizin im Flavius Josephus*, Reichenhall, 1919.—Joseph Jacobs: Jewish Contributions to Civilization, Phila., 1919.—R. Landau: *Geschichte der jüdischen Aerzte*, Berlin, 1895.—S. Scherbel: *Jüdische Aerzte*, Berlin, 1905.—M. Steinschneider: *Jüdische Aerzte*, Frankfurt a. M., 1914.—I. Münz: *Die jüdischen Aerzte im Mittelalter*, Frankfurt a. M., 1922.—H. Rosin: *Die Juden in der Medizin*, Berlin, 1926.—S. R. Bennett: Diseases of the Bible, London 1887.—Also: C. D. Spivak and F. T. Haneman in Jewish Encycl., N. Y., 1904, viii, 409–422.

Jurisprudence (Medical): Handb. d. gerichtl. Med. (Maschka), Tübingen, 1881, i, 1–32 (V. Janowsky), with bibliography.—Cycloped. Am. Med. Biog. (Kelly), Phila.. 1912, pp. lxxv–lxxxv (T. H. Shastid).

King's Evil: Monograph by Raymond Crawfurd, Oxford, 1911.—M. Bloch: *Les rois thaumaturges*, Strasbourg, 1924.—Also: Proc. Charaka Club, N. Y., 1906, ii, 58–71 (J. S. Billings).

Laboratories (Scientific): Johns Hopkins Hosp. Bull., Balt., 1896, vii, 19–24 (W. H. Welch).

Laryngology and Rhinology (History of): Jonathan Wright's History of Laryngology and Rhinology (2. ed., Phila., 1914) is the best account in English, a very valuable and accurate work. The history by Gordon Holmes (Med. Press & Circ., London, 1885) was translated into French and German (1887). Paul Heymann's monographs in Handbuch d. Laryngol. und Rhinol., Vienna, 1896, and in the Puschmann Handbuch (1905, iii, 573–600) are worthy of note. See, also: Centralbl. f. Laryngol., Berl., 1908, xxiv, 221; 476: 1909, xxv, 227 (Sir F. Semon).—For history of laryngoscopy, see Verneuil (Gaz. hebd. de méd., Paris, 1863, x, 201–205) and Louis Elsberg (Phila. Med. Times, 1873–4, iv, 129–134), who has also left the best account of laryngology in America (Tr. Am. Laryngol. Ass., 1879, St. Louis, 1882, i, 33–90). Chauveau's *Histoire des maladies du pharynx* (1901–6) is an exhaustive work in five volumes. The history of rhinology by Karl Kassel (Würzburg, 1914) is a recent and reliable work.

Leprosy: Apart from such contributions as the monograph of G. Sticker (Wien, 1924), the articles of Sudhoff in his *Archiv* (1910–15), H. M. Fay's Paris dissertation of 1907, C. A. Mercier's Leper Houses (London, 1915) and the books of Danielssen and Boeck or Zambaco pacha, the subject has been mainly treated with reference to its distribution in space, *e. g.*, Hirsch in Creighton's (Sydenham Society) translation, Lond., 1885, ii, 1–58.

Libraries (Medical): Ref. Handb. Med. Sc. (Stedman), 3. ed., N. Y., 1915, v, 901–910 (F. H. Garrison). —E. Edwards: Memoirs of Libraries, 2 v., London, 1859.—J. W. Clark: The Care of Books, Cambridge, 1909.—J. W. Farlow: History of the Boston Medical Library, Norwood, Mass., 1918.—Bull. M. Library Ass., Balt., 1918, viii, 41–50 (J. Ruhräh).—Sudhoff's "chat" on *Medizinische Bibliotheken*, Leipzig, 1921.

Magic: G. Naudé: *Apologie*, Paris, 1625.—J. C. Adelung: *Geschichte der menschlichen Narrheit*, 1785–9.—J. Ennemoser: History of Magic, 2 v., 1854.—F. Lenormant: *La magie chez les Chaldéens*, Paris, 1874.—J.-E. J. Regnault: *La sorcellerie*, Bordeaux, 1806.—Sir E. A. T. Wallis Budge; Egyptian Magic (1899). 2. ed., London, 1901.—W. W. Skeat: Malay Magic, London, 1900.—Sir J. G. Frazer: The Golden Bough, London, 1913–15.—C. Singer: Early English Magic and Medicine, London, 1920.—W. H. R. Rivers: Medicine, Magic, and Religion, London, 1924.— Lynn Thorndike: History of Magic, 2 v., New York, 1923.—Dict. encycl. d. sc. méd., Par., 1881, 3. s., x, 455–482 (A. Chéreau).

Magnetism: Deutsches Arch. f. Gesch. d. Med., Leipz., 1878, i, 320, 381 (W. Waldmann).

Manuscripts (Medical): Daremberg: *Notices et extracts* (Paris, 1853).—Arch. f. Gesch. d. Med., Leipz., 1908–9, ii, 1; 385 (P. Pansier).—*Ibid.*, 1909–10, iii, 273–303 (Sudhoff).—H. Diels: Abhandl. d. k. preuss. Akad. d. Wissensch., Berl., phil.-hist. cl, 1905, 1–158: 1906, 1–115: 1907, 1–72.— Arch. f. Gesch. d. Med., Leipz., 1908–9, i, 1; 385 (P. Pansier); 1918–19, xi, 213–215 (K. Sudhoff) ; 1925, xvii, 205–240 (H. E. Sigerist).

Massage: Handb. d. Gesch. d. Med., Jena, 1903–5, iii, 327–340 (L. Ewer).

Mechanotherapy: Janus, Amst., 1914, xix, 178–240 (R. J. Cyriax).

Medicine (Internal): See, Clinical Medicine.

Medieval Medicine: G. F. Fort: Medical Economy During the Middle Ages, New York, 1883.— E. Dupouy: *Le moyen âge médical* (Paris, 1888).—Sir T. C. Allbutt: Science and Medieval Thought (Lond., 1901); his Historical Relations of Medicine and Surgery (etc.) (Lond., 1905); H. M. Ferrari da Grado: *Une chaire de médecine au XVe siècle* (Paris thesis No. 333, 1899) and Allbutt's account of the same in Med. Chron., Manchester, 1903, 4. s., v, 1–15.—J. J. Walsh: The Popes in Science (N. Y., 1908), and M. Neuburger: *Geschichte der Medizin*, Pagel-Sudhoff, Berlin, 1915, 152–195, also: Proc. Roy. Soc. Med., Lond., 1916–17, x, sect. Hist. Med., 107–160, Conrad Brunner's study of medieval Swiss medicine (Veröffentl. d. schweiz. Gesellsch. f. Gesch. d. med., Zürich, 1922, i, 1–158).—See also: Benedicenti: *Malati, medici e farmacisti*, Milano, 1925, and numerous contributions of Sudhoff in his Archiv. für Geschichte der Medizin, Leipzig, 1907–20, *passim*.

Mexican Medicine: F. A. Flores: *Historia de la medicina en México* (3 vols., Mexico, 1886–8).— Wien. med. Presse, 1905, xlvi, 1897–1905 (M. Neuburger).—Gac. med. de Mexico (1915), 1916, x, 3: 466 (1916), 1918, xi, 210 (N. Leon).

Microscopy (Medical): Proc. Roy. Soc. Med., Lond., 1914–15, vii, Sect. Hist. Med., 247–279 (C. Singer).—J. Roy. Micr. Soc., Lond., 1915, 317–340 (C. Singer).

Military Medicine: The prolegomena to Hermann Frölich's *Militärmedicin* (Brunswick, 1887) constitute the authoritative source for bibliographical references up to 1887, and his many essays on the subject (1869–1901) should be collected, bound and read. For Roman medico-military administration see J. Marquardt: *Handb. d. römisch. Alterthümer* (Marquardt & Mommsen). 2. Aufl., Leipz., 1884, v, 317–362 and W. Haberling: Veröffentl. a. d. Geb. d. Mil.-San.-Wesens, Berl., 1910, 19–76. For the Roman military hospitals: Meyer-Steineg: Jena med.-hist. Beitr., 1912, Heft 3, 31–34. For care of the wounded in the Middle Ages: W. Haberling: Jena med.-hist. Beitr., 1917, Heft 10. For the priority of the Swiss in state care of the wounded: Conrad Brunner: *Die Verwundeten in den Kriegen der alten Eidgenossenschaft*, Tübingen, 1903. The history of the Prussian medico-military organization was exhaustively handled by A. L. Richter (Erlangen, 1860), C. J. Prager (Berlin, 1864. 2. ed., 1875), and F. Loeffler (Berlin, 1868); that of the different European countries by Emil Knorr (Hannover, 1880), and Paul Myrdacz (Vienna, 1898). For biographies of German army surgeons of the 17th–19th centuries, see A. Köhler [*et al.*]: Veröffentl. a. d. Geb. d. Mil.-San.-Wesens, Berl., 1899, Heft 13: 1901, Heft 18: 1904, Heft 24, 27. See, also: J. Monéry: *La musée du Val de Grâce*, Paris, 1923. Gurlt's history of international and voluntary nursing in war-time (1873–9), his history of military surgery in Prussia (1875), and the military portions of his history of surgery (1898) are very important, as also J. S. Billings' reports on the American Army hospitals and posts (Circulars No. 4 and 8, 1870–75), the Medical and Surgical History of the War of the Rebellion (1870–88), Virchow's review of the progress of military medicine (1874), **A. A.** Woodhull's report upon the medical department of the British Army (1894), A. von Coler's history of military surgery (1901) and the medical histories of the Revolutionary, Mexican and Civil Wars by Louis C. Duncan (1914–20). The transportation and surgical treatment of the wounded has been exhaustively handled by Cabanès in *Chirurgiens et blessés à travers l'histoire* (Paris, 1918), with many historic illustrations. For medico-military administration during the 16th–18th centuries, see: Ann. Med. History, N. Y., 1917–18, i, 281–300 (C. L. Heizmann). See, also: F. H. Garrison: Notes on the History of Military Medicine, Washington, 1922. For bibliographies of campaigns by title, see Index Catalogue, viii, 1055–1072 and 2. s., x, 500–517; also the bibliographies of Surgery (Military).

Muscle (Physiology of): J. F. Fulton: Muscular Contraction, Baltimore, 1926, 3–55 (with chronologica bibliography).

Nature (Healing Power): Max Neuburger: *Die Lehre von der Heilkraft der Natur*, Stuttgart, 1926.

Neurology: Sketch by F. H. Garrison in C. L. Dana: Text-book Nerv. Dis., 10. ed., N. Y., 1925, pp. iv–liii.—S. E. Jelliffe: Fifty Years of American Neurology (New York, 1925).—Arch. f. Psychiat., Berl., 1925, lxxvi, 6–20 (Nonne); 21–46 (Wallenburg); 47–57 (Spielmeyer).—Psychiat.-Neurol. Wochenschr., 1907–8, ix, 110; 117; 128; 134 (Mönkemöller): 1918–19, xx, 113–132 (Obersteiner).—Klin. Wochenschr., Berlin, 1928, vii, 169; 222 (Wartenburg), and the many valuable studies of Max Neuburger (1899–1921).

Numismatics (Medical): J. C. W. Moehsen: *Beschreibung einer Berlinischen Medaillen-Sammlung* (2 vols., Berl. & Leipz., 1773–1781).—C. A. Rudolph: *Index numismatum* (Berl., 1823, with the emendations of C. L. von Duisberg, 1862–8).—L. J. Renaudier: *Études historiques* [etc.], Paris 1851.—H. Kluyskens: *Des hommes célèbres* [etc.] (2 vols., Gand, 1859).—E. Rüppell in Numismat. Ztschr., Wien, 1876, vi.—Pfeiffer & Ruland: *Pestilentia in nummis* (Tübingen, 1882).—H. R. Storer in Am. J. Numismatics, Boston, 1887–1912, *passim*.—F. Parkes Weber: Death in Art (3 ed., Lond., 1918).—Helen Farquhar: Royal Charities, Lond., 1916–22.—O. Bernhard: *Griechische und römische Münzbilder*, Zürich, 1926.—Ann. Med. Hist., N. Y., 1925, viii, 128–135 (F. H. Garrison).—Arch. f. Gesch. d. Med., Leipz., 1909–10, iii, 227: 1915–16, viii, 290 (A. M. Pachinger).

Nursing: H. Haeser: *Geschichte christlicher Krankenpflege und Pflegerschaften* (Berlin, 1857).—Mary A. Nutting & Lavinia L. Dock: A History of Nursing (4 v., N. Y., 1907–12).—Minnie Goodnow Outlines (1916), 4 ed., Philadelphia, 1928.—Arch. f. Gesch. d. Med., Leipz., 1914–15, viii, 147–164 (K. Bass).

Oath (Physician's): W. H. S. Jones: The Doctor's Oath, Cambridge, 1924.

Obstetrics: Heinrich Fasbender's *Geschichte der Geburtshülfe* (Jena, 1906) is one of those extraordinarily exhaustive and accurate monographs such as only a German scholar could turn out, occupying 1028 pages of closely woven narrative, with full bibliographic data. It is the most valuable reference work. Siebold's *Geschichte* (2. Aufl., Tübingen, 1901–2), with the supplements on the modern period by Rudolf Dohrn (1903) and on American obstetrics by J. Whitridge Williams, is the most readable. Max Wegscheider's monograph in the Puschmann Handbuch (1905, iii, 878–952) is excellent for reference purposes. E. Ingerslev's *Fragmenter* (Copenhagen, 1906–7) is noteworthy. Witkowski's *Histoire des accouchements* (Paris, 1887) and his various monographs on the cultural aspects of pregnancy and labor, the female breast, etc., are full of curious and amusing facts. A notable contribution on the graphic side is Felice La Torre's *L'utero attraverso i secoli* (Castello, 1917), which is replete with portraits, reproductions of title-pages and plates from the earlier works and MSS., including all known pictures of recumbent *gravidæ*, etc. Engelmann's Labor among Primitive Peoples (St. Louis, 1882) is an anthropological classic, and his historical sketch in Hirst's System of Obstetrics (1888, i, 17–67) is very valuable. Aveling's studies of English Midwives (1872) and of the Chamberlens (1882), Ingerslev on Röslin's Rosegarten (1902), Sinclair's life of Semmelweis (1909), R. A. Monpin's *L'avortement provoqué dans l'antiquité* (Paris diss. 111, 1918), W. H. Allport's study of the 17th century *Hebammenbücher*, and Ibrahim Menascha on Egyptian obstetrics (Arch. f. Gynäk., Berl., 1928, cxxx, 425–461) are all of them fascinating monographs showing the close relationship between obstetrics and the cultural history of mankind. The history of obstetrics in Mexico has been ably and exhaustively treated by Nicolas Leon (Mexico, 1910), with many unique illustrations. Herbert N. Spencer's History of British Midwifery (London, 1927) is a recent work.

Ophthalmology: Julius Hirschberg's *Geschichte der Augenheilkunde* in the new edition of the Graefe-Saemisch Handbuch, *passim*, is the authoritative work for reading and reference. It is a wonderful monument of German thoroughness. The shorter histories of August Hirsch (Graefe-Saemisch Handbuch, 1st ed., 1877, vii, 235–554), Pansier (in the Lagrange & Valude Encyclopédie, 1903, i, 1–86), Horstmann (Puschmann's Handbuch d. Gesch. d. Med., 1905, iii, 489–572) and (in English) that of T. H. Shastid in Am. Encycl. & Dict. Ophth. (Wood, Chicago, 1917, xi, 8524–8904, with supplement by Edward Jackson in the literature, *Ibid.*, 8905–8925, are also valuable. Special studies of worth are H. Magnus on the history of cataract (Leipzig, 1876) and ancient ophthalmology (Breslau, 1901), Victor Deneffe on the Gallo-Roman oculists (Antwerp, 1896), Pansier

(1901), Emil Bock (1903), and K. K. Lundsgaard (Copenhagen, 1913) on the history of spec-tacles, Mortimer Frank on representative ophthalmic surgeons (Wood's System of Ophth. Operat. Chicago, 1911, i, 17-41), B. Laufer on optical lenses (Leiden, 1915), and Alvin A. Hubbell on The Development of Ophthalmology in America (Chicago, 1908). See also: The articles of Hirschberg on Greek ophthalmology in Arch. f. Ophth., Berl., 1918, xcvii, 301-345 and Arch. f. Augenh., Wiesb., 1919, lxxxv, 146-183; also Univ. Penn. Lect., Phila., 1917, i, 99-123. See also: Japanese Medicine; Spectacles.

Opotherapy: Arch. f. Gesch. d. Med. Leipz., 1910-11, iv, 138-156 (H. Schelenz).

Orthodontia: B. W. Weinberger, Orthodontics, St. Louis, 1926.

Orthopedics: J. K. Young: Manual and Atlas of Orthopedic Surgery, Phila., 1905, 1-14. Sir A. Keith: Menders of the Maimed (1919), 2 ed., London, 1925.—R. B. Osgood: The Evolution of Orthopedic Surgery, St. Louis, 1925.—V. Putti: *Protesi antichi*, Bologna, 1925.—O. Neustätter: *Bilderatlas* (160 pl.), Munich, 1926.—Annual reports of R. B. Osgood and others in Boston Med-ical and Surgical Journal.

Otology: Adam Politzer's *Geschichte der Ohrenheilkunde* (v. i, Stuttgart, F. Enke, 1907-13), now com-pleted, is the authoritative and standard work. Michael Sachs in Puschmann's Handbuch (1905, iii, 464-488) gives a good shorter account. For ancient otology, see H. Werner: Arch. f. Gesch. d. Med., Leipz., 1926, xviii, 151-171.

Palæopathology: Roy L. Moodie: The Antiquity of Disease, Chicago, 1923.

Papal Physicians: P. Mandosius: Θέατρον (etc.), Rome, 1784.—G. Narini: *Degli archiatri pontifici*, 2 v. Rome, 1784. For history of the Papal physicians at Avignon (1308-1403), see Janus, Amst., 1909, xiv, 405-434 (P. Pansier).

Parasitology: Arch. de parasitol., Par., 1908, xiii, 251; 1913, xv, 543 (L. Moulé).—Handb. d. Gesch. d. Med., Jena, 1903, ii, 648-665 (H. Vierordt).—Paris thesis by H. Rémignard (1902).

Pathology: The best modern history is that of Hans Chiari in Puschmann's Handbuch (1903, ii, 473-559). Earlier sketches, as cited by Chiari, were given by Morgagni (1761), Rayer (Paris thesis, 1815), Cruveilhier (Ann. de l'anat. et physiol. path., Paris, 1846, i), Eugene Boeckel (N. dict. de méd. et de chir. prat., Paris, 1865, ii), and Rudolf Virchow (*Hundert Jahre Pathologie* Berlin, 1895).—Edgar Goldschmid's history of pathological illustration (Leipzig, 1925) is a new departure. See also: H. L. Joseph Freiburg diss., 1912.—Arch. f. Gesch. d. Med., Leipz., 1926, xviii, 302-327 (P. Diepgen). Esmond R. Long: A History of Pathology, Baltimore, 1928.

Pathology (Vegetable): H. H. Whetzel: An Outline of the History of Phytopathology, Philadelphia, 1918.

Pediatrics: Wolf Becher in Puschmann's Handbuch, 1905, iii, 982-1060. Also: Handb. d. Kinder-krankheiten (Gerhardt), Tübingen, 1877, i, 1-50 (C. Hennig).—Syst. Pediat. (Abt.), Phila., 1923, i, 1-170 (F. H. Garrison).—Janos Bokai: *Geschichte der Pädiatrik*, Berlin, 1922.—John Ruhräh: Pediatrics of the Past (New York, 1925).—Handb. d. Kinderheilk. (Pfaundler & Schloss-mann), Leipz., 1923, i, 1-11 (H. Brüning).—T. Kroner on Greek pediatrics (Jahrb. f. Kinderh., Leipz., 1876, x, 340; 1877, xi, 83; 236).—J. W. Troitzky: *Hippocrates als Kinderarzt* (Arch. f. Kinderh., Stuttg., 1900, xxix, 228-247).—Sister Mary Rosaria: The Nurse in Greek Life, Boston, 1917.—The address of Abraham Jacobi (Am. Med., Phila., 1904, viii, 795-805) and his history of American pediatrics in Arch. f. Kinderh., Stuttg., 1913 (Baginsky-Festschrift), 413-426.

Percussion and Auscultation: Handb. d. Gesch. d. Med., Jena, 1903, ii, 604-611 (H. Vierordt).—Arch. f. Gesch. d. Med., Leipz., 1907-8, i, 329; 403 (B. Noltenius).—*Ibid.*, 1910-11, iv, 43-78 (E. Ebstein).

Periodicals (Medical): Ref. Handb. Med. Sc. (Stedman), 3. ed., N. Y., 1915, v, 706-712 (F. H. Garrison).—Dublin Quart. J. Med. Sc., 1846, i, pp. i-xlviii (W. R. Wilde).—Union méd., Par., 1867, 3. s., ii, 151; 179; 193; 229; 474 (A. Chéreau).—Boston M. & S. J., 1879, c, 1; 108 (J. S. Billings).—München. med. Wchnschr., 1903, l, 455-463 (K. Sudhoff).—Piccioni: *Storia del giornalismo medico in Italia* (Turin, 1894).—Bibliog. moderne, Par., 1908, 58-96 (E. Wicker-sheimer).—A. Castiglioni: *Gli albori del giornalismo medico italiano*, Trieste, 1923.—Riedel: Arch., Berl., 1925, Sonderheft, 1-50 (W. von Brunn).—Jour. Am. Med. Ed. Assoc., N. Y., 1925, v, 39-48 (V. Robinson).—Vrach. Dielo, Kharkhov, 1925, viii, 2023-2028 (V. Kugan).—Nederl. Tijdschr. v. Geneesk., Amst., 1927, pt. 1, 3; 1711: pt. 2, 13 (C. C. Delprat).

Persian Medicine: A. M. Fonahn: *Zur Quellenkunde der persischen Medizin* (Leipzig, 1910).—H. Fichtner: *Die Medizin im Avesta*, Leipzig diss., 1914.—G. Sticker: Sudhoff-Festschrift, Zürich, 1924, 8-23.

Pest: G. Sticker: *Die Pest* (Giessen, 1908, 1. Th., 1-478).—F. A. Gasquet: The Black Death, 1893.—R. Crawfurd: Plague and Pestilence in Literature and Art, London, 1914.—K. O. Meinsma: *De zwarte dood*, Zutphen, 1924.—Joh. Nohl: The Black Death, London, 1926.—A. C. Klebs & K. Sudhoff: *Die ersten gedruckten Pestschriften*, Munich, 1926.—Also, Sudhoff on the pest tracts of 1348–1498, in his Archiv, 1910–23. i–xv. *passim*; and Dorothea Singer in Proc. Roy. Soc. Med., Lond., 1915–16, ix, Sect. Hist. Med. 159–212.—F. P. Wilson: The Plague in Shakespeare's London (Oxford, 1927).

Pharmacy: Hermann Schelenz's *Geschichte der Pharmacie* (Berlin, 1904) and A. C. Wootton's "Chronicles of Pharmacy" (London, 1910) are the best works for reading and reference. Adrien Philippe's *Histoire des apothicaires* (Paris, 1853), enlarged and translated into German by Hermann Ludwig (2. Aufl., Jena, 1859) is an earlier work, of solid character, on the history of druggists. Herman Peter's *Aus pharmazeutischer Vorzeit in Bild und Wort* (2 vols., Berlin, 1889–91) takes up the cultural side of the subject, with many interesting pictures. J. Berendes' *Die Pharmacie bei den alten Kulturvölkern* (2 v., Halle, 1891), his history of pharmacy (Leipzig, 1898), his translation of Dioscorides (Stuttgart, 1902) and the *Histoire de la pharmacie* of L. André-Pointier (Paris, 1900) are all valuable. An excellent history of American pharmacy by Edward Kremers has recently appeared in Am. Druggist, N. Y., 1920, lxviii, No. 3, 9; No. 4, 9; No. 5, 13. A. Bilancioni, *Malati, medici e farmacisti* (2 v., Milano, 1924) is very learned.—Of histories of particular pharmacies, Plough Court by E. C. Cripps (London, 1927) is typical. See, also, Drugs.

Physiology: The most readable work on this subject in English is Sir Michael Foster's Lectures on the History of Physiology (Cambridge, 1901), which is based upon original research and full of atmosphere and color. John Call Dalton's Doctrines of the Circulation (Philadelphia, 1884), William Marcet's History of Respiration in Man (London, 1897), Max Neuburger on the development of experimental physiology of the brain and spinal cord before the time of Flourens (Stuttgart, 1897), and William Stirling's Some Apostles of Physiology (London, 1902) are works of a similar character. Stirling's work is a beautiful folio, filled with fine pictures of the great masters, and, like Foster's book, inspired with enthusiasm. The text-books of Sir E. A. Schäfer (London, 1898) and Luigi Luciani (Milano, 1901–11, 5. ed., 1919–21, English translation, London, 1911–21), as also the Principles of Sir W. M. Bayliss (4. ed., London, 1924) are invaluable, and illustrate Goethe's dictum that "the history of a science is the science itself." See, also: P. A. Robin: The Old Physiology in English Literature, New York, 1911. Heinrich Boruttau's *Geschichte* (Puschmann's Handbuch, 1903, ii, 327–456) and John C. Cardwell's Development of Animal Physiology (Med. Library & Histor. Jour., New York, 1904–6, ii–iv, *passim*) may be consulted for the whole subject in its bibliographical relations. See, also, Nature, Lond., 1896, liv, 580; 600: 1897, lvi, 435 (Sir M. Foster).

Poets (Medical): T. Bartholinus: *De medicis poetis*, Copenhagen, 1669.—Janus, Bresl., 1847, ii, 772–812 (O. Seidenschnur).—Dict. encycl. d. sc. méd. (Dechambre), Par., 1877, 2. s., v, 715–727 (A. Chéreau).—C. L. Dana: Poetry and the Doctors, Woodstock, Vt., 1918.—Ann. Med. History N. Y., 1919–20, ii, 213–227 (J. Foote).

Portuguese Medicine: M. Lemos: *Historia*, 2 v., Lisbon, 1891.

Printers (Old): The subject needs special handling and has to be pieced out from such books as R. A. Peddie's Short History of Printing (London, 1927), T. L. De Vinne on the Italian printers of the 15th Century (New York, 1910), H. E. Plomer's Short History of English Printing (London, 1900), E. Voullième's *Die deutschen Drucker des 15ten Jahrhunderts* (Berlin, 1916) and *Der Buchdruck Kölns* (Bonn, 1903), Konrad Haebler (London, 1897), and K. Burger (Leipzig, 1913) on the early printers of Spain and Portugal, Haebler's *Tipografia iberica* (The Hague, 1902), and on 15th Century German printers in foreign countries (München, 1924), C. W. Zapf on the Augsburg printers (MM), Karl Schottenlohr on Ratisbon publishers in the 15th and 16th Centuries (Mainz, 1920), Robert Proctor on the printing of Greek in the 15th century (Oxford, 1900), Ph. Renouard's Documents on Paris printers of 1450–1600 (Paris, 1901), F. Madan's Early Oxford Press (Oxford, 1925), G. M. Panzer on early Nuremberg printing (Nürnberg, 1789), M.-L. Potain on printers' trademarks of 15th century France (Paris, E. Droz, 1926), and C. M. Bricquet on watermarks (*Les filigranes*, 4. v., Leipzig, 1923).

Prognosis: Wien. med. Presse, 1907, xlviii, 1–7 (M. Neuburger).—Arch. f. Gesch. d. Naturw., vi, 163–178 (T. Meyer-Steineg).

Prostitution: Handwörterb. d. Sex.-Wissensch. (Marcuse), Bonn, 1923, 365–371 (K. Sudhoff). For prostitution in armies: W. Haberling: Ztschr. f. Bekämpf. d. Geschlechtskr., Leipz., 1914, xv, 63; 103; 143; 169; 312; 323.

Protein Therapy: Bull. N. Y. Acad. Med., 1927, iii, 555–560 (F. H. Garrison).

Psychiatry: The subject has been almost entirely in the hands of German writers. Heinrich Laehr, to begin with, has made a complete history of psychiatry in the form of a calendar, now in its fourth edition (Berlin, 1893) and is the author of an unsurpassable bibliography of the literature of psychiatry, neurology, and psychology from 1459 to 1799 (Berlin, 1900). The history of J. B. Friedreich (1830) was translated by Smith Ely Jelliffe (Alienist & Neurologist, St. Louis, 1910–17, xxxi–xxxviii, *passim*). For short histories of psychiatry see the text-books of Heinroth (1818), von Feuchtersleben (1845), Flemming (1859), Leidesdorf (1865), von Krafft-Ebing (1879, or

8th ed., 1903) and Schüle (1878). Also: S. Kornfeld in Puschmann's Handbuch (1905, iii, 601–728) and Th. Kirchhoff on the history of German psychiatry (Berlin, 1890) and his general sketch in: Handb. d. Psychiat. (Aschaffenburg), Leipz. & Berl., 1912, Allg. Th., 4. Abth., 1–48. Also: R. Pophal: *Die Krankheitsbegriff in der Psychiatrie*, Berlin, 1925.—Otto Mönkemöller's history of psychiatry in Hannover (Halle, 1903), his studies of German psychiatry in the 18th (1902) and early 19th centuries (1905), and his book on the satirical and humorous aspects of the subject (1906) are of great cultural value. See, also, E. Kraepelin: *Hundert Jahre Psychiatrie* (Ztschr. f. d. ges. Neurol., Berl,. 1917–18, xxxviii, 161–275) and Traité internat. de psychol. path. (Marie), Par., 1910, i, 31–93 (F. del Greco).

Psychoanalysis: S. Freud: History (Nerv. & Ment. Dis. Monogr. Ser., No. 25), New York, 1916.

Quackery: H. Magnus: *Das Kurpfuscherthum* (Breslau, 1903).—A. Corsini: *Medici ciarlatani* (Bologna, 1922).—Brit. M. J., Lond., 1911, i, 1250–1263.—Arch. f. Gesch. d. Med., Leipz., 1908–9, ii, 285–300 (C. Sticker).

Quarantine: Johns Hopkins Hosp. Bull., Balt., 1914, xxv, 80–86 (W. W. Ford).

Roman Medicine: A. M. Birkholz: *Cicero medicus* (Leipzig, 1806).—G. Ritter von Rittershain: *Die Heilkünstler des alten Roms* (Berlin, 1875).—M. Albert: *Les médecins gracs à Rome*, Paris, 1894.—Th. Meyer: *Geschichte des römischen Aerztestandes* (Kiel, 1907).—Handb. d. Gesch. d. Med. (Puschmann), Jena, 1901–2, i, 403–414 (I. Bloch).—Brit. Med. Jour., Lond., 1909, ii, 1449; 1515; 1598 (Sir T. C. Allbutt).—Prosper Ménière (1858) and Edmond Dupouy (1885) on medicine in the Latin poets.—M. Meyer: Theodorus Priscianus, Jena, 1909.—W. Schönack: Scribonius Largus, Jena, 1912.—A. Söllner: Vitruvius (Jena med.-hist. Beitr., 1913, Heft 4).

Russian Medicine: W. M. von Richter: *Geschichte der Medicin in Russland*, 3 v., Moscow, 1813–17.—Janus, Amst., 1901, vi, 430; 475; 1906, xi, 314: 1912, xvii, 485 (F. Herrmann).—*Ibid.*, 1902, vii, 352; 404; 568; 635 (M. Lachtin).—Lancet, Lond., 1897, ii, 343–374.—Arch. f. Gesch. d. Med., Leipz., 1908–9, ii, 404–418 (F. Dorbeck). See, also: Index Catalogue, 1887, viii, 924; 1905, 2 s., x, 461.

Saint-S˙mon (Medicine in): Suzanne Thery, Paris diss., 1923, No. 299.—Chron. méd., Par., 1912, xix, 705; 737 (J. Rieux).

Saints (Medical): D. H. Kerler: *Die Patronate der Heiligen*, Ulm, 1905.—L. Deubner: *Kosmas und Damian* (Leipzig & Berlin, 1907).—Bristol M.-Chir. J., 1912, xxx, 289–294 (R. Fletcher).

Salerno (School of): Collectio Salernitana (S. De Renzi), 5 v., Naples, 1852–9.—P. Giacosa, *Magistri Salernitani* (etc.), Turin, 1901.—H. E. Handerson: The School of Salernum, N. Y., 1883.—Med. Chron., Manchester, 1904–5, 4. s., viii, 67–93, 1 pl. (W. Stirling).—Arch. f. Gesch. d. Med., Leipz., 1913–14, vii, 360; 1914–15, viii, 292; 352: 1915–16, ix, 221: 1916–17, x, 91: 1919–20, xii, 149 (K. Sudhoff).—F. R. Packard: The School of Salerno, New York, 1920.—Prometheus, Leipz., 1921 253–260 (K. Sudhoff).—Sudhoff-Festschr. (Essays, etc.), Zürich, 1924, 121–138 (C. & D. Singer).

Scandinavian Medicine: Janus, Amst., 1907, xii (665); 1908, xiii (631) *passim* (F. Grön).—S. Laache: *Norsk Medicin i hundrede Aar* (Kristiania, 1911).

Schematic Eye: Janus, Amst., 1909, xiv, 435–456 (E. Pergens).

Science: Ed. Fournié: *Application des sciences à la médecine*, Paris, 1878.—F. C. Müller: *Geschichte der organischen Naturwissenschaften in 19ten Jahrhundert*, Berlin, 1902.—Rudolf Eisler: *Geschichte der Wissenschaften* (Leipzig, 1906).—F. Dannemann: *Die Naturwissenschaften*, 2 v., Leipzig, 1910. —A. Mieli: *Manuale*, Rome, 1925.—Studies, ed. C. Singer, 2 v., Oxford, 1917.—A. E. Garrod: Harveian Oration, London, 1924.—G. Sarton: Introduction to the History of Science, v. 1, Baltimore, 1927.—C. Singer: From Magic to Science, London, 1928.—Also, the briefer history of W. T. Sedgwick & H. W. Tyler (Boston, 1917).—Bibliography by Aksel Josephson (John Crerar Library, Chicago, 1911).—Science, N. Y., 1908, n. s., xxvii, 49–64 (W. H. Welch).

Scottish Medicine: J. D. Comrie: History, London (1927), 1928.

Scurvy: A. F. Hess: Scurvy, Past and Present, Philadelphia, 1921.

Shakespeare (Medicine in): J. C. Bucknill: The Medical Knowledge of Shakespeare (London, 1860).—T. E. Thiselton-Dyer: Folk-lore of Shakespeare (London, 1883).—J. Moyes: Medicine & Kindred Arts (etc.) (Glasgow, 1896).—Ber. d. deutsch. pharm. Gesellsch., Berl., 1911, xxi, 373: 1912, xxii, 268; 359 (H. Schelenz).—Tr. Med. Soc., Lond., 1915–16, xxxix, 257–325, Toronto 1919, lii, 546–574 (Sir St. Clair Thomson).—Discovery, Lond., 1927, iii, 132; 160 (D. F. Harris).

South American Medicine: F. H. Martin's Survey, New York, 1927.—R. Schiaffino: *Historia de la medicina en el Uruguay*, v. 1, Montevideo, 1927.

Spanish Medicine: The histories of A. Chinchilla (4 v., Valencia, 1841–8), A. H. Morejon (7 v., Madrid, 1842–52), and E. Garcia del Rio (Madrid, 1921).

Spectacles: D. M. Manni: *Degli occhiali da naso* [etc.], Florence, 1738.—P. Pansier: *Histoire des lunettes* (Paris, 1901).—E. Bock: *Die Brille und ihre Geschichte* (Wien, 1903).—R. Greeff: *Die*

Erfindung der Augengläser, Berlin, 1921.—Ber. ü. d. Versamml. d. ophth. Gesellsch., 1912, Wiesb., 1913, xxxix, 419–451 (R. Greeff).—Ztschr. f. ophthal. Optik., Berl., 1913–14, i, 46: 1916, iv, 142: 1917, v, 42; 65: 1918, vi, 1; 36; 97 (R. Greeff). *Ibid.*, 1917, v, 1; 33; 78 (M. von Rohr).

Surgery: For prehistoric surgery the essays of H. Tillmanns (1883), R. Lehmann-Nitsche (1896–8), G. Buschan (1902), and K. Jäger (1907), Robert Fletcher on prehistoric trephining (Washington, 1882) and Lucas-Championnière: *Les origines de la trépanation* (Paris, 1912).—Up to the end of the 16th century Gurlt's *Geschichte der Chirurgie* (1898) and Malgaigne's *Histoire de chirurgie* (1840) are the authoritative sources, the former unrivalled for accuracy, and containing many interesting plates of surgical instruments. See also, Friedrich Helfreich in Puschmann's Handbuch (v. iii, 1–306), a valuable source of reference. Walter von Brunn's recent book (1927) is a reliable, well illustrated presentation. Karl Sudhoff's splendid volumes on medieval surgery (Stud. z. Gesch. d. Med. (Puschmann Stiftung), Leipz., 1914–18, Heft 10–12) open up a vast amount of new material on horoscopic surgery, unprinted texts of the older writers, history of instrumentation, etc., with many wonderful pictures from the MSS. Kurt Sprengel's *Geschichte* (Halle, 1805–19) gives histories of the different operations. George J. Fisher's essay (Internat. Encycl. Surg. (Ashhurst), N. Y., 1886, vi, 1146–1202) gives a very accurate and full account of the earlier writers up to the 18th century. The best history of the whole subject of surgery in English is that of John S. Billings, forming the introductory chapter to Dennis's System of Surgery (New York, 1895, i, 1–444). It is not only wonderfully accurate in respect of facts and dates, but imbued with a genuinely critical spirit. In the same class are Sir William Fergusson's Lectures of 1867, and the important monograph of Sir Clifford Allbutt on "The Historical Relations of Medicine and Surgery to the End of the Sixteenth Century," the best history of medieval surgery in English. See also Zeis's history of plastic surgery (Leipzig, 1863), George Fischer on the cultural aspects of 18th century surgery (*Chirurgie vor 100 Jahren*, 1876), also translated into English by Carl H. von Klein in J. Am. M. Ass., Chicago, 1897, xxviii, 308–1898, xxx, 211, *passim;* J. S. Milne (Oxford, 1897) and Th. Meyer-Steineg (Jena, 1912) on surgical instruments, and the excellent article by Charles Creighton in Encycl. Britan., 11 ed., Cambridge, 1911, xxvi, 125–129. English surgery is ably specialized in John Flint South's Memorials of the Craft of Surgery in England (1886), Sidney Young's Annals of the Barber-Surgeons of London (1890), and the interesting monographs of D'Arcy Power. German surgery may be studied in Rohlfs' *Die chirurgischen Klassiker Deutschlands* (Leipzig, 1883–5), in Georg Fischer (1876), H. Tillmann's *Hundert Jahre Chirurgie* (1898) and Ernst Becker's essay on old-time Hildesheimer surgeons (1902). For biographies and achievements of recent German surgeons, see *Deutscher-Chirugenkalender* (Fr. Michelsson), 2. Aufl., Leipzig, 1926. American surgery up to 1876 is exhaustively treated by Samuel D. Gross in Am. Jour. Med. Sc., Phila., 1876, n. s., lxxi, 431–484. The essays of James Evelyn Pilcher (Jour. Am. Med. Assoc., 1890, xiv, suppl. No. 18, 629–636) and Frederick S. Dennis (Med. Rec., N. Y., xlii, 637–648) are also valuable for reference.—P. De Vecchi: Modern Italian Surgery, New York, 1921.

Symbolism (Medical): T. S. Sozinskey: Medical Symbolism (Phila., 1891).—H. Bayley: The Lost Language of Symbolism, 2 vols. (Lond., 1912).

Technics: F. M. Feldhaus: *Die Technik der Vorzeit* (Leipz. & Berl., 1914).—L. Darmstaedter: *Handbuch zur Geschichte der Naturwissenschaften* (Berlin, 1908).—H. Diels: *Antike Technik*, Leipzig, 1924.

Teratology: J. W. Ballantyne: Teratogenesis, Edinburgh, 1897.—A. Sonderegger: *Missgeburten und Wundergestalten*, Zürich, 1927.

Test-types: Janus, Amst., 1905, x, 419; 1906, xi, 360 (E. Pergens).

Therapeutics: R. Lépine: *La thérapeutique sous les premiers Césars* (Paris, 1890).—J. Petersen: *Hauptmomente in der geschichtlichen Entwicklung der medicinischen Therapie* (Kopenhagen, 1877). —E. J. Waring: *Bibliotheca therapeutica* (London, 1878).—Ch. Fiessinger: *La thérapeutique des vieux maitres* (Paris, 1897).—Fischer: *Zur Geschichte der Therapie*, Wien, 1925.—J. J. Walsh: Cures, New York, 1923.

Theriac: Janus, Amst., 1911, xvi, 371; 457 (C. E. Daniëls).—Johns Hopkins Hosp. Bull., Balt., 1915, xxvi, 222–226 (G. W. Corner).—Bull. Soc. d'hist. de pharm., Par., mars, 1920 (E. Wickersheimer).

Thermometry: H. C. Bolton: Evolution of the Thermometer (Easton, Pa., 1900).—F. Burckhardt: *Zur Geschichte des Thermometers* (Basel, 1902).—Mitt. z. Gesch. d. Med. u. d. Naturw., Hamb. & Leipzig, 1902, i, 5; 57; 143; 282 (E. Wohlwill).—Ztschr. f. phys. u. diät. Therap., Leipz., 191–2, v, 388–403 (C. E. Daniëls).—Lancet, Lond., 1816, i, 173; 281; 338; 450; 495 (G. Sims Woodhead and P. C. Varrier-Jones).

Theurgic Therapy: Ad. Franz: *Die kirchlichen Benediktionen im Mittelalter*, 2 v. (Freiburg i. B., 1909).

Thibetan Medicine: H. Laufer: *Beiträge zur Kenntnis der tibetischen Medicin* (Leipz., 1900).

Toxicology: L. Lewin: *Die Gifte in der Weltgeschichte*, Berlin, 1920; and his *Phantastica*, 2. Aufl., Berlin, 1927.

Transfusion: G. W. Crile, Hæmorrhage and Transfusion, N. Y., 1909, 151–158.

Tuberculosis: A. Predöhl: *Zur Geschichte der Tuberkulose* (Hamburg, 1888).

Universities (Medieval): G. Rashdall: The Universities in Europe during the Middle Ages, Oxford, 1925.

Urology (History of): The monograph by E. Desnos in Encycl. franç. d'urol., Par., 1914, i, 1–294, distances every other publication on this theme. It is very exhaustive and its many interesting illustrations include rare illuminated pictures from old MS. never before reproduced. See, also: C. Viellard: *L'urologie et les médecins urologiques* (Paris, 1903).—Ztschr. f. Heilk., Berl., 1894, xv, 53–74 (J. Neumann).—Ztschr. f. Urol., Leipz., 1915, ix, 201; 241; 281 (E. Ebstein).—Bull. Johns Hopkins Hosp., Balt., 1916, xxvii, 327–331 (H. H. Young).

Vaccination: E. M. Crookshank: History and Pathology of Vaccination, 2 v., London, 1889.

Variolation: Johns Hopkins Hosp. Bull., Balt., 1913, xxiv, 69–83 (A. C. Klebs).—Also his: *Die Variolation im 18ten Jahrhundert* (Giessen, 1914).

Venereal Diseases: C. Girtanner: *Abhandlung über die venerischen Krankheiten*, 3 v., Göttingen, 1788–9; 2. Aufl., 1793.—C. G. Gruner: *Spicilegium scriptorum de morbo gallico*, Jena, 1799–1802.— J. Rosenbaum: *Geschichte der Lustseuche im Alterthume*, 7. Aufl., Berlin, 1904.—J. Proksch: *Die Litteratur über die venerischen Krankheiten*, Bonn, 1898–1900 and his *Geschichte* (Bonn, 1895–1900).—I. Bloch: *Die Ursprung der Syphilis*, Jena, 1900–11.—K. Sudhoff: *Mal franzoso in Italien*, Giessen, 1912; also, *Aus der Frühgeschichte der Syphilis*, Leipzig, 1912, and *Der Ursprung der Syphilis*, Leipzig, 1913.—G. Vorberg: *Über den Ursprung der Syphilis*, Stuttgart, 1924, and the many periodical contributions of Sudhoff's followers.

Veterinary Medicine: L. Moulé: *Histoire de la médecine vétérinaire*, Paris, 1891–1911.—H. Neffgen: *Das Veterinär-Papyrus von Kahun*, Berl., 1904.—C. P. Lyman: A History of Veterinary Medicine (etc.) (Cambridge, Mass., 1898).—Bull. Soc. centr. de méd. vét., Par., 1890, 7. s., vii, 519, *passim.*—Sir F. Smith: The Early History of Veterinary Literature, v. 1. [to 1700], Lond., 1919.

Whooping-cough: G. Sticker: *Der Keuchhusten* (Wien, 1896).

Witchcraft: J. Weyer: *Histoires, disputes et discours*, 2 v., Paris, 1885.—J. Wickwar: Witchcraft London, 1925.—Fac. de méd. de Par., Confér. histor., 1866, 383–443 (Axenfeld).—Arch. Neurol. & Psychiat., Chicago, 1920, iii, 465–484 (C. A. Potts).

Women in Medicine: C. F. Harless: *Die Verdienste der Frauen*, Göttingen, 1830.—H. Schelenz: *Frauen im Reiche Aeskulaps*, Leipz., 1900.—M. Lipinski: *Histoire des femmes médecins*, Paris diss., 1900.—Louisa Martindale: The Woman Doctor, London, 1922.

Zoölogy: Bibliography of Zoölogy by J. V. Carus and W. Engelmann (Leipzig, 1861).—V. Carus: *Geschichte der Zoölogie*, 1853.

IV. QUESTIONS AND EXERCISES

1. Translate into idiomatic English:
    (a) Hyrtl's address over a box of cigars. (Allg. Wien. Med. Ztg., 1880, xxv, 521.)
    (b) Charcot: *La foie qui guérit.* (Arch. de neurol., Par., 1893, xxv, 72–87.)
    (c) Stossgebet eines practischen Arztes. (Med. Woche, Berl., 1903, 243–247.)
    (d) E. and J. de Goncourt: Une visite à la Charité. (Chronique méd., Par., 1796, iii, 460–464.)

2. Write brief sketches (ten-minute expositions) of any of the following: Achille Chéreau; K. F. H. Marx; Vulpian; Florian Heller; Oviedo; Bence Jones; Lorenzo Bellini; La Mettrie; Romeo Seligmann; Gideon Harvey; Adamantios Coray; Maximiano Lemos; Guido Baccelli; Pierre Rouanet; Pravaz; Oswaldo Cruz; Ludwig Choulant; Julius Wolff; Venel; Oken; Raphael Blanchard; Sir William Gull; Symphorien Champier; Albers-Schönberg; Hideyo Noguchi.

3. Expand any one of the above into a full-length biographical study, with complete references and full bibliography (using S. G. O. or A. M. A. models).

4. Write out a critical discussion of Max Wellmann's changes of viewpoint with reference to the authorship of Celsus.

5. Make as complete a list as you can of modern dramas in which medicine is a leading motive.

6. Explain: bezoars; *parabolani;* Bestiaries; psora; wound-suckers; hypocras; Occam's razor; derivative blood-letting; moxa; St. Anthony's fire; Galenicals; weapon-salve; *Bertillonage;* sympathetic powder; couvade; *genius epidemicus;* Daltonism; *medici condotti;* cruentation; Geneva Convention; *xenodochia;* Baunscheidtism; infibulation; Rosicrucians; phlogiston; *Hollandgeherei;* odic force; azote; falling sickness; vomica; *rhizotomi; loi Roussel;* Eck's fistula; charcoal model; *Kurierfreiheit; la graine;* schizoids; synthalin; genotype; sublimation; sex-linked inheritance; panmixia; pallium; effort syndrome; sublimation; *Gestalt* psychology; emergent evolution.

7. What were the remoter origins of the humoral pathology? Trace the alternations of humoral and solidist doctrine from Hippocrates to Besredka.

8. Name as many medical men as you can who published poetry before 1850; after 1850.

9. Prepare brief histories of: fo cal infection; town-planning; decompression of the brain; hemostasis; valvular diseases of the heart; industrial hygiene; vesicovaginal fistula; disposal of the dead; dengue; inspection of food and drugs; phototherapy; physiological chemistry; medical libraries.

10. What was Huxley's reaction to Buddhism? What does it signify?

11. Discuss the history of the shuttle-wise (ebb and flow) doctrine of the circulation and the trend toward the circle-wise concept up to Harvey's demonstration.

12. Make a list of the Papal physicians.

13. Why did Goethe dislike Haller?

14. What was the Hindu method of teaching surgical procedure?

15. What changes have been rung upon the neurogenic and myogenic theories of cardiac action from Harvey to Gaskell?

16. Why are schools of thought injurious to medicine?

17. What important works of Malpighi were printed at the expense of the Royal Society?

18. How did Descartes acquire his knowledge of anatomy?

19. Prepare complete bibliographies of the writings of: Achille Chéreau; Ephraim McDowell; Carl Ernst von Baer; Oliver Wendell Holmes; William Hunter; Daremberg; Johann Peter Frank; Georges Hayem; Lancisi; Emile Littré; Ramazzini; Semmelweis; Thomas Hodgkin; Friedrich Hoffmann.

20. Who were the successive owners of the Gold Headed Cane?

21. What books are of fundamental importance in the history of dentistry?

22. What painters have represented chlorosis? bubonic plague? insanity? idiocy? leprosy? pregnancy? syphilis? rhinophyma? the gaits and attitudes in hysteria and paralysis?

23. Write a review (500–1000 words) of any of the following: W. T. Porter: Shock at the Front, Boston, 1918.—Howard Kelly and W. L. Burrage: American Medical Biographies, 3 ed., New York, 1928.—Hans Much: *Hippocrates der Grosse*, Stuttgart, 1926.—W. C. Curry: Chaucer and the Medieval Sciences, New York, 1926.—Charles Singer: Greek Biology and Greek Medicine, Oxford, 1922.—H. O. Taylor: Greek Biology and Medicine, Boston, 1922.— F. P. Wilson: The Plague in Shakespeare's London, Oxford, 1927.

24. What improvements (if any) in evacuating the wounded from the battlefield were made by Larrey? Percy? Goercke? Sax? Brambilla? Letterman?

25. Who discovered the pathogenic parasites of favus? dysentery? hook-worm infection? African sleeping sickness? yaws? Texas fever?

26. What ideas, fallacies or medical superstitions are implicit in the following?
"O, fools, and slow of heart, to believe all that the prophet has spoken." Luke, xxiv, 25.

"Curiosus nemo est quin idem sit malevolus."   Plautus.

"Non est cardiacus" (Craterum dixisse putato).
"Hic aeger."   Horace. Sat ii, 3, 161–162.
"Le cœur a ses raisons que la raison ne connait pas."   Pascal.
"Es ist der Geist der sich den Körper baut."   Schiller.

"Verum ambitiosus et audax:
Naviget Anticyram."   Horace. Sat ii, 3, 165–166.

"Swift to their several quarters hasted then
The cumbrous elements, earth, flood, air, fire."   Milton.

"Un corps débile affaiblit l'âme."   Rousseau.

"Im engen Kreis verengert sich der Sinn."   Schiller.

"Ferme acerrima proximorum odia sunt."   Tacitus.

"Through all thy veins shall run
A cold and drowsy humor, which shall seize
Each vital spirit."   Romeo and Juliet, iv, 1.

"Quando fu l'aer si pien di malizia,
Che gli animali, infino al picciol vermo,
Cascaron tutti."   Dante.   Paradiso, xxix, 5.

"Why universal plodding poisons up
The nimble spirits in the arteries."   Love's Labour's Lost, iv, 3.

"Curatio ipsa et contactus aegrorum vulgabat morbos."   Livy, xxv, 26.

"The white cold virgin snow upon my heart
Abates the action of my liver."   Tempest, iv, 1.

"I feel my liver pierced, and all my veins,
That there begin and nourish every part,
Mangl'd and torn."   Marlowe.   Tamburlaine, pt. 2, iii, iv.

"But I am pigeon-livered and lack gall."   Hamlet, ii, 2.

"Reason and respect
Make livers pale and lustihood deject."   Troilus and Cressida, ii, 2.

"Nec porro augendis rebus spatio foret usus
Seminis ad coitum, si e nilo crescere possent."   Lucretius, i, 184–185.

"And well observe Hippocrates' old rule,
The only medicine for the foot is rest."   Thomas Nash.

"*Jeune chirurgien, vieux médecin.*" French proverb.

"Look to thy mouth: diseases enter there." George Herbert.

"*Mature fieri senem, si diu velis esse senex.*" Cicero.

"That such a crafty devil as his mother
Should yield the world this ass!" Cymbeline, ii, 1.

"*Un sot n'a pas assez d'étoffe pour être bon.*" La Rochefoucauld.

"Evil is wrought by want of Thought, as well as by want of Heart." Thomas
Hood.

"*Hysterica passio!*—down thou climbing sorrow,
Thy element's below!" King Lear, ii, 4.

"*Praeterea nobis veratrum est acre venenum,
Et capris adipes et coturnicibus auget.*" Lucretius, iv, 637.

"Meantime she quenched her fury at the flood,
And with a lenten salad cooled her blood." Dryden.

"*Imago, animi vultus indices oculi.*" Cicero.

"These words of yours draw life-blood from my heart." Henry VI, pt. 4.

"Or if that surly spirit, melancholy,
Had baked thy blood and made it heavy thick,
Which else runs tickling up and down thy veins." King John, iii, 3.

"*Turpe senex miles; turpe senilis amor.*" Ovid.

"The circling streams, once thought but pools of blood." Dryden.

"*Materies igitur, solido quae corpore constat,
Esse aeterna posset, cum cetera dissoluantur.*" Lucretius, i, 518.

"Would heart of man once think it?" Hamlet, i, 5.

"*Quin etiam morbis in corporis avius errat
Saepe animus, dementet, enim deliraque fatur.*" Lucretius, iii, 463.

"*Quare animum quoque dissolui fateare necesse est
Quandoquidem penetrant in eum contagia morbi.*" Lucretius, iii, 470.

"Death, having preyed upon the outward parts,
Leaves them insensible; and his siege is now
Against the mind." King John, v, 7.

"*Aut alio possis animi traducere motus.*" Lucretius, iv, 1072.

"It is certain that either wise bearing, or ignorant carriage, is caught, as men
take diseases, of one another, therefore let men take heed of their company."
II. Henry IV, v, 1.

"*Decidit abscissum, cum mens tamen atque hominis vis
Mobilitate mali non quit sentire dolorem.*" Lucretius, iii, 645.

"The sense of death is most in apprehension." Measure for Measure, iii, 1

"You believ'd her arteries
Grew as they do in your anatomies,
. . . If you had seen
Penelope dissected, or the Queen
Of Sheba, then you might have found a way,
To have preserved her from that fatal day." Francis Beaumont.

"*Cette maladie qui s'appelle la vie.*" Mademoiselle de l'Espinasse.

"The labor we delight in physics pain." Macbeth, ii, 3.

"*Odi et amo; quare id faciam fortasse requiris;
Nescio, sed fieri sentio et excrucior.*" Catullus.

"I stand, and to the gods and to the dead
Do reverence without prayer or praise, and shed
Offering to these unknown, the gods of gloom,
And what of honey and spice my seed-lands bear,
And what I may of fruits in this chilled air,
And lay, Orestes like, across the tomb
A curl of severed hair." Swinburne: Ave atque Vale.

"*Et come a lume acuta si dissona
Per lo spirto visivo che ricorre
Allo splendor che va di gonna in gonna.*" Dante. Paradiso, xxvi, 70.

"The cause of love can never be assigned;
'Tis in no face, but in the lover's mind."   Dryden.

"*Multaque tum interiisse animantum saecla necesse est
Nec potuisse propaganda procudere prolem
Nam quaecumque vides vesci viialibus auris,
Aut dolus aut virtus aut denique mobilitas est
Ex ineunte aevo genus id tutata reservans.*"   Lucretius, v, 855.

"There's language in her eye, her cheek, her lip,
Nay her foot speaks, her wanton spirits look out
At every joint and motive of her body."   Troilus and Cressida, iv, 5.

"*Genio y figura hasta la muerte.*"   Juan Valera.

"But where the greater malady is fixed
The lesser is scarcely felt."   King Lear, iii, 4.

"They burnt old shoes, goose-feathers, asafœtida,
A few horn-shavings, with a bone or two,
And she is well again about the house."   Ben Jonson. Magnetic Lady, v, 1.

"*Sentit enim vim quisque suam quoad possit abuli.
Cornua nata prius vitulo quam frontibus extent
Illis iratus petit atque infestus inurget.*"   Lucretius, v, 1033.

"Carry his water to the wise woman."   Twelfth Night, iii, 4.

"*Tête de fous ne blanchit jamais.*"   French proverb.

"What with Venus and other oppresioun
Of houses, Mars his venim is adoun,
That Ypermnistra dar not handle a knyf
In malice, thogh she sholde lese her lyf."   Chaucer.

"*Amor est titillatio, concomitante idea externae causae.*"   Spinoza.

"Not always actions show the man; we find
Who does a kindness is not therefore kind.

. . . .

Who combats bravely is not therefore brave,
He dreads a death-bed like the meanest slave;
Who reasons wisely is not always wise;
His pride in reasoning, not in acting, lies."   Pope.

"First Physician: A pleurisy I see it.
Second Physician: I rather hold it for *tremor cordis.*"   Beaumont and
Fletcher. Monsieur Thomas, ii, 4.

"When humors rise, they eat a sovereign herb,
Whereby what clogs their stomach they cast up;
And as some writers of experience tell,
They were the first invented vomiting."   Thomas Nash (1593).

"*Enfant malade et douze fois impure.*"   Alfred de Vigny.

"*Milites a medicis gratis curentur.*"   Aurelian.

"All the infections that the sun sucks up
From bogs, fens, flats on Prosper fall and make him
By inch-meal a disease."   Tempest, ii, 2.

"*Sic in amore Venus simulacris ludit amantes.*"   Lucretius, iv, 1101.

"For once to marry
Is honorable in woman, and her ignorance
Stands for a virtue, coming new and fresh."   Thomas Middleton.

"*Ne Saturnus cum malis mandaret adeptus
Aeternumque daret matri sub pectore vulnus.*"   Lucretius, ii, 636.

"'Tis time to give them physic; their diseases
Are grown so catching."   Henry VIII, i, 3.

"*Huic accedit uti quicque in sua corpora rursum
Dissoluat natura neque ad nilum interemat res.*"   Lucretius, i, 215.

"In poison there is physic." II. Henry IV, i, 1.

"*Ich sag' es dir; ein Kerl der speculirt*
Ist wie ein Tier auf dürrer Heide,
Von einem bösen Geist herumgefuhrt,
Und rings herum liegt schöne, grüne Weide." Goethe.

"Virtue itself turns vice, being misapplied;
And vice sometime's by action dignified." Romeo and Juliet, ii, 3.

"*Est deus in nobis, et sunt commercia coeli.*" Ovid.

"*Nil igitur mors est ad nos neque pertinet hilum*
Quandoquidem natura animi mortalis habetur." Lucretius, iii, 830.

"*Nec tamen omni modis poterat concordia gigni,*
Sed bona magnaque pars servabat fœdera caste;
Aut genus humanum jam tum foret omne peremptum
Nec potuisse adhuc perducere saecla propago." Lucretius, v, 1024.

27. What modern orchestral composition attempts to dramatize the onset and course of an acute, fatal disease?

28. In what way has the ethical spirit of medicine influenced modern civilization?

29. Who first advanced the idea of the socialization of medicine and its absorption into the general body of scientific knowledge? What fallacies and pitfalls are implicit in this notion?

30. Criticize Naunyn's argument in denying that the practice of medicine is an art.

31. Who first devised methods for cataloguing the incunabula? What new ideas did Sudhoff bring to the study of the medical incunabula? Why did he call it a "sport for bibliophiles"?

32. What was Weigert's Siva-theory? What is its bearing upon recent therapeutics?

33. Who predicted that the pathogen of yellow fever would be a flagellate protozoön?

34. What was the effect of the window-tax upon disease-incidence and social welfare in the 17th–18th centuries?

35. What are the best editions of Hippocrates and Galen:
    (a) For medical philologists?
    (b) For students and practitioners?

36. State Crookshank's theory of the causation of epidemics in space and time? What were its origins? How does it conflict with the bacterial theory of communicable diseases?

37. Who originated the following expressions: protoplasm? eugenics? pneumothorax? phagocytosis? conservation of energy? dissipation of energy? pin-hole pupil? ægophony? metabolism (*Stoffwechsel*)? medical police? diphtheria? typhoid fever? enteric fever? tabes dorsalis? locomotor ataxia? erythromelalgia? anesthesia? opsonic index? coma vigil? internal secretions? aphasia? neurons? hormones? synapse? autonomic system? vagotonia? entelechies?

38. Who were Ctesias? Oporinus? Caelius Aurelianus? Stannius? Caius? Scultetus? Simon Colinæus? Sanctorius? Anutius Fœsius? Nicholas Culpeper? Louise Bourgeois? the Chamberlens? the Chevalier Taylor? Valentine Greatrakes? John St. John Long? Antommarchi? La Peyronie? Struensee?

39. Who discovered the mammalian ovum? the spermatozoa? the red blood-corpuscles? the gastric juice? chyle? the cerebrospinal fluid?

40. Who were the prime movers of experimental epidemiology? What are its lines of approach and attack?

41. What Galenic texts did Linacre translate?

42. What names are associated with the introduction of clinical thermometry?

43. What chapter in Carlyle hinges upon a proprietary medicine?

44. Explain: "The Reve was a sclendre colerick man

. . . .

> Ful longe were his legges, and ful lene,
> Y-lyk a staf, there was no calf y-sene."   Chaucer.   Prologue.

> "Dead Henry's wounds
> Open their congeal'd mouths and bleed afresh!
> Blush, blush, thou lump of foul deformity;
> For 'tis thy presence that exhales this blood
> From cold and empty veins where no blood dwells."   Richard III, i, 2

> "He gives the web and the pin, squints the eye,
> And makes the hare-lip."   King Lear, iii, 4.

> "And she is herself in the tub."   Measure for Measure, iii, 2.

> "There nas quik-silver, litarge, ne brimstoon,
> Boras, Ceruce, ne oille of tartre noon,
> Ne oyntement that wolde clense and lyte,
> That him mighte helpen of his whelkes Whyte,
> Nor of the Knobbes Sittinge on his chekes."   Chaucer.   Prologue.

> "Light is an effect of fire and fire will burn: *ergo*, light wenches will
>   burn."   Comedy of Errors, iv, 3.

> "He plays well the physition,
> With licking tongue he cures."   Timothy Kendall (1577).

45. What did Frederick the Great do for the development of medicine in Prussia?

46. Explain: archæus; *gisants;* embrocations; "the tub-fast and the diet"; *chirurgiens de robe courte; coqueluche;* setons; Winchester goose; Jesuit's bark; green water; spitting pill; spagyric medicine; imposthumes; plica Polonica; temple sleep; making medicine; *trousse-galante;* uromancy; *doctores bullati;* polypragmatism; judicial astrology; medical constitutions; "all or none."

47. What is the medical interest in: Phineas Fletcher: The Purple Island? Campanella: *Civitas solis?* Samuel Butler: Erewhon? Molière: *Monsieur de Porceaugnac?* Charles Brocken Brown: Arthur Mervyn? Ibsen: An Enemy of Society? Diderot: *Entretien entre d'Alembert et Diderot (Le rêve de d'Alembert)?* Thomas Mann: *Zauberburg?*

48. What changes in medical practice were made by Brissot? Broussais? Corvisart? John Brown? Skoda? Brand of Stettin? Sir James Mackenzie?

49. Who introduced the following drugs: cinchona bark? calomel? strychnine? digitalis? morphine? ether? chloral? chloroform? sulphonal? veronal?

50. In what subjects did the Arabian physicians excel?

51. Who made the first experiments on decerebrated animals?

52. Who first devised an alphabet for deaf-mutes?

53. What English physicians in the 18th century possessed expensive museums and botanic gardens?

54. Write out a brief abstract (1000–5000 words) of the more interesting features in any of the following medical autobiographies: Von Baer (1865); Charles Caldwell (1855); Kussmaul (1899–1903); Leyden (1910); Pirogoff (1894); Felix Platter: Marion Sims (1884); Sir Ronald Ross (1923); Strümpell (1925); Winslow (1912); Ramón y Cajal (1901–17).

55. What is the earliest recorded instance of the use of iron as a tonic?

56. What modern cities have erected monuments to Servetus?

57. Who wrote the authoritative life of Vesalius? In what respects is it a model for medical biographers?

58. Who were the best pupils of: Boerhaave? Monro *primus?* John Hunter? Magendie? Johannes Müller? Louis? Carl Ludwig? Sir Astley Cooper? Billroth? Frerichs? Virchow? Naunyn? Sir Michael Foster? J. N. Langley? Pavloff?

59. What are the leading medical names of Spain? Russia? Norway? Sweden? Switzerland? Denmark? Japan?

60. What is the historical significance of the equations: $CaCO_3 = CaO + CO_2$? $CaO + H_2O = Ca(OH)_2$? $NH_4CNO = CO(NH_2)_2$? $C_6H_5COOH + NH_2\text{-}CH_2COOH = NH(C_6H_5CO).CH_2.COOH + H_2O$?

61. What mathematical laws of physical chemistry are now fundamental in physiology?

62. What army surgeons have achieved distinction in other fields of activity?

63. What was the first medical tract to be printed? What was the first medical book to be printed?

64. What great writers of antiquity described the plagues of Athens and Ægina?

65. With what do you associate the following dates: 1348? 1453? 1543? 1628? 1775? 1798? 1832? 1847? 1849? 1850? 1859? 1867?

66. What did Ivan the Terrible do for Russian medicine?

67. Devise courses of reading and prepare historical essays on any of the following subjects:

"Wise women" up to the 17th Century. Vulpian. Medicine in English Novels of the 18th Century. Wound-suckers. Medical Lexicography. Hypnotism and Psychotherapy in the 16th and 17th Centuries. The Fortunes of D'Aquin and Fagon at the Court of Louis XIV. Status of the Executioner in the Surgery of the 18th Century. Contribution of the South to American Medicine. Bedside Reasoning in the Middle Ages. Public Health in the United States before 1850. The Early Printers of Medical Books. Tobias Smollett. The Medical Humoresques of Fechner.

68. Who made the earliest experiments in anaphylaxis, and who originated the term?

69. What medical men have been prominent in combating the doctrine of spontaneous generation?

70. What opinions about medicine and the medical profession were entertained by the following celebrities: Petrarch? Molière? Montaigne? Frederick the Great? Goethe? Napoleon? Lord Beaconsfield? Tolstoi?

71. What important scientific ideas are adumbrated in the poetic fragments of Empedocles (Monist, Chicago, 1907, xvii, 451–474).

72. What pathologists and surgeons have classified tumors?

73. Who made the first botany? the first materia medica? the first formulary? the first pharmacopœia?

74. What was the difference between the "Nature-Philosophy" and "Natural History" schools of German medicine?

75. Why did *Life* (New York) satirize medicine during the decade 1908–1918?

76. Who first described paralysis agitans? emphysema of the lungs? heart-block? aortic insufficiency? leukemia? syringomyelia? rheumatic gout? poliomyelitis? facial neuralgia? beriberi? ascending neuritis? hemolytic jaundice? myxedema? presbyophrenia? bubonic plague?

77. What light does the "Wundenmann" throw upon medieval surgery? What do you understand by "wound surgery"?

78. Who were the pioneers in vital statistics? Who originated medical statistics?

79. What American surgeons were associated with the rise of modern gynecology?

80. What was the earliest medical periodical of France? England? Germany? Italy? Holland? Russia? Spain? United States? Mexico?

81. Who first successfully ligated the following arteries: the external iliac? the innominate? the vertebral? the subclavian? the common carotid? the femoral? the gluteal?

82. Who devised the following procedures: frozen sections? litholapaxy? ophthalmoscopy? laryngoscopy? rhinoscopy? bronchoscopy? intra-vital staining? extra-vital tissue cultures? test-breakfasts? intubation of the larynx? symphysiotomy? rest cure? intratracheal insufflation? sterilization by ultra-violet rays? diazo reaction? fixation of the complement? deviation of the complement? suspension laryngoscopy? psychoanalysis?

59

83. What physicians did much to advance geology.

84. How are physicians described in the novels of Smollett? Le Sage? Dickens? Balzac? Charles Reade? Wilkie Collins?

85. Name the principal medical botanists.

86. What were the first printed books or tracts on ophthalmology? pediatrics? dentistry? gynecology? otology? anatomy? pathology?

87. What distinguished men were victims of angina pectoris?

88. What was the favorite English text-book on the practice of medicine in the first half of the 19th century?

89. With what do you associate the following localities: Cos? Epidaurus? Stagira? Monte Cassino? Great Windmill Street? Nauheim? Jullundur? Kaiserswerth? Görbersdorf? Gheel? Scutari? Saranac Lake? Rochester? Cergnat?

90. What prominent physicians and surgeons have illustrated their own works?

91. What were the first American books or pamphlets on anatomy? physiology? surgery? pathology? dentistry? gynecology? psychiatry? medical education? medical ethics? history of medicine?

92. What are the modern equivalents of: the āaā disease? morbus Hungaricus? cynanche trachealis? West Indian dry gripes? peripneumonia notha? the mother? tabes mesaraica? the marbles? the vapors? the purples? Devonshire colic? spleen? throat distemper? jail-fever?

93. Who were the discoverers of oxygen?

94. Name the principal neurological discoveries of Sir Charles Bell; Romberg; Duchenne of Boulogne; Erb; Charcot; Marie; Weir Mitchell.

95. Name some celebrated persons who were victims of phthisis.

96. Why does the Talmud throw more light upon ancient Jewish medicine than the Bible?

97. Who made chemistry a quantitative science?

98. Why did Naunyn decline the chair of internal medicine at Vienna?

99. What physicians or students of medicine wrote the following: Essay on Human Understanding? *Discours de la Méthode?* The History of John Bull? Humphrey Clinker? The Good Natured Man? Elsie Venner? Ten Thousand a Year? *Causeries du Lundi?* Hugh Wynne? *Der Geisterseher?* Tom Burke of Ours? *L'Abbé Tigrane? El Gran Galeoto?* The Assaying of Brabantius?

100. What different maladies have been called by the name of the "English disease"?

101. What medical journals were founded by Reil? Johannes Müller? Desault? Langenbeck? Virchow? Friedreich? A. von Graefe? Kölliker? Pflüger? Lombroso? Gegenbaur? Naunyn? Hoppe-Seyler? Schaudinn? Freud?

102. Who introduced the idea of reflex action? Who demonstrated it experimentally?

103. What physicians signed the Declaration of Independence?

104. What was Galen's crucial experiment to demonstrate the motor power of the heart?

105. Who wrote the following: Arcana naturæ? Biblia naturæ? De motu cordis? Les passions de l'ame? On airs, waters, and places? De usu partium? Avis au peuple? Micrographia? Sepulchretum? Systema naturæ? L'homme machine? Hortus sanitatis? The Metamorphosis of Ajax? Antitheriaka? Inventum novum? Rosa Anglica? Novum lumen? Lilium medicinæ?

106. Why does Mesmer fall into the group of 18th century quacks? What were Charcot's reasons for abandoning hypnotism?

107. What effect did the return of Halley's comet have upon medicine?

108. Why is Mott's translation of Velpeau's Surgery more valuable for reference than the original?

109. What did the following politicians and publicists do for medicine: Napoleon III? Gambetta? Lord Warburton? Théophile Roussel? Sir Robert Peel?

110. What physicians opposed the persecution of witches?

111. What anatomists were accused of vivisecting human beings?

112. What were the temperamental peculiarities of Billroth? Charcot? William Hunter? Daniel Drake? Naunyn? Lawson Tait? Virchow? Frerichs? Victor Horsley? Broussais? Heim? Dupuytren?

113. In respect of what pathological theories was Virchow at variance with the following authorities: Cruveilhier? Rokitansky? Hughes Bennett? Cohnheim? Charcot? Koch? Behring?

114. Who were instrumental in abolishing judicial torture?

115. What pathological lesions have been found in Egyptian mummies?

116. What diseases were originally described by: Benjamin Rush? Laennec? Willis? Heberden? Fothergill? Aretæus? Parry? Sydenham? Virchow? F. von Hebra? Kussmaul? Hodgkin? Bright? Alibert? Sir Samuel Wilks?

117. What physicians have paid severe penalties for infraction of the Hippocratic vow to silence?

118. Give the references to Cheyne-Stokes respiration before the time of Stokes.

119. What arguments have been advanced for and against the supposed American origin of syphilis?

120. What is the derivation of: Dum Dum fever? hysteria? phthisis? typhoid? colica Pictonum? la grippe? Thomsen's disease? nyctalopia? ague? incunabula? Stoffordshire knot? angula Ludovici? measles? influenza? Hutchinson's triad? Merseburg triad? stovaine?

121. Who conceived the idea of representing embryonic relations in three dimensions?

122. Why should the date of Werlhof's description of purpura be 1735, instead of 1775, as sometimes given?

123. State your views as to editorial revision of titles of medical papers. Why should ambiguous, misleading, cryptic or redundant titles be rejected?

124. How do you explain the remarkable proliferation of medical (periodical) literature since the World War? Is mass-production advantageous to the best interests of medicine?

125. What are the proper qualifications of a medical editor? a medical librarian? a medical amanuensis? a research-worker in medical literature? an instructor in medical history?

INDEX OF PERSONAL NAMES

[Entries in heavy type refer to biographical data.]

INDEX OF SUBJECTS

[Entries in heavy type refer to complete data]